PROFESSIONAL GUIDE TO

Diagnostic Tests

PROFESSIONAL GUIDE TO
Diagnostic Tests

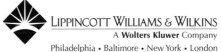

LIPPINCOTT WILLIAMS & WILKINS
A **Wolters Kluwer** Company

Philadelphia • Baltimore • New York • London
Buenos Aires • Hong Kong • Sydney • Tokyo

**Library of Congress
Cataloging-in-Publication Data**

Professional guide to diagnostic tests.
   p. ; cm.
Includes index.
   1. Diagnosis, Laboratory. I. Lippincott
Williams & Wilkins.
   [DNLM: 1. Diagnostic Tests, Routine. 2.
Hematologic Tests. 3. Urinalysis. WB 200 P965
2004]
RB37.P735 2004
616.07'56—dc22
ISBN 1-58255-304-1 (alk. paper)   2003024865

Contents

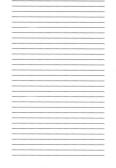

Contributors and consultants

Lee (Haralee) Abramo, RN, MSN
Director of Education
Los Robles Regional Medical Center
Thousand Oaks, Calif.
Part-time nursing faculty
California State University, Dominguez
  Hills
Carson

Ivy M. Alexander, RN, BSN, PhD, CANP
Assistant Professor
Yale University
New Haven, Conn.

Deborah Bastien, RN, BSN, MS, C
Professor of Nursing
College of the Mainland
Texas City, Tex.

Eric W. Bussear, MPH, PA-C
Assistant Professor
Nova Southeastern University
Ft. Lauderdale, Fla.

Deborah T. Castellucci, RN, PhD, CRNP
Assistant Professor/Acting Chair
Millersville University of Pennsylvania
Geriatric Nurse Practitioner
Center for Urologic Care
Wyomissing, Pa.

Janie C. Choate, MAT, PA-C
Director, Physician Assistant Studies
University of the Sciences
Philadelphia

Wendy Tagan Conroy, RN, MSN, FNP, BC
Advanced Practice Registered Nurse
Saint Francis Hospital and Medical
  Center
Hartford, Conn.

Sandra Davis, RN, MSN, CRNP
Assistant Professor
Drexel University
Philadelphia

Ellen Digan, MA, MT(ASCP)
Professor of Biology, Coordinator MLT
  Program
Manchester (Conn.) Community College

Diane Dixon, MA, MMSc, PhD(c), PA-C,
Assistant Professor
University of South Alabama
Mobile

Shelba Durston, RN, MSN, CCRN
Adjunct Faculty
San Joaquin Delta College
Stockton, Calif.
Staff Nurse
San Joaquin General Hospital
French Camp, Calif.

Ken W. Edmisson, RNC, ND, EdD, FNP
Associate Professor
Middle Tennessee State University
Murfreesboro

Carmel A. Esposito, RN, MSN, EdD
Consultant
Follansbee, W.Va.

Margaret Fried, RN, MA
Instructional Faculty
Pima Community College
Tucson, Ariz.

William F. Galvin, BA, MSEd, CRT, RRT, CPFT
Assistant Professor, School of Allied Health Professions
Program Director, Respiratory Care Program
Gwynedd Mercy College
Gwynedd Valley, Pa.

James J. Greco, MSN, ARNP-BC
Instructor
University of Florida
Gainesville

Teri Hamill, PhD, FAAA
Associate Professor of Audiology
Nova Southeastern University
Ft. Lauderdale, Fla.

Katherine Purgatorio Howard, RN, MS, BC
Instructor of Nursing
Charles E. Gregory School of Nursing
Raritan Bay Medical Center
Perth Amboy, N.J.

Nathan Kindig, BS, PA-C
Physician Assistant (Sports Medicine & Reconditioning Team)
U.S. Navy Medical Clinic
Pearl Harbor, Hawaii

Julie E. London, RN, MSN
Associate Professor Nursing
Community College Allegheny Co.
Boyce Campus
Monroeville, Pa.

Cecilia Jane Maier, RN, MS, CCRN
Assistant Professor
Mount Carmel College of Nursing
Columbus, Ohio

Karen S. March, RN, MSN, CCRN, APRN-BC
Assistant Professor of Nursing
York College of Pennsylvania

Barbara Maxwell, RNC, MSN, CNS
Assistant Professor of Nursing
State University of New York Ulster
Stone Ridge

E. Ann Myers, MD
Physician
Golden Gate Endocrine Specialists, Inc.
San Francisco

Mary Jane Nottoli, RN, MSN, CNS
Nursing Faculty
Ursuline College
Cleveland
Nursing Supervisor
MetroHealth Skilled Facility
Cleveland

Mary Jean Rutherford, MEd, MT(ASCP)SC, CLS(NCA)
CLS Programs Director, Associate Professor
Arkansas State University
State University

Barbara L. Sauls, EdD, PA-C
Clinical Director, Physician Assistant Program
King's College
Wilkes-Barre, Pa.

David B. Toub, MD, FACOG
Medical Director
MedCases, Inc.
Philadelphia

Dan Vetrosky, PA-C, MEd, PhD(c)
Assistant Professor
University of South Alabama
Mobile

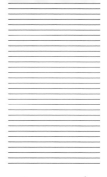

Foreword

Today's medical landscape revolves around technology that's ever changing. New diagnostic tests are constantly being introduced while tried-and-true testing procedures are being updated to accommodate the latest technological advances. As a health care professional, you have to keep up with these changes to ensure that you're delivering quality patient care. Your ability to provide your patients with detailed information regarding procedures, perform proper patient preparation and test administration, and differentiate normal test findings from abnormal ones is inherent upon your overall knowledge of today's testing procedures.

Of course, with the hundreds of diagnostic tests currently in use, you can't be expected to know everything, which is why reference materials that present information in a clear, concise format are essential to your daily practice. *Professional Guide to Diagnostic Tests* was designed with this thought in mind. With more than 550 laboratory and diagnostic tests and hundreds of photos, charts, and tables, this comprehensive guide gives you all the information you need to discuss and administer today's most commonly used tests.

Professional Guide to Diagnostic Tests is organized into six major sections broken down by test type. Section I (Chapters 1 through 11) discusses laboratory tests that are performed on whole blood,

serum, or plasma. These chapters provide information on routine tests such as hemoglobin determination as well as new procedures such as the B-type natriuretic peptide assay. Chapter 5 provides a particularly extensive review of hormone testing.

Section II (Chapters 12 through 17) provides an in-depth look at the tests that can be performed on a urine specimen. Section III (Chapters 18 and 19) details histologic and microbiologic procedures, including tests for ova and parasites. Section IV (Chapters 20 through 22) on organ tests breaks down tests specific to the thyroid, eye, and ear. In particular, chapter 22 includes overviews of several new audiologic and vestibular tests that every health care practitioner should become familiar with.

Section V (Chapters 23 through 29) covers diagnostic procedures for all body systems. You'll find the overview of the deoxyribonucleic acid-based cervical cancer screening test in Chapter 25 and the extensive listing of GI system tests in Chapter 27 especially useful.

Finally, Section VI (Chapter 30) encompasses tests that resist easy classification, such as skin tests, radiology and nuclear medicine procedures, and miscellaneous assays, including the D-xylose absorption test, which uses both urine and serum samples to detect the cause of malabsorption syndrome.

To add to the title's comprehensiveness, each chapter begins with an introduction that discusses the tests that follow, including explanations of their uses, summaries of test methods, and additional information where applicable, such as anatomy and physiology.

Each test entry starts with a general description of the test, including its purpose, then moves onto patient preparation, special equipment necessary to perform the procedure, the steps of the procedure, posttest care, precautions, normal findings and reference values, abnormal findings (and their interpretation), and factors that can interfere with proper test administration and accuracy. Stand-out logos, such as *Alert* and *Age issue,* call attention to important clinical points.

Each entry in *Professional Guide to Diagnostic Tests* eliminates the fluff to give you only what you need.

The book continues with 10 indispensable appendices. The appendix on blood and urine collection techniques provides information essential to obtaining optimum samples for evaluation. The chart on color-top collection tubes is an invaluable guide for selecting the appropriate container to use during venipunctures. The guide to selected reagent strip tests answers all your questions when it comes to this tricky subject. The fourth appendix summarizes various changes that occur in laboratory values in elderly patients. The fifth appendix addresses drugs that can interfere with laboratory test results.

An especially useful section for all health care professionals is the quick-reference guide to laboratory test results; this appendix is a quick and easy source for normal values in several age groups. Another extraordinary appendix is the illustrated guide to home testing. With its ready-to-copy format, it will become an indispensable part of your instructional materials library.

The remaining appendices, covering patient preparation for specific testing procedures, crisis values of laboratory tests, and blood tests that require immediate transport of the sample, provide even more valuable information.

Professional Guide to Diagnostic Tests is a comprehensive and convenient book that should be in the library of every health care professional. Whether referencing commonly performed tests or complex diagnostic procedures, this is the book to depend on.

Karen A. Brown, MS, MT (ASCP), CLS (NCA)
Associate Professor and MLT Program Director
Department of Pathology
University of Utah
School of Medicine
Salt Lake City

SECTION I.
BLOOD TESTS

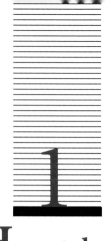

Hematology

Introduction

Blood is a continuously circulating tissue that performs many vital functions. Most important is its ability to transport oxygen (bound to hemoglobin in red blood cells [RBCs]) from the lungs to the body tissues and to return carbon dioxide from the tissues to the lungs. Blood contains white blood cells (WBCs), called leukocytes, which produce antibodies and consume pathogens by phagocytosis. Blood also contains complement, a group of immunologically significant protein substances.

Other functions performed by blood include maintenance of hemostasis with platelets and with coagulation factors, which repair tissue injuries and prevent bleeding; regulation of body temperature and of acid-base and fluid balances; movement of nutrients and regulatory hormones to body tissues; and disposal of metabolic wastes through the kidneys, lungs, and skin. Abnormalities of either RBCs or WBCs can result in various disorders.

2

Blood is three times as viscous as water, tastes slightly salty, and has an alkaline pH of 7.35 to 7.45. Oxygenated arterial blood is bright red; oxygen-poor venous blood is dark red.

Blood has two major components: plasma, the clear, straw-colored liquid portion; and the formed elements, erythrocytes (RBCs), leukocytes (WBCs), and thrombocytes (platelets).

Red cells
Also known as erythrocytes and red corpuscles, RBCs appear in the embryonic yolk sac during the first weeks of fetal development. During the second trimester, the fetal liver and spleen produce most RBCs. Starting just before birth, the marrow of all bones produces RBCs. The total quantity of active marrow decreases as the person grows. By adulthood, the marrow of membranous bones (sternum, ribs, vertebrae, and pelvis) become the primary source of red cells. Red cell production declines with advancing age.

Current theory states that hemocytoblasts are the progenitors of red cells. Hemocytoblasts repeatedly change shape and function until they become mature red cells. Most circulating red cells are vioconcave and disk-shaped, range in color from pale pink at the center to deep pink at the periphery, and are normally 7 microns in diameter. Abnormal red cells may vary in size (anisocytosis) or in color (anisochromia) or may assume permanent changes in shape (poikilocytosis). In *anisochromia,* RBC color ranges from insufficient (hypochromic) to excessive (hyperchromic). In *poikilocytosis,* bizarre shapes, such as teardrop, sickle, or pear, generally reflect abnormal cell formation and development in the bone marrow.

The number of red cells in an adult varies according to sex, age, and geographic location. Men usually have higher counts than women, and elderly persons have fewer red cells than young adults. Persons living at high altitudes generally have more red cells than those living at sea level—a compensatory adaptation to the thinner air.

Red cell function
A primary function of red cells is to maintain a high concentration of circulatory hemoglobin (Hb). The main component of the red cell, Hb is a conjugated protein that enables red cells to carry oxygen from the lungs to the tissues and to carry carbon dioxide from the tissues back to the lungs for excretion. Red cells also transport large quantities of carbon dioxide through the activity of carbonic anhydrase, a red cell enzyme. By accelerating the reaction between carbon dioxide and water, this enzyme promotes absorption into the blood of large quantities of carbon dioxide. Thus, red cells help maintain the body's acid-base balance.

Mature red cells circulate in the blood for about 120 days. As they age, these cells become fragile, finally rupture and decompose, and then are removed by the spleen and liver.

Hemoglobin
Hb, which constitutes about 90% of the mature red cell's dry weight, is composed of 4% heme—an iron and porphyrin complex that colors it—and 96% globin—a simple water-soluble protein. Hb synthesis depends on the metabolism of the porphyrin complex, globin, and iron.

The body contains about 4 g of iron; more than half this amount is in the Hb of red cells. Iron is absorbed from food in the upper intestine, primarily the duodenum, through the blood; the amount ab-

CLASSIFYING ABNORMAL HEMOGLOBINS

Abnormal hemoglobins can be classified as homozygous or heterozygous. This chart lists some abnormal hemoglobins and their clinical effects.

Classification	Abnormal hemoglobin	Clinical effects
Homozygous (double complement of genes)	S	Sickle cell anemia
	C	Three variants, two of which cause sickling
	D, E	Mild hemolytic anemia
	M	Methemoglobinemia and cyanosis
Heterozygous (bearing a single gene)	Chesapeake, Hiroshima, Capetown, Bethesda	Increased oxygen affinity and polycythemia
	Kansas, Seattle, Bristol, Yoshizuka	Decreased oxygen affinity, cyanosis, and anemia
	Torino, Ann Arbor, Hasharon	Congenital Heinz body hemolytic anemia
	H, Bart's	Thalassemias

sorbed is normally in response to the amount lost daily. For transport, iron combines with a glycoprotein, transferrin. Some iron is transported to the bone marrow for Hb synthesis; some goes to needy tissues, such as muscle, for myoglobin synthesis; and unused iron is converted to ferritin and is stored in the liver, spleen, bone marrow, and reticuloendothelial system. The iron in the Hb of destroyed red cells is recycled by the spleen, either for inclusion in new red cells or for storage in the liver. Normally, less than 1 mg of iron is lost daily through the skin, stool, and urine.

Three major types of Hb are found in normal blood: Hb A, Hb A_2, and Hb F. Hb A accounts for more than 95% of adult Hb, with Hb A_2 comprising 2% to 3%. Although traces of Hb F appear in adult blood, this type appears predominately in the fetus and neonate, thereafter decreasing to 2% to 3% of the infant's blood at age 6 months.

Hemoglobin variants

Each heme molecule is attached to a *globin* molecule. Each of these combinations represents a subunit of Hb, and each Hb molecule contains four subunits. One molecule of Hb can carry four molecules of oxygen. The globins are present as two identical pairs. Variations occur, however, creating abnormal hemoglobins. Because the heme portion of all Hb is identical, variations are possible only in these polypeptide globins, resulting from substitutions in any of the amino acid chains. Such substitutions may result in structurally unstable Hb. An identical substitution in both polypeptide pairs produces a *homozygous* variation; a substitution in one pair or nonidentical changes in both pairs result in *heterozygous* variation.

Overall, genetic and acquired variations account for more than 200 abnormal hemoglobins. (See *Classifying abnormal hemoglobins.*)

Abnormal hemoglobins were initially identified using capital letters — for example, Hb S for the abnormal Hb in sickle cell anemia. As the alphabet was nearly exhausted, new abnormal hemoglobins were identified with place names, such as Hb D Punjab. (A letter plus a place name means identical mobility on Hb electrophoresis, but different substitution.) In addition, the Greek letters alpha and beta are used to identify a known abnormal polypeptide chain.

Abnormal red cell production

Erythropoietin, a glycoprotein of low molecular weight originating in the kidneys, stimulates production (erythropoiesis), maturation, and release of red cells from the bone marrow and other blood-forming tissues. Low oxygen levels in the kidneys and in other tissues (hypoxia) causes increased secretion of this glycoprotein, which accelerates red cell production. (See *How hypoxia stimulates erythropoiesis.*) Hypoxia can result from severe anemia, heart failure, pulmonary disease, or living at high altitudes.

Anemias, defined by abnormally low Hb concentration, red cell count, and hematocrit (HCT), may reflect acute or chronic blood loss, excessive hemolysis, or deficient blood production. Anemias are classified by their causes or by the structural changes they produce in the red cells — normocytic (normal), microcytic (small), or macrocytic (large) — and by Hb content as normochromic or hypochromic (normal color or pale).

Together these classifications can describe anemia accurately. If the size, shape, and Hb content of RBCs are nor-

HOW HYPOXIA STIMULATES ERYTHROPOIESIS

Hypoxia provides a compensatory increase in red cell production that allows the cells to absorb and transport more oxygen per unit of inspired air, as shown in the flowchart below.

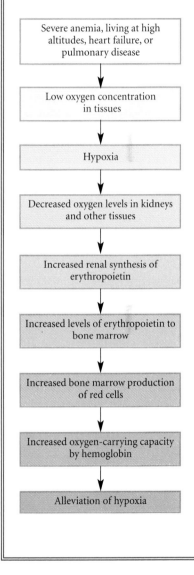

Severe anemia, living at high altitudes, heart failure, or pulmonary disease

↓

Low oxygen concentration in tissues

↓

Hypoxia

↓

Decreased oxygen levels in kidneys and other tissues

↓

Increased renal synthesis of erythropoietin

↓

Increased levels of erythropoietin to bone marrow

↓

Increased bone marrow production of red cells

↓

Increased oxygen-carrying capacity by hemoglobin

↓

Alleviation of hypoxia

mal, but RBC production is depressed, *normocytic normochromic anemia,* commonly associated with vitamin B_{12} or folic acid deficiency, is diagnosed. If RBCs are small and pale from Hb deficiency, the patient has *microcytic hypochromic anemia,* which typically results from iron deficiency.

Hemolytic anemia, with red cell destruction, may result from a congenital defect (such as sickle cell anemia or thalassemia) or as an acquired response to certain drugs (such as methyldopa), to certain disorders (Hodgkin's disease, lupus erythematosus, or lymphomas), or to foreign red cells (transfusion reaction).

Similarly, reduced erythropoiesis may result from various diseases and deficiencies. For example, prolonged X-ray therapy can cause chromic bone marrow hypoplasia and varying degrees of pancytopenia (aplastic anemia). Impairment or destruction of bone marrow by cancer, thymic tumor, or chloramphenicol creates deficiency of hemocytoblasts, causing anemia.

Deficient erythropoiesis also results from deficiency of iron, folic acid, or vitamin B_{12}. Another major cause, particularly in renal failure, is impaired secretion of erythropoietin, the hormone that stimulates bone marrow production.

Erythropoietin levels drop markedly when the kidneys are removed or damaged, but this condition can now be treated with recombinant erythropoietin.

Polycythemias

The body reacts to hypoxia by a compensatory increase in red cell production. Severe and chronic hypoxia, which may result from congenital heart disease and pulmonary disease, can lead to overcompensation and overproduction of RBCs, a condition called polycythemia.

Polycythemias may be relative or absolute and either primary or secondary. In *relative* (or *spurious*) *polycythemia,* HCT is elevated because circulating plasma volume is decreased, but total red cell mass is normal. Relative polycythemia follows dehydration from vomiting, diarrhea, or heatstroke and massive fluid loss from extensive burns.

In *absolute polycythemia,* the RBC count may rise to 8 million/μl as the circulating mass of RBCs increases and HCT rises to 70% to 80%. The cause of *primary polycythemia* (polycythemia vera) is unknown, but the bone marrow produces many more RBCs than necessary and perhaps more WBCs and platelets.

Secondary (or *reactive*) *polycythemia* develops in people who live at altitudes higher than 14,000 feet; to compensate for less atmospheric oxygen, the blood needs more RBCs. Secondary polycythemia may also result from disorders that cause increased erythropoietin production, including certain hemoglobinopathies, cardiopulmonary disease, and certain renal cysts and tumors.

White cells

The five types of WBCs are known as neutrophils, eosinophils, basophils, monocytes, and lymphocytes. *Neutrophils* are so named because they accept acidic and basic stains. White cells that develop an orange-red cytoplasm when stained with the acid dye eosin are called *eosinophils* (eosin-loving cells), and the cytoplasm of *basophils* readily accepts a basic dye. These three cell types are collectively known as *granulocytes* because they characteristically display irregularly shaped nuclei and granules dispersed in their cytoplasm.

Monocytes and *lymphocytes* are mononuclear cells. Monocytes are phagocytic and develop into macrophages. Most lymphocytes are formed in lymphoid tissue, but some of them—and all neutrophils, basophils, eosinophils, and monocytes—are formed only in bone marrow.

The special function of white cells, particularly neutrophils, is to protect the body against infection. WBCs respond to inflammation by chemotaxis, a process of chemical attraction or repulsion. Inflamed tissue causes positive chemotaxis, a biochemical alarm that draws white cells to the infected area. White cells move about by ameboid motion or diapedesis. In ameboid motion, one end of the cell alternately protrudes and pulls the remainder of the cell along with it. In diapedesis, the cell squeezes itself through pores or interstitial spaces in the capillary endothelium. When at the infection site, white cells engulf and digest any foreign matter by a process called phagocytosis. (See *Understanding phagocytosis,* pages 8 and 9.)

Granulocytes

Produced in the bone marrow and stored there until the body needs them, granulocytes normally circulate for about 12 hours, but during severe stress, they survive only 2 or 3 hours. The following abnormal cellular inclusions can appear in granulocytes:

■ *Döhle's inclusion bodies:* A patient with severe burns, bacterial infection, malignant disease, or extensive cytolysis may have neutrophils with large, round, blue cytoplasmic masses. These bodies reflect a too-rapid proliferation of neutrophils, but they may also occur in normal pregnancy.

■ *Azurophil granules:* Small, smoothly rounded granules that contain diverse lysosomal enzymes, azurophil granules appear in lymphocytes, monocytes, and immature granulocytes. After such cells mature and specific granulation develops, a few azurophil granules persist in the cells but reflect no pathology.

■ *Auer bodies (Auer rods):* Composed of slender, rodlike masses of pink or purple cytoplasmic material, Auer bodies indicate abnormal cellular development of granulocytes or monocytes. Because these bodies never appear in lymphocytes, their presence makes possible the classification of very immature, undifferentiated leukemic cells as belonging to the myelomonocytic series.

■ *Hypersegmentation and macropolycytes:* Abnormal metabolism of folic acid and vitamin B_{12} may induce production of abnormally large granulocytes and erythrocytes. Hypersegmented neutrophils may have seven or eight lobes in their nuclei, instead of the normal three to five.

Neutrophils

More than half the white cells in the peripheral circulation are neutrophils. Because they quickly phagocytize significant quantities of microorganisms, neutrophils are the body's first line of defense against infection. Each mature neutrophil can inactivate 5 to 20 bacteria.

A small number of slightly immature neutrophils, known as *band cells,* normally appears in peripheral blood. In a differential count, the presence of many band cells and their precursors is known as a shift to the left and indicates infection. A shift to the right describes the presence of mature, hypersegmented neutrophils that have more nuclear segments than normal; this commonly occurs with pernicious anemia and hepatic disease. Increased band cells and a low total WBC count reflect bone marrow depression (as in typhoid fever), known as a degenerative

UNDERSTANDING PHAGOCYTOSIS

With the help of neutrophils (polymorphonuclear leukocytes), macrophages (mononuclear leukocytes) remove microorganisms and other foreign material (antigens) that invade the skin and mucous membranes in a process called *phagocytosis.* Here's how they do it.

1. Chemotaxis
Chemotactic factors attract macrophages to the infection site.

2. Opsonization
Antibody (immunoglobulin G) or complement fragment (C3b) coats the microorganism.

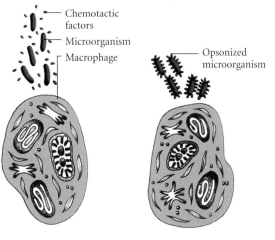

Chemotactic factors
Microorganism
Macrophage

Opsonized microorganism

shift. A regenerative shift implies stimulation of the bone marrow (as in pneumonia and appendicitis) and may be noted by increased band cells, metamyelocytes, and myelocytes, together with a high WBC count.

Eosinophils
Although eosinophils are phagocytic, they proliferate in response to allergic conditions rather than to bacterial infection. In allergic reactions, eosinophils pour into the blood and collect at the site of tissue inflammation; they detoxify foreign protein matter and ingest antigen-antibody complexes before these complexes can damage the body. The most common causes of eosinophilia are allergic disorders and parasitic infections.

Basophils
Basophils contain large amounts of histamine. Their most important role is in immediate hypersensitivity reactions. Basophils have specific immunoglobulin E receptors that cause degranulation when the appropriate antigens are present. This reaction may be recognized as anaphylaxis brought on by drugs or insect stings and as some form of bronchial asthma, hives, or allergic rhinitis.

Monocytes to macrophages
The body's second line of defense, monocytes arrive at infection sites in smaller numbers than do neutrophils. Bone marrow releases immature monocytes into the circulation. Within a few hours, they enter the tissue, where they perform their phagocytic function. As a monocyte matures into a macrophage, it enlarges; its

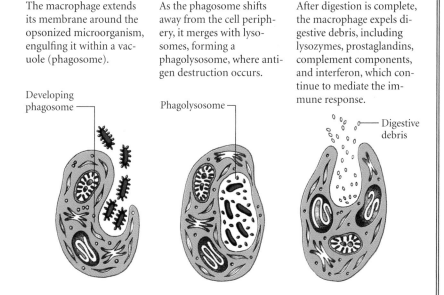

3. Ingestion
The macrophage extends its membrane around the opsonized microorganism, engulfing it within a vacuole (phagosome).

Developing phagosome

4. Digestion
As the phagosome shifts away from the cell periphery, it merges with lysosomes, forming a phagolysosome, where antigen destruction occurs.

Phagolysosome

5. Release
After digestion is complete, the macrophage expels digestive debris, including lysozymes, prostaglandins, complement components, and interferon, which continue to mediate the immune response.

Digestive debris

lysosome and hydrolytic enzymes increase, enhancing its bactericidal activity. These macrophages ingest debris; depending on the amount ingested, they may eventually become so engorged that they die. Immature monocytes that become fixed in the tissue are called *tissue macrophages,* or *histiocytes;* they become part of the reticuloendothelial system and establish themselves in the lymph nodes, lung alveoli, the spleen, the bone marrow, and the hepatic sinuses (known as *Kupffer's cells*).

Lymphocytes
Important in humoral and cell-mediated immunity, lymphocytes are produced in the lymph nodes, spleen, thymus, tonsils, and lymphoid tissue of the gut. Together with neutrophils, they make up the majority of white cells in the peripheral blood. In cellular immunity, sensitized T lymphocytes (thymus-derived) attach to and destroy specific foreign antigens. Humoral immunity refers to the production of circulating antibodies by B lymphocytes (bone marrow-derived) that attack invading microorganisms.

Immune reactions to viral infections may cause changes in the appearance of mature lymphocytes, which are then called *variant reactive* (or *atypical*) *lymphocytes.* These cells may appear in infectious mononucleosis, hepatitis, viral pneumonia, and allergic conditions.

Plasma cells
Usually found in the lymphoid tissue and bone marrow, but rarely in the peripheral circulation, plasma cells produce antibodies to help fight disease. Contact with a specific antigen causes certain lympho-

cytes to become plasma cells and stimulates their immune activity. Plasma cells may appear in the circulation during severe infection to reinforce immunity when sufficient antibodies aren't available. The presence of such cells in the blood may also indicate multiple myeloma, plasma cell leukemia, scarlet fever, muscles, or chickenpox.

Reticuloendothelial system
The reticuloendothelial system (RES) is made up of tissue histiocytes, macrophages, and lymphatic tissue. Although RES cells are much less mobile than circulating white cells, they're also responsible for removing foreign matter and endogenous debris from the blood, lymph, and interstitial spaces of the body. For example, when Hb is released from ruptured red cells, cells from this system digest it.

Abnormal white cell production
Malignant mutation of the blood-forming tissues can cause unrestrained white cell production, better known as *leukemia*. This condition is marked by a sharp rise in the number of abnormal white cells, first in the tissues of origin and then throughout the body.

Leukemias are classified according to the type of white cell proliferation: lymphocytic, granulocytic, or monocytic. The more immature the blood cell — that is, the more primitive its development — the more severe the disease; the older the cell, the more chronic the disease. For example, abnormal, excessive granulocyte production results in *chronic granulocytic leukemia*. Abnormally high levels of immature lymphocytes and their precursors (lymphoblasts) predominate in *acute lymphoblastic leukemia.*

In *agranulocytosis,* bone marrow stops producing granulocytes, leaving the body virtually defenseless against infection. Acute agranulocytosis, which is fatal if untreated, may result from infection or may be the result of exposure to certain antibodies or certain drugs (such as clindamycin, sulfonamides, melphalan, other chemotherapeutic agents, and barbiturates).

Blood platelets
Derived from megakaryocytes in bone marrow and also known as thrombocytes, platelets protect vascular surfaces and help the blood clot to stop bleeding. Abnormal platelet function (thrombasthenia), increased platelet counts (thrombocythemia), and decreased platelet counts (thrombocytopenia) can interfere with hemostasis. (See chapter 2 for more information about platelets.)

Complete blood count
This commonly requested test gives a fairly complete picture of all the blood's formed elements. The complete blood count (CBC) generally is composed of two sections: direct measurement of cellular components, including Hb and erythrocyte indices, and differentiation of WBCs, with an assessment of WBC, RBC, and platelet morphology. The following tests are usually included: Hb concentration, HCT, red and white cell counts, differential white cell count, and stained smear for red cell and platelet examination. Besides pointing the way toward further definitive studies, CBC data have proven extremely valuable in themselves.

CBC data can detect anemias, determine their severity, and compare the status of specific blood elements. Thus, the CBC is especially useful for evaluating conditions in which HCT doesn't parallel the RBC count. Normally, as the RBC count rises, so does HCT. However, in a patient with microcytic or macrocytic anemia, this natural correlation may not hold true. For example, the patient with iron deficiency anemia has undersized red cells that cause his HCT to decrease, even though his RBC count may be reported as near-normal. Conversely, the patient with pernicious anemia has many oversized red cells that cause his HCT to be higher than his RBC count.

White cell differential

Although the WBC count alone can suggest infection, a white cell differential adds a detailed evaluation of white cell distribution and morphology that can help confirm the possibility of an infection and suggest the type of organism (bacterial or viral). A differential may also indicate that the cause of the WBC count change is something other than infection such as leukemia.

The stained red cell examination commonly accompanies the white cell differential as part of the CBC. After the differential, the same stained slide is evaluated for RBC distribution and morphology, including changes in cell contents, color, size, and shape, providing additional information for detecting leukemia, anemia, and thalassemia. Variations in size and shape are reported as the number of immature or nucleated RBCs/100 WBCs, noting cell inclusions.

RED BLOOD CELL TESTS

Red blood cell count

The red blood cell (RBC) count, also called an *erythrocyte count,* is part of a complete blood count. It's used to detect the number of RBCs in a microliter (μl), or cubic millimeter (mm^3), of whole blood. The RBC count itself provides no qualitative information regarding the size, shape, or concentration of hemoglobin (Hb) within the corpuscles, but it may be used to calculate two erythrocyte indices: mean corpuscular volume (MCV) and mean corpuscular hemoglobin (MCH).

Purpose

- To provide data for calculating MCV and MCH, which reveal RBC size and Hb content
- To support other hematologic tests for diagnosing anemia or polycythemia

Patient preparation

- Explain to the patient that the RBC count is used to evaluate the number of RBCs and to detect possible blood disorders.
- Tell the patient that a blood sample will be taken. Explain who will perform the venipuncture and when.
- Explain to the patient that he may feel slight discomfort from the needle puncture and the tourniquet.
- **AGE ISSUE** *If the patient is a child, explain to him (if he's old enough) and his parents that a small amount of blood will be taken from his finger or earlobe.*
- Inform the patient that he need not restrict food and fluids.

Procedure and posttest care

■ For adults and older children, draw venous blood into a 3- or 4.5-ml EDTA sodium metabisulfite solution tube.
■ For younger children, collect capillary blood in a microcollection device.
■ Ensure that subdermal bleeding has stopped before removing pressure.
■ If a hematoma develops at the venipuncture site, apply warm soaks.

Precautions

■ Fill the collection tube completely.
■ Invert the tube gently several times to mix the sample and the anticoagulant.
■ Handle the sample gently to prevent hemolysis.

Reference values

Normal RBC values vary, depending on the type of sample and on the patient's age and sex, as follows:
■ adult males: 4.5 to 5.5 million RBCs/µl (SI, 4.5 to 5.5 $\times$ 10^{12}/L) of venous blood
■ adult females: 4 to 5 million RBCs/µl (SI, 4 to 5 $\times$ 10^{12}/L) of venous blood.

AGE ISSUE *Reference values for infants and children also vary depending on age:*
– *full-term neonates: 4.4 to 5.8 million/µl (SI, 4.4 to 5.8 $\times$ 10^{12}/L) of capillary blood at birth, decreasing to 3 to 3.8 million /µl (SI, 3 to 3.8 $\times$ 10^{12}/L) at age 2 months, and increasing slowly thereafter*
– *children: 4.6 to 4.8 million/µl (SI, 4.6 to 4.8 2 10^{12}/L) of venous blood.*

Normal values may exceed these levels in patients living at high altitudes or those who are very active.

Abnormal findings

An elevated RBC count may indicate absolute or relative polycythemia. A depressed count may indicate anemia, fluid overload, or hemorrhage beyond 24 hours. Further tests, such as stained cell examination, hematocrit, Hb, red cell indices, and white cell studies, are needed to confirm the diagnosis.

Interfering factors

■ Failure to use the proper anticoagulant or to adequately mix the sample and the anticoagulant
■ Hemoconcentration due to prolonged tourniquet constriction
■ Hemodilution due to drawing the sample from the same arm used for I.V. infusion of fluids
■ High white blood cell count (false-high test results in semiautomated and automated counters)
■ Diseases that cause RBCs to agglutinate or form rouleaux (false decrease)
■ Hemolysis due to rough handling of the sample or drawing the blood through a small-gauge needle for venipuncture

Hematocrit

A hematocrit (HCT) test may be done separately or as part of a complete blood count. It measures percentage by volume of packed red blood cells (RBCs) in a whole blood sample; for example, an HCT of 40% indicates that a 100-ml sample of blood contains 40 ml of packed RBCs. Packing is achieved by centrifuging anticoagulated whole blood in a capillary tube so that red cells are tightly packed without hemolysis. Test results may be used to calculate two erythrocyte indices; mean corpuscular volume and mean corpuscular hemoglobin concentration.

Purpose

■ To aid diagnosis of polycythemia, anemia, or abnormal states of hydration
■ To aid calculation of erythrocyte indices

Patient preparation

- Explain to the patient that HCT is tested to detect anemia and other abnormal blood conditions.
- Tell the patient that the test requires a blood sample. Explain who will perform the venipuncture and when.
- Explain to the patient that he may feel slight discomfort from the needle puncture and the tourniquet.
- Inform the patient that he need not restrict food and fluids.

AGE ISSUE *If the patient is a child, explain to him (if he's old enough) and his parents that a small amount of blood will be taken from his finger or earlobe.*

Procedure and posttest care

- Perform a fingerstick using a heparinized capillary tube with a red band on the anticoagulant end.
- Fill the capillary tube from the red-banded end to about two-thirds capacity; seal this end with clay.
- Alternatively, perform a venipuncture and fill a 3- or 4.5-ml EDTA tube.
- Ensure subdermal bleeding has stopped before removing pressure.
- If a hematoma develops at the venipuncture site, apply warm soaks. If the hematoma is large, monitor pulses distal to the venipuncture site.

Precautions

- Send the sample to the laboratory immediately.
- If you perform the test, place the tube in the centrifuge with the red end pointing outward.
- Fill the collection tube completely.
- Invert the tube gently several times to mix the sample.

Reference values

HCT is usually measured electronically. The results are 3% lower than manual measurements, which trap plasma in the column of packed RBCs.

Reference values for adults vary, depending on the type of sample, the laboratory performing the test, and the patient's age and sex, as follows:
- adult males: 42% to 52% (SI, 0.42 to 0.52)
- adult females: 36% to 48% (SI, 0.36 to 0.48).

AGE ISSUE *Reference values for children also vary depending on age:*
- *neonates 55% to 68% (SI, 0.55 to 0.68)*
- *neonates age 1 week: 47% to 65% (SI, 0.47 to 0.65)*
- *infants age 1 month: 37% to 49% (SI, 0.37 to 0.49)*
- *infants age 3 months: 30% to 36% (SI, 0.3 to 0.36)*
- *age 1 year: 29% to 41% (SI, 0.29 to 0.41)*
- *age 10 years: 36% to 40% (SI, 0.36 to 0.4).*

Abnormal findings

Low HCT suggests anemia, hemodilution, or massive blood loss. High HCT indicates polycythemia or hemoconcentration due to blood loss and dehydration.

Interfering factors

- Failure to fill the tube properly, to use the proper anticoagulant, or to adequately mix the sample and the anticoagulant
- Hemolysis due to rough handling of the sample or drawing the blood through a small-gauge needle for venipuncture
- Hemoconcentration due to tourniquet constriction for longer than 1 minute (increase, typically 2.5% to 5%)
- Hemodilution due to drawing the blood from the arm above an I.V. infusion

Red cell indices

Using the results of the red blood cell (RBC) count, hematocrit (HCT), and total hemoglobin (Hb) tests, red cell indices (erythrocyte indices) provide important information about the size, Hb concentration, and Hb weight of an average RBC.

Purpose
■ To aid diagnosis and classification of anemias

Patient preparation
■ Explain to the patient that red cell indices help determine if he has anemia.
■ Tell the patient that a blood sample will be taken. Explain who will perform the venipuncture and when.
■ Explain to the patient that he may feel slight discomfort from the needle puncture and the tourniquet.

Procedure and posttest care
■ Perform a venipuncture and collect the sample in a 3- or 4.5-ml EDTA tube.
■ Ensure subdermal bleeding has stopped before removing pressure.
■ If a hematoma develops at the venipuncture site, apply warm soaks. If the hematoma is large, monitor pulses distal to the phlebotomy site.

Precautions
■ Completely fill the collection tube and invert it gently several times to adequately mix the sample and the anticoagulant.
■ Handle the sample gently to prevent hemolysis.

Reference values
The indices tested include mean corpuscular volume (MCV), mean corpuscular hemoglobin (MCH), and mean corpuscular hemoglobin concentration (MCHC).

MCV, the ratio of HCT (packed cell volume) to the RBC count, expresses the average size of the erythrocytes and indicates whether they're undersized (microcytic), oversized (macrocytic), or normal (normocytic). MCH, the Hb-RBC ratio, gives the weight of Hb in an average red cell. MCHC, the ratio of Hb weight to HCT, defines the concentration of Hb in 100 ml of packed RBCs. It helps to distinguish normally colored (normochromic) RBCs from paler (hypochromic) RBCs.

The range of normal red cell indices is as follows:
■ MCV: 84 to 99 μm^3
■ MCH: 26 to 32 pg/cell
■ MCHC: 30 to 36 g/dl.

Abnormal findings
Low MCV and MCHC indicate microcytic, hypochromic anemias caused by iron deficiency anemia, pyridoxine-responsive anemia, or thalassemia. A high MCV suggests macrocytic anemias caused by megaloblastic anemias, folic acid or vitamin B_{12} deficiency, inherited disorders of deoxyribonucleic acid synthesis, or reticulocytosis. Because the MCV reflects the average volume of many cells, a value within the normal range can encompass RBCs of varying size, from microcytic to macrocytic. (See *Comparative red cell indices in anemias.*)

Interfering factors
■ Failure to use the proper anticoagulant or to adequately mix the sample and the anticoagulant
■ Hemolysis due to rough handling of the sample or use of a small-gauge needle for blood aspiration
■ Hemoconcentration due to prolonged tourniquet constriction

COMPARATIVE RED CELL INDICES IN ANEMIAS

	Normal values (Normocytic, normochromic)	Iron deficiency anemia (Microcytic, hypochromic)	Pernicious anemia (Macrocytic, normochromic)
MCV	84 to 99 μm^3	60 to 80 μm^3	96 to 150 μm^3
MCH	26 to 32 pg/cell	5 to 25 pg/cell	33 to 53 pg/cell
MCHC	30 to 36 g/dl	20 to 30 g/dl	33 to 38 g/dl

Key:
MCV = Mean corpuscular volume
MCH = Mean corpuscular hemoglobin
MCHC = Mean corpuscular hemoglobin concentration

■ High white blood cell count (false-high RBC count in semiautomated and automated counters, invalidating MCV and MCHC results)
■ Falsely elevated Hb values, invalidating MCH and MCHC results
■ Diseases that cause RBCs to agglutinate or form rouleaux (false-low RBC count)

Erythrocyte sedimentation rate

The erythrocyte sedimentation rate (ESR) measures the degree of erythrocyte settling in a blood sample during a specified period. The ESR is a sensitive but nonspecific test that's commonly the earliest indicator of disease when other chemical or physical signs are normal. The ESR usually increases significantly in widespread inflammatory disorders; elevations may be prolonged in localized inflammation and malignant disease.

Purpose
■ To monitor inflammatory or malignant disease
■ To aid detection and diagnosis of occult disease, such as tuberculosis, tissue necrosis, or connective tissue disease

Patient preparation
■ Explain to the patient that the ESR test is used to evaluate the condition of red blood cells.
■ Tell the patient that a blood sample will be taken. Explain who will perform the venipuncture and when.
■ Explain to the patient that he may feel slight discomfort from the needle puncture and the tourniquet.
■ Inform the patient that he need not restrict food and fluids.

Procedure and posttest care
■ Perform a venipuncture and collect the sample in a 4.5-ml tube with EDTA added or a tube with sodium citrate added. (Check with the laboratory to determine its preference.)
■ Ensure subdermal bleeding has stopped before removing pressure.
■ If a hematoma develops at the venipuncture site, apply warm soaks. If

the hematoma is large, monitor pulses distal to the phlebotomy site.

Precautions
- Completely fill the collection tube and invert it gently several times to thoroughly mix the sample and the anticoagulant.
- Because prolonged standing decreases the ESR, examine the sample for clots or clumps and send it to the laboratory immediately. It must be tested within 2 to 4 hours.
- Handle the sample gently to prevent hemolysis.

Reference values
The ESR normally ranges from 0 to 10 mm/hour (SI, 0 to 10 mm/hour) in males, and 0 to 20 mm/hour (SI, 0 to 20 mm/hour) in females. Rates gradually increase with age.

Abnormal findings
The ESR rises in pregnancy, anemia, acute or chronic inflammation, tuberculosis, paraproteinemias (especially multiple myeloma and Waldenström's macroglobulinemia), rheumatic fever, rheumatoid arthritis, and some cancers.

Polycythemia, sickle cell anemia, hyperviscosity, and low plasma fibrinogen or globulin levels tend to depress the ESR.

Interfering factors
- Failure to use the proper anticoagulant, to adequately mix the sample and the anticoagulant, or to send the sample to the laboratory immediately
- Use of a small-gauge needle for blood aspirations
- Hemolysis due to rough handling or excessive mixing of the sample
- Hemoconcentration due to prolonged tourniquet constriction

Reticulocyte count

Reticulocytes are nonnucleated, immature red blood cells (RBCs) that remain in the peripheral blood for 24 to 48 hours while maturing. They're generally larger than mature RBCs. In the reticulocyte count test, reticulocytes in a whole blood sample are counted and expressed as a percentage of the total RBC count. Because the manual method of reticulocyte counting uses only a small sample, values may be imprecise and should be compared with the RBC count or hematocrit. The reticulocyte count is useful for evaluating anemia and is an index of effective erythropoiesis and bone marrow response to anemia.

Purpose
- To aid in distinguishing between hypoproliferative and hyperproliferative anemias
- To help assess blood loss, bone marrow response to anemia, and therapy for anemia

Patient preparation
- Explain to the patient that the reticulocyte count is used to detect anemia or to monitor its treatment.
- Tell the patient that a blood sample will be taken. Explain who will perform the venipuncture and when.
- Explain to the patient that he may feel slight discomfort from the needle puncture and the tourniquet.

🔹 **AGE ISSUE** *If the patient is an infant or child, explain to the parents that a small amount of blood will be taken from his finger or earlobe.*

- Notify the laboratory and physician of medications the patient is taking that may affect test results; they may need to be restricted.

- Inform the patient that he need not restrict food and fluids.

Procedure and posttest care
- Perform a venipuncture and collect the sample in a 3- or 4.5-ml EDTA tube.
- Ensure subdermal bleeding has stopped before removing pressure.
- If a hematoma develops at the venipuncture site, apply warm soaks. If the hematoma is large, monitor pulses distal to the phlebotomy site.
- Instruct the patient that he may resume medications discontinued before the test, as ordered.
- Monitor the patient with an abnormal reticulocyte count for trends or significant changes in repeated tests.

Precautions
- Completely fill the collection tube and invert it gently several times to mix the sample and the anticoagulant.
- Handle the sample gently.

Reference values
Reticulocytes compose 0.5% to 2.5% (SI, 0.005 to 0.025) of the total RBC count.

AGE ISSUE *In infants, the normal reticulocyte count ranges from 2% to 6% (SI, 0.002 to 0.006) at birth, decreasing to adult levels in 1 to 2 weeks.*

Abnormal findings
A low reticulocyte count indicates hypoproliferative bone marrow (hypoplastic anemia) or ineffective erythropoiesis (pernicious anemia).

A high reticulocyte count indicates a bone marrow response to anemia caused by hemolysis or blood loss. The reticulocyte count may also increase after therapy for iron deficiency anemia or pernicious anemia.

Interfering factors
- Failure to use the proper anticoagulant or to adequately mix the sample and the anticoagulant
- Prolonged tourniquet constriction
- Azathioprine, chloramphenicol, dactinomycin, and methotrexate (possible false-low)
- Corticotropin, antimalarials, antipyretics, furazolidone (in infants), levodopa (possible false-high)
- Sulfonamides (possible false-low or false-high)
- Recent blood transfusion
- Hemolysis caused by rough handling of the sample or use of a small-gauge needle for blood aspiration

Osmotic fragility

Osmotic fragility measures red blood cell (RBC) resistance to hemolysis when exposed to a series of increasingly dilute saline solutions. The sooner hemolysis occurs, the greater the osmotic fragility of the cells. Osmotic fragility is based on osmosis — movement of water across a membrane from a less concentrated one, in a natural tendency to correct the imbalance.

Red cells suspended in an isotonic saline solution — one with the same salt concentration (osmotic pressure) as normal plasma (0.85 g/dl) — keep their shape. If red cells are added to a hypotonic (less concentrated) solution, they take up water until they burst; if placed in a hypertonic solution, they shrink. (See *Understanding concentration and fluid flow,* page 18.)

The degree of hypotonicity needed to produce hemolysis varies inversely with the red cell's osmotic fragility; the closer the saline tonicity is to normal physiologic values when hemolysis occurs, the

UNDERSTANDING CONCENTRATION AND FLUID FLOW

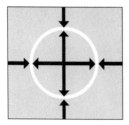 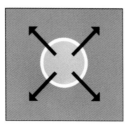 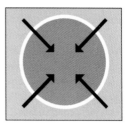

Isotonic

An isotonic fluid has a concentration of dissolved particles, or tonicity, equal to that of intracellular fluid. When isotonic fluids, such as 5% dextrose in water and normal saline solution, enter the circulation, they cause no net movement of water across the semipermeable cell membrane. And because the osmotic pressure is the same inside and outside the cells, they neither swell nor shrink.

Hypertonic

A hypertonic fluid has a concentration greater than that of intracellular fluid. When a hypertonic solution, such as 50% dextrose or 3% sodium chloride, is rapidly infused into the body, water rushes out of the cells to the area of greater concentration, and the cells shrivel. Dehydration can also make extracellular fluid hypertonic, leading to the same kind of cellular shrinking.

Hypotonic

A hypotonic fluid has a concentration less than that of intracellular fluid. When a hypotonic solution, such as 2.5% dextrose or half-normal saline solution, surrounds a cell, water diffuses into the intracellular fluid, causing the cell to swell. Inappropriate use of I.V. fluids or severe electrolyte loss makes body fluids hypotonic.

---

more fragile the cells. In some cases, red cells don't hemolyze immediately and their incubation in solution for 24 hours improves test sensitivity.

Osmotic fragility offers quantitative confirmation of red cell morphology and should supplement the stained cell examination.

Purpose

■ To aid diagnosis of hereditary spherocytosis

■ To confirm morphologic RBC abnormalities

Patient preparation

■ Explain to the patient that osmotic fragility is used to identify the cause of anemia.

■ Tell the patient that a blood sample will be taken. Explain who will perform the venipuncture and when.

■ Explain to the patient that he may feel slight discomfort from the needle puncture and the tourniquet.

■ Inform the patient that he need not restrict food and fluids.

Procedure and posttest care

■ Perform a venipuncture, collecting the sample in a 4.5-ml heparinized tube.

- If a hematoma develops at the venipuncture site, apply warm soaks.

Precautions
- Because this test isn't routinely performed, notify the laboratory before drawing the sample. Reference laboratories have certain guidelines and testing dates that you'll need to follow.
- Completely fill the collection tube and invert it gently several times to mix the sample and the anticoagulant thoroughly.
- Handle the sample gently to prevent accidental hemolysis.

Reference values
Osmotic fragility values (percentage of RBCs hemolyzed) that have been obtained photometrically are plotted against decreasing saline tonicity to produce an S-shaped curve with a slope characteristic of the disorder. Reference values differ with tonicities.

Abnormal findings
Low osmotic fragility (increased resistance to hemolysis) is characteristic of thalassemia, iron deficiency anemia, sickle cell anemia, and other RBC disorders in which target cells are found. Low osmotic fragility also occurs after splenectomy.

High osmotic fragility (increased tendency to hemolysis) occurs in hereditary spherocytosis; in spherocytosis associated with autoimmune hemolytic anemia, severe burns, or chemical poisoning.

AGE ISSUE *High osmatic fragility may also be found in hemolytic disease of the newborn (erythroblastosis fetalis).*

Interfering factors
- Failure to use the proper anticoagulant in the collection tube, to fill the tube

completely, or to adequately mix the sample and the anticoagulant
- Hemolysis due to rough handling of the sample
- Presence of hemolytic organisms in the sample
- Conditions, such as severe anemia, that provide fewer RBCs for testing
- Recent blood transfusion

HEMOGLOBIN TESTS

Total hemoglobin

Total hemoglobin (Hb) is used to measure the amount of Hb found in a deciliter (dl, or 100 ml) of whole blood. It's usually part of a complete blood count. Hb concentration correlates closely with the red blood cell (RBC) count and affects the Hb-RBC ratio (mean corpuscular hemoglobin [MCH] and mean corpuscular hemoglobin concentration [MCHC]).

Purpose
- To measure the severity of anemia or polycythemia and to monitor response to therapy
- To obtain data for calculating the MCH and MCHC

Patient preparation
- Explain to the patient that the Hb test is used to detect anemia or polycythemia or to assess his response to treatment.
- Tell the patient that a blood sample will be taken. Explain who will perform the venipuncture and when.
- Explain to the patient that he may feel slight discomfort from the needle puncture and the tourniquet.

AGE ISSUE *If the patient is an infant or child, explain to the parents that a small amount of blood will be taken from his finger or earlobe.*

■ Inform the patient that he need not restrict food and fluids.

Procedure and posttest care

■ For adults and older children, perform a venipuncture and collect the sample in a 3- or 4.5-ml EDTA tube.

AGE ISSUE *For younger children and infants, collect the sample by fingerstick or heelstick in a microcollection device with EDTA.*

■ If a hematoma develops at the venipuncture site, apply warm soaks. If the hematoma is large, monitor pulses distal to the venipuncture site.

■ Ensure subdermal bleeding has stopped before removing pressure.

Precautions

■ Completely fill the collection tube and invert it gently several times to thoroughly mix the sample and the anticoagulant.

■ Handle the sample gently to prevent hemolysis.

Reference values

Hb concentration varies depending on the type of sample drawn and the patient's age and sex:

■ adult males: 14 to 17.4 g/dl (SI, 140 to 174 g/L)

■ males after middle age: 12.4 to 14.9 g/dl (SI, 124 to 149 g/L)

■ adult females: 12 to 16 g/dl: (SI, 120 to 160 g/L)

■ females after middle age: 11.7 to 13.8 g/dl (SI, 117 to 138 g/L).

AGE ISSUE *Reference values for infants and children also vary depending on age:*

– neonates: 17 to 22 g/dl (SI, 170 to 220 g/L)

– 1 week: 15 to 20 g/dl (SI, 150 to 200 g/L)

– 1 month: 11 to 15 g/dl (SI, 110 to 150 g/L)

– children: 11 to 13 g/dl (SI, 110 to 130 g/L).

Those who are more active or who live in high altitudes may have higher values.

Abnormal findings

Low Hb concentration may indicate anemia, recent hemorrhage, or fluid retention, causing hemodilution.

Elevated Hb suggests hemoconcentration from polycythemia or dehydration.

Interfering factors

■ Failure to use the proper anticoagulant or to adequately mix the sample and the anticoagulant

■ Hemolysis due to rough handling of the sample

■ Hemoconcentration due to prolonged tourniquet constriction

■ Very high white blood cell counts, lipemia, or RBCs that are resistant to lysis (false-high)

Fetal hemoglobin

Fetal hemoglobin (Hb), or Hb F, is a normal Hb produced in the red blood cells of a fetus and in smaller amounts in infants. It constitutes 50% to 90% of the Hb in a neonate; the remaining Hb consists of Hb A_1 and Hb A_2, the Hb in adults.

Under normal conditions, the body ceases to manufacture Hb F during the first years of life and begins to manufacture adult Hb. If this changeover doesn't occur and Hb F continues to constitute more than 5% of the Hb after age 6 months, an abnormality should be suspected, particularly thalassemia.

Purpose
- To diagnose thalassemia

Patient preparation
- Explain to the patient that the Hb test is used to detect thalassemia disease.
- Tell the patient that a blood sample will be taken. Explain who will perform the venipuncture and when.
- Reassure the patient that drawing the sample will take less than 3 minutes.
- Explain to the patient that he may feel slight discomfort from the needle puncture and the tourniquet.

AGE ISSUE *If the patient is a child, explain to his parents that a small amount of blood will be taken from his finger or earlobe.*

- Inform the patient or his parents that he need not restrict food and fluids.

Procedure and posttest care
- Perform a venipuncture and collect the sample of blood in a 4.5-ml EDTA tube.

AGE ISSUE *For a young child, collect capillary blood in a microcollection device.*

- If a hematoma develops at the venipuncture site, apply warm soaks. If the hematoma is large, monitor pulses distal to the venipuncture site.
- Ensure subdermal bleeding has stopped before removing pressure.

Precautions
- Completely fill the collection tube and invert it gently several times to mix the sample and the anticoagulant thoroughly.
- Handle the sample gently to prevent hemolysis.

Reference values
Normal values for Hb F range as follows:
- age 0 to 30 days: 60% to 90% (SI, 0.60 to 0.90)
- age 1 to 23 months: 2% (SI, 0.02)
- age 24 months to adult: 0% to 2% (SI, 0 to 0.02).

Abnormal findings
In beta-thalassemia major, Hb F may be 30% or more of the total Hb. Slight increases in Hb F concentration appear in many unrelated hematologic disorders, such as aplastic anemia, homozygous sickle cell disease, and myeloproliferative disorders. Fetal Hb commonly increases to as much as 5% during normal pregnancy.

Interfering factors
- Hemolysis due to rough handling of the sample
- Delay in analyzing the specimen for more than 2 to 3 hours (possible false-high)

Hemoglobin electrophoresis

Hemoglobin (Hb) electrophoresis is probably the most useful laboratory method for separating and measuring normal and abnormal Hb. Through electrophoresis, different types of Hb are separated to form a series of distinctly pigmented bands in a medium. Results are then compared with those of a normal sample.

Hb A, A_2, S, and C are routinely checked, but the laboratory may change the medium or its pH to expand the range of this test.

Purpose
- To measure the amount of Hb A and to detect abnormal Hb
- To aid diagnosis of thalassemia

VARIATIONS OF HEMOGLOBIN TYPE AND DISTRIBUTION

Hemoglobin	Percentage of total hemoglobin	Clinical implications
Hb A	95% to 100% (SI, 0.95 to 1.0)	Normal
Hb A$_2$	4% to 5.8% (SI, 0.04 to 0.058)	ß-thalassemia minor
	1.5% to 3% (SI, 0.015 to 0.03)	Normal
	Under 1.5% (SI, <0.015)	Hb H disease
Hb F	Under 1% (SI, <0.01)	Normal
	2% to 5% (SI, 0.02 to 0.05)	ß-thalassemia minor
	10% to 90% (SI, 0.1 to 0.9)	ß-thalassemia major
	5% to 15% (SI, 0.05 to 0.15)	ß-δ-thalassemia minor
	5% to 35% (SI, 0.05 to 0.35)	Heterozygous hereditary persistence of fetal Hb (HPFH)
	100% (SI, 1.0)	Homozygous HPFH
	15% (SI, 0.15)	Homozygous Hb S
Homozygous Hb S	70% to 98% (SI, 0.7 to 0.98)	Sickle cell disease
Homozygous Hb C	90% to 98% (SI, 0.9 to 0.98)	Hb C disease
Heterozygous Hb C	24% to 44% (SI, 0.24 to 0.44)	Hb C trait

Patient preparation

- Explain to the patient that Hb electrophoresis is used to evaluate Hb.
- Tell the patient that a blood sample will be taken. Explain who will perform the venipuncture and when.
- Explain to the patient that he may feel slight discomfort from the needle puncture and the tourniquet.

🌀 AGE ISSUE *If the patient is an infant or child, explain to the parents that a small amount of blood will be taken from his finger.*

- Inform the patient that he need not restrict food and fluids.

Procedure and posttest care

- Ask the patient if he has received a blood transfusion within the past 4 months.
- Perform a venipuncture and collect the sample in a 3- or 4.5-ml EDTA tube.

🌀 AGE ISSUE *For young children, collect capillary blood in a microcollection device.*

- If a hematoma develops at the venipuncture site, apply warm soaks. If the hematoma is large, monitor pulses distal to the venipuncture site.
- Ensure subdermal bleeding has stopped before removing pressure.

Precautions

- Completely fill the collection tube and invert it gently several times to mix the sample and the anticoagulant.
- Don't shake the tube vigorously.

INHERITANCE PATTERNS IN SICKLE CELL ANEMIA

When both parents have sickle cell anemia (left), childbearing — if possible at all — is dangerous for the mother, and all offspring will have sickle cell anemia. When one parent has sickle cell anemia and one is normal (right), all offspring will be carriers of sickle cell anemia.

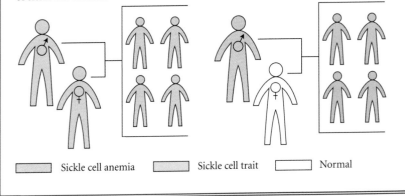

Sickle cell anemia   Sickle cell trait   Normal

Reference values

In adults, Hb A accounts for 95% (SI, 0.95) of all Hb; Hb A_2, 1.5% to 3% (SI, 0.15 to 0.030); and Hb F, < 2% (SI, < 0.02).

AGE ISSUE *In neonates, Hb F normally accounts for half the total. Hb S and Hb C are normally absent.*

Abnormal findings

Hb electrophoresis allows identification of various types of Hb. Certain types may indicate a hemolytic disease. (See *Variations of hemoglobin type and distribution.*)

Interfering factors

■ Failure to fill the tube completely, to use the proper anticoagulant, or to adequately mix the sample and the anticoagulant
■ Hemolysis due to rough handling of the sample
■ Blood transfusion within the past 4 months

Sickle cells

The sickle cell test, also known as the hemoglobin (Hb) S test, is used to detect sickle cells, which are severely deformed, rigid erythrocytes that may slow blood flow. Sickle cell trait (characterized by heterozygous Hb S) is found almost exclusively in blacks — 0.2% of blacks born in the United States have sickle cell disease. (See *Inheritance patterns in sickle cell anemia.*)

Although the sickle cell test is useful as a rapid screening procedure, it may produce erroneous results. Hb electrophoresis should be performed to confirm the diagnosis if sickle cell disease is strongly suspected.

Purpose

■ To identify sickle cell disease and sickle cell trait (See *Identifying sickle cell trait,* page 24.)

IDENTIFYING SICKLE CELL TRAIT

This relatively benign condition results from heterozygous inheritance of the abnormal hemoglobin (Hb) S-producing gene. Like sickle cell anemia, it's most common in blacks.

In persons with sickle cell trait, 20% to 40% of their total Hb is Hb S; the rest is normal. Such persons, called carriers, usually have no symptoms. They have normal Hb and hematocrit values and can expect a normal life span. Nevertheless, they must avoid situations that provoke hypoxia, which occasionally causes a sickling crisis similar to that in sickle cell anemia.

Genetic counseling is essential for sickle cell carriers. Every child of two sickle cell carriers has a 25% chance of inheriting sickle cell anemia and a 50% chance of being a carrier.

Patient preparation

■ Explain to the patient that the Hb S test is used to detect sickle cell disease.
■ Tell the patient that a blood sample will be taken. Explain who will perform the venipuncture and when.
■ Explain to the patient that he may feel slight discomfort from the needle puncture and the tourniquet.

 AGE ISSUE *If the patient is an infant or child, explain to his parents that a small amount of blood will be taken from his finger or earlobe.*
■ Check the patient's history for a blood transfusion within the past 3 months.
■ Inform the patient that he need not restrict food and fluids.

Procedure and posttest care

■ Perform a venipuncture and collect the sample in a 3- or 4.5-ml EDTA tube.

 AGE ISSUE *For young children, collect capillary blood in a microcollection device.*
■ If a hematoma develops at the venipuncture site, apply warm soaks. If the hematoma is large, monitor pulses distal to the phlebotomy site.
■ Ensure subdermal bleeding has stopped before removing pressure.

Precautions

■ Completely fill the collection tube and invert it gently several times to thoroughly mix the sample and the anticoagulant.
■ Don't shake the tube vigorously.

Normal findings

Results of the Hb S test are reported as positive or negative. A negative result suggests the absence of Hb S.

Abnormal findings

A positive result may indicate the presence of sickle cells, but Hb electrophoresis is needed to further diagnose the sickling tendency of cells. Rarely, in the absence of Hb S, other abnormal Hb may cause sickling.

Interfering factors

■ Failure to fill the tube completely, to use the proper anticoagulant in the collection tube, or to adequately mix the sample and the anticoagulant
■ Hemolysis due to rough handling of the sample or use of a small-gauge needle for blood aspiration
■ Hb concentration <10%, elevated Hb S levels in infants under age 6 months, or transfusion within 3 months of the test (possible false-negative)

Unstable hemoglobin

Unstable hemoglobin (Hb) is a rare, congenital defect caused by amino acid substitutions in the structure of Hb. It's called "unstable" because of the ease with which the Hb decomposes. The presence of unstable Hb may lead to the formation of small masses called *Heinz bodies,* which accumulate on red blood cell membranes. Although Heinz bodies are usually removed by the spleen or liver, they may cause mild to severe hemolysis. (See *Signs and symptoms of unstable hemoglobin.*) Unstable Hb is best detected by precipitation tests (heat stability or isopropanol solubility).

Purpose
■ To detect unstable Hb

Patient preparation
■ Explain to the patient that the unstable Hb test is used to detect abnormal Hb in the blood.
■ Tell the patient that a blood sample will be taken. Explain who will perform the venipuncture and when.
■ Explain to the patient that he may feel slight discomfort from the needle puncture and the tourniquet.
■ Notify the laboratory and physician of medications the patient is taking that may affect test results; they may need to be restricted.
■ Inform the patient that he need not restrict food and fluids.

Procedure and posttest care
■ Perform a venipuncture and collect the sample in a 3- or 4.5-ml EDTA tube.
■ If a hematoma develops at the venipuncture site, apply warm soaks. If the hematoma is large, monitor pulses distal to the venipuncture site.

SIGNS AND SYMPTOMS OF UNSTABLE HEMOGLOBIN

More than 60 varieties of unstable hemoglobin (Hb) exist, each named after the city in which it was discovered. Their effects vary according to their number, the degree of instability, the condition of the spleen, and the oxygen-binding abilities of the unstable Hb.

Patients with unstable Hb typically exhibit pallor, jaundice, splenomegaly and, with severely unstable Hb, cyanosis, pigmenturia, and hemoglobinuria. Thalassemia commonly causes similar signs and symptoms, but the molecular bases of the two diseases differ greatly.

■ Ensure subdermal bleeding has stopped before removing pressure.
■ Instruct the patient that he may resume medications discontinued before the test, as ordered.

Precautions
■ Completely fill the collection tube and invert it gently several times to mix the sample and the anticoagulant thoroughly.
■ To avoid hemolysis, don't shake the tube vigorously.

Normal findings
When no unstable Hb appears in the sample, the heat stability test result is negative; the isopropanol solubility test result is reported as stable.

Abnormal findings
A positive heat stability test result or unstable solubility test result, especially with hemolysis, strongly suggests the presence of unstable Hb.

IDENTIFYING HEINZ BODIES

After special supravital staining, Heinz bodies (particles of denatured hemoglobin that are usually attached to the cell membrane) appear as small, purple inclusions at cell margins. Heinz bodies are present in certain hemolytic anemias.

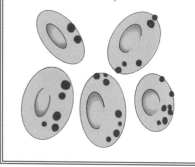

RBCs, the presence of unstable Hb, unbalanced globin chain synthesis due to thalassemia, or a red cell enzyme deficiency (such as glucose-6-phosphate dehydrogenase deficiency). Although Heinz bodies are removed from RBCs by the spleen, they're a major cause of hemolytic anemias. (See *Identifying Heinz bodies*.)

Heinz bodies can be detected in a whole blood sample using phase microscopy or supravital stains; when they don't form spontaneously, various oxidant drugs may be added to the sample to induce their formation.

Purpose
■ To help detect causes of hemolytic anemia

Patient preparation
■ Explain to the patient that this test is used to determine the cause of anemia.
■ Tell the patient that a blood sample will be taken. Explain who will perform the venipuncture and when.
■ Explain to the patient that he may feel slight discomfort from the needle puncture and the tourniquet.
■ Notify the laboratory and physician of medications the patient is taking that may affect test results; they may need to be restricted.
■ Inform the patient that he need not restrict food and fluids.

Procedure and posttest care
■ Perform a venipuncture and collect the sample in a 3- or 4.5-ml EDTA tube.
■ If a hematoma develops at the venipuncture site, apply warm soaks. If the hematoma is large, monitor pulses distal to the venipuncture site.
■ Ensure subdermal bleeding has stopped before removing pressure.

Interfering factors
■ Failure to fill the tube completely, to use the proper anticoagulant, or to adequately mix the sample and the anticoagulant
■ Hemoconcentration due to prolonged tourniquet constriction
■ Hemolysis due to rough handling of the sample
■ Hemolysis due to antimalarials, furazolidone (in infants), nitrofurantoin, phenacetin, procarbazine, and sulfonamides (possible false-positive or unstable results)
■ High levels of Hb F (possible false-positive isopropanol)
■ Recent blood transfusion

Heinz bodies

Heinz bodies are particles of decomposed hemoglobin (Hb) that precipitate from the cytoplasm of red blood cells (RBCs) and accumulate on RBC membranes. They form as a result of drug injury to

- Instruct the patient that he may resume medications discontinued before the test, as ordered.

Precautions
- Fill the sample collection tube completely.
- Invert the tube gently several times to mix the sample and the anticoagulant.

Normal findings
A negative test result indicates an absence of Heinz bodies.

Abnormal findings
The presence of Heinz bodies—a positive test result—may indicate an inherited RBC enzyme deficiency, the presence of unstable Hb, thalassemia, or drug-induced RBC injury. Heinz bodies may also be present after splenectomy.

Interfering factors
- Failure to fill the collection tube completely, to use the appropriate anticoagulant, to adequately mix the sample and the anticoagulant, or to send the sample to the laboratory immediately
- Antimalarials, furazolidone (in infants), nitrofurantoin, phenacetin, procarbazine, and sulfonamides (possible false-positive)
- Recent blood transfusion

Serum iron and total iron-binding capacity

Iron is essential to the formation and function of hemoglobin as well as many other heme and nonheme compounds. After iron is absorbed by the intestine, it's distributed to various body compartments for synthesis, storage, and transport. (See *Normal iron metabolism,* page 28.) Serum iron concentration is normally highest in the morning and declines progressively during the day; therefore, the sample should be drawn in the morning.

An iron assay is used to measure the amount of iron bound to transferrin in blood plasma. Total iron-binding capacity (TIBC) measures the amount of iron that would appear in plasma if all the transferrin were saturated with iron.

Serum iron and TIBC are of greater diagnostic usefulness when performed with the serum ferritin assay, but together these tests may not accurately reflect the state of other iron compartments, such as myoglobin iron and the labile iron pool. Bone marrow or liver biopsy and iron absorption or excretion studies may yield more information.

Purpose
- To estimate total iron storage
- To aid diagnosis of hemochromatosis
- To help distinguish iron deficiency anemia from anemia of chronic disease (For information on another test used to differentiate anemias, see *Siderocyte stain,* page 29.)
- To help evaluate nutritional status

Patient preparation
- Explain to the patient that this test evaluates the body's capacity to store iron.
- Tell the patient that a blood sample will be taken. Explain who will perform the venipuncture and when.
- Explain to the patient that he may feel slight discomfort from the needle puncture and the tourniquet.
- Notify the laboratory and physician of medications the patient is taking that may affect test results; they may need to be restricted.
- Inform the patient that he need not restrict food and fluids.

NORMAL IRON METABOLISM

Ingested iron, absorbed and oxidated in the bowel, bonds with the protein transferrin for circulation to bone marrow, where hemoglobin (Hb) synthesis occurs, and to all iron-hungry body cells. In the spleen, Hb breakdown recycles iron back to the bone marrow or into storage. The body conserves iron, losing small amounts through skin, stool, urine, and menses. Storage areas in the liver, spleen, bone marrow, and reticuloendothelial system hold iron as ferritin until the body needs it; the liver alone stores about 60%.

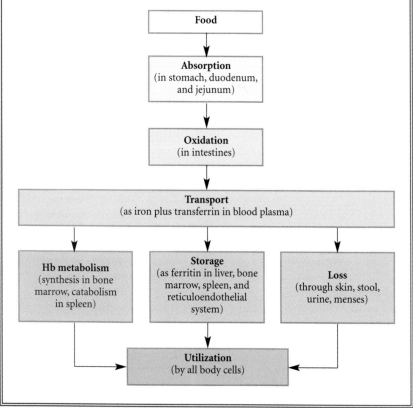

Procedure and posttest care

■ Perform a venipuncture and collect the sample in a 4.5-ml clot-activator tube.
■ If a hematoma develops at the venipuncture site, apply warm soaks. If the hematoma is large, monitor pulses distal to the venipuncture site.
■ Ensure subdermal bleeding has stopped before removing pressure.
■ Instruct the patient that he may resume medications discontinued before the test, as ordered.

Precautions

■ Handle the sample gently to prevent hemolysis.
■ Send the sample to the laboratory immediately.

SIDEROCYTE STAIN

Siderocytes are red blood cells (RBCs) containing particles of nonhemoglobin iron known as siderocytic granules. In neonates, siderocytic granules are normally present in normoblasts and reticulocytes during hemoglobin synthesis. However, the spleen removes most of these granules from normal RBCs, and they disappear rapidly with age.

In adults, an elevated siderocyte level usually indicates abnormal erythropoiesis, which may occur in congenital spherocytic anemia, chronic hemolytic anemias (such as the thalassemias), pernicious anemia, hemochromatosis, toxicities (such as lead poisoning), infection, or severe burns. Elevated levels may also follow splenectomy because the spleen normally removes siderocytic granules.

Performing the test

The siderocyte stain test measures the number of circulating siderocytes. Venous blood is drawn into a 3- or 4.5-ml EDTA tube or, for infants and children, collected in a Microtainer or pipette and smeared directly on a 3″ x 5″ glass slide. When the blood smear is stained, siderocytic granules appear as purple-blue specks clustered around the periphery of mature erythrocytes. Cells containing these granules are counted as a percentage of total RBCs. The results aid differential diagnosis of the anemias and hemochromatosis and help detect toxicities.

Interpreting results

Normally, neonates have a slightly elevated siderocyte level that reaches the normal adult value of 0.5% (SI, 0.05) of total RBCs in 7 to 10 days. In patients with pernicious anemia, the siderocyte level is 8% to 14% (SI, 0.08 to 0.14); in chronic hemolytic anemia, 20% to 100% (SI, 0.2 to 1.0); in lead poisoning, 10% to 30% (SI, 0.1 to 0.3); and in hemochromatosis, 3% to 7% (SI, 0.03 to 0.07). A high siderocyte level calls for additional testing (including bone marrow examination) to determine the cause of abnormal erythropoiesis.

Reference values

Normal serum iron and TIBC values are as follows:

- Serum iron
- Males: 60 to 170 µg/dl (SI, 10.7 to 30.4 µmol/L)
- Females: 50 to 130 µg/dl (SI, 9 to 23.3 µmol/L)
- TIBC
- Males and females: 300 to 360 µg/dl (SI, 54 to 64 µmol/L)
- Saturation
- Males and females: 20% to 50% (SI, 0.2 to 0.5).

Abnormal findings

In iron deficiency, serum iron levels decrease and TIBC increases, decreasing saturation. In cases of chronic inflammation (such as in rheumatoid arthritis), serum iron may be low in the presence of adequate body stores, but TIBC may remain unchanged or may decrease to preserve normal saturation. Iron overload may not alter serum levels until relatively late but, in general, serum iron increases and TIBC remains the same, which increases the saturation.

Interfering factors

- Hemolysis due to rough handling of the sample or failure to send the sample to the laboratory immediately
- Chloramphenicol and hormonal contraceptives (possible false-positive)
- Corticotropin (possible false-negative)

■ Iron supplements (possible false-positive serum iron values but false-negative TIBC)

Serum ferritin

Ferritin, a major iron-storage protein, normally appears in small quantities in serum. In healthy adults, serum ferritin levels are directly related to the amount of available iron stored in the body and can be measured accurately by radio-immunoassay.

Purpose
■ To screen for iron deficiency and iron overload
■ To measure iron storage
■ To distinguish between iron deficiency (a condition of low iron storage) and chronic inflammation (a condition of normal storage)

Patient preparation
■ Explain to the patient that the serum ferritin test is used to assess the available iron stored in the body.
■ Tell the patient that a blood sample will be taken. Explain who will perform the venipuncture and when.
■ Explain to the patient that he may feel slight discomfort from the needle puncture and the tourniquet.
■ Review the patient's history for transfusion within the past 4 months.
■ Inform the patient that he need not restrict food and fluids.

Procedure and posttest care
■ Perform a venipuncture, collecting the sample in a 10-ml tube without additives.
■ If a hematoma develops at the venipuncture site, apply warm soaks. If the hematoma is large, monitor pulses distal to the venipuncture site.

■ Ensure subdermal bleeding has stopped before removing pressure.

Reference values
Normal serum ferritin values in adults vary with age and sex, as follows:
■ adult males: 20 to 300 ng/ml (SI, 20 to 300 µg/L)
■ adult females: 20 to 120 ng/ml (SI, 20 to 120 µg/L).

AGE ISSUE Normal values in infants and children also vary with age:
– neonates: 25 to 200 ng/ml (SI, 25 to 200 µg/L)
– age 1 month: 200 to 600 ng/ml (SI, 200 to 600 µg/L)
– age 2 to 5 months: 50 to 200 ng/ml (SI, 50 to 200 µg/L)
– age 6 months to 15 years: 7 to 140 ng/ml (SI, 7 to 140 µg/L).

Abnormal findings
High serum ferritin levels may indicate acute or chronic hepatic disease, iron overload, leukemia, acute or chronic infection or inflammation, Hodgkin's disease, or chronic hemolytic anemias. In these disorders, iron stores in the bone marrow may be normal or significantly increased. Serum ferritin levels are characteristically normal or slightly elevated in patients with chronic renal disease.

Low serum ferritin levels indicate chronic iron deficiency.

Interfering factors
■ Recent blood transfusion (possible false-high)

Methemoglobin

Methemoglobin (MetHb, Hb M) is a structural hemoglobin (Hb) variant, which is formed when the heme portion of deoxygenated Hb is oxidized to a ferric state. When this occurs, the heme is incapable of combining with oxygen and transporting it to the tissues, and the patient becomes cyanotic.

Purpose
■ To detect acquired methemoglobinemia, which is caused by excessive radiation or the toxic effects of chemicals or drugs
■ To detect congenital methemoglobinemia

Patient preparation
■ If possible, obtain a history of the patient's hematologic status and Hb disorder, conditions that produce nitrite, and exposure to sources of nitrites in drugs.
■ Explain to the patient that this test is used to detect abnormal Hb in the blood.
■ Tell the patient that a blood sample will be taken. Explain who will perform the venipuncture and when.
■ Explain to the patient that he may feel slight discomfort from the needle puncture and the tourniquet.
■ Notify the laboratory and physician of medications the patient is taking that may affect test results; they may need to be restricted.

Procedure and posttest care
■ Perform a venipuncture and collect the sample in a 4.5-ml heparinized tube.
■ If a hematoma develops at the venipuncture site, apply warm soaks. If the hematoma is large, monitor pulses distal to the venipuncture site.
■ Ensure subdermal bleeding has stopped before removing pressure.

Precautions
■ Fill the collection tube completely and invert it gently several times.
■ To avoid hemolysis, don't shake the tube vigorously.

■ Place the collection tube on ice and send it to the laboratory immediately.

Reference values
Normal MetHb levels are 0% to 1.5% (SI, 0 to 0.015) of total Hb.

Abnormal findings
Increased MetHb levels may indicate acquired or hereditary methemoglobinemia or carbon monoxide poisoning. These levels can also be caused by taking certain drugs or being exposed to certain substances.

Decreased MetHb levels may occur in pancreatitis.

Interfering factors
■ Aniline dyes, nitroglycerin, benzocaine, chlorates, lidocaine, nitrates, nitrites, phenacetin, sulfonamides, radiation, primaquine, and resorcinol (possible increase)
■ Nitrite toxicity in breast-feeding infants (increase due to conversion of inorganic nitrate to nitrite ion)

WHITE BLOOD CELL TESTS

White blood cell count

A white blood cell (WBC) count, also called a leukocyte count, is part of a complete blood count. It indicates the number of white cells in a microliter (µl, or cubic millimeter) of whole blood.

WBC counts may vary by as much as 2,000 cells/µl (SI, 2×10^9/L) on any given day due to strenuous exercise, stress, or digestion. The WBC count may increase or decrease significantly in certain diseases, but is diagnostically useful only when the patient's white cell differential and clinical status are considered.

Purpose
- To determine infection or inflammation
- To determine the need for further tests, such as the WBC differential or bone marrow biopsy
- To monitor response to chemotherapy or radiation therapy

Patient preparation
- Explain to the patient that the WBC test is used to detect an infection or inflammation.
- Tell the patient that a blood sample will be taken. Explain who will perform the venipuncture and when.
- Explain to the patient that he may feel slight discomfort from the needle puncture and the tourniquet.
- Inform the patient that he should avoid strenuous exercise for 24 hours before the test. Also tell him that he should avoid eating a heavy meal before the test.
- If the patient is being treated for an infection, advise him that this test will be repeated to monitor his progress.
- Notify the laboratory and physician of medications the patient is taking that may affect test results; they may need to be restricted.

Procedure and posttest care
- Perform a venipuncture and collect the sample in a 3- or 4.5-ml EDTA tube.
- If a hematoma develops at the venipuncture site, apply warm soaks. If the hematoma is large, monitor pulses distal to the venipuncture site.
- Ensure subdermal bleeding has stopped before removing pressure.

- Instruct the patient that he may resume his usual diet, activity, and medications discontinued before the test, as ordered.
- A patient with severe leukopenia may have little or no resistance to infection and requires protective isolation.

Precautions
- Completely fill the sample collection tube.
- Invert the sample gently several times to mix the sample and the anticoagulant.

Reference values
The WBC count ranges from 4,000 to 10,000/µl (SI, 4 to 10 $\times$ 10^9/L).

Abnormal findings
An elevated WBC count (leukocytosis) commonly signals infection, such as an abscess, meningitis, appendicitis, or tonsillitis. A high count may also result from leukemia and tissue necrosis due to burns, myocardial infarction, or gangrene.

A low WBC count (leukopenia) indicates bone marrow depression that may result from viral infections or from toxic reactions, such as those following treatment with antineoplastics, ingestion of mercury or other heavy metals, or exposure to benzene or arsenicals. Leukopenia characteristically accompanies influenza, typhoid fever, measles, infectious hepatitis, mononucleosis, and rubella.

Interfering factors
- Hemolysis due to rough handling of the sample
- Exercise, stress, or digestion
- Most antineoplastics; anti-infectives, such as metronidazole and flucytosine; anticonvulsants, such as phenytoin derivatives; thyroid hormone antagonists; and

PERFORMING A LAP STAIN

Levels of leukocyte alkaline phosphatase (LAP), an enzyme found in neutrophils, may be altered by infection, stress, chronic inflammatory diseases, Hodgkin's disease, and hematologic disorders. Most of these conditions elevate LAP levels; only a few—notably chronic myelogenous leukemia (CML)—depress them. Thus, this test is usually used to differentiate CML from other disorders that produce an elevated white blood cell count.

Procedure
To perform the LAP stain, a blood sample is obtained by venipuncture or fingerstick. The venous blood sample is collected in a 7-ml *green-top* tube and transported immediately to the laboratory, where a blood smear is prepared; the peripheral blood sample is smeared on a 3″ glass slide and fixed in cold formalin-methanol. The blood smear is then stained to show the amount of LAP present in the cytoplasm of the neutrophils. One hundred neutrophils are counted and assessed; each is assigned a score of 0 to 4, according to the degree of LAP staining. Normally, values for LAP range from 40 to 100, depending on the laboratory's standards.

Implications of results
Depressed LAP values typically indicate CML; however, values may also be low in paroxysmal nocturnal hemoglobinuria, aplastic anemia, and infectious mononucleosis. Elevated levels may indicate Hodgkin's disease, polycythemia vera, or a neutrophilic leukemoid reaction—a response to such conditions as infection, chronic inflammation, or pregnancy.

After a diagnosis of CML, the LAP stain may also be used to help detect onset of the blastic phase of the disease, when LAP levels typically rise. However, LAP levels also increase toward normal in response to therapy; because of this, test results must be correlated with the patient's condition.

nonsteroidal anti-inflammatory drugs such as indomethacin (decrease)

White blood cell differential

The white blood cell (WBC) differential is used to evaluate the distribution and morphology of WBCs, providing more specific information about a patient's immune system than the WBC count alone.

WBCs are classified as one of five major types of leukocytes—neutrophils, eosinophils, basophils, lymphocytes, and monocytes—and the percentage of each type is determined. The differential count is the percentage of each type of WBC in the blood. The total number of each type of WBC is obtained by multiplying the percentage of each type by the total WBC count.

High levels of these leukocytes are associated with various allergic diseases and reactions to parasites. An eosinophil count is sometimes ordered as a follow-up test when an elevated or depressed eosinophil level is reported.

Purpose
- To evaluate the body's capacity to resist and overcome infection
- To detect and identify various types of leukemia (See *Performing a LAP stain*.)
- To determine the stage and severity of an infection

INTERPRETING WBC DIFFERENTIAL VALUES

The differential count measures the types of white blood cells (WBCs) as a percentage of the total WBC count (the relative value). The absolute value is obtained by multiplying the relative value of each cell type by the total WBC count. The relative and absolute values must be considered to obtain an accurate diagnosis.

For example, consider a patient whose WBC count is 6,000/µl (SI, 6×10^9/L) and whose differential shows 30% (SI, 0.3) neutrophils and 70% (SI, 0.7) lymphocytes. His relative lymphocyte count seems to be quite high (lymphocytosis), but when this figure is multiplied by his WBC count (6,000 × 70% = 4,200 lymphocytes/µl), (SI, [6×10^9/L] × 9.79 = 4.2×10^9/L lymphocytes), it's well within the normal range.

However, this patient's neutrophil count (30%; SI, 0.3) is low; when this figure is multiplied by the WBC count (6,000 × 30% = 1,800 neutrophils/ml) (SI, [6×10^9/L] × 0.30 = 1.8×10^9/L neutrophils), the result is a low absolute number, which may mean depressed bone marrow.

The normal percentages of WBC type in adults are:
Neutrophils: 54% to 75% (SI, 0.54 to 0.75)
Eosinophils: 1% to 4% (SI, 0.01 to 0.04)
Basophils: 0% to 1% (SI, 0 to 0.01)
Monocytes: 2% to 8% (SI, 0.02 to 0.08)
Lymphocytes: 25% to 40% (SI, 0.25 to 0.4).

■ To detect allergic reactions and parasitic infections and assess their severity (eosinophil count)

■ To distinguish viral from bacterial infections

Patient preparation

■ Explain to the patient that the WBC differential test is used to evaluate the immune system.

■ Tell the patient that a blood sample will be taken. Explain who will perform the venipuncture and when.

■ Explain to the patient that he may feel slight discomfort from the needle puncture and the tourniquet.

■ Notify the laboratory and physician of medications the patient is taking that may affect test results; they may need to be restricted.

■ Inform the patient that he need not restrict food and fluids, but should refrain from strenuous exercise for 24 hours before the test.

Procedure and posttest care

■ Perform a venipuncture and collect the sample in a 3- or 4.5-ml EDTA tube.

■ If a hematoma develops at the venipuncture site, apply warm soaks. If the hematoma is large, monitor pulses distal to the venipuncture site.

■ Ensure subdermal bleeding has stopped before removing pressure.

Precautions

■ Completely fill the collection tube.

■ Invert the sample gently several times to thoroughly mix the sample and the anticoagulant.

■ To prevent hemolysis, don't shake the tube.

Reference values

For normal values for the five types of WBCs classified in the differential for adults and children, see *Interpreting WBC differential values*. For an accurate diagnosis, differential test results must always

INFLUENCE OF DISEASE ON BLOOD CELL COUNT

The white blood cell (WBC) differential aids diagnosis because some disorders affect only one WBC type. Below, each type is listed as well as the corresponding effect and its cause.

Cell type	How affected
Neutrophils	*Increased by:* ■ Infections: osteomyelitis, otitis media, salpingitis, septicemia, gonorrhea, endocarditis, smallpox, chickenpox, herpes, Rocky Mountain spotted fever ■ Ischemic necrosis due to myocardial infarction, burns, carcinoma ■ Metabolic disorders: diabetic acidosis, eclampsia, uremia, thyrotoxicosis ■ Stress response due to acute hemorrhage, surgery, excessive exercise, emotional distress, third trimester of pregnancy, childbirth ■ Inflammatory diseases: rheumatic fever, rheumatoid arthritis, acute gout, vasculitis, myositis *Decreased by:* ■ Bone marrow depression due to radiation or cytotoxic drugs ■ Infections: typhoid, tularemia, brucellosis, hepatitis, influenza, measles, mumps, rubella, infectious mononucleosis ■ Hypersplenism: hepatic disease and storage diseases ■ Collagen vascular disease such as systemic lupus erythematosus (SLE) ■ Folic acid or vitamin B_{12} deficiency
Eosinophils	*Increased by:* ■ Allergic disorders: asthma, hay fever, food or drug sensitivity, serum sickness, angioneurotic edema ■ Parasitic infections: trichinosis, hookworm, roundworm, amebiasis ■ Skin diseases: eczema, pemphigus, psoriasis, dermatitis, herpes ■ Neoplastic diseases: chronic myelocytic leukemia (CML), Hodgkin's disease, metastases and necrosis of solid tumors *Decreased by:* ■ Stress response ■ Cushing's syndrome
Basophils	*Increased by:* ■ CML, Hodgkin's disease, ulcerative colitis, chronic hypersensitivity states *Decreased by:* ■ Hyperthyroidism ■ Ovulation, pregnancy ■ Stress
Lymphocytes	*Increased by:* ■ Infections: tuberculosis (TB), hepatitis, infectious mononucleosis, mumps, rubella, cytomegalovirus ■ Thyrotoxicosis, hypoadrenalism, ulcerative colitis, immune diseases, lymphocytic leukemia *Decreased by:* ■ Severe debilitating illnesses: heart failure, renal failure, advanced TB ■ Defective lymphatic circulation, high levels of adrenal corticosteroids, immunodeficiency due to immunosuppressives

(continued)

INFLUENCE OF DISEASE ON BLOOD CELL COUNT *(continued)*

Cell type	How affected
Monocytes	*Increased by:*

Monocytes

Increased by:
- Infections: subacute bacterial endocarditis, TB, hepatitis, malaria
- Collagen vascular disease: SLE, rheumatoid arthritis
- Carcinomas
- Monocytic leukemia
- Lymphomas

be interpreted in relation to the total WBC count.

Abnormal findings

Abnormal differential patterns provide evidence for many disease states and other conditions. (See *Influence of disease on blood cell count,* pages 35 and 36.)

Interfering factors

- Failure to completely fill the collection tube, to use the proper anticoagulant, or to adequately mix the sample and the anticoagulant
- Hemolysis due to rough handling of the sample
- Methysergide, desipramine (increase or decrease eosinophil count), indomethacin, procainamide (decrease eosinophil count), anticonvulsants, capreomycin, cephalosporins, D-penicillamine, gold compounds, isoniazid, nalidixic acid, novobiocin, para-aminosalicylic acid, paromomycin, penicillins, phenothiazines, rifampin, streptomycin, sulfonamides, and tetracyclines (increase count by provoking an allergic reaction)

Selected readings

Anderson, S.C., and Poulsen, K.B. *Anderson's Atlas of Hematology.* Philadelphia: Lippincott Williams & Williams, 2003.

Cavanaugh, B.M. *Nurse's Manual of Laboratory and Diagnostic Tests,* 4th ed. Philadelphia: F.A. Davis Co., 2003.

Diseases, 3rd ed. Springhouse, Pa.: Springhouse Corp., 2001.

Fischbach, F. *A Manual of Laboratory and Diagnostic Tests,* 7th ed. Philadelphia: Lippincott Williams & Wilkins, 2004.

Guyton, A.C., and Hall, J.E. *Textbook of Medical Physiology,* 10th ed. Philadelphia: W.B. Saunders Co., 2001.

McClatchey, K.D. *Clinical Laboratory Medicine,* 2nd ed. Philadelphia: Lippincott Williams & Wilkins, 2002.

Nursing2004 Drug Handbook, 24th ed. Philadelphia: Lippincott Williams & Wilkins, 2004.

Pagana, K.D., and Pagana, T.J. *Mosby's Diagnostic and Laboratory Test Reference,* 6th ed. St. Louis: Mosby–Year Book, Inc., 2003.

Schnell, Z., et al. *Davis's Comprehensive Handbook of Laboratory and Diagnostic Tests with Nursing Implications.* Philadelphia: F.A. Davis Co., 2003.

Hemostasis

Introduction

The circulatory system protects itself from excessive blood loss or blood clotting by hemostasis. In this process, vascular injury activates a complex chain of events — vasoconstriction, platelet aggregation, and coagulation — that leads to clotting, which stops bleeding. This clotting must be localized to the injury site, and ultimately the clot must be removed.

Vasoconstriction:
Primary response
Within seconds of vascular injury, neural reflexes and local smooth-muscle spasms cause the walls of the damaged vessel to contract, aided by secretion of serotonin, epinephrine, and lipoproteins. Constriction lasts about 10 minutes in a small vessel and up to 30 minutes in a larger one. The extent of tissue damage determines the extent of vasospasm; for example, a blood vessel that suffers a clean cut bleeds more than one that's crushed. However, vasoconstriction slows blood flow only briefly in small vessels and is insufficient to prevent blood loss from large ones.

37

Permanent repair requires a hemostatic plug formed of platelet aggregates and a fibrin clot.

Aggregation of platelets

Circulating platelets converge on the wound site, first touching and then adhering to the collagen fibers of the torn vessel lining (endothelium). This contact of platelets with collagen stimulates the platelets to secrete adenosine diphosphate (ADP), which causes them to change shape and aggregate, sticking together in clumps. Additional ADP activates more platelets, which also collect at the site. This aggregation loosely plugs the wound to help prevent further blood loss.

Coagulation

When platelet aggregation is underway, blood loses its fluidity and forms a gelatinous clot. More than a score of agents in blood and in tissues influence this process. Some promote coagulation (procoagulants) and others inhibit it (anticoagulants). When vascular injury causes bleeding, procoagulants gather at the injury site and stimulate formation of a stable fibrin clot.

Clotting begins within 60 seconds of injury and proceeds through the interaction of two parallel pathways—extrinsic and intrinsic. The *extrinsic pathway* is activated when tissue thromboplastin is released at the injury site. At the same time, procoagulants in the blood are activated in the *intrinsic pathway* to produce plasma thromboplastin and several other factors. Both systems then interact to continue activating other coagulation factors until a meshwork of fibrin strands is built that traps blood cells, more platelets, and plasma to form a clot.

Three crucial steps

Clotting normally proceeds in three stages:
- Trauma to blood vessels or tissues triggers thromboplastin activity through intrinsic and extrinsic pathways.
- Next, these pathways converge to convert prothrombin to thrombin.
- Thrombin converts fibrinogen in the surrounding plasma to a fibrin plug.

Formation of thromboplastin

When blood contacts injured tissue, the tissue frees factor III (tissue thromboplastin), an ill-defined, clot-promoting substance. Because factor III alone is ineffective, it interacts with factor VII (proconvertin) in the presence of calcium ions. Factor IV (calcium ions [Ca^{++}]) and tissue phospholipids form a complex that initiates the reactions of the extrinsic pathway. This complex then activates factor X (Stuart-Prower factor) at the end of the extrinsic pathway.

In intrinsic clotting, plasma thromboplastin results from progressive activation of several procoagulants. When stimulated by surface contact or vascular injury, factor XII (Hageman factor) activates factor XI (plasma thromboplastin antecedent), which, in the presence of calcium, initiates activity of factor IX (Christmas factor). The activated form of this plasma protein, in the presence of platelet phospholipids, converts factor VIII (antihemophilic factor) to its active state and forms a complex that activates factor X.

Almost simultaneously, factor X reacts with factor V (proaccelerin), in the presence of Ca^{++} and platelet phospholipids, to form a prothrombin-converting complex. Within 15 seconds of its formation, this protein begins to split factor II (prothrombin) to form thrombin. (See *Blood coagulation factors.*)

BLOOD COAGULATION FACTORS

Factor	Synonym	Profile	Site of synthesis
I	Fibrinogen	Precursor of fibrin	Liver
II	Prothrombin	Precursor of thrombin	Liver
III	Tissue thromboplastin	Activator of prothrombin	All tissues
IV	Ca^{++}	Essential for prothrombin activation and formation of fibrin	From diet
V	Proaccelerin	Accelerates conversion of prothrombin to thrombin	Liver
VII	Serum prothrombin (proconvertin)	Accelerates conversion of prothrombin to thrombin	Liver
VIII	Antihemophilic factor (AHF, hemophilic factor A)	Associated with factors IX, XI, and XII; aids in forming activated factor X via intrinsic system and conversion of prothrombin to thrombin	Reticuloendothelial system
IX	Christmas factor (hemophilic factor B, plasma thromboplastin component [PTC])	Activated by factor XI; essential to formation of activated factor X through intrinsic system; associated with factors VIII, XI, and XII	Liver
X	Stuart-Prower factor	Triggers prothrombin conversion; requires vitamin K	Liver
XI	Plasma thromboplastin antecedent (PTA)	Activated by factor XII; associated with factors VIII, IX, and XII in formation of activated factor X through intrinsic system	Unknown
XII	Hageman factor	First factor activated in the intrinsic pathway; activates factor XI	Unknown
XIII	Fibrin stabilizing factor (FSF)	Produces stronger urea-insoluble fibrin clot	Unknown

Conversion of prothrombin to thrombin

Prothrombin splits into two parts: One is inert and the other is thrombin. Thrombin is a potent enzyme that converts fibrinogen to fibrin, helps stabilize the final clot, and starts clot breakdown (fibrinolysis) after healing.

Conversion of fibrinogen to fibrin

After thrombin is formed in adequate amounts, it hydrolyzes fibrinogen (factor

I), splitting two low-molecular-weight peptides from each fibrinogen molecule. The remaining peptides are fibrin monomers, which automatically combine end to end and side by side to form fibrin threads that eventually build a weak, soluble polymer meshwork.

To strengthen this weak fibrin clot, thrombin activates another plasma enzyme called factor XIII (fibrin stabilizing factor). In the presence of Ca++, this enzyme strengthens the fibrin polymer by forming covalent bonds and causing cross-linkage of peptide bonds. This action results in a firm, insoluble clot.

Coagulation defects and bleeding disorders

Coagulation defects due to *factor I (fibrinogen) deficiency* may be hereditary or acquired. Hereditary errors are classified as quantitative (afibrinogenemia or hypofibrinogenemia) or qualitative (dysfibrinogenemia). Afibrinogenemia causes severe bleeding that may be life-threatening. This disorder, thought to be transmitted as an autosomal recessive trait, first occurs in the neonate as umbilical bleeding. Acquired hypofibrinogenemia can result from conditions such as disseminated intravascular coagulation (DIC), primary fibrinogenolysis, and hepatic disease.

Factor II deficiency, or hypoprothrombinemia, can also be hereditary or acquired. Hereditary transmission, as an autosomal recessive trait, is rare. This defect can be acquired from vitamin K deficiency, warfarin therapy, or hepatic disease. It's frequently associated with deficiencies of factor VII, IX, and X.

Factor VII deficiency can also be inherited as an autosomal recessive trait. Although the clinical effects of this hereditary defect may vary, it commonly causes overt symptoms of abnormal coagulation, such as epistaxis, easy bruising, and bleeding from the gums. An acquired form of factor VII deficiency can result from vitamin K deficiency, warfarin therapy, or hepatic disease.

A *defect of factor VIII* causes two congenital disorders: hemophilia A (classic hemophilia) and von Willebrand's disease. Hemophilia A, a sex-linked recessive disorder transmitted by females that occurs almost exclusively in males, is marked by severe bleeding (hemarthroses and muscular and GI bleeding). Von Willebrand's disease, which causes a milder coagulation dysfunction than hemophilia A, is characterized by abnormal platelet function and a mild-to-moderate deficiency of factor VIII and is transmitted to both sexes as an autosomal dominant trait. Symptoms of this disorder include epistaxis, ecchymoses, and oozing after tooth extraction. Both DIC and fibrinolysis may induce acquired factor VIII deficiency.

Congenital *deficiency of factor IX* can cause hemophilia B (Christmas disease), a severe bleeding disorder transmitted as a sex-linked recessive trait from mothers to sons. Because factor IX is formed in the liver and depends on the presence of sufficient vitamin K, an acquired deficiency of this factor can result from lack of vitamin K or from warfarin therapy and hepatic disease.

A *factor X deficiency,* inherited as an autosomal recessive trait (rare), is generally associated with depressed levels of vitamin K, hepatic disease, and anticoagulant therapy.

Congenital *factor XII deficiency,* also transmitted as an autosomal recessive trait, is similarly unlikely to cause symptoms.

COMMON COAGULATION SCREENING TESTS

Test	Implications of abnormal findings
Bleeding time	*Prolonged bleeding time:* thrombocytopenia, disseminated intravascular coagulation (DIC), or von Willebrand's disease; *Abnormal bleeding time with normal platelet count:* platelet function disorder
Capillary fragility	*Excessive number of petechiae in 2" (5-cm) circle of skin:* capillary wall weakness or platelet disorder
Partial thromboplastin time (PTT)	*Prolonged PTT:* presence of anticoagulant, FSP, fibrinolysins, or antibodies to specific clotting factors; or deficiency of clotting factor other than factor VII or XIII
Prothrombin time (PT)	*Prolonged PT:* deficiency of fibrinogen (factor I), prothrombin (factor II), or factors V, VII, or X; hepatic disease; vitamin K deficiency; or ongoing anticoagulant therapy
Plasma thrombin time (TT)	*Prolonged TT:* hepatic disease, fibrin degradation products, effective heparin therapy, hypofibrinogenemia, or dysfibrinogenemia
Fibrin split products (FSP)	*Elevated FSP:* pulmonary embolus, myocardial infarction, deep vein thrombosis, DIC, or primary fibrinogenolysis syndrome.

A small number of patients (5% to 10%) with systemic lupus erythematosus (SLE) develop inhibitors known as lupus-like anticoagulants. These inhibitors appear to be directed at the phospholipids that activate the clotting factors. The presence of these anticoagulants is rarely linked to a clinical bleeding tendency unless another abnormality in hemostasis is present. In the case of SLE, this abnormality is a low platelet count (thrombocytopenia).

Various tests are used to help detect coagulation disorders. (See *Common coagulation screening tests.* See also *Collecting specimens for coagulation testing,* page 42.)

Platelet disorders

Platelets, oval or discoid cytoplasmic fragments about 2 to 4 microns in diameter, are derived from bone marrow megakaryocytes. Platelet disorders stemming from abnormalities of number (thrombocytopenia and thrombocytosis) or function (thrombasthenia and thrombocytopathia) impair vascular integrity and the coagulation mechanism. However, serious coagulopathy is likely only when large numbers of platelets are dysfunctional or deficient.

In *thrombocytopenia,* the most common platelet deficiency, the number of platelets is abnormally low (less than $150,000/\mu l$); nevertheless, overt bleeding doesn't generally develop until the count drops below $50,000/\mu l$. Thrombocytopenia may result from decreased bone marrow production of platelets related to aplastic anemia, leukemia, and vitamin B_{12} or folic acid deficiency; from accelerated destruction of platelets by the spleen; from exaggerated destruction of platelets caused by antiplatelet or drug-induced antibodies; from severe blood loss; or from accelerated consumption of plate-

COLLECTING SPECIMENS FOR COAGULATION TESTING

Proper specimen collection and handling is especially important when collecting blood samples for coagulation testing because damage to the vessel wall during venipuncture can cause coagulation to begin, thus affecting test results. Keep in mind the following guidelines for venipuncture and specimen collection.

Timing
Collect samples for coagulation testing at approximately the same time each day, if possible, to eliminate the circadian variations of the different coagulation proteins.

Venipuncture equipment
Avoid using small-bore (large-gauge [> 21G]) needles to collect coagulation test samples because this size needle may mechanically disrupt platelets and activate the coagulation cascade.

Collection technique
A clean venipuncture with a minimum of tissue trauma is essential to obtain a good quality plasma specimen for coagulation testing. Any trauma to the tissue can stimulate the release of tissue thromboplastin, which can contaminate the needle. Therefore, when drawing blood for several laboratory tests, don't draw the coagulation test sample first. If no other tests will be performed, first draw a *red-top* discard tube to negate the effect of tissue thromboplastin on test results. If you're drawing from an intermittent access device, discard 20 ml of blood before collecting the coagulation test sample (for a heparinized line, discard 30 ml). Make sure that the coagulation test tube is filled with blood to the appropriate level to achieve a whole blood-anticoagulant ratio of 9:1.

In addition, avoid prolonged application of the tourniquet because this can stimulate the release of tissue thromboplastin and elevate levels of coagulation factor VII, fibrin monomer, and tissue plasminogen activator.

Specimen handling and transport
Coagulation specimens should be kept capped during transport and storage before testing because uncapped specimens lose carbon dioxide. Loss of carbon dioxide would result in a pH increase, which would affect coagulation test results.

---

lets, as seen in DIC and idiopathic thrombocytopenic purpura.

Antiplatelet antibodies stimulate the reticuloendothelial system to sequester circulating platelets. Proliferation of antibodies may result from treatment with such medications as quinidine, quinine, and thiazide derivatives. Sulfonamides and phenylbutazone may exert a direct toxic effect on platelets through an unknown mechanism. Drug toxicity is likely to induce bleeding from capillaries rather than from larger vessels. This tendency causes small hemorrhages that appear on the skin as purple discolorations (purpura).

In *thrombocytosis,* which is usually secondary to other disorders, the platelet count is abnormally high (more than $400,000/\mu l$) and is associated with inflammatory response, iron deficiency, or splenectomy. Abnormally elevated platelet counts also appear in myeloproliferative disorders, such as polycythemia vera, myelofibrosis, and chronic granulocytic leukemia. Thrombocytosis doesn't generally cause symptoms, but may occasionally lead to bleeding or thrombosis.

Qualitative platelet disorders may be congenital or acquired. Congenital disorders include *thrombasthenia,* a rare autosomal recessive trait; *storage-pool disease,* typified by decreased ADP levels in blood platelets; and *Bernard-Soulier (giant platelet) disease,* marked by abnormally large platelets that fail to aggregate with the reagent ristocetin. Acquired defects may result from aspirin ingestion, uremia, dysproteinemias, and chronic hepatic disease.

Vascular defects

Bleeding due to vascular defects results from abnormal vascular permeability (as in vitamin C deficiency) or fragility (as in purpura senilis). Blood vessels can also rupture and bleed after certain abrupt movements because blood vessels are lightly anchored to surrounding tissue. In allergic purpura, increased vascular permeability and tissue hemorrhage result from an inflammatory capillary reaction.

PLATELET ACTIVITY TESTS

Bleeding time

Bleeding time is used to measure the duration of bleeding after a measured skin incision. Bleeding time may be measured by one of three methods: template, Ivy, or Duke. The template method is the most commonly used and the most accurate because the incision size is standardized. Bleeding time depends on the elasticity of the blood vessel wall and on the number and functional capacity of platelets.

Although the bleeding time test is usually performed on the patient with a personal or family history of bleeding disorders, it's also useful — along with a platelet count — for preoperative screening. The test isn't usually recommended for the patient with a platelet count of less than 75,000/µl (SI, 75 × 10⁹/L).

Purpose
- To assess overall hemostatic function (platelet response to injury and functional capacity of vasoconstriction)
- To detect congenital and acquired platelet function disorders

Patient preparation
- Explain to the patient that the bleeding time test is used to measure the time required to form a clot and stop bleeding.
- Tell the patient who will be performing the test and when it will take place.
- Inform the patient that he need not restrict food and fluids.
- Inform the patient that he may feel some discomfort from the incisions, the antiseptic, and the tightness of the blood pressure cuff. Also inform the patient that depending on the method used, incisions or punctures may leave tiny scars that should be barely visible when healed.
- Notify the laboratory and physician of medications the patient is taking that may affect test results; they may need to be restricted.

Procedure and posttest care
- *Template method:* Wrap the pressure cuff around the upper arm and inflate the cuff to 40 mm Hg. Select an area on the forearm with no superficial veins and clean it with antiseptic. Allow the skin to dry completely before making the incision. Apply the appropriate template lengthwise to the forearm. Use the lancet to make two incisions 1 mm deep and 9 mm long. Start the stopwatch. Without touching the cuts, gently blot the drops of

blood with filter paper every 30 seconds until the bleeding stops in both cuts. Average the time of the two cuts and record the result.

■ *Ivy method:* After applying the pressure cuff and preparing the test site, make three small punctures with a disposable lancet. Start the stopwatch immediately. Taking care not to touch the punctures, blot each site with filter paper every 30 seconds until the bleeding stops. Average the bleeding time of the three punctures and record the result.

■ *Duke method:* Drape the patient's shoulder with a towel. Clean the earlobe and let the skin air-dry. Make a puncture wound 2 to 4 mm deep on the earlobe with a disposable lancet. Start the stopwatch. Being careful not to touch the ear, blot the site with filter paper every 30 seconds until bleeding stops. Record bleeding time.

■ In a patient with a bleeding tendency (hemophilia), maintain a pressure bandage over the incision for 24 to 48 hours to prevent further bleeding. Check the test area frequently; keep the edges of the cuts aligned to minimize scarring.

■ In other patients, a piece of gauze held in place by an adhesive bandage is sufficient.

■ Instruct the patient that he may resume any medications discontinued before the test, as ordered.

Precautions

■ Be sure to maintain a cuff pressure of 40 mm Hg throughout the test.

■ If the bleeding doesn't diminish after 15 minutes, discontinue the test.

■ Apply direct pressure to the test site until bleeding ceases.

Reference values

The normal range of bleeding time is from 3 to 6 minutes (SI, 3 to 6 min) in the template method; from 3 to 6 minutes in the Ivy method; and from 1 to 3 minutes (SI, 1 to 3 min) in the Duke method.

Abnormal findings

Prolonged bleeding time may indicate the presence of disorders associated with thrombocytopenia, such as Hodgkin's disease, acute leukemia, disseminated intravascular coagulation, hemolytic disease of the newborn, Schönlein-Henoch purpura, severe hepatic disease (cirrhosis, for example), or severe deficiency of factors I, II, V, VII, VIII, IX, and XI. Prolonged bleeding time in a patient with a normal platelet count suggests a platelet function disorder (thrombasthenia, thrombocytopathia) and requires further investigation with clot retraction, prothrombin consumption, and platelet aggregation tests.

Interfering factors

■ Sulfonamides, thiazide diuretics, antineoplastics, anticoagulants, nonsteroidal anti-inflammatory drugs, vitamin E supplementation, aspirin and aspirin compounds, and some nonnarcotic analgesics (prolonged bleeding time)

Platelet count

Platelets, or thrombocytes, are the smallest formed elements in blood. They promote coagulation and the formation of a hemostatic plug in vascular injury.

Platelet count is one of the most important screening tests of platelet function. Accurate counts are vital.

Purpose
- To evaluate platelet production
- To assess the effects of chemotherapy or radiation therapy on platelet production
- To diagnose and monitor severe thrombocytosis or thrombocytopenia
- To confirm a visual estimate of platelet number and morphology from a stained blood film

Patient preparation
- Explain to the patient that the platelet count test is used to determine if the patient's blood clots normally.
- Tell the patient that a blood sample will be taken. Explain who will perform the venipuncture and when.
- Inform the patient that he need not restrict food and fluids.
- Explain to the patient that he may feel slight discomfort from the needle puncture and the tourniquet.
- Notify the laboratory and physician of medications the patient is taking that may affect test results; they may need to be restricted.

Procedure and posttest care
- Perform a venipuncture and collect the sample in a 3- or 4.5-ml EDTA tube.
- If a hematoma develops at the venipuncture site, apply warm soaks. If the hematoma is large, monitor pulses distal to the venipuncture site.
- Ensure subdermal bleeding has stopped before removing pressure.
- Instruct the patient that he may resume any medications discontinued before the test, as ordered.

Precautions
- To prevent hemolysis, avoid excessive probing at the venipuncture site and handle the sample gently.

- Completely fill the collection tube and invert it gently several times to mix the sample and the anticoagulant thoroughly.

Reference values
Normal platelet counts range from 140,000 to 400,000/μl (SI, 140 to 400 $\times$ 10^9/L) in adults.

AGE ISSUE *In children, normal platelet counts range from 150,000 to 450,000/μl (SI, 150 to 450 $\times$ 10^9/L) in children.*

Abnormal findings
A platelet count below 50,000/μl can cause spontaneous bleeding; when the count is below 5,000/μl, fatal central nervous system bleeding or massive GI hemorrhage is possible. A decreased platelet count (thrombocytopenia) can result from aplastic or hypoplastic bone marrow; infiltrative bone marrow disease, such as leukemia, or disseminated infection; megakaryocytic hypoplasia; ineffective thrombopoiesis due to folic acid or vitamin B_{12} deficiency; pooling of platelets in an enlarged spleen; increased platelet destruction due to drugs or immune disorders; disseminated intravascular coagulation; Bernard-Soulier syndrome; or mechanical injury to platelets.

An increased platelet count (thrombocytosis) can result from hemorrhage, infectious disorders, iron deficiency anemia, recent surgery, pregnancy, splenectomy, or inflammatory disorders. In such cases, the platelet count returns to normal after the patient recovers from the primary disorder. However, the count remains elevated in primary thrombocythemia, myelofibrosis with myeloid metaplasia, polycythemia vera, and chronic myelogenous leukemia.

When the platelet count is abnormal, diagnosis usually requires further studies, such as complete blood count, bone marrow biopsy, direct antiglobulin test (direct Coombs' test), and serum protein electrophoresis.

Interfering factors
- Failure to use the proper anticoagulant or to mix the sample and anticoagulant promptly and adequately
- Hemolysis due to rough handling of the sample or excessive probing at the venipuncture site
- Heparin (decrease)
- Acetazolamide, acetohexamide, antineoplastics, brompheniramine maleate, carbamazepine, chloramphenicol, ethacrynic acid, furosemide, gold salts, hydroxychloroquine, indomethacin, isoniazid, mephenytoin, mefenamic acid, methazolamide, methimazole, methyldopa, oral diazoxide, penicillamine, penicillin, phenylbutazone, phenytoin, pyrimethamine, quinidine sulfate, quinine, salicylates, streptomycin, sulfonamides, thiazide and thiazide-like diuretics, and tricyclic antidepressants (possible decrease)
- High altitudes, persistent cold temperatures, strenuous exercise, or excitement (increase)

Capillary fragility

Also called the *positive-pressure test,* the *tourniquet test ,*and the *Rumpel-Leede test,* the capillary fragility test is a nonspecific method for evaluating bleeding tendencies. This test is used to measure the capillaries' ability to remain intact under increased intracapillary pressure. The pressure is controlled by a blood pressure cuff placed around the patient's upper arm and inflated to 70 to 90 mm Hg or midway between the diastolic and systolic pressure. The pressure is maintained for

5 minutes. This temporary increase in pressure may cause rhexis bleeding of the capillaries and formation of petechiae on the arm, wrist, or hand. The number of petechiae within a given circular space is recorded as the test result.

Purpose
- To assess the fragility of capillary walls
- To identify a platelet deficiency (thrombocytopenia)

Patient preparation
- Explain to the patient that the capillary fragility test is used to identify abnormal bleeding tendencies.
- Tell the patient who will be performing the procedure and when.
- Inform the patient that he need not restrict food and fluids.
- Explain to the patient that he may feel discomfort from the pressure of the blood pressure cuff.

Procedure and posttest care
- The patient's skin temperature and the room temperature should be normal to ensure accurate results.
- Select and mark a 2″ (5-cm) space on the patient's forearm. Ideally, the site should be free from petechiae; otherwise, record the number of petechiae before starting the test.
- Fasten the cuff around the arm and raise the pressure to a point midway between the systolic and diastolic blood pressures. Maintain this pressure for 5 minutes, then release the cuff.
- Count the number of petechiae that appear in the 2″ space.
- Record the test results.
- Encourage the patient to open and close his hand a few times to hasten return of blood to the forearm.

Precautions
- Don't repeat this test on the same arm within 1 week.
- This test is contraindicated in patients with disseminated intravascular coagulation (DIC) or other bleeding disorders and in those with significant petechiae already present.

Reference values
A few petechiae may normally be present before the test. Less than 10 petechiae on the forearm 5 minutes (SI, 5 m) after the test is considered normal, or negative; more than 10 petechiae is considered a positive result. The following scale may also be used to report test results.

Number of petechiae/5 cm	Score
0 to 10	1+
11 to 20	2+
21 to 50	3+
Over 50	4+

Abnormal findings
A positive finding (more than 10 petechiae, or a score of 2+ to 4+) indicates weakness of the capillary walls (vascular purpura) or a platelet defect. It may occur in such conditions as thrombocytopenia, thrombasthenia, purpura senilis, scurvy, DIC, von Willebrand's disease, vitamin K deficiency, dysproteinemia, and polycythemia vera and in severe deficiencies of factor VII, fibrinogen, or prothrombin. Conditions unrelated to bleeding defects, such as scarlet fever, measles, influenza, chronic renal disease, hypertension, and diabetes with coexisting vascular disease, may also increase capillary fragility.

AGE ISSUE *An abnormal number of petechiae sometimes appear before menstruation and at other times in some healthy persons, especially in women over age 40.*

Interfering factors
- Decreasing estrogen levels in postmenopausal women (possible increase)
- Glucocorticoids (possible decrease)
- Repeating the test on the same arm within 1 week, causing errors in counting the number of petechiae

Platelet aggregation

After vascular injury, platelets gather at the injury site and clump together to form an aggregate or plug that helps maintain hemostasis and promotes healing. The platelet aggregation test, an in vitro procedure, is used to measure the rate at which the platelets in a plasma sample form a clump after the addition of an aggregating reagent.

Purpose
- To assess platelet aggregation
- To detect congenital and acquired platelet bleeding disorders

Patient preparation
- Explain to the patient that the platelet aggregation test is used to determine if blood clots properly.
- Tell the patient that the test requires a blood sample. Explain who will perform the venipuncture and when. (See *Aspirin and platelet aggregation,* page 48.)
- Explain to the patient that he may feel slight discomfort from the needle puncture and the tourniquet.
- Instruct the patient to fast or to maintain a nonfat diet for 8 hours before the test because lipemia can affect the test results.

ASPIRIN AND PLATELET AGGREGATION

Unlike other salicylates, aspirin inhibits platelet aggregation. The inhibition occurs in the second phase of platelet aggregation, when it prevents the release of adenosine diphosphate from platelets. Mean bleeding time may double in healthy individuals after ingestion of aspirin. In children or in patients with bleeding disorders, such as hemophilia, bleeding time may be even more prolonged.

Effect on platelets
The effect of aspirin on platelets seems to result from the inhibition of prostaglandin synthesis. A single 325-mg oral dose of aspirin results in about 90% inhibition of the enzyme cyclooxygenase in circulating platelets, preventing the synthesis of compounds that induce platelet aggregation. The inhibition of cyclooxygenase is irreversible; thus, its effect lasts for 4 to 6 days — the life span of platelets. Bleeding time peaks within 12 hours. Altered hemostasis persists about 36 hours after the last dose of aspirin, sometimes longer for the patient receiving long-term therapy.

Effect on blood vessels
Aspirin's action on blood vessels may oppose that seen in platelets because cyclooxygenase plays a different role in the vascular endothelium. Here, the enzyme produces prostacyclin, a compound that inhibits platelet aggregation and causes vasodilation. Inhibition of cyclooxygenase in the vascular endothelium, in effect, reverses aspirin's antithrombotic effect on platelets. However, studies suggest that cyclooxygenase in the platelets is more sensitive than that in the vascular endothelium and that, therefore, a low aspirin dosage (for example, 80 mg daily or 325 mg every other day) may prove more effective in preventing thrombosis than higher dosages.

■ Notify the laboratory and physician of medications the patient is taking that may affect test results; they may need to be restricted.

Procedure and posttest care
■ Perform a venipuncture and collect the sample in a 4.5-ml siliconized tube.
■ Completely fill the collection tube and invert it gently several times to mix the sample and the anticoagulant thoroughly.
■ Apply pressure to the venipuncture site for 5 minutes or until bleeding stops.
■ If a hematoma develops at the venipuncture site, apply warm soaks.
■ Instruct the patient that he may resume his usual diet and medications discontinued before the test, as ordered.

Precautions
■ Because the list of medications known to alter the results of this test is long and continually growing, the patient should be as drug-free as possible before the test.
■ If the patient has taken aspirin within the past 14 days and the test can't be postponed, ask the laboratory to verify the presence of aspirin in the plasma. If test results are abnormal for such a sample, the use of aspirin must be discontinued and the test repeated in 2 weeks.
■ Avoid excessive probing at the venipuncture site.
■ Remove the tourniquet promptly to avoid bruising.
■ Handle the sample gently to prevent hemolysis and keep it between 71.6° F

and 98.6° F (22° C and 37° C) to prevent aggregation.

Reference values

Normal aggregation occurs in 3 to 5 minutes (SI, 3 to 5 min), but findings are temperature-dependent and vary with the laboratory. Aggregation curves obtained by using different reagents help to distinguish various qualitative platelet defects.

Abnormal findings

Abnormal findings may indicate von Willebrand's disease, Bernard-Soulier syndrome, storage pool disease, Glanzmann's thrombasthenia, polycythemia vera, severe liver disease, or uremia.

Interfering factors

■ Failure to observe pretest restrictions
■ Failure to use the proper anticoagulant or to adequately mix the sample and the anticoagulant
■ Hemolysis due to rough handling of the sample or to excessive probing at the venipuncture site
■ Aspirin and aspirin compounds, phenylbutazone, sulfinpyrazone, phenothiazines, anti-inflammatory drugs, antihistamines, and tricyclic antidepressants (decrease)
■ Ingestion of large amounts of garlic (inhibits platelet aggregation)

COAGULATION TESTS

Partial thromboplastin time

The partial thromboplastin time (PTT) is used to evaluate all the clotting factors of the intrinsic pathway — except platelets — by measuring the time required for formation of a fibrin clot after the addition of calcium and phospholipid emulsion to a plasma sample. An activator, such as kaolin, is used to shorten clotting time.

Purpose

■ To screen for deficiencies of the clotting factors in the intrinsic pathways
■ To monitor response to heparin therapy

Patient preparation

■ Explain to the patient that the PTT test is used to determine if blood clots normally.
■ Tell the patient that a blood sample will be taken. Explain who will perform the venipuncture and when.
■ Explain to the patient that he may feel slight discomfort from the needle puncture and the tourniquet.
■ When appropriate, tell the patient receiving heparin therapy that this test may be repeated at regular intervals to assess his response to treatment.
■ Inform the patient that he need not restrict food and fluids.

Procedure and posttest care

■ Perform a venipuncture and collect the sample in a 7-ml tube with sodium citrate added.
■ If a hematoma develops at the venipuncture site, apply warm soaks. If the hematoma is large, monitor pulses distal to the venipuncture site.
■ Ensure subdermal bleeding has stopped before removing pressure.

Precautions

■ Completely fill the collection tube, invert it gently several times, and send it to the laboratory on ice.

■ To prevent hemolysis, avoid excessive probing at the venipuncture site and handle the sample gently.

■ For a patient on anticoagulant therapy, additional pressure may be needed at the venipuncture site to control bleeding.

Reference values

Normally, a fibrin clot forms 21 to 35 seconds (SI, 21 to 35 s) after adding reagents. For a patient on anticoagulant therapy, ask the physician to specify the reference values for the therapy being delivered.

Abnormal findings

A prolonged PTT may indicate a deficiency of certain plasma clotting factors, the presence of heparin, or the presence of fibrin split products, fibrinolysins, or circulating anticoagulants that are antibodies to specific clotting factors.

Interfering factors

■ Failure to fill the collection tube completely, to use the proper anticoagulant, or to adequately mix the sample and the anticoagulant

■ Hemolysis due to rough handling of the sample or to excessive probing at the venipuncture site

■ Failure to send the sample to the laboratory immediately or to place it on ice

Prothrombin time

Prothrombin time (PT) measures the time required for a fibrin clot to form in a citrated plasma sample after addition of calcium ions and tissue thromboplastin (factor III).

Purpose

■ To evaluate the extrinsic coagulation system (factors V, VII, and X and prothrombin and fibrinogen)

■ To monitor response to oral anticoagulant therapy

Patient preparation

■ Explain to the patient that the PT test is used to determine if the blood clots normally.

■ Notify the laboratory and physician of medications the patient is taking that may affect test results; they may need to be restricted.

■ Tell the patient that a blood sample will be taken. Explain who will perform the venipuncture and when.

■ Explain to the patient that he may feel slight discomfort from the needle puncture and the tourniquet.

■ When appropriate, explain that this test is used to monitor the effects of oral anticoagulants; the test will be performed daily when therapy begins and will be repeated at longer intervals when medication levels stabilize.

■ Inform the patient that he need not restrict food and fluids.

Procedure and posttest care

■ Perform a venipuncture and collect the sample in a 3- or 4.5-ml siliconized tube.

■ If a hematoma develops at the venipuncture site, apply warm soaks. If the hematoma is large, monitor pulses distal to the venipuncture site.

■ Ensure subdermal bleeding has stopped before removing pressure.

■ Instruct the patient that he may resume his usual diet and medications discontinued before the test, as ordered.

Precautions

■ Completely fill the collection tube and invert it gently several times to mix the sample and the anticoagulant thoroughly. If the tube isn't filled to the correct volume, an excess of citrate appears in the sample.

■ To prevent hemolysis, avoid excessive probing during venipuncture and handle the sample gently.

Reference values

Normally, PT values range from 10 to 14 seconds (SI, 10 to 14 s). Values vary, however, depending on the source of tissue thromboplastin and the type of sensing devices used to measure clot formation. In a patient receiving oral anticoagulants, PT is usually maintained between 1 and 2½ times the normal control value.

Abnormal findings

Prolonged PT may indicate deficiencies in fibrinogen; prothrombin; factors V, VII, or X (specific assays can pinpoint such deficiencies); or vitamin K. It may also result from ongoing oral anticoagulant therapy. A prolonged PT that exceeds 2½ times the control value is commonly associated with abnormal bleeding.

Interfering factors

■ Failure to fill the collection tube completely (possible false-high)

■ Failure to adequately mix the sample and the anticoagulant or to send the sample to the laboratory promptly

■ Hemolysis due to rough handling of the sample

■ Salicylates, more than 1 g/day (increase)

■ Fibrin or fibrin split products in the sample or plasma fibrinogen levels >100 mg/dl (possible prolonged PT)

■ Antihistamines, chloral hydrate, corticosteroids, digoxin, diuretics, glutethimide, griseofulvin, progestin-estrogen combinations, pyrazinamide, vitamin K, and xanthines, such as caffeine and theophylline (possible decrease)

■ Corticotropin, anabolic steroids, cholestyramine resin, heparin I.V. (within 5 hours of sample collection), indomethacin, mefenamic acid, para-aminosalicylic acid, methimazole, oxyphenbutazone, phenylbutazone, phenytoin, propylthiouracil, quinidine, quinine, thyroid hormones, vitamin A, or alcohol in excess (prolonged PT)

■ Antibiotics, barbiturates, hydroxyzine, sulfonamides, mineral oil, or clofibrate (possible increase or decrease)

Activated clotting time

Activated clotting time, or automated coagulation time, measures whole blood clotting time. It's commonly performed during procedures that require extracorporeal circulation, such as cardiopulmonary bypass, ultrafiltration, hemodialysis, and extracorporeal membrane oxygenation (ECMO), and during invasive procedures, such as cardiac catheterization and percutaneous transluminal coronary angioplasty.

Purpose

■ To monitor the effect of heparin

■ To monitor the effect of protamine sulfate in heparin neutralization

■ To detect severe deficiencies in clotting factors (except factor VII)

Patient preparation

■ Explain to the patient that the activated clotting time test is used to monitor the effect of heparin on the blood's ability to coagulate.

■ Tell the patient that the test requires a blood sample, which is usually drawn from an existing vascular access site; therefore, no venipuncture will be needed.

- Explain who will perform the test and that it's usually done at the bedside.
- Explain that two blood samples will be drawn. The first one will be discarded so that any heparin in the tubing doesn't interfere with the results.
- If the sample is drawn from a line with a continuous infusion, stop the infusion before drawing the sample.

Procedure and posttest care
- Withdraw 5 to 10 ml of blood from the line and discard it.
- Withdraw a clean sample of blood into the special tube containing celite provided with the activated clotting time unit.
- Start the activated clotting time unit and wait for the signal to insert the tube.
- Flush the vascular access site according to your facility's policy.

Precautions
- Guard against contamination with heparin if drawn from an access site containing heparin.

Reference values
In a non-anticoagulated patient, normal activated clotting time is 107 seconds plus or minus 13 seconds (SI, 107 ± 13 s). During cardiopulmonary bypass, heparin is titrated to maintain an activated clotting time between 400 and 600 seconds (SI, 400 to 600 s). During ECMO, heparin is titrated to maintain the activated clotting time between 220 and 260 seconds (SI, 220 to 260 s).

Interfering factors
- Failure to fill the collection tube completely, to use the proper anticoagulant, to adequately mix the sample and the anticoagulant, or to send the sample to the laboratory immediately or place it on ice

- Hemolysis due to rough handling of the sample or to excessive probing at the venipuncture site
- Failure to draw at least 5 ml waste to avoid sample contamination when drawing the sample from a venous access device that's used for heparin infusion

One-stage factor assay: Extrinsic coagulation system

When prothrombin time (PT) and partial thromboplastin time (PTT) are prolonged, a one-stage assay is used to detect a deficiency of factor II, V, or X. If PT is abnormal, but PTT is normal, factor VII may be deficient.

Purpose
- To identify a specific factor deficiency in a person with prolonged PT or PTT
- To study the patient with congenital or acquired coagulation defects
- To monitor the effects of blood component therapy in the factor-deficient patient

Patient preparation
- Explain to the patient that the one-stage assay test is used to assess the function of the blood coagulation mechanism.
- Tell the patient that a blood sample will be taken. Explain who will perform the venipuncture and when.
- Explain to the patient that he may feel slight discomfort from the needle puncture and the tourniquet.
- When the patient is factor deficient and receiving blood component therapy, tell him that he may need a series of tests. (See *Factor XIII assay: The missing link.*)
- Notify the laboratory and physician of medications the patient is taking that may

FACTOR XIII ASSAY: THE MISSING LINK

When a patient shows poor wound healing and other symptoms of a bleeding disorder despite normal coagulation test results, a factor XIII assay is recommended. In this test, a plasma sample is incubated with either chloracetic acid or a urea solution after normal clotting takes place. The clot is observed for 24 hours; if it dissolves, a severe factor XIII deficiency exists.

Factor XIII is responsible for stabilizing the fibrin clot, the final step in the clotting process. If the clot is unstable, it breaks loose, resulting in scarring and poor wound healing. Deficiency of this factor is usually transmitted as an autosomal recessive trait, but may result from hepatic disease or tumors.

Effects of deficiency
The clinical effects of factor XIII deficiency include umbilical bleeding in the neonate, prolonged bleeding after trauma, hemarthrosis, spontaneous abortion (rarely), intraovarial bleeding (more common in factor XIII deficiency than in other bleeding disorders), and recurrent ecchymoses, hematomas, and poor wound healing. Bleeding after trauma may begin immediately or may be delayed as long as 12 to 36 hours.

Improving prognosis
Treatment with infusions of plasma or cryoprecipitate has improved the prognosis of the patient with factor XIII deficiency; in some cases, the patient may even live a normal life. However, before appropriate treatment can begin, diagnostic evaluation must rule out other bleeding disorders. Dysfibrinogenemia, hyperfibrinogenemia, and disseminated intravascular coagulation also cause rapid clot dissolution in this assay, but unlike factor XIII deficiency, they also cause an abnormal fibrinogen level and thrombin time.

---

affect test results; they may need to be restricted.
■ Inform the patient that he need not restrict food and fluids.

Procedure and posttest care
■ Perform a venipuncture and collect the sample in a 3- or 4.5-ml siliconized tube.
■ Apply direct pressure to the venipuncture site until bleeding stops.
■ If a hematoma develops at the venipuncture site, apply warm soaks. A patient with a bleeding disorder may require a pressure bandage to stop bleeding at the venipuncture site.
■ Instruct the patient that he may resume his usual diet and medications discontinued before the test, as ordered.

Precautions
■ If the patient has a suspected coagulation defect, avoid excessive probing during venipuncture, don't leave the tourniquet on too long (it will cause bruising), and apply pressure to the puncture site for 5 minutes or until the bleeding stops.
■ Completely fill the collection tube and invert it gently several times to mix the sample and the anticoagulant.
■ Handle the sample gently to prevent hemolysis, and send it to the laboratory immediately or place it on ice.

Reference values
The reference ranges for most factors is 50% to 150% of normal (SI, 0.5 to 1.5).

Abnormal findings

Deficiency of factor X may also indicate disseminated intravascular coagulation (DIC). A factor V deficiency suggests severe hepatic disease, DIC, or fibrinogenolysis. Deficiencies of all four factors may be congenital; absence of factor II is lethal.

Interfering factors

■ Failure to mix the sample and the anticoagulant adequately or to send the sample to the laboratory immediately or place it on ice

■ Hemolysis due to rough handling of the sample

■ Oral anticoagulants (possible increase due to inhibition of vitamin K-dependent synthesis and activation of clotting factors II, VII, and X, which form in the liver)

One-stage factor assay: Intrinsic coagulation system

When prothrombin time is normal but partial thromboplastin time is abnormal, a one-stage assay is used to identify a deficiency in the intrinsic coagulation system: factor VIII, IX, XI, or XII.

Purpose

■ To identify a specific factor deficiency

■ To study a patient with a congenital or an acquired coagulation defect

■ To monitor the effects of blood component therapy in the factor-deficient patient

Patient preparation

■ Explain to the patient that the one-stage assay test is used to assess the function of the blood coagulation mechanism.

■ Tell the patient that a blood sample will be taken. Explain who will perform the venipuncture and when.

■ Explain to the patient that he may feel slight discomfort from the needle puncture and the tourniquet.

■ Notify the laboratory and physician of medications the patient is taking that may affect test results; they may need to be restricted.

■ When the patient is factor deficient and receiving blood component therapy, tell him that a series of tests may be needed to monitor therapeutic progress.

■ Inform the patient that he need not restrict food and fluids.

Procedure and posttest care

■ Perform a venipuncture and collect the sample in a 3- or 4.5-ml siliconized tube.

■ Apply direct pressure to the venipuncture site until bleeding subsides.

■ If a hematoma develops at the venipuncture site, apply warm soaks. A patient with a bleeding disorder may require a pressure bandage to stop bleeding at the venipuncture site.

■ Instruct the patient that he may resume any medications discontinued before the test, as ordered.

Precautions

■ If a coagulation defect is suspected, avoid excessive probing during venipuncture, don't leave the tourniquet on too long (it will cause bruising), and apply pressure to the puncture site for 5 minutes or until the bleeding stops.

■ Completely fill the collection tube and invert it gently several times to mix the sample and the anticoagulant thoroughly.

■ Handle the sample gently to prevent hemolysis and send it to the laboratory immediately or place it on ice.

UNDERSTANDING THE ANTITHROMBIN III TEST

The antithrombin III test helps detect the cause of impaired coagulation, especially hypercoagulation, by measuring levels of antithrombin III (AT III), a protein that inactivates thrombin and inhibits coagulation. AT III may be evaluated by a functional clotting assay or synthetic substrates. Exogenous heparin is added to a fresh, citrated blood sample to accelerate activity, then excess thrombin (factor Xa) is added to the plasma. The amount of factor Xa not activated by AT III is quantitated and com-

pared to a normal control sample. Reference values may vary for each laboratory, but should lie between 80% and 120% of normal.

Decreased AT III levels can indicate disseminated intravascular coagulation or thromboembolic, hypercoagulation, or hepatic disorders. Slightly decreased levels can result from hormonal contraceptives. Elevated levels can result from kidney transplantation and the use of oral anticoagulants or anabolic steroids.

Reference values

Reference ranges for most factors are 50% to 150% of normal activity (SI, 0.5 to 1.5).

Abnormal findings

A factor VIII deficiency may indicate hemophilia A, von Willebrand's disease, or a factor VIII inhibitor. An acquired deficiency of factor VIII may result from disseminated intravascular coagulation or fibrinolysis. Factor VIII antigen and ristocetin cofactor tests distinguish between hemophilia A (and its carrier state) and von Willebrand's disease.

A factor IX deficiency may suggest hemophilia B, or it may be acquired as a result of hepatic disease, a factor IX inhibitor, a vitamin K deficiency, or coumarin therapy. Factor VIII and IX inhibitors occur after blood transfusions in a patient deficient in either factor and are antibodies specific to each factor.

A factor XI deficiency may appear after the stress of trauma or surgery or transiently in a neonate. A factor XII deficiency may be inherited or acquired (such as nephrosis) and may also appear transiently in a neonate.

Interfering factors

■ Failure to adequately mix the sample and the anticoagulant or to send the sample to the laboratory immediately
■ Hemolysis due to rough handling of the sample
■ Oral anticoagulants (decrease in factor IX)
■ Pregnancy (increase in factor VIII)

Plasma thrombin time

Plasma thrombin time, or thrombin clotting time, measures how quickly a clot forms when a standard amount of bovine thrombin is added to a platelet-poor plasma sample from the patient and to a normal plasma control sample. After thrombin is added, the clotting time for each sample is compared and recorded. This test allows a quick but imprecise estimation of plasma fibrinogen levels, which are a function of clotting time. (See *Understanding the antithrombin III test*, for information about another test that helps determine the cause of coagulation disorders.)

Purpose
- To detect a fibrinogen deficiency or defect
- To aid the diagnosis of disseminated intravascular coagulation (DIC) and hepatic disease
- To monitor the effectiveness of treatment with heparin or thrombolytic agents

Patient preparation
- Explain to the patient that the plasma thrombin time test is used to determine if blood clots normally.
- Notify the laboratory and physician of medications the patient is taking that may affect test results; they may need to be restricted.
- Tell the patient that a blood sample will be taken. Explain who will perform the venipuncture and when.
- Explain to the patient that he may feel slight discomfort from the needle puncture and the tourniquet.
- Inform the patient that he need not restrict food and fluids.

Procedure and posttest care
- Perform a venipuncture and collect the sample in a 3- to 4.5-ml siliconized tube.
- If a hematoma develops at the venipuncture site, apply warm soaks. If the hematoma is large, monitor pulses distal to the phlebotomy site.
- Ensure bleeding has stopped before removing pressure.
- Instruct the patient that he may resume any medications discontinued before the test, as ordered.

Precautions
- If the tube isn't filled to the correct volume, an excess of citrate appears in the sample. Completely fill the collection tube and invert it gently several times to mix the sample and the anticoagulant thoroughly.
- To prevent hemolysis, avoid excessive probing during venipuncture and rough handling of the sample.
- Immediately put the sample on ice and send it to the laboratory.

Reference values
Normal thrombin times range from 10 to 15 seconds (SI, 10 to 15 s). Test results are usually reported with a normal control value.

Abnormal findings
A prolonged thrombin time may indicate heparin therapy, hepatic disease, DIC, hypofibrinogenemia, or dysfibrinogenemia. The patient with a prolonged thrombin time may require measurement of fibrinogen levels; in suspected DIC, the test for fibrin split products is also necessary.

Interfering factors
- Failure to use the proper anticoagulant, to adequately mix the sample and the anticoagulant, or to send the sample to the laboratory properly
- Hemolysis due to rough handling of the sample or to excessive probing at the venipuncture site
- Heparin, fibrinogen, or fibrin degradation products (possible increase)

Plasma fibrinogen

Fibrinogen (factor I) originates in the liver and is converted to fibrin by thrombin during clotting. Because fibrin is necessary for clot formation, fibrinogen deficiency can produce mild to severe bleeding disorders.

Purpose
- To aid the diagnosis of suspected clotting or bleeding disorders caused by fibrinogen abnormalities

Patient preparation
- Explain to the patient that the plasma fibrinogen test is used to determine if blood clots normally.
- Tell the patient that a blood sample will be taken. Explain who will perform the venipuncture and when.
- Explain to the patient that he may feel slight discomfort from the needle puncture and the tourniquet.
- Notify the laboratory and physician of medications the patient is taking that may affect test results; they may need to be restricted.
- Inform the patient that he need not restrict food and fluids.

Procedure and posttest care
- Perform a venipuncture and collect the sample in a 3- or 4.5-ml tube with sodium citrate added.
- If a hematoma develops at the site, apply warm soaks. If the hematoma is large, monitor pulses distal to the phlebotomy site.
- Ensure that subdermal bleeding has stopped before removing pressure.
- Instruct the patient that he may resume any medications discontinued before the test, as ordered.

Precautions
- This test is contraindicated in the patient with active bleeding or acute infection or illness and in a patient who has had a blood transfusion within 4 weeks.
- Avoid excessive probing during venipuncture and handle the sample gently.
- Completely fill the collection tube, invert it gently several times, and send it to the laboratory immediately or place it on ice.

Reference values
Fibrinogen levels normally range from 200 to 400 mg/dl (SI, 2 to 4 g/L).

Abnormal findings
Depressed fibrinogen levels may indicate congenital afibrinogenemia; hypofibrinogenemia or dysfibrinogenemia; disseminated intravascular coagulation; fibrinolysis; severe hepatic disease; cancer of the prostate, pancreas, or lung; or bone marrow lesions. Obstetric complications or trauma may cause low levels.

Markedly decreased fibrinogen levels impede the accurate interpretation of coagulation tests that have a fibrin clot as an end point.

Elevated levels may indicate cancer of the stomach, breast, or kidney or inflammatory disorders, such as pneumonia or membranoproliferative glomerulonephritis.

Prolonged partial thromboplastin time, prothrombin time, and thrombin time may also indicate a fibrinogen deficiency.

Interfering factors
- Failure to fill the collection tube completely, to adequately mix the sample and anticoagulant, or to send the sample to the laboratory promptly
- Hemolysis due to excessive probing at the venipuncture site or to rough handling of the sample
- Heparin or hormonal contraceptives
- Third trimester of pregnancy and postoperative status (possible increase)

Fibrin split products

After a fibrin clot forms in response to vascular injury, the clot is eventually de-

CAUSES OF DISSEMINATED INTRAVASCULAR COAGULATION

Obstetric	Amniotic fluid embolism, eclampsia, retained dead fetus, retained placenta, abruptio placentae, and toxemia
Neoplastic	Sarcoma, metastatic carcinoma, acute leukemia, prostate cancer, and giant hemangioma
Infectious	Acute bacteremia, septicemia, and rickettsemia; viral, fungal, or protozoal infection
Necrotic	Trauma, destruction of brain tissue, extensive burns, heatstroke, rejection of transplant, and hepatic necrosis
Cardiovascular	Fat embolism, acute venous thrombosis, cardiopulmonary bypass surgery, hypovolemic shock, cardiac arrest, and hypotension
Other	Snakebite, cirrhosis, transfusion of incompatible blood, purpura, and glomerulonephritis

graded by plasmin, a fibrin-dissolving enzyme. The resulting fragments are known as fibrin split products (FSP), or fibrinogen degradation products. In the FSP test, they are detected in the diluted serum that's left in a blood sample after clotting.

Purpose
- To detect FSP in the circulation
- To help determine the presence and the approximate severity of a hyperfibrinolytic state (such as disseminated intravascular coagulation [DIC]) that may result in primary fibrinogenolysis or hypercoagulability (See *Causes of disseminated intravascular coagulation*.)

Patient preparation
- Explain to the patient that the FSP test is used to determine if blood clots normally.
- Tell the patient that a blood sample will be taken. Explain who will perform the venipuncture and when.
- Explain to the patient that he may feel slight discomfort from the needle puncture and the tourniquet.

- Notify the laboratory and physician of medications the patient is taking that may affect test results; they may need to be restricted.
- Inform the patient that he need not restrict food and fluids.

Procedure and posttest care
- Perform a venipuncture and draw 2 ml of blood into a plastic syringe.
- Transfer the sample to the tube provided by the laboratory, which contains a soybean trypsin inhibitor and bovine thrombin.
- If a hematoma develops at the venipuncture site, apply warm soaks. If the hematoma is large, monitor pulses distal to the phlebotomy site.
- Ensure subdermal bleeding has stopped before removing pressure.
- Instruct the patient that he may resume any medications discontinued before the test, as ordered.

Precautions
- Draw the sample before administering heparin to avoid false-positive test results.

- Gently invert the collection tube several times to mix the contents thoroughly.
- The blood clots within 2 seconds; after clotting, the sample must be sent immediately to the laboratory to be incubated at 98.6° F (37° C) for 30 minutes before testing proceeds.

Reference values

Serum contains < 10 µg/ml (SI, < 10 mg/L) of FSP. A quantitative assay shows levels of < 3 µg/ml (SI, < 3 mg/L).

Abnormal findings

FSP levels increase in primary fibrinolytic states due to increased levels of circulating profibrinolysin; in secondary states due to DIC and subsequent fibrinolysis; and in alcoholic cirrhosis, preeclampsia, abruptio placentae, congenital heart disease, sunstroke, burns, intrauterine death, pulmonary embolus, deep vein thrombosis (transient increase), and myocardial infarction (after 1 or 2 days). FSP levels usually exceed 100 µg/ml (SI, greater than 100 mg/L) in active renal disease or renal transplant rejection.

Interfering factors

- Pretest administration of heparin (false-high)
- Failure to fill the collection tube completely, to adequately mix the sample and additive, or to send the sample to the laboratory immediately
- Hemolysis due to rough handling of the sample
- Fibrinolytic drugs, such as urokinase, streptokinase, and tissue plasminogen activator, and large doses of barbiturates (increase)

Plasma plasminogen

Plasma plasminogen testing is used to assess plasminogen levels in a plasma sample. During fibrinolysis, plasmin dissolves fibrin clots to prevent excessive coagulation and impaired blood flow. Plasmin doesn't circulate in active form, however, so it can't be directly measured. Its circulating precursor, plasminogen, can be measured and used to evaluate the fibrinolytic system.

Purpose

- To assess fibrinolysis
- To detect congenital and acquired fibrinolytic disorders

Patient preparation

- Explain to the patient that the plasma plasminogen test is used to evaluate blood clotting.
- Tell the patient that a blood sample will be taken. Explain who will perform the venipuncture and when.
- Explain to the patient that he may feel slight discomfort from the needle puncture and the tourniquet.
- Notify the laboratory and physician of medications the patient is taking that may affect test results; they may need to be restricted.
- Inform the patient that he need not restrict food and fluids.

Procedure and posttest care

- Perform a venipuncture and collect the sample in a 4.5-ml siliconized tube.
- If a hematoma develops at the venipuncture site, apply warm soaks. If the hematoma is large, monitor pulses distal to the venipuncture site.
- Ensure bleeding has stopped before removing pressure.

■ Instruct the patient that he may any resume medications discontinued before the test, as ordered.

Precautions
■ Collect the sample as quickly as possible to prevent stasis, which can slow blood flow, causing coagulation and plasminogen activation.
■ To prevent hemolysis, avoid excessive probing during venipuncture and rough handling of the sample.
■ Invert the tube gently several times and immediately send the sample to the laboratory. If testing must be delayed, plasma must be separated and frozen at –94° F (–67.8° C).

Reference values
Normal plasminogen levels range from 10 to 20 mg/dl (0.1 to 0.2 g/L) by immunologic methods.

Abnormal findings
Diminished plasminogen levels can result from disseminated intravascular coagulation, tumors, preeclampsia, and eclampsia, which accelerate plasminogen conversion to plasmin and increase fibrinolysis. Some liver diseases prevent formation of sufficient plasminogen, decreasing fibrinolysis.

Interfering factors
■ Failure to use the proper collection tube, to adequately mix the sample and citrate, to send the sample to the laboratory immediately, or to have the sample separated and frozen
■ Hemolysis due to excessive probing during venipuncture or to rough handling of the sample
■ Hemoconcentration due to prolonged tourniquet use before venipuncture (possible false-low)

■ Hormonal contraceptives (possible slight increase)
■ Thrombolytic drugs, such as streptokinase and urokinase (possible decrease)

Protein C

Vitamin K-dependent, protein C is produced in the liver and circulates in the plasma. It acts as a potent anticoagulant by suppressing activated factors V and VIII. Deficiencies of protein C may be acquired or congenital.

If a deficiency of protein C is identified, further immunologic tests may be needed to determine the type of deficiency. Identifying the role of protein C deficiency in idiopathic venous thrombosis may help prevent thromboembolism.

Purpose
■ To investigate the mechanism of idiopathic venous thrombosis

Patient preparation
■ Explain to the patient that the protein C test evaluates blood clotting.
■ Tell the patient that a blood sample will be taken. Explain who will perform the venipuncture and when.
■ Explain to the patient that he may feel slight discomfort from the needle puncture and the tourniquet.
■ Inform the patient that he need not restrict food and fluids.
■ Notify the laboratory and physician of medications the patient is taking that may affect test results; they may need to be restricted.

Procedure and posttest care
■ Perform a venipuncture. Collect a 3-ml sample in a siliconized vacuum specimen tube or in a special syringe with anticoagulant provided by the laboratory.

- If a hematoma develops at the venipuncture site, apply warm soaks. Apply direct pressure to the venipuncture site until bleeding stops.
- Instruct the patient that he may resume any medications discontinued before the test, as ordered.

Precautions
- Avoid excessive probing during venipuncture.
- Completely fill the collection tube and invert it several times to mix the sample and anticoagulant thoroughly; handle the sample gently.
- Send the sample to the laboratory immediately.

Reference values
The normal range is 70% to 140% (SI, 0.7 to 1.4).

Abnormal findings
Rare, homozygous protein C deficiency is characterized by rapidly fatal thrombosis in the perinatal period, a condition known as *purpura fulminans.*

The more common heterozygous deficiency is associated with genetic susceptibility to venous thromboembolism before age 30 and continuing throughout life. The patient may require long-term treatment with warfarin therapy or protein C supplements from plasma fractions.

Protein C deficiency is also seen in a patient with liver cirrhosis and vitamin K deficiency and in a patient taking warfarin.

Interfering factors
- Hemolysis due to excessive probing at the venipuncture site or to rough handling of the sample
- Anticoagulant therapy

Euglobulin lysis time

Euglobulin lysis time measures the interval between clot formation and clot dissolution in plasma. A precipitated plasma extract is clotted with thrombin, and the time required for the clot to lyse is measured.

Purpose
- To assess the fibrinolytic system
- To help detect abnormal fibrinolytic states

Patient preparation
- Explain to the patient that the euglobulin lysis time test is used to evaluate the blood clotting mechanism.
- Tell the patient that a blood sample will be taken. Explain who will perform the venipuncture and when.
- Explain to the patient that he may feel slight discomfort from the needle puncture and the tourniquet.
- Inform the patient that he need not restrict food and fluids.

Procedure and posttest care
- Perform a venipuncture. Collect a 4.5-ml sample in a tube with sodium citrate or in a chilled tube with 0.5 ml of sodium oxalate.
- Apply direct pressure to the venipuncture site until bleeding stops.
- If a hematoma develops at the venipuncture site, apply warm soaks.

Precautions
- When drawing the sample, be careful not to rub the area over the vein too vigorously, pump the fist excessively, or leave the tourniquet in place too long.
- Avoid excessive probing during venipuncture and handle the sample gently.

■ If a tube with sodium citrate is used, mix the sample and anticoagulant thoroughly. If a chilled tube containing 0.5 ml of sodium oxalate is used, mix the sample and preservative thoroughly, pack the sample in ice, and send it to the laboratory immediately.

Reference values
Lysis normally occurs within 2 to 4 hours (SI, 2 to 4 h).

Abnormal findings
Clot lysis within 1 hour (SI, 1 h) indicates increased plasminogen activator activity. In pathologic fibrinolysis, lysis time only may be 5 to 10 minutes (SI, 5 to 10 m).

Interfering factors
■ Prolonged tourniquet constriction, vigorous vein preparation, or excessive pumping of the fist (decrease)
■ Hemolysis due to excessive probing at the venipuncture site or to rough handling of the sample
■ Failure to place the collection tube and sample on ice
■ Thrombolytic therapy, dextran, and clofibrate (decrease)

D-dimer

A D-dimer is an asymmetrical carbon compound fragment formed after thrombin converts fibrinogen to fibrin, factor XIIIa stabilizes it into a clot, and plasma acts on the cross-linked, or clotted, fibrin. The test is specific for fibrinolysis because it confirms the presence of fibrin split products.

Purpose
■ To diagnose disseminated intravascular coagulation (DIC)

■ To differentiate subarachnoid hemorrhage from a traumatic lumbar puncture in spinal fluid analysis

Patient preparation
■ Obtain the patient's history of hematologic diseases, recent surgery, and the results of other tests performed.
■ Explain to the patient that the D-dimer test is used to determine if the blood is clotting normally.
■ Tell the patient that the test requires a blood sample. Explain who will perform the venipuncture and when.
■ Explain to the patient that he may feel slight discomfort from the needle puncture and the tourniquet.

Procedure and posttest care
■ Perform a venipuncture and collect the sample in a 4.5-ml tube with sodium citrate added.
■ For a spinal fluid analysis, the sample is collected during a lumbar puncture and placed in a plastic vial. See "Cerebrospinal fluid analysis," pages 732 to 736, for details of the procedure.
■ Apply pressure to the venipuncture site for 5 minutes or until bleeding stops.
■ If a hematoma develops at the venipuncture site, apply warm soaks.

Precautions
■ Completely fill the collection tube, invert it gently several times, and send it to the laboratory immediately.
■ For a patient with coagulation problems, you may need to apply additional pressure at the venipuncture site to control bleeding.

Reference values
Normal D-dimer test results are negative or < 250 μg/L (SI, < 250 μg/L).

Abnormal findings

Increased D-dimer values may indicate DIC, pulmonary embolism, arterial or venous thrombosis, neoplastic disease, pregnancy (late and postpartum), surgery occurring up to 2 days before testing, subarachnoid hemorrhage (spinal fluid only), or secondary fibrinolysis.

Interfering factors

■ Failure to fill the collection tube completely or to send the sample to the laboratory immediately
■ Hemolysis due to rough handling of the sample
■ High rheumatoid factor titers or increased CA-125 levels (possible false-positive)
■ Spinal fluid analysis in an infant under age 6 months (possible false-negative)

International Normalized Ratio

The International Normalized Ratio (INR) system is viewed as the best means of standardizing measurement of prothrombin time to monitor oral anticoagulant therapy. It isn't used as a screening test for coagulopathies.

Purpose

■ To evaluate the effectiveness of oral anticoagulant therapy

Patient preparation

■ Explain to the patient that the INR test is used to determine the effectiveness of his oral anticoagulant therapy.
■ Tell the patient that a blood sample will be taken. Explain who will perform the venipuncture and when.
■ Explain to the patient that he may feel slight discomfort from the needle puncture and the tourniquet.

Procedure and posttest care

■ Perform a venipuncture and collect the sample in a 4.5-ml tube with sodium citrate added.
■ If a hematoma develops at the venipuncture site, apply warm soaks. If the hematoma is large, monitor pulses distal to the venipuncture site.
■ Ensure subdermal bleeding has stopped before removing pressure.

Precautions

■ Completely fill the collection tube; otherwise, an excess of citrate appears in the sample.
■ Gently invert the tube several times to thoroughly mix the sample and the anticoagulant.
■ To prevent hemolysis, avoid excessive probing during venipuncture and handle the sample gently.
■ Put the sample on ice and send it to the laboratory promptly.

Reference values

A normal INR for those receiving warfarin therapy is 2.0 to 3.0 (SI, 2.0 to 3.0). For those with mechanical prosthetic heart valves, an INR of 2.5 to 3.5 (SI, 2.5 to 3.5) is suggested.

Abnormal findings

Increased INR values may indicate disseminated intravascular coagulation, cirrhosis, hepatitis, vitamin K deficiency, salicylate intoxication, uncontrolled oral anticoagulation, or massive blood transfusion.

Interfering factors

■ Failure to fill the collection tube completely, to adequately mix the sample and the anticoagulant, or to send the sample to the laboratory immediately

- Hemolysis due to excessive probing at the venipuncture site or to rough handling of the sample

Selected readings

Anderson, S.C., and Poulsen, K.B. *Anderson's Atlas of Hematology.* Philadelphia: Lippincott Williams & Wilkins, 2003.

Cavanaugh, B.M. *Nurse's Manual of Laboratory and Diagnostic Tests,* 4th ed. Philadelphia: F.A. Davis Co., 2003.

Diseases, 3rd ed. Springhouse, Pa.: Springhouse Corp., 2001.

Fischbach, F. *A Manual of Laboratory and Diagnostic Tests,* 7th ed. Philadelphia: Lippincott Williams & Wilkins, 2004.

Fuse, I., et al. "DDAVP Normalized the Bleeding Time in Patients with Congenital Platelet TxA2 Receptor Abnormality," *Transfusion* 43(5):563-67, May 2003.

Guyton, A.C., and Hall, J.E. *Textbook of Medical Physiology,* 10th ed. Philadelphia: W.B. Saunders Co., 2001.

McClatchey, K.D. *Clinical Laboratory Medicine,* 2nd ed. Philadelphia: Lippincott Williams & Wilkins, 2002.

Nursing2004 Drug Handbook. Philadelphia: Lippincott Williams & Wilkins, 2004.

Pagana, K.D., and Pagana, T.J. *Mosby's Diagnostic and Laboratory Test Reference,* 6th ed. St. Louis: Mosby Year–Book, Inc., 2003.

Schnell, Z., et al. *Davis's Comprehensive Handbook of Laboratory and Diagnostic Tests with Nursing Implications.* Philadelphia: F.A. Davis Co., 2003.

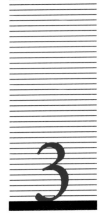

Blood gases and electrolytes

Introduction

Laboratory analysis of blood gases and electrolytes helps evaluate the body's respiratory and metabolic status. Arterial blood gas (ABG) values provide important information about the adequacy of gas exchange in the lungs, the integrity of the ventilatory control system, and blood pH and acid-base balance. Serum electrolyte levels also supply valuable data about the body's acid-base balance and fluid balance.

Metabolic processes continually form acids, which must be eliminated to maintain acid-base balance. To maintain this balance, the lungs and kidneys interact to maintain pH within an acceptable range. Blood gas studies measure the lungs' capacity to regulate carbon dioxide concentration in the blood; serum electrolyte assays determine the kidneys' capacity to retain or excrete metabolic acids and bases. Because these functions are so closely interwoven, accurate assessment of homeostasis requires simultaneous interpretation of blood gas and electrolyte studies.

Arterial blood gases

Blood gas studies are usually performed on arterial blood, which contains oxygen (O_2) and carbon dioxide (CO_2). ABG values are measurements of the partial pressure that oxygen (PaO_2) and carbon dioxide ($PaCO_2$) exert in the blood. As the concentration of the gas rises, so does its partial pressure. To understand the clinical significance of ABG values, one must first understand how gas exchange in the lungs occurs.

Environmental oxygen, about 21% of inspired air, travels through the airways into the lungs; the waste product, carbon dioxide, travels from the lungs to the surrounding air. Consequently, the alveoli in the lungs contain a mixture of inspired oxygen moving through the capillaries and into circulation and carbon dioxide (waste product of metabolism) moving through the capillaries for exhalation.

Oxygen taken up in the lungs is transported to the tissues through the circulatory system. Only a small amount of inspired oxygen can dissolve in arterial blood; how much dissolves depends on the PaO_2. The remainder combines chemically with hemoglobin. *Oxygen content* (O_2CT) measures the amount of oxygen combined with hemoglobin; this value is used infrequently. *Oxygen saturation* (SaO_2) is the ratio of the amount of oxygen in the blood combined with hemoglobin to the total amount of oxygen that the hemoglobin could carry. (See *Important definitions.*)

Carbon dioxide is produced by cellular metabolism and is released into the bloodstream. Because it's more soluble than oxygen, it dissolves in the blood, mostly forming bicarbonate (HCO_3^-) and carbamino compounds (bound to hemoglobin).

Acid-base balance

Enzymes that control vital cellular functions perform most efficiently when the body's pH ranges between 7.35 and 7.45. The carbonic acid–HCO_3^- buffer system helps maintain body pH at this desirable level. The system may be represented by these equations:

$$CO_2 + H_2O \rightarrow H_2CO_3$$

(carbon dioxide + water → carbonic acid).

In turn, carbonic acid can undergo the following change:

$$H_2CO_3 \rightarrow H^+ + HCO_3^-$$

(carbonic acid → hydrogen ion + bicarbonate).

Bicarbonate and carbonic acid normally exist in a 20:1 ratio. A change in this ratio causes a blood pH that's abnormally acid or alkaline.

The lungs control carbonic acid levels by converting carbonic acid to carbon dioxide and water for excretion. By changing the rate and depth of respiration, the lungs can adjust the amount of carbon dioxide lost to maintain the normal ratio. This compensatory mechanism is rapidly effective. For example, in metabolic acidosis, the lungs increase their rate and depth to "blow off" excess carbon dioxide (carbonic acid), thus raising the pH to acceptable levels.

When the lungs are functioning inadequately, they can actually produce an acid-base imbalance. For example, they cause *respiratory acidosis* by hypoventilation and excessive retention of carbon dioxide (carbonic acid excess); they cause *respiratory alkalosis* by hyperventilation and excessive exhalation of carbon dioxide (carbonic acid deficit).

The kidneys — primary regulators of HCO_3^- — excrete, reabsorb, or regenerate the amount of HCO_3^- needed to maintain the normal carbonic acid– HCO_3^- ratio. This can effectively compensate for

IMPORTANT DEFINITIONS

Partial pressure	A measure of the force that a gas exerts on the fluid in which it's dissolved
PaO_2	Partial pressure of oxygen in arterial blood
$PaCO_2$	Partial pressure of carbon dioxide in arterial blood
pH	A measure of acid-base balance, or the concentration of free hydrogen ions in the blood
O_2CT	Oxygen content, or the volume of oxygen combined with hemoglobin in arterial blood
SaO_2	Arterial oxygen saturation, a measure of the percentage of oxygen combined with hemoglobin compared to the total amount of oxygen with which hemoglobin could combine
Electrolytes	Substances that dissociate into ions when fused or in solution and that thus conduct electricity
Cations	Positively charged ions
Anions	Negatively charged ions
Acidosis	Metabolic or respiratory changes that result in a loss of base or an accumulation of acid
Alkalosis	Metabolic or respiratory changes that result in a loss of acid or an accumulation of base

an imbalance that results from pulmonary dysfunction. However, this compensatory response is notably slower than pulmonary compensation and usually occurs over a 3- to 4-day period.

The kidneys have another important role to play: Because the acids resulting from metabolic processes — with the exception of carbonic acid — can't be converted to gases for exhalation by the lungs, they must be excreted by the kidneys. Thus, renal dysfunction can cause metabolic acid-base imbalance. Summarized briefly, metabolic acidosis results when the body loses too much base (HCO_3-) or retains excessive acid; metabolic alkalosis results when the body retains too much base or loses too much acid.

Clinical significance of ABG values

Abnormal variations in ABG values may result from respiratory or metabolic causes. Compensatory mechanisms, such as those in the lungs and kidneys, automatically attempt to correct an imbalance. But compensation isn't correction, and compensatory mechanisms are limited.

Although valuable in assessing overall respiratory and metabolic status, ABG measurements aren't diagnostically specific. For example, taken alone, ABG values don't distinguish between pulmonary and cardiac disorders. These values are most useful when considered with other factors, such as cardiac output, regional blood flow, and tissue oxygen consumption.

FUNCTIONS OF SERUM ELECTROLYTES

CATIONS	Sodium (Na+)	■ Maintains osmotic pressure of extracellular fluid ■ Helps regulate neuromuscular activity ■ Influences acid-base balance and chloride and potassium levels ■ Helps regulate water excretion
	Potassium (K+)	■ Maintains cellular osmotic equilibrium ■ Helps regulate neuromuscular and enzymatic activity and acid-base balance ■ Influences kidney function
	Calcium (Ca++)	■ Helps regulate and promote neuromuscular activity, skeletal development, and blood coagulation
	Magnesium (Mg++)	■ Helps regulate intracellular activity and sodium, potassium, calcium, and phosphorus levels
ANIONS	Chloride (Cl−)	■ Influences acid-base balance ■ Helps maintain blood osmotic pressure and arterial pressure
	Bicarbonate (HCO3−)	■ Acts with carbonic acid in buffer system that regulates blood pH
	Phosphate (HPO4−)	■ Helps regulate calcium levels, energy metabolism, and acid-base balance

The significance of ABG analysis is also limited by the fact that these studies don't necessarily detect disease. For example, the lungs may continue to function properly with unchanged ABG values. Therefore, other diagnostic screening tests, such as spirometry or chest X-ray, must be performed. When dealing with ABG values, make sure you check the accepted values for your facility. Normal ranges may vary according to the laboratory method used.

Serum electrolytes

Electrolytes are substances that dissociate into ions when dissolved in the blood. Electrolytes that carry a positive charge are called cations; those that carry a negative charge are called anions. Sodium, calcium, chloride, and bicarbonate are the major extracellular electrolytes. Sodium is the most abundant extracellular cation;

chloride, the most abundant anion. Potassium, magnesium, and phosphate are the major intracellular electrolytes. Potassium is the most abundant intracellular cation; phosphate, the most abundant anion. Note that hemolyzed blood samples will show a false increase in potassium levels because of the way potassium is released from red blood cells.

Serum concentrations of electrolytes influence movement of fluid within and between body compartments. (See *Functions of serum electrolytes.*) Such movement depends on osmolality—the concentration of electrolytes in the respective fluid compartments. Total electrolyte concentration (usually expressed in milliequivalents [mEq] per liter of serum) plus other dissolved substances, such as glucose, determine the osmolality of a

UNDERSTANDING BODY FLUIDS

Fluids — mainly water — account for 60% of an adult's total body weight. Body fluids contain substances that dissociate in solutions and conduct a weak electric current (electrolytes) as well as substances that don't break down into smaller substances. Electrolytes with a positive charge are called *cations;* those carrying a negative charge are called *anions.* A cation-anion balance results in electric neutrality.

Two main compartments house the body's fluids. With its 100 trillion cells, the *intracellular compartment* accounts for 40% of the total body weight (approximately 25 L of fluid). In the spaces between the cells, the *extracellular com-*

partment constitutes 15% of the total body weight (approximately 15 L of interstitial fluid). Intravascular fluid, or plasma, accounts for the final 5%. A change in the amount or composition of these compartments can be fatal.

Electrolytes play a crucial role in the body's water distribution, osmolality, acid-base balance, and neuromuscular irritability. Potassium (K^+) is the principal cation, and phosphate (HPO_4^-) is the dominant anion in the intracellular compartment. Like plasma, the interstitial fluid contains high concentrations of sodium (Na^+) and chloride (Cl^-). Together, fluids and electrolytes nourish and maintain the body.

given compartment. During osmosis, water flows from a compartment of lower osmolality to one of higher osmolality until the osmotic pressure in the two compartments is equal. (See *Understanding body fluids.*)

Electrolytes and homeostasis

The body can function properly only if the kidneys and lungs (with the aid of endocrine hormones) maintain electrolyte balance between intracellular and extracellular compartments. The hypothalamus and the pituitary control osmolality by regulating antidiuretic hormone, which promotes water reabsorption by the kidneys. The kidneys govern fluid and electrolytes through filtration, reabsorption, and excretion.

Electrolytes also help maintain acid-base balance. The kidneys may exchange potassium or sodium for hydrogen and absorb or excrete bicarbonate or chloride ions to maintain a proper pH. Serum electrolyte concentrations affect all metabolic activity in some way. Also, elec-

trolyte concentration differences between intracellular fluid and extracellular fluid regulate neuromuscular function. Consequently, serum electrolyte studies are essential to routine medical evaluation in all hospitalized patients. Abnormal electrolyte values may reflect fluid or acid-base imbalance or kidney, neuromuscular, endocrine, or skeletal dysfunction.

ARTERIAL BLOOD GAS TESTS

Arterial blood gas analysis

Arterial blood gas (ABG) analysis is used to measure the partial pressure of arterial oxygen (PaO_2), the partial pressure of arterial carbon dioxide ($PaCO_2$), and the pH of an arterial sample. Oxygen content (O_2CT), arterial oxygen saturation (SaO_2), and bicarbonate (HCO_3^-) values are also measured. A blood sample for

ABG analysis may be drawn by percutaneous arterial puncture or from an arterial line.

The PaO_2 indicates how much oxygen the lungs are delivering to the blood. The $PaCO_2$ indicates how efficiently the lungs eliminate carbon dioxide. The pH indicates the acid-base level of the blood, or the hydrogen ion (H^+) concentration. Acidity indicates H^+ excess; alkalinity, H^+ deficit. (See *Balancing pH*.) O_2CT, SaO_2, and HCO_3^- values also aid diagnosis.

Purpose
- To evaluate the efficiency of pulmonary gas exchange
- To assess the integrity of the ventilatory control system
- To determine the acid-base level of the blood
- To monitor respiratory therapy

Patient preparation
- Explain to the patient that ABG analysis is used to evaluate how well the lungs are delivering oxygen to blood and eliminating carbon dioxide.
- Tell the patient that the test requires a blood sample. Explain who will perform the arterial puncture and when, and which site — radial, brachial, or femoral artery — has been selected for the puncture.
- Inform the patient that he need not restrict food and fluids.
- Instruct the patient to breathe normally during the test, and warn him that he may experience a brief cramping or throbbing pain at the puncture site.

Procedure and posttest care
- Perform an arterial puncture or draw blood from an arterial line. Use a heparinized blood gas syringe to draw the sample. Eliminate air from the sample,

place it on ice immediately, and transport it for analysis.
- After applying pressure to the puncture site for 3 to 5 minutes or until bleeding has stopped, tape a gauze pad firmly over it. (If the puncture site is on the arm, don't tape the entire circumference; this may restrict circulation.)
- If the patient is receiving anticoagulants or has a coagulopathy, apply pressure to the puncture site longer than 5 minutes if necessary.
- Monitor vital signs and observe for signs of circulatory impairment, such as swelling, discoloration, pain, numbness, and tingling in the bandaged arm or leg.
- Watch for bleeding from the puncture site.

Precautions
- Wait at least 20 minutes before drawing arterial blood when starting, changing, or discontinuing oxygen therapy; after initiating or changing settings of mechanical ventilation; or after extubation.
- Before sending the sample to the laboratory, note on the laboratory request whether the patient was breathing room air or receiving oxygen therapy when the sample was collected.
- If the patient was receiving oxygen therapy, note the flow rate and method of delivery. If he's on a ventilator, note the fraction of inspired oxygen, tidal volume mode, respiratory rate, and positive-end expiratory pressure.
- Note the patient's rectal temperature.

Reference values
Normal ABG values fall within these ranges:
- PaO_2: 80 to 100 mm Hg (SI, 10.6 to 13.3 kPa)
- $PaCO_2$: 35 to 45 mm Hg (SI, 4.7 to 5.3 kPa)

BALANCING PH

To measure the acidity or alkalinity of a solution, chemists use a pH scale of 1 to 15 that measures hydrogen ion concentrations. As hydrogen ions and acidity increase, pH falls below 7.0, which is neutral. Conversely, when hydrogen ions decrease, pH and alkalinity increase. Acid-base balance, or homeostasis of hydrogen ions, is necessary if the body's enzyme systems are to work properly.

The slightest change in ionic hydrogen concentration alters the rate of cellular chemical reactions; a sufficiently severe change can be fatal. To maintain a normal blood pH — generally between 7.35 and 7.45 — the body relies on three mechanisms.

Buffers

Chemically composed of two substances, buffers prevent radical pH changes by replacing strong acids added to a solution (such as blood) with weaker ones. For example, strong acids capable of yielding many hydrogen ions are replaced by weaker ones that yield fewer hydrogen ions. Because of the principal buffer coupling of bicarbonate and carbonic acid — normally in a ratio of 20:1 — the plasma acid-base level rarely fluctuates. Increased bicarbonate, however, indicates alkalosis, whereas decreased bicarbonate points to acidosis. Increased carbonic acid indicates acidosis, and decreased carbonic acid indicates alkalosis.

Respiration

Respiration is important in maintaining blood pH. The lungs convert carbonic acid to carbon dioxide and water. With every expiration, carbon dioxide and water leave the body, decreasing the carbonic acid content of the blood. Consequently, fewer hydrogen ions are formed, and blood pH increases. When the blood's hydrogen ion or carbonic acid content increases, neurons in the respiratory center stimulate respiration.

Hyperventilation eliminates carbon dioxide and hence carbonic acid from the body, reduces hydrogen ion formation, and increases pH. Conversely, increased blood pH from alkalosis — decreased hydrogen ion concentration — causes hypoventilation, which restores blood pH to its normal level by retaining carbon dioxide and thus increasing hydrogen ion formation.

Urinary excretion

The third factor in acid-base balance is urine excretion. Because the kidneys excrete varying amounts of acids and bases, they control urine pH, which in turn affects blood pH. For example, when blood pH is decreased, the distal and collecting tubules remove excessive hydrogen ions (carbonic acid forms in the tubular cells and dissociates into hydrogen and bicarbonate) and displaces them in urine, thereby eliminating hydrogen from the body. In exchange, basic ions in the urine — usually sodium — diffuse into the tubular cells, where they combine with bicarbonate. This sodium bicarbonate is then reabsorbed in the blood, resulting in decreased urine pH and, more important, increased blood pH.

- pH: 7.35 to 7.45 (SI, 7.35 to 7.45)
- O_2CT: 15% to 23% (SI, 0.15 to 0.23)
- SaO_2: 94% to 100% (SI, 0.94 to 1)
- HCO_3^-: 22 to 25 mEq/L (SI, 22 to 25 mmol/L).

Abnormal findings

Low PaO_2, O_2CT, and SaO_2 levels and a high $PaCO_2$ may result from conditions that impair respiratory function, such as respiratory muscle weakness or paralysis, respiratory center inhibition (from head injury, brain tumor, or drug abuse), and airway obstruction (possibly from mucus plugs or a tumor). Similarly, low readings may result from bronchiole obstruction caused by asthma or emphysema, from an abnormal ventilation-perfusion ratio due to partially blocked alveoli or pulmonary capillaries, or from alveoli that are damaged or filled with fluid because of disease, hemorrhage, or near-drowning.

When inspired air contains insufficient oxygen, PaO_2, O_2CT, and SaO_2 decrease, but $PaCO_2$ may be normal. Such findings are common in pneumothorax, impaired diffusion between alveoli and blood (due to interstitial fibrosis, for example), or an arteriovenous shunt that permits blood to bypass the lungs.

Low O_2CT — with normal PaO_2, SaO_2 and, possibly, $PaCO_2$ values — may result from severe anemia, decreased blood volume, and reduced hemoglobin oxygen-carrying capacity.

In addition to clarifying blood oxygen disorders, ABG values can give considerable information about acid-base disorders. (See *Acid-base disorders*.)

Interfering factors

■ Failure to heparinize syringe, place sample in an iced bag, or send the sample to the laboratory immediately
■ Exposing the sample to air (increase or decrease in PaO_2 and $PaCO_2$)
■ Venous blood in the sample (possible decrease in PaO_2 and increase in $PaCO_2$)
■ HCO_3^-, ethacrynic acid, hydrocortisone, metolazone, prednisone, and thiazides (possible increase in $PaCO_2$)
■ Acetazolamide, methicillin, nitrofurantoin, and tetracycline (possible decrease in $PaCO_2$)
■ Fever (possible false-high PaO_2 and $PaCO_2$)

ACID-BASE DISORDERS

Disorders and ABG findings

Respiratory acidosis (excess CO_2 retention)
pH < 7.35 (SI, < 7.35)
HCO_3^- >26 mEq/L (SI, > 26 mmol/L) (if compensating)
$PaCO_2$ > 45 mm Hg (SI, > 5.3 kPa)

Respiratory alkalosis (excess CO_2 excretion)
pH > 7.45 (SI, > 7.45)
HCO_3^- < 22 mEq/L (SI, < 22 mmol/L) (if compensating)
$PaCO_2$ < 35 mm Hg (SI, < 4.7 kPa)

Metabolic acidosis (HCO_3^- loss, acid retention)
pH < 7.35 (SI, < 7.35)
HCO_3^- < 22 mEq/L < (SI, < 22 mmol/L)
$PaCO_2$ < 35 mm Hg (SI, < 4.7 kPa) (if compensating)

Metabolic alkalosis (HCO_3^- retention, acid loss)
pH > 7.45 (SI, > 7.45)
HCO_3^- > 26 mEq/L (SI, > 26 mmol/L)
$PaCO_2$ > 45 mm Hg (SI, > 5.3 kPa)

Total carbon dioxide content

When carbon dioxide (CO_2) pressure in red blood cells exceeds 40 mm Hg, CO_2 spills out of the cells and dissolves in plasma. There it may combine with water to form carbonic acid, which in turn may dissociate into hydrogen and bicarbonate ions.

The total CO_2 content test is used to measure the total concentration of all forms of CO_2 in serum, plasma, or whole blood samples. It's commonly ordered for patients with respiratory insufficiency and is usually included in an assessment

Possible causes	Signs and symptoms
■ Central nervous system depression from drugs, injury, or disease ■ Asphyxia ■ Hypoventilation due to pulmonary, cardiac, musculoskeletal, or neuromuscular disease ■ Obesity ■ Postoperative pain ■ Abdominal distention	Diaphoresis, headache, tachycardia, confusion, restlessness, apprehension
■ Hyperventilation due to anxiety, pain, or improper ventilator settings ■ Respiratory stimulation caused by drugs, disease, hypoxia, fever, or high room temperature ■ Gram-negative bacteremia ■ Compensation for metabolic acidosis (chronic renal failure)	Rapid, deep breathing; paresthesia; light-headedness; twitching; anxiety; fear
■ HCO_3^- depletion due to renal disease, diarrhea, or small-bowel fistulas ■ Excessive production of organic acids due to hepatic disease; endocrine disorders, including diabetes mellitus, hypoxia, shock, and drug intoxication ■ Inadequate excretion of acids due to renal disease	Rapid, deep breathing; fruity breath; fatigue; headache; lethargy; drowsiness; nausea; vomiting; coma (if severe)
■ Loss of hydrochloric acid from prolonged vomiting or gastric suctioning ■ Loss of potassium due to increased renal excretion (as in diuretic therapy) or steroid overdose ■ Excessive alkali ingestion ■ Compensation for chronic respiratory acidosis	Slow, shallow breathing; hypertonic muscles; restlessness; twitching; confusion; irritability; apathy; tetany; seizures; coma (if severe)

of electrolyte balance. Test results are most significant when considered with pH and arterial blood gas values.

Since about 90% of CO_2 in serum is in the form of bicarbonate, this test closely assesses bicarbonate levels. Total CO_2 content reflects the adequacy of gas exchange in the lungs and the efficiency of the carbonic acid–bicarbonate buffer system, which maintains acid-base balance and normal pH.

Purpose
■ To help evaluate acid-base balance

Patient preparation
■ Explain to the patient that the total CO_2 content test is performed to measure the amount of CO_2 in the blood.
■ Tell the patient that the test requires a blood sample. Explain who will perform the venipuncture and when.
■ Explain to the patient that he may experience discomfort from the needle puncture and the tourniquet.
■ Inform the patient that he need not restrict food and fluids.
■ Notify the laboratory and physician of medications the patient is taking that may affect test results; they may need to be restricted.

Procedure and posttest care
- Perform a venipuncture.
- When CO_2 content is measured along with electrolytes, a 3- or 4-ml clot activator tube may be used.
- When this test is performed alone, a heparinized tube is appropriate.
- Apply direct pressure to the venipuncture site until the bleeding has stopped.
- If a hematoma develops at the venipuncture site, apply warm soaks.
- Instruct the patient that he may resume any medications discontinued before the test, as ordered.

Precautions
- Fill the tube completely to prevent diffusion of CO_2 into the vacuum.

Reference values
Normally, total CO_2 levels range from 22 to 26 mEq/L (SI, 22 to 26 mmol/L). Levels may vary, depending on the patient's sex and age.

Abnormal findings
High CO_2 levels may occur in metabolic alkalosis, respiratory acidosis, primary aldosteronism, and Cushing's syndrome. CO_2 levels may also increase after excessive loss of acids, such as severe vomiting and continuous gastric drainage.

Decreased CO_2 levels are common in metabolic acidosis. Decreased total CO_2 levels in metabolic acidosis also result from loss of bicarbonate. Levels may decrease in respiratory alkalosis.

Interfering factors
- Underfilling the collection tube, allowing CO_2 to escape, which results in inaccurate levels
- Excessive use of corticotropin, cortisone, or thiazide diuretics; excessive ingestion of alkali or licorice (increase)

- Salicylates, paraldehyde, methicillin, dimercaprol, ammonium chloride, and acetazolamide; ingestion of ethylene glycol or methyl alcohol (decrease)

Alveolar-to-arterial oxygen gradient

Using calculations based on the patient's laboratory values, the alveolar-to-arterial oxygen gradient (A-aDO_2) test can help identify the cause of hypoxemia and intrapulmonary shunting by providing an approximation of the partial pressure of oxygenation of the alveoli and arteries. It may help differentiate the cause as ventilated alveoli but no perfusion, unventilated alveoli with perfusion, or collapse of the alveoli and capillaries.

Purpose
- To evaluate the efficiency of gas exchange
- To assess the integrity of the ventilatory control system
- To monitor respiratory therapy

Patient preparation
- Explain to the patient that the A-aDO_2 test is used to evaluate how well the lungs are delivering oxygen to the blood and eliminating carbon dioxide.
- Tell the patient that the test requires a blood sample. Explain who will perform the arterial puncture and when.
- Inform the patient that he need not restrict food and fluids.
- Instruct the patient to breathe normally during the test, and warn him that he may experience cramping or throbbing pain at the puncture site.

Procedure and posttest care
- Perform an arterial puncture or draw blood from an arterial line using a heparinized blood gas syringe.

- Eliminate all air from the sample and place it on ice immediately.
- Apply pressure to the puncture for 3 to 5 minutes or until bleeding has stopped.
- Place a gauze pad over the site and tape it in place, but don't tape the entire circumference.
- Monitor vital signs and observe for signs of circulatory impairment, such as swelling, discoloration, pain, numbness, and tingling in the bandaged arm or leg.
- Watch for bleeding from the puncture site.
- The arterial sample is analyzed for partial pressure of arterial oxygen (PaO_2) and partial pressure of arterial carbon dioxide ($PaCO_2$). Also examined are barometric pressure (PB), water vapor pressure (PH_2O), and fraction of inspired oxygen (FIO_2) (21% for room air). From these values, the alveolar oxygen tension (PAO_2), the arterial-to-oxygen ratio (a/A ratio), and the $A\text{-}aDO_2$ are derived by solving these mathematical formulas:

$$PAO_2 = FIO_2 \, (PB - PH_2O) - 1.25 \, (PaCO_2)$$
$$\text{a/A ratio} = PaO_2 \text{ divided by } PAO_2$$
$$A\text{-}aDO_2 = PAO_2 - PaO_2$$

- Based on the results of the formulas, appropriate interventions to correct patient problems are initiated.

Precautions

- Before sending the sample to the laboratory, note on the laboratory request whether the patient was breathing room air or receiving oxygen therapy when the sample was collected.
- If the patient was receiving oxygen therapy, note the flow rate and method of delivery. If he was on a ventilator, note the FIO_2, tidal volume, mode, respiratory rate, and positive end-expiratory pressure.
- Note the patient's rectal temperature.

Reference values

Normal values on room air for $A\text{-}aDO_2$ at rest is < 10 mm Hg and at maximum exercise is 20 to 30 mm Hg.

Abnormal findings

- Increased values may be caused by mucus plugs, bronchospasm, or airway collapse (asthma, bronchitis, emphysema).
- Hypoxemia results in increased $A\text{-}aDO_2$ and may be caused by arterial septal defects, pneumothorax, atelectasis, emboli, or edema.

Interfering factors

- Failure to heparinize the syringe, place the sample in an iced bag, or send the sample to the laboratory immediately
- Exposing the sample to air (increase or decrease)
- Age and increasing oxygen concentration (increase)

Arterial-to-alveolar oxygen ratio

Using calculations based on the patient's laboratory values, the arterial-to-alveolar oxygen ratio (a/A ratio) test can help identify the cause of hypoxemia and intrapulmonary shunting by providing an approximation of the partial pressure of oxygenation of the alveoli and arteries. It may help differentiate the cause as ventilated alveoli but no perfusion, unventilated alveoli with perfusion, or collapse of the alveoli and capillaries.

Purpose

- To evaluate the efficiency of gas exchange
- To assess the integrity of the ventilatory control system
- To monitor respiratory therapy

Patient preparation

- Explain to the patient that the a/A ratio test is used to evaluate how well the lungs are delivering oxygen to the blood and eliminating carbon dioxide.
- Tell the patient that the test requires a blood sample. Explain who will perform the arterial puncture and when.
- Inform the patient that he need not restrict food and fluids.
- Instruct the patient to breathe normally during the test, and warn him that he may experience cramping or throbbing pain at the puncture site.

Procedure and posttest care

- Perform an arterial puncture or draw blood from an arterial line using a heparinized blood gas syringe.
- Eliminate all air from the sample and place it on ice immediately.
- Apply pressure to the puncture for 3 to 5 minutes or until bleeding has stopped.
- Place a gauze pad over the site and tape it in place, but don't tape the entire circumference.
- Monitor vital signs and observe for signs of circulatory impairment, such as swelling, discoloration, pain, numbness, and tingling in the bandaged arm or leg.
- Watch for bleeding from the puncture site.
- The arterial sample is analyzed for partial pressure of arterial oxygen (PaO_2) and partial pressure of arterial carbon dioxide ($PaCO_2$). Also examined are barometric pressure (PB), water vapor pressure (PH_2O), and fractional concentration of inspired oxygen (FIO_2) (21% for room air). From these values, the alveolar oxygen tension (PAO_2), the a/A ratio, and the alveolar-to-arterial oxygen gradient (A-aDO_2) are derived by solving these mathematical formulas:

$$PaO_2 = FIO_2 (PB - PH_2O) - 1.25 (PaCO_2)$$
$$a/A \text{ ratio} = PaO_2 \text{ divided by } PAO_2$$
$$A\text{-}aDO_2 = PAO_2 - PaO_2$$

- Based on the results of the formulas, appropriate interventions to correct patient problems are initiated.

Precautions

- Before sending the sample to the laboratory, note on the laboratory request whether the patient was breathing room air or receiving oxygen therapy when the sample was collected.
- If the patient was receiving oxygen therapy, note the flow rate and method of delivery. If he was on a ventilator, note the FIO_2, tidal volume, mode, respiratory rate, and positive end-expiratory pressure.
- Note the patient's rectal temperature.

Reference values

A normal a/A ratio is 75%.

Abnormal findings

- Increased values may be caused by mucus plugs, bronchospasm, or airway collapse (asthma, bronchitis, emphysema).
- Hypoxemia results in increased A-aDO_2 and may be caused by arterial septal defects, pneumothorax, atelectasis, emboli, or edema.

Interfering factors

- Failure to heparinize the syringe, place the sample in an iced bag, or send the sample to the laboratory immediately
- Exposing the sample to air (increase or decrease)
- Age and increasing oxygen concentration (increase)

ELECTROLYTE TESTS

Calcium

About 99% of the body's calcium is found in the teeth. Approximately 1% of total calcium in the body circulates in the blood. Of this, about 50% is bound to plasma proteins and 40% is ionized, or free. Evaluation of serum calcium levels measures the total amount of calcium in the blood, and ionized calcium measures the fraction of serum calcium that's in the ionized form.

Purpose
■ To evaluate endocrine function, calcium metabolism, and acid-base balance
■ To guide therapy in patients with renal failure, renal transplant, endocrine disorders, malignancies, cardiac disease, and skeletal disorders

Patient preparation
■ Explain to the patient that the serum calcium test is used to determine blood calcium levels.
■ Tell the patient that the test requires a blood sample. Explain who will perform the venipuncture and when.
■ Explain to the patient that he may experience slight discomfort from the needle puncture and the tourniquet.
■ Inform the patient that he need not restrict food and fluids.

Procedure and posttest care
■ Perform a venipuncture (without a tourniquet if possible) and collect the sample in a 3- or 4-ml clot-activator tube.
■ Apply direct pressure to the venipuncture site until bleeding stops.
■ If a hematoma develops at the venipuncture site, apply warm soaks.

Reference values
Normally, total calcium levels range from 8.2 to 10.2 mg/dl (SI, 2.05 to 2.54 mmol/L) in adults. Ionized calcium levels are 4.65 to 5.28 mg/dl (SI, 1.1 to 1.25 mmol/L).

AGE ISSUE *In children, total calcium levels range from 8.6 to 11.2 mg/dl (SI, 2.15 to 2.79 mmol/L).*

Abnormal findings
Abnormally high serum calcium levels (hypercalcemia) may occur in hyperparathyroidism and parathyroid tumors, Paget's disease of the bone, multiple myeloma, metastatic carcinoma, multiple fractures, and prolonged immobilization. Elevated levels may also result from inadequate excretion of calcium, such as adrenal insufficiency and renal disease; from excessive calcium ingestion; and from overuse of antacids such as calcium carbonate.

CLINICAL ALERT *Observe the patient with hypercalcemia for deep bone pain, flank pain due to renal calculi, and muscle hypotonicity. Hypercalcemic crisis begins with nausea, vomiting, and dehydration, leading to stupor and coma, and can end in cardiac arrest.*

Low calcium levels (hypocalcemia) may result from hypoparathyroidism, total parathyroidectomy, and malabsorption. Decreased serum calcium levels may also occur with Cushing's syndrome, renal failure, acute pancreatitis, peritonitis, malnutrition with hypoalbuminemia, and blood transfusions (due to citrate).

In the patient with hypocalcemia, be alert for circumoral and peripheral numbness and tingling, muscle twitching, Chvostek's sign (facial muscle spasm), tetany, muscle cramping, Trousseau's sign (carpopedal spasm), seizures, arrhythmias, laryngeal spasm, decreased cardiac output, prolonged bleeding time, fractures, and prolonged Q interval.

Interfering factors
- Venous stasis due to prolonged tourniquet application (possible false-high)
- Excessive ingestion of vitamin D or its derivatives (dihydrotachysterol, calcitriol) or use of androgens, calciferol-activated calcium salts, progestins-estrogens, and thiazide diuretics (increase)
- Acetazolamide, corticosteroids, plicamycin, chronic laxative use, and excessive transfusions of citrated blood (possible increase or decrease)

Chloride

The chloride test is used to measure serum levels of chloride, the major extracellular fluid anion. Chloride helps maintain osmotic pressure of blood and, therefore, helps regulate blood volume and arterial pressure. Chloride levels also affect acid-base balance. Chloride is absorbed from the intestines and excreted primarily by the kidneys.

Purpose
- To detect acid-base imbalance (acidosis or alkalosis) and to aid evaluation of fluid status and extracellular cation-anion balance

Patient preparation
- Explain to the patient that the serum chloride test is used to evaluate the chloride content of blood.
- Tell the patient that the test requires a blood sample. Explain who will perform the venipuncture and when.
- Explain to the patient that he may experience slight discomfort from the needle puncture and the tourniquet.
- Inform the patient that he need not restrict food and fluids.

- Notify the laboratory and physician of medications the patient is taking that may affect test results; they may need to be restricted.

Procedure and posttest care
- Perform a venipuncture and collect the sample in a 3- or 4-ml clot-activator tube.
- Apply direct pressure to the venipuncture site until bleeding stops.
- If a hematoma develops at the venipuncture site, apply warm soaks.
- Instruct the patient to resume any medications discontinued before the test, as ordered.

Precautions
- Handle the sample gently to prevent hemolysis.

Reference values
Normally, serum chloride levels range from 100 to 108 mEq/L (SI, 100 to 108 mmol/L) in adults.

Abnormal findings
Chloride levels are inversely related to bicarbonate levels, reflecting acid-base balance. Excessive loss of gastric juices or other secretions containing chloride may cause hypochloremic metabolic alkalosis; excessive chloride retention or ingestion may lead to hyperchloremic metabolic acidosis.

An increase in chloride levels may be evident in severe dehydration, complete renal shutdown, head injury (producing neurogenic hyperventilation), and primary aldosteronism.

Decreased levels of chloride may result from low sodium and potassium levels due to prolonged vomiting, gastric suctioning, intestinal fistula, chronic renal failure, and Addison's disease. Heart failure or edema resulting in excess extracellular fluid can cause dilutional hypochloremia.

> **CLINICAL ALERT** *Observe the patient with hypochloremia for hypertonicity of muscles, tetany, depressed respirations, and decreased blood pressure with dehydration. In the patient with hyperchloremia, be alert for signs of developing stupor, rapid deep breathing, and weakness, which may lead to coma.*

Interfering factors
- Hemolysis due to rough handling of the sample
- Use of ammonium chloride, cholestyramine, boric acid, oxyphenbutazone, or phenylbutazone and excessive I.V. infusion of sodium chloride (possible increase)
- Use of thiazide diuretics, ethacrynic acid, furosemide, or bicarbonates and prolonged I.V. infusion of dextrose 5% in water (decrease)

Magnesium

The magnesium test is used to measure serum levels of magnesium, an electrolyte that's vital to neuromuscular function. It also helps in intracellular metabolism, activates many essential enzymes, and affects the metabolism of nucleic acids and proteins. Magnesium also helps transport sodium and potassium across cell membranes and influences intracellular calcium levels. Most magnesium is found in bone and intracellular fluid; a small amount is found in extracellular fluid. Magnesium is absorbed by the small intestine and excreted in urine and stool.

Purpose
- To evaluate electrolyte status
- To assess neuromuscular and renal function

Patient preparation
- Explain to the patient that the serum magnesium test is used to determine the magnesium content of the blood.
- Instruct the patient not to use magnesium salts (such as milk of magnesia or Epsom salt) for at least 3 days before the test, but tell him that he need not restrict food and fluids.
- Tell the patient that the test requires a blood sample. Explain who will perform the venipuncture and when.
- Explain to the patient that he may experience slight discomfort from the needle puncture and the tourniquet.

Procedure and posttest care
- Perform a venipuncture without a tourniquet, if possible, and collect the sample in a 3- or 4-ml clot-activator tube.
- Apply pressure to the venipuncture site until bleeding stops.
- If a hematoma develops at the venipuncture site, apply warm soaks.

Precautions
- Handle the sample gently to prevent hemolysis.

Reference values
Serum magnesium levels range from 1.3 to 2.1 mg/dl (SI, 0.65 to 1.05 mmol/L).

Abnormal findings
Elevated serum magnesium levels (hypermagnesemia) most commonly occur in renal failure, when the kidneys excrete inadequate amounts of magnesium, and also by magnesium administration or ingestion. Adrenal insufficiency (Addison's disease) can also increase serum magnesium levels.

In suspected or confirmed hypermagnesemia, observe the patient for lethargy; flushing; diaphoresis; decreased blood pressure; slow, weak pulse; muscle weakness; diminished deep tendon reflexes; slow, shallow respiration, and electrocardiogram (ECG) changes (prolonged PR interval, wide QRS complex, elevated T waves, atrioventricular block, premature ventricular contractions [PVCs]).

Decreased serum magnesium levels (hypomagnesemia) most commonly result from chronic alcoholism. Other causes include malabsorption syndrome, diarrhea, faulty absorption after bowel resection, prolonged bowel or gastric aspiration, acute pancreatitis, primary aldosteronism, severe burns, hypercalcemic conditions (including hyperparathyroidism), malnutrition, and certain diuretic therapy.

In hypomagnesemia, watch for leg and foot cramps, hyperactive deep tendon reflexes, arrhythmias, muscle weakness, seizures, twitching, tetany, tremors, and ECG changes (PVCs and ventricular fibrillation).

Interfering factors
■ Venous stasis due to tourniquet use
■ Obtaining a sample above an I.V. site that's receiving a solution containing magnesium
■ Excessive use of antacids or cathartics or excessive infusion of magnesium sulfate (increase)
■ Prolonged I.V. infusions without magnesium; excessive use of diuretics (decrease)
■ I.V. administration of calcium gluconate (possible false-low if measured using the Titan yellow method)
■ Hemolysis of the sample (false-high)

Phosphates

The phosphate test is used to measure serum levels of phosphates, the primary anion in intracellular fluid. Phosphates

are essential in the storage and utilization of energy, calcium regulation, red blood cell function, acid-base balance, formation of bone, and the metabolism of carbohydrates, protein, and fat. The intestines absorb most phosphates from dietary sources; the kidneys excrete phosphates and serve as a regulatory mechanism. Abnormal concentrations of serum phosphates usually result from improper excretion rather than faulty ingestion or absorption from dietary sources.

Normally, calcium and phosphates have an inverse relationship; if one is increased, the other is decreased.

Purpose
■ To aid diagnosis of renal disorders and acid-base imbalance
■ To detect endocrine, skeletal, and calcium disorders

Patient preparation
■ Explain to the patient that the serum phosphate test is used to measure phosphate levels in the blood.
■ Tell the patient that the test requires a blood sample. Explain who will perform the venipuncture and when.
■ Explain to the patient that he may experience slight discomfort from the needle puncture and the tourniquet.
■ Inform the patient that he need not restrict food and fluids.
■ Notify the laboratory and physician of medications the patient is taking that may affect test results; they may need to be restricted.

Procedure and posttest care
■ Perform a venipuncture without using a tourniquet, if possible, and collect the sample in 3- or 4-ml clot-activator tube.
■ Apply pressure to the venipuncture site until bleeding stops.

- If a hematoma develops at the venipuncture site, apply warm soaks.
- Instruct the patient that he may resume any medications discontinued before the test, as ordered.

Precautions
- Handle the sample gently to prevent hemolysis.

Reference values
Normally, serum phosphate levels in adults range from 2.7 to 4.5 mg/dl (SI, 0.87 to 1.45 mmol/L).

⚙ **AGE ISSUE** *In children, the normal range is 4.5 to 6.7 mg/dl (SI, 1.45 to 1.78 mmol/L).*

Abnormal findings
Decreased phosphate levels (hypophosphatemia) may result from malnutrition, malabsorption syndromes, hyperparathyroidism, renal tubular acidosis, and treatment of diabetic ketoacidosis (DKA). In children, hypophosphatemia can suppress normal growth. Symptoms of hypophosphatemia include anemia, prolonged bleeding, bone demineralization, decreased white blood cell count, and anorexia.

Increased levels (hyperphosphatemia) may result from skeletal disease, healing fractures, hypoparathyroidism, acromegaly, DKA, high intestinal obstruction, lactic acidosis (due to hepatic impairment), and renal failure. Hyperphosphatemia is seldom clinically significant, but it can alter bone metabolism in prolonged cases. Symptoms of hyperphosphatemia include tachycardia, muscular weakness, diarrhea, cramping, and hyperreflexia.

Interfering factors
- Venous stasis due to tourniquet use

- Sample obtained above an I.V. site that's receiving a solution containing phosphate
- Excessive vitamin D intake or therapy with anabolic steroids or androgens (possible increase)
- Use of acetazolamide, insulin, epinephrine, or phosphate-binding antacids; excessive excretion due to prolonged vomiting or diarrhea; vitamin D deficiency; and extended I.V. infusion of dextrose 5% in water (possible decrease)
- Hemolysis of the sample (false-high)

Potassium

The potassium test is used to measure serum levels of potassium, the major intracellular cation. Potassium helps to maintain cellular osmotic equilibrium and to regulate muscle activity, enzyme activity, and acid-base balance. It also influences renal function.

The body has no efficient method for conserving potassium; the kidneys excrete nearly all ingested potassium, even when the body's supply is depleted.

Potassium levels are affected by variations in the secretions of adrenal steroid hormones and by fluctuations in pH, serum glucose levels, and serum sodium levels. A reciprocal relationship appears to exist between potassium and sodium; a substantial intake of one element causes a corresponding decrease in the other. Although it readily conserves sodium, the body has no efficient method for conserving potassium. Even in potassium depletion, the kidneys continue to excrete potassium; therefore, potassium deficiency can develop rapidly and is quite common.

Because the kidneys excrete nearly all ingested potassium daily, a dietary intake of at least 40 mEq/day is essential. A nor-

DIETARY SOURCES OF POTASSIUM

A healthy person needs to consume at least 40 mEq of potassium daily. The chart here highlights foods and beverages, their serving size, and the amount of potassium each contains.

Foods and beverages	Serving size	Amount of potassium (mEq)
Meats		
Beef	4 oz (112 g)	11.2
Chicken	4 oz	12.0
Scallops	5 large	30.0
Veal	4 oz	15.2
Vegetables		
Artichokes	1 large bud	7.7
Asparagus (frozen, cooked)	½ cup	5.5
Asparagus (raw)	6 spears	7.7
Beans (dried, cooked)	½ cup	10.0
Beans (lima)	½ cup	9.5
Broccoli (cooked)	½ cup	7.0
Carrots (cooked)	½ cup	5.7
Carrots (raw)	1 large	8.8
Mushrooms (raw)	4 large	10.6
Potatoes (baked)	1 small	15.4
Spinach (raw or cooked)	½ cup	8.5
Squash (winter and baked)	½ cup	12.0
Tomatoes (raw)	1 medium	10.4
Fruits		
Apricots (dried)	4 halves	5.0
Apricots (raw)	3 small	8.0
Bananas	1 medium	12.8
Cantaloupe	6 oz	13.0
Figs (dried)	7 small	17.5
Peaches (raw)	1 medium	6.2
Pears (raw)	1 medium	6.2
Beverages		
Apricot nectar	1 cup (240 ml)	9.0
Grapefruit juice	1 cup	8.2
Orange juice	1 cup	11.4
Pineapple juice	1 cup	9.0
Prune juice	1 cup	14.4
Tomato juice	1 cup	11.6
Milk (whole or skim)	1 cup	8.8

TREATING POTASSIUM IMBALANCE

Hypokalemia and hyperkalemia can cause serious problems if not treated promptly.

Hypokalemia
A patient with a potassium deficiency can be treated with oral potassium chloride replacement and increased dietary intake. In severe cases, potassium can be replaced by I.V. infusion at a rate not exceeding 20 mEq/hour and at a concentration of no more than 80 mEq/L of I.V. fluid. Mix the potassium well in the I.V. solution because it can settle near the neck of the bottle or plastic bag. Failure to mix the solution adequately or to infuse it properly can cause a burning sensation at the I.V. site and possibly even fatal hyperkalemia.

Monitor the electrocardiogram, urine output, and serum potassium levels frequently during the infusion. Never administer I.V. potassium replacement to a patient with inadequate urine flow because diminished excretion can rapidly lead to hyperkalemia.

Hyperkalemia
Dangerously high potassium levels may be reduced with sodium polystyrene sulfonate — a potassium-removing resin — administered orally, rectally, or through a nasogastric tube. Hyperkalemia may also be treated with an I.V. infusion of sodium bicarbonate or of glucose and insulin, which lowers blood potassium by causing it to move into cells.

A calcium I.V. infusion provides fast but transient relief from the cardiotoxic effects of hyperkalemia; however, it doesn't directly lower serum potassium levels. In renal failure, dialysis may help remove excess potassium, but this corrects the imbalance much more slowly.

---

mal diet usually includes 60 to 100 mEq of potassium. (See *Dietary sources of potassium* and *Treating potassium imbalance*.)

Purpose
- To evaluate clinical signs of potassium excess (hyperkalemia) or potassium depletion (hypokalemia)
- To monitor renal function, acid-base balance, and glucose metabolism
- To evaluate neuromuscular and endocrine disorders
- To detect the origin of arrhythmias

Patient preparation
- Explain to the patient that the serum potassium test is used to determine the potassium content of blood.
- Tell the patient that the test requires a blood sample. Explain who will perform the venipuncture and when.
- Explain to the patient that he may experience slight discomfort from the needle puncture and the tourniquet.
- Inform the patient that he need not restrict food and fluids.
- Notify the laboratory and physician of medications the patient is taking that may affect test results; they may need to be restricted.

Procedure and posttest care
- Perform a venipuncture and collect the sample in a 3- or 4-ml clot-activator tube.
- Apply direct pressure to the venipuncture site until bleeding stops.
- If a hematoma develops at the venipuncture site, apply warm soaks.
- Instruct the patient to resume any medications discontinued before the test, as ordered.

Precautions

■ Draw the sample immediately after applying the tourniquet because a delay may increase the potassium level by allowing intracellular potassium to leak into the serum.

■ Handle the sample gently to avoid hemolysis.

Reference values

Normally, serum potassium levels range from 3.5 to 5 mEq/L (SI, 3.5 to 5 mmol/L).

Abnormal findings

Abnormally high serum potassium levels are common in conditions in which excess cellular potassium enters the blood, such as burn injuries, crush injuries, diabetic ketoacidosis, transfusions of large amounts of blood, and myocardial infarction. Hyperkalemia may also indicate reduced sodium excretion, possibly due to renal failure (preventing normal exchange of sodium and potassium) or Addison's disease (due to potassium buildup and sodium depletion).

▶ **CLINICAL ALERT** *Observe the patient with hyperkalemia for weakness, malaise, nausea, diarrhea, colicky pain, muscle irritability progressing to flaccid paralysis, oliguria, and bradycardia. The electrocardiogram (ECG) reveals flattened P waves; a prolonged PR interval; a wide QRS complex; tall, tented T waves; and ST-segment depression. Cardiac arrest may occur without warning.*

Below-normal potassium values commonly result from aldosteronism or Cushing's syndrome, loss of body fluids (such as long-term diuretic therapy, vomiting, or diarrhea), and excessive licorice ingestion. Although serum values and clinical symptoms can indicate a potassium imbalance, an ECG allows a definitive diagnosis.

▶ **CLINICAL ALERT** *Observe the patient with hypokalemia for decreased reflexes; a rapid, weak, irregular pulse; mental confusion; hypotension; anorexia; muscle weakness; and paresthesia. The ECG shows a flattened T wave, ST-segment depression, and U-wave elevation. In severe cases, ventricular fibrillation, respiratory paralysis, and cardiac arrest can develop.*

Interfering factors

■ Repeated clenching of the fist before venipuncture (possible increase)

■ Delay in drawing blood after applying a tourniquet or excessive hemolysis of the sample (increase)

■ Excessive or rapid potassium infusion, spironolactone or penicillin G potassium therapy, and renal toxicity from administration of amphotericin B, methicillin, or tetracycline (increase)

■ Insulin and glucose administration; diuretic therapy (especially with thiazides but not with triamterene, amiloride, or spironolactone); and I.V. infusions without potassium (decrease)

Sodium

The sodium test is used to measure serum levels of sodium in relation to the amount of water in the body. Sodium, the major extracellular cation, affects body water distribution, maintains osmotic pressure of extracellular fluid, and helps promote neuromuscular function. It also helps maintain acid-base balance and influences chloride and potassium levels.

Because extracellular sodium concentration helps the kidneys to regulate body water (decreased sodium levels promote water excretion and increased levels promote retention), serum levels of sodium are evaluated in relation to the amount of water in the body. For example, a sodium

FLUID IMBALANCES

This chart lists the causes, signs and symptoms, and diagnostic test findings associated with hypervolemia (increased fluid volume) and hypovolemia (decreased fluid volume).

Causes	Signs and symptoms	Laboratory findings
Hypervolemia		
■ Increased water intake ■ Decreased water output due to renal disease ■ Heart failure ■ Excessive ingestion or infusion of sodium chloride ■ Long-term administration of adrenocortical hormones ■ Excessive infusion of isotonic solutions	■ Increased blood pressure, pulse rate, body weight, and respiratory rate ■ Bounding peripheral pulses ■ Moist pulmonary crackles ■ Moist mucous membranes ■ Moist respiratory secretions ■ Edema ■ Weakness ■ Seizures and coma due to swelling of brain cells	■ Decreased red blood cell (RBC) count, hemoglobin concentration, packed cell volume, serum sodium concentration (dilutional decrease), and urine specific gravity
Hypovolemia		
■ Decreased water intake ■ Fluid loss due to fever, diarrhea, or vomiting ■ Systemic infection ■ Impaired renal concentrating ability ■ Fistulous drainage ■ Severe burns ■ Hidden fluid in body cavities	■ Increased pulse and respiratory rates ■ Decreased blood pressure and body weight ■ Weak and thready peripheral pulses ■ Thick, slurred speech ■ Thirst ■ Oliguria ■ Anuria ■ Dry skin	■ Increased RBC count, hemoglobin concentration, packed cell volume, serum sodium concentration, and urine specific gravity

deficit (hyponatremia) refers to a decreased level of sodium in relation to the body's water level. (See *Fluid imbalances*.) The body normally regulates this sodium-water balance through aldosterone, which inhibits sodium excretion and promotes its resorption (with water) by the renal tubules to maintain balance. Low sodium levels stimulate aldosterone secretion; elevated sodium levels depress it.

Purpose
■ To evaluate fluid-electrolyte and acid-base balance and related neuromuscular, renal, and adrenal functions

Patient preparation
■ Explain to the patient that the serum sodium test is used to determine the sodium content of the blood.
■ Tell the patient that the test requires a blood sample. Explain who will perform the venipuncture and when.

- Explain to the patient that he may experience slight discomfort from the needle puncture and the tourniquet.
- Inform the patient that he need not restrict food and fluids.
- Notify the laboratory and physician of medications the patient is taking that may affect test results; they may need to be restricted.

Procedure and posttest care
- Perform a venipuncture and collect the sample in a 3- or 4-ml clot-activator tube.
- Apply direct pressure to the venipuncture site until bleeding stops.
- If a hematoma develops at the venipuncture site, apply warm soaks.
- Instruct the patient to resume any medications discontinued before the test, as ordered.

Precautions
- Handle the sample gently to prevent hemolysis.

Reference values
Normally, serum sodium levels range from 135 to 145 mEq/L (SI, 135 to 145 mmol/L).

Abnormal findings
Sodium imbalance can result from a loss or gain of sodium or from a change in the patient's state of hydration. Increased serum sodium levels (hypernatremia) may be due to inadequate water intake, water loss in excess of sodium (such as diabetes insipidus, impaired renal function, prolonged hyperventilation and, occasionally, severe vomiting or diarrhea), and sodium retention (such as aldosteronism). Hypernatremia can also result from excessive sodium intake.

▶ **CLINICAL ALERT** *In the patient with hypernatremia and associated loss of water, observe for signs of thirst, rest-*

lessness, dry and sticky mucous membranes, flushed skin, oliguria, and diminished reflexes. If increased total body sodium causes water retention, observe for hypertension, dyspnea, edema, and heart failure.

Abnormally low serum sodium levels (hyponatremia) may result from inadequate sodium intake or excessive sodium loss due to profuse sweating, GI suctioning, diuretic therapy, diarrhea, vomiting, adrenal insufficiency, burns, and chronic renal insufficiency with acidosis. Urine sodium determinations are usually more sensitive to early changes in sodium balance and should be evaluated simultaneously with serum sodium findings.

▶ **CLINICAL ALERT** *In the patient with hyponatremia, watch for apprehension, lassitude, headache, decreased skin turgor, abdominal cramps, and tremors that may progress to seizures.*

Interfering factors
- Hemolysis due to rough handling of the sample
- Most diuretics (decrease by promoting sodium excretion)
- Lithium, chlorpropamide, and vasopressin (decrease by inhibiting water excretion)
- Corticosteroids (increase by promoting sodium retention)
- Antihypertensives, such as methyldopa, hydralazine, and reserpine (possible increase due to sodium and water retention)

Anion gap

Total concentrations of cations and anions are usually equal, making serum electrically neutral. Measuring the gap between measured cation and anion levels provides information about the level of anions (including sulfate, phosphate, organic acids such as ketone bodies and lactic acid, and proteins) that are not routinely measured in laboratory tests. In metabolic acidosis, measuring the anion gap helps to identify the type of acidosis and possible causes. Further tests are usually needed to determine the specific cause of metabolic acidosis.

Purpose
- To distinguish types of metabolic acidosis
- To monitor renal function and total parenteral nutrition

Patient preparation
- Explain to the patient that the anion gap test is used to determine the cause of acidosis.
- Tell the patient that the test requires a blood sample. Explain who will perform the venipuncture and when.
- Explain to the patient that he may experience slight discomfort from the needle puncture and the tourniquet.
- Inform the patient that he need not restrict food and fluids.
- Notify the laboratory and physician of medications the patient is taking that may affect test results; they may need to be restricted.

Procedure and posttest care
- Perform a venipuncture and collect the sample in a 3- or 4-ml clot-activator tube.
- Apply direct pressure to the venipuncture site until bleeding stops.
- If a hematoma develops at the venipuncture site, apply warm soaks.
- Instruct the patient to resume medications discontinued before the test, as ordered.

Precautions
- Handle the sample gently to prevent hemolysis.

ANION GAP AND METABOLIC ACIDOSIS

Metabolic acidosis with a normal anion gap (8 to 14 mEq/L) occurs in conditions characterized by loss of bicarbonate, such as:
- hypokalemic acidosis due to renal tubular acidosis, diarrhea, or ureteral diversions
- hyperkalemic acidosis due to acidifying agents (for example, ammonium chloride, hydrochloric acid), hydronephrosis, or sickle cell nephropathy.

Metabolic acidosis with an *increased anion gap* (>14 mEq/L) occurs in conditions characterized by accumulation of organic acids, sulfates, or phosphates, such as:
- renal failure
- ketoacidosis due to starvation, diabetes mellitus, or alcohol abuse
- lactic acidosis
- ingestion of toxins, such as salicylates, methanol, ethylene glycol (antifreeze), and paraldehyde.

Reference values
Normally, the anion gap ranges from 8 to 14 mEq/L (SI, 8 to 14 mmol/L).

Abnormal findings
A normal anion gap doesn't rule out metabolic acidosis. It may occur in hyperchloremic acidosis, renal tubular acidosis, and severe bicarbonate-wasting conditions, such as biliary or pancreatic fistulas and poorly functioning ileal loops.

When acidosis results from loss of bicarbonate in the urine or other body fluids, the anion gap remains unchanged. This is known as *normal anion gap acidosis.* (See *Anion gap and metabolic acidosis.*)

An increased anion gap indicates an increase in one or more of the unmeasured anions (sulfate, phosphates, organic acids such as ketone bodies and lactic acid, and proteins). This may occur with acidoses that are characterized by excessive organic or inorganic acids, such as lactic acidosis or ketoacidosis.

When acidosis results from an accumulation of metabolic acids — as occurs in lactic acidosis, for example — the anion gap increases (>14 mEq/L) with the increase in unmeasured anions. Metabolic acidosis caused by such an accumulation is known as *high anion gap acidosis*.

A decreased anion gap is rare, but may occur with hypermagnesemia and paraproteinemic states, such as multiple myeloma and Waldenström's macroglobulinemia.

Interfering factors

■ Hemolysis due to rough handling of the sample
■ Diuretics, lithium, chlorpropamide, and vasopressin (possible decrease due to decreased serum sodium levels)
■ Corticosteroids and antihypertensives (possible increase due to increased serum sodium levels)
■ Salicylates, paraldehyde, methicillin, dimercaprol, ammonium chloride, acetazolamide, ethylene glycol, and methyl alcohol (possible increase due to decreased serum bicarbonate levels)
■ Adrenocorticotropic hormone, cortisone, mercurial or chlorthiazide diuretics, and excessive ingestion of alkali or licorice (possible decrease due to increased serum bicarbonate levels)
■ Ammonium chloride, cholestyramine, boric acid, oxyphenbutazone, phenylbutazone, and excessive I.V. infusion of sodium chloride (possible decrease due to increased serum chloride levels)
■ Thiazide diuretics, ethacrynic acid, furosemide, bicarbonates, and prolonged I.V. infusion of dextrose 5% in water (possible increase due to decreased serum chloride levels)
■ Iodine absorption from wounds packed with povidone-iodine or excessive use of magnesium-containing antacids, especially by patients with renal failure (possible false-low)

Selected readings

Anderson, S.C., and Poulsen, K.B. *Anderson's Atlas of Hematology.* Philadelphia: Lippincott Williams & Wilkins, 2003.

Cavanaugh, B.M. *Nurse's Manual of Laboratory and Diagnostic Tests,* 4th ed. Philadelphia: F.A. Davis Co., 2003.

Diseases, 3rd ed. Springhouse, Pa.: Lippincott Williams & Wilkins, 2001.

Fischbach, F. *A Manual of Laboratory and Diagnostic Tests,* 7th ed. Philadelphia: Lippincott Williams & Wilkins, 2004.

Guyton, A.C., and Hall, J.E. *Textbook of Medical Physiology,* 10th ed. Philadelphia: W.B. Saunders Co., 2001.

Lynes, D. "An Introduction to Blood Gas Analysis," *Nursing Times* 99(11):54-55, March 2003.

McClatchey, K.D. *Clinical Laboratory Medicine,* 2nd ed. Philadelphia: Lippincott Williams & Wilkins, 2002.

Nursing 2004 Drug Handbook. Philadelphia: Lippincott Williams & Wilkins, 2004.

Pagana, K.D., and Pagana, T.J. *Mosby's Diagnostic and Laboratory Test Reference,* 6th ed. St. Louis: Mosby Year–Book, Inc., 2003.

Schnell, Z., et al. *Davis's Comprehensive Handbook of Laboratory and Diagnostic Tests with Nursing Implications.* Philadelphia: F.A. Davis Co., 2003.

Walton, H.G., et al. "Comparison of Blood Gas and Electrolyte Test Results from the Gem-Premier and the ABL-70 Versus a Conventional Laboratory Analyzer," *Journal of Extracorporeal Technology* 35(1):24-27, March 2003.

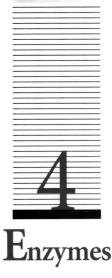

Enzymes

HOW ENZYMES WORK

According to current theory, enzymes work as catalysts because of their surface activity. Because each reactant has its own unique three-dimensional surface, an enzyme combines with reactants whose molecular surfaces fit its own (top). To initiate a reaction, the reactants and an enzyme specific to them combine briefly (middle). At the end of the reaction, the enzyme and the reactants separate, leaving the enzyme unchanged (bottom).

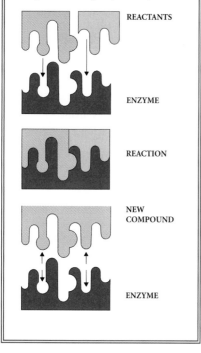

REACTANTS

ENZYME

REACTION

NEW COMPOUND

ENZYME

Introduction

Enzymes are reusable proteins that catalyze the thousands of chemical reactions needed to keep a single cell alive and functioning. They accelerate and control reaction rates without being destroyed in the process.

Different kinds of cells produce different enzymes, and most tissues contain many different enzymes. When tissue cells are damaged by disease or some other defect, they release enzymes specific to that area into the bloodstream, where they can be readily detected. For example, leakage from dying cells is the source of elevated serum enzyme levels in myocardial infarction (MI), infectious hepatitis, and other disease states.

Although serum levels of any one enzyme may not identify its tissue of origin, comparing serum levels of several enzymes may provide important diagnostic information because individual enzymes are present in different tissues in different ratios. Such analysis may reveal the extent of pathology and monitor the progress of healing. (See *How enzymes work.*)

Sensitivity and specificity

Because certain diseases that produce similar symptoms cause distinctively different enzyme abnormalities, enzyme tests can be used to separate them. The diagnostic value of these tests depends on their sensitivity and specificity. Sensitivity indicates how reliably the test gives a positive result when a particular disease is present; specificity indicates how often the test is "normal" when the disease is absent. Thus, enzyme tests with low sensitivity produce negative readings when the disease is present; tests with low specificity show positive readings when the disease is absent.

Some enzymes, such as *creatine kinase* (CK) and *lactate dehydrogenase* (LD), occur in multiple forms — isoenzymes — that differ in molecular details while retaining their basic identities. CK also appears in isoenzyme subunits called isoforms. Certain organs or tissues contain more or less of one isoenzyme than another; therefore, testing for isoenzymes may provide better sensitivity or specificity than measuring an entire enzyme group.

CK is present in heart muscle, skeletal muscle, and brain tissue. CK isoenzymes are combinations of the subunits M (muscle) and B (brain). For example, CK-BB is found primarily in brain and nerve tissue, CK-MB in heart muscle, and CK-MM in skeletal muscle. Therefore, in a suspected acute MI, elevated CK-MB levels reliably indicate cardiac damage.

LD has five isoenzymes that are formed from different combinations of two subunits: M (muscle) and H (heart). The patterns of LD_1 and LD_2 levels are monitored—along with other serum enzyme levels—to trace the progress of an MI. LD_3 levels are elevated primarily in patients with pulmonary infarction, whereas LD_4 and LD_5 elevations are characteristic of skeletal muscle and hepatic disorders. (See *Isoenzymes of lactate dehydrogenase*.)

Enzyme test batteries

Isoenzymes may be separated and assayed by several laboratory methods, including electrophoresis, column chromatography, difference in heat stability, substrate alterations, and the use of chemical inhibitors. These techniques take advantage of physical or chemical properties of the isoenzyme molecule.

Some enzymes and isoenzymes are routinely tested in groups to help identify disorders, such as an MI and hepatic and pancreatic disease. Nevertheless, because some enzymes are present in many organs and disease states, positive test results are meaningful only in light of the patient's overall clinical status.

ISOENZYMES OF LACTATE DEHYDROGENASE

Individual monomers of the five lactate dehydrogenase (LD) isoenzymes carry the letter H, for those subunits that appear most consistently in heart tissue, or the letter M, for those predominant in skeletal muscle tissue. Injury to almost any tissue stimulates the release of isoenzymes with a tetrametric pattern peculiar to the injured tissue and roughly parallel to the degree of damage. For instance, in myocardial infarction, blood levels of LD_1 (HHHH) and LD_2 (HHHM) are elevated. Damage to pulmonary tissue causes the release of LD_3 (HHMM); injury to the liver and skeletal muscle causes the release of LD_4 (HMMM) and LD_5 (MMMM).

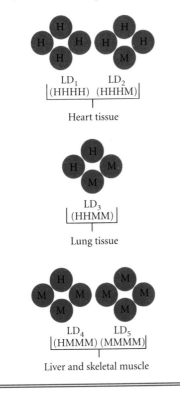

HYDROXYBUTYRIC DEHYDROGENASE

Hydroxybutyric dehydrogenase (HBD), or alpha-hydroxybutyric dehydrogenase, is actually total lactate dehydrogenase (LD) that's tested using a hydroxybutyric acid substrate instead of lactic or pyruvic acid. With this substrate, the electrophoretically fast-moving LD_1 and LD_2 (cardiac) isoenzymes exhibit more activity than the slow-moving LD_5 (liver) fraction, so that HBD activity roughly parallels LD_1 and LD_2 activity. Measurement of serum HBD is sometimes used as a substitute for LD isoenzyme fractionation because this analysis is easier to perform and less expensive than LD electrophoresis.

Although HBD concentration primarily reflects LD_1 and LD_2 activity, it may also show LD_5 activity if enough of this isoenzyme is present (as it is in some forms of hepatic disease). Therefore, this test isn't consistently reliable in distinguishing between myocardial and hepatic cellular damage and is used infrequently.

Cardiac enzymes and isoenzymes

CK-MB levels rise 4 to 8 hours after onset of infarction, peak at 18 to 24 hours, and may remain elevated for as long as 72 hours. LD_1 and LD_2 levels usually rise within 24 hours after an episode, tapering off 72 to 96 hours later.

Some laboratories also measure hydroxybutyric dehydrogenase (HBD) in a suspected acute MI when electrophoresis equipment isn't available or when the total LD isn't sufficient to confirm diagnosis. Serum HBD levels rise 8 to 10 hours after an MI, peak in 48 to 96 hours, and return to normal in 16 to 18 days. (See *Hydroxybutyric dehydrogenase.*)

Recent studies have indicated that there are additional cardiac markers that, when elevated, may indicate an MI. They include serum myoglobin and serum protein troponin.

Myoglobin is a hemoprotein found in cardiac and skeletal muscles that's released from cells when muscle damage occurs. Myoglobin levels rise 1 to 3 hours after an MI. Performing serial measurements of myoglobin levels increases test specificity and sensitivity. These levels are most helpful when used in conjunction with other cardiac markers, such as CK and troponin.

Measurement of a cardiac protein called troponin is the most precise way to determine if a patient has experienced an MI. Some 6 hours after an MI, a blood test can detect two forms of troponin: T and I. Troponin T levels peak about 2 days after an MI and return to normal about 16 days later. Troponin I levels reach their peak in less than 1 day after an MI and return to normal in about 7 days.

The detection of either form of troponin provides conclusive evidence of an MI. Higher troponin levels have been associated with an increased risk of mortality.

Aspartate aminotransferase (AST) also rises during an acute MI, increasing 6 to 8 hours after and peaking in 18 to 24 hours. The AST level may increase to 4 to 10 times normal, but returns to normal in 4 to 5 days. Because AST is also found in other tissues, such as liver and muscle, an increase isn't sufficient to diagnose an MI. Thus, correct interpretation of enzyme analyses always requires careful comparison with the patient's clinical status and correlation to other enzyme assays.

Because the diagnostic value of some enzyme tests depends on the comparison of sequential test results, *each* blood sample must be labeled with the date and the hour it was collected. For example, in an acute MI, the first set of tests is ordered to obtain a baseline. Subsequent sets of tests are ordered serially (perhaps at 6, 12, and 24 hours after the episode and daily thereafter) to monitor changes in enzyme concentrations, particularly elevations. However, decreases can also be important in evaluating the patient's prognosis. Adding "Rule out MI" to the laboratory request will aid the diagnostician, but it's also essential to record the time that the sample was drawn.

C-reactive protein (CRP) is a substance produced by the liver that increases when there's inflammation in the body. A high level of CRP indicates an inflammation at some location in the body. Other diagnostic tests will be needed to determine where the inflammation is located and the cause. Elevated CRP levels can indicate conditions such as MI, angina, systemic lupus erythematosus, postoperative infection, trauma, and heatstroke.

The CRP test is being used to predict heart attack risk along with other tests, including lipid profiles. Normally, CRP isn't present in the blood.

B-type natriuretic peptide (BNP) is an FDA-approved blood test that's being used as a marker in helping accurately diagnose heart failure. BNP is a hormone polypeptide that's secreted by ventricular tissues in the heart. The substance is secreted as a response to increased ventricular volume and pressure. This test not only diagnoses heart failure but can grade the severity of it. An accurate diagnosis is important in the management and treatment of heart failure, which in the past has been underdiagnosed and undertreated.

Hepatic enzymes and isoenzymes

The liver is the site of many biochemical reactions that are controlled by numerous enzymes. Many of these reactions occur at diagnostically significant levels in the serum in a spectrum of hepatobiliary disorders ranging from minute changes within hepatic cells (hepatitis) to extrahepatic disorders such as biliary obstruction.

A deficiency of the liver enzyme *alpha-$_1$ antitrypsin* (AAT) causes other enzymes to damage tissues in the lungs and liver. An AAT deficiency is a hereditary disease that can lead to a rare form of emphysema in adults and a rare form of cirrhosis in children.

Although neither AST nor *alanine aminotransferase* (ALT) is confined to the liver, both can reliably identify hepatic disease. In severe necrosis (as in viral hepatitis), AST levels may rise as high as 100 times the reference range because of massive tissue destruction. ALT levels may rise even higher and remain elevated longer than AST. These enzymes become detectable early in the disease and persist longer than changes in other liver function studies.

Gamma glutamyl transferase (GGT) is a sensitive indicator of early hepatocellular damage, obstruction, or alcohol-induced hepatic disease; it's usually measured with other enzymes to confirm hepatic disease. Elevated levels rise in patterns similar to those of serum alkaline phosphatase.

The enzyme *alkaline phosphatase* (ALP) can be separated into several isoenzymes, each of which is found in different tissues. Isoenzyme type 1 is specific to hepatic disorders; serum levels rise dramatically in biliary cirrhosis and in bile duct obstruction that impedes phosphatase excretion.

When ALP levels are elevated, measuring another phosphatase enzyme — *5′-nucleotidase* (5′NT), which is formed mostly in the liver — can determine whether ALP elevations are liver- or bone-related. Usually, 5′NT and ALP levels are elevated in hepatic disease, whereas only ALP levels rise in skeletal disease.

Two isoenzymes of LD — LD_4 and LD_5 — occur predominantly in the liver. Their serum levels are commonly elevated even before jaundice appears and return to normal while clinical symptoms are still evident.

Leucine aminopeptidase, a proteolytic enzyme, is found in liver cells. It's released into the blood after damage to the liver cells. Other enzymes, such as ALT, AST, ALP, and GGT, are more sensitive indicators of liver problems.

Pancreatic enzymes

Amylase and *lipase* are produced by the pancreas and secreted into the small intestine, where they break down starches and fats, respectively. Both appear in serum after acute pancreatitis. Serum amylase levels rise rapidly in acute pancreatitis, reaching twice the normal values just 4 hours after the onset of symptoms; however, levels also drop quickly, returning to normal 48 to 72 hours later. Serum lipase levels rise similarly, but remain elevated for as long as 14 days.

Prostatic and other enzymes

Acid phosphatase is found mainly in the adult prostate gland. Elevated levels of this enzyme usually indicate prostate cancer that has penetrated the prostatic capsule.

Miscellaneous enzyme tests

Special enzyme tests that aren't part of specific organ test profiles include plasma renin activity, cholinesterase, glucose-6-phosphate dehydrogenase (G6PD), pyruvate kinase (PK), hexosaminidase A and B, uroporphyrinogen I synthase, galactose-1-phosphate uridyltransferase, and angiotensin-converting enzyme (ACE).

Plasma renin testing helps identify primary aldosteronism. Pseudocholinesterase may aid in the diagnosis of pesticide poisonings and succinylcholine hypersensitivity. Assays for G6PD, PK, uroporphyrinogen I synthase, and galactose-1-phosphate uridyltransferase can help detect inherited enzyme deficiencies. Hexosaminidase A and B testing is used to diagnose Tay-Sachs disease. The ACE test is used mainly to detect sarcoidosis.

CARDIAC ENZYME TESTS

Creatine kinase and isoforms

Creatine kinase (CK) is an enzyme that catalyzes the creatine-creatinine metabolic pathway in muscle cells and brain tissue. Because of its intimate role in energy production, CK reflects normal tissue catabolism; increased serum levels indicate trauma to cells.

Fractionation and measurement of three distinct CK isoenzymes — CK-BB (CK_1), CK-MB (CK_2), and CK-MM (CK_3) — have replaced the use of total CK levels to accurately localize the site of increased tissue destruction. CK-BB is most commonly found in brain tissue. CK-MM and CK-MB are found primarily in skeletal and heart muscle. In addition, subunits of CK-MB and CK-MM, called isoforms or isoenzymes, can be assayed to increase the test's sensitivity.

Purpose

- To detect and diagnose an acute myocardial infarction (MI) and reinfarction (CK-MB primarily used)
- To evaluate possible causes of chest pain and to monitor the severity of myocardial ischemia after cardiac surgery, cardiac catheterization, and cardioversion (CK-MB primarily used)
- To detect early dermatomyositis and musculoskeletal disorders that aren't neurogenic in origin such as Duchenne's muscular dystrophy (total CK primarily used)

Patient preparation

- Explain to the patient that this test is used to assess myocardial and musculoskeletal function and that multiple blood samples are required to detect fluctuations in serum levels.
- Tell the patient who will be performing the venipunctures and when.
- Explain to the patient that he may experience slight discomfort from the needle puncture and the tourniquet.
- If the patient is being evaluated for musculoskeletal disorders, advise him to avoid exercising for 24 hours before the test.
- Notify the laboratory and physician of medications the patient is taking that may affect test results; they may need to be restricted.

Procedure and posttest care

- Perform a venipuncture and collect the sample in a 4-ml tube without additives.
- Apply direct pressure to the venipuncture site until bleeding stops.

- If a hematoma develops at the venipuncture site, apply warm soaks.
- Instruct the patient that he may resume exercise and medications discontinued before the test, as ordered.

Precautions

- Draw the sample before giving I.M. injections or 1 hour after giving them because muscle trauma increases the total CK level.
- Obtain the sample on schedule. Note on the laboratory request the time the sample was drawn and the hours elapsed since the onset of chest pain.
- Handle the sample gently to prevent hemolysis.
- Send the sample to the laboratory immediately because CK activity diminishes significantly after 2 hours at room temperature.

Reference values

Total CK values determined by ultraviolet or kinetic measurement range from 55 to 170 U/L (SI, 0.94 to 2.89 µkat/L) for men and from 30 to 135 U/L (SI, 0.51 to 2.3 µkat/L) for women. CK levels may be significantly higher in muscular people.

AGE ISSUE *Infants up to age 1 have levels two to four times higher than adult levels, possibly reflecting birth trauma and striated muscle development.*

Normal ranges for isoenzyme levels are as follows: CK-BB, undetectable; CK-MB, < 5% (SI, < 0.05); CK-MM, 90% to 100% (SI, 0.9 to 1.0).

Abnormal findings

CK-MM makes up 99% of total CK normally present in serum. Detectable CK-BB isoenzyme may indicate, but doesn't confirm, a diagnosis of brain tissue injury, widespread malignant tumors, severe shock, or renal failure.

RELEASE OF CARDIAC ENZYMES AND PROTEINS

Because they're released by damaged tissue, serum proteins and isoenzymes (catalytic proteins that vary in concentration in specific organs) can help identify the compromised organ and assess the extent of damage. After an acute myocardial infarction, cardiac enzymes and proteins rise and fall in a characteristic pattern, as shown in the graph below.

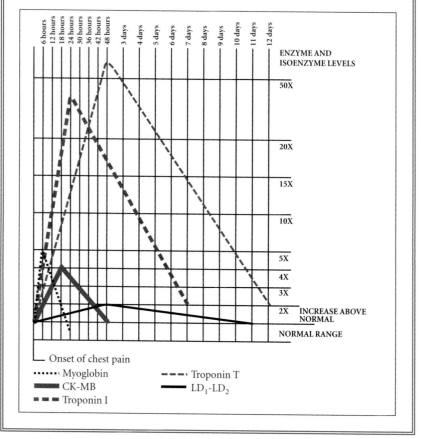

CK-MB levels greater than 5% of the total CK level indicate an MI, especially if the lactate dehydrogenase (LD) isoenzyme ratio is more than 1 (flipped LD). In an acute MI and after cardiac surgery, CK-MB begins to increase within 2 to 4 hours, peaks within 12 to 24 hours, and usually returns to normal within 24 to 48 hours; persistent elevations and increasing levels indicate ongoing myocardial damage. Total CK follows roughly the same pattern, but increases slightly later. CK-MB levels may not increase in heart failure or during angina pectoris not accompanied by myocardial cell necrosis. Serious skeletal muscle injury that occurs in certain muscular dystrophies, polymyositis, and severe myoglobinuria may produce a mild CK-MB increase because a small amount of this isoenzyme is present in some skeletal muscles.

Increasing CK-MM values follow skeletal muscle damage from trauma, such as surgery and I.M. injections, and from diseases, such as dermatomyositis and muscular dystrophy (values may be 50 to 100 times normal). A moderate increase in CK-MM levels develops in a patient with hypothyroidism; sharp increases occur with muscle activity caused by agitation such as during an acute psychotic episode.

Total CK levels may be increased in patients with severe hypokalemia, carbon monoxide poisoning, malignant hyperthermia, and alcoholic cardiomyopathy. They may also be increased after seizures and, occasionally, in patients who have suffered pulmonary or cerebral infarctions. Troponin I and cardiac troponin C are present in the contractile cells of cardiac myocardial tissue, and are released with injury to the myocardial tissue. Troponin levels increase within 1 hour of the infarction and may remain elevated for up to 14 days. (See *Release of cardiac enzymes and proteins.*)

Interfering factors
■ Hemolysis due to rough handling of the sample
■ Failure to send the sample to the laboratory immediately or to refrigerate the serum if testing will be delayed more than 2 hours (possible decrease in concentration)
■ Failure to draw the samples at the scheduled time (may miss peak levels)
■ Halothane and succinylcholine, alcohol, lithium, large doses of aminocaproic acid, I.M. injections, cardioversion, invasive diagnostic procedures, recent vigorous exercise or muscle massage, severe

coughing, and trauma (increase in total CK)
■ Surgery through skeletal muscle (increase in total CK)

Lactate dehydrogenase

Lactate dehydrogenase (LD) catalyzes the reversible conversion of muscle lactic acid into pyruvic acid, an essential step in the metabolic process that ultimately produces cellular energy. Because LD is present in almost all body tissues, cellular damage increases total serum LD, limiting its diagnostic usefulness.

However, five tissue-specific isoenzymes can be identified and measured, using immunochemical separation and quantitation or electrophoresis. Two of these isoenzymes, LD_1 and LD_2, appear primarily in the heart, red blood cells (RBCs), and kidneys; LD_3, primarily in the lungs; and LD_4 and LD_5, in the liver and the skeletal muscles. Also, the midzone fractions (LD_2, LD_3, LD_4) can be elevated in granulocytic leukemia, lymphomas, and platelet disorders.

The specificity of LD isoenzymes and their distribution pattern is useful in diagnosing hepatic, pulmonary, and erythrocyte damage. But their widest clinical application is in aiding diagnosis of acute myocardial infarction (MI). An LD isoenzyme assay is useful when creatine kinase (CK) hasn't been measured within 24 hours of an acute MI. The myocardial LD level rises later than CK (12 to 48 hours after infarction begins), peaks in 2 to 5 days, and drops to normal in 7 to 10 days if tissue necrosis doesn't persist. (See *LD isoenzyme variations in disease,* page 98.)

LD ISOENZYME VARIATIONS IN DISEASE

Disease	LD$_1$	LD$_2$	LD$_3$	LD$_4$	LD$_5$
Cardiovascular					
Myocardial infarction (MI)					
MI with hepatic congestion					
Rheumatic carditis					
Myocarditis					
Heart failure (decompensated)					
Shock					
Angina pectoris					
Pulmonary					
Pulmonary embolism					
Pulmonary infarction					
Hematologic					
Pernicious anemia					
Hemolytic anemia					
Sickle cell anemia					
Hepatobiliary					
Hepatitis					
Active cirrhosis					
Hepatic congestion					

NORMAL   DIAGNOSTIC   NOT DIAGNOSTIC

Adapted with permission from information from Helena Laboratories, 1513 Lindberg Drive, Beaumont, Tex.

Purpose
- To aid differential diagnosis of an MI, pulmonary infarction, anemias, and hepatic disease
- To support CK isoenzyme test results in diagnosing an MI or to provide diagnosis when CK-MB samples are drawn too late to display increase

■ To monitor the patient's response to some forms of chemotherapy

Patient preparation
■ Explain to the patient that this test is used primarily to detect tissue alterations.
■ Tell the patient that the test requires a blood sample. Explain who will perform the venipuncture and when.
■ Explain to the patient that he may experience slight discomfort from the needle puncture and the tourniquet.
■ Inform the patient that he need not restrict food and fluids.
■ If an MI is suspected, tell the patient that the test will be repeated on the next two mornings to monitor progressive changes.

Procedure and posttest care
■ Perform a venipuncture and collect the sample in a 4-ml clot-activator tube.
■ Apply direct pressure to the venipuncture site until bleeding stops.
■ If a hematoma develops at the venipuncture site, apply warm soaks.

Precautions
■ Draw the samples on schedule to avoid missing peak levels, and mark the collection time on the laboratory request.
■ Handle the sample gently to prevent artifact blood sample hemolysis because RBCs contain LD_1.
■ Send the sample to the laboratory immediately or, if transport is delayed, keep the sample at room temperature. Changes in temperature reportedly inactivate LD_5, thus altering isoenzyme patterns.

Reference values
Total LD levels normally range from 71 to 207 U/L (SI, 1.2 to 3.52 µkat/L). Normal distribution is as follows:

■ LD_1: 14% to 26% (SI, 0.14 to 0.26) of total
■ LD_2: 29% to 39% (SI, 0.29 to 0.39) of total
■ LD_3: 20% to 26% (SI, 0.20 to 0.26) of total
■ LD_4: 8% to 16% (SI, 0.08 to 0.16) of total
■ LD_5: 6% to 16% (SI, 0.06 to 0.16) of total.

Abnormal findings
Because many common diseases increase total LD levels, isoenzyme electrophoresis is usually necessary for diagnosis. In some disorders, total LD may be within normal limits, but abnormal proportions of each enzyme indicate specific organ tissue damage. For instance, in an acute MI, the concentration of LD_1 is greater than LD_2 within 12 to 48 hours after the onset of symptoms; therefore, the LD_1/LD_2 ratio is greater than 1. This reversal of the normal isoenzyme pattern is typical of myocardial damage and is known as flipped LD.

Midzone fractions (LD_2, LD_3, LD_4) can be increased in granulocytic leukemia, lymphomas, and platelet disorders.

Interfering factors
■ Hemolysis due to rough handling of the sample
■ For diagnosis of an acute MI, failure to draw the sample on schedule
■ Failure to send the sample to the laboratory immediately (may obscure LD isoenzyme patterns)
■ Failure to centrifuge the sample and separate the cells from the serum
■ Recent surgery or pregnancy (possible increase)
■ Prosthetic heart valve (possible increase due to chronic hemolysis)
■ Anabolic steroids, anesthetics, alcohol, narcotics, and procainamide (increase)

Myoglobins

Myoglobin, which is usually found in skeletal and cardiac muscle, functions as an oxygen-binding muscle protein. It's released into the bloodstream in ischemia, trauma, and inflammation of the muscle.

The release of myoglobin into the bloodstream is especially important when trying to determine damaged cardiac muscle. Creatine kinase and its isoform CK-MB are released more slowly than myoglobin during a myocardial infarction (MI). Therefore, myoglobin, which can be detected as soon as 2 hours after the onset of chest pain and peaks in 4 hours, can be useful as an early indicator of an MI.

Purpose
■ As a nonspecific test, to estimate damage to skeletal or cardiac muscle tissue
■ To predict flareups of polymyositis
■ Specifically, to determine if an MI has occurred

Patient preparation
■ Explain the purpose of the test to the patient.
■ Obtain a patient history, including disorders that may be associated with increased myoglobin levels.
■ Tell the patient that the test requires a blood sample. Explain who will be performing the venipuncture and when.
■ Explain to the patient that he may experience slight discomfort from the needle puncture and the tourniquet.
■ Inform the patient that the results need to be correlated with other tests for a definitive diagnosis.

Procedure and posttest care
■ Perform a venipuncture and collect the sample in a 4-ml tube with no additives.

■ Apply direct pressure to the venipuncture site until bleeding stops.
■ If a hematoma develops at the venipuncture site, apply warm soaks.

Precautions
■ Expect to collect blood samples 4 to 8 hours after the onset of an acute MI.
■ Handle the sample gently to avoid hemolysis.
■ Send the sample to the laboratory immediately.

Reference values
Normal myoglobin values are 0 to 0.09 µg/ml (SI, 5 to 70 µ/L).

Abnormal findings
Besides MI, increased myoglobin levels may occur in acute alcohol intoxication, dermatomyositis, hypothermia (with prolonged shivering), muscular dystrophy, polymyositis, rhabdomyelitis, severe burns, trauma, severe renal failure, and systemic lupus erythematosus.

Interfering factors
■ Hemolysis or radioactive scans performed within 1 week of the test
■ Recent angina, cardioversion, or improper timing of the test (possible increase)
■ I.M. injection (possible false-positive)

Troponin

Cardiac troponin I (cTnI) and cardiac troponin T (cTnT) are proteins in the striated cells that are extremely specific markers of cardiac damage. When injury occurs to the myocardial tissue, these proteins are released into the bloodstream. Elevations in troponin levels can be seen within 1 hour of myocardial infarction (MI) and will persist for a week or longer.

Purpose
- To detect and diagnose acute MI and reinfarction
- To evaluate possible causes of chest pain

Patient preparation
- Explain to the patient that this test helps assess myocardial injury and that multiple samples may be drawn to detect fluctuations in serum levels.
- Inform the patient he need not restrict foods and fluids.
- Tell the patient that the test requires a blood sample. Explain who will be performing the venipuncture and when.
- Explain to the patient that he may feel slight discomfort from the needle puncture and the tourniquet.

Procedure and posttest care
- Perform a venipuncture and collect the specimen in a 7-ml clot-activator tube.
- If a hematoma develops at the venipuncture site, apply warm soaks.

Precautions
- Obtain each specimen on schedule and note the date and collection time on each.

Reference values
Laboratory results may vary. Some laboratories may call a test positive if it shows any detectable levels, and others may give a range for abnormal results. Normally, cTnI levels are < 0.35 µg/L (SI, < 0.35 µg/L). cTnT levels are < 0.1 µg/L (SI, < 0.1 µg/L). cTnI levels > 2.0 µg/L (SI, > 2.0 µg/L) suggest cardiac injury. Results of a qualitative cTnT rapid immunoassay that are > 0.1 µg/L (SI, > 0.1 µg/L) are considered positive for cardiac injury. As long as tissue injury continues, the troponin levels will remain high.

Abnormal findings
Troponin levels rise rapidly and are detectable within 1 hour of myocardial cell injury. cTnI levels aren't detectable in a person without cardiac injury.

Interfering factors
- Sustained vigorous exercise (increase in absence of significant cardiac damage)
- Cardiotoxic drugs such as doxorubicin (increase)
- Renal disease and certain surgical procedures (possible increase)

C-reactive protein

C-reactive protein (CRP) is an abnormal protein that appears in the blood during an inflammatory process. It's absent from the blood of healthy people. This nonspecific protein is mainly synthesized in the liver and is found in many body fluids (pleural, peritoneal, pericardial, synovial). It appears in the blood 18 to 24 hours after the onset of tissue damage with levels that increase up to a thousandfold and then decline rapidly when the inflammatory process regresses. CRP has been found to rise before increases in antibody titers and erythrocyte sedimentation rate (ESR) levels occur. It also decreases sooner than ESR levels.

Purpose
- To evaluate the inflammatory disease course and severity in conditions, including tissue necrosis (myocardial infarction [MI], malignancy, rheumatoid arthritis)
- To monitor acute inflammatory phases of rheumatoid arthritis and rheumatic fever, so early treatment can be initiated
- To monitor the patient's response to treatment or determine if the acute phase is declining
- To help interpret the ESR

- To monitor the wound healing process of internal incisions, burns, and organ transplantation

Patient preparation
- Explain to the patient that this test is used to identify the presence of infection or to monitor treatment.
- Inform the patient that he needs to restrict all fluids except for water for 8 to 12 hours before the test.
- Tell the patient that the test requires a blood sample. Explain who will perform the venipuncture and when.
- Explain to the patient that he may experience slight discomfort from the needle puncture and the tourniquet.
- Notify the laboratory and physician of medications the patient is taking that may affect test results; they may need to be restricted.

Procedure and posttest care
- Perform a venipuncture and collect the sample in a 5-ml clot-activator tube.
- Apply direct pressure to the venipuncture site until bleeding stops.
- If a hematoma develops at the venipuncture site, apply warm soaks.
- Instruct the patient that he may resume his usual diet and medications discontinued before the test, as ordered.

Precautions
- Keep the blood sample away from heat.

Reference values
CRP usually isn't present in the blood. In adults, results may be reported as < 0.8 mg/dl (SI, < 8 mg/L).

Abnormal findings
An elevated CRP level may be present in rheumatoid arthritis, rheumatic fever, MI, cancer (active, widespread), acute bacterial and viral infections, and inflammatory bowel disease, Hodgkin's disease, systemic lupus erythematosus, and postoperatively (declines after the fourth day).

Interfering factors
- Steroids and salicylates (false normal level)
- Hormonal contraceptives (false increase)
- Pregnancy (third trimester) and intrauterine contraceptive devices (increase)

B-type natriuretic peptide assay

B-type natriuretic peptide (BNP) is a neurohormone produced predominantly by the heart ventricle. BNP is released from the heart in response to blood volume expansion or pressure overload.

Plasma BNP increases with the severity of heart failure. Studies have demonstrated that the heart is the major source of circulating BNP. It's an excellent hormonal marker of ventricular systolic and diastolic dysfunction.

Purpose
- To aid in the diagnosis and severity of heart failure

Patient preparation
- Explain to the patient that the BNP assay is used to identify the presence and severity of heart failure.
- Tell the patient that the assay requires a blood sample. Explain who will perform the venipuncture and when.
- Explain to the patient that he may experience slight discomfort from the needle puncture and the tourniquet.
- Inform the patient that he need not restrict food and fluids.

LINKING BNP LEVELS TO HEART FAILURE SYMPTOM SEVERITY

The following table shows the level of B-type natriuretic peptide (BNP) levels and the correlation with symptoms of heart failure. The higher the level of BNP, the more severe the symptoms.

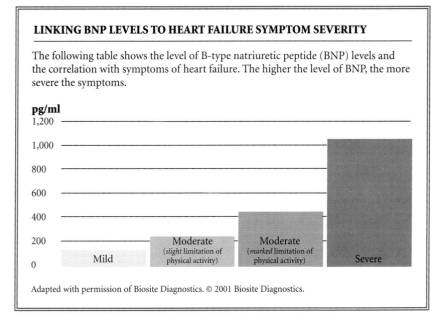

Adapted with permission of Biosite Diagnostics. © 2001 Biosite Diagnostics.

Procedure and posttest care
- Perform a venipuncture and collect the sample in a 3.5-ml EDTA tube.
- Apply direct pressure to the venipuncture site until bleeding stops.
- If a hematoma develops at the venipuncture site, apply warm soaks.

Precautions
- Handle the sample gently to prevent hemolysis.

Reference values
The normal value is < 100 pg/ml.

Abnormal findings
Blood concentrations greater than 100 pg/ml are an accurate predictor of heart failure. The level of BNP in the blood is related to the severity of heart failure. The higher the level, the worse the symptoms of heart failure. (See *Linking BNP levels to heart failure symptom severity.*)

Interfering factors
- Hemolysis due to rough handling of the sample

HEPATIC ENZYME TESTS

Alpha₁-antitrypsin

A protein produced by the liver, alpha₁-antitrypsin (also known as AAT or alpha₁-AT) is believed to inhibit the release of protease into body fluids by dying cells and is a major component of alpha₁-globulin. AAT is measured using radioimmunoassay or isoelectric focusing. Congenital absence or deficiency of AAT has been linked to high susceptibility to emphysema in adults and cirrhosis in children.

Purpose
- To screen the patient at high risk for emphysema
- To use as a nonspecific method of detecting inflammation, severe infection, and necrosis
- To test for congenital AAT deficiency

Patient preparation
AGE ISSUE Explain to the patient or child's parents that this test is used to diagnose respiratory or liver disease as well as inflammation, infection, or necrosis.
- Tell the patient that the test requires a blood sample. Explain who will be performing the venipuncture and when.
- Explain to the patient that he may experience slight discomfort from the needle puncture and the tourniquet.
- Tell the patient to avoid smoking because irritants in tobacco stimulate leukocytes in the lungs to release protease.
- Tell the patient to avoid hormonal contraceptives and steroids for 24 hours before the test.
- Tell the patient to fast for at least 8 hours before the test.

Procedure and posttest care
- Perform a venipuncture and collect the sample in a 4-ml tube without additives.
AGE ISSUE In a child, puncture the clean area with a sharp needle or lancet, then collect the blood sample in a pipette, small container, or onto a slide.
- Apply direct pressure to the venipuncture site until bleeding stops.
- Instruct the patient that he may resume his usual diet and medications discontinued before the test, as ordered.

Precautions
- Handle the sample gently to avoid hemolysis.

- Send the sample to the laboratory promptly.
- If clinically indicated, the patient with AAT levels lower than 125 mg/dl (SI, 1.25 g/L) should be phenotyped to confirm homozygous and heterozygous deficiencies. (The heterozygous patient doesn't appear to be at increased risk for early emphysema.)

Reference values
AAT levels vary by age, but the normal range is 110 to 200 mg/dl (SI, 1.1 to 2.0 g/L).

Abnormal findings
Decreased AAT levels may occur in early-onset emphysema and cirrhosis, nephrotic syndrome, malnutrition, congenital alpha$_1$-globulin deficiency and, transiently, in the neonate.

Increased AAT levels can occur in chronic inflammatory disorders, necrosis, pregnancy, acute pulmonary infections, hyaline membrane disease in infants, hepatitis, systemic lupus erythematosus, and rheumatoid arthritis.

Interfering factors
- Hormonal contraceptives and corticosteroids (possible false-high)
- Smoking or failure to fast for 8 hours before the test (possible false-high)

Aspartate aminotransferase

Aspartate aminotransferase (AST) is one of two enzymes that catalyze the conversion of the nitrogenous portion of an amino acid to an amino acid residue. It's essential to energy production in the Krebs cycle. AST is found in the cytoplasm and mitochondria of many cells, primarily in the liver, heart, skeletal muscles, kidneys, pancreas, and red blood cells. It's released into serum in proportion to cellular damage.

Although a high correlation exists between myocardial infarction (MI) and elevated AST levels, this test is sometimes considered superfluous for diagnosing an MI because of its relatively low organ specificity; it doesn't allow differentiation between acute MI and the effects of hepatic congestion due to heart failure.

Purpose
- To aid detection and differential diagnosis of acute hepatic disease
- To monitor patient progress and prognosis in cardiac and hepatic diseases
- To aid diagnosis of an MI in correlation with creatine kinase and lactate dehydrogenase levels

Patient preparation
- Explain to the patient that this test is used to assess heart and liver function.
- Inform the patient that the test usually requires three venipunctures (one on admission and one each day for the next 2 days).
- Tell the patient that he need not restrict food and fluids.
- Explain to the patient that he may experience slight discomfort from the needle puncture and the tourniquet.
- Notify the laboratory and physician of medications the patient is taking that may affect test results; they may need to be restricted.

Procedure and posttest care
- Perform a venipuncture and collect the sample in a 4-ml clot-activator tube.
- Apply direct pressure to the venipuncture site until bleeding stops.
- If a hematoma develops at the venipuncture, apply warm soaks.

- Instruct the patient that he may resume medications discontinued before the test, as ordered.

Precautions
- To avoid missing peak AST levels, draw serum samples at the same time each day.
- Handle the sample gently to prevent hemolysis and send it to the laboratory immediately.

Reference values
AST levels range from 8 to 46 U/L (SI, 0.14 to 0.78 µkat/L) in males and from 7 to 34 U/L (SI, 0.12 to 0.5 µkat/L) in females.

 AGE ISSUE *Normal values for infants are typically higher.*

Abnormal findings
AST levels fluctuate in response to the extent of cellular necrosis, being transiently and minimally increased early in the disease process and extremely increased during the most acute phase. Depending on when the initial sample is drawn, AST levels may increase, indicating increasing disease severity and tissue damage, or decrease, indicating disease resolution and tissue repair.

Maximum elevations (more than 20 times normal) may indicate acute viral hepatitis, severe skeletal muscle trauma, extensive surgery, drug-induced hepatic injury, or severe passive liver congestion.

High levels (10 to 20 times normal) may indicate a severe MI, severe infectious mononucleosis, or alcoholic cirrhosis. High levels also occur during the prodromal or resolving stages of conditions that cause maximum elevations.

Moderate to high levels (5 to 10 times normal) may indicate dermatomyositis, Duchenne's muscular dystrophy, or chronic hepatitis. Moderate to high levels also occur during prodromal and resolving stages of diseases that cause high elevations.

Low to moderate levels (2 to 5 times normal) occur at some time during the preceding conditions or diseases or may indicate hemolytic anemia, metastatic hepatic tumors, acute pancreatitis, pulmonary emboli, delirium tremens, or fatty liver. AST levels rise slightly after the first few days of biliary duct obstruction.

Interfering factors

- Hemolysis due to rough handling of the sample
- Failure to draw the sample as scheduled (may miss peak)
- Chlorpropamide, opioids, methyldopa, erythromycin, sulfonamides, pyridoxine, dicumarol, and antitubercular agents; large doses of acetaminophen, salicylates, or vitamin A; and many other drugs known to affect the liver (increase)
- Strenuous exercise and muscle trauma due to I.M. injections (increase)

Alanine aminotransferase

The alanine aminotransferase (ALT) test is used to measure serum levels of ALT, one of two enzymes that catalyze a reversible amino group transfer reaction in the Krebs cycle. ALT is necessary for tissue energy production. It's found primarily in the liver, with lesser amounts in the kidneys, heart, and skeletal muscles, and is a sensitive indicator of acute hepatocellular disease.

When such damage occurs, ALT is released from the cytoplasm into the bloodstream, typically before jaundice appears, resulting in abnormally high serum levels that may not return to normal for days or weeks. This test measures serum ALT levels using the spectrophotometric method.

Purpose

- To detect and evaluate treatment of acute hepatic disease, especially hepatitis and cirrhosis without jaundice
- To distinguish between myocardial and hepatic tissue damage (used with aspartate aminotransferase)
- To assess the hepatotoxicity of some drugs

Patient preparation

- Explain to the patient that this test is used to assess liver function.
- Tell the patient that the test requires a blood sample. Explain who will perform the venipuncture and when.
- Explain to the patient that he may experience slight discomfort from the needle puncture and the tourniquet.
- Inform the patient that he need not restrict food and fluids.
- Notify the laboratory and physician of medications the patient is taking that may affect test results; they may need to be restricted.

Procedure and posttest care

- Perform a venipuncture and collect the sample in a 4-ml tube without additives.
- Apply direct pressure to the venipuncture site until bleeding stops.
- If a hematoma develops at the venipuncture site, apply warm soaks.
- Instruct the patient that he may resume medications discontinued before the test, as ordered.

Precautions

- Handle the sample gently to prevent hemolysis.
- ALT activity is stable in serum for up to 3 days at room temperature.

Reference values

Serum ALT levels range from 8 to 50 IU/L (SI, 0.14 to 0.85 μkat/L).

Abnormal findings

Very high ALT levels (up to 50 times normal) suggest viral or severe drug-induced hepatitis or other hepatic disease with extensive necrosis. Moderate to high levels may indicate infectious mononucleosis, chronic hepatitis, intrahepatic cholestasis or cholecystitis, early or improving acute viral hepatitis, or severe hepatic congestion due to heart failure.

Slight to moderate elevations of ALT may appear in any condition that produces acute hepatocellular injury, such as active cirrhosis and drug-induced or alcoholic hepatitis. Marginal elevations occasionally occur in acute myocardial infarction, reflecting secondary hepatic congestion or the release of small amounts of ALT from myocardial tissue.

Interfering factors

■ Hemolysis due to rough handling of the sample

■ Barbiturates, griseofulvin, isoniazid, nitrofurantoin, methyldopa, phenothiazines, phenytoin, salicylates, tetracycline, chlorpromazine, para-aminosalicylic acid, and other drugs that cause hepatic injury by competitively interfering with cellular metabolism (false-high)

■ Narcotic analgesics, such as morphine, codeine, and meperidine (possible false-high due to increased intrabiliary pressure)

■ Ingestion of lead or exposure to carbon tetrachloride (sharp increase due to direct injury to hepatic cells)

Alkaline phosphatase

The alkaline phosphatase (ALP) test is used to measure serum levels of ALP, an enzyme that influences bone calcification as well as lipid and metabolite transport. ALP measurements reflect the combined activity of several ALP isoenzymes found in the liver, bones, kidneys, intestinal lining, and placenta. Bone and liver ALP are always present in adult serum, with liver ALP most prominent, except during the third trimester of pregnancy (when the placenta originates about half of all ALP). The intestinal variant of ALP can be a normal component (in less than 10% of normal patterns; almost exclusively in the sera of blood groups B and O), or it can be an abnormal finding associated with hepatic disease.

The ALP test is particularly sensitive to mild biliary obstruction and is a primary indicator of space-occupying hepatic lesions. Although skeletal and hepatic diseases can raise ALP levels, this test is most useful for diagnosing metabolic bone disease. Additional liver function studies are usually required to identify hepatobiliary disorders.

Purpose

■ To detect and identify skeletal diseases primarily characterized by marked osteoblastic activity

■ To detect focal hepatic lesions causing biliary obstruction, such as a tumor or an abscess

■ To assess the patient's response to vitamin D in the treatment of rickets

■ To supplement information from other liver function studies and GI enzyme tests

Patient preparation

■ Explain to the patient that this test is used to assess liver and bone function.

■ Instruct the patient to fast for at least 8 hours before the test because fat intake stimulates intestinal ALP secretion.
■ Tell the patient that this test requires a blood sample. Explain who will perform the venipuncture and when.
■ Inform the patient that he may experience slight discomfort from the needle puncture and the tourniquet.

Procedure and posttest care
■ Perform a venipuncture and collect the sample in a 4-ml clot-activator tube.
■ Apply direct pressure to the venipuncture site until bleeding stops.
■ If a hematoma develops at the venipuncture site, apply warm soaks.
■ Instruct the patient that he may resume his usual diet.

Precautions
■ Handle the sample gently to prevent hemolysis.
■ Send the sample to the laboratory immediately; ALP activity increases at room temperature because of a rise in pH.

Reference values
Total ALP levels normally range from 30 to 85 IU/ml (SI, 42 to 128 U/L).

Abnormal findings
Although significant ALP elevations are possible with diseases that affect many organs, they usually indicate skeletal disease or extrahepatic or intrahepatic biliary obstruction causing cholestasis. Many acute hepatic diseases cause ALP elevations before they affect serum bilirubin levels.

Moderate increases in ALP levels may reflect acute biliary obstruction from hepatocellular inflammation in active cirrhosis, mononucleosis, and viral hepatitis. Moderate increases are also seen in osteomalacia and deficiency-induced rickets.

Sharp elevations in ALP levels may indicate complete biliary obstruction by malignant or infectious infiltrations or fibrosis, most common in Paget's disease and, occasionally, in biliary obstruction, extensive bone metastasis, and hyperparathyroidism. Metastatic bone tumors resulting from pancreatic cancer raise ALP levels without a concomitant rise in serum alanine aminotransferase levels.

Isoenzyme fractionation and additional enzyme tests (gamma glutamyl transferase, lactate dehydrogenase, 5′-nucleotidase, and leucine aminopeptidase) are sometimes performed when the cause of ALP elevations is in doubt. Rarely, low levels of serum ALP are associated with hypophosphatasia and protein or magnesium deficiency.

Interfering factors
■ Hemolysis due to rough handling of the sample
■ Failure to analyze the sample within 4 hours
■ Recent ingestion of vitamin D (possible increase due to the effect on osteoblastic activity)
■ Recent infusion of albumin prepared from placental venous blood (marked increase)
■ Drugs that influence liver function or cause cholestasis, such as barbiturates, chlorpropamide, hormonal contraceptives, isoniazid, methyldopa, phenothiazines, phenytoin, and rifampin (possible mild increase)
■ Halothane sensitivity (possible drastic increase)
■ Clofibrate (decrease)
■ Healing long-bone fractures and the third trimester of pregnancy (possible increase)

- Age and sex (increase in infants, children, adolescents, and individuals over age 45)

Leucine aminopeptidase

The leucine aminopeptidase (LAP) test is used to measure serum levels of LAP, an isoenzyme of alkaline phosphatase (ALP) that's widely distributed in body tissues. The greatest concentrations appear in the hepatobiliary tissues, pancreas, and small intestine. Serum LAP levels parallel serum ALP levels in hepatic disease.

Purpose
- To provide information about suspected liver, pancreatic, and biliary diseases
- To differentiate skeletal disease from hepatobiliary or pancreatic disease
- To evaluate neonatal jaundice

Patient preparation
- Explain to the patient that this test is used to evaluate liver and pancreatic function.
- Tell the patient that the test requires a blood sample. Explain who will perform the venipuncture and when.
- Explain to the patient that he may experience slight discomfort from the needle puncture and the tourniquet.
- Tell the patient to fast for at least 8 hours before the test.
- Notify the laboratory and physician of medications the patient is taking that may affect test results; they may need to be restricted.

Procedure and posttest care
- Perform a venipuncture and collect the sample in a 4-ml clot-activator tube.
- Apply direct pressure to the venipuncture site until bleeding stops.

- Instruct the patient that he may resume his usual diet and medications discontinued before the test, as ordered.

Precautions
- Handle the sample gently to avoid hemolysis.
- Transport the sample to the laboratory immediately.

Reference values
Normal values are 80 to 200 U/ml (SI, 80 to 200 kU/L) in men and 75 to 185 U/ml (SI, 75 to 185 kU/L) in women.

Abnormal findings
Elevated levels can occur in biliary obstruction, tumors, strictures, and atresia; advanced pregnancy; and therapy with drugs containing estrogen or progesterone.

Interfering factors
- Advanced pregnancy (false-high)
- Estrogen or progesterone (false-high)

Gamma glutamyl transferase

Also called *gamma glutamyl transpeptidase,* gamma glutamyl transferase (GGT) participates in the transfer of amino acids across cellular membranes and, possibly, in glutathione metabolism. The highest concentrations of GGT exist in the renal tubules, but the enzyme also appears in the liver, biliary tract, epithelium, pancreas, lymphocytes, brain, and testes. The GGT test is used to measure serum GGT levels.

Because GGT isn't elevated in bone growth or pregnancy, this test is a somewhat more sensitive indicator of hepatic necrosis than the aspartate aminotransferase assay and is as sensitive as or more sensitive than the alkaline phosphatase (ALP) assay. However, the test is nonspecific, providing little data about the type of hepatic disease, because increased levels also occur in renal, cardiac, and prostatic disease and with the use of certain medications. GGT is particularly sensitive to the effects of alcohol on the liver, and levels may be elevated after moderate alcohol intake and in chronic alcoholism, even without clinical evidence of hepatic injury.

Purpose
■ To provide information about hepatobiliary diseases, to assess liver function, and to detect alcohol ingestion
■ To distinguish between skeletal and hepatic disease when the serum ALP level is elevated (A normal GGT level suggests that such elevation stems from skeletal disease.)

Patient preparation
■ Explain to the patient that this test is used to evaluate liver function.
■ Tell the patient that the test requires a blood sample. Explain who will perform the venipuncture and when.
■ Explain to the patient that he may experience slight discomfort from the needle puncture and the tourniquet.
■ Inform the patient that he need not restrict food and fluids.

Procedure and posttest care
■ Perform a venipuncture and collect the sample in a 4-ml tube without additives.
■ Apply direct pressure to the venipuncture site until bleeding stops.
■ If a hematoma develops at the venipuncture site, apply warm soaks.

Precautions
■ Handle the sample gently to prevent hemolysis.
■ GGT activity is stable in serum at room temperature for 2 days.

Reference values
Normal serum GTT levels range as follows:
■ children: 3 to 30 U/L (SI, 0.05 to 0.51 µkat/L)
■ males: age 16 and older, 6 to 38 U/L (SI, 0.10 to 0.63 µkat/L)
■ females: ages 16 to 45, 4 to 27 U/L (SI, 0.08 to 0.46 µKat/L); age 45 and older, 6 to 37 U/L (SI, 0.10 to 0.63 µkat/L).

Abnormal findings
Serum GGT levels rise in acute hepatic disease because enzyme production increases in response to hepatocellular injury. Moderate increases occur in acute pancreatitis, renal disease, and prostatic metastases; postoperatively; and in some patients with epilepsy or brain tumors. Levels also increase after alcohol ingestion because of enzyme induction. The sharpest elevations occur in patients with obstructive jaundice and hepatic metastatic infiltrations.

GGT levels may also increase 5 to 10 days after acute myocardial infarction, either as a result of tissue granulation and healing or as an indication of the effects of cardiac insufficiency on the liver.

Interfering factors
■ Hemolysis due to rough handling of the sample
■ Clofibrate and hormonal contraceptives (decrease)
■ Aminoglycosides, barbiturates, phenytoin glutethimide, and methaqualone (increase)

- Moderate alcohol intake (increase for at least 60 hours)

5′-nucleotidase

The enzyme 5′-nucleotidase (5′NT) is a phosphatase formed almost entirely in the hepatobiliary tract. Unlike alkaline phosphatase (ALP), it hydrolyzes nucleoside 5′-phosphate groups only. Measurement of serum 5′NT levels helps to determine whether ALP elevation is due to skeletal or hepatic disease. Because 5′NT remains normal in skeletal disease and pregnancy, it's more specific for assessing hepatic dysfunction than ALP or leucine aminopeptidase.

This test, which measures serum 5′NT levels, is technically more difficult than the ALP assay. It hasn't been widely used as a liver function study, although some authorities consider it more sensitive than ALP to diagnose cholangitis, biliary cirrhosis, and malignant infiltrations of the liver. However, 5′NT is most commonly used to determine whether ALP elevation is due to skeletal or hepatic disease.

Purpose
- To distinguish between hepatobiliary and skeletal disease when the source of increased ALP levels is uncertain
- To help differentiate biliary obstruction from acute hepatocellular damage
- To detect hepatic metastasis in the absence of jaundice

Patient preparation
- Explain to the patient that this test is used to evaluate liver function.
- Tell the patient that the test requires a blood sample. Explain who will perform the venipuncture and when.

- Explain to the patient that he may experience slight discomfort from the needle puncture and the tourniquet.
- Tell the patient that he need not restrict food and fluids.

Procedure and posttest care
- Perform a venipuncture and collect the sample in a 4-ml tube without additives.
- Apply direct pressure to the venipuncture site until bleeding stops.
- If a hematoma develops at the venipuncture site, apply warm soaks.

Precautions
- Handle the sample gently to prevent hemolysis.

Reference values
Serum 5′NT values for adults range from 2 to 17 U/L (SI, 0.03 to 0.29 μkat/L); values for children may be lower.

Abnormal findings
Extremely high levels of 5′NT occur in common bile duct obstruction by calculi or tumors in diseases that cause severe intrahepatic cholestasis such as neoplastic infiltrations of the liver. Slight to moderate increases may reflect acute hepatocellular damage or active cirrhosis.

Interfering factors
- Hemolysis due to rough handling of the sample
- Cholestatic drugs, such as phenothiazines, morphine, meperidine, and codeine as well as aspirin, acetaminophen, and phenytoin (increase)

PANCREATIC ENZYME TESTS

Serum amylase

An enzyme that's synthesized primarily in the pancreas and salivary glands and is secreted in the GI tract, amylase (alpha-amylase or AML) helps to digest starch and glycogen in the mouth, stomach, and intestine. In cases of suspected acute pancreatic disease, measurement of serum or urine AML is the most important laboratory test.

Purpose
- To diagnose acute pancreatitis
- To distinguish between acute pancreatitis and other causes of abdominal pain that require immediate surgery
- To evaluate possible pancreatic injury caused by abdominal trauma or surgery

Patient preparation
- Explain to the patient that this test is used to assess pancreatic function.
- Tell the patient that this test requires a blood sample. Explain who will perform the venipuncture and when.
- Inform the patient that he may experience slight discomfort from the needle puncture and the tourniquet.
- Inform the patient that he need not fast before the test, but must abstain from alcohol.
- Notify the laboratory and physician of medications the patient is taking that may affect test results; they may need to be restricted.

Procedure and posttest care
- Perform a venipuncture and collect the sample in a 4-ml clot-activator tube.
- Apply direct pressure to the venipuncture site until bleeding stops.
- If a hematoma develops at the venipuncture site, apply warm soaks.
- Instruct the patient that he may resume medications discontinued before the test, as ordered.

Precautions
- If the patient has severe abdominal pain, draw the sample before diagnostic or therapeutic intervention. For accurate results, it's important to obtain an early sample.
- Handle the sample gently to prevent hemolysis.

Reference values
Normal serum amylase levels range from 25 to 85 U/L (SI, 0.39 to 1.45 µkat/L) for adults age 18 and older.

Abnormal findings
After the onset of acute pancreatitis, AML levels begin to rise within 2 hours, peak within 12 to 48 hours, and return to normal within 3 to 4 days. Determination of urine levels should follow normal serum AML results to rule out pancreatitis. Moderate serum elevations may accompany obstruction of the common bile duct, pancreatic duct, or ampulla of Vater; pancreatic injury from a perforated peptic ulcer; pancreatic cancer; and acute salivary gland disease. Impaired kidney function may increase serum levels.

Levels may be slightly elevated in a patient who's asymptomatic or responding unusually to therapy.

Decreased levels can occur in chronic pancreatitis, pancreatic cancer, cirrhosis, hepatitis, and toxemia of pregnancy.

Interfering factors
- Hemolysis due to rough handling of the sample

- Ingestion of ethyl alcohol in large amounts (possible false-high)
- Aminosalicylic acid, asparaginase, azathioprine, corticosteroids, cyproheptadine, narcotic analgesics, hormonal contraceptives, rifampin, sulfasalazine, and thiazide or loop diuretics (possible false-high)
- Recent peripancreatic surgery, perforated ulcer or intestine, abscess, spasm of the sphincter of Oddi or, rarely, macroamylasemia (possible false-high) (See *Understanding macroamylasemia*.)

Serum lipase

Lipase is produced in the pancreas and secreted into the duodenum, where it converts triglycerides and other fats into fatty acids and glycerol. The destruction of pancreatic cells, which occurs in acute pancreatitis, causes large amounts of lipase to be released into the blood. (See *Blocked enzyme pathway*, page 114.) The lipase test is used to measure serum lipase levels; it's most useful when performed with a serum or urine amylase test.

Purpose
- To aid diagnosis of acute pancreatitis

Patient preparation
- Explain to the patient that this test is used to evaluate pancreatic function.
- Tell the patient that the test requires a blood sample. Explain who will perform the venipuncture and when.
- Inform the patient that he may experience slight discomfort from the needle puncture and the tourniquet.
- Instruct the patient to fast overnight before the test.
- Notify the laboratory of medications the patient is taking that may affect test results; they may need to be restricted.

> **UNDERSTANDING MACROAMYLASEMIA**
>
> An uncommon, benign condition, macroamylasemia doesn't cause any symptoms, but it occasionally causes elevated serum amylase (AML) levels. This condition occurs when macroamylase — a complex of AML and an immunoglobulin or other protein — is present in a patient's serum.
>
> A typical patient with macroamylasemia has an elevated serum AML level and a normal or slightly decreased urine AML level. This characteristic pattern helps differentiate macroamylasemia from conditions in which serum and urine AML levels rise such as pancreatitis. But it doesn't differentiate macroamylasemia from hyperamylasemia due to impaired renal function, which may raise serum AML levels and lower urine AML levels. Chromatographic, ultracentrifugation, or precipitation tests are necessary to detect macroamylase in serum and definitively confirm macroamylasemia.

Procedure and posttest care
- Perform a venipuncture and collect the sample in a 4-ml clot-activator tube.
- Apply direct pressure to the venipuncture site until bleeding stops.
- If a hematoma develops at the venipuncture site, apply warm soaks.
- Instruct the patient that he may resume his usual diet and medications discontinued before the test, as ordered.

Precautions
- Handle the sample gently to prevent hemolysis.

BLOCKED ENZYME PATHWAY

The pancreas secretes lipase, amylase, and other enzymes that pass through the pancreatic duct into the duodenum. In pancreatitis and obstruction of the pancreatic duct by a tumor or calculus (shown below), these enzymes can't reach their intended destination. Instead, they're diverted into the bloodstream by a mechanism that's not fully understood.

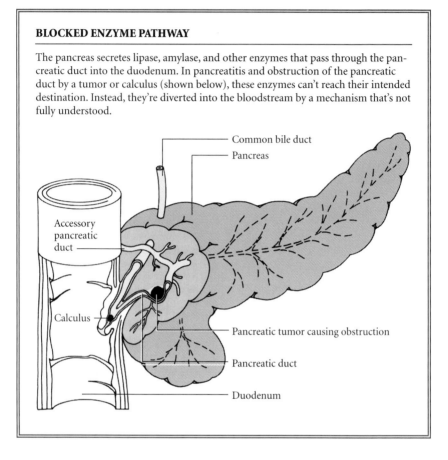

Reference values

Serum lipase levels are normally < 160 U/L (SI, < 2.72 μkat/L).

Abnormal findings

High lipase levels suggest acute pancreatitis or pancreatic duct obstruction. After an acute attack, levels remain elevated for up to 14 days. Lipase levels may also increase in other pancreatic injuries, such as perforated peptic ulcer with chemical pancreatitis due to gastric juices, and in a patient with high intestinal obstruction, pancreatic cancer, or renal disease with impaired excretion.

Interfering factors

■ Hemolysis due to rough handling of the sample

■ Cholinergics, codeine, meperidine, and morphine (false-high due to spasm of the sphincter of Oddi)

SPECIAL ENZYME TESTS

Acid phosphatase

Acid phosphatase — a group of phosphatase enzymes most active at a pH of about 5.0 — is found primarily in the prostate gland and semen and, to a lesser extent, in the liver, spleen, red blood cells, bone marrow, and platelets. The acid phosphatase test is used to measure total acid phosphatase and the prostatic fraction in serum.

Prostatic and erythrocytic enzymes are this group's two major isoenzymes, which can be separated in the laboratory. The prostatic isoenzyme is more specific for prostate cancer.

The more widespread the cancer is, the more likely that serum acid phosphatase levels will be increased.

Purpose

- To detect prostate cancer
- To monitor the patient's response to therapy for prostate cancer (successful treatment decreases acid phosphatase levels)

Patient preparation

- Explain to the patient that this test is used to evaluate prostate function.
- Tell the patient that the test requires a blood sample. Explain who will perform the venipuncture and when.
- Explain to the patient that he may experience slight discomfort from the needle puncture and the tourniquet.
- Inform the patient that he need not restrict food and fluids.
- Notify the laboratory and physician of medications the patient is taking that may affect test results; they may need to be restricted.

Procedure and posttest care

- Perform a venipuncture and collect the sample in a 4-ml tube without additives.
- Apply direct pressure to the venipuncture site until bleeding stops.

- If a hematoma develops at the venipuncture site, apply warm soaks.
- Instruct the patient that he may resume medications discontinued before the test, as ordered.

Precautions

- Don't draw the sample within 48 hours of prostate manipulation (rectal examination).
- Handle the sample gently to prevent hemolysis.
- Send the sample to the laboratory immediately. Acid phosphatase levels decrease by 50% within 1 hour if the sample remains at room temperature without a preservative or if it isn't packed in ice.

Reference values

Serum values for total acid phosphatase depend on the assay method and range from 0 to 3.7 U/L (SI, 0 to 3.7 U/L).

Abnormal findings

High prostatic acid phosphatase levels generally indicate the presence of a tumor that has spread beyond the prostatic capsule. If the tumor has metastasized to bone, high acid phosphatase levels are accompanied by high alkaline phosphatase (ALP) levels, reflecting increased osteoblastic activity.

Acid phosphatase levels rise moderately in prostatic infarction, Paget's disease (some cases), Gaucher's disease and, occasionally, other conditions such as multiple myeloma. False results may occur if ALP levels are high because acid phosphatase and ALP are similar, differing mainly in their optimum pH ranges.

Interfering factors

- Hemolysis due to rough handling of the sample or improper sample storage

- Delayed delivery of the sample to the laboratory (possible false-low or false-normal)
- Fluorides, phosphates, and oxalates (possible false-low)
- Clofibrate (possible false-high)
- Prostate massage, catheterization, or rectal examination within 48 hours of the test

Prostate-specific antigen

Until recently, digital rectal examination and measurement of prostatic acid phosphatase were the primary methods of monitoring the progression of prostate cancer. Now measurement of prostate-specific antigen (PSA) helps track the course of this disease and evaluate the patient's response to treatment.

PSA appears in normal, benign hyperplastic, and malignant prostatic tissue as well as metastatic prostatic carcinoma. Serum PSA levels are used to monitor the spread or recurrence of prostate cancer and to evaluate the patient's response to treatment. Measurement of serum PSA levels along with a digital rectal examination is now recommended as a screening test for prostate cancer in men over age 50. (See *Controversy over PSA screening.*) It's also useful in assessing response to treatment in a patient with stage B3 to D1 prostate cancer and in detecting tumor spread or recurrence.

Purpose

- To screen for prostate cancer in men over age 50
- To monitor prostate cancer's course and evaluate treatment

Patient preparation

- Explain to the patient that this test is used to screen for prostate cancer or, if

appropriate, to monitor the course of treatment.
- Tell the patient that the test requires a blood sample. Explain who will perform the venipuncture and when.
- Explain to the patient that he may experience slight discomfort from the needle puncture and the tourniquet.
- Inform the patient that he need not restrict food and fluids.

Procedure and posttest care

- Perform a venipuncture and collect the sample in a 7-ml clot-activator tube.
- Apply direct pressure to the venipuncture site until bleeding stops.
- If a hematoma develops at the venipuncture site, apply warm soaks.

Precautions

- Collect the sample either before digital prostate examination or at least 48 hours after examination to avoid falsely elevated PSA levels.
- Handle the sample gently to prevent hemolysis.
- Immediately put the sample on ice and send it to the laboratory.

Reference values

AGE ISSUE *Normal values are as follows:*
- *ages 40 to 50: 2 to 2.8 ng/ml (SI, 2 to 2.8 µg/L)*
- *ages 51 to 60: 2.9 to 3.8 ng/ml (SI, 2.9 to 3.8 µg/L)*
- *ages 61 to 70: 4 to 5.3 ng/ml (SI, 4 to 5.3 µg/L)*
- *ages 71 and older: 5.6 to 7.2 ng/ml (SI, 5.6 to 7.2 µg/L).*

Abnormal findings

About 80% of patients with prostate cancer have pretreatment PSA values greater than 4 ng/ml. However, PSA results alone

CONTROVERSY OVER PSA SCREENING

Measurement of prostate-specific antigen (PSA) allows earlier detection of prostate cancer than digital rectal examination (DRE) alone. Accordingly, the American Cancer Society and the American Urological Association currently recommend that PSA screening begin at age 40 (in combination with DRE) in black men and any man who has a father or brother with prostate cancer, and at age 50 in all other men.

But does this test actually reduce mortality from prostate cancer? The answer to that question remains unknown. Some specialists question the value of all prostate cancer screening tests because of the costs involved, the uncertain benefits, and the known risks associated with current treatments.

Before undergoing a PSA test, the patient should understand that controversy surrounds nearly every aspect of prostate cancer screening and treatment. Among the issues he'll face may include:
■ Even if cancer is detected, treatment may not be advisable, either because of the patient's advanced age or because the physician believes the tumor is so slow-growing that it won't result in death.

■ The current treatments for prostate cancer—surgery and radiation therapy—may not be as effective as experts formerly believed, and no effective chemotherapy protocol is currently available.
■ Surgery and radiation therapy carry a high risk of impotence, incontinence, and other problems, which the patient must weigh against the uncertain benefits of therapy.
■ Screening tests sometimes yield false-positive results, requiring transrectal ultrasonography or a biopsy to confirm the diagnosis.
■ A mildly elevated PSA level may be the result of normal age-related increases. (Data from a study of more than 9,000 men showed that PSA levels increase about 30% per year in men under age 70 and more than 40% per year in men over age 70.)

In summary, the value of prostate cancer screening in general and PSA testing in particular won't be clearly established until studies show a definitive link between early treatment and reduced mortality.

don't confirm a diagnosis of prostate cancer. About 20% of patients with benign prostatic hyperplasia also have levels greater than 4 ng/ml. Further assessment and testing, including tissue biopsy, are needed to confirm cancer.

Interfering factors
■ Hemolysis due to rough handling of the sample
■ Excessive doses of chemotherapeutic drugs, such as cyclophosphamide, di-

ethylstilbestrol, and methotrexate (possible increase or decrease)

Plasma renin activity

Renin secretion from the kidneys is the first stage of the renin-angiotensin-aldosterone cycle, which controls the body's sodium-potassium balance, fluid volume, and blood pressure. Renin is released into the renal veins in response to sodium depletion and blood loss. It catalyzes the conversion of angiotensinogen, an alpha$_2$-globulin plasma protein, to angiotensin I, which in turn is converted by hydrolysis into angiotensin II, a vasoconstrictor that stimulates aldosterone production in the adrenal cortex. (See *Renin-angiotensin feedback system.*) When present in excessive amounts, angiotensin II causes renal hypertension.

The plasma renin activity (PRA) test is a screening procedure for renovascular hypertension, but doesn't unequivocally confirm it. When supplemented by other special tests, the PRA test can help establish the cause of hypertension. For instance, sampling blood obtained from the renal veins by renal vein catheterization and analyzing the renal venous renin ratio can identify renovascular disorders. Indexing renin levels against urinary sodium excretion can help identify primary aldosteronism. A sodium-depleted PRA test can then confirm this.

Some experts believe that the type of treatment chosen for essential hypertension should depend on whether renin levels are low, normal, or high; the PRA test can categorize the disease to allow for appropriate therapy.

PRA is measured by radioimmunoassay of a peripheral or renal blood sample; results are expressed as the rate of angiotensin I formation per unit of time. Patient preparation is crucial and may take up to 1 month.

Purpose
- To screen for renal origin of hypertension
- To help plan treatment of essential hypertension, a genetic disease commonly aggravated by excess sodium intake
- To help identify hypertension linked to unilateral (sometimes bilateral) renovascular disease by renal vein catheterization
- To help identify primary aldosteronism (Conn's syndrome) resulting from an aldosterone-secreting adrenal adenoma
- To confirm primary aldosteronism (sodium-depleted plasma renin test)

Patient preparation
- Explain to the patient that this test is used to determine the cause of hypertension.
- Notify the laboratory and physician of medications the patient is taking that may affect test results; they may need to be restricted.
- Tell the patient to maintain a normal sodium diet (3 g/day) during this period.
- For the sodium-depleted plasma renin test, tell the patient that he'll receive furosemide (or, if he has angina or cerebrovascular insufficiency, chlorthiazide) and will follow a specific low-sodium diet for 3 days.
- The patient shouldn't receive radioactive treatments for several days before the test.
- Tell the patient that the test requires a blood sample. Explain who will perform the venipuncture and when.
- Explain to the patient that he may experience slight discomfort from the needle puncture and the tourniquet. Collect a morning sample, if possible.
- If a recumbent sample is ordered, instruct the patient to remain in bed at least 2 hours before the sample is obtained. (Posture influences renin secretion.) If an upright sample is ordered, instruct him to stand or sit upright for 2 hours before the test is performed.
- If renal vein catheterization is ordered, make sure the patient has signed an informed consent form. Tell the patient that the procedure will be done in the X-ray department and that he'll receive a local anesthetic.

RENIN-ANGIOTENSIN FEEDBACK SYSTEM

The renin-angiotensin-aldosterone system, sometimes known as the juxtaglomerular apparatus, is an important homeostatic device for regulating the body's sodium and water levels and blood pressure. It works this way:

Juxtaglomerular cells (1) in each of the kidney's glomeruli secrete the enzyme renin into the blood. The rate of renin secretion depends on the rate of perfusion in the afferent renal arterioles (2) and on the amount of sodium in the serum. A low sodium load and low perfusion pressure (as in hypovolemia) increase renin secretion; high sodium and high perfusion pressure decrease it.

Renin circulates throughout the body. In the liver, renin converts angiotensino-gen to angiotensin I (3), which passes to the lungs. There it's converted by hydrolysis to angiotensin II (4), a potent vasoconstrictor that acts on the adrenal cortex to stimulate production of the hormone aldosterone (5). Aldosterone acts on the juxtaglomerular cells to stimulate or depress renin secretion, completing the feedback cycle that automatically readjusts homeostasis.

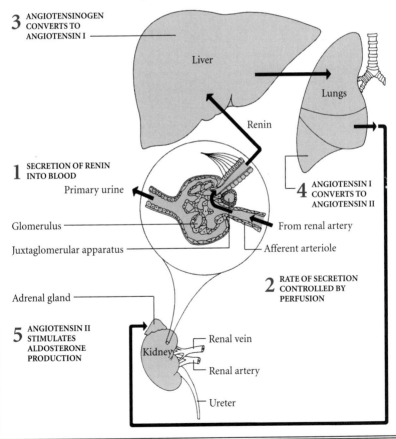

3 ANGIOTENSINOGEN CONVERTS TO ANGIOTENSIN I

Liver

Lungs

Renin

1 SECRETION OF RENIN INTO BLOOD

Primary urine

Glomerulus

Juxtaglomerular apparatus

4 ANGIOTENSIN I CONVERTS TO ANGIOTENSIN II

From renal artery

Afferent arteriole

2 RATE OF SECRETION CONTROLLED BY PERFUSION

Adrenal gland

5 ANGIOTENSIN II STIMULATES ALDOSTERONE PRODUCTION

Kidney

Renal vein

Renal artery

Ureter

Procedure and posttest care
Peripheral vein sample
- Perform a venipuncture and collect the sample in a 4-ml EDTA tube.
- Note on the laboratory request if the patient was fasting and whether he was upright or supine during sample collection.
- Apply direct pressure to the venipuncture site until bleeding stops.
- If a hematoma develops at the venipuncture site, apply warm soaks.

Renal vein catheterization
- A catheter is advanced to the kidneys through the femoral vein under fluoroscopic control and samples are obtained from the renal veins and vena cava.
- After renal vein catheterization, apply pressure to the catheterization site for 10 to 20 minutes to prevent extravasation.
- Monitor vital signs and check the catheterization site every 30 minutes for 2 hours and then every hour for 4 hours to ensure that the bleeding has stopped. Check the patient's distal pulse for signs of thrombus formation and arterial occlusion (cyanosis, loss of pulse, cool skin).

Both methods
- Instruct the patient that he may resume his usual diet and medications discontinued before the test, as ordered.

Precautions
- Because renin is unstable, the sample must be drawn into a chilled syringe and collection tube, placed on ice, and sent to the laboratory immediately.
- Completely fill the collection tube and invert it gently several times to mix the sample and the anticoagulant.

Reference values
✱ AGE ISSUE *Plasma renin activity and aldosterone levels decrease with age.*
- *Sodium-depleted, upright, peripheral vein: For ages 18 to 39, the range is 2.9 to 24 ng/ml/hour; mean, 10.8 ng/ml/hour. For age 40 and over, the range is 2.9 to 10.8 ng/ml/hour; mean, 5.9 ng/ml/hour.*
- *Sodium-replete, upright, peripheral vein: For ages 18 to 39, the range is less than or equal to 0.6 to 4.3 ng/ml/hour; mean, 1.9 ng/ml/hour. For age 40 and over, the range is less than or equal to 0.6 to 3.0 ng/ml/hour; mean, 1 ng/ml/hour.*
- *Renal vein catheterization: The renal venous renin ratio (the renin level in the renal vein compared to the level in the inferior vena cava) is less than 1.5 to 1.*

Abnormal findings
Elevated renin levels may occur in essential hypertension (uncommon), malignant and renovascular hypertension, cirrhosis, hypokalemia, hypovolemia due to hemorrhage, renin-producing renal tumors (Bartter's syndrome), and adrenal hypofunction (Addison's disease). High renin levels may also be found in chronic renal failure with parenchymal disease, end-stage renal disease, and transplant rejection.

Decreased renin levels may indicate hypervolemia due to a high-sodium diet, salt-retaining steroids, primary aldosteronism, Cushing's syndrome, licorice ingestion syndrome, or essential hypertension with low renin levels.

High serum and urine aldosterone levels with low plasma renin activity help identify primary aldosteronism. In the sodium-depleted renin test, low plasma renin confirms this and differentiates it from secondary aldosteronism (characterized by increased renin).

ROLE OF ACETYLCHOLINESTERASE IN NERVE IMPULSE TRANSMISSION

Each time a nerve impulse arrives at the neuromuscular junction (between a myelinated nerve fiber and a skeletal muscle fiber), the nerve terminals release about 300 vesicles (bubbles) of acetylcholine into the synaptic clefts. Then acetylcholinesterase (one component of cholinesterase) inactivates acetylcholine by hydrolyzing it to acetate and choline. This action is necessary to allow the muscle fiber to recover between excitation by acetylcholine. Without acetylcholinesterase, muscle excitation would be continuous.

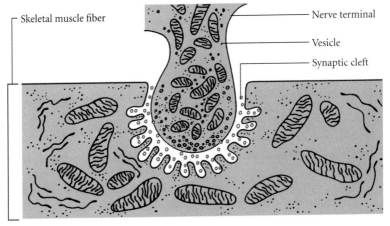

Adapted with permission from Fawcett, D. *Textbook of Histology*, 12th ed. New York: Chapman & Hall, 1994.

Interfering factors

- Failure to observe pretest restrictions
- Improper patient position
- Failure to use the proper anticoagulant in the collection tube, to completely fill it, or to adequately mix the sample and the anticoagulant (EDTA helps preserve angiotensin I; heparin doesn't.)
- Failure to chill the collection tube, syringe, and sample or to send the sample to the laboratory immediately
- Salt intake, severe blood loss, licorice ingestion, hormonal contraceptives, pregnancy, and therapy with diuretics, antihypertensives, or vasodilators (increase)
- Salt-retaining corticosteroid therapy and antidiuretic therapy (decrease)
- Radioisotope use within several days before the test

Cholinesterase

The cholinesterase test is used to measure the amounts of two similar enzymes that hydrolyze acetylcholine: acetylcholinesterase and pseudocholinesterase. Acetylcholinesterase is present in nerve tissue, red cells of the spleen, and the gray matter of the brain. It inactivates acetylcholine at nerve junctions and helps transmit impulses across nerve endings to muscle fibers. (See *Role of acetylcholinesterase in nerve impulse transmission*.)

Pseudocholinesterase is produced primarily in the liver and appears in small amounts in the pancreas, intestines, heart, and white matter of the brain. Although pseudocholinesterase has no known function, its measurement is significant because certain chemicals that inactivate acetylcholinesterase also affect pseudocholinesterase.

Two groups of anticholinesterase chemicals — organophosphates and muscle relaxants — are important. Organophosphates, which are used by the military as nerve gases and are common ingredients in many insecticides, inactivate acetylcholinesterase directly. Muscle relaxants (such as succinylcholine), which interfere with acetylcholine-mediated transmission across nerve endings, are normally destroyed by pseudocholinesterase.

When poisoning by an organophosphate is suspected, either cholinesterase may be measured. For technical reasons, pseudocholinesterase is generally tested, although this analysis is less sensitive than for acetylcholinesterase.

In suspected poisoning by muscle relaxants, the patient lacks adequate pseudocholinesterase, which usually inactivates the muscle relaxant. In this case, measurement of pseudocholinesterase is required.

Purpose
- To evaluate before surgery or electroconvulsive therapy the patient's potential response to succinylcholine, which is hydrolyzed by cholinesterase
- To screen for adverse reactions to muscle relaxants
- To assess overexposure to insecticides containing organophosphate compounds
- To assess liver function and aid diagnosis of hepatic disease (a rare purpose)

Patient preparation
- Explain to the patient that this test is used to assess muscle function or the extent of poisoning.
- Tell the patient that the test requires a blood sample. Explain who will perform the venipuncture and when.
- Explain to the patient that he may experience slight discomfort from the needle puncture and the tourniquet.
- Inform the patient that he need not restrict food and fluids.
- Notify the laboratory and physician of medications the patient is taking that may affect test results; they may need to be restricted.

Procedure and posttest care
- Perform a venipuncture and collect the sample in a 7-ml clot-activator tube.
- Apply direct pressure to the venipuncture site until bleeding stops.
- If a hematoma develops at the venipuncture site, apply warm soaks.
- Instruct the patient that he may resume medications discontinued before the test, as ordered.

Precautions
- Handle the sample gently to prevent hemolysis.
- If the sample can't be sent to the laboratory within 6 hours after being drawn, refrigerate it.

Reference values
Pseudocholinesterase levels range from 204 to 532 IU/dl (SI, 2.04 to 5.32 kU/L).

Abnormal findings
Severely decreased pseudocholinesterase levels suggest a congenital deficiency or organophosphate insecticide poisoning; levels near zero necessitate emergency treatment.

Pseudocholinesterase levels are usually normal in early extrahepatic obstruction and variably decreased in hepatocellular diseases, such as hepatitis and cirrhosis (especially cirrhosis with ascites and jaundice). Levels also drop in acute infections, chronic malnutrition, anemia, myocardial infarction, obstructive jaundice, and metastasis.

Interfering factors
- Hemolysis due to rough handling of the sample
- Pregnancy or recent surgery
- Cyclophosphamide, echothiophate iodide, monoamine oxidase inhibitors, succinylcholine, neostigmine, quinine, quinidine, chloroquine, caffeine, theophylline, epinephrine, ether, barbiturates, atropine, morphine, codeine, phenothiazines, vitamin K, and folic acid (possible false-low)

Glucose-6-phosphate dehydrogenase

An enzyme found in most body cells, glucose-6-phosphate dehydrogenase (G6PD) is involved in metabolizing glucose. The G6PD test is used to detect G6PD deficiency, a hereditary, sex-linked condition that impairs stability of the red cell membrane and allows red cells to be destroyed by strong oxidizing agents.

Red cell enzyme levels normally decrease as cells age, but G6PD deficiency accelerates this process, making older red cells more prone to destruction than younger ones. In mild deficiency, young red cells retain enough G6PD to survive; in severe deficiency, all red cells are destroyed.

About 10% of Black males in the United States inherit a mild G6PD deficiency; some people of Mediterranean origin inherit a severe deficiency. In some White individuals, fava beans may produce hemolytic episodes. Although a deficiency of G6PD provides partial immunity to falciparum malaria, it precipitates an adverse reaction to antimalarials.

Purpose
- To detect hemolytic anemia caused by G6PD deficiency
- To aid differential diagnosis of hemolytic anemia

Patient preparation
- Explain to the patient that this test is used to detect an inherited enzyme deficiency that may affect red blood cells.
- Tell the patient that the test requires a blood sample. Explain who will perform the venipuncture and when.
- Explain to the patient that he may experience slight discomfort from the needle puncture and the tourniquet.
- Inform the patient that he need not restrict food and fluids.
- Check the patient's history and report recent blood transfusion or ingestion of aspirin, sulfonamides, phenacetin, nitrofurantoin, vitamin K derivatives, antimalarials, or fava beans, which cause hemolysis in someone who's G6PD-deficient.

Procedure and posttest care
- Perform a venipuncture and collect the sample in a 4-ml EDTA tube.
- Apply direct pressure to the venipuncture site until bleeding stops.
- If a hematoma develops at the venipuncture site, apply warm soaks.

Precautions
- Completely fill the collection tube and invert it gently several times to mix the sample and the anticoagulant.

- Handle the sample gently to prevent hemolysis.
- Refrigerate the sample if you can't send it to the laboratory immediately.

Reference values
Serum G6PD values vary with the measurement method used, but usually range from 4.3 to 11.8 U/G (SI, 0.28 to 0.76 mU/mol) of hemoglobin.

Abnormal findings
Fluorescent spot testing or staining for Heinz bodies or erythrocytes can test for G6PD deficiency. If results are positive, the kinetic quantitative assay for G6PD may be performed. Electrophoretic techniques assess genetic variants of deficiencies (which may cause lifelong, mild, or asymptomatic anemia). Some variants are symptomatic only when the patient experiences stress or illness or has been exposed to drugs or agents that elicit hemolytic episodes.

Interfering factors
- Performing the test after a hemolytic episode or a blood transfusion (possible false-negative)
- Failure to use the proper anticoagulant or to adequately mix the sample and the anticoagulant
- Hemolysis due to rough handling of the sample
- Aspirin, sulfonamides, nitrofurantoin, vitamin K derivatives, primaquine, and fava beans (decreased G6PD enzyme activity, precipitating a hemolytic episode)

Homocysteine, total, plasma

Homocysteine (tHcy), a sulfur-containing amino acid, is a transmethylation product of methionine. It's an intermediate in the synthesis of cysteine, which is produced by the enzymatic or acid hydrolysis of proteins. The test is useful for the biochemical diagnosis of inborn errors of methionine, folate, and vitamins B_6 and B_{12} metabolism.

Purpose
- Biochemical diagnosis of inborn errors of methionine, folate, and vitamins B_6 and B_{12} metabolism
- Indicator of acquired folate or cobalamin deficiency
- Evaluation of risk factors for atherosclerotic vascular disease
- Evaluation as a contributing factor in the pathogenesis of neural tube defects
- Evaluation of cause of recurrent spontaneous abortions.
- Evaluation of delayed child development or failure to thrive in infants

Patient preparation
- Inform the patient that this test detects homocysteine levels in plasma.
- Advise him to fast for 12 to 14 hours before the test.
- Tell him that this test requires a blood sample, who will perform the venipuncture and when, and that he may experience transient discomfort from the needle puncture and the pressure of the tourniquet.

Procedure and posttest care
- Perform a venipuncture, and collect the sample in a 5-ml tube with EDTA added.
- If a hematoma develops at the venipuncture site, apply warm soaks.

Precautions
- Handle the sample gently to prevent hemolysis.

- Immediately put the sample on ice and send it to the laboratory.

Reference values

Normal total homocysteine levels are 4 to 17 μmol/L.

Abnormal findings

- Low homocysteine levels are associated with inborn or acquired folate or cobalamine deficiency and inborn B_6 or B_{12} deficiency.
- Elevated homocysteine levels are associated with a higher incidence of atherosclerotic vascular disease. In patients with type 2 diabetes mellitus, studies have shown that homocysteine levels increase with even a modest deterioration in renal function.

Interfering factors

- Failure to adhere to dietary restrictions will alter test results.
- Failure to immediately freeze the specimen will alter test results
- Penicillamine reduces the plasma levels of homocysteine.
- Azauridine, nitrous oxide and a methotrexate deficiency will cause increased plasma levels of homocysteine.

Pyruvate kinase

An erythrocyte enzyme, pyruvate kinase (PK) takes part in the anaerobic metabolism of glucose. An abnormally low PK level is an inherited autosomal recessive trait that may cause a red cell membrane defect associated with congenital hemolytic anemia. PK assay confirms PK deficiency when red cell enzyme deficiency is the suspected cause of anemia.

Purpose

- To differentiate PK-deficient hemolytic anemia from other congenital hemolytic anemias or from acquired hemolytic anemia
- To detect PK deficiency in asymptomatic, heterozygous inheritance

Patient preparation

- Explain to the patient that this test is used to detect inherited enzyme deficiencies.
- Tell the patient that the test requires a blood sample. Explain who will perform the venipuncture and when.
- Explain to the patient that he may experience slight discomfort from the needle puncture and the tourniquet.
- Inform the patient that he need not restrict food and fluids.
- Check the patient's history for recent blood transfusion and note it on the laboratory request.

Procedure and posttest care

- Perform a venipuncture and collect the sample in a 4-ml EDTA tube.
- Apply direct pressure to the venipuncture site until bleeding stops.
- If a hematoma develops at the venipuncture site, apply warm soaks.

Precautions

- Completely fill the collection tube and invert it gently several times to mix the sample and the anticoagulant.
- Handle the sample gently to prevent hemolysis.
- Refrigerate the sample if you can't send it to the laboratory immediately.

Reference values

Serum PK levels range from 9 to 22 U/g of hemoglobin (Hb); in the low substrate assay, they range from 1.7 to 6.8 U/g of hemoglobin.

Abnormal findings

Low serum PK levels confirm a diagnosis of PK deficiency and allow differentiation between PK-deficient hemolytic anemia and other inherited disorders.

Interfering factors

- Failure to use the proper anticoagulant or to adequately mix the sample and the anticoagulant
- Hemolysis due to rough handling of the sample
- Failure to remove white cells from sample (possible false results)
- Recent blood transfusion or recent hemolytic event

Serum hexosaminidase A and B

This fluorometric test measures the hexosaminidase A and B content of serum samples drawn by venipuncture or collected from a neonate's umbilical cord or of amniotic fluid obtained by amniocentesis. Hexosaminidase deficiency can also be identified by testing cultured skin fibroblasts; however, this procedure is costly and technically complex. A reference center for congenital disease should be consulted for the preferred screening method and specimen.

Hexosaminidase is a group of enzymes that are necessary for metabolism of gangliosides, water-soluble glycolipids found primarily in brain tissue. The hexosaminidase A and B test is used to measure the hexosaminidase A and B content of serum and amniotic fluid.

Deficiency of hexosaminidase A indicates Tay-Sachs disease, which affects people of eastern European Jewish ances-

try about 100 times more often than the general population. Both parents must carry the defective gene to transmit Tay-Sachs disease to their children. Sandhoff's disease, which results from deficiency of hexosaminidase A and B, is uncommon and not prevalent in any ethnic group.

Purpose

- To confirm or rule out Tay-Sachs disease in the neonate
- To screen for a Tay-Sachs carrier
- To establish prenatal diagnosis of hexosaminidase A deficiency

Patient preparation

- Explain to the patient that this test is used to identify carriers of Tay-Sachs disease.
- Tell the patient that the test requires a blood sample. Explain who will perform the venipuncture and when.
- Explain to the patient that he may experience slight discomfort from the needle puncture and the tourniquet.
- Inform the patient that he need not restrict food and fluids.

AGE ISSUE *When testing a neonate, explain to the parents that this test is used to detect Tay-Sachs disease. Tell them that blood will be drawn from the neonate's arm, neck, or umbilical cord; that the procedure is safe and quickly performed; and that the neonate will have a small bandage on the venipuncture site. Inform them that no pretest restrictions of food or fluid are needed.*

- If the test is being performed prenatally, advise the patient of preparations for amniocentesis.

Procedure and posttest care

- Perform a venipuncture, collect cord blood, or assist with amniocentesis, as appropriate. Collect the sample in a 7-ml clot-activator tube.

■ Apply direct pressure to the venipuncture site until bleeding stops.

■ If a hematoma develops at the venipuncture site, apply warm soaks.

■ When testing a neonate, follow laboratory procedure for collecting serum samples.

Precautions

■ Handle the sample gently to prevent hemolysis.

■ This test can't be done on a pregnant woman's serum (but her leukocytes or amniotic fluid may be tested, if necessary); if the father's blood test result is negative, Tay-Sachs disease won't be transmitted to the child.

■ If the test can't be performed immediately, freeze the sample.

Reference values

Total serum levels of hexosaminidase range from 5 to 12.9 U/L; hexosaminidase A accounts for 55% to 76% of the total.

Abnormal findings

Absence of hexosaminidase A indicates Tay-Sachs disease (total hexosaminidase levels can be normal). Absence of hexosaminidase A and B indicates Sandhoff's disease, an uncommon, virulent variant of Tay-Sachs disease in which deterioration occurs more rapidly.

Interfering factors

■ Hemolysis due to rough handling of the sample

■ Hormonal contraceptives (false-high)

■ Rifampin and isoniazid (increase)

Uroporphyrinogen I synthase

The uroporphyrinogen I synthase test is used to measure blood levels of uroporphyrinogen I synthase, an enzyme involved in heme biosynthesis. This enzyme is usually present in erythrocytes, fibroblasts, lymphocytes, hepatic cells, and amniotic fluid cells. A hereditary deficiency that can reduce uroporphyrinogen I synthase levels by 50% or more results in acute intermittent porphyria (AIP). This disorder can be latent indefinitely until certain factors (some sex hormones and drugs, a low-carbohydrate diet, or an infection) precipitate active disease.

An improvement over traditional urine tests that can detect AIP only during an acute episode, the uroporphyrinogen I synthase test can detect AIP even during its latent phase. Thus, it can identify an affected individual before an acute episode occurs. Because it's specific for AIP, this test can also differentiate AIP from other types of porphyria.

Enzyme activity is determined by fluorometrically measuring the conversion rate of porphobilinogen to uroporphyrinogen. If levels are indeterminate, urine and stool tests for aminolevulinic acid (ALA) and porphobilinogen may be ordered to support the diagnosis because excretion of these porphyrin precursors increases substantially during an acute episode of AIP and may increase slightly during the latent phase.

Purpose

■ To aid diagnosis of latent or active AIP

■ To differentiate AIP from other types of porphyria

Patient preparation

- Explain to the patient that this test is used to detect a red blood cell disorder.
- Inform the patient that he'll need to fast for 12 to 14 hours before the test and to abstain from alcohol for 24 hours, but that he may drink water.
- Tell the patient that the test requires a blood sample. Explain who will perform the venipuncture and when.
- Explain to the patient that he may experience slight discomfort from the needle puncture and the tourniquet.
- If the patient's hematocrit is available, note it on the laboratory request.
- Notify the laboratory and physician of medications the patient is taking that may affect test results; they may need to be restricted.

Procedure and posttest care

- Perform a venipuncture and collect the sample in a 10-ml heparinized tube.
- Apply direct pressure to the venipuncture site until bleeding stops.
- If a hematoma develops at the venipuncture site, apply warm soaks.
- Instruct the patient that he may resume his usual diet and medications discontinued before the test, as ordered.
- If AIP is present, refer the patient for nutrition and genetic counseling. Advise him to avoid low-carbohydrate diets, alcohol, and drugs that may trigger an acute episode and to seek prompt care for all infections.

Precautions

- Handle the sample gently to prevent hemolysis.
- Place the sample on ice and send it to the laboratory immediately.

Reference values

Normal values for uroporphyrinogen I synthase are ≥ 7 nmol/sec/L.

Abnormal findings

Decreased uroporphyrinogen I synthase levels generally indicate latent or active AIP; symptoms differentiate these phases. Levels that are < 6 nmol/sec/L confirm AIP. Levels between 6 and 6.9 nmol/sec/L are indeterminate, in which case urine and stool tests for the porphyrin precursors ALA and porphobilinogen may be ordered to support the diagnosis.

Interfering factors

- Failure to observe pretest restrictions or to freeze the sample (false-positive)
- Hemolysis due to rough handling of the sample
- Hemolytic and hepatic diseases (possible increase)
- Alcohol and use of drugs, such as steroid hormones, estrogens, barbiturates, sulfonamides, phenytoin, griseofulvin, chlordiazepoxide, meprobamate, glutethimide, and ergot alkaloids (possible decrease)

Galactose-1-phosphate uridyl transferase

Galactose-1-phosphate uridyl transferase (GPUT) is involved in the conversion of galactose to glucose during lactose metabolism. Deficiency may lead to galactosemia, a hereditary disorder marked by elevated serum galactose levels and decreased serum glucose levels. Unless detected and treated soon after birth, galactosemia can impair eye, brain, and liver development, causing irreversible cataracts, mental retardation, and cirrhosis.

The qualitative test, a simple screening test for deficiency of GPUT, is required in some facilities for all neonates. The quantitative test requires a blood sample and measures the amount of a fluorescent substance generated during a coupled enzyme reaction. This is generally ordered as soon as possible after a positive screening test and may occasionally be ordered for an adult to detect a carrier state.

Prenatal testing of amniotic fluid can also detect GPUT deficiency, but it's rarely performed because neonatal screening can detect the deficiency in time to prevent irreversible damage.

Purpose
- To screen the infant for galactosemia
- To detect a heterozygous carrier of galactosemia

Patient preparation
- When testing a neonate, explain to the parents that the test screens for galactosemia, a potentially dangerous enzyme deficiency.
- If a blood sample wasn't taken from the umbilical cord at birth, tell the parents that a small amount of blood will be drawn from the infant's heel. Explain that the procedure is safe and quickly performed.
- When testing an adult, explain that this test is used to identify carriers of galactosemia, a genetic disorder that may be transmitted to offspring.
- Tell the patient that the test requires a blood sample. Explain who will perform the venipuncture and when.
- Explain to the patient that he may experience slight discomfort from the needle puncture and the tourniquet.
- Inform the patient that he need not restrict food and fluids.

Procedure and posttest care
- For a qualitative (screening) test, collect cord blood or blood from a heelstick on special filter paper, saturating all three circles.
- For a quantitative test, perform a venipuncture and collect a 4-ml sample in a heparinized or EDTA tube, depending on the laboratory method used.
- Indicate the patient's age on the laboratory request.
- Check the patient's history for a recent exchange transfusion. Note this on the laboratory request or postpone the test.
- Apply direct pressure to the venipuncture site until bleeding stops.
- If a hematoma develops at the venipuncture site, apply warm soaks.
- If test results indicate galactosemia, refer the parents for nutrition counseling, and provide a galactose- and lactose-free diet for their infant. A soybean- or meat-based formula may be substituted for formulas based on cow's milk.

Precautions
- Handle the sample gently to prevent hemolysis.
- Send the sample to the laboratory on wet ice.

Reference values
Normally, the qualitative test is negative. The normal range for the quantitative test is 18.5 to 28.5 U/g of hemoglobin (Hb); confirm the normal range with the laboratory in case a different method is used.

Abnormal findings
A positive qualitative test may indicate a transferase deficiency. A follow-up quantitative test should be performed as soon as possible. Quantitative test results showing less than 5 U/g of Hb indicate galac-

tosemia. Levels between 5 and 18.5 U/g of Hb may indicate a carrier state.

Interfering factors
- Hemolysis due to rough handling of the sample
- Failure to use the proper collection tube or to send the sample to the laboratory on wet ice (possible false-positive because heat inactivates transferase)
- Total exchange transfusion (transient false-negative because normal blood contains enzyme)

Angiotensin-converting enzyme

The angiotensin-converting enzyme (ACE) test is used to measure serum levels of ACE, which is found in lung capillaries and, in lesser concentrations, blood vessels and kidney tissue. Its primary function is to help regulate arterial pressure by converting angiotensin I to angiotensin II. Despite ACE's role in blood pressure regulation, this test is of little use in diagnosing hypertension. Instead, it's primarily used to diagnose sarcoidosis because of the high correlation between elevated serum ACE levels and this disease. Presumably, elevated serum levels reflect macrophage activity. This test also monitors response to treatment in sarcoidosis and helps confirm a diagnosis of Gaucher's disease or leprosy.

Purpose
- To aid diagnosis of sarcoidosis, especially pulmonary sarcoidosis
- To monitor the patient's response to therapy in sarcoidosis
- To help confirm Gaucher's disease or Hansen's disease

Patient preparation
- Explain to the patient that this test is used to diagnose sarcoidosis, Gaucher's disease, or Hansen's disease or, if appropriate, to check his response to treatment for sarcoidosis.
- Tell the patient that the test requires a blood sample. Explain who will perform the venipuncture and when.
- Explain to the patient that he may experience slight discomfort from the needle puncture and the tourniquet.
- Inform the patient that he must fast for 12 hours before the test.
- Note the patient's age on the laboratory request. If he's under age 20, the test may have to be postponed because a person under age 20 has variable ACE levels.

Procedure and posttest care
- Perform a venipuncture and collect the sample in a 7-ml clot-activator tube.
- Apply direct pressure to the venipuncture site until bleeding stops.
- If a hematoma develops at the venipuncture site, apply warm soaks.

Precautions
- Avoid using a tube with EDTA because this can decrease ACE levels, altering test results.
- Handle the sample gently to prevent hemolysis.
- Send the sample to the laboratory immediately or freeze it and place it on dry ice until the test can be performed.

Reference values
In the colorimetric assay, normal values for serum ACE in patients age 20 and older range from 8 to 52 U/L (SI, 0.14 to 0.88 μkat/L).

Abnormal findings

Elevated serum ACE levels may indicate sarcoidosis, Gaucher's disease, or Hansen's disease, but results must be correlated with the patient's clinical condition. In some cases, elevated ACE levels may result from hyperthyroidism, diabetic retinopathy, or hepatic disease.

Serum ACE levels decline as the patient responds to steroid or prednisone therapy for sarcoidosis.

Interfering factors

■ Failure to fast before the test (may cause significant lipemia of the sample)
■ Use of a collection tube with EDTA (possible decrease)
■ Hemolysis due to rough handling of the sample
■ Failure to send the sample to the laboratory at once or to freeze it and place it on dry ice (possible false-low due to ACE degradation)

Selected readings

Braunwald, E., et al., eds. *Harrison's Principles of Internal Medicine,* 15th ed. New York: McGraw-Hill Book Co., 2001.

Cavanaugh, B.M. *Nurse's Manual of Laboratory and Diagnostic Tests,* 4th ed. Philadelphia: F.A. Davis Co., 2003.

Fischbach, F. *A Manual of Laboratory and Diagnostic Tests,* 7th ed. Philadelphia: Lippincott Williams & Wilkins, 2004.

Guyton, A.C., and Hall, J.E. *Textbook of Medical Physiology,* 10th ed. Philadelphia: W.B. Saunders Co., 2001.

Henry, J.B., ed. *Clinical Diagnosis and Management by Laboratory Methods,* 20th ed. Philadelphia: W.B. Saunders Co., 2001.

Pagana, K.D., and Pagana, T. J. *Mosby's Diagnostic and Laboratory Test Reference,* 6th ed. Philadelphia: Mosby Year–Book, Inc., 2003.

Schnell, Z., et al. *Davis's Comprehensive Handbook of Laboratory and Diagnostic Tests with Nursing Implications.* Philadelphia: F.A. Davis Co., 2003.

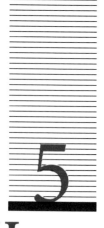

Hormones

Introduction

Hormones are powerful, complex chemicals that are normally produced by the endocrine system and transported through the bloodstream to stimulate or inhibit the metabolic activity of target glands or organs. Some hormones, such as epinephrine, have profound and widespread effects on body tissues; others regulate the production and release of another hormone by the target cell and are referred to as trophic hormones — thyroid-stimulating hormone (TSH) is an example. Hormones continuously interact in complicated feedback systems, negative and positive, to maintain hormonal homeostasis. Thus, a change in the circulating blood level of one hormone eventually changes the secretion of others. Consequently, the circulating blood levels of hormones have enormous diagnostic significance, and numerous tests have been devised to detect and evaluate abnormal secretion.

In chemical terms, hormones can be divided into three classes of compounds: polypeptides, amines, and steroids. The polypeptides include hormones, such as antidiuretic hormone (ADH) and gastrin; the amines include hormones, such as thyroxine and the catecholamines; and the steroids include the gonadal hormones estrogen and testosterone.

Chemical transmitters

Basically, hormones are chemical transmitters, or messengers. Most hormones attach to specific receptor sites on cell membranes, activating adenyl cyclase, an enzyme responsible for producing cyclic adenosine monophosphate (cAMP) within the cell. Just as the hormone travels through the blood with a chemical message for its target gland, cAMP acts as the third messenger within the cell itself.

Prostaglandins have been implicated as the second messenger in the response system. The end result of this delicate and intricate communications network is a change in cellular function — increased protein synthesis, for example, or the release of more metabolic fuel such as glycogen. Hormones are thus indispensable to the maintenance of homeostasis and to the growth or repair of body tissues.

Sites of secretion

Most hormones are secreted by the ductless glands or organs of the endocrine system: the pituitary, thyroid, parathyroid, and adrenal glands, and the pancreas, gonads (ovaries and testes), and placenta. (See *Sites of hormonal secretion*, page 134.) Most of these glands and organs are controlled — directly or indirectly — by the hypothalamus, the clearinghouse or message coordinator for the endocrine and autonomic nervous systems. Some hormones are secreted by nonendocrine organs; gastrin, for example, is secreted by the stomach.

The *pituitary gland* (or hypophysis) is situated within the sella turcica of the sphenoid bone, inside the skull. This small gland dominates and regulates most of the secretory activity of the endocrine system. It has an anterior lobe (adenohypophysis) and a posterior lobe (neurohypophysis).

The *anterior pituitary* consists of glandular tissue connected to the hypothalamus by a vascular network called the hypothalamic-pituitary portal venous system. It secretes many hormones whose bloodstream levels have diagnostic significance. The basophilic cells of the anterior pituitary secrete four polypeptide hormones that affect other endocrine glands: corticotropin, follicle-stimulating hor-

SITES OF HORMONAL SECRETION

Powerful, complex chemicals, hormones circulate through the bloodstream to stimulate or inhibit the activity of target glands or organs. In coordination with the nervous system, these target glands secrete the hormones that maintain homeostasis.

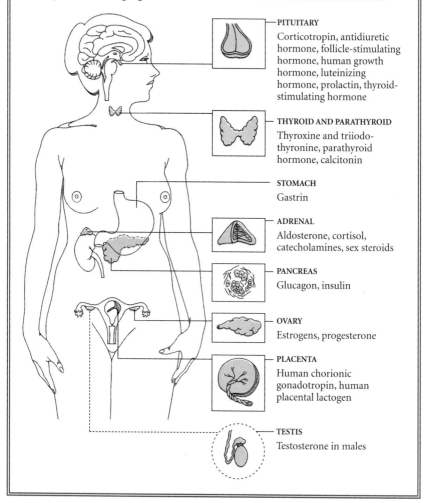

PITUITARY
Corticotropin, antidiuretic hormone, follicle-stimulating hormone, human growth hormone, luteinizing hormone, prolactin, thyroid-stimulating hormone

THYROID AND PARATHYROID
Thyroxine and triiodo-thyronine, parathyroid hormone, calcitonin

STOMACH
Gastrin

ADRENAL
Aldosterone, cortisol, catecholamines, sex steroids

PANCREAS
Glucagon, insulin

OVARY
Estrogens, progesterone

PLACENTA
Human chorionic gonadotropin, human placental lactogen

TESTIS
Testosterone in males

mone, luteinizing hormone, and TSH. The acidophilic cells secrete two hormones that directly affect peripheral tissues: prolactin and growth hormone. Hyposecretion or hypersecretion of these hormones leads to serious disorders, such as Cushing's syndrome, sterility, and dwarfism.

The *posterior pituitary* comprises neural tissue or neuroepithelial cells and is continuous with the hypothalamus. It releases stored ADH on neural stimulation by the hypothalamus, where ADH is formed.

The *thyroid gland* consists of two lobes, straddling the trachea and connected by an isthmus, that lie just below the cricoid cartilage. A primary regulator of body metabolism, the thyroid secretes two vital hormones — thyroxine (T_4) and triiodothyronine (T_3) — to maintain the proper metabolic rate for cellular function. The thyroid hormones have a stimulatory effect on calorigenesis (increased oxygen consumption in body tissues) and affect the growth and development of the nervous and musculoskeletal systems. They also regulate the synthesis, storage, and use of carbohydrates, fats, proteins, vitamins, and body fluids.

Serum T_4 and T_3 — probably the most commonly evaluated hormones — are measured to detect hyperthyroidism or hypothyroidism. If confirming tests are needed, free forms of T_4 and T_3 (FT_4 and FT_3 — unbound to thyroxine-binding globulin [TBG]) — can be measured. Tests of protein binding, such as serum TBG electrophoresis and T_3 resin uptake, also help assess thyroid function.

The *parathyroids* — four small glands usually located behind the thyroid — release parathyroid hormone (PTH), which maintains calcium and phosphorus homeostasis. PTH, with vitamin D, stimulates the osteocytes to release calcium from the bones to raise the serum calcium level. In contrast, calcitonin — a polypeptide hormone secreted by the parafollicular cells of the thyroid gland — and high levels of phosphate stimulate absorption of calcium ions into the bones to lower the calcium level.

The *adrenal glands* secrete mineralocorticoids (primarily aldosterone) to maintain sodium and water balance; glucocorticoids (primarily cortisol) to regulate carbohydrate, fat, and protein metabolism; sex steroids (androgens and estrogens); and catecholamines (mainly epinephrine, norepinephrine, and dopamine) to regulate reactions to stress. The adrenal cortex secretes mineralocorticoids, glucocorticoids, and sex steroids. The adrenal medulla secretes catecholamines — this is part of the body's fight-or-flight response to stress.

In the *pancreas*, the islets of Langerhans (beta cells) secrete insulin and the alpha cells secrete glucagon; both hormones have a marked effect on total body metabolism but especially on carbohydrate metabolism. The *stomach* secretes gastrin, a hormone that plays an indispensable role in facilitating digestion.

The *ovaries* and *testes* secrete the gonadal hormones estrogen and testosterone, respectively, which govern development of secondary sex characteristics and reproductive function. The ovaries also secrete progesterone, which serves primarily to prepare the endometrium for the implantation of a fertilized ovum. During pregnancy, the *placenta* serves as a temporary endocrine organ, secreting the hormones human chorionic gonadotropin and human placental lactogen.

Hormonal "watchdog" mechanisms

Because hormones are so powerful, despite the minute quantities in which they appear in the blood, the body monitors their activities closely to prevent unwanted physiologic effects. Two important "watchdog" mechanisms to control hormonal levels are *neurohumoral regulation* and a closed-loop *feedback system*. In neurohumoral regulation, certain releasing or inhibiting factors produced in the supraoptic hypothalamic nuclei travel to

CLINICAL INDICATIONS FOR HORMONE TESTS

Disease or disorder	Hormones tested
Acromegaly, gigantism	Corticotropin, human growth hormone (hGH), follicle-stimulating hormone (FSH), luteinizing hormone (LH), thyroid-stimulating hormone (TSH)
Addison's disease	Corticotropin, cortisol
Aldosteronism	Aldosterone
Anemia	Erythropoietin
Congenital adrenal hyperplasia	Corticotropin, cortisol, androgens, estrogens, human chorionic gonadotropin (hCG), androstenedione
Cushing's syndrome	Corticotropin, cortisol, androstenedione, dehydroepiandrosterone
Diabetes insipidus	Antidiuretic hormone
Diabetes mellitus	Insulin, cortisol, glucagon, C-peptide
Dwarfism	Corticotropin, hGH, FSH, LH, TSH
Gigantism	hGH
Hyperparathyroidism and hypoparathyroidism	Parathyroid hormone
Hyperthyroidism and hypothyroidism	Thyroxine (T_4) and triiodothyronine (T_3), free T_4 and free T_3, TSH, thyroxine-binding globulin, T_3 resinuptake
Hypogonadism	Estrogens, testosterone, FSH, LH, androstenedione
Hypopituitarism	Corticotropin, hGH, FSH, LH, TSH, T_4, T_3, alpha-subunit of the pituitary glycoprotein hormones
Medullary thyroid carcinoma	Calcitonin
Performance enhancers, suspected use of	Erythropoietin, anabolic steroids, androgens
Pituitary tumors	Corticotropin, hGH, prolactin, FSH, LH
Polycythemia	Erythropoietin
Precocious puberty	FSH, LH, estrogens, androgens, androstenedione
Specific tumors	Erythropoietin, hCG
Zollinger-Ellison syndrome	Gastrin

the pituitary gland, where they regulate hormone secretion.

The positive loop of the feedback system, which is constantly at work within the endocrine system, encompasses the initial stimulus, such as an elevated blood glucose level, that results in the secretion of the controlling hormone — in this case, insulin. The negative loop goes into action when the desired secretory response or hormonal concentration is achieved. For example, decreased blood glucose levels cause the pancreas to curtail its secretion of insulin.

Hormone assay methods

Radioimmunoassay and enzyme immunoassay are two testing methods used by laboratories to measure hormone levels. But the assay method is just one consideration that affects the reliability of test results. For example, diurnal variations in hormone secretion require careful scheduling of the sample collection to coincide with or avoid times of peak secretion.

Other important considerations in evaluating hormone levels are age, gender, exercise, emotional stress, nutritional status, and medication use, all of which may affect the hormone level to be tested.

Assessment crucial

Remember to assess the patient accurately for endocrine disorders, such as hypothyroidism or diabetes. In a child, watch especially for indications of abnormal growth patterns, such as absent or delayed puberty, irregular bone structure, muscular atrophy, or weight changes. (See *Clinical indications for hormone tests.*)

Remember, careful observation, accurate history taking, and patient teaching are essential to the care of the patient scheduled for hormone tests.

PITUITARY HORMONE TESTS

Plasma corticotropin

The corticotropin test measures the plasma levels of corticotropin by radioimmunoassay. Corticotropin stimulates the adrenal cortex to secrete cortisol and, to a lesser degree, androgens and aldosterone. It also has some melanocyte-stimulating activity, increases the uptake of amino acids by muscle cells, promotes lipolysis by fat cells, stimulates pancreatic beta cells to secrete insulin, and may contribute to the release of growth hormone. Corticotropin levels vary diurnally, peaking between 6 a.m. and 8 a.m. and ebbing between 6 p.m. and 11 p.m. Through a negative feedback mechanism, plasma cortisol levels control corticotropin secretion — for example, high cortisol levels suppress corticotropin secretion. Emotional and physical stress (pain, surgery, insulin-induced hypoglycemia) stimulate secretion and can override the effects of plasma cortisol levels.

The corticotropin test may be ordered for a patient with signs of adrenal hypofunction (insufficiency) or hyperfunction (Cushing's syndrome). Corticotropin suppression or stimulation testing is usually necessary to confirm diagnosis. The instability and unavailability of corticotropin greatly limit this test's diagnostic significance and reliability.

Purpose

- To facilitate differential diagnosis of primary and secondary adrenal hypofunction
- To aid differential diagnosis of Cushing's syndrome

Patient preparation

- Explain to the patient that this test helps determine if his hormonal secretion is normal.
- Advise the patient that he must fast and limit his physical activity for 10 to 12 hours before the test.
- Tell the patient that the test requires a blood sample. Explain who will perform the venipuncture and when.
- Explain to the patient that he may experience slight discomfort from the needle puncture and the tourniquet.
- Check the patient's history for medications that may affect the accuracy of test results, as ordered. Withhold these medications for 48 hours or longer before the test. If they must be continued, note this on the laboratory request.
- Arrange with the dietary department to provide a low-carbohydrate diet for 2 days before the test. This requirement may vary, depending on the laboratory.

Procedure and posttest care

- For a patient with suspected adrenal hypofunction, perform the venipuncture for a baseline level between 6 a.m. and 8 a.m. (peak secretion).
- For a patient with suspected Cushing's syndrome, perform the venipuncture between 6 p.m. and 11 p.m. (low secretion).
- Collect the sample in a plastic EDTA tube (corticotropin may adhere to glass). The tube must be full because excess anticoagulant will affect results.
- Pack the sample in ice and send it to the laboratory immediately, where plasma must be rapidly separated from blood cells at 39.2° F (4° C). The collection technique may vary, depending on the laboratory.
- Apply direct pressure to the venipuncture site until bleeding stops.

- If a hematoma develops at the venipuncture site, apply warm soaks.
- Instruct the patient that he may resume his usual diet, activities, and medications discontinued before the test, as ordered.

Precautions

- Because proteolytic enzymes in plasma degrade corticotropin, a temperature of 39.2° F is necessary to retard enzyme activity.
- Immediate transfer of the sample, packed in ice, to the laboratory is essential for reliable test results.

Reference values

Mayo Medical Laboratories sets baseline values at less than 120 pg/ml (SI, < 26.4 pmol/L at 6 a.m. to 8 a.m.), but these values may vary, depending on the laboratory.

Abnormal findings

A higher-than-normal corticotropin level may indicate primary adrenal hypofunction (Addison's disease), in which the pituitary gland attempts to compensate for the unresponsiveness of the target organ by releasing excessive corticotropin. The underlying cause of adrenocortical hypofunction may be idiopathic atrophy of the adrenal cortex or partial destruction of the gland by granuloma, neoplasm, amyloidosis, or inflammatory necrosis.

A low-normal corticotropin level suggests secondary adrenal hypofunction resulting from pituitary or hypothalamic dysfunction. The primary determinant may be panhypopituitarism, absence of corticotropin-releasing hormone in the hypothalamus, or chronic blunting of corticotropin levels by long-term corticosteroid therapy.

In suspected Cushing's syndrome, an elevated corticotropin level suggests

Cushing's disease, in which pituitary dysfunction (due to adenoma) causes continuous hypersecretion of corticotropin and, consequently, continuously elevated cortisol levels without diurnal variations. Moderately elevated corticotropin levels suggest pituitary-dependent adrenal hyperplasia and nonadrenal tumors such as oat cell carcinoma of the lungs.

A low-normal corticotropin level implies adrenal hyperfunction due to adrenocortical tumor or hyperplasia.

Interfering factors

- Failure to observe pretest restrictions
- Corticosteroids, including cortisone and its analogues (decrease)
- Drugs that increase endogenous cortisol secretion, such as estrogens, calcium gluconate, amphetamines, spironolactone, and ethanol (decrease)
- Lithium carbonate (decreases cortisol levels and may interfere with corticotropin secretion)
- Menstrual cycle and pregnancy
- Radioactive scan performed within 1 week before the test
- Acute stress (including hospitalization and surgery) and depression (increase)

Rapid corticotropin

The rapid corticotropin test (also known as the cosyntropin test) is gradually replacing the 8-hour corticotropin stimulation test as the most effective diagnostic tool for evaluating adrenal hypofunction. Using cosyntropin, the rapid corticotropin test provides faster results and causes fewer allergic reactions than the 8-hour test, which uses natural corticotropin from animal sources.

This test requires prior determination of baseline cortisol levels to evaluate the effect of cosyntropin administration on cortisol secretion. An unequivocally high morning cortisol level rules out adrenal hypofunction and makes further testing unnecessary.

Purpose

- To aid in identification of primary and secondary adrenal hypofunction

Patient preparation

- Explain to the patient that this test helps determine if his condition is due to a hormonal deficiency.
- Inform him that he may be required to fast for 10 to 12 hours before the test and must be relaxed and resting quietly for 30 minutes before the test.
- Tell him that the test takes at least 1 hour to perform.
- If the patient is an inpatient, withhold corticotropin and all steroid medications, as ordered. If he's an outpatient, tell him to refrain from taking these drugs, if instructed by his physician. If the drugs must be continued, note this on the laboratory request.
- Explain to the patient that he may experience slight discomfort from the needle puncture and the tourniquet.

Procedure and posttest care

- Draw 5 ml of blood for a baseline value. Collect the sample in a 5-ml heparinized tube. Label this sample "preinjection" and send it to the laboratory.
- Inject 250 μg (0.25 mg) of cosyntropin I.V. or I.M. (I.V. administration provides more accurate results because ineffective absorption after I.M. administration may cause wide variations in response.) Direct I.V. injection should take about 2 minutes.
- Draw another 5 ml of blood at 30 and 60 minutes after the cosyntropin injection. Collect the samples in 5-ml hep-

arinized tubes. Label the samples "30 minutes postinjection" and "60 minutes postinjection" and send them to the laboratory. Include the collection times on the laboratory request.

■ Apply direct pressure to the venipuncture site until bleeding stops.

■ If a hematoma develops at the venipuncture site, apply warm soaks.

■ Observe the patient for signs of a rare allergic reaction to cosyntropin, such as hives, itching, and tachycardia.

■ Instruct the patient that he may resume his usual diet, activities, and medications discontinued before the test, as ordered.

Precautions

■ Handle the samples gently to prevent hemolysis. They require no special precautions other than avoiding stasis.

Reference values

Normally, cortisol levels rise after 30 to 60 minutes to a peak of 18 mg/dl (SI, 500 mmol/L) or more 60 minutes after the cosyntropin injection. Generally, doubling the baseline value indicates a normal response.

Abnormal findings

A normal result excludes adrenal hypofunction (insufficiency). In the patient with primary adrenal hypofunction (Addison's disease), cortisol levels remain low. Thus, the rapid corticotropin test provides an effective method of screening for adrenal hypofunction. If test results show subnormal increases in cortisol levels, prolonged stimulation of the adrenal cortex may be required to differentiate between primary and secondary adrenal hypofunction.

Interfering factors

■ Failure to observe pretest restrictions

■ Hemolysis due to rough handling of the sample

■ Estrogens and amphetamines (increase in plasma cortisol)

■ Smoking and obesity (possible increase in plasma cortisol)

■ Lithium carbonate (decrease in plasma cortisol)

■ Radioactive scan performed within 1 week before the test

Serum human growth hormone

Human growth hormone (hGH), also called somatotropin, is a protein secreted by acidophils of the anterior pituitary gland. It's the primary regulator of human growth. Unlike other pituitary hormones, hGH has no easily defined feedback mechanism or single target gland — it affects many body tissues. Like insulin, hGH promotes protein synthesis and stimulates amino acid uptake by cells. It also raises plasma glucose levels by inhibiting glucose uptake and utilization by cells, and increases free fatty acid concentrations by enhancing lipolysis.

Secretion of hGH appears to be regulated by the hypothalamus by means of a growth hormone-releasing factor and a growth hormone release-inhibiting factor (somatostatin). Secretion of hGH is diurnal and varies with such factors as exercise, sleep, stress, and nutritional status. Hyposecretion or hypersecretion of this hormone may induce pathologic states (such as dwarfism or gigantism). Altered hGH levels are common in the patient with pituitary dysfunction.

This test, a quantitative analysis of plasma hGH levels, is usually performed as part of an anterior pituitary stimulation or suppression test. Such testing is crucial because clinical manifestations of an hGH deficiency can rarely be reversed by therapy.

Purpose

- To aid differential diagnosis of dwarfism because growth retardation can result from pituitary or thyroid hypofunction
- To confirm diagnosis of acromegaly and gigantism in the adult
- To aid diagnosis of pituitary and hypothalamic tumors
- To help evaluate hGH therapy

Patient preparation

- Explain to the patient, or his parents if the patient is a child, that this test measures hormone levels and helps determine the cause of abnormal growth.
- Instruct the patient to fast and limit activity for 10 to 12 hours before the test.
- Tell the patient that the test requires a blood sample. Explain who will perform the venipuncture and when. Inform him that another sample may have to be drawn the next day for comparison.
- Explain to the patient that he may experience slight discomfort from the needle puncture and the tourniquet.
- Withhold all medications that affect hGH levels such as pituitary-based steroids. If they must be continued, note this on the laboratory request.
- Make sure the patient is relaxed and recumbent for 30 minutes before the test; stress and activity elevate hGH levels.

Procedure and posttest care

- Between 6 a.m. and 8 a.m. on 2 consecutive days, or as ordered, perform a venipuncture and collect at least 7 ml of blood in a clot-activator tube.
- Apply direct pressure to the venipuncture site until bleeding stops.
- If a hematoma develops at the venipuncture site, apply warm soaks.

- Instruct the patient that he may resume his usual diet, activities, and medications discontinued before the test, as ordered.

Precautions

- Handle the sample gently to prevent hemolysis.
- Send it to the laboratory immediately because hGH has a half-life of only 20 to 25 minutes.

Reference values

Normal hGH levels for males range from undetectable to 5 ng/ml (SI, 5 µg/L); for females, from undetectable to 10 ng/ml (SI, 10 µg/L).

AGE ISSUE *Children's values may range from undetectable to 16 ng/ml (SI, 16 µg/L), and are usually higher.*

Abnormal findings

Increased hGH levels may indicate a pituitary or hypothalamic tumor, frequently an adenoma, which causes gigantism in children and acromegaly in adults and adolescents. Some patients with diabetes mellitus have elevated hGH levels without acromegaly. Suppression testing is necessary to confirm diagnosis.

Pituitary infarction, metastatic disease, and tumors may decrease hGH levels. Dwarfism may be due to low hGH levels, although only 15% of all cases of growth failure relate to endocrine dysfunction. Confirming the diagnosis requires stimulation testing with arginine or insulin.

Interfering factors

- Failure to observe pretest restrictions
- Hemolysis due to rough handling of the sample
- Arginine, beta-adrenergic blockers such as propranolol, and estrogens (increase)

- Amphetamines, bromocriptine, levodopa, dopamine, pituitary-based steroids, methyldopa, and histamine (increase)
- Insulin (induced hypoglycemia), glucagon, and nicotinic acid (increase)
- Phenothiazines (such as chlorpromazine) and corticosteroids (decrease)
- Radioactive scan performed within 1 week before the test

Growth hormone suppression

Also called glucose loading, the growth hormone suppression test evaluates excessive baseline levels of human growth hormone (hGH) from the anterior pituitary gland. Normally, hGH raises plasma glucose and fatty acid concentrations; in response, insulin secretion increases to counteract these effects. Consequently, a glucose load should suppress hGH secretions. In a patient with excessive hGH levels, failure of suppression indicates anterior pituitary dysfunction and confirms a diagnosis of acromegaly or gigantism.

Purpose
- To assess elevated baseline levels of hGH
- To confirm diagnosis of gigantism in children and acromegaly in adults and adolescents

Patient preparation
- Explain to the patient, or his parents if the patient is a child, that this test helps determine the cause of his abnormal growth.
- Instruct the patient to fast and limit physical activity for 10 to 12 hours before the test.
- Tell him that two blood samples will be drawn. Warn him that he may experience nausea after drinking the glucose solution and some discomfort from the needle punctures and the tourniquet.
- Withhold all steroids and other pituitary-based hormones. If they or other medications must be continued, note this on the laboratory request.
- Tell the patient to lie down and relax for 30 minutes before the test.

Procedure and posttest care
- Perform a venipuncture and collect 6 ml of blood (basal sample) in a 7-ml clot-activator tube between 6 a.m. and 8 a.m.
- Administer 100 g of glucose solution by mouth. To prevent nausea, advise the patient to drink the glucose slowly.
- About 1 hour later, draw venous blood into a 7-ml clot-activator tube. Label the tubes appropriately, and send them to the laboratory immediately.
- Apply direct pressure to the venipuncture site until bleeding stops.
- If a hematoma develops at the venipuncture site, apply warm soaks.
- Instruct the patient that he may resume his usual diet, activities, and medications discontinued before the test, as ordered.

Precautions
- Handle the samples gently to prevent hemolysis.
- Send each sample to the laboratory immediately because hGH has a half-life of only 20 to 25 minutes.

Reference values
Normally, glucose suppresses hGH to levels ranging from undetectable to 3 ng/ml (SI, 3 µg/L) in 30 minutes to 2 hours.

AGE ISSUE *In children, rebound stimulation may occur after 2 to 5 hours.*

Abnormal findings

In a patient with active acromegaly, elevated baseline hGH levels (5 ng/ml [SI, 5 µg/L]) aren't suppressed to less than 5 ng/ml during the test. Unchanged or rising hGH levels in response to glucose loading indicate hGH hypersecretion and may confirm suspected acromegaly and gigantism. This response may be verified by repeating the test after a 1-day rest.

Interfering factors

- Failure to observe pretest restrictions
- Hemolysis due to rough handling of the sample
- Corticosteroids and phenothiazines such as chlorpromazine (possible decrease in hGH secretion)
- Arginine, levodopa, amphetamines, glucagon, niacin, and estrogens (possible increase in hGH secretion)
- Radioactive scan performed within 1 week before the test
- Delay in sending the specimen to the laboratory

Insulin tolerance

The insulin tolerance test measures serum levels of human growth hormone (hGH) and corticotropin after administration of a loading dose of insulin and is more reliable than direct measurement of hGH and corticotropin because many healthy people have undetectable fasting levels of these hormones. Insulin-induced hypoglycemia stimulates hGH and corticotropin secretion in persons with an intact hypothalamic-pituitary-adrenal axis. Failure of stimulation indicates anterior pituitary or adrenal hypofunction and helps confirm an hGH or a corticotropin deficiency.

Because the insulin tolerance test stimulates an adrenergic response, it isn't recommended for patients with cardiovascular or cerebrovascular disorders, epilepsy, or low basal plasma cortisol levels.

Purpose

- To aid diagnosis of hGH and corticotropin deficiency
- To identify pituitary dysfunction
- To aid differential diagnosis of primary and secondary adrenal hypofunction

Patient preparation

- Explain to the patient, or his parents if the patient is a child, that this test evaluates hormonal secretion.
- Instruct the patient to fast and restrict physical activity for 10 to 12 hours before the test.
- Explain that the test involves I.V. infusion of insulin and the collection of multiple blood samples.
- Warn the patient that he may experience an increased heart rate, diaphoresis, hunger, and anxiety after administration of insulin. Reassure him that these symptoms are transient, and that if they become severe, the test will be discontinued.
- Tell the patient to lie down and relax for 90 minutes before the test.

Procedure and posttest care

- Between 6 a.m. and 8 a.m., perform a venipuncture and collect three 5-ml samples of blood for basal levels: one in a gray-top tube (for blood glucose) and two in green-top tubes (for hGH and corticotropin).
- Administer an I.V. bolus of U-100 regular insulin (0.15 U/kg, or as ordered) over 1 to 2 minutes.
- Use an indwelling venous catheter to avoid repeated venipunctures. Collect additional blood samples 15, 30, 45, 60, 90, and 120 minutes after insulin administration. At each interval, collect three sam-

ples: one in a tube with sodium fluoride and potassium oxidate and two in heparinized tubes. Label the tubes appropriately and send them to the laboratory immediately.

■ Apply direct pressure to the venipuncture site until bleeding stops.

■ If a hematoma develops at the I.V. or venipuncture site, apply warm soaks.

■ Instruct the patient that he may resume his usual diet, activities, and medications discontinued before the test, as ordered.

Precautions

■ Be sure to have concentrated glucose solution readily available in the event that the patient has a severe hypoglycemic reaction to insulin.

■ Label the tubes appropriately, including the collection times on the laboratory request, and send all samples to the laboratory immediately.

■ Handle the samples gently to prevent hemolysis.

Reference values

Normally, blood glucose falls to 50% of the fasting level 20 to 30 minutes after insulin administration. This stimulates a 10- to 20-ng/dl (SI, 10 to 20 µg/L) increase in baseline values for hGH and corticotropin, with peak levels occurring 60 to 90 minutes after insulin administration.

Abnormal findings

Failure of stimulation or a blunted response suggests dysfunction of the hypothalamic-pituitary-adrenal axis. An hGH increase of less than 10 ng/dl (SI, < 10 µg/L) above baseline suggests hGH deficiency. A definitive diagnosis of hGH deficiency requires a supplementary stimulation test such as the arginine test. Ad-

ditional testing is necessary to determine the site of the abnormality.

An increase in corticotropin levels of less than 10 ng/dl above baseline suggests adrenal insufficiency. The metyrapone or corticotropin stimulation test then confirms the diagnosis and determines whether the insufficiency is primary or secondary.

Interfering factors

■ Failure to observe pretest restrictions

■ Hemolysis due to rough handling of the sample

■ Corticosteroids and pituitary-based drugs (increase in hGH)

■ Glucocorticoids and beta-adrenergic blockers (decrease in hGH)

■ Glucocorticoids, estrogens, calcium gluconate, amphetamines, methamphetamines, spironolactone, and ethanol (decrease in corticotropin)

Arginine

The arginine test, also known as the human growth hormone (hGH) stimulation test, measures hGH levels after I.V. administration of arginine, an amino acid that normally stimulates hGH secretion. It's commonly used to identify pituitary dysfunction in infants and children with growth retardation and to confirm hGH deficiency. This test may be performed concomitantly with an insulin tolerance test or after administration of other hGH stimulants, such as glucagon, vasopressin, and levodopa.

Purpose

■ To aid diagnosis of pituitary tumors

■ To confirm hGH deficiency in infants and children with low baseline levels

Patient preparation

- Explain to the patient, or his parents if the patient is a child, that this test identifies hGH deficiency.
- Instruct the patient to fast and limit physical activity for 10 to 12 hours before the test.
- Explain to the patient that this test requires I.V. infusion of a drug and collection of several blood samples. Tell him that the test takes at least 2 hours to perform.
- Withhold all steroid medications, including pituitary-based hormones, as ordered. If they must be continued, record this on the laboratory request.
- Tell the patient to lie down and relax for at least 90 minutes before the test.

Procedure and posttest care

- Between 6 a.m. and 8 a.m., perform a venipuncture and collect 6 ml of blood (basal sample) in a clot-activator tube.
- Use an indwelling venous catheter to avoid repeated venipunctures. Start I.V. infusion of arginine (0.5 g/kg of body weight) in normal saline solution, and continue for 30 minutes.
- Discontinue the I.V. infusion, and then draw a total of three 6-ml samples at 30-minute intervals. Collect each sample in a clot-activator tube, and label it appropriately.
- Apply direct pressure to the venipuncture site until bleeding stops.
- If a hematoma develops at the I.V. or venipuncture site, apply warm soaks.
- Instruct the patient that he may resume his usual diet, activities, and medications discontinued before the test, as ordered.

Precautions

- Collect each sample at the scheduled time, and specify the collection time on the laboratory request.

- Send each sample to the laboratory immediately because hGH has a half-life of only 20 to 25 minutes.
- Handle the samples gently to prevent hemolysis.

Reference values

Arginine should raise hGH levels to more than 10 ng/ml (SI, > 10 µg/L) in men, more than 15 ng/ml (SI, > 15 µg/L) in women, and more than 48 ng/ml (SI, > 48 µg/L) in children. Such an increase may appear in the first sample collected 30 minutes after arginine infusion is discontinued or in the samples collected 60 and 90 minutes afterward.

Abnormal findings

Levels that are elevated during fasting or that rise during sleep help to rule out hGH deficiency. Failure of hGH levels to rise after arginine infusion indicates decreased anterior pituitary hGH reserve. In children, this deficiency causes dwarfism; in adults, it can indicate panhypopituitarism. When hGH levels fail to reach 10 ng/ml, retesting is required at the same time of day as the original test.

Interfering factors

- Failure to observe pretest restrictions
- Hemolysis due to rough handling of the sample
- Radioactive scan performed within 1 week before the test

Serum follicle-stimulating hormone

The follicle-stimulating hormone (FSH) test of gonadal function, performed more commonly on women than on men, measures FSH levels and is vital in infertility studies. Its overall diagnostic significance typically depends on the results of related hormone tests (for luteinizing hormone, estrogen, or progesterone, for example).

A glycoprotein secreted by the anterior pituitary gland, FSH stimulates gonadal activity in both sexes. In females, it spurs development of primary ovarian follicles into graafian follicles for ovulation. Secretion varies diurnally and fluctuates during the menstrual cycle, peaking at ovulation. In males, continuous secretion of FSH (and testosterone) stimulates and maintains spermatogenesis. Plasma levels fluctuate widely in females; to obtain a true baseline level, daily testing may be necessary (for 3 to 5 days), or multiple samples may be drawn on the same day.

Purpose
■ To aid in the diagnosis and treatment of infertility and disorders of menstruation such as amenorrhea
■ To aid in the diagnosis of precocious puberty in girls (before age 9) and in boys (before age 10)
■ To aid in the differential diagnosis of hypogonadism

Patient preparation
■ Explain to the patient, or her parents if she's a minor, that this test helps determine if her hormonal secretion is normal.
■ Tell the patient that the test requires a blood sample. Explain who will perform the venipuncture and when.
■ Explain to the patient that she may experience slight discomfort from the needle puncture and the tourniquet.
■ Withhold medications that may interfere with accurate determination of test results for 48 hours before the test, as ordered. If they must be continued (for example, for infertility treatment), note this on the laboratory request.
■ Make sure the patient is relaxed and recumbent for 30 minutes before the test.

Procedure and posttest care
■ Perform a venipuncture, preferably between 6 a.m. and 8 a.m., and collect the sample in a 7-ml clot-activator tube. Send the sample to the laboratory immediately.
■ Apply direct pressure to the venipuncture site until bleeding stops.
■ If a hematoma develops at the venipuncture site, apply warm soaks.
■ Instruct the patient that she may resume medications discontinued before the test, as ordered.

Precautions
■ Handle the sample gently to prevent hemolysis.
■ If the patient is female, indicate the phase of her menstrual cycle on the laboratory request. If she's menopausal, note this on the laboratory request.

Reference values
Reference values vary greatly, depending on the patient's age, stage of sexual development, and — for a female — phase of her menstrual cycle. For the menstruating female, approximate FSH values are as follows:
■ follicular phase: 5 to 20 mIU/ml (SI, 5 to 20 IU/L)
■ ovulatory phase: 15 to 30 mIU/ml (SI, 15 to 30 IU/L)
■ luteal phase: 5 to 15 mIU/ml (SI, 5 to 15 IU/L).

Approximate FSH values for men range from 5 to 20 mIU/ml (SI, 5 to 20 IU/L); for menopausal women, 50 to 100 mIU/ml (SI, 50 to 100 IU/L).

Abnormal findings
Decreased FSH levels may cause male or female infertility: aspermatogenesis in men and anovulation in women. Low FSH levels may indicate secondary hypogonadotropic states, which can result

from anorexia nervosa, panhypopituitarism, or hypothalamic lesions.

High FSH levels in women may indicate ovarian failure associated with Turner's syndrome (primary hypogonadism) or Stein-Leventhal syndrome (polycystic ovary syndrome). Elevated levels may occur in patients with precocious puberty (idiopathic or with central nervous system lesions) and in postmenopausal women. In men, abnormally high FSH levels may indicate destruction of the testes (from mumps orchitis or X-ray exposure), testicular failure, seminoma, or male climacteric. Congenital absence of the gonads and early-stage acromegaly may cause FSH levels to rise in both sexes.

Interfering factors
- Failure to observe pretest restrictions
- Hemolysis due to rough handling of the sample
- Ovarian steroid hormones, such as estrogen and progesterone, related compounds, and phenothiazines such as chlorpromazine (possible decrease through negative feedback by inhibiting FSH flow from the hypothalamus and pituitary gland)
- Radioactive scan performed within 1 week before the test

Plasma luteinizing hormone

The plasma luteinizing hormone (LH) test, usually ordered for anovulation and infertility studies in women, is a quantitative analysis of plasma LH or interstitial cell-stimulating hormone levels. Performed most commonly on females, it's usually ordered for anovulation and infertility studies. For accurate diagnosis, results must be evaluated in light of findings obtained from related hormone tests

(follicle-stimulating hormone [FSH], estrogen, and testosterone, for example).

LH is a glycoprotein secreted by basophilic cells of the anterior pituitary gland. In women, cyclic LH secretion (with FSH) causes ovulation and transforms the ovarian follicle into the corpus luteum, which in turn secretes progesterone. (See *LH secretion peaks at ovulation,* pages 148 and 149.) In males, continuous LH secretion stimulates the interstitial (Leydig) cells of the testes to release testosterone, which stimulates and maintains spermatogenesis (with FSH).

Purpose
- To detect ovulation
- To assess male or female infertility
- To evaluate amenorrhea
- To monitor therapy designed to induce ovulation

Patient preparation
- Explain to the patient that this test helps determine if her secretion of female hormones is normal.
- Because there's no evidence that plasma LH levels are affected by fasting, eating, or exercise, such pretest restrictions may be unnecessary.
- Tell the patient that this test requires a blood sample. Explain who will perform the venipuncture and when.
- Inform the patient that she may experience slight discomfort from the needle puncture and the tourniquet.
- Withhold drugs that may interfere with plasma LH levels, such as steroids (including estrogens and progesterone), for 48 hours before the test, as ordered. If they must be continued, note this on the laboratory request.

LH SECRETION PEAKS AT OVULATION

The menstrual cycle is divided into three distinct phases: the menstrual phase (days 1 to 5); the proliferative, or follicular, phase (days 6 to 13); and after ovulation on day 14, the secretory, or luteal, phase (days 15 to 28).

The menstrual phase
This phase of the normal cycle is characterized by endometrial sloughing, corpus luteum degeneration, and new follicle growth. During this stage, the concentra-

tion of estrogen and progesterone is low, triggering increased follicle-stimulating hormone (FSH) and luteinizing hormone (LH) secretion.

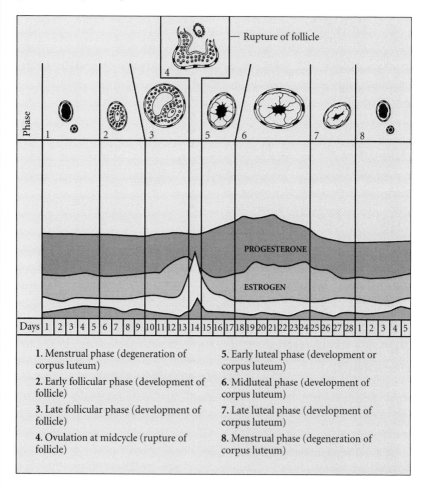

1. Menstrual phase (degeneration of corpus luteum)

2. Early follicular phase (development of follicle)

3. Late follicular phase (development of follicle)

4. Ovulation at midcycle (rupture of follicle)

5. Early luteal phase (development or corpus luteum)

6. Midluteal phase (development of corpus luteum)

7. Late luteal phase (development of corpus luteum)

8. Menstrual phase (degeneration of corpus luteum)

The follicular phase

During the follicular phase, the follicle stimulated by FSH reaches full size and increase its secretion of estrogen. Simultaneously with increased estrogen, FSH decreases while LH increases slowly but steadily. During the late follicular phase, LH rises sharply and FSH rises slightly. At about the 14th day, within hours of this abrupt surge in LH, estrogen levels in the plasma drop and ovulation occurs. After ovulation, the concentration of LH and FSH falls rapidly.

The secretory phase

During the final, or luteal, phase, the follicle reorganizes as the corpus luteum secretes progesterone and estrogen. Within 7 to 8 days after ovulation, if fertilization hasn't occurred, the corpus luteum regresses and progesterone and estrogen levels decrease. The endometrium sloughs, and the menstrual cycle begins again.

Procedure and posttest care

- Perform a venipuncture, and collect the sample in a 7-ml clot-activator tube.
- Apply direct pressure to the venipuncture site until bleeding stops.
- If a hematoma develops at the venipuncture site, apply warm soaks.
- Instruct the patient that she may resume medications discontinued before the test, as ordered.

Precautions

- Handle the sample gently to prevent hemolysis.
- If the patient is a female, indicate the phase of her menstrual cycle on the laboratory request. Make a note if the patient is menopausal.

Reference values

AGE ISSUE *Normal LH values may have a wide range, as follows:*
– *adult females: follicular phase — 5 to 15 mIU/ml (SI, 5 to 15 IU/L); ovulatory phase — 30 to 60 mIU/ml (SI, 30 to 60 IU/L); luteal phase — 5 to 15 mIU/ml (SI, 5 to 15 IU/L)*
– *postmenopausal females: 50 to 100 mIU/ ml (SI, 50 to 100 IU/L)*
– *adult males: 5 to 20 mIU/ml (SI, 5 to 20 IU/L)*
– *children: 4 to 20 mIU/ml (SI, 4 to 20 IU/L).*

Abnormal findings

In women, absence of a midcycle peak in plasma LH levels may indicate anovulation. Decreased or low-normal plasma LH levels may indicate hypogonadism; these findings are commonly associated with amenorrhea. High plasma LH levels may indicate congenital absence of ovaries or ovarian failure associated with

Stein-Leventhal syndrome (polycystic ovary syndrome), Turner's syndrome (ovarian dysgenesis), menopause, or early-stage acromegaly. Infertility can result from primary or secondary gonadal dysfunction.

In men, low plasma LH values may indicate secondary gonadal dysfunction (of hypothalamic or pituitary origin); high values may indicate testicular failure (primary hypogonadism) or destruction or congenital absence of testes.

Interfering factors
- Failure to observe pretest restrictions
- Hemolysis due to rough handling of the sample
- Steroids, including estrogens, progesterone, and testosterone (possible decrease)
- Radioactive scan performed within 1 week before the test

Serum prolactin

Similar in molecular structure and biological activity to growth hormone (hGH), prolactin is a polypeptide hormone secreted by the anterior pituitary gland. Prolactin is essential for the development of the mammary glands for lactation during pregnancy and for stimulating and maintaining lactation postpartum. (See *Physiology of lactation.*) Like hGH, prolactin acts directly on tissues, and its levels rise in response to sleep and physical or emotional stress.

This radioimmunoassay is a quantitative analysis of serum prolactin levels, which normally rise 10- to 20-fold during pregnancy, corresponding to concomitant elevations in human placental lactogen levels. After delivery, prolactin secretion falls to basal levels in mothers who don't breast-feed. However, prolactin secretion increases during breast-feeding, apparently as a result of a stimulus triggered by suckling that curtails the release of prolactin-inhibiting factor by the hypothalamus. This, in turn, allows transient elevations of prolactin secretion by the pituitary gland.

This test is considered useful in patients suspected of having pituitary tumors, which are known to secrete prolactin in excessive amounts. Another test used to evaluate hypothalamic dysfunction is the thyrotropin-releasing hormone (TRH) stimulation test. (See *TRH stimulation test,* page 152.)

Purpose
- To facilitate diagnosis of pituitary dysfunction, possibly due to pituitary adenoma
- To aid in the diagnosis of hypothalamic dysfunction regardless of cause
- To evaluate secondary amenorrhea and galactorrhea

Patient preparation
- Tell the patient that this test helps evaluate hormonal secretion.
- Advise the patient to restrict food and fluids and limit physical activity for 12 hours before the test. Encourage her to relax for about 30 minutes before the test.
- Tell the patient the test requires a blood sample. Explain who will perform the venipuncture and when.
- Explain to the patient that she may experience slight discomfort from the needle puncture and the tourniquet.
- Withhold drugs that may interfere with test results, as ordered. If they must be continued, note this on the laboratory request.

PHYSIOLOGY OF LACTATION

During pregnancy, progesterone and estrogen normally interact to suppress milk secretion while developing the breasts for lactation. Estrogen causes the breasts to grow by increasing their fat content; progesterone causes lobule growth and develops the alveolar cells' secretory capacity.

After childbirth, the mother's anterior pituitary gland secretes prolactin (suppressed during pregnancy), which helps the alveolar epithelium produce and release colostrum. Usually, within 3 days of prolactin release, the breasts secrete large amounts of milk rather than colostrum. The infant's sucking stimu-lates nerve endings at the nipple, initiating the let-down reflex that allows the expression of milk from the mother's breasts. Sucking also stimulates the release of another pituitary hormone, oxytocin, into the mother's bloodstream. This hormone causes alveolar contraction, which forces milk into the ducts and the lactiferous sinuses beneath the alveolar surface, making milk available to the infant. (It also promotes normal involution of the uterus.) Because the infant's suckling stimulates milk production and expression, the more the infant breast-feeds, the more milk the breast produces.

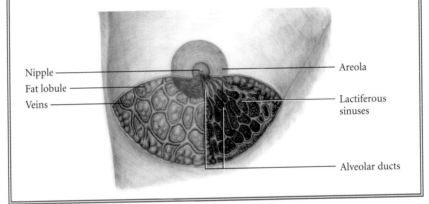

Nipple — Areola
Fat lobule — Lactiferous sinuses
Veins — Alveolar ducts

Procedure and posttest care

■ Perform a venipuncture at least 3 hours after the patient wakes; samples collected earlier are likely to show sleep-induced peak levels. Collect the sample in a 7-ml clot-activator tube.

■ Apply direct pressure to the venipuncture site until bleeding stops.

■ If a hematoma develops at the venipuncture site, apply warm soaks.

■ Instruct the patient that she may resume her usual diet, activities, and medications discontinued before the test, as ordered.

Precautions

■ Handle the sample gently to prevent hemolysis.

■ Confirm slight elevations with repeat measurements on two other occasions.

Reference values

Normal values range from undetectable to 23 ng/ml (SI, 23 µg/L) in nonlactating females. Levels normally rise ten- to twentyfold during pregnancy and, after delivery, fall to basal levels in mothers who don't breast-feed. Prolactin secretion increases during breast-feeding.

TRH STIMULATION TEST

The thyrotropin-releasing hormone (TRH) test evaluates hypothalamic dysfunction and pituitary tumors by stimulating the release of prolactin. The procedure is as follows: perform a venipuncture in the basal state to obtain a baseline prolactin level, and then place the patient in the supine position. Administer an I.V. bolus dose (500 mcg) of synthetic TRH over 15 to 30 seconds. Take blood samples at 15- and 30-minute intervals to measure prolactin.

A baseline prolactin reading greater than 200 ng/ml (SI, 200 IU/L) indicates a pituitary tumor, but levels between 30 and 200 ng/ml (SI, 30 to 200 IU/L) are also consistent with this condition. Normally, patients show at least a twofold increase in prolactin after injection with TRH. If the prolactin level fails to rise, hypothalamic dysfunction or adenoma of the pituitary gland is likely.

Abnormal findings

Abnormally high prolactin levels (100 to 300 ng/ml [SI, 100 to 300 µg/L]) suggest autonomous prolactin production by a pituitary adenoma, especially when amenorrhea or galactorrhea is present (Forbes-Albright syndrome). Rarely, hyperprolactinemia may also result from severe endocrine disorders such as hypothyroidism. Idiopathic hyperprolactinemia may be associated with anovulatory infertility. Confirm slight elevations with repeat measurements on two other occasions.

Decreased prolactin levels in a lactating mother cause failure of lactation and may be associated with postpartum pituitary infarction (Sheehan's syndrome). Abnormally low prolactin levels have also been found in the patient with empty-sella syndrome. In these cases, a flattened pituitary gland makes the pituitary fossa look empty.

Interfering factors

- Failure to take into account physiologic variations related to sleep or stress
- Ethanol, morphine, methyldopa, and estrogens (increase)
- Apomorphine, ergot alkaloids, and levodopa (decrease)
- Radioactive scan performed within 1 week before the test or recent surgery
- Breast stimulation
- Hemolysis due to rough handling of the sample

Serum thyroid-stimulating hormone

Thyroid-stimulating hormone (TSH), or thyrotropin, promotes increases in the size, number, and activity of thyroid cells and stimulates the release of triiodothyronine and thyroxine. These hormones affect total body metabolism and are essential for normal growth and development.

This test measures serum TSH levels by radioimmunoassay. It can detect primary hypothyroidism and determine whether the hypothyroidism results from thyroid gland failure or from pituitary or hypothalamic dysfunction. Normal serum TSH levels rule out primary hypothyroidism. This test may not distinguish between low-normal and subnormal levels, especially in secondary hypothyroidism.

Purpose

- To confirm or rule out primary hypothyroidism and distinguish it from secondary hypothyroidism
- To monitor drug therapy in the patient with primary hypothyroidism

Patient preparation

- Explain to the patient that this test helps assess thyroid gland function.
- Tell the patient that the test requires a blood sample. Explain who will perform the venipuncture and when.
- Explain to the patient that he may experience slight discomfort from the needle puncture and the tourniquet.
- Withhold steroids, thyroid hormones, aspirin, and other medications that may influence test results, as ordered. If they must be continued, note this on the laboratory request.
- Keep the patient relaxed and recumbent for 30 minutes before the test.

Procedure and posttest care

- Between 6 a.m. and 8 a.m., perform a venipuncture and collect the sample in a 5-ml clot-activator tube.
- Apply direct pressure to the venipuncture site until bleeding stops.
- If a hematoma develops at the venipuncture site, apply warm soaks.
- Instruct the patient that he may resume medications discontinued before the test, as ordered.

Precautions

- Handle the sample gently to prevent hemolysis.

Reference values

Normal TSH values range from undetectable to 15 µIU/ml (SI, 15 mU/L).

Abnormal findings

TSH levels may be slightly elevated in euthyroid patients with thyroid cancer. Levels that exceed 20 µIU/ml (SI, 20 mU/L) suggest primary hypothyroidism or, possibly, endemic goiter.

Low or undetectable TSH levels may be normal, but occasionally indicate secondary hypothyroidism (with inadequate

---

TRH CHALLENGE TEST

The thyrotropin-releasing hormone (TRH) challenge test, which evaluates thyroid function and is the first direct test of pituitary reserve, is a reliable diagnostic tool in thyrotoxicosis (Graves' disease). The challenge test requires an injection of TRH.

How it's done

After a venipuncture is performed to obtain a baseline thyroid-stimulating hormone (TSH) reading, synthetic TRH (protirelin) is administered by I.V. bolus in a dose of 200 to 500 mcg. As many as five samples (5 ml each) are then drawn at 5, 10, 15, 20, and 60 minutes after the TRH injection to assess thyroid response. To facilitate blood collection, an indwelling catheter can be used to obtain the required samples.

What the test shows

A sudden spike above the baseline TSH reading indicates a normally functioning pituitary, but suggests hypothalamic dysfunction. If the TSH level fails to rise or remains undetectable, pituitary failure is likely. In thyrotoxicosis and thyroiditis, TSH levels fail to rise when challenged by TRH.

---

secretion of TSH or thyrotropin-releasing hormone [TRH]). Low TSH levels may also result from hyperthyroidism (Graves' disease) and thyroiditis; both are marked by hypersecretion of thyroid hormones, which suppresses TSH release. Provocative testing with TRH is necessary to confirm the diagnosis. (See *TRH challenge test.*)

Interfering factors

- Failure to observe pretest restrictions

- Hemolysis due to rough handling of the sample

Neonatal thyroid-stimulating hormone

The neonatal thyroid-stimulating hormone (TSH) test is an immunoassay that confirms congenital hypothyroidism after an initial screening test detects low thyroxine (T_4) levels. Normally, TSH levels surge after birth, triggering a rise in thyroid hormone that's essential for neurologic development. In primary congenital hypothyroidism, the thyroid gland doesn't respond to TSH stimulation, resulting in diminished thyroid hormone levels and elevated TSH levels. Early detection and treatment of congenital hypothyroidism is critical to prevent mental retardation and cretinism.

Purpose

- To confirm diagnosis of congenital hypothyroidism

Patient preparation

- Explain to the infant's parents that this test helps confirm the diagnosis of congenital hypothyroidism. Emphasize the importance of detecting the disorder early so that prompt therapy can prevent irreversible brain damage.

Equipment
Filter paper sample

- Alcohol or povidone-iodine swabs, sterile lancet, specially marked filter paper, 2″ x 2″ sterile gauze pads, adhesive bandage, labels, gloves

Serum sample

- Venipuncture equipment

Procedure and posttest care
Filter paper sample

- Assemble the necessary equipment, wash your hands thoroughly, and put on gloves.
- Wipe the infant's heel with an alcohol or povidone-iodine swab, and then dry it thoroughly with a gauze pad.
- Perform a heelstick.
- Squeezing the infant's heel gently, fill the circles on the filter paper with blood. Make sure the blood saturates the paper.
- Gently apply pressure with a gauze pad to ensure hemostasis at the puncture site.
- Allow the filter paper to dry, label it appropriately, and send it to the laboratory.

Serum sample

- Perform a venipuncture, and collect the sample in a 3-ml clot-activator tube. Label the sample and send it to the laboratory immediately.
- Apply direct pressure to the venipuncture or heelstick site until bleeding stops.
- If a hematoma develops at the venipuncture site, apply warm soaks.

Precautions

- Handle the samples carefully to prevent hemolysis.

Reference values

At age 1 to 2 days, TSH levels are normally 25 to 30 µIU/ml (SI, 25 to 30 mU/L). Thereafter, levels are normally less than 25 µIU/ml (SI, < 25 mU/L).

Abnormal findings

Neonatal TSH levels must be interpreted in light of the T_4 concentration. Elevated TSH levels accompanied by decreased T_4 levels indicates primary congenital hypothyroidism (thyroid gland dysfunction). Low TSH and T_4 levels may be present in secondary congenital hypothyroidism (pituitary or hypothalamic dysfunction). Normal TSH levels accompanied by low T_4 levels may indicate hypothyroidism due to a congenital defect in T_4-binding globulin or transient congenital hypothyroidism due to prematurity or prenatal hypoxia. A complete thyroid workup must be done to confirm the cause of hypothyroidism before treatment can begin.

Interfering factors
- Failure to let a filter paper sample dry completely
- Hemolysis due to rough handling of the sample
- Corticosteroids, triiodothyronine, and T_4 (decrease)
- Lithium carbonate, potassium iodide, excessive topical resorcinol, and TSH injection (increase)

Serum antidiuretic hormone

Antidiuretic hormone (ADH), also called vasopressin, promotes water reabsorption in response to increased osmolality (water deficiency with high concentration of sodium and other solutes). In response to decreased osmolality (water excess), reduced secretion of ADH allows increased excretion of water to maintain fluid balance. (See *ADH release and regulation,* page 156.) Along with aldosterone, ADH helps regulate sodium, potassium, and fluid balance. It also stimulates vascular smooth-muscle contraction, causing an increase in arterial blood pressure.

This relatively rare test, a quantitative analysis of serum ADH levels, may identify diabetes insipidus and other causes of severe homeostatic imbalance. It may be ordered as part of dehydration or hypertonic saline infusion testing, which determines the body's response to states of hyperosmolality.

Purpose
- To aid in the differential diagnosis of pituitary diabetes insipidus, nephrogenic diabetes insipidus (congenital or familial), and syndrome of inappropriate antidiuretic hormone (SIADH)

Patient preparation
- Explain to the patient that this test, used to measure hormonal secretion levels, may aid in identifying the cause of his symptoms.
- Instruct the patient to fast and limit physical activity for 10 to 12 hours before the test.
- Tell the patient that the test requires a blood sample. Explain who will perform the venipuncture and when.
- Explain to the patient that he may experience slight discomfort from the needle puncture and the tourniquet.
- Withhold medications that may cause SIADH before the test, as ordered. If they must be continued, note this on the laboratory request.
- Make sure the patient is relaxed and recumbent for 30 minutes before the test.

Procedure and posttest care
- Perform a venipuncture and collect the sample in a plastic collection tube (without additives) or a chilled EDTA tube.
- Immediately send the sample to the laboratory, where serum must be separated from the clot within 10 minutes.
- Perform a serum osmolality test at the same time to help interpret the results.
- Apply direct pressure to the venipuncture site until bleeding stops.
- If a hematoma develops at the venipuncture site, apply warm soaks.

ADH RELEASE AND REGULATION

Neural impulses signal the supraoptic nuclei of the hypothalamus to produce antidiuretic hormone (ADH). After it's formed, ADH moves along the hypothalamicohypophysial tract to the posterior pituitary, where it's stored until needed by the kidneys to maintain fluid balance. In the kidneys, ADH acts on the collecting tubules to retain water.

Homeostasis is maintained by a negative feedback mechanism: Ample water or water excess inhibits further ADH secretion by the supraoptic nuclei of the hypothalamus or ADH release from the posterior pituitary. A similar negative feedback mechanism that's vital to hormonal homeostasis prevents oversecretion of other hormones.

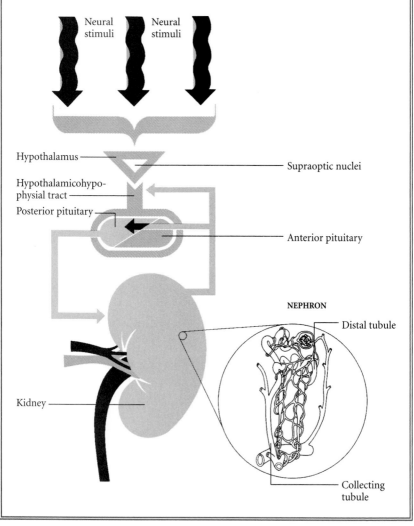

- Instruct the patient that he may resume his usual diet, activities, and medications discontinued before the test, as ordered.

Precautions
- Make sure you use a syringe and collection tube made of plastic because the fragile ADH degrades on contact with glass.

Reference values
ADH values range from 1 to 5 pg/ml (SI, 1 to 5 mg/L). It may also be evaluated in light of serum osmolality; if serum osmolality is less than 285 mOsm/kg, ADH is normally less than 2 pg/ml (SI, < 2 mg/L); if it's greater than 290 mOsm/kg, ADH may range from 2 to 12 pg/ml (SI, 2 to 12 mg/L).

Abnormal findings
Absent or below-normal ADH levels indicate pituitary diabetes insipidus, resulting from a neurohypophyseal or hypothalamic tumor, viral infection, metastatic disease, sarcoidosis, tuberculosis, Hand-Schüller-Christian disease, syphilis, neurosurgical procedures, or head trauma.

Normal ADH levels in the presence of signs of diabetes insipidus (such as polydipsia, polyuria, and hypotonic urine) may indicate the nephrogenic form of the disease, marked by renal tubular resistance to ADH; however, levels may rise if the pituitary gland tries to compensate.

Elevated ADH levels may also indicate SIADH, possibly as a result of bronchogenic carcinoma, acute porphyria, hypothyroidism, Addison's disease, cirrhosis of the liver, infectious hepatitis, severe hemorrhage, or circulatory shock.

Interfering factors
- Failure to observe pretest restrictions

- Morphine, anesthetics, estrogen, oxytocin, chlorpropamide, vincristine, carbamazepine, cyclophosphamide, tranquilizers, hypnotics, lithium carbonate, and chlorothiazide (increase)
- Stress, pain, and positive-pressure ventilation (increase)
- Alcohol and negative-pressure ventilation (decrease)
- Radioactive scan performed within 1 week before the test
- Delay in sending sample to the laboratory

Alpha-subunit of pituitary glycoprotein hormones

Using radioimmunoassay, the alpha-subunit of pituitary glycoprotein hormone test measures the alpha-subunit of the pituitary glycoprotein hormones (alpha-PGH). These hormones—thyroid-stimulating hormone (TSH) and human chorionic gonadotropin—contain similar alpha-subunits but differ in their beta-subunits. Alpha-PGH measurement assesses total pituitary production of these hormones.

Purpose
- To aid diagnosis of recurrent pituitary tumors in the patient who has undergone resection

Patient preparation
- Explain to the patient that this test helps assess pituitary function.
- Inform the patient that he need not fast.
- Tell the patient that the test requires a blood sample. Explain who will perform the venipuncture and when.

- Explain to the patient that he may experience slight discomfort from the needle puncture and the tourniquet.

Procedure and posttest care
- Perform a venipuncture and collect the sample in a 5-ml clot-activator tube.
- Send the sample to the laboratory immediately.
- Apply direct pressure to the venipuncture site until bleeding stops.
- If a hematoma develops at the venipuncture site, apply warm soaks.

Precautions
- Handle the sample gently to prevent hemolysis.
- Indicate the patient's sex on the laboratory request.

Reference values
Normal alpha-PGH values are up to 1.2 ng/ml (SI, 1.2 µg/L).

Abnormal findings
Low levels of alpha-PGH appear in the patient with inadequate pituitary hormone production. Hypopituitarism results in reduced follicle-stimulating hormone, luteinizing hormone, and TSH levels.

Elevated alpha-PGH levels indicate recurrent pituitary tumors or ineffective treatment.

Interfering factors
- Hemolysis due to rough handling of the sample.

THYROID AND PARATHYROID HORMONE TESTS

Serum thyroxine

Thyroxine (T_4) is an amine secreted by the thyroid gland in response to thyroid-stimulating hormone (TSH) and, indirectly, thyrotropin-releasing hormone. The rate of secretion is normally regulated by a complex system of negative and positive feedback involving the thyroid, anterior pituitary, and hypothalamus. The suspected precursor, or prohormone, of triiodothyronine (T_3), T_4 is believed to convert to T_3 by monodeiodination, which occurs mainly in the liver and kidneys.

Only a fraction of T4 (about 0.05%) circulates freely in the blood; the rest binds strongly to plasma proteins, primarily thyroxine-binding globulin (TBG). This minute fraction is responsible for the clinical effects of thyroid hormone. TBG binds so tenaciously that T4 survives in the plasma for a relatively long time, with a half-life of about 6 days. This immunoassay, one of the most common thyroid diagnostic tools, measures the total circulating T4 level when TBG is normal. An alternative test is the Murphy-Pattee or T4 (D), based on competitive protein binding.

Purpose
- To evaluate thyroid function
- To aid diagnosis of hyperthyroidism and hypothyroidism
- To monitor the patient's response to antithyroid medication in hyperthyroidism or to thyroid replacement therapy in hypothyroidism (TSH estimates are needed to confirm hypothyroidism.)

Patient preparation
- Explain to the patient that this test helps evaluate thyroid gland function.
- Inform the patient that he need not fast or restrict activity.
- Tell the patient that the test requires a blood sample. Explain who will perform the venipuncture and when.
- Withhold medications that may interfere with test results, as ordered. If they must be continued, note this on the laboratory request. If this test is being performed to monitor thyroid therapy, the patient should continue to receive daily thyroid supplements.

Procedure and posttest care
- Perform a venipuncture and collect the sample in a 7-ml clot-activator tube.
- Send the sample to the laboratory immediately so that the serum can be separated.
- Apply direct pressure to the venipuncture site until bleeding stops.
- If a hematoma develops at the venipuncture site, apply warm soaks.
- Instruct the patient that he may resume medications discontinued before the test, as ordered.

Precautions
- Handle the sample gently to prevent hemolysis.

Reference values
Normally, total T_4 levels range from 5 to 13.5 µg/dl (SI, 60 to 165 mmol/L).

Abnormal findings
Abnormally elevated T_4 levels are consistent with primary and secondary hyperthyroidism, including excessive T_4 (levothyroxine) replacement therapy (factitious or iatrogenic hyperthyroidism). Subnormal levels suggest primary or secondary hypothyroidism or may be due to T_4 suppression by normal, elevated, or replacement T_3 levels. In doubtful cases of hypothyroidism, TSH levels may be indicated.

Normal T_4 levels don't guarantee euthyroidism; for example, normal readings occur in T_3 toxicosis. Overt signs of hyperthyroidism require further testing.

Interfering factors
- Hemolysis due to rough handling of the sample
- Hereditary factors and hepatic disease (possible increase or decrease in TBG)
- Protein-wasting disease (such as nephrotic syndrome) and androgens (possible decrease in TBG)
- Estrogens, progestins, levothyroxine, and methadone (increase)
- Free fatty acids, heparin, iodides, liothyronine sodium, lithium, methylthiouracil, phenylbutazone, phenytoin, propylthiouracil, salicylates (high doses), steroids, sulfonamides, and sulfonylureas (decrease)
- Clofibrate (possible increase or decrease)

Serum triiodothyronine

The triiodothyronine (T_3) test is highly specific radioimmunoassay that measures total (bound and free) serum content of T_3 to investigate clinical indications of thyroid dysfunction. T_3, the more potent thyroid hormone, is an amine derived primarily from thyroxine (T_4) through the process of monodeiodination. At least 50% and as much as 90% of T_3 is thought to be derived from T_4 as a result of this pivotal transformation, during which T_4 loses one of its iodine atoms to become T_3. The remaining 10% or more is secreted directly by the thyroid gland. Like T_4

secretion, T_3 secretion occurs in response to thyroid-stimulating hormone (TSH) and, secondarily, thyrotropin-releasing hormone.

Although T_3 is present in the bloodstream in minute quantities and is metabolically active for only a short time, its impact on body metabolism dominates that of T_4. Another significant difference between the two major thyroid hormones is that T_3 binds less firmly to thyroxine—binding globulin (TBG). Consequently, T_3 persists in the bloodstream for a short time; half disappears in about 1 day, whereas half of T_4 disappears in 6 days.

Purpose
■ To aid diagnosis of T_3 toxicosis
■ To aid diagnosis of hypothyroidism and hyperthyroidism
■ To monitor the patient's response to thyroid replacement therapy in hypothyroidism

Patient preparation
■ Explain to the patient that this test helps to evaluate thyroid gland function and determine the cause of his symptoms.
■ Withhold medications, such as steroids, propranolol, and cholestyramine, which may influence thyroid function, as ordered. If they must be continued, record this information on the laboratory request.
■ Tell the patient that the test requires a blood sample. Explain who will perform the venipuncture and when.
■ Explain to the patient that he may experience slight discomfort from the needle puncture and the tourniquet.

Procedure and posttest care
■ Perform a venipuncture and collect the sample in a 7-ml clot-activator tube.
■ Send the sample to the laboratory as soon as possible to avoid stasis and to allow early separation of serum from the clotted blood.
■ Apply direct pressure to the venipuncture site until bleeding stops.
■ If a hematoma develops at the venipuncture site, apply warm soaks.
■ Instruct the patient that he may resume medications discontinued before the test, as ordered.

Precautions
■ Handle the sample gently to prevent hemolysis.
■ If the patient must receive thyroid preparations, such as T_3 (liothyronine), note the administration time on the laboratory request. Otherwise, T_3 levels aren't reliable.

Reference values
Normal serum T_3 levels range from 80 to 200 ng/dl (SI, 1.2 to 3 nmol/L).

Abnormal findings
Serum T_3 and T_4 levels usually rise and fall in tandem. However, in T_3 toxicosis, T_3 levels rise while total and free T_4 levels remain normal. T_3 toxicosis occurs in the patient with Graves' disease, toxic adenoma, or toxic nodular goiter. T_3 levels also surpass T_4 levels in the patient receiving thyroid replacement therapy containing more T_3 than T_4. In iodine-deficient areas, the thyroid may produce larger amounts of the more cellularly active T_3 than of T_4 in an effort to maintain the euthyroid state.

Generally, T_3 levels appear to be a more accurate diagnostic indicator of hyperthyroidism. Although T_3 and T_4 levels are increased in about 90% of patients with hyperthyroidism, there's a disproportionate increase in T_3. In some patients with hypothyroidism, T_3 levels may fall within the normal range and not be diagnostically significant.

A rise in serum T_3 levels normally occurs during pregnancy. Low T_3 levels may appear in the euthyroid patient with systemic illness (especially hepatic or renal disease), during severe acute illness, and after trauma or major surgery; in such cases, TSH levels are within normal limits. Low serum T_3 levels are sometimes found in the euthyroid patient with malnutrition.

Interfering factors
- Hemolysis due to rough handling of the sample
- Markedly increased or decreased TBG levels, regardless of cause
- Failure to take into account medications that affect T_3 levels, such as steroids, clofibrate, cholestyramine, and propranolol (See *Drugs that interfere with T_3 tests.*)

Serum thyroxine-binding globulin

The thyroxine-binding globulin (TBG) test measures the serum level of TBG, the predominant protein carrier for circulating thyroxine (T_4) and triiodothyronine (T_3). TBG values may be identified by saturating the sample for TBG determination with radioactive T_4, then subjecting this to electrophoresis and measuring the amount of TBG by the amount of radioactive T_4 by radioimmunoassay.

Any condition that affects TBG levels and subsequent binding capacity also affects the amount of free T_4 (FT_4) in circulation. An underlying TBG abnormality

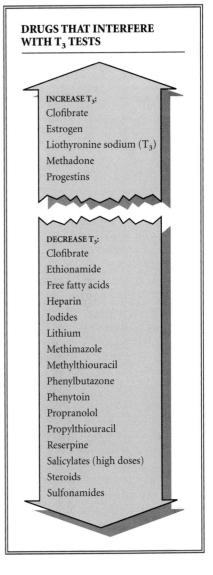

DRUGS THAT INTERFERE WITH T_3 TESTS

INCREASE T_3:
Clofibrate
Estrogen
Liothyronine sodium (T_3)
Methadone
Progestins

DECREASE T_3:
Clofibrate
Ethionamide
Free fatty acids
Heparin
Iodides
Lithium
Methimazole
Methylthiouracil
Phenylbutazone
Phenytoin
Propranolol
Propylthiouracil
Reserpine
Salicylates (high doses)
Steroids
Sulfonamides

renders tests for total T_3 and T_4 inaccurate, but doesn't affect the accuracy of tests for free T_3 (FT_3) and FT_4.

Purpose
- To evaluate abnormal thyrometabolic states that don't correlate with thyroid hormone (T_3 or T_4) values (for example,

a patient with overt signs of hypothyroidism and a low FT_4 level with a high total T_4 level due to a marked increase of TBG secondary to hormonal contraceptives)

■ To identify TBG abnormalities

Patient preparation
■ Explain to the patient that this test helps evaluate thyroid function.
■ Tell the patient that the test requires a blood sample. Explain who will perform the venipuncture and when.
■ Explain to the patient that he may experience slight discomfort from the needle puncture and the tourniquet.
■ Withhold medications that may affect the accuracy of test results, such as estrogens, anabolic steroids, phenytoin, salicylates, or thyroid preparations, as ordered. If they must be continued, note this on the laboratory request. (They may be continued to determine if prescribed drugs are affecting TBG levels.)

Procedure and posttest care
■ Perform a venipuncture, and collect the sample in a 7-ml clot activator tube.
■ Apply direct pressure to the venipuncture site until bleeding stops.
■ If a hematoma develops at the venipuncture site, apply warm soaks.
■ Instruct the patient that he may resume medications discontinued before the test, as ordered.

Precautions
■ Handle the sample gently to prevent hemolysis.

Reference values
Normal values for TBG by immunoassay range from 16 to 32 µg/dl (SI, 120 to 180 mg/ml).

Abnormal findings
Elevated TBG levels may indicate hypothyroidism or congenital (genetic) excess, some forms of hepatic disease, or acute intermittent porphyria. TBG levels normally rise during pregnancy and are high in neonates. Suppressed levels may indicate hyperthyroidism or congenital deficiency and can occur in active acromegaly, nephrotic syndrome, and malnutrition associated with hypoproteinemia, acute illness, or surgical stress.

Patients with TBG abnormalities require additional testing, such as the serum FT_3 and T_4 tests, to evaluate thyroid function more precisely.

Interfering factors
■ Hemolysis due to rough handling of the sample
■ Estrogens, including hormonal contraceptives, and phenothiazines such as perphenazine (increase)
■ Androgens, prednisone, phenytoin, and high doses of salicylates (decrease)

T_3 uptake

Also called triiodothyronine (T_3) uptake, the T_3 uptake test indirectly measures free thyroxine (FT_4) levels by demonstrating the availability of serum protein-binding sites for thyroxine (T_4). The results of T_3 uptake are frequently combined with a T_4 radioimmunoassay or T_4 (D) (competitive protein-binding test) to determine the FT_4 index, a mathematical calculation thought to reflect FT_4 by correcting for thyroxine-binding globulin (TBG) abnormalities.

The T_3 uptake test has become less popular recently because rapid tests for T_3, T_4, and thyroid-stimulating hormone are readily available.

Purpose
- To aid diagnosis of hypothyroidism and hyperthyroidism when TBG is normal
- To aid diagnosis of primary disorders of TBG levels

Patient preparation
- Explain to the patient that this test helps evaluate thyroid function.
- Tell the patient that the test requires a blood sample. Explain who will perform the venipuncture and when.
- Explain to the patient that he may experience slight discomfort from the needle puncture and the tourniquet.
- Tell the patient that the laboratory requires several days to complete the analysis.
- Withhold medications that may interfere with test results, such as estrogens, androgens, phenytoin, salicylates, and thyroid preparations, as ordered. If they must be continued, note this on the laboratory request.

Procedure and posttest care
- Perform a venipuncture and collect the sample in a 7-ml clot-activator tube.
- Apply direct pressure to the venipuncture site until bleeding stops.
- If a hematoma develops at the venipuncture site, apply warm soaks.
- Instruct the patient that he may resume medications discontinued before the test, as ordered.

Precautions
- Handle the sample gently to prevent hemolysis.

Reference values
Normal T$_3$ uptake values are 25% to 35%.

Abnormal findings
A high T$_3$ uptake percentage in the presence of elevated T$_4$ levels indicates hyperthyroidism (implying few TBG free binding sites and high FT$_4$ levels). A low uptake percentage, together with low T$_4$ levels, indicates hypothyroidism (implying more TBG free binding sites and low FT$_4$ levels). Thus, in primary thyroid disease, T$_4$ and T$_3$ uptake vary in the same direction; availability of binding sites varies inversely.

Discordant variance in T$_4$ and T$_3$ uptake suggests a TBG abnormality. For example, a high T$_3$ uptake percentage and a low or normal FT$_4$ level suggest decreased TBG levels. Such decreased levels may result from protein loss (as in nephrotic syndrome), decreased production (due to androgen excess or genetic or idiopathic causes), or competition for T$_4$ binding sites by certain drugs (salicylates, phenylbutazone, and phenytoin). Conversely, a low T$_3$ uptake percentage and a high or normal FT$_4$ level suggest increased TBG levels. Such increased levels may be due to exogenous or endogenous estrogen (pregnancy) or result from idiopathic causes. Thus, in primary disorders of TBG levels, measured T$_4$ and free sites change in the same direction.

Interfering factors
- Radioisotope scans performed before sample collection
- Anabolic steroids, heparin, phenytoin, salicylates (high dose), thyroid preparations, and warfarin (possible increase in TBG and thyroxine-binding protein electrophoresis)
- Antithyroid agents, clofibrate, estrogen, hormonal contraceptives, and thiazide diuretics (decreased uptake)

Free thyroxine and free triiodothyronine

The free thyroxine (FT_4) and free triiodothyronine (FT_3) tests, commonly done simultaneously, measure serum levels of FT_4 and FT_3, the minute portions of T_4 and T_3 not bound to thyroxine-binding globulin (TBG) and other serum proteins. These unbound hormones are responsible for the thyroid's effects on cellular metabolism. Measurement of free hormone levels is the best indicator of thyroid function.

Because of disagreement as to whether FT_4 or FT_3 is the better indicator, laboratories commonly measure both. The disadvantages of these tests include a cumbersome and difficult laboratory method, inaccessibility, and cost. This test may be useful in the 5% of patients in whom the standard T_3 or T_4 tests fail to produce diagnostic results.

Purpose
- To measure the metabolically active form of the thyroid hormones
- To aid diagnosis of hyperthyroidism and hypothyroidism when TBG levels are abnormal

Patient preparation
- Explain to the patient that this special test helps evaluate thyroid function.
- Tell the patient that the test requires a blood sample. Explain who will perform the venipuncture and when.
- Explain to the patient that he may experience slight discomfort from the needle puncture and the tourniquet.

Procedure and posttest care
- Perform a venipuncture and collect the sample in a 7-ml clot-activator tube.

- Apply direct pressure to the venipuncture site until bleeding stops.
- If a hematoma develops at the venipuncture site, apply warm soaks.

Precautions
- Handle the sample gently to prevent hemolysis.

Reference values
Normal range for FT_4 is 0.9 to 2.3 ng/dl (SI, 10 to 30 nmol/L); for FT_3, 0.2 to 0.6 ng/dl (SI, 0.003 to 0.009 nmol/L). Values vary, depending on the laboratory.

Abnormal findings
Elevated FT_4 and FT_3 levels indicate hyperthyroidism, unless peripheral resistance to thyroid hormone is present. T_3 toxicosis, a distinct form of hyperthyroidism, yields high FT_3 levels with normal or low FT_4 values. Low FT_4 levels usually indicate hypothyroidism, except in patients receiving replacement therapy with T_3. Patients receiving thyroid therapy may have varying levels of FT_4 and FT_3, depending on the preparation used and the time of sample collection.

Interfering factors
- Hemolysis due to rough handling of the sample
- Thyroid therapy, depending on dosage (possible increase)

Screening test for congenital hypothyroidism

The screening test for congenital hypothyroidism measures serum thyroxine (T_4) levels in the neonate to detect congenital hypothyroidism. Characterized by low or absent levels of T_4, congenital hypothyroidism affects roughly 1 in 5,000 neonates, occurring in girls three times more often than in boys. This disorder can result from thyroid dysgenesis or hypoplasia, congenital goiter, or maternal use of thyroid inhibitors during pregnancy. If untreated, it can lead to irreversible brain damage by age 3 months.

Because clinical signs are few, in the past, most cases of congenital hypothyroidism went undetected until cretinism became apparent or death followed respiratory distress. Recently, radioimmunoassays for T_4 and thyroid-stimulating hormone (TSH) have been used effectively to screen neonates for congenital hypothyroidism. This test is now mandatory in some states.

Purpose

- To screen neonates for congenital hypothyroidism

Patient preparation

- Explain to the parents that although hypothyroidism is uncommon in infants, this screening test detects the disorder early enough to begin therapy before irreversible brain damage occurs.
- Tell the parents that the test will be performed before the infant is discharged from the facility and again 4 to 6 weeks later.
- Emphasize the importance of the screening and the need for following the test protocol.
- Because false-positive findings can result from variations in the test procedure or from a congenital thyroxine-binding globulin (TBG) defect, inform the parents that a second test may be done before the infant is discharged.

Equipment

Gloves, alcohol or povidone-iodine swabs, sterile lancet, specially marked filter paper, 2″ × 2″ sterile gauze pads, small adhesive bandage strip, labels for infant's and mother's names, physician's name, room number, and date

Procedure and posttest care

- After assembling the necessary equipment and washing your hands, put on gloves.
- Wipe the infant's heel with an alcohol or a povidone-iodine swab, and then dry it thoroughly with a gauze pad.
- Perform a heelstick.
- Squeezing the heel gently and fill the circles on the filter paper with blood. Make sure the blood saturates the paper. Apply gentle pressure with a gauze pad to ensure hemostasis at the puncture site.
- When the filter paper is dry, label it appropriately and send it to the laboratory.
- Heelsticks heal readily and require no special care.
- If results of the screening test indicate congenital hypothyroidism, tell the parents that additional testing is necessary to determine the cause of the disorder.
- If the sample isn't processed in the facility's laboratory, make sure the parents are notified when test results are available.

Reference values

AGE ISSUE *Immediately after birth, neonatal T_4 levels are considerably higher than normal adult levels. By the end of the first week, T_4 values decrease markedly:*
- *1 to 5 days: 4.9 µg/dl (SI, 58.8 nmol/L)*
- *6 to 8 days: 4 µg/dl (SI, 48 nmol/L)*
- *9 to 11 days: 3.5 µg/dl (SI, 42 nmol/L)*
- *12 to 120 days: 3 µg/dl (SI, 36 nmol/L).*

Abnormal findings

Low serum T_4 levels in the neonate require TSH testing for clarification of the

CALCITONIN STIMULATION TESTS

Stimulation testing is typically necessary in patients with medullary thyroid carcinoma when baseline calcitonin levels fail to rise high enough to confirm the diagnosis. The most common test is a 4-hour I.V. calcium infusion (15 mg/kg) to provoke calcitonin secretion. Samples are taken just before the infusion and at 3 and 4 hours postinfusion. Calcitonin levels rise rapidly after the infusion in patients with medullary thyroid carcinoma.

Another test involves I.V. infusion of pentagastrin (0.5 mcg/kg over 5 to 10 seconds). A blood sample is drawn just before the I.V. infusion and at 90 seconds, 5 minutes, and 10 minutes postinfusion. In patients with medullary thyroid carcinoma, calcitonin levels rise markedly over the baseline reading.

diagnosis. Decreased T_4 levels accompanied by elevated TSH readings (> 25 µU/ml [SI, 300 nmol/L]) indicate primary congenital hypothyroidism (thyroid gland dysfunction). If T_4 and TSH levels are depressed, secondary congenital hypothyroidism (resulting from pituitary or hypothalamic dysfunction) should be suspected.

If T_4 levels are subnormal in the presence of normal TSH readings, further testing is required. Serum TBG levels must be analyzed to identify infants with hypothyroidism resulting from congenital defects in TBG. This low T_4–normal TSH pattern also occurs in a transient form of congenital hypothyroidism, which may accompany prematurity, or prenatal hypoxia.

A complete thyroid workup, including serum T_3, TBG, and free T_4 levels, is necessary for unequivocal diagnosis of congenital hypothyroidism before treatment begins.

Interfering factors
■ Failure to allow filter paper to dry completely
■ Failure to follow special directions for obtaining the sample

Plasma calcitonin

The plasma calcitonin test is a radioimmunoassay that measures plasma levels of calcitonin (thyrocalcitonin). The exact role of calcitonin in normal human physiology hasn't been fully defined. However, calcitonin is known to act as an antagonist to parathyroid hormone and to lower serum calcium levels.

The usual clinical indication for this test is suspected medullary carcinoma of the thyroid, which causes hypersecretion of calcitonin (without associated hypocalcemia). Equivocal results require provocative testing with I.V. pentagastrin or calcium to rule out disease. (See *Calcitonin stimulation tests.*)

Purpose
■ To aid diagnosis of thyroid medullary carcinoma and ectopic calcitonin-producing tumors (rare)

Patient preparation
■ Explain to the patient that this test helps evaluate thyroid function.
■ Instruct the patient to fast overnight because food may interfere with calcium homeostasis and, subsequently, calcitonin levels.

- Tell the patient that the test requires a blood sample. Explain who will perform the venipuncture and when.
- Explain to the patient that he may experience slight discomfort from the needle puncture and the tourniquet.
- Tell him that the laboratory requires several days to complete the analysis.

Procedure and posttest care
- Perform a venipuncture and collect the sample in a 7-ml heparinized tube.
- Apply direct pressure to the venipuncture site until bleeding stops.
- If a hematoma develops at the venipuncture site, apply warm soaks.
- Instruct the patient that he may resume his usual diet.

Precautions
- Handle the sample gently to prevent hemolysis.
- Send the sample to the laboratory immediately.

Reference values
Serum calcitonin levels (basal) normally are 40 pg/ml (SI, 40 ng/L) for males and 20 pg/ml (SI, 20 ng/L) for females.

Reference values after 4-hour calcium infusion are:
- males: 190 pg/ml (SI, 190 ng/L)
- females: 130 pg/ml (SI, 130 ng/L).

Values after testing with pentagastrin infusion are:
- males: 110 pg/ml (SI, 110 ng/L)
- females: 30 pg/ml (SI, 30 ng/L).

Abnormal findings
Elevated serum calcitonin levels in the absence of hypocalcemia usually indicate medullary carcinoma of the thyroid. Transmitted as an autosomal dominant trait, thyroid medullary carcinoma may occur as part of multiple endocrine neo-

plasia. Occasionally, increased calcitonin levels may be due to ectopic calcitonin production by oat cell carcinoma of the lung or by breast carcinoma.

Interfering factors
- Failure to fast overnight before the test
- Hemolysis due to rough handling of the sample

Parathyroid hormone

Parathyroid hormone (PTH), also known as parathormone, regulates plasma concentration of calcium and phosphorus. Normally, PTH release is regulated by a negative feedback mechanism involving serum calcium. Normal or elevated circulating calcium levels (especially the ionized form) inhibit PTH release; decreased levels stimulate PTH release. The overall effect of PTH is to raise plasma levels of calcium while lowering phosphorus levels.

Circulating PTH exists in three distinct molecular forms: the intact PTH molecule, which originates in the parathyroid glands, and two smaller circulating forms, N-terminal fragments and C-terminal fragments. Two radioimmunoassays are available to detect intact PTH and the N- and C-terminal fragments. Both tests can be used to confirm diagnosis of hyperparathyroidism and hypoparathyroidism.

Each test has other specific applications as well. The C-terminal PTH assay is more useful in diagnosing chronic disturbances in PTH metabolism, such as secondary and tertiary hyperparathyroidism; it also better differentiates ectopic from primary hyperparathyroidism. The assay for intact PTH and the N-terminal fragment (both forms are measured concomitantly) more accurately reflects acute

CLINICAL IMPLICATIONS OF ABNORMAL PARATHYROID SECRETION

Conditions	Causes	PTH levels	Ionized calcium levels
Primary hyperparathyroidism	■ Parathyroid adenoma or carcinoma	(High)	(High) to (Low)
Secondary hyperparathyroidism	■ Chronic renal disease ■ Severe vitamin D deficiency ■ Calcium malabsorption ■ Pregnancy and lactation	(High)	(Low)
Tertiary hyperparathyroidism	■ Progressive secondary hyperparathyroidism	(High)	(High) to (Low)
Hypoparathyroidism	■ Accidental removal of the parathyroid glands ■ Autoimmune disease	(Low)	(Low)
Malignant tumors	■ Squamous cell carcinoma of the lung ■ Renal, pancreatic, or ovarian carcinoma	(High) to (Normal)	(High)

Key:

High ●   Normal ◐   Low ○

changes in PTH metabolism and thus is useful in monitoring a patient's response to PTH therapy.

The clinical and diagnostic effects of PTH excess or deficiency are directly related to the effects of PTH on bone and the renal tubules and to its interaction with ionized calcium and biologically active vitamin D. Therefore, measuring serum calcium, phosphorus, and creatinine levels with serum PTH is helpful when trying to understand the causes and effects of pathologic parathyroid function. Suppression or stimulation tests may help confirm findings.

Purpose
■ To aid the differential diagnosis of parathyroid disorders

Patient preparation
■ Explain to the patient that this test helps evaluate parathyroid function.
■ Instruct the patient to observe an overnight fast because food may affect PTH levels and interfere with results.
■ Tell the patient that the test requires a blood sample. Explain who will perform the venipuncture and when.
■ Explain to the patient that he may experience slight discomfort from the needle puncture and the tourniquet.

Procedure and posttest care
- Perform a venipuncture and collect 3 ml of blood into two separate 7-ml clot-activator tubes.
- Apply direct pressure to the venipuncture site until bleeding stops.
- If a hematoma develops at the venipuncture site, apply warm soaks.
- Instruct the patient that he may resume his usual diet.

Precautions
- Handle the sample gently to prevent hemolysis.
- Send the sample to the laboratory immediately so the serum can be separated and frozen for assay.

Reference values
Normal serum PTH levels vary, depending on the laboratory, and must be interpreted in association with serum calcium levels. Typical values for intact PTH range from 10 to 50 pg/ml (SI, 1.1 to 5.3 pmol/L); N-terminal fraction is 8 to 24 pg/ml (SI, 0.8 to 2.5 pmol/L); C-terminal fraction, 0 to 340 pg/ml (SI, 0 to 35.8 pmol/L).

Abnormal findings
Measured concomitantly with serum calcium levels, abnormally elevated PTH values may indicate primary, secondary, or tertiary hyperparathyroidism. Abnormally low PTH levels may result from hypoparathyroidism and from certain malignant diseases. (See *Clinical implications of abnormal parathyroid secretion.*)

Interfering factors
- Failure to fast overnight before the test
- Hemolysis due to rough handling of the sample

ADRENAL AND RENAL HORMONE TESTS

Aldosterone

The aldosterone test measures serum aldosterone levels by quantitative analysis and radioimmunoassay. Aldosterone — the principal mineralocorticoid secreted by the zona gomerulosa of the adrenal cortex — regulates ion transport across cell membranes in the renal tubules to promote reabsorption of sodium and chloride in exchange for potassium and hydrogen ions. (See *Sites of adrenal hormone production,* page 170.) Consequently, aldosterone helps to maintain blood pressure and volume and to regulate fluid and electrolyte balance.

Aldosterone secretion is controlled primarily by the renin-angiotensin concentration of potassium. Thus, high serum potassium levels elicit secretion of aldosterone through a potent feedback system; similarly, hyponatremia, hypovolemia, and other disorders that provoke the release of renin stimulate aldosterone secretion.

This test identifies aldosteronism and, when supported by plasma renin levels, distinguishes between the primary and secondary forms of this disorder.

Purpose
- To aid diagnosis of primary and secondary aldosteronism, adrenal hyperplasia, hypoaldosteronism, and salt-losing syndrome

Patient preparation
- Explain to the patient that this test helps determine if his symptoms are due to improper hormonal secretion.

SITES OF ADRENAL HORMONE PRODUCTION

The adrenal glands are paired structures located retroperitoneally, one atop each kidney. Each gland consists of the cortex, composed of three layers, and the medulla. The outer layer of the cortex, the zona glomerulosa, produces aldosterone; the first inner layer, the zona fasciculata, produces cortisol; the next inner layer, the zona reticularis, secretes sex hormones (primarily androgens); and the medulla stores catecholamines (epinephrine and norepinephrine).

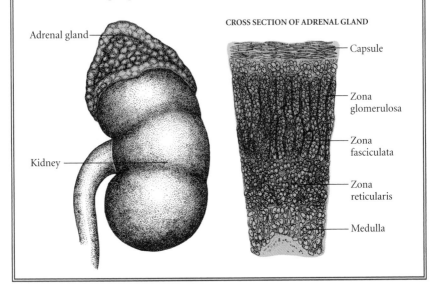

CROSS SECTION OF ADRENAL GLAND

- Tell the patient that the test requires a blood sample. Explain who will perform the venipuncture and when.
- Explain to the patient that he may experience slight discomfort from the needle puncture and the tourniquet.
- Instruct the patient to maintain a low-carbohydrate, normal-sodium diet (135 mEq or 3 g/day) for at least 2 weeks or, preferably, for 30 days before the test.
- Withhold drugs that alter fluid, sodium, and potassium balance—especially diuretics, antihypertensives, steroids, hormonal contraceptives, and estrogens—for at least 2 weeks or, preferably, for 30 days before the test, as ordered.
- Withhold all renin inhibitors for 1 week before the test, as ordered. If they must be continued, note this on the laboratory request.
- Tell the patient to avoid licorice for at least 2 weeks before the test because it produces an aldosterone-like effect.

Procedure and posttest care
- Perform a venipuncture while the patient is still supine after a night's rest.
- Collect the sample in a 7-ml clot-activator tube and send it to the laboratory immediately.
- Draw another sample 4 hours later, while the patient is standing and after he has been up and about, to evaluate the effect of postural change.

- Collect the second sample in a 7-ml clot-activator tube and send it to the laboratory immediately.
- Apply direct pressure to the venipuncture site until bleeding stops.
- If a hematoma develops at the venipuncture site, apply warm soaks.
- Instruct the patient that he may resume his usual diet and medications discontinued before the test, as ordered.

Precautions
- Handle the sample gently to prevent hemolysis.
- Record on the laboratory request whether the patient was supine or standing during the venipuncture.
- If the patient is a premenopausal female, specify the phase of her menstrual cycle because aldosterone levels may fluctuate.
- Send the sample to the laboratory immediately.

Reference values
Laboratory values vary with time of day and posture — upright postures have higher values. In upright individuals, normal values are 7 to 30 ng/dl (SI, 190 to 832 pmol/L). In supine individuals, values are 3 to 16 ng/dl (SI, 80 to 440 pmol/L).

Abnormal findings
Excessive aldosterone secretion may indicate primary or secondary disease. Primary aldosteronism (Conn's syndrome) may result from adrenocortical adenoma or carcinoma or from bilateral adrenal hyperplasia. Secondary aldosteronism can result from renovascular hypertension, heart failure, cirrhosis of the liver, nephrotic syndrome, idiopathic cyclic edema, and the third trimester of pregnancy.

Low serum aldosterone levels may indicate primary hypoaldosteronism, salt-losing syndrome, eclampsia, or Addison's disease.

Interfering factors
- Failure to observe pretest restrictions
- Hemolysis due to rough handling of the sample
- Some antihypertensives, such as methyldopa, that promote sodium and water retention (possible decrease)
- Diuretics (possible increase)
- Some corticosteroids, such as fludrocortisone, that mimic mineralocorticoid activity (possible decrease)
- Radioactive scan performed within 1 week before the test

Plasma cortisol

Cortisol — the principal glucocorticoid secreted by the zona fasciculata of the adrenal cortex — helps metabolize nutrients, mediate physiologic stress, and regulate the immune system. Cortisol secretion normally follows a diurnal pattern: Levels rise during the early morning hours and peak around 8 a.m., and then decline to very low levels in the evening and during the early phase of sleep. (See *Diurnal variations in cortisol secretion,* page 172.) Intense heat or cold, infection, trauma, exercise, obesity, and debilitating disease influence cortisol secretion.

This radioimmunoassay, a quantitative analysis of plasma cortisol levels, is usually ordered for patients with signs of adrenal dysfunction. Dynamic tests, suppression tests for hyperfunction, and stimulation tests for hypofunction are generally required to confirm the diagnosis.

Purpose
- To aid in the diagnosis of Cushing's disease, Cushing's syndrome, Addison's

DIURNAL VARIATIONS IN CORTISOL SECRETION

Cortisol secretion rises in the early morning, peaking after the patient awakens. Levels decline sharply in the evening and during the early phase of sleep. They rise again during the night and peak by the next morning.

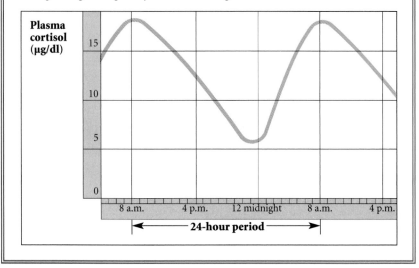

disease, and secondary adrenal insufficiency

Patient preparation

■ Explain to the patient that this test helps determine if his symptoms are due to improper hormonal secretion.
■ Instruct the patient to maintain a normal salt diet (2 to 3 g/day) for 3 days before the test and to fast and limit physical activity for 10 to 12 hours before the test.
■ Tell the patient that the test requires a blood sample. Explain who will perform the venipuncture and when.
■ Explain to the patient that he may experience slight discomfort from the needle puncture and the tourniquet.
■ Withhold all medications that may interfere with plasma cortisol levels, such as estrogens, androgens, and phenytoin, for 48 hours before the test, as ordered. If the patient is receiving replacement therapy

and is dependent on exogenous steroids for survival, note this on the laboratory request as well as other medications that must be continued.
■ Make sure the patient is relaxed and recumbent for at least 30 minutes before the test.

Procedure and posttest care

■ Perform a venipuncture between 6 a.m. and 8 a.m.
■ Collect the sample in a 7-ml heparinized tube, label it appropriately, and send it to the laboratory immediately.
■ For diurnal variation testing, draw another sample between 4 p.m. and 6 p.m.
■ Collect the second sample in a 7-ml heparinized tube, label it appropriately, and send it to the laboratory immediately.
■ Apply direct pressure to the venipuncture site until bleeding stops.

- If a hematoma develops at the venipuncture site, apply warm soaks.
- Instruct the patient that he may resume his usual diet, activities, and medications discontinued before the test, as ordered.

Precautions
- Handle the sample gently to prevent hemolysis.
- Record the collection time on the laboratory request.

Reference values
Normally, plasma cortisol levels range from 9 to 35 μg/dl (SI, 250 to 690 nmol/L) in the morning and from 3 to 12 μg/dl (SI, 80 to 330 nmol/L) in the afternoon. The afternoon level is usually half the morning level.

Abnormal findings
Increased plasma cortisol levels may indicate adrenocortical hyperfunction in Cushing's disease (a rare disease due to basophilic adenoma of the pituitary gland) or Cushing's syndrome (glucocorticoid excess from any cause). In most patients with Cushing's syndrome, the adrenal cortex secretes independently of a natural rhythm. Thus, absence of diurnal variation in cortisol secretion is a significant finding in almost all patients with Cushing's syndrome; in these patients, little difference in values is found between morning and afternoon samples. Diurnal variations may also be absent in otherwise healthy people who are under considerable emotional or physical stress.

Decreased cortisol levels may indicate primary adrenal hypofunction (Addison's disease), usually due to idiopathic glandular atrophy (a presumed autoimmune process). Tuberculosis, fungal invasion, and hemorrhage can cause adrenocortical destruction. Low cortisol levels resulting from secondary adrenal insufficiency may occur in conditions of impaired corticotropin secretion, such as hypophysectomy, postpartum pituitary necrosis, craniopharyngioma, and chromophobe adenoma.

Interfering factors
- Failure to observe pretest restrictions
- Hemolysis due to rough handling of the sample
- Pregnancy or use of hormonal contraceptives because of increase in cortisol-binding plasma proteins (false-high)
- Obesity, stress, and severe hepatic or renal disease (possible increase)
- Androgens and phenytoin due to decrease in cortisol-binding plasma proteins (possible decrease)
- Radioactive scan performed within 1 week before the test

Plasma catecholamines

The plasma catecholamines test, a quantitative (total or fractionated) analysis of plasma catecholamines, has clinical importance in the patient with hypertension and signs of adrenal medullary tumor as well as in the patient with a neural tumor that affects endocrine function. Elevated plasma catecholamine levels necessitate supportive confirmation by urinalysis.

Major catecholamines include the hormones epinephrine, norepinephrine, and dopamine. When secreted into the bloodstream, catecholamines produced in the adrenal medulla prepare the body for the fight-or-flight response. They increase heart rate and contractility, constrict blood vessels and redistribute circulating blood toward the skeletal and coronary muscles, mobilize carbohydrate and lipid reserves, and sharpen alertness. Excessive catecholamine secretion by tumors causes hypertension, weight loss, episodic sweating, headache, palpitations, and anxiety.

Plasma levels commonly fluctuate in response to temperature, stress, postural change, diet, smoking, anoxia, volume depletion, renal failure, obesity, and many drugs.

Purpose

- To rule out pheochromocytoma (adrenal medullary or extra-adrenal) in the patient with hypertension
- To help identify neuroblastoma, ganglioneuroblastoma, and ganglioneuroma
- To distinguish between adrenal medullary tumors and other catecholamine-producing tumors through fractional analysis (Urinalysis for catecholamine degradation products is recommended to support the diagnosis.)
- To aid diagnosis of autonomic nervous system dysfunction such as idiopathic orthostatic hypotension

Patient preparation

- Explain to the patient that this test helps determine if hypertension or other symptoms are related to improper hormonal secretion.
- As ordered, instruct the patient to refrain from using self-prescribed medications, especially cold and allergy remedies that may contain sympathomimetics, for 2 weeks before the test.
- Tell the patient to exclude amine-rich foods and beverages, such as bananas, avocados, cheese, coffee, tea, cocoa, beer, and Chianti, from his diet for 48 hours; to maintain vitamin C intake, which is necessary for formation of catecholamines; to abstain from smoking for 24 hours; and to fast for 10 to 12 hours before the test.

- Tell the patient that the test requires one or two blood samples. Explain who will perform the venipuncture and when.
- Explain to the patient that he may experience slight discomfort from the needle puncture and the tourniquet.
- If the patient is in your facility, withhold medications that affect catecholamine levels, such as amphetamines, phenothiazines (chlorpromazine), sympathomimetics, and tricyclic antidepressants, as ordered.
- Insert an indwelling venous catheter (heparin lock) 24 hours before the test because the stress of the venipuncture itself may significantly raise catecholamine levels.
- Make sure the patient is relaxed and recumbent for 45 to 60 minutes before the test.
- If necessary, provide blankets to keep the patient warm; low temperatures stimulate catecholamine secretion.

Procedure and posttest care

- Perform a venipuncture between 6 a.m. and 8 a.m.
- Collect the sample in a 10-ml chilled EDTA tube (sodium metabisulfite solution), which can be obtained from the laboratory on request.
- If a second sample is requested, have the patient stand for 10 minutes and draw the sample into another tube exactly like the first.
- If a heparin lock is used, it may be necessary to discard the first 1 or 2 ml of blood. Check with the laboratory for the preferred procedure.
- Apply direct pressure to the venipuncture site until bleeding stops.
- If a hematoma develops at the venipuncture site, apply warm soaks.

■ Instruct the patient that he may resume his usual diet and medications discontinued before the test, as ordered.

Precautions
■ After collecting each sample, roll the tube slowly between your palms to distribute the EDTA without agitating the blood.
■ Pack the tube in crushed ice to minimize deactivation of catecholamines and send it to the laboratory immediately.
■ Indicate on the laboratory request whether the patient was supine or standing during the venipuncture and the time the sample was drawn.

Reference values
In fractional analysis, catecholamine levels range as follows:
■ supine: epinephrine, undetectable to 110 pg/ml (SI, undetectable to 600 pmol/L); norepinephrine, 70 to 750 pg/ml (SI, 413 to 4,432 pmol/L)
■ standing: epinephrine, undetectable to 140 pg/ml (SI, undetectable to 764 pmol/L); norepinephrine, 200 to 1,700 pg/ml (SI, 1,182 to 10,047 pmol/L).

Abnormal findings
High catecholamine levels may indicate pheochromocytoma, neuroblastoma, ganglioneuroblastoma, or ganglioneuroma. Elevations are possible, but don't directly confirm thyroid disorders, hypoglycemia, and cardiac disease. Electroconvulsive therapy, shock resulting from hemorrhage, endotoxins, and anaphylaxis also raise catecholamine levels.

In the patient with normal or low baseline catecholamine levels, failure to show an increase in the sample taken after standing suggests autonomic nervous system dysfunction.

Fractional analysis helps identify the cause of elevated catecholamine levels. For example, adrenal medullary tumors secrete epinephrine, whereas ganglioneuromas, ganglioblastomas, and neuroblastomas secrete norepinephrine.

Interfering factors
■ Failure to observe pretest restrictions
■ Epinephrine, levodopa, amphetamines, phenothiazines, sympathomimetics, decongestants, and tricyclic antidepressants (increase)
■ Reserpine (decrease)
■ Radioactive scan performed within 1 week before the test

Androstenedione

The androstenedione test helps identify disorders related to altered hormone levels, such as female virilization syndromes and polycystic ovary (Stein-Leventhal) syndrome. Androstenedione is a precursor of cortisol, aldosterone, estrogen, and testosterone. Tumors of the ovaries or adrenal glands can secrete excessive amounts of androstenedione, which then converts to testosterone, resulting in virilizing symptoms, such as hirsutism and sterility.

Increased androstenedione production may induce premature sexual development in children. It may produce renewed ovarian stimulation, endometriosis, bleeding, and polycystic ovaries in postmenopausal women. In obese women, increased levels of estrogen can lead to menstrual irregularities. In men, overproduction of androstenedione may cause feminizing signs such as gynecomastia.

Purpose
■ To help determine the cause of gonadal dysfunction, menstrual or menopausal ir-

regularities, virilizing symptoms, and premature sexual development

Patient preparation

- Explain to the patient that this test determines the cause of her symptoms.
- Tell the patient that the test requires a blood sample. Explain who will perform the venipuncture and when.
- Explain to the patient that she may experience slight discomfort from the needle puncture and the tourniquet.
- Explain that the test should be done 1 week before or after her menstrual period and that it may be repeated.
- Withhold steroid and pituitary-based hormones, as ordered. If they must be continued, note this on the laboratory request.

Procedure and posttest care

- Perform a venipuncture and collect a serum sample in a 7-ml clot-activator tube or collect a plasma sample in a green-top tube. (If a plasma sample is taken, refrigerate it or place it on ice.)
- Label the sample appropriately and send it to the laboratory immediately.
- Apply direct pressure to the venipuncture site until bleeding stops.
- If a hematoma develops at the venipuncture site, apply warm soaks.
- Instruct the patient that she may resume medications discontinued before the test, as ordered.

Precautions

- Handle the sample gently to prevent hemolysis.
- Refrigerate plasma samples or place them on ice.
- Record the patient's age, sex, and (if appropriate) phase of her menstrual cycle on the laboratory request.

Reference values

Normal values by radioimmunoassay are:
- females: 85 to 275 ng/dl (SI, 3.0 to 9.6 nmol/L)
- males: 75 to 205 ng/dl (SI, 2.6 to 7.2 nmol/L).

Abnormal findings

Elevated androstenedione levels are associated with polycystic ovary (Stein-Leventhal) syndrome; Cushing's syndrome; ovarian, testicular, and adrenocortical tumors; ectopic corticotropin-producing tumors; late-onset congenital adrenal hyperplasia; and ovarian stromal hyperplasia. Elevated levels result in increased estrone levels, causing premature sexual development in children; menstrual irregularities in premenopausal women; bleeding, endometriosis, and polycystic ovaries in postmenopausal women; and feminizing signs, such as gynecomastia, in men. Decreased levels occur in hypogonadism.

Interfering factors

- Hemolysis due to rough handling of the sample
- Steroids and pituitary hormones (possible increase)

Erythropoietin

The erythropoietin (EPO) test of renal hormone production measures EPO by immunoassay. It's used to evaluate anemia, polycythemia, and kidney tumors. It's also used to evaluate abuse of commercially prepared EPO by athletes who believe that the drug enhances performance.

A glycoprotein hormone, EPO is secreted by the liver of fetuses, but by the kidneys in adults. The hormone acts on stem cells in the bone marrow to stimulate production of red blood cells (RBCs). It's regulated by a feedback loop involving red cell volume and oxygen saturation of the blood, especially in the brain.

Purpose
- To aid diagnosis of anemia and polycythemia
- To aid diagnosis of kidney tumors
- To detect EPO abuse by athletes

Patient preparation
- Explain to the patient that this test determines if hormonal secretion is causing changes in his RBCs.
- Instruct the patient to fast for 8 to 10 hours before the test.
- Tell the patient that the test requires a blood sample. Explain who will perform the venipuncture and when.
- Explain to the patient that he may experience slight discomfort from the needle puncture and the tourniquet.
- Keep the patient relaxed and recumbent for 30 minutes before the test.

Procedure and posttest care
- Perform a venipuncture and collect the sample in a 5-ml clot-activator tube.
- If requested, a hematocrit may be drawn at the same time by collecting an additional sample in a 2-ml EDTA tube.
- Apply direct pressure to the venipuncture site until bleeding stops.
- If a hematoma develops at the venipuncture site, apply warm soaks.

Precautions
- Handle the sample gently to prevent hemolysis.

Reference values
The reference range for EPO is 5 to 36 mU/ml (SI, 5 to 36 IU/L).

Abnormal findings
Low levels of EPO appear in the patient with anemia who has inadequate or absent hormone production. Congenital absence of EPO can occur. Severe renal disease may decrease EPO production.

Elevated EPO levels occur in anemias as a compensatory mechanism in the reestablishment of homeostasis. Inappropriate elevations (when the hematocrit is normal to high) are seen in polycythemia and EPO-secreting tumors.

Some athletes use EPO to enhance performance. The increased RBC volume conveys additional oxygen-carrying capacity to the blood. Adverse reactions include clotting abnormalities, headache, seizures, hypertension, nausea, vomiting, diarrhea, and rash.

Interfering factors
- Failure to collect a sample in the fasting state
- Hemolysis due to rough handling of the sample

Plasma atrial natriuretic factor

The plasma atrial natriuretic factor (ANF) is a radioimmunoassay that measures the plasma level of ANF, also known as atrial natriuretic peptides or atriopeptins. An extremely potent natriuretic agent and vasodilator, ANF rapidly produces diuresis and increases the glomerular filtration rate. ANF's role in regulating extracellular fluid volume, blood pressure, and sodium metabolism appears critical. It promotes sodium excretion, inhibits the renin-angiotensin system's effect on aldosterone secretion, and decreases atrial pressure by decreasing venous return, thereby reducing blood pressure and volume.

The patient with overt heart failure has highly elevated plasma levels of ANF. The patient with cardiovascular disease and elevated cardiac filling pressure but without heart failure also has markedly elevated ANF levels. ANF may provide a marker for early asymptomatic left ventricular dysfunction and increased cardiac volume.

Purpose
- To confirm heart failure
- To identify asymptomatic cardiac volume overload

Patient preparation
- As appropriate, explain the purpose of the test to the patient.
- Inform the patient that he must fast for 12 hours before the test.
- Tell the patient that the test requires a blood sample. Explain who will perform the venipuncture and when.
- Explain to the patient that he may experience slight discomfort from the needle puncture and the tourniquet.
- Explain that the test results will be available within 4 days.
- Check the patient's history for medications that can influence test results.
- Withhold beta-adrenergic blockers, calcium antagonists, diuretics, vasodilators, and cardiac glycosides for 24 hours before collection, as ordered.

Procedure and posttest care
- Perform a venipuncture and collect the sample in a prechilled potassium-EDTA tube.
- After chilled centrifugation, the EDTA plasma should be promptly frozen and sent to the laboratory.
- Apply direct pressure to the venipuncture site until bleeding stops.

- If a hematoma develops at the venipuncture site, apply warm soaks.
- Instruct the patient that he may resume his usual diet and medications discontinued before the test, as ordered.

Precautions
- Handle the sample gently to prevent hemolysis.

Reference values
Normal ANF levels range from 20 to 77 pg/ml.

Abnormal findings
Markedly elevated levels of ANF occur in the patient with frank heart failure and significantly elevated cardiac filling pressure.

Interfering factors
- Cardiovascular drugs, including beta-adrenergic blockers, calcium antagonists, diuretics, vasodilators, and cardiac glycosides

PANCREATIC AND GASTRIC HORMONE TESTS

Insulin

The insulin test, a radioimmunoassay, is a quantitative analysis of serum insulin levels. Insulin is usually measured concomitantly with glucose levels because glucose is the primary stimulus for insulin release from pancreatic islet cells. (See *How the pancreas produces insulin.*)

Insulin regulates the metabolism and transport or mobilization of carbohydrates, amino acids, proteins, and lipids. Stimulated by increased plasma levels of

HOW THE PANCREAS PRODUCES INSULIN

The pancreas is composed of an exocrine portion—acinar cells, which secrete digestive enzymes—and an endocrine portion—the islets of Langerhans, which secrete insulin and glucagon into the bloodstream in response to changes in blood glucose levels. The islets of Langerhans contain two principal types of cells—beta cells, which produce insulin when blood glucose increases, and alpha cells, which produce glucagon when blood glucose decreases.

Splenic arteries transport oxygenated blood to the pancreas; mesenteric veins transport insulin and glucagon, contained in deoxygenated blood, from the pancreas.

Insulin lowers blood glucose levels by facilitating transport of glucose into cells and by increasing the conversion of glucose into liver and muscle glycogen; it also prevents breakdown of liver glycogen to yield glucose. Glucagon exerts the opposite effect.

CROSS SECTION OF PANCREAS

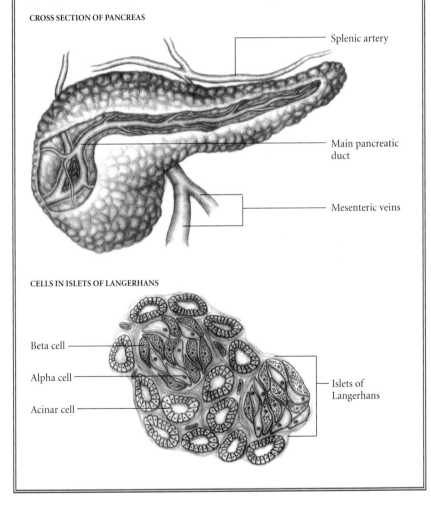

Splenic artery

Main pancreatic duct

Mesenteric veins

CELLS IN ISLETS OF LANGERHANS

Beta cell

Alpha cell

Acinar cell

Islets of Langerhans

glucose, insulin secretion reaches peak levels after meals, when metabolism and food storage are greatest.

Purpose
- To aid diagnosis of hyperinsulinemia as well as hypoglycemia resulting from a tumor or hyperplasia of pancreatic islet cells, glucocorticoid deficiency, or severe hepatic disease
- To aid diagnosis of diabetes mellitus and insulin-resistant states

Patient preparation
- Explain to the patient that this test helps determine if the pancreas is functioning normally.
- Instruct the patient to fast for 10 to 12 hours before the test.
- Tell the patient that the test requires a blood sample. Explain who will perform the venipuncture and when.
- Explain to the patient that he may experience slight discomfort from the needle puncture and the tourniquet.
- Explain that questionable results may require a repeat test or a simultaneous glucose tolerance test, which requires that the patient drink a glucose solution.
- Withhold corticotropin, corticosteroids (including hormonal contraceptives), thyroid supplements, epinephrine, and other medications that may interfere with test results, as ordered. If they must be continued, note this on the laboratory request.
- Make sure the patient is relaxed and recumbent for 30 minutes before the test.

Procedure and posttest care
- Perform a venipuncture and collect one sample for insulin level in a 7-ml EDTA tube.

- Collect a sample for glucose level in a tube with sodium fluoride and potassium oxalate.
- Apply direct pressure to the venipuncture site until bleeding stops.
- If a hematoma develops at the venipuncture site, apply warm soaks.
- Instruct the patient that he may resume his usual activities, diet, and medications discontinued before the test, as ordered.

Precautions
- Pack the insulin sample in ice, and send it, along with the glucose sample, to the laboratory immediately.
- In the patient with an insulinoma, fasting for this test may precipitate dangerously severe hypoglycemia. Keep an ampule of dextrose 50% available to counteract possible hypoglycemia.
- Handle the samples gently to prevent hemolysis.

Reference values
Serum insulin levels normally range from 0 to 35 µU/ml (SI, 144 to 243 pmol/L).

Abnormal findings
Insulin levels are interpreted in light of the prevailing glucose concentration. A normal insulin level may be inappropriate for the glucose results. High insulin and low glucose levels after a significant fast suggest the presence of an insulinoma. Prolonged fasting or stimulation testing may be required to confirm the diagnosis. In insulin-resistant diabetes mellitus, insulin levels are elevated; in non–insulin-resistant diabetes, they're low.

Interfering factors
- Failure to observe pretest restrictions
- Agitation and stress
- Hemolysis due to rough handling of the sample

- Failure to pack the insulin sample in ice and send it to the laboratory promptly
- Corticotropin, corticosteroids (including hormonal contraceptives), thyroid hormones, and epinephrine (possible increase)
- Use of insulin by the patient with type 2 diabetes mellitus (possible increase)
- High levels of insulin antibodies in the patient with type 1 diabetes mellitus

Gastrin

Gastrin is a polypeptide hormone produced and stored primarily in the antrum of the stomach and to a lesser degree in the islets of Langerhans. Its main function is to facilitate food digestion by triggering gastric acid secretion. It also stimulates the release of pancreatic enzymes and the gastric enzyme pepsin, increases gastric and intestinal motility, and stimulates bile flow from the liver. Abnormal secretion of gastrin can result from tumors (gastrinomas) and pathologic disorders that affect the stomach, pancreas and, less commonly, the esophagus and small bowel.

This radioimmunoassay, a quantitative analysis of gastrin levels, is especially useful in patients suspected of having gastrinomas (Zollinger-Ellison syndrome). In doubtful situations, provocative testing may be necessary.

Purpose
- To confirm a diagnosis of gastrinoma, the gastrin-secreting tumor in Zollinger-Ellison syndrome
- To aid differential diagnosis of gastric and duodenal ulcers and pernicious anemia (Gastrin estimation has limited value in the patient with a duodenal ulcer.)

Patient preparation
- Explain to the patient that this test helps determine the cause of GI symptoms.
- Instruct the patient to abstain from alcohol for at least 24 hours before the test and to fast and avoid caffeinated drinks for 12 hours before the test, although he may drink water.
- Tell the patient that the test requires a blood sample. Explain who will perform the venipuncture and when.
- Explain to the patient that he may experience slight discomfort from the needle puncture and the tourniquet.
- Withhold all drugs that may interfere with test results, especially insulin and anticholinergics, such as atropine and belladonna, as ordered. If they must be continued, note this on the laboratory request.
- Tell the patient to lie down and relax for at least 30 minutes before the test.

Procedure and posttest care
- Perform a venipuncture and collect the sample in a 10- to 15-ml clot-activator tube.
- Apply direct pressure to the venipuncture site until bleeding stops.
- If a hematoma develops at the venipuncture site, apply warm soaks.
- Instruct the patient that he may resume his usual diet and medications discontinued before the test, as ordered.

Precautions
- Handle the sample gently to avoid hemolysis.
- To prevent destruction of serum gastrin by proteolytic enzymes, immediately send the sample to the laboratory to have the serum separated and frozen.

Reference values

Normal serum gastrin levels are 50 to 150 pg/ml (SI, 50 to 150 ng/L).

Abnormal findings

Strikingly high serum gastrin levels (> 1,000 pg/ml [SI, > 1,000 ng/L]) confirm Zollinger-Ellison syndrome. (Levels as high as 450,000 pg/ml [SI, 450,000 ng/L] have been reported.)

Increased serum levels of gastrin may occur in a few patients with duodenal ulceration (< 1 %) and in patients with achlorhydria (with or without pernicious anemia) or extensive stomach carcinoma (because of hyposecretion of gastric juices and hydrochloric acid).

Interfering factors

- Failure to observe pretest restrictions
- Hemolysis due to rough handling of the sample
- Amino acids (especially glycine), calcium carbonate, acetylcholine, calcium chloride, and ethanol (increase)
- Anticholinergics, such as atropine, as well as hydrochloric acid and secretin, a strongly basic polypeptide (decrease)
- Insulin-induced hypoglycemia (increase)

Plasma glucagon

Glucagon, a polypeptide hormone secreted by the alpha cells of the islets of Langerhans in the pancreas, acts primarily on the liver to promote glucose production and control glucose storage. Glucogan is secreted in response to hypoglycemia; secretion is inhibited by the other pancreatic hormones, insulin and somatostatin. Normally, the coordinating release of glucagon, insulin, and somatostatin ensures an adequate and constant fuel supply while maintaining blood glucose levels within relatively stable limits.

This test, a quantitative analysis of plasma glucagon by radioimmunoassay, evaluates patients suspected of having glucagonoma (alpha cell tumor) or hypoglycemia due to idiopathic glucagon deficiency or pancreatic dysfunction. Glucagon is usually measured concomitantly with serum glucose and insulin because glucose and insulin levels influence glucagon secretion.

Purpose

- To aid diagnosis of glucagonoma and hypoglycemia due to chronic pancreatitis or idiopathic glucagon deficiency

Patient preparation

- Explain to the patient that this test helps to evaluate pancreatic function.
- Instruct the patient to fast for 10 to 12 hours before the test.
- Tell the patient that the test requires a blood sample. Explain who will perform the venipuncture and when.
- Explain to the patient that he may experience slight discomfort from the needle puncture and the tourniquet.
- Withhold insulin, catecholamines, and other drugs that could influence the test results, as ordered. If they must be continued, note this on the laboratory request.
- Have the patient lie down and relax for 30 minutes before the test.

Procedure and posttest care

- Perform a venipuncture and collect the sample in a chilled 10-ml EDTA tube.
- Apply direct pressure to the venipuncture site until bleeding stops.
- If a hematoma develops at the venipuncture site, apply warm soaks.

■ Instruct the patient that he may resume his usual diet and medications discontinued before the test, as ordered.

Precautions
■ Place the sample on ice and send it to the laboratory immediately.
■ Handle the sample gently to prevent hemolysis.

Reference values
Fasting glucagon levels are normally less than 60 pg/ml (SI, < 60 ng/L).

Abnormal findings
Elevated fasting glucagon levels (900 to 7,800 pg/ml [SI, 900 to 7,800 ng/L]) can occur in glucagonoma, diabetes mellitus, acute pancreatitis, and pheochromocytoma.

Abnormally low glucagon levels are associated with idiopathic glucagon deficiency and hypoglycemia due to chronic pancreatitis.

Interfering factors
■ Failure to observe pretest restrictions
■ Hemolysis due to rough handling of the sample
■ Failure to pack the sample in ice and send it to the laboratory immediately
■ Exercise, stress, prolonged fasting, insulin, or catecholamines (increase)
■ Radioactive scans and tests performed within 48 hours of the test

C-peptide

Connecting peptide (C-peptide) is a biologically inactive chain formed during the proteolytic conversion of proinsulin to insulin in the pancreatic beta cells. It has no insulin effect either biologically or immunologically. Circulating insulin is measured by immunologic assay. As insulin is released into the bloodstream, the C-peptide chain splits off from the hormone.

Purpose
■ To determine the cause of hypoglycemia
■ To indirectly measure insulin secretion in the presence of circulating insulin antibodies
■ To detect residual tissue after total pancreatectomy for carcinoma
■ To determine beta-cell function in the patient with diabetes mellitus

Patient preparation
■ Explain to the patient that this test helps to evaluate pancreatic function and determine the cause of hypoglycemia.
■ Instruct the patient to fast for 8 to 12 hours before the test, except for water.
■ Tell the patient that the test requires a blood sample. Explain who will perform the venipuncture and when.
■ Explain to the patient that he may experience slight discomfort from the needle puncture and the tourniquet.
■ If the patient is scheduled for radioisotope testing, it should take place after blood is drawn for C-peptide levels. Blood glucose levels are usually drawn at the same time as C-peptide levels.
■ If the C-peptide stimulation test is done, I.V. glucagon is administered, as ordered, after a baseline blood sample is drawn.
■ Withhold drugs that may interfere with test results, as ordered. If they must be continued, note this on the laboratory request.

Procedure and posttest care
■ Perform a venipuncture and collect a 1-ml sample in a chilled clot-activator

tube. The blood is separated and frozen to be tested later.

■ Collect a sample for glucose level in a tube with sodium fluoride and potassium oxalate, if ordered.

■ Apply direct pressure to the venipuncture site until bleeding stops.

■ If a hematoma develops at the venipuncture site, apply warm soaks.

■ Instruct the patient that he may resume his usual activities, diet, and medications discontinued before the test, as ordered.

Precautions

■ Pack the sample in ice and send it, along with the glucose sample, to the laboratory immediately.

■ Handle the samples gently to prevent hemolysis.

Reference values

Serum C-peptide levels generally parallel those of insulin. Normal fasting values range between 0.78 and 1.89 ng/ml (SI, 0.26 to 0.63 mmol/L). An insulin:C-peptide ratio may be performed to differentiate insulinoma from factitious hypoglycemia. A ratio of 1.0 or less indicates increased, endogenous insulin secretion; a ratio of 1.0 or more indicates exogenous insulin.

Abnormal findings

Elevated levels may indicate endogenous hyperinsulinism (insulinemia), oral hypoglycemic drug ingestion, pancreas or B-cell transplantation, renal failure, or type 2 diabetes mellitus. Decreased levels may indicate factitious hypoglycemia (surreptitious insulin administration), radical pancreatectomy, or type 1 diabetes.

Interfering factors

■ Failure to observe pretest restrictions

■ Hemolysis due to rough handling of the sample

■ Failure to pack the sample in ice and send it to the laboratory

GONADAL HORMONE TESTS

Estrogens

Estrogens (and progesterone) are secreted by the ovaries under the influence of the pituitary gonadotropins, follicle-stimulating hormone (FSH), and luteinizing hormone (LH). Estrogens—in particular, estradiol, the most potent estrogen— interact with the hypothalamic-pituitary axis through negative and positive feedback mechanisms. Slowly rising or sustained high levels inhibit secretion of FSH and LH (negative feedback), but a rapid rise in estrogen just before ovulation seems to stimulate LH secretion (positive feedback).

Estrogens are responsible for the development of secondary female sexual characteristics and for normal menstruation; levels are usually undetectable in children. These hormones are secreted by ovarian follicular cells during the first half of the menstrual cycle and by the corpus luteum during the luteal phase and during pregnancy. In menopause, estrogen secretion drops to a constantly low level.

This radioimmunoassay measures serum levels of estradiol, estrone, and estriol (the only estrogens that appear in serum in measurable amounts) and has diagnostic significance in evaluating female gonadal dysfunction. (See *Predicting premature labor.*) Tests of hypothalamic-pituitary function may be required to confirm the diagnosis.

Purpose
- To determine sexual maturation and fertility
- To aid diagnosis of gonadal dysfunction, such as precocious or delayed puberty, menstrual disorders (especially amenorrhea), and infertility
- To determine fetal well-being
- To aid diagnosis of tumors known to secrete estrogen

Patient preparation
- Explain to the patient that this test helps determine if secretion of female hormones is normal and that the test may be repeated during the various phases of the menstrual cycle.
- Tell the patient that she need not restrict food and fluids.
- Tell the patient that the test requires a blood sample. Explain who will perform the venipuncture and when.
- Explain to the patient that she may experience slight discomfort from the needle puncture and the tourniquet.
- Withhold all steroid and pituitary-based hormones, as ordered. If they must be continued, note this on the laboratory request.

Procedure and posttest care
Care may vary slightly, depending on whether plasma or serum is being measured.
- Perform a venipuncture and collect the sample in a 10-ml clot-activator tube.
- If the patient is premenopausal, indicate the phase of her menstrual cycle on the laboratory request.
- Apply direct pressure to the venipuncture site until bleeding stops.
- If a hematoma develops at the venipuncture site, apply warm soaks.

PREDICTING PREMATURE LABOR

A simple salivary test can now help determine whether a pregnant woman is at risk for premature labor, a complication that's detrimental to the health of the premature infant. The test, known as the SalEst test, measures salivary levels of estriol, an estrogen that increases a thousandfold during pregnancy. For women determined to be at risk, the SalEst test is 98% accurate in ruling out premature labor and delivery.

The test is performed on women between 22 and 36 weeks' gestation, using their saliva and the SalEst test kit. Estriol has been found to increase 2 to 3 weeks before the spontaneous onset of labor and delivery. A positive test indicates that the patient is at risk for premature labor. With this knowledge and evaluation by a physician, precautions can be instituted to decrease the risk of preterm labor and maintain fetal viability.

- Instruct the patient that she may resume medications discontinued before the test, as ordered.

Precautions
- Handle the sample gently to prevent hemolysis.
- Send the sample to the laboratory immediately.

Reference values
Normal serum estrogen levels for premenopausal women vary widely during the menstrual cycle, ranging from 26 to 149 pg/ml (SI, 90 to 550 pmol/L). The range for postmenopausal women is 0 to 34 pg/ml (SI, 0 to 125 pmol/L).

Serum estrogen levels in men range from 12 to 34 pg/ml (SI, 40 to 125 pmol/ L).

AGE ISSUE *In children younger than age 6, the normal level of serum estrogen is 3 to 10 pg/ml (SI, 10 to 36 pmol/ L). Estriol is secreted in large amounts by the placenta during pregnancy. Levels range from 2 ng/ml (SI, 7 nmol/L) by 30 weeks' gestation to 30 ng/ml (SI, 105 nmol/L) by week 40.*

Abnormal findings

Decreased estrogen levels may indicate primary hypogonadism, or ovarian failure, as in Turner's syndrome or ovarian agenesis; secondary hypogonadism, such as in hypopituitarism; or menopause.

Abnormally high estrogen levels may occur with estrogen-producing tumors, in precocious puberty, and in severe hepatic disease, such as cirrhosis, that prevents clearance of plasma estrogens. High estrogen levels may also result from congenital adrenal hyperplasia, which is the increased conversion of androgens to estrogen.

Interfering factors

- Hemolysis due to rough handling of the sample
- Pregnancy and pretest use of estrogens such as hormonal contraceptives (possible increase)
- Clomiphene, an estrogen antagonist (possible decrease)
- Steroids and pituitary-based hormones such as dexamethasone

Plasma progesterone

Progesterone, an ovarian steroid hormone secreted by the corpus luteum, causes thickening and secretory development of the endometrium in preparation for implantation of the fertilized ovum.

Progesterone levels, therefore, peak during the midluteal phase of the menstrual cycle. If implantation doesn't occur, progesterone (and estrogen) levels drop sharply and menstruation begins about 2 days later. (See *Understanding the menstrual cycle*.)

During pregnancy, the placenta releases about 10 times the normal monthly amount of progesterone to maintain the pregnancy. Increased secretion begins toward the end of the first trimester and continues until delivery. Progesterone prevents abortion by decreasing uterine contractions. Along with estrogen, progesterone helps prepare the breasts for lactation.

This radioimmunoassay is a quantitative analysis of plasma progesterone levels and provides reliable information about corpus luteum function in fertility studies and placental function in pregnancy. Serial determinations are recommended. Although plasma levels provide accurate information, progesterone can also be monitored by measuring urine pregnanediol, a catabolite of progesterone.

Purpose

- To assess corpus luteum function as part of infertility studies
- To evaluate placental function during pregnancy
- To aid in confirming ovulation; test results support basal body temperature readings

Patient preparation

- Explain to the patient that this test helps determine if her female sex hormone secretion is normal.
- Inform the patient that she need not restrict food and fluids.

UNDERSTANDING THE MENSTRUAL CYCLE

The menstrual cycle is divided into three distinct phases.

■ During the menstrual phase, which starts on the first day of menstruation, the top layer of the endometrium breaks down and flows out of the body. This flow, the menses, consists of blood, mucus, and unneeded tissue.
■ During the proliferative (follicular) phase, the endometrium begins to thicken, and the level of estrogen in the blood increases, surging at midcycle. Then es-

trogen production decreases, the follicle matures, and ovulation occurs.
■ During the secretory (luteal) phase, the endometrium begins to thicken to nourish an embryo should fertilization occur. Without fertilization, the top layer of the endometrium breaks down and the menstrual phase of the cycle begins again.

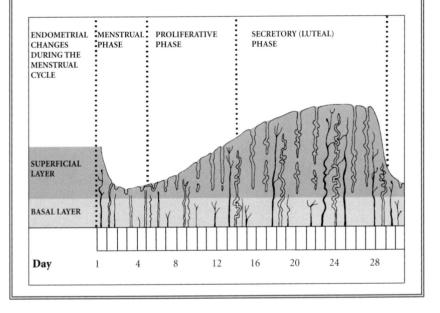

ENDOMETRIAL CHANGES DURING THE MENSTRUAL CYCLE

MENSTRUAL PHASE | PROLIFERATIVE PHASE | SECRETORY (LUTEAL) PHASE

SUPERFICIAL LAYER

BASAL LAYER

Day 1 4 8 12 16 20 24 28

■ Tell the patient that the test requires a blood sample. Explain who will perform the venipuncture and when.
■ Explain to the patient that she may experience slight discomfort from the needle puncture and the tourniquet.
■ Inform the patient that the test may be repeated at specific times coinciding with phases of her menstrual cycle or with each prenatal visit.

■ Check the patient's history to determine if she's taking drugs that may interfere with test results, including progesterone and estrogen. Note your findings on the laboratory request.

Procedure and posttest care
■ Perform a venipuncture and collect the sample in a 7-ml heparinized tube.

- Apply direct pressure to the venipuncture site until bleeding stops.
- If a hematoma develops at the venipuncture site, apply warm soaks.

Precautions
- Handle the sample gently to prevent hemolysis.
- Completely fill the collection tube; then invert it gently at least 10 times to mix the sample and the anticoagulant adequately.
- Indicate the date of the patient's last menstrual period and the phase of her cycle on the laboratory request. If the patient is pregnant, also indicate the month of gestation.
- Send the sample to the laboratory immediately.

Reference values
During menstruation, normal progesterone values are:
- follicular phase: < 150 ng/dl (SI, < 5nmol/L)
- luteal phase: 300 to 1,200 ng/dl (SI, 10 to 40 nmol/L).

During pregnancy, normal progesterone values are:
- first trimester: 1,500 to 5,000 ng/dl (SI, 50 to 160 nmol/L)
- second and third trimester: 8,000 to 20,000 ng/dl (SI, 250 to 650 nmol/L).

Normal values in menopausal women are 10 to 22 ng/dl (SI, 0 to 2 nmol/L).

Abnormal findings
Elevated progesterone levels may indicate ovulation, luteinizing tumors, ovarian cysts that produce progesterone, or adrenocortical hyperplasia and tumors that produce progesterone along with other steroidal hormones.

Low progesterone levels are associated with amenorrhea due to several causes (such as panhypopituitarism and gonadal dysfunction), eclampsia, threatened abortion, and fetal death.

Interfering factors
- Hemolysis due to rough handling of the sample
- Progesterone or estrogen therapy
- Radioactive scans performed within 1 week of the test

Testosterone

The principal androgen secreted by the interstitial cells of the testes (Leydig cells), testosterone induces puberty in the male and maintains male secondary sex characteristics. (See *Sites of testosterone secretion.*) Prepubertal levels of testosterone are low. Increased testosterone secretion during puberty stimulates growth of the seminiferous tubules and sperm production; it also contributes to the enlargement of external genitalia, accessory sex organs (such as prostate glands), and voluntary muscles and to the growth of facial, pubic, and axillary hair.

Testosterone production begins to increase at the onset of puberty and continues to rise during adulthood. Production begins to taper off at about age 40 and eventually drops to about one-fifth the peak level by age 80. In women, the adrenal glands and ovaries secrete small amounts of testosterone.

This competitive protein-binding test measures plasma or serum testosterone levels. When combined with measurement of plasma gonadotropin levels (follicle-stimulating hormone and luteinizing hormone), it's a reliable aid in the evaluation of gonadal dysfunction in men and women.

SITES OF TESTOSTERONE SECRETION

In the testis, several hundred pyramid-shaped lobules contain one or several seminiferous tubules. Within the tissue connecting the tubules, large polygonal Leydig cells secrete testosterone, the most potent androgenic hormone.

CROSS SECTION OF A TESTIS

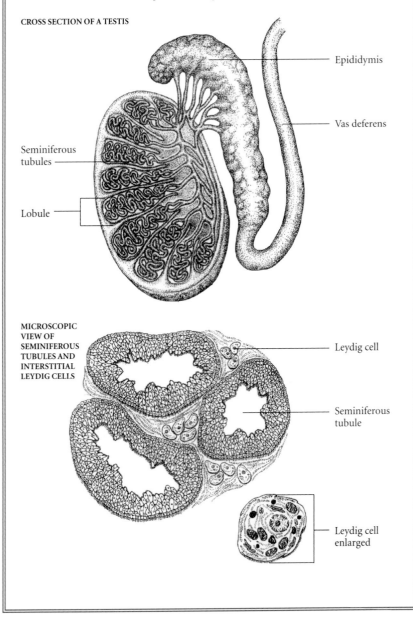

Epididymis

Vas deferens

Seminiferous tubules

Lobule

MICROSCOPIC VIEW OF SEMINIFEROUS TUBULES AND INTERSTITIAL LEYDIG CELLS

Leydig cell

Seminiferous tubule

Leydig cell enlarged

Purpose

- To facilitate differential diagnosis of male sexual precocity in boys under age 10 (True precocious puberty must be distinguished from pseudoprecocious puberty.)
- To aid differential diagnosis of hypogonadism (Primary hypogonadism must be distinguished from secondary hypogonadism.)
- To evaluate male infertility or other sexual dysfunction
- To evaluate hirsutism and virilization in women

Patient preparation

- Explain to the patient that this test helps determine if male sex hormone secretion is adequate.
- Inform the patient that he need not restrict food and fluids.
- Tell the patient that the test requires a blood sample. Explain who will perform the venipuncture and when.
- Explain to the patient that he may experience slight discomfort from the needle puncture and the tourniquet.

Procedure and posttest care

- Perform a venipuncture and collect a serum sample in a 7-ml clot-activator tube.
- If plasma is to be collected, use a heparinized tube.
- Indicate the patient's age, sex, and history of hormone therapy on the laboratory request.
- Apply direct pressure to the venipuncture site until bleeding stops.
- If a hematoma develops at the venipuncture site, apply warm soaks.

Precautions

- Handle the sample gently to prevent hemolysis and send it to the laboratory promptly.
- The sample is stable and requires no refrigeration or preservative for up to 1 week. Frozen samples are stable for at least 6 months.

Reference values

Normal testosterone levels are (laboratory values may vary slightly):

- males: 300 to 1,200 ng/dl (SI, 10.4 to 41.6 nmol/L)
- females: 20 to 80 ng/dl (SI, 0.7 to 2.8 nmol/L).

AGE ISSUE *Prepubertal children have lower values than adult levels.*

Abnormal findings

Increased testosterone levels can occur with a benign adrenal tumor or cancer, hyperthyroidism, and incipient puberty. In women with ovarian tumors or polycystic ovary syndrome, testosterone levels may rise, leading to hirsutism.

Low testosterone levels can indicate primary hypogonadism (as in Klinefelter's syndrome) or secondary hypogonadism (hypogonadotropic eunuchoidism) from hypothalamic-pituitary dysfunction. Low levels can also follow orchiectomy, testicular or prostate cancer, delayed male puberty, estrogen therapy, and cirrhosis of the liver.

AGE ISSUE *Elevated testosterone levels in prepubertal boys may indicate true sexual precocity due to excessive gonadotropin secretion or pseudoprecocious puberty due to male hormone production by a testicular tumor. They can also indicate congenital adrenal hyperplasia, which results in precocious puberty in boys (from ages 2 to 3) and pseudohermaphroditism and milder virilization in girls.*

Interfering factors

- Hemolysis due to rough handling of the sample
- Exogenous sources of estrogens and androgens, thyroid and growth hormones, and other pituitary-based hormones
- Estrogens (decrease in free testosterone levels, increasing sex hormone-binding globulin, which binds testosterone)
- Androgens (possible increase)

PLACENTAL HORMONE TESTS

Human chorionic gonadotropin

Human chorionic gonadotropin (hCG) is a glycoprotein hormone produced in the placenta. If conception occurs, a specific assay for hCG—commonly called the beta-subunit assay—may detect this hormone in the blood 9 days after ovulation. This interval coincides with the implantation of the fertilized ovum into the uterine wall. Although the precise function of hCG is still unclear, it appears that hCG, with progesterone, maintains the corpus luteum during early pregnancy.

Production of hCG increases steadily during the first trimester, peaking around 10 weeks' gestation. Levels then fall to less than 10% of first-trimester peak levels during the remainder of the pregnancy. About 2 weeks after delivery, the hormone may no longer be detectable. (See *Production of hCG during pregnancy,* page 192.)

This serum immunoassay, a quantitative analysis of hCG beta-subunit level, is more sensitive (and costlier) than the routine pregnancy test using a urine sample.

Purpose

- To detect early pregnancy
- To determine adequacy of hormonal production in high-risk pregnancies (for example, habitual abortion)
- To aid diagnosis of trophoblastic tumors, such as hydatidiform mole and choriocarcinoma, and tumors that ectopically secrete hCG
- To monitor treatment for induction of ovulation and conception

Patient preparation

- Explain to the patient that this test determines if she's pregnant. If detection of pregnancy isn't the diagnostic objective, offer the appropriate explanation.
- Inform the patient that she need not restrict food and fluids.
- Tell the patient that the test requires a blood sample. Explain who will perform the venipuncture and when.
- Explain to the patient that she may experience slight discomfort from the needle puncture and the tourniquet.

Procedure and posttest care

- Perform a venipuncture and collect the sample in a 7-ml clot-activator tube.
- Apply direct pressure to the venipuncture site until bleeding stops.
- If a hematoma develops at the venipuncture site, apply warm soaks.

Precautions

- Handle the sample gently to prevent hemolysis.
- Send the sample to the laboratory immediately.

PRODUCTION OF HCG DURING PREGNANCY

Production of human chorionic gonadotropin (hCG) increases steadily during the first trimester, peaking around 10 weeks' gestation, as shown below. Levels then fall to less than 10% of first-trimester levels during the rest of the pregnancy.

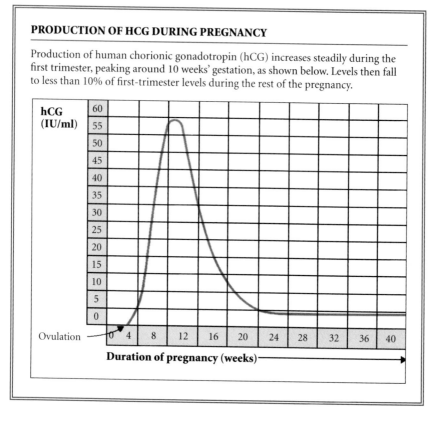

Reference values

Normally, hCG levels are less than 4 IU/L. During pregnancy, hCG levels vary widely, depending partly on the number of days after the last normal menstrual period.

Abnormal findings

Elevated hCG beta-subunit levels indicate pregnancy; significantly higher concentrations are present in a multiple pregnancy. Increased levels may also suggest hydatidiform mole, trophoblastic neoplasms of the placenta, and nontrophoblastic carcinomas that secrete hCG (including gastric, pancreatic, and ovarian adenocarcinomas). Low hCG beta-subunit levels can occur in ectopic pregnancy or pregnancy of less than 9 days. Beta-subunit levels can't differentiate between pregnancy and tumor recurrence because they're high in both conditions.

Interfering factors

■ Hemolysis due to rough handling of the sample
■ Heparin anticoagulants and EDTA (decrease; ask laboratory whether test will be performed on plasma or serum)

Human placental lactogen

A polypeptide hormone, human placental lactogen (hPL) — also known as *human chorionic somatomammotropin* — displays lactogenic and somatotropic (growth hormone) properties in a pregnant female. In combination with prolactin, hPL prepares the breasts for lactation. It also indirectly provides energy for maternal metabolism and fetal nutrition. It facilitates protein synthesis and mobilization essential to fetal growth. Secretion is autonomous, beginning at about 5 weeks' gestation and declining rapidly after delivery. According to some evidence, this hormone may not be essential for a successful pregnancy.

This radioimmunoassay measures plasma hPL levels, which are roughly proportional to placental mass. Such assays may be required in high-risk pregnancies (patients with diabetes mellitus or hypertension) and suspected placental tissue dysfunction. Because values vary widely during the latter half of pregnancy, serial determinations over several days provide the most reliable test results. This test, when combined with the measurement of estriol levels, is a reliable indicator of placental function and fetal well-being. It may also be useful as a tumor marker in certain malignant states such as ectopic tumors that secrete hPL.

Purpose
■ To assess placental function and fetal well-being (combined with measurement of estriol levels)
■ To aid diagnosis of hydatidiform mole and choriocarcinoma (human chorionic gonadotropin levels may be more useful in diagnosing these conditions)
■ To aid diagnosis and monitor treatment of nontrophoblastic tumors that ectopically secrete hPL

Patient preparation
■ Explain to the patient that this test helps assess placental function and fetal well-being. If assessing fetal well-being isn't the diagnostic objective, offer an appropriate explanation.
■ Tell the patient that the test requires a blood sample. Explain who will perform the venipuncture and when.
■ Explain to the patient that she may experience slight discomfort from the needle puncture and the tourniquet.
■ Inform the pregnant patient that this test may be repeated during her pregnancy.

Procedure and posttest care
■ Perform a venipuncture and collect the sample in a 7-ml clot-activator tube.
■ Apply direct pressure to the venipuncture site until bleeding stops.
■ If a hematoma develops at the venipuncture site, apply warm soaks.

Precautions
■ Handle the sample gently to prevent hemolysis.
■ Send the sample to the laboratory immediately.

Reference values
For pregnant women, normal hPL levels vary with the gestational phase and slowly increase throughout pregnancy, reaching 8.6 μg/ml at term.
■ 5 to 27 weeks: < 4.6 μg/ml
■ 28 to 31 weeks: 2.4 to 6.1 μg/ml
■ 32 to 35 weeks: 3.7 to 7.7 μg/ml
■ 36 weeks to term: 5.0 to 8.6 μg/ml
At term, patients with diabetes may have mean levels of 9 to 11 μg/ml. Normal levels for males and nonpregnant females are less than 0.5 μg/ml.

Abnormal findings
For reliable interpretation, hPL levels must be correlated with gestational age; for example, after 30 weeks' gestation, lev-

els below 4 µg/ml may indicate placental dysfunction. Low hPL concentrations are also characteristically associated with postmaturity syndrome, intrauterine growth retardation, preeclampsia, and eclampsia. Declining concentrations may help differentiate incomplete abortion from threatened abortion.

Be aware that low hPL concentrations don't confirm fetal distress. Conversely, concentrations over 4 µg/ml after 30 weeks' gestation don't guarantee fetal well-being because elevated levels have been reported after fetal death.

An hPL value above 6 µg/ml after 30 weeks' gestation may suggest an unusually large placenta, commonly occurring in a patient with diabetes mellitus, multiple pregnancy, or Rh isoimmunization. The test's usefulness in predicting fetal death in a patient with diabetes mellitus and in managing Rh isoimmunization during pregnancy is limited.

Below-normal concentrations of hPL may be associated with trophoblastic neoplastic disease, such as hydatidiform mole and choriocarcinoma. Abnormal concentrations of hPL have been found in the sera of patients with other neoplastic disorders, including bronchogenic carcinoma, hepatoma, lymphoma, and pheochromocytoma. In these patients, hPL levels are used as tumor markers for evaluating chemotherapy, monitoring tumor growth and recurrence, and detecting residual tissue after excision.

Interfering factors
■ Hemolysis due to rough handling of the sample

Selected readings

Behrman, R.E., et al., eds. *Nelson Textbook of Pediatrics*, 17th ed. Philadelphia: W.B. Saunders Co., 2004.

Braunwald, E., et al., eds. *Harrison's Principles of Internal Medicine*, 15th ed. New York: McGraw-Hill Book Co., 2001.

Cunningham, F.G., et al. *Williams Obstetrics*, 21st ed. New York: McGraw-Hill Book Co., 2001.

Fischbach, F. *A Manual of Laboratory and Diagnostic Tests*, 7th ed. Philadelphia: Lippincott Williams & Wilkins, 2004.

Goldman, L., and Ausiello, D., eds. *Cecil Textbook of Medicine*, 22nd ed. Philadelphia: W.B. Saunders Co., 2004.

Guyton, A.C., and Hall, J.E. *Textbook of Medical Physiology*, 10th ed. Philadelphia: W.B. Saunders Co., 2001.

Henry, J.B., ed. *Clinical Diagnosis and Management by Laboratory Methods*, 20th ed. Philadelphia: W.B. Saunders Co., 2001.

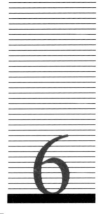

6

Lipids and lipoproteins

Introduction

Lipids, also called *fats,* are organic substances with a hydrophobic side chain or a steroid nucleus (or with both of these molecular features) that causes them to be insoluble in water. The major lipids are the triglycerides, free cholesterol, cholesteryl esters, and phospholipids. For transportation through the body, lipids must combine with plasma proteins into a lipid-protein molecular complex called *lipoproteins:* nonesterified fatty acids (free fatty acids) bind to albumin; other blood lipids (free and esterified cholesterol, triglycerides, and phospholipids) bind to globulin.

Lipid differences
Lipoproteins can be described as an inner core of hydrophobic lipids (triglycerides and cholesteryl esters) within a surface membrane of proteins (apoproteins), free cholesterol, and phospholipids. Lipoproteins differ based on density, lipid composition, and apoprotein surface components.

Lipoproteins are classified by ultracentrifugation density and electrophoretic mobility as follows:

- *Chylomicrons,* the lowest density lipoproteins consisting mostly of triglycerides, are the form in which long-chain fats and cholesterol are transported from the intestine to the blood. Eventually, chylomicrons break down into other lipids and free fatty acids.
- *Very-low-density (prebeta) lipoproteins* (VLDLs) consist mostly of triglycerides and smaller amounts of phospholipids, cholesterol, and protein. They are synthesized in the liver from free fatty acids formed in the catabolism of chylomicrons, or from exogenous triglyceride production.
- *Intermediate-density lipoproteins* are short-lived and contain almost equal amounts of cholesterol and triglycerides and smaller amounts of phospholipids and protein. They're composed of the lipid portion that remains after synthesis of VLDLs and are converted to low-density lipoproteins by lipase.
- *Low-density (beta) lipoproteins* (LDLs) are about half cholesterol and half protein, phospholipids, and triglycerides. They carry most of the cholesterol found in the blood, thus supplying cholesterol to peripheral cells.
- *High-density (alpha) lipoproteins* (HDLs) are about half protein and half phospholipids, cholesterol, and triglycerides. They facilitate the transfer of cholesterol from peripheral tissues and atherogenic lipoproteins to the liver.

Clinical implications

Lipoprotein phenotyping—classifying the patient by the pattern of his lipoprotein levels—is an important procedure for diagnosing and treating hyperlipoproteinemias and hypolipoproteinemias. These disorders produce many symptoms ranging from mild (such as xanthomas) to severe (such as pancreatitis).

Lipoprotein determinations are also useful in evaluating the risk of coronary artery disease (CAD). At one time, total blood cholesterol—the amount of cholesterol in all lipoproteins—was considered the major indicator of CAD for patients younger than age 50. However, the Framingham Heart Study found that high levels of HDL actually help prevent CAD, whereas high levels of LDL increase the risk. Lecithin–cholesterol acyltransferase, a circulating enzyme, helps HDLs absorb cholesterol through esterification. Further studies have shown that patients with angina pectoris or myocardial infarction generally have lower HDL levels than healthy persons and that low HDL levels—which can be hereditary—aren't just associated with CAD, but precede it. Low HDL levels are also connected with diabetes mellitus, hypertension, cigarette smoking, obesity, and lack of exercise.

The higher incidence of heart disease among men and postmenopausal women—compared with premenopausal women—may result from low levels of estrogen, a hormone that helps regulate HDL synthesis. Paradoxically, hormonal contraceptives and pregnancy elevate HDL levels. However, because HDL levels are only 5% to 8% lower in premenopausal women than in men of the same age, the potentially protective action of estrogens against atherosclerosis remains controversial.

Although HDL and LDL levels are good indicators of potential CAD, a full lipoprotein profile is a more useful measure. This battery of tests includes total cholesterol, total triglycerides, and lipoprotein phenotyping.

Antilipemic regimen

Care for the patient with elevated LDL levels consists of teaching diet and lifestyle changes and pharmacologic therapy, if indicated, to reduce the risk of heart disease. For example, exercise (especially running), a low-fat diet, and reducing high blood pressure may raise levels of beneficial HDLs.

LIPID TESTS

Triglycerides

Serum triglyceride analysis provides quantitative analysis of triglycerides — the main storage form of lipids — which constitute about 95% of fatty tissue. Although not in itself diagnostic, the triglyceride test permits early identification of hyperlipidemia and the risk of coronary artery disease (CAD).

Purpose

- To screen for hyperlipidemia or pancreatitis
- To help identify nephrotic syndrome and the individual with poorly controlled diabetes mellitus
- To assess the risk of CAD
- To calculate the low-density lipoprotein cholesterol level using the Freidewald equation

Patient preparation

- Explain to the patient that the triglyceride test is used to detect fat metabolism disorders.
- Tell the patient that the test requires a blood sample. Explain who will perform the venipuncture and when.
- Explain to the patient that he may experience slight discomfort from the needle puncture and the tourniquet.

- Instruct the patient to fast for at least 12 hours before the test and to abstain from alcohol for 24 hours. Tell him that he can drink water.
- Notify the laboratory and physician of medications the patient is taking that may affect test results; they may need to be restricted.

Procedure and posttest care

- Perform a venipuncture and collect a sample in a 4-ml EDTA tube.
- Apply direct pressure to the venipuncture site until bleeding stops.
- If a hematoma develops at the venipuncture site, apply warm soaks.
- Instruct the patient that he may resume his usual diet and medications discontinued before the test, as ordered.

Precautions

- Send the sample to the laboratory immediately.
- Avoid prolonged venous occlusion; remove the tourniquet within 1 minute of application.

Reference values

Triglyceride values vary with age and sex. There's some controversy about the most appropriate normal ranges, but values of 44 to 180 mg/dl (SI, 0.44 to 2.01 mmol/L) for adult men and 10 to 190 mg/dl (SI, 0.11 to 2.21 mmol/L) for adult women are widely accepted.

Abnormal findings

Increased or decreased serum triglyceride levels suggest a clinical abnormality; additional tests are required for a definitive diagnosis.

A mild to moderate increase in serum triglyceride levels indicates biliary obstruction, diabetes mellitus, nephrotic syndrome, endocrinopathies, or overconsumption of alcohol. Markedly increased levels without an identifiable cause reflect congenital hyperlipoproteinemia and necessitate lipoprotein phenotyping to confirm the diagnosis.

Decreased serum triglyceride levels are rare and occur mainly in malnutrition and abetalipoproteinemia.

Interfering factors
- Failure to observe pretest restrictions
- Use of a glycol-lubricated collection tube
- Failure to send the sample to the laboratory immediately
- Antilipemics (decreased serum lipid levels)
- Cholestyramine and colestipol (decreased cholesterol levels, but increased or having no effect on triglyceride levels)
- Corticosteroids (long-term use), hormonal contraceptives, estrogen, ethyl alcohol, furosemide, and miconazole (increase)
- Clofibrate, dextrothyroxine, gemfibrozil, and niacin (decreased cholesterol and triglyceride levels)
- Probucol (decreased cholesterol levels, but variable effect on triglyceride levels)

Total cholesterol

The total cholesterol test, the quantitative analysis of serum cholesterol, is used to measure the circulating levels of free cholesterol and cholesterol esters; it reflects the level of the two forms in which this biochemical compound appears in the body. High serum cholesterol levels may be associated with an increased risk of coronary artery disease (CAD). A 3-minute skin test is now available for use in physician offices. (See *Skin test for cholesterol*).

Purpose
- To assess the risk of CAD

- To evaluate fat metabolism
- To aid in the diagnosis of nephrotic syndrome, pancreatitis, hepatic disease, hypothyroidism, and hyperthyroidism
- To assess the efficacy of lipid-lowering drug therapy

Patient preparation
- Explain to the patient that the total cholesterol test is used to assess the body's fat metabolism.
- Tell the patient that the test requires a blood sample. Explain who will perform the venipuncture and when.
- Explain to the patient that he may experience slight discomfort from the needle puncture and the tourniquet.
- Instruct the patient not to eat or drink for 12 hours before the test, but that he may have water.
- Notify the laboratory and physician of medications the patient is taking that may affect test results; they may need to be restricted.

Procedure and posttest care
- Perform a venipuncture and collect the sample in a 4-ml EDTA tube. The patient should be in a sitting position for 5 minutes before the blood is drawn. Fingersticks can also be used for initial screening when using an automated analyzer.
- Apply direct pressure to the venipuncture site until bleeding stops.
- Instruct the patient that he may resume his usual diet and medications discontinued before the test, as ordered.

Precautions
- Send the sample to the laboratory immediately.

Reference values
Total cholesterol concentrations vary with age and sex. Total cholesterol values are:

- adults males: (desirable) < 205 mg/dl (SI, < 5.3 mmol/L)
- adults females: (desirable) < 190mg/dl (SI, < 4.9 mmol/L).

AGE ISSUE Desirable total cholesterol levels in children ages 12 to 18 are < 170 mg/dl (SI, < 4.4 mmol/L).

Abnormal findings

Elevated serum cholesterol levels (hypercholesterolemia) may indicate a risk of CAD as well as incipient hepatitis, lipid disorders, bile duct blockage, nephrotic syndrome, obstructive jaundice, pancreatitis, and hypothyroidism.

Low serum cholesterol levels (hypocholesterolemia) are commonly associated with malnutrition, cellular necrosis of the liver, and hyperthyroidism. Abnormal cholesterol levels commonly necessitate further testing to pinpoint the cause.

Interfering factors

- Failure to observe pretest restrictions
- Failure to send the sample to the laboratory immediately
- Cholestyramine, clofibrate, colestipol, dextrothyroxine, haloperidol, neomycin, niacin, and chlortetracycline (decrease)
- Epinephrine, chlorpromazine, trifluoperazine, hormonal contraceptives, and trimethadione (increase)
- Androgens (possible variable effect)

Phospholipids

The phospholipid test is a quantitative analysis of phospholipids, the major form of lipids in cell membranes. Phospholipids are involved in cellular membrane composition and permeability and help control enzyme activity within the membrane. They aid the transport of fatty acids and lipids across the intestinal barrier and from the liver and other fat stores to other body tissues. Phospholipids are essential for pulmonary gas exchange.

SKIN TEST FOR CHOLESTEROL

A new 3-minute test that measures the amount of cholesterol in the skin rather than in the blood is the first noninvasive test of its kind. It measures how much cholesterol is present in other tissues in the body and provides additional data about a person's risk of heart disease.

The test, which doesn't require patients to fast, involves placing a bandage-like applicator pad on the palm of the hand. Drops of a special solution that reacts to skin cholesterol are then added to the pad; 3 minutes later a handheld computer interprets the information into a skin cholesterol reading.

Because the test measures the amount of cholesterol that has accumulated in the tissues over time, results don't correlate with blood cholesterol levels; therefore, the test isn't meant to be a substitute or surrogate for a cholesterol test that measures the amount of cholesterol in the blood. In addition, the Food and Drug Administration cautions that the test isn't intended for use as a screening tool for heart disease in the general population. Instead, it has been approved for use among adults with severe heart disease — those with at least a 50% blockage of two or more heart arteries.

Purpose

- To aid in the evaluation of fat metabolism
- To aid in the diagnosis of hypothyroidism, diabetes mellitus, nephrotic syndrome, chronic pancreatitis, obstructive jaundice, and hypolipoproteinemia

Patient preparation

- Explain to the patient that the phospholipid test is used to determine how the body metabolizes fats.

■ Tell the patient that the test requires a blood sample. Explain who will perform the venipuncture and when.

■ Explain to the patient that he may experience slight discomfort from the needle puncture and the tourniquet.

■ Instruct the patient to abstain from drinking alcohol for 24 hours before the test and not to eat or drink anything after midnight before the test.

■ Notify the laboratory and physician of medications the patient is taking that may affect test results; they may need to be restricted.

Procedure and posttest care

■ Perform a venipuncture and collect the sample in a 10- to 15-ml tube without additives.

■ Apply direct pressure to the venipuncture site until bleeding stops.

■ If a hematoma develops at the venipuncture site, apply warm soaks.

■ Instruct the patient that he may resume his usual diet and medications discontinued before the test, as ordered.

Precautions

■ Send the sample to the laboratory immediately because spontaneous redistribution may occur among plasma lipids.

Reference values

Normal phospholipid levels range from 180 to 320 mg/dl (SI, 1.8 to 3.2 g/L). Although men usually have higher levels than women, values in pregnant women exceed those of men.

Abnormal findings

Elevated phospholipid levels may indicate hypothyroidism, diabetes mellitus, nephrotic syndrome, chronic pancreatitis, or obstructive jaundice. Decreased levels may indicate primary hypolipoproteinemia.

Interfering factors

■ Failure to observe pretest restrictions

■ Antilipemics (possible decrease)

■ Estrogens, epinephrine, and some phenothiazines (increase)

LIPOPROTEIN TESTS

Lipoprotein-cholesterol fractionation

Cholesterol fractionation tests are used to isolate and measure the types of cholesterol in serum: low-density lipoproteins (LDLs) and high-density lipoproteins (HDLs). The HDL level is inversely related to the risk of coronary artery disease (CAD); the higher the HDL level, the lower the incidence of CAD. Conversely, the higher the LDL level, the higher the incidence of CAD.

Purpose

■ To assess the risk of CAD

■ To assess the efficacy of lipid-lowering drug therapy

Patient preparation

■ Tell the patient that the lipoprotein-cholesterol fractionation test is used to determine his risk of CAD.

■ Tell the patient that the test requires a blood sample. Explain who will perform the venipuncture and when.

■ Explain to the patient that he may experience slight discomfort from the needle puncture and the tourniquet.

■ Instruct the patient to maintain his normal diet for 2 weeks before the test, to abstain from alcohol for 24 hours before the test, and to fast and avoid exercise for 12 to 14 hours before the test.

■ Notify the laboratory and physician of medications the patient is taking that may affect test results; they may need to be restricted.

Procedure and posttest care

- Perform a venipuncture and collect the sample in a 7-ml EDTA tube.
- Apply direct pressure to the venipuncture site until bleeding stops.
- If a hematoma develops at the venipuncture site, apply warm soaks.
- Instruct the patient that he may resume his usual diet and medications discontinued before the test, as ordered.

Precautions

- Send the sample to the laboratory immediately to avoid spontaneous redistribution among the lipoproteins.
- If the sample can't be transported immediately, refrigerate it but don't freeze it.

Reference values

Normal lipoprotein values vary by age, sex, geographic area, and ethnic group; check the laboratory for reference values. HDL levels range from 37 to 70 mg/dl (SI, 0.96 to 1.8 mmol/L) for males and from 40 to 85 mg/dl (SI, 1.03 to 2.2 mmol/L) for females. LDL levels are less than 130 mg/dl (SI, < 3.36 mmol/L) in individuals who don't have CAD. Borderline high levels are greater than 160 mg/dl (SI, > 4.1 mmol/L).

The American College of Cardiology recommends an HDL of 40 mg/dl or higher with women maintaining an HDL cholesterol of at least 45 mg/dl. HDL levels greater than 60 mg/dl are considered heart healthy. LDL levels should optimally be less than 100 mg/dl, with levels of 60 mg/dl or more considered high.

Abnormal findings

High LDL levels increase the risk of CAD. Elevated HDL levels generally reflect a healthy state, but can also indicate chron-

---

PLAC TEST

The PLAC test, a new blood test that can help determine who might be at risk for coronary heart disease, was recently approved by the Food and Drug Administration (FDA). The FDA's decision was based on a recent study of more than 1,300 patients, which was a part of a large multicenter study sponsored by the National Heart, Lung, and Blood Institute.

The PLAC test works by measuring lipoprotein-associated phospholipase A2, an enzyme produced by macrophages, a type of white blood cell. When heart disease is present, macrophages increase production of the enzyme. According to the FDA, an elevated PLAC test result, in conjunction with a low-density-lipoprotein (LDL) cholesterol level of less than 130 mg/dl, generally indicates that a patient has two to three times the risk of coronary heart disease compared to similar patients with lower PLAC test results. The study also found that those people with the highest PLAC test results and LDL cholesterol levels lower than 130mg/dL had the greatest risk of heart disease.

---

ic hepatitis, early-stage primary biliary cirrhosis, and alcohol consumption. Increased HDL levels can occur as a result of long-term aerobic and vigorous exercise. Rarely, a sharp rise (to as high as 100 mg/dl [SI, 2.58 mmol/L]) in a second type of HDL (alpha$_2$-HDL) may signal CAD. (See *PLAC test*.)

Interfering factors

- Concurrent illness, especially if accompanied by fever, recent surgery, or myocardial infarction
- Collecting the sample in a heparinized tube (possible false-high due to activation

of the enzyme lipase, which causes release of fatty acids from triglycerides)

■ Failure to send the sample to the laboratory immediately

■ Antilipemic medications, such as clofibrate, cholestyramine, colestipol, dextrothyroxine, niacin, probucol, and gemfibrozil (decrease)

■ Hormonal contraceptives, disulfiram, alcohol, miconazole, and high doses of phenothiazines (possible increase)

■ Estrogens (possible increase or decrease)

■ The presence of bilirubin, hemoglobin, salycilates, iodine, and vitamins A and D

Lipoprotein phenotyping

Lipoprotein phenotyping is used to determine levels of the four major lipoproteins: chylomicrons, very-low-density (prebeta) lipoproteins, low-density (beta) lipoproteins, and high-density (alpha) lipoproteins. (See *Familial hyperlipoproteinemias.*) Detecting altered lipoprotein patterns is essential in identifying hyperlipoproteinemia and hypolipoproteinemia.

Purpose
■ To determine the classification of hyperlipoproteinemia and hypolipoproteinemia

Patient preparation
■ Explain to the patient that lipoprotein typing is used to determine how the body metabolizes fats.

■ Tell the patient that the test requires a blood sample. Explain who will perform the venipuncture and when.

■ Explain to the patient that he may experience slight discomfort from the needle puncture and the tourniquet.

■ Instruct the patient to abstain from alcohol for 24 hours before the test and to

fast after midnight before the test. Provide a low-fat meal the night before the test.

■ Check the patient's drug history for heparin use. As ordered, withhold antilipemics, such as cholestyramine, about 2 weeks before the test.

■ Notify the laboratory if the patient is receiving treatment for another condition that might significantly alter lipoprotein metabolism, such as diabetes mellitus, nephrosis, or hypothyroidism.

Procedure and posttest care
■ Perform a venipuncture and collect the sample in a 4-ml EDTA tube.

■ If a hematoma develops at the venipuncture site, apply warm soaks.

■ Instruct the patient to resume his usual diet and medications discontinued before the test, as ordered.

Precautions
■ When drawing multiple samples, collect the sample for lipoprotein phenotyping first because venous obstruction for 2 minutes can affect test results.

■ Fill the collection tube completely and invert it gently several times to mix the sample and the anticoagulant thoroughly.

■ Handle the sample gently to prevent hemolysis.

Findings
The types of hyperlipoproteinemias and hypolipoproteinemias are identified by characteristic electrophoretic patterns.

Familial lipoprotein disorders are classified as either hyperlipoproteinemias or hypolipoproteinemias. There are six types of hyperlipoproteinemias: I, IIa, IIb, III, IV, and V. Types IIa, IIb, and IV are relatively common. All hypolipoproteinemias are rare, including hypobetalipoproteinemia, betalipoproteinemia, and alphalipoprotein deficiency.

FAMILIAL HYPERLIPOPROTEINEMIAS

Type	Causes and incidence	Clinical signs	Laboratory findings
I	▪ Deficient lipoprotein lipase, resulting in increased chylomicrons ▪ May be induced by alcoholism ▪ Incidence: rare	▪ Eruptive xanthomas ▪ Lipemia retinalis ▪ Abdominal pain	▪ Increased chylomicron, total cholesterol, and triglyceride levels ▪ Normal or slightly increased very-low-density lipoproteins (VLDLs) ▪ Normal or decreased low-density lipoproteins (LDLs) and high-density lipoproteins ▪ Cholesterol-triglyceride ratio < 0.2
IIa	▪ Deficient cell receptor, resulting in increased LDL and excessive cholesterol synthesis ▪ May be induced by hypothyroidism ▪ Incidence: common	▪ Premature coronary artery disease (CAD) ▪ Arcus cornea ▪ Xanthelasma ▪ Tendinous and tuberous xanthomas	▪ Increased LDL ▪ Normal VLDL ▪ Cholesterol-triglyceride ratio > 2.0
IIb	▪ Deficient cell receptor, resulting in increased LDL and excessive cholesterol synthesis ▪ May be induced by dysgammaglobulinemia, hypothyroidism, uncontrolled diabetes mellitus, and nephrotic syndrome ▪ Incidence: common	▪ Premature CAD ▪ Obesity ▪ Possible xanthelasma	▪ Increased LDL, VLDL, total cholesterol, and triglycerides
III	▪ Unknown cause, resulting in deficient VLDL-to-LDL conversion ▪ May be induced by hypothyroidism, uncontrolled diabetes mellitus, and paraproteinemia ▪ Incidence: rare	▪ Premature CAD ▪ Arcus cornea ▪ Eruptive tuberous xanthomas	▪ Increased total cholesterol, VLDL, and triglycerides ▪ Normal or decreased LDL ▪ Cholesterol-triglyceride ratio of > 0.4 ▪ Broad beta band observed on electrophoresis

(continued)

FAMILIAL HYPERLIPOPROTEINEMIAS *(continued)*

Type	Causes and incidence	Clinical signs	Laboratory findings
IV	■ Unknown cause, resulting in decreased levels of lipase ■ May be induced by uncontrolled diabetes mellitus, alcoholism, pregnancy, steroid or estrogen therapy, dysgammaglobulinemia, and hyperthyroidism ■ Incidence: common	■ Possible premature CAD ■ Obesity ■ Hypertension ■ Peripheral neuropathy	■ Increased VLDL and triglycerides ■ Normal LDL ■ Cholesterol-triglyceride ratio of < 0.25
V	■ Unknown cause, resulting in defective triglyceride clearance ■ May be induced by alcoholism, dysgammaglobulinemia, uncontrolled diabetes mellitus, nephrotic syndrome, pancreatitis, and steroid therapy ■ Incidence: rare	■ Premature CAD ■ Abdominal pain ■ Lipemia retinalis ■ Eruptive xanthomas ■ Hepatosplenomegaly	■ Increased VLDL, total cholesterol, and triglyceride levels ■ Chylomicrons present ■ Cholesterol-triglyceride ratio < 0.6

Interfering factors

■ Recent use of antilipemics (lower levels)
■ Failure to observe pretest restrictions
■ Hemolysis due to rough handling of the sample
■ Administration of heparin (which activates the enzyme lipase, producing fatty acids from triglycerides) or collection of the sample in a heparinized tube (possible false-high)

Selected readings

Anderson, S.C., and Poulsen, K.B. *Anderson's Atlas of Hematology.* Philadelphia: Lippincott Williams & Wilkins, 2003.

Cavanaugh, B.M. *Nurse's Manual of Laboratory and Diagnostic Tests,* 4th ed. Philadelphia: F.A. Davis Co., 2003.

Elisaf, M. "Effects of Fibrate on Serum Metabolic Parameters," *Current Medical Research and Opinion* 18(5):269-76, August 2002.

Goldman, L., and Ausiello, D., eds. *Cecil Textbook of Medicine,* 22nd ed. Philadelphia: W.B. Saunders Co., 2004.

Guyton, A.C., and Hall, J.E. *Textbook of Medical Physiology,* 10th ed. Philadelphia: W.B. Saunders Co., 2001.

Henry, J.B., et al. *Clinical Diagnosis and Management by Laboratory Methods,* 20th ed. Philadelphia: W.B. Saunders Co., 2001.

McClatchey, K.D. *Clinical Laboratory Medicine,* 2nd ed. Philadelphia: Lippincott Williams & Wilkins, 2002.

Mensink, R.P., et al. "Effects of Dietary Fatty Acids and Carbohydrates on the Ratio of Serum Total to HDL Cholesterol and on Serum Lipids and Apolipoprotein: A Meta-analysis of 60 Controlled Trials," *American Journal of Clinical Nutrition* 77(5):1146-55, May 2003.

Pagana, K.D., and Pagana, T.J., *Mosby's Diagnostic and Laboratory Test Reference,* 6th ed. St. Louis: Mosby Year–Book, Inc., 2003.

Schnell, Z., et al. *Davis's Comprehensive Handbook of Laboratory and Diagnostic Tests with Nursing Implications.* Philadelphia: F.A. Davis Co., 2003.

7

Protein, protein metabolites, and pigments

Introduction

Serum proteins, the most abundant compounds in serum, have great diagnostic significance because of their vital functions: binding and detoxifying drugs and other potentially toxic substances; performing as antibodies, enzymes, and hormones; sustaining the oncotic pressure of blood; maintaining acid-base balance through their buffering action; and serving as a reserve source of nutrition for tissues.

One protein — *albumin* — the most abundant, comprises almost 54% of the plasma proteins; *globulins* account for approximately 38% of plasma proteins. Fibrinogen accounts for approximately 7% of plasma proteins and is converted to fibrin during coagulation. The remaining 1% of circulating proteins consists of hormones, enzymes, complements, and carriers for lipids.

Serum protein formation

The major serum proteins are albumin, the globulins (alpha$_1$, alpha$_2$, beta, and gamma), and fibrinogen. The liver forms most of the albumin as well as the alpha and beta globulins. The reticuloendothelial system and immature plasma cells in the spleen, lymph nodes, and bone marrow produce gamma globulin.

Albumin is primarily responsible for maintaining the oncotic pressure of plasma, which in turn maintains normal water distribution in blood volume. Albumin also acts as a blood buffer and helps transport many drugs, dyes, and fatty acids by combining with them in the plasma.

The alpha globulins are responsible for transporting bilirubin and steroids, the beta globulins transport iron and copper, and the gamma globulins make up the antibodies of the immune system. For example, ceruloplasmin is a blue, copper-containing alpha globulin involved in copper transport and regulation. Ceruloplasmin is absent in the rare, inherited congenital form of Wilson's disease. Haptoglobulin comprises a group of alpha$_2$-globulins in human plasma and has the ability to combine with hemoglobin. Levels are decreased in hemolytic diseases and increased in inflammatory conditions, diabetes mellitus, or with tissue damage. Transferrin, a nonheme beta$_1$-globulin, acts as an iron-transporting protein.

The laboratory measurement of plasma proteins provides an extremely significant clinical assesment tool for detecting, diagnosing, and monitoring diseases and certain pathophysiological processes. An abnormality in the intricate relationship between these proteins may be indicative of varying disease states (for example, in-fection, inflammation, malnutrition, or autoimmune disorders). Plasma protein determinations early in the course of a disease may lead to improved patient outcome and decreased patient costs.

Protein metabolism

Approximately three-fourths of body solids are proteins. Unlike carbohydrates and fats, proteins aren't stored by the body. Instead, they're continuously broken down into amino acids in the intestinal mucosa and other sites such as the liver (also the site of gluconeogenesis). These amino acids form a common reserve for the synthesis of new proteins, hormones, enzymes, and nonprotein nitrogenous compounds such as creatine. Certain genetic disorders, such as phenylketonuria, can result from lack of a specific enzyme or inadequate transport activity, which alters the metabolic function of one or more amino acids.

The major end product of protein metabolism is *urea,* which is formed in the liver by deamination of amino acids. Urea is excreted in urine and is the primary method of nitrogen elimination. Blood levels of urea, measured as blood urea nitrogen (BUN), begin to rise with impaired glomerular excretion and are an important index of renal function.

Another important protein metabolite is *ammonia,* most of which is ultimately metabolized to urea in the liver and then excreted. Because impaired hepatic function inhibits such conversion of ammonia, serum ammonia levels rise in severe hepatic disease and can lead to hepatic coma.

Creatine is a nonprotein nitrogenous compound that combines with phosphate to form phosphocreatine, an important storage form of high-energy phosphate.

This compound is particularly prevalent in muscles. *Creatinine,* the end product of creatine metabolism, is excreted in urine and, like BUN levels, reflects the efficiency of renal excretory function.

Uric acid is the end product of purine metabolism and is excreted in urine. Serum uric acid levels and urate crystal deposits in synovial fluid are significant in diagnosing gout. Excessive levels in urine can lead to kidney calculi.

Bile pigments

Bile pigments are waste products of heme degradation, initiated by the breakdown of erythrocytes at the end of their life cycle. The five major steps in bile pigment metabolism include formation, plasma transport, hepatic uptake, conjugation, and biliary excretion. In humans, the bone marrow and spleen are the main sites of normal red cell destruction and heme degradation.

Although bile pigments have no known function, abnormalities in their overall transformation are significant in diagnosing hepatobiliary disease and conditions marked by excessive hemolysis. Conjugated bilirubin is converted into pigments responsible for the characteristic color of bile and stool; unconjugated bilirubin migrates in normal plasma, largely combined with albumin. Serum bilirubin levels may rise in hemolytic anemia, hepatocellular injury, and biliary duct occlusion.

PROTEIN TESTS

Protein electrophoresis

Protein electrophoresis is used to measure serum albumin and globulin, the major blood proteins, by separating the proteins into five distinct fractions: albumin and alpha$_1$, alpha$_2$, beta, and gamma globulin proteins.

Purpose
■ To aid in the diagnosis of hepatic disease, protein deficiency, renal disorders, and GI and neoplastic diseases

Patient preparation
■ Explain to the patient that protein electrophoresis is used to determine the protein content of blood.
■ Tell the patient that the test requires a blood sample. Explain who will perform the venipuncture and when.
■ Explain to the patient that he may experience slight discomfort from the needle puncture and the tourniquet.
■ Inform the patient that he need not restrict food and fluids.
■ Notify the laboratory and physician of medications the patient is taking that may affect test results; they may need to be restricted.

Procedure and posttest care
■ Perform a venipuncture and collect the sample in a 7-ml clot-activator tube.
■ Apply direct pressure to the venipuncture site until bleeding stops.
■ If a hematoma develops at the venipuncture site, apply warm soaks.
■ Inform the patient that he may resume his usual medications discontinued before the test, as ordered.

Precautions
■ This test must be performed on a serum sample to avoid measuring the fibrinogen fraction.

Reference values
Normally, total serum protein levels range from 6.4 to 8.3 g/dl (SI, 64 to 83 g/L), and

CLINICAL IMPLICATIONS OF ABNORMAL PROTEIN LEVELS

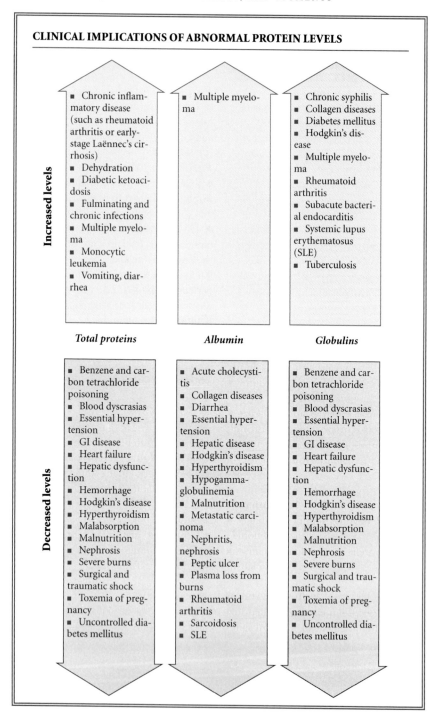

Increased levels

Total proteins

- Chronic inflammatory disease (such as rheumatoid arthritis or early-stage Laënnec's cirrhosis)
- Dehydration
- Diabetic ketoacidosis
- Fulminating and chronic infections
- Multiple myeloma
- Monocytic leukemia
- Vomiting, diarrhea

Albumin

- Multiple myeloma

Globulins

- Chronic syphilis
- Collagen diseases
- Diabetes mellitus
- Hodgkin's disease
- Multiple myeloma
- Rheumatoid arthritis
- Subacute bacterial endocarditis
- Systemic lupus erythematosus (SLE)
- Tuberculosis

Decreased levels

Total proteins

- Benzene and carbon tetrachloride poisoning
- Blood dyscrasias
- Essential hypertension
- GI disease
- Heart failure
- Hepatic dysfunction
- Hemorrhage
- Hodgkin's disease
- Hyperthyroidism
- Malabsorption
- Malnutrition
- Nephrosis
- Severe burns
- Surgical and traumatic shock
- Toxemia of pregnancy
- Uncontrolled diabetes mellitus

Albumin

- Acute cholecystitis
- Collagen diseases
- Diarrhea
- Essential hypertension
- Hepatic disease
- Hodgkin's disease
- Hyperthyroidism
- Hypogammaglobulinemia
- Malnutrition
- Metastatic carcinoma
- Nephritis, nephrosis
- Peptic ulcer
- Plasma loss from burns
- Rheumatoid arthritis
- Sarcoidosis
- SLE

Globulins

- Benzene and carbon tetrachloride poisoning
- Blood dyscrasias
- Essential hypertension
- GI disease
- Heart failure
- Hepatic dysfunction
- Hemorrhage
- Hodgkin's disease
- Hyperthyroidism
- Malabsorption
- Malnutrition
- Nephrosis
- Severe burns
- Surgical and traumatic shock
- Toxemia of pregnancy
- Uncontrolled diabetes mellitus

the albumin fraction ranges from 3.5 to 5 g/dl (SI, 35 to 50 g/L). The alpha$_1$-globulin fraction ranges from 0.1 to 0.3 g/dl (SI, 1 to 3 g/L); alpha$_2$-globulin ranges from 0.6 to 1 g/dl (SI, 6 to 10 g/L). Beta globulin ranges from 0.7 to 1.1 g/dl (SI, 7 to 11 g/L); gamma globulin ranges from 0.8 to 1.6 g/dl (SI, 8 to 16 g/L).

Abnormal findings
For common abnormal findings, see *Clinical implications of abnormal protein levels.*

Interfering factors
■ Pretest administration of a contrast agent, such as sulfobromophthalein (false-high total protein)
■ Pregnancy or cytotoxic drugs (possible decrease in serum albumin)
■ Use of plasma instead of serum

Ceruloplasmin

The ceruloplasmin test is used to measure serum levels of ceruloplasmin, an alpha$_2$-globulin that binds about 95% of serum copper, usually in the liver. Ceruloplasmin is thought to regulate iron uptake by transferrin, making iron available to reticulocytes for heme synthesis.

Purpose
■ To aid in the diagnosis of Wilson's disease, Menkes' syndrome, and copper deficiency

Patient preparation
■ Explain to the patient that this test is used to determine the copper content of blood.
■ Tell the patient that the test requires a blood sample. Explain who will perform the venipuncture and when.

■ Explain to the patient that he may experience slight discomfort from the needle puncture and the tourniquet.
■ Notify the laboratory and physician of medications the patient is taking that may affect test results; they may need to be restricted.

Procedure and posttest care
■ Perform a venipuncture and collect the sample in a 7-ml clot-activator tube.
■ Apply direct pressure to the venipuncture site until bleeding stops.
■ If a hematoma develops at the venipuncture site, apply warm soaks.
■ Inform the patient that he may resume his usual medications discontinued before the test, as ordered.

Precautions
■ Send the sample to the laboratory immediately.

Reference values
Serum ceruloplasmin levels normally range from 22.9 to 43.1 g/dl (SI, 0.22 to 0.43 g/L).

Abnormal findings
Low ceruloplasmin levels usually indicate Wilson's disease. Low levels may also occur in Menkes' syndrome, nephrotic syndrome, and hypocupremia caused by total parenteral nutrition. Elevated levels may indicate certain hepatic diseases and infections.

Interfering factors
■ Estrogen, methadone, phenytoin, and pregnancy (possible increase)

Haptoglobin

The haptoglobin test is used to measure serum levels of haptoglobin, a glycoprotein produced in the liver. In acute intravascular hemolysis, the haptoglobin concentration decreases rapidly and may remain low for 5 to 7 days, until the liver synthesizes more glycoprotein.

Purpose
- To serve as an index of hemolysis
- To distinguish between hemoglobin and myoglobin in plasma because haptoglobin doesn't bind with myoglobin
- To investigate hemolytic transfusion reactions
- To establish proof of paternity using genetic (phenotypic) variations in haptoglobin structure

Patient preparation
- Explain to the patient that this test is used to determine the condition of red blood cells.
- Tell the patient that the test requires a blood sample. Explain who will perform the venipuncture and when.
- Explain to the patient that he may experience slight discomfort from the needle puncture and the tourniquet.
- Inform the patient that he need not restrict food and fluids.
- Notify the laboratory and physician of medications the patient is taking that may affect test results; they may need to be restricted.

Procedure and posttest care
- Perform a venipuncture and collect the sample in a 7-ml clot-activator tube.
- Apply direct pressure to the venipuncture site until bleeding stops.
- If a hematoma develops at the venipuncture site, apply warm soaks.
- Inform the patient that he may resume his usual medications discontinued before the test, as ordered.

Precautions
- Handle the sample gently to prevent hemolysis.

Reference values
Normally, serum haptoglobin concentrations, measured in terms of the protein's hemoglobin-binding capacity, range from 40 to 180 mg/dl (SI, 0.4 to 1.8 g/L). Nephelometric procedures yield lower results.

⚙ **AGE ISSUE** *Haptoglobin is absent in 90% of neonates, but in most cases, levels gradually increase to normal by age 4 months.*

Abnormal findings
Markedly decreased serum haptoglobin levels are characteristic in acute and chronic hemolysis, severe hepatocellular disease, infectious mononucleosis, and transfusion reactions. Hepatocellular disease inhibits haptoglobin synthesis. In hemolytic transfusion reactions, haptoglobin levels begin decreasing after 6 to 8 hours and drop to 40% of pretransfusion levels after 24 hours.

If serum haptoglobin values are very low, watch for symptoms of hemolysis: chills, fever, back pain, flushing, distended jugular veins, tachycardia, tachypnea, and hypotension.

In about 1% of the population, including 4% of blacks, haptoglobin is permanently absent; this disorder is known as congenital ahaptoglobinemia.

Strikingly elevated serum haptoglobin levels occur in diseases marked by chronic inflammatory reactions or tissue destruction, such as rheumatoid arthritis and malignant neoplasms.

Interfering factors
- Hemolysis due to rough handling of the sample

- Corticosteroids and androgens (possible increase; may mask hemolysis in patients with inflammatory disease)

Transferrin

A quantitative analysis of serum transferrin (siderophilin) levels is used to evaluate iron metabolism. Transferrin is a glycoprotein formed in the liver. It transports circulating iron obtained from dietary sources or the breakdown of red blood cells by reticuloendothelial cells to bone marrow for use in hemoglobin synthesis or to the liver, spleen, and bone marrow for storage. A serum iron level is usually obtained simultaneously.

Purpose
- To determine the iron-transporting capacity of the blood
- To evaluate iron metabolism in iron deficiency anemia

Patient preparation
- Explain to the patient that the transferrin test is used to determine the cause of anemia.
- Tell the patient that the test requires a blood sample. Explain who will perform the venipuncture and when.
- Explain to the patient that he may experience slight discomfort from the needle puncture and the tourniquet.
- Inform the patient that he need not restrict food and fluids.
- Notify the laboratory and physician of medications the patient is taking that may affect test results; they may need to be restricted.

Procedure and posttest care
- Perform a venipuncture and collect the sample in a 4-ml clot-activator tube.
- Apply direct pressure to the venipuncture site until bleeding stops.

- If a hematoma develops at the venipuncture site, apply warm soaks.
- Inform the patient that he may resume his usual medications discontinued before the test, as ordered.

Precautions
- Handle the sample gently to prevent hemolysis.
- Send the sample to the laboratory immediately.

Reference values
Normal serum transferrin values range from 200 to 400 mg/dl (SI, 2 to 4 g/L).

Abnormal findings
Inadequate transferrin levels may lead to impaired hemoglobin synthesis and, possibly, anemia. Low serum levels may indicate inadequate transferrin production due to hepatic damage or excessive protein loss from renal disease. Decreased transferrin levels may also result from acute or chronic infection and cancer.

Increased serum transferrin levels may indicate severe iron deficiency.

Interfering factors
- Hemolysis due to rough handling of the sample
- Hormonal contraceptives and late pregnancy (possible increase)

PROTEIN METABOLITE TESTS

Plasma amino acid screening

Plasma amino acid screening is a qualitative screen for inborn errors of amino acid metabolism. Amino acids are the chief component of all proteins and polypeptides. The body contains at least 20 amino acids; 10 of these aren't formed in the body and must be acquired by diet. Certain congenital enzyme deficiencies interfere with normal metabolism of these amino acids, resulting in amino acid accumulation or deficiency.

Purpose
■ To screen for inborn errors of amino acid metabolism

Patient preparation
■ Explain to the parents that plasma and amino acid screening is used to determine how well their infant metabolizes amino acids.
■ Instruct the parents that the infant must fast for 4 hours before the test.
■ Tell the parents that a small amount of blood will be drawn from the infant's heel, but that collecting the sample only takes a few minutes.

Procedure and posttest care
■ Perform a heelstick and collect 0.1 ml of blood in a heparinized capillary tube.
■ Apply direct pressure to the venipuncture site until bleeding stops.
■ If a hematoma develops at the heelstick site, apply warm soaks.
■ Tell the parents to resume their infant's usual diet.

Precautions
■ Handle the sample gently to prevent hemolysis.

Normal findings
Chromatography shows a normal plasma amino acid pattern.

Abnormal findings
Excessive accumulation of amino acids typically produces overflow amino-

acidurias. Congenital abnormalities of the amino acid transport system in the kidneys produce a second group of disorders called renal aminoacidurias. Comparisons of blood and urine chromatography can help distinguish between the two types of aminoacidurias. The plasma amino acid pattern is normal in renal aminoacidurias and abnormal in overflow aminoacidurias.

Interfering factors
■ Failure to observe pretest restrictions
■ Hemolysis due to rough handling of the sample

Phenylalanine screening

The phenylalanine screening test, also called the Guthrie screening test, is used to screen infants for elevated serum phenylalanine levels, a possible indication of phenylketonuria (PKU). Phenylalanine is a naturally occurring amino acid essential to growth and nitrogen balance; an accumulation of this amino acid may indicate a serious enzyme deficiency. This test detects abnormal phenylalanine levels through the growth rate of *Bacillus subtilis,* an organism that needs phenylalanine to thrive. To ensure accurate results, the test must be performed after 3 full days (preferably 4 days) of milk or formula feeding.

Purpose
■ To screen the infant for possible PKU

Patient preparation
■ Explain to the parents that the test is a routine screening measure for possible PKU and is required in many states.
■ Tell the parents that a small amount of blood will be drawn from the infant's

heel, and that collecting the sample only takes a few minutes.

Procedure and posttest care
■ Perform a heelstick and collect three drops of blood — one in each circle — on the filter paper.
■ Reassure the parents of a child who may have PKU that although this disease is a common cause of congenital mental deficiency, early detection and continuous treatment with a low-phenylalanine diet can prevent permanent mental retardation.

Precautions
■ Note the infant's name and birth date and the date of the first milk or formula feeding on the laboratory request.
■ Send the sample to the laboratory immediately.

Reference values
A negative test result indicates normal phenylalanine levels (< 2 mg/dl [SI, < 121 µmol/L]) and no appreciable danger of PKU.

Abnormal findings
At birth, a neonate with PKU usually has normal phenylalanine levels, but after milk or formula feeding begins, levels gradually increase because of a deficiency of the liver enzyme that converts phenylalanine to tyrosine. A positive test result suggests the *possibility* of PKU. A definitive diagnosis requires exact serum phenylalanine measurement and urine testing. A positive test result may also indicate hepatic disease, galactosemia, or delayed development of certain enzyme systems. (See *Confirming PKU*.)

CONFIRMING PKU

If phenylalanine screening detects the possible presence of phenylketonuria (PKU), serum phenylalanine and tyrosine levels are measured to confirm the diagnosis. Phenylalanine hydroxylase is the enzyme that converts phenylalanine to tyrosine. If this enzyme is absent, increasing phenylalanine levels and falling tyrosine levels indicate PKU.

Samples are obtained by venipuncture (femoral or external jugular) and measured by fluorometry. Elevated serum phenylalanine levels (> 4 mg/dl [SI, > 242 µmol/L]) and low tyrosine levels — with urinary excretion of phenylpyruvic acid — confirm the diagnosis of PKU.

Interfering factors
■ Performing the test before the infant has received at least 3 full days of milk or formula feeding (false-negative)

Plasma ammonia

The plasma ammonia test measures plasma levels of ammonia, a nonprotein nitrogen compound that helps maintain acid-base balance. In such diseases as cirrhosis of the liver, ammonia can bypass the liver and accumulate in the blood. Plasma ammonia levels may help indicate the severity of hepatocellular damage.

Purpose
■ To help monitor the progression of severe hepatic disease and the effectiveness of therapy
■ To recognize impending or established hepatic coma

Patient preparation

- Explain to the patient (or to a family member if the patient is comatose) that the plasma ammonia test is used to evaluate liver function.
- Tell the patient that the test requires a blood sample. Explain who will perform the venipuncture and when.
- Inform the patient that he may experience slight discomfort from the needle puncture and the tourniquet.
- Notify the laboratory and physician of medications the patient is taking that may affect test results; they may need to be restricted.

Procedure and posttest care

- Perform a venipuncture and collect the sample in a 10-ml heparinized tube.
- Apply direct pressure to the venipuncture site until bleeding stops.
- If a hematoma develops at the venipuncture site, apply warm soaks.
- Watch for signs of impending or established hepatic coma if plasma ammonia levels are high.

Precautions

- Notify the laboratory before performing the venipuncture so that preliminary preparations can begin.
- Handle the sample gently to prevent hemolysis, pack it in ice, and send it to the laboratory immediately.
- Do *not* use a chilled container.

Reference values

Plasma ammonia levels in adults usually range from 15 to 45 µg/dl (SI, 11 to 32 µmol/L).

Abnormal findings

Elevated plasma ammonia levels are common in severe hepatic disease, such as cirrhosis and acute hepatic necrosis, and can lead to hepatic coma. Elevated levels may also occur in Reye's syndrome, severe heart failure, GI hemorrhage, and erythroblastosis fetalis.

Interfering factors

- Hemolysis due to rough handling of the sample
- Delay in testing
- Acetazolamide, thiazides, ammonium salts, and furosemide (increase)
- Parenteral nutrition or a portacaval shunt (possible increase)
- Lactulose, neomycin, and kanamycin (decrease)
- Smoking, poor venipuncture technique, and exposure to ammonia cleaners in the laboratory (possible increase)

Blood urea nitrogen

The blood urea nitrogen (BUN) test is used to measure the nitrogen fraction of urea, the chief end product of protein metabolism. Formed in the liver from ammonia and excreted by the kidneys, urea constitutes 40% to 50% of the blood's nonprotein nitrogen. The BUN level reflects protein intake and renal excretory capacity, but is a less reliable indicator of uremia than the serum creatinine level.

Purpose

- To evaluate kidney function and aid in the diagnosis of renal disease
- To aid in the assessment of hydration

Patient preparation

- Tell the patient that this test is used to evaluate kidney function.
- Inform the patient that he need not restrict food and fluids, but should avoid a diet high in meat.

- Tell the patient that the test requires a blood sample. Explain who will perform the venipuncture and when.
- Explain to the patient that he may experience slight discomfort from the needle puncture and the tourniquet.
- Notify the laboratory and physician of medications the patient is taking that may affect test results; they may need to be restricted.

Procedure and posttest care
- Perform a venipuncture and collect the sample in a 3- to 4-ml clot-activator tube.
- Apply direct pressure to the venipuncture site until bleeding stops.
- If a hematoma develops at the venipuncture site, apply warm soaks.
- Inform the patient that he may resume his usual medications discontinued before the test, as ordered.

Precautions
- Handle the sample gently to prevent hemolysis.

Reference values
BUN values normally range from 8 to 20 mg/dl (SI, 2.9 to 7.5 mmol/L).

AGE ISSUE *BUN will show slightly higher values in the elderly patient.*

Abnormal findings
Elevated BUN levels occur in renal disease, reduced renal blood flow (due to dehydration, for example), urinary tract obstruction, and increased protein catabolism (such as burns).

Low BUN levels occur in severe hepatic damage, malnutrition, and overhydration.

Interfering factors
- Hemolysis due to rough handling of the sample

- Chloramphenicol (possible decrease)
- Aminoglycosides, amphotericin B, and methicillin (increased due to nephrotoxicity)

Creatinine

Analysis of serum creatinine levels provides a more sensitive measure of renal damage than blood urea nitrogen levels. Creatinine is a nonprotein end product of creatine metabolism that appears in serum in amounts proportional to the body's muscle mass.

Purpose
- To assess glomerular filtration
- To screen for renal damage

Patient preparation
- Explain to the patient that the serum creatinine test is used to evaluate kidney function.
- Tell the patient that the test requires a blood sample. Explain who will perform the venipuncture and when.
- Explain to the patient that he may experience slight discomfort from the needle puncture and the tourniquet.
- Instruct the patient that he need not restrict food and fluids.
- Notify the laboratory and physician of medications the patient is taking that may affect test results; they may need to be restricted.

Procedure and posttest care
- Perform a venipuncture and collect the sample in a 3- or 4-ml clot-activator tube.
- Apply direct pressure to the venipuncture site until bleeding stops.
- If a hematoma develops at the venipuncture site, apply warm soaks.

- Inform the patient that he may resume his usual medications discontinued before the test, as ordered.

Precautions
- Handle the sample gently to prevent hemolysis.
- Send the sample to the laboratory immediately.

Reference values
Creatinine concentrations normally range from 0.8 to 1.2 mg/dl (SI, 62 to 115 µmol/L) in males and 0.6 to 0.9 mg/dl (SI, 53 to 97 µmol/L) in females.

Abnormal findings
Elevated serum creatinine levels generally indicate renal disease that has seriously damaged 50% or more of the nephrons. Elevated levels may also be associated with gigantism and acromegaly.

Interfering factors
- Ascorbic acid, barbiturates, and diuretics (possible increase)
- Exceptionally large muscle mass, such as that found in athletes (possible increase despite normal renal function)
- Hemolysis due to rough handling of the sample
- Phenosulfonphthalein (given within the previous 24 hours can elevate creatinine levels if the test is based on the Jaffé reaction)

Uric acid

The uric acid test is used to measure serum levels of uric acid, the major end metabolite of purine. Disorders of purine metabolism, rapid destruction of nucleic acids, and conditions marked by impaired renal excretion characteristically raise serum uric acid levels.

Purpose
- To confirm the diagnosis of gout
- To help detect renal dysfunction

Patient preparation
- Explain to the patient that the uric acid test is used to detect gout and kidney dysfunction.
- Tell the patient that the test requires a blood sample. Explain who will perform the venipuncture and when.
- Explain to the patient that he may experience slight discomfort from the needle puncture and the tourniquet.
- Instruct the patient to fast for 8 hours before the test.
- Notify the laboratory and physician of medications the patient is taking that may affect test results; they may need to be restricted.

Procedure and posttest care
- Perform a venipuncture and collect the sample in a 3- or 4-ml clot-activator tube.
- Apply direct pressure to the venipuncture site until bleeding stops.
- If a hematoma develops at the venipuncture site, apply warm soaks.
- Inform the patient that he may resume his usual diet and medications discontinued before the test, as ordered.

Precautions
- Handle the sample gently to prevent hemolysis.

Reference values
Uric acid concentrations in men normally range from 3.4 to 7 mg/dl (SI, 202 to 416 µmol/L); in women, normal levels range from 2.3 to 6 mg/dl (SI, 143 to 357 µmol/L).

Abnormal findings

Increased uric acid levels may indicate gout or impaired kidney function. Levels may also rise in heart failure, glycogen storage disease (type I, von Gierke's disease), infections, hemolytic and sickle cell anemia, polycythemia, neoplasms, and psoriasis.

Low uric acid levels may indicate defective tubular absorption (such as Fanconi's syndrome) or acute hepatic atrophy.

Interfering factors

- Failure to observe pretest restrictions
- Loop diuretics, ethambutol, vincristine, pyrazinamide, thiazides, and low doses of aspirin (possible increase)
- Acetaminophen, ascorbic acid, and levodopa (possible false-high if using colorimetric method)
- Aspirin in high doses (possible decrease)
- Starvation, high-purine diet, stress, and alcohol abuse (possible increase)

PIGMENT TESTS

Bilirubin

The bilirubin test is used to measure serum levels of bilirubin, the predominant pigment in bile. Bilirubin is the major product of hemoglobin catabolism. Serum bilirubin measurements are especially significant in neonates because elevated unconjugated bilirubin can accumulate in the brain, causing irreparable damage.

Purpose

- To evaluate liver function
- To aid in the differential diagnosis of jaundice and monitor its progress

- To aid in the diagnosis of biliary obstruction and hemolytic anemia
- To determine whether a neonate requires an exchange transfusion or phototherapy because of dangerously high unconjugated bilirubin levels

Patient preparation

- Explain to the patient that the bilirubin test is used to evaluate liver function and the condition of red blood cells.
- Tell the patient that the test requires a blood sample. Explain who will perform the venipuncture and when.

AGE ISSUE *If the patient is an infant, tell the parents that a small amount of blood will be drawn from his heel. Tell them who will be performing the heelstick and when.*

- Explain to the patient that he may experience slight discomfort from the needle puncture and the tourniquet.
- Inform the adult patient that he need not restrict fluids, but should fast for at least 4 hours before the test.

AGE ISSUE *Fasting isn't necessary for the neonate.*

Procedure and posttest care

- If the patient is an adult, perform a venipuncture and collect the sample in a 3- or 4-ml clot-activator tube.

AGE ISSUE *If the patient is an infant, perform a heelstick and fill the microcapillary tube to the designated level with blood.*

- Apply direct pressure to the venipuncture site until bleeding stops.
- If a hematoma develops at the venipuncture or heelstick site, apply warm soaks.

Precautions

- Protect the sample from strong sunlight and ultraviolet light.

■ Handle the sample gently and send it to the laboratory immediately.

Reference values

In adults, normal indirect serum bilirubin levels are 1.1 mg/dl (SI, 19 µmol/L), and direct serum bilirubin levels are less than 0.5 mg/dl (SI, < 6.8 µmol/L).

AGE ISSUE *In neonates, total serum bilirubin levels are 2 to 12 mg/dl (SI, 34 to 205 µmol/L).*

Abnormal findings

Elevated indirect serum bilirubin levels usually indicate hepatic damage. High levels of indirect bilirubin are also likely in severe hemolytic anemia. If hemolysis continues, direct and indirect bilirubin levels may rise. Other causes of elevated indirect bilirubin levels include congenital enzyme deficiencies such as Gilbert syndrome.

Elevated direct serum bilirubin levels usually indicate biliary obstruction. If obstruction continues, direct and indirect bilirubin levels may rise. In severe chronic hepatic damage, direct bilirubin concentrations may return to normal or near-normal levels, but indirect bilirubin levels remain elevated.

In neonates, total bilirubin levels of 15 mg/dl (SI, 257 µmol/L) or more indicate the need for an exchange transfusion.

Interfering factors

■ Exposure of the sample to direct sunlight or ultraviolet light (possible decrease)
■ Hemolysis due to rough handling of the sample

Fractionated erythrocyte porphyrins

The fractionated erythrocyte porphyrin test is used to measure erythrocyte porphyrins (also called erythropoietic porphyrins): protoporphyrin, coproporphyrin, and uroporphyrin. Porphyrins are present in all protoplasm and are significant in energy storage and use. They're produced during heme biosynthesis and usually appear in small amounts in blood, urine, and stool. The production and excretion of porphyrins or their precursors increase in porphyria.

Purpose

■ To aid in the diagnosis of congenital and acquired erythropoietic porphyrias
■ To help confirm the diagnosis of disorders affecting red blood cell (RBC) activity

Patient preparation

■ Explain to the patient that the fractionated erythrocyte porphyrin test is used to detect RBC disorders.
■ Tell the patient that the test requires a blood sample. Explain who will perform the venipuncture and when.
■ Explain to the patient that he may experience slight discomfort from the needle puncture and the tourniquet.

Procedure and posttest care

■ Perform a venipuncture and collect the sample in a 5-ml or larger heparinized tube.
■ Label the sample, place it on ice, and send it to the laboratory immediately.
■ Apply direct pressure to the venipuncture site until bleeding stops.
■ If a hematoma develops at the venipuncture site, apply warm soaks.

Precautions

- Handle the sample gently to prevent hemolysis.
- Send the sample to the laboratory promptly.

Reference values

Total porphyrin levels range from 16 to 60 µg/dl (SI, 0.25 to 1.062 µmol/L) of packed RBCs. Protoporphyrin levels range from 16 to 60 µg/dl. Coproporphyrin and uroporphyrin levels are normally less than 2 µg/dl (SI, < 0.035 µmol/L).

Abnormal findings

Elevated total porphyrin levels suggest the need for further enzyme testing to identify the specific porphyria. Elevated protoporphyrin levels may indicate erythropoietic protoporphyria, infection, increased erythropoiesis, thalassemia, sideroblastic anemia, iron deficiency anemia, or lead poisoning.

Increased coproporphyrin levels may indicate congenital erythropoietic porphyria, erythropoietic protoporphyria or coproporphyria, or sideroblastic anemia.

Elevated uroporphyrin levels may indicate congenital erythropoietic porphyria or erythropoietic protoporphyria.

Interfering factors

- Hemolysis due to rough handling of the sample
- Exposure of the sample to direct sunlight or ultraviolet light

Selected readings

Anderson, S.C., and Poulsen, K.B. *Anderson's Atlas of Hematology.* Philadelphia: Lippincott Williams & Wilkins, 2003.

Cavanaugh, B.M. *Nurse's Manual of Laboratory and Diagnostic Tests,* 4th ed. Philadelphia: F.A. Davis Co., 2003.

Elisaf, M. "Effects of Fibrate on Serum Metabolic Parameters," *Current Medical Research and Opinion* 18(5):269-76, August 2002.

Goldman, L., and Ausiello, D., eds. *Cecil Textbook of Medicine,* 22nd ed. Philadelphia: W.B. Saunders Co., 2004.

Guyton, A.C., and Hall, J.E. *Textbook of Medical Physiology,* 10th ed. Philadelphia: W.B. Saunders Co., 2001.

Henry, J.B., et al. *Clinical Diagnosis and Management by Laboratory Methods,* 20th ed. Philadelphia: W.B. Saunders Co., 2001.

McClatchey, K.D. *Clinical Laboratory Medicine,* 2nd ed. Philadelphia: Lippincott Williams & Wilkins, 2002.

Pagana, K.D., and Pagana, T.J. *Mosby's Diagnostic and Laboratory Test Reference,* 6th ed. St Louis: Mosby Year–Book, Inc., 2003.

Schnell, Z., et al. *Davis's Comprehensive Handbook of Laboratory and Diagnostic Tests with Nursing Implications.* Philadelphia: F.A. Davis Co., 2003.

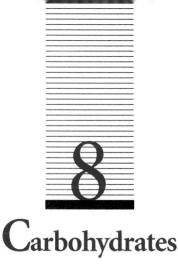

8

Carbohydrates

Introduction

Tests that measure the body's tolerance for carbohydrates — that is, the capacity to metabolize carbohydrates — have great clinical significance and rank among the most commonly performed laboratory tests. Clinical trials have proven the association between the development of diabetic complications and elevated plasma glucose (hyperglycemia). Blood glucose determinations are also useful for evaluating the function of hormone-secreting organs that help regulate blood glucose, for assessing intestinal absorption of glucose, and for evaluating liver function.

Such tests actually measure the capacity for conversion of carbohydrates by insulin. Because the direct assay of insulin is technically difficult and costly, the most useful tests measure insulin activity indirectly — by measuring blood glucose concentration.

These tests encompass many techniques for measuring blood glucose and differ greatly in specificity and sensitivity. The type of sample used also varies; normal values given in many common reference sources represent values derived from analysis of whole blood, which includes all reducing substances present in blood, such as fructose and other sugars and some drugs. However, most current automated laboratory equipment is specific for true glucose. (Reference values listed in this book are for plasma and for true glucose, unless otherwise specified.)

Why measure glucose?

Glucose, a 6-carbon monosaccharide, is the body's major source of energy. Blood glucose derives from the conversion of ingested carbohydrates to glucose and to other simple sugars by enzymatic activity in the digestive tract, from the metabolic conversion of noncarbohydrate sources in the liver and kidneys, and from the breakdown of hepatic glycogen (a major storage form of glucose).

Insulin and glucagon are the two chief regulators of glucose levels, but several other hormones influence glucose levels and are vital to normal carbohydrate metabolism. Growth hormone and corticotropin, secreted by the anterior pituitary gland, raise glucose levels by promoting glucose formation from fat and protein. Cortisol and similar 11-oxysteroids, secreted by the adrenal cortex, produce the same effect. Epinephrine and thyroxine raise blood levels by stimulating the conversion of glycogen to glucose.

Metabolism after eating and fasting

Carbohydrate metabolism is most easily explained by examining the body's response to food ingestion and to fasting. Ingestion of food causes a modest rise in blood glucose levels, triggering secretion of the hormone insulin by the beta cells of the islets of Langerhans, located in the pancreas.

Insulin, a simple protein, acts as a hypoglycemic by stimulating cellular absorption of glucose and promoting its conversion to storage forms. In the liver, insulin increases the synthesis of glucose to glycogen (glycogenesis) and thus inhibits the breakdown of hepatic glycogen to glucose. Normally, the liver stores 60% or more of ingested glucose as glycogen; peripheral tissues receive the rest. In the muscles, insulin enhances protein synthesis and amino acid storage and promotes the conversion of glucose to glycogen or fat. In adipose tissue, most of the absorbed glucose acts to synthesize triglycerides, inhibiting their breakdown to free fatty acids and glycerol. The two major determinants of hepatic and peripheral glucose uptake are prompt secretion of insulin and a normal tissue response to insulin.

In the fasting state, the body derives energy from stored sources. In response to diminishing levels of circulating carbohydrates, insulin secretion decreases and the glucagon concentration increases. *Glucagon* is a hyperglycemic, a small protein secreted by the alpha cells of the islets of Langerhans. When dietary carbohydrates — the body's preferred source of energy — are in short supply, glucagon stimulates glucose formation from protein and fat catabolized in the liver and kidneys (glyconeogenesis) and from the breakdown of hepatic glycogen stores (glycogenolysis). In adipose tissue, glucagon stimulates the breakdown of triglycerides to free fatty acids and glycerol (lipolysis); in the muscles, glucagon breaks down protein into amino acids (proteolysis).

Effects of abnormal insulin secretion

Insulin deficiency, as occurs in diabetes mellitus, causes profound abnormalities in carbohydrate, lipid, and protein metabolism that ultimately affect all body tissues, especially skeletal muscle, adipose tissue, and the liver. Without adequate insulin, the body can't use ingested carbohydrates efficiently. The resulting deficiency of carbohydrate energy sources causes the body to metabolize fat. Consequently, ketone bodies — intermediate products of fat metabolism — accumulate in the blood. The end result of this abnormal metabolic pattern is marked hyperglycemia, osmotic diuresis, severe dehydration, electrolyte imbalance, metabolic acidosis, and severe weight loss.

Excessive insulin secretion, as occurs in insulinoma, causes similarly disruptive metabolic effects. Insulin excess produces *hypoglycemia* (low blood glucose levels), characterized by diaphoresis, nervousness, weakness, nausea, and tachycardia. In the patient without diabetes, insulinoma is one cause of severe episodes of hypoglycemia. Unlike other causes of hypoglycemia, in which excessive insulin secretion follows immediately after eating (functional or reactive hypoglycemia), insulin secretion in insulinoma follows no distinct pattern. Hypoglycemia may develop long after eating (fasting hypoglycemia).

Although *hyper*glycemia is usually characteristic of diabetes, *hypo*glycemia may result from kidney failure, hepatic disease, alcoholism, decreased food intake, or excessive insulin administration. Brain tissue is most vulnerable to hypoglycemia because it doesn't synthesize glucose or store it in significant amounts. Thus, hypoglycemia is likely to impair cerebral function.

Glucagon imbalance rare
Primary glucagon imbalance is rare. Primary causes of elevated glucagon levels include familial hyperglucagonemia (an autosomal dominant disorder) and glucagonoma (islet alpha-cell tumor). Because abnormal islet alpha cells and abnormal beta cells may appear simultaneously, glucagonoma is characteristically associated with mild diabetes.

Elevated glucagon levels are usually linked to diabetes and insulin deficiency. Because insulin inhibits glucagon secretion, its absence or deficiency allows secretion of glucagon to continue, even in the presence of hyperglycemia. Another factor that enhances glucagon activity is unresponsiveness to insulin of the hepatic cells. Thus, glucagon may contribute to hyperglycemia, especially in hypoinsulinemia diabetes.

Glucose screening tests
Various tests screen for diabetes mellitus by measuring the body's response to fasting and to carbohydrate ingestion. The *fasting plasma glucose test* measures plasma glucose levels after a 12- to 14-hour fast. A patient with diabetes will have consistently high glucose levels because of insufficient insulin levels.

The *2-hour postprandial plasma glucose test,* performed 2 hours after the patient has eaten a high-carbohydrate meal, measures immediate insulin response to carbohydrate ingestion.

The *oral glucose tolerance test* (OGTT), the most sensitive method of evaluating borderline diabetes in selected patients, measures carbohydrate metabolism after ingestion of a challenge dose of glucose. This test is used to confirm diabetes and to aid in the diagnosis of hypoglycemia. It has significant limitations, however. Because no universal agreement exists regarding what values indicate an abnormal OGTT curve, the test allows no absolute distinction between a healthy person and one with mild diabetes. Moreover, this test has been known to suggest diabetes in a significant percentage of healthy people. Thus, an OGTT-confirmed diagnosis of latent or asymptomatic diabetes isn't necessarily significant.

Another limitation of this test is that different test methods provide different sets of values. Moreover, even when the same values are used for repeated testing, test results aren't consistently reproducible. Because of these limitations, the trend in laboratory testing is away from the OGTT and toward the fasting plasma glucose test for diagnosing diabetes mellitus.

Other useful tests

The *beta-hydroxybutyrate assay* helps detect carbohydrate deprivation resulting from dietary imbalances, digestive disturbances, frequent vomiting, or starvation. This test, which measures one of the three ketone bodies, is especially helpful in monitoring the effect of insulin therapy during treatment of diabetic ketoacidosis. It's also helpful during emergency care of hypoglycemia, acidosis, and alcohol ingestion.

The *glycosylated hemoglobin test* measures the reactive amount of glucose in hemoglobin and evaluates carbohydrate status for up to 120 days. This test is useful because patients with diabetes are known to have abnormal concentrations of hemoglobins A_{1a}, A_{1b}, and A_{1c} in the red blood cells — about twice the level in people without diabetes. In patients with poorly controlled diabetes, the abnormal concentrations of these hemoglobins may rise to three times the normal levels.

The *oral lactose tolerance test,* which measures plasma glucose levels after a challenge dose of lactose, helps diagnose lactose intolerance due to lactase deficiency.

Levels of *blood lactate,* the reduction product of pyruvate, are measured by enzymatic methods using lactate dehydrogenase. These methods are recommended for evaluating patients with symptoms of lactic acidosis such as Kussmaul's respirations. Either arterial or venous blood can be used for this test, but venous samples are easily obtained and so are more commonly used.

CARBOHYDRATE METABOLISM TESTS

Fasting plasma glucose

The fasting plasma glucose (or fasting blood sugar) test is used to measure plasma glucose levels after a 12- to 14-hour fast. This test is commonly used to screen for diabetes mellitus, in which absence or deficiency of insulin allows persistently high glucose levels.

Purpose
- To screen for diabetes mellitus
- To monitor drug or diet therapy in the patient with diabetes mellitus

Patient preparation
- Explain to the patient that this test is used to detect disorders of glucose metabolism and aids in the diagnosis of diabetes.
- Tell the patient that the test requires a blood sample. Explain who will perform the venipuncture and when.
- Explain to the patient that he may experience slight discomfort from the needle puncture and the tourniquet.
- Instruct the patient to fast for 12 to 14 hours before the test.

■ Notify the laboratory and physician of medications the patient is taking that may affect test results; they may need to be restricted.

■ Alert the patient to the symptoms of hypoglycemia (weakness, restlessness, nervousness, hunger, and sweating) and tell him to report such symptoms immediately.

Procedure and posttest care

■ Perform a venipuncture and collect the sample in a 5-ml clot-activator tube.

■ Apply direct pressure to the venipuncture site until bleeding stops.

■ If a hematoma develops at the venipuncture site, apply warm soaks.

■ Provide a balanced meal or a snack.

■ Instruct the patient that he may resume his usual medications discontinued before the test, as ordered.

Precautions

■ Send the sample to the laboratory immediately. If transport is delayed, refrigerate the sample.

■ Note on the laboratory request when the patient last ate, the sample collection time, and when the last pretest dose of insulin or oral antidiabetic drug (if applicable) was given.

Reference values

The normal range for fasting plasma glucose varies according to the laboratory procedure. Generally, normal values after at least an 8-hour fast are 70 to 110 mg (SI, 3.9 to 6.1 mmol/L) of true glucose per deciliter of blood.

Abnormal findings

Confirmation of diabetes mellitus requires fasting plasma glucose levels of 126 mg/dl (SI, 7 mmol/L) or more obtained on two or more occasions. In the patient with borderline or transient elevated levels, a 2-hour postprandial plasma glucose test or oral glucose tolerance test may be performed to confirm the diagnosis.

Increased fasting plasma glucose levels can also result from pancreatitis, recent acute illness (such as myocardial infarction), Cushing's syndrome, acromegaly, and pheochromocytoma. Hyperglycemia may also stem from hyperlipoproteinemia (especially type III, IV, or V), chronic hepatic disease, nephrotic syndrome, brain tumor, sepsis, or gastrectomy with dumping syndrome and is typical in eclampsia, anoxia, and seizure disorders.

Low plasma glucose levels can result from hyperinsulinism, insulinoma, von Gierke's disease, functional and reactive hypoglycemia, myxedema, adrenal insufficiency, congenital adrenal hyperplasia, hypopituitarism, malabsorption syndrome, and some cases of hepatic insufficiency.

Interfering factors

■ Failure to observe pretest restrictions (possible increase)

■ Recent illness, infection, or pregnancy (possible increase)

■ Glycolysis due to failure to refrigerate the sample or to send it to the laboratory immediately (possible false-negative)

■ Acetaminophen, if using the glucose oxidase or hexokinase method (possible false-positive)

■ Chlorthalidone, thiazide diuretics, furosemide, triamterene, hormonal contraceptives, benzodiazepines, phenytoin, phenothiazines, lithium, epinephrine, arginine, phenolphthalein, dextrothyroxine, diazoxide, large doses of nicotinic acid, corticosteroids, and recent I.V. glucose infusions (increase)

- Ethacrynic acid (may cause hyperglycemia); large doses in patients with uremia (can cause hypoglycemia)
- Beta-adrenergic blockers, ethanol, clofibrate, insulin, oral antidiabetic agents, and monoamine oxidase inhibitors (possible decrease)
- Strenuous exercise (decrease)

Two-hour postprandial plasma glucose

Also called the 2-hour postprandial blood sugar test, the 2-hour postprandial plasma glucose procedure is a valuable screening tool for detecting diabetes mellitus. The test is performed when the patient demonstrates symptoms of diabetes (polydipsia and polyuria) or when results of the fasting plasma glucose test suggest diabetes.

Purpose
- To aid in the diagnosis of diabetes mellitus
- To monitor drug or diet therapy in the patient with diabetes mellitus

Patient preparation
- Explain to the patient that the 2-hour postprandial plasma glucose test is used to evaluate glucose metabolism and to detect diabetes.
- Tell the patient that the test requires a blood sample. Explain who will perform the venipuncture and when.
- Explain to the patient that he may experience slight discomfort from the needle puncture and the tourniquet.
- Tell the patient to eat a balanced meal or one containing 100 g of carbohydrates before the test and then fast for 2 hours. Instruct him to avoid smoking and strenuous exercise after the meal.

- Notify the laboratory and physician of medications the patient is taking that may affect test results; they may need to be restricted.

Procedure and posttest care
- Perform a venipuncture and collect the sample in a 5-ml clot-activator tube.
- Apply direct pressure to the venipuncture site until bleeding stops.
- If a hematoma develops at the venipuncture site, apply warm soaks.
- Instruct the patient that he may resume his usual diet, medications, and activity discontinued before the test, as ordered.

Precautions
- Send the sample to the laboratory immediately or refrigerate it.
- Specify on the laboratory request when the patient last ate, the sample collection time, and when the last pretest dose of insulin or oral antidiabetic drug was given.
- If the sample is to be drawn by a technician, tell the patient the exact time the venipuncture must be performed.

Reference values
AGE ISSUE In the patient who doesn't have diabetes, postprandial glucose values are less than 145 mg/dl (SI, <8 mmol/L) by the glucose oxidase or hexokinase method; levels are slightly elevated in people over age 50. (See Two-hour postprandial plasma glucose levels by age, page 226.)

Abnormal findings
Two-hour postprandial blood glucose values of 200 mg/dl (SI, 11.1 mmol/L) or above indicate diabetes mellitus. High levels may also occur with pancreatitis, Cushing's syndrome, acromegaly, and pheochromocytoma. Hyperglycemia may also be caused by hyperlipoproteinemia

TWO-HOUR POSTPRANDIAL PLASMA GLUCOSE LEVELS BY AGE

The greatest difference in normal and diabetic insulin responses, and thus in plasma glucose concentration, occurs about 2 hours after a glucose challenge. Test values can fluctuate according to the patient's age. After age 50, for example, normal levels rise markedly and steadily, sometimes reaching 160 mg/dl (SI, 8.82 mmol/L) or higher. In a younger patient, a glucose concentration of more than 145 mg/dl (SI > 8 mmol/L) suggests incipient diabetes and requires further evaluation.

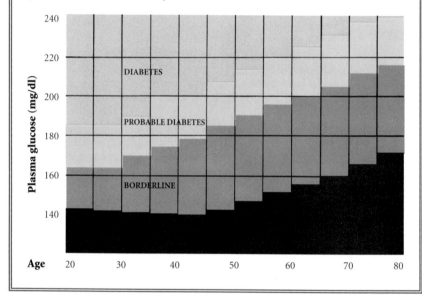

(especially type III, IV, or V), chronic hepatic disease, nephrotic syndrome, brain tumor, sepsis, gastrectomy with dumping syndrome, eclampsia, anoxia, and seizure disorders.

Low glucose levels occur in hyperinsulinism, insulinoma, von Gierke's disease, functional and reactive hypoglycemia, myxedema, adrenal insufficiency, congenital adrenal hyperplasia, hypopituitarism, malabsorption syndrome, and some cases of hepatic insufficiency.

Interfering factors

- Recent illness, infection, or pregnancy (possible increase)
- Acetaminophen, if using the glucose oxidase or hexokinase method (possible false-positive)
- Chlorthalidone, thiazide diuretics, furosemide, triamterene, hormonal contraceptives, benzodiazepines, phenytoin, phenothiazines, lithium, epinephrine, arginine, phenolphthalein, dextrothyroxine, diazoxide, large doses of nicotinic acid, corticosteroids, and recent I.V. glucose infusions (increase)

- Ethacrynic acid (possible increase); large doses in patients with uremia (possible decrease)
- Beta-adrenergic blockers, amphetamines, ethanol, clofibrate, insulin, oral antidiabetic drugs, and monoamine oxidase inhibitors (possible decrease)
- Strenuous exercise or stress (possible decrease)
- Glycolysis caused by failure to refrigerate the sample or to send it to the laboratory immediately (possible decrease)

Oral glucose tolerance

The oral glucose tolerance test (OGTT) is the most sensitive method of evaluating borderline cases of diabetes mellitus. Plasma and urine glucose levels are monitored for 3 hours after ingestion of a challenge dose of glucose to assess insulin secretion and the body's ability to metabolize glucose.

The OGTT isn't generally used in patients with fasting plasma glucose values greater than 140 mg/dl (SI, > 7.7 mmol/L) or postprandial plasma glucose values greater than 200 mg/dl (SI, > 11 mmol/L).

Purpose
- To confirm diabetes mellitus in selected patients
- To aid in the diagnosis of hypoglycemia and malabsorption syndrome

Patient preparation
- Explain to the patient that the OGTT is used to evaluate glucose metabolism.
- Instruct the patient to maintain a high-carbohydrate diet for 3 days and then to fast for 10 to 16 hours before the test, as instructed by the physician.
- Tell the patient not to smoke, drink coffee or alcohol, or exercise strenuously for 8 hours before or during the test.

- Tell the patient that this test requires five blood samples and usually five urine samples. Explain who will perform the venipunctures and when and that the patient may experience slight discomfort from the needle punctures and the tourniquet.
- Suggest to the patient that he bring a book or other quiet diversion with him to the test. The procedure usually takes 3 hours, but can last as long as 6 hours.
- Notify the laboratory and physician of medications the patient is taking that may affect test results; they may need to be restricted.
- Alert the patient to the symptoms of hypoglycemia (weakness, restlessness, nervousness, hunger, and sweating) and tell him to report such symptoms immediately.

Procedure and posttest care
- Between 7 a.m. and 9 a.m., perform a venipuncture to obtain a fasting blood sample. Draw this sample into a 7-ml clot-activator tube. A saline lock may be inserted and used to collect the multiple blood samples needed, as per facility protocol.
- Collect a urine sample at the same time if your facility includes this as part of the test.
- After collecting these samples, administer the test load of oral glucose and record the time of ingestion. Encourage the patient to drink the entire glucose solution within 5 minutes.
- Draw blood samples 30 minutes, 1 hour, 2 hours, and 3 hours after giving the loading dose using 7-ml clot-activator tubes.
- Collect urine samples at the same intervals.
- Tell the patient to lie down if he feels faint from the numerous venipunctures.

- Encourage the patient to drink water throughout the test to promote adequate urine excretion.
- Apply direct pressure to the venipuncture site until bleeding stops.
- If a hematoma develops at the venipuncture site, apply warm soaks.
- Provide a balanced meal or a snack, but observe for a hypoglycemic reaction.
- Instruct the patient that he may resume his usual medications discontinued before the test, as ordered.

Precautions
- Send blood and urine samples to the laboratory immediately or refrigerate them.
- Specify when the patient last ate and the blood and urine sample collection times.
- As appropriate, record the time the patient received his last pretest dose of insulin or oral antidiabetic drug.
- If the patient develops severe hypoglycemia, notify the physician. Draw a blood sample, record the time on the laboratory request, and discontinue the test. Have the patient drink a glass of orange juice with sugar added or administer I.V. glucose to reverse the reaction.

Reference values
Normal plasma glucose levels peak at 160 to 180 mg/dl (SI, 8.8 to 9.9 mmol/L) within 30 minutes to 1 hour after administration of an oral glucose test dose and return to fasting levels or lower within 2 to 3 hours. Urine glucose tests remain negative throughout.

Abnormal findings
Decreased glucose tolerance, in which levels peak sharply before falling slowly to fasting levels, may confirm diabetes mellitus or may result from Cushing's disease,

hemochromatosis, pheochromocytoma, or central nervous system lesions.

Increased glucose tolerance, in which levels may peak at less than normal levels, may indicate insulinoma, malabsorption syndrome, adrenocortical insufficiency (Addison's disease), hypothyroidism, or hypopituitarism.

Interfering factors
- Recent infection, fever, pregnancy, or acute illness such as myocardial infarction (possible increase)
- Failure to observe pretest restrictions
- Carbohydrate deprivation before the test (causing a diabetic response [abnormal increase with a delayed decrease] because the pancreas is unaccustomed to responding to high-carbohydrate load)
- Chlorthalidone, thiazide diuretics, furosemide, triamterene, hormonal contraceptives, benzodiazepines, phenytoin, phenothiazines, lithium, epinephrine, phenolphthalein, caffeine, arginine, dextrothyroxine, diazoxide, corticosteroids, large doses of nicotinic acid, and recent I.V. glucose infusions (possible increase)
- Beta-adrenergic blockers, amphetamines, ethanol, clofibrate, insulin, oral antidiabetic drugs, and monoamine oxidase inhibitors (possible decrease)

AGE ISSUE *Patients age 50 or older experience decreasing carbohydrate tolerance, which causes increasing glucose tolerance to upper limits of about 1 mg/dl for every year over age 50.*

β-hydroxybutyrate

The β-hydroxybutyrate test is used to measure serum levels of β-hydroxybutyric acid (beta-hydroxybutyrate), one of the three ketone bodies. The other two ketone bodies are acetoacetate and acetone. An accumulation of all three ketone bodies is referred to as ketosis; excessive formation of ketone bodies in the blood is called ketonemia.

Purpose
- To diagnose carbohydrate deprivation, which may result from starvation, digestive disturbances, dietary imbalances, or frequent vomiting
- To aid in the diagnosis of diabetes mellitus resulting from decreased carbohydrate intake
- To aid in the diagnosis of glycogen storage diseases, specifically von Gierke's disease
- To diagnose or monitor the treatment of metabolic disorders, such as diabetic ketoacidosis or lactic acidosis

Patient preparation
- Explain to the patient that this test is used to evaluate ketones in the blood.
- Tell the patient that the test requires a blood sample. Explain who will perform the venipuncture and when.
- Explain to the patient that he may experience slight discomfort from the needle puncture and the tourniquet.
- Inform the patient that he need not restrict food and fluids.

Procedure and posttest care
- Perform a venipuncture and collect the sample in a 5-ml clot-activator tube.
- Allow the sample to clot.
- Centrifuge the sample and remove the serum.
- If an acetone level is requested, have this analysis performed first.
- Keep in mind that serum β-hydroxybutyrate remains stable for at least 1 week at 25.6° to 46.4° F (−3.5° to 8° C). Plasma is also an acceptable sample for β-hydroxybutyrate analysis.

- Apply direct pressure to the venipuncture site until bleeding stops.
- If a hematoma develops at the venipuncture site, apply warm soaks.

Precautions
- Send the sample to the laboratory immediately.

Reference values
The normal value for serum or plasma β-hydroxybutyrate levels is less than 0.4 mmol/L (SI, < 0.4 mmol/L).

Abnormal findings
Elevated β-hydroxybutyrate levels may suggest worsening ketosis. Reference values greater than 2 mmol/L (SI, > 2 mmol/L) should be reported to the patient's physician immediately.

Interfering factors
- Presence of lactate dehydrogenase at high concentrations and lactic acid at concentrations greater than 10 mmol/L (SI, > 10 mmol/L) (possible increase)
- Increased sodium fluoride concentrations (possible decrease)
- Fasting (increase with extended fasting time)

Glycosylated hemoglobin

Also called total fasting hemoglobin (Hb), the glycosylated Hb test is a tool for monitoring diabetes therapy. Measurement of glycosylated Hb levels provides information about the average blood glucose level during the preceding 2 to 3 months. This test requires only one venipuncture every 6 to 8 weeks and can therefore be used for evaluating the long-term effectiveness of diabetes therapy.

Purpose
■ To assess control of diabetes mellitus

Patient preparation
■ Explain to the patient that the glycosylated Hb test is used to evaluate diabetes therapy.
■ Tell the patient that the test requires a blood sample. Explain who will perform the venipuncture and when.
■ Explain to the patient that he may experience slight discomfort from the needle puncture and the tourniquet.
■ Inform the patient that he need not restrict food and fluids, and instruct him to maintain his prescribed medication and diet regimens.

Procedure and posttest care
■ Perform a venipuncture and collect the sample in a 5-ml EDTA tube.
■ Apply direct pressure to the venipuncture site until bleeding stops.
■ If a hematoma develops at the venipuncture site, apply warm soaks.
■ Schedule the patient for an appointment in 6 to 8 weeks for appropriate follow-up testing.

Precautions
■ Completely fill the collection tube.
■ Invert the sample gently several times to mix the sample and the anticoagulant adequately.

Reference values
Glycosylated Hb values are reported as a percentage of the total Hb within an erythrocyte. Glycosylated Hb accounts for 4% to 7%.

Abnormal findings
In diabetes, the patient has good control of blood glucose concentrations when the glycosylated Hb value is less than 8%. A glycosylated Hb value greater than 10% indicates poor control.

Interfering factors
■ Failure to adequately mix the sample and the anticoagulant
■ Hemolytic anemia (decreased)
■ Hyperglycemia, thalassemia, chronic renal failure, the patient receiving dialysis, the patient that has a splenectomy, and the patient with elevated triglycerides or Hb F levels (increased)

Oral lactose tolerance

The oral lactose tolerance test is used to measure plasma glucose levels after ingestion of a challenge dose of lactose. It's used to screen for lactose intolerance due to lactase deficiency.

Absence or deficiency of lactase causes undigested lactose to remain in the intestinal lumen, producing such symptoms as abdominal cramps and watery diarrhea. True congenital lactase deficiency is rare. Usually, lactose intolerance is acquired because lactase levels generally decrease with age.

Purpose
■ To detect lactose intolerance

Patient preparation
■ Explain to the patient that this test is used to determine if his symptoms are due to an inability to digest lactose.
■ Instruct the patient to fast and to avoid strenuous activity for 8 hours before the test.
■ Inform the patient that this test requires four blood samples. Tell the patient who will be performing the venipunctures and when.
■ Explain to the patient that he may experience slight discomfort from the nee-

dle punctures and the tourniquet. Tell the patient that the entire procedure may take up to 2 hours.

■ Notify the laboratory and physician of medications the patient is taking that may affect test results; they may need to be restricted.

Procedure and posttest care

■ After the patient has fasted for 8 hours, perform a venipuncture and collect a blood sample in a 4-ml tube with sodium fluoride and potassium oxalate added.

■ Administer the test load of lactose: for an adult, 50 g of lactose dissolved in 400 ml of water; for a child, 50 g/m² of body surface area. Record the time of ingestion.

■ Draw a blood sample 30, 60, and 120 minutes after giving the loading dose. Use a 4-ml tube with sodium fluoride and potassium oxalate added.

■ If ordered, collect a stool sample 5 hours after giving the loading dose.

■ Apply direct pressure to the venipuncture site until bleeding stops.

■ If a hematoma develops at the venipuncture site, apply warm soaks.

■ Instruct the patient to resume his usual diet, medications, and activity discontinued before the test, as ordered.

Precautions

■ Send blood and stool samples to the laboratory immediately or refrigerate them if transport is delayed.

■ Specify the collection time on the laboratory requests.

■ Watch for symptoms of lactose intolerance — abdominal cramps, nausea, bloating, flatulence, and watery diarrhea — caused by the loading dose.

Reference values

Normally, plasma glucose levels rise over 20 mg/dl (SI, > 1.1 mmol/L) over fasting levels within 15 to 60 minutes after ingestion of the lactose loading dose.

Abnormal findings

A rise in plasma glucose of less than 20 mg/dl (SI, < 1.1 mmol/L) indicates lactose intolerance, as does stool acidity (pH of 5.5 or less) and high glucose content (> 1+ on the dipstick). Accompanying signs and symptoms provoked by the test also suggest, but don't confirm, the diagnosis because such symptoms may appear in the patient with normal lactase activity after a loading dose of lactose. Small-bowel biopsy with lactase assay may be performed to confirm the diagnosis.

Interfering factors

■ Failure to observe pretest restrictions

■ Thiazide diuretics, hormonal contraceptives, benzodiazepines, propranolol, and insulin (possible false-low)

■ Delayed emptying of stomach contents (possible decrease)

■ Glycolysis (possible false-negative)

TISSUE OXIDASE TEST

Lactic acid and pyruvic acid

Lactic acid, present in blood as lactate ion, is derived primarily from muscle cells and erythrocytes. It's an intermediate product of carbohydrate metabolism and is usually metabolized by the liver. Blood lactate concentration depends on the rates of production and metabolism; levels may increase significantly during exercise.

Lactate and pyruvate together form a reversible reaction that's regulated by oxygen supply. When oxygen levels are deficient, pyruvate converts to lactate; when they're adequate, lactate converts to pyruvate. When the hepatic system fails to metabolize lactose sufficiently or when excess pyruvate converts to lactate, lactic acidosis may result. Measurement of blood lactate levels is recommended for all patients with symptoms of lactic acidosis such as Kussmaul's respirations.

Comparison of pyruvate and lactate levels provides reliable information about tissue oxidation, but measurement of pyruvate is technically difficult and infrequently performed.

Purpose
■ To assess tissue oxidation
■ To help determine the cause of lactic acidosis

Patient preparation
■ Explain to the patient that this blood test is used to evaluate the oxygen level in tissues.
■ Tell the patient that the test requires a blood sample. Explain who will perform the venipuncture and when.
■ Explain to the patient that he may experience slight discomfort from the needle puncture and the tourniquet.
■ Withhold food overnight and make sure the patient rests for at least 1 hour before the test.

Procedure and posttest care
■ Perform a venipuncture and collect the sample in a 5-ml tube with sodium fluoride and potassium oxalate added.
■ Apply direct pressure to the venipuncture site until bleeding stops.
■ If a hematoma develops at the venipuncture site, apply warm soaks.

■ Instruct the patient that he may resume his usual diet and activity discontinued before the test, as ordered.

Precautions
■ Because venostasis may raise blood lactate levels, tell the patient that he must not clench his fist during the venipuncture.
■ Avoid using a tourniquet; however, if one must be used, release it at least 2 minutes before collecting the sample so blood can circulate.
■ Because lactate and pyruvate are extremely unstable, place the sample container in an ice-filled cup and send it to the laboratory immediately.

Reference values
Blood lactate values normally range from 0.93 to 1.65 mEq/L (SI, 0.93 to 1.65 mmol/L); pyruvate levels, from 0.08 to 0.16 mEq/L (SI, 0.08 to 0.16 mmol/L). The lactate-pyruvate ratio is normally less than 10:1.

Abnormal findings
Elevated blood lactate levels associated with hypoxia may result from strenuous muscle exercise, shock, hemorrhage, septicemia, myocardial infarction, pulmonary embolism, and cardiac arrest. When no reason for diminished tissue perfusion is apparent, increased lactate levels may result from systemic disorders, such as diabetes mellitus, leukemias and lymphomas, hepatic disease, and renal failure, or from enzymatic defects, such as von Gierke's disease (glycogen storage disease) and fructose 1,6-diphosphatase deficiency.

Lactic acidosis can follow ingestion of large doses of acetaminophen and ethanol as well as I.V. infusion of epinephrine, glucagon, fructose, or sorbitol.

Interfering factors
- Failure to observe pretest restrictions
- Failure to pack the sample in ice and to transport it to the laboratory immediately (possible increase)

Selected readings

Anderson, S.C., and Poulsen, K.B. *Anderson's Atlas of Hematology.* Philadelphia: Lippincott Williams & Wilkins, 2003.

Cavanaugh, B.M. *Nurse's Manual of Laboratory and Diagnostic Tests,* 4th ed. Philadelphia: F.A. Davis Co., 2003.

Greci, L.S., et al. "Utility of HbA$_{1c}$ Levels for Diabetes Case Finding in Hospitalized Patients with Hyperglycemia," *Diabetes Care* 26(4):1064-68, April 2003.

Goldman, L., and Ausiello, D., eds. *Cecil Textbook of Medicine,* 22nd ed. Philadelphia: W.B. Saunders Co., 2004.

Greenspan, F.S., and Gardner, D.G. *Basic and Clinical Endocrinology,* 7th ed. Stamford, Conn.: Appleton & Lange, 2004.

Guyton, A.C., and Hall, J.E. *Textbook of Medical Physiology,* 10th ed. Philadelphia: W.B. Saunders, Co., 2001.

Henry, J.B., et al. *Clinical Diagnosis and Management by Laboratory Methods,* 20th ed. Philadelphia: W.B. Saunders Co., 2001.

McClatchey, K.D. *Clinical Laboratory Medicine,* 2nd ed. Philadelphia: Lippincott Williams & Wilkins, 2002.

Pagana, K.D., and Pagana, T.J. *Mosby's Diagnostic and Laboratory Test Reference,* 6th ed. St. Louis: Mosby Year–Book, Inc., 2003.

Schnell, Z., et al. *Davis's Comprehensive Handbook of Laboratory and Diagnostic Tests with Nursing Implications.* Philadelphia: F.A. Davis Co., 2003.

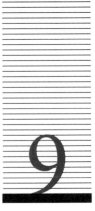

9

Vitamins and trace elements

Introduction

Vitamins and trace elements — organic and inorganic nutrients, respectively — are indispensable to normal metabolism and proper nutrition. Because the body can't synthesize most of these compounds, an adequate intake from nutritional sources is essential to maintain normal concentrations in the body. This is rarely a problem, except in people with very inadequate diets, because generous amounts of vitamins and trace elements are found in the basic food groups. Although food processing and cooking can reduce or destroy some of the nutrients in food, a balanced diet usually provides sufficient amounts to maintain health. Supplements are recommended only for a severely inadequate diet or a known deficiency.

Today, a far greater danger than trace element deficiency is toxic excess — through industrial exposure to potentially toxic levels of trace elements. Fortunately, sophisticated diagnostic techniques have been developed to detect minute concentrations of trace elements in serum. One such technique is atomic absorption spectroscopy. Equally sensitive bioassays and chemical assays are available to investigate vitamin toxicity or deficiency. For example, radioisotopes have been used to measure minute amounts of a specific vitamin such as vitamin B_{12} in serum.

Vitamins: Vital to support life
Originally classified as "vital amines," vitamins differ in chemical composition and aren't, in fact, all amines. However, they are vital for body maintenance, growth, and reproduction. Laboratory animals fed vitamin-depleted diets of carbohydrates, fats, minerals, and proteins failed to survive; only the animals fed diets containing adequate vitamins survived.

Because vitamins are generously prevalent in so many foods, absence of a vitamin, or *avitaminosis,* is rare indeed. A more common condition is *hypovitaminosis,* in which serum levels of a particular vitamin are below normal and may produce adverse clinical reactions. (See *Signs and symptoms of nutritional imbalances,* pages 236 and 237.)

Classification
Vitamins are classified as fat soluble or water soluble. *Fat-soluble vitamins,* which include vitamins A, D, E, and K, are associated with lipids in food sources and are similarly absorbed. Although these vitamins are necessary for survival, excessive or prolonged ingestion of most fat-soluble vitamins — especially in doses that exceed the recommended daily allowance — can have toxic effects because the body stores them in varying amounts and doesn't readily excrete them.

Unlike fat-soluble vitamins, which tend to be stored and accumulate in the body, *water-soluble vitamins,* including vitamin C and the B complex vitamins, are readily excreted in the urine. Consequently, excessive dietary ingestion doesn't produce toxicity, and deficiency of these vitamins is more common.

The vitamins and trace elements that will be discussed in detail in this chapter are vitamins A (and carotene), B_2, B_{12}, C, D_3, and folic acid.

Trace elements
Trace elements are minerals found in the body in minute quantities. Vital to health, many trace elements are an integral part of intracellular enzyme systems necessary for energy metabolism and other important biological processes. Although more than 20 trace elements have been identified, only a few (including manganese, cobalt, chromium, and zinc) are known to be essential to body functions. Manganese and zinc, for example, figure prominently in enzyme activation; cobalt is a critical factor in hepatopoiesis; and chromium is essential in amino acid transport. (Copper, another essential trace element, is commonly measured indirectly [See "Ceruloplasmin," page 209.])

Trace elements are found throughout nature in water, plants, and soil. Their concentrations in plant and animal food sources can lead to deficiencies or toxicity. However, because amounts required are so small and available from so many food sources, trace element deficiencies are rare. They're most likely to develop during long-term total parenteral nutrition unless the feeding solution contains trace element supplements.

Excessive accumulations and toxicity are becoming a more common problem. For example, heavy industrial use of such minerals as chromium and zinc can result in overexposure through inhalation, skin contact, or accidental ingestion. Similarly,
(Text continues on page 238.)

SIGNS AND SYMPTOMS OF NUTRITIONAL IMBALANCES

Vitamin or trace element	Deficiency	Toxicity
Vitamin A and carotene	■ Night blindness ■ Xerophthalmia ■ Bitot's spots ■ Skin and mucous membrane infections ■ Follicular hyperkeratosis	■ Hyperirritability ■ Yellow skin ■ Alopecia ■ Bone and joint pain ■ Headaches, vertigo ■ Hepatosplenomegaly, elevated liver enzyme levels ■ Malaise, fatigue ■ Abdominal pain, anorexia ■ Transient hydrocephalus and vomiting (in infants) ■ Dry skin, brittle nails
Vitamin B$_{12}$	*Megaloblastic anemia with:* ■ Yellow skin ■ Anorexia and weight loss ■ Dyspnea ■ Prolonged bleeding time ■ Abdominal pain, constipation, anorexia, and weight loss ■ Glossitis ■ Peripheral neuropathy ■ Ataxia ■ Weakness	■ Nontoxic (even in high doses)
Vitamin C	■ Bleeding gums, loose teeth, bruising ■ Joint pain ■ Irritability ■ Retarded growth ■ Dyspnea ■ Poor wound healing ■ Increased susceptibility to infection ■ Weight loss ■ Fever ■ Vomiting and diarrhea ■ Anemia	*Only after prolonged ingestion of massive doses (5,000 to 15,000 mg daily):* ■ Nausea and vomiting ■ Diarrhea ■ Possible formation of urinary tract calculi, especially uric acid calculi
Folic acid	*Megaloblastic anemia with:* ■ Yellow skin ■ Dyspnea ■ Prolonged bleeding ■ Abnormal pain, anorexia, and weight loss ■ Peripheral neuropathy ■ Ataxia ■ Weakness	■ Nontoxic (even in high doses)

SIGNS AND SYMPTOMS OF NUTRITIONAL IMBALANCES *(continued)*

Vitamin or trace element	Deficiency	Toxicity
Vitamin D$_3$	*Rickets in infants and children, characterized by:* ■ In early stages, profuse sweating, restlessness, and irritability ■ In late stages, bony malformations due to bone softening, delayed closing of fontanels, poorly developed muscles, and tetany *Osteomalacia in adults, characterized by:* ■ Bone malformation due to softening of bones in pelvis, spine, legs, and thorax ■ Rheumatic pain in lower back and legs ■ Spontaneous fractures	*Early:* ■ Anorexia ■ Nausea ■ Vomiting ■ Diarrhea ■ Headache *Late:* ■ Hypercalcemia leading to metastatic calcification and renal failure ■ Osteoporosis due to increased mobilization from bone
Chromium	■ Possible impaired glucose tolerance	■ Dermatitis ■ Vertigo ■ Abdominal pain ■ Anuria ■ Shock, seizures, coma
Manganese	■ Retarded growth ■ Bone abnormalities ■ Reproductive dysfunction ■ Ataxia	■ Pulmonary dysfunction ■ Early-stage encephalitis-like syndrome: anorexia, weakness, headache, impotence ■ Late-stage parkinsonian syndrome: masklike facies, monotone voice, tremor, muscle rigidity, spastic gait, clonus
Zinc	■ Sparse hair growth ■ Hepatosplenomegaly ■ Severe anemia ■ Impaired taste and smell acuity ■ Foul odor in nasopharynx ■ Anorexia ■ Pica (in children) ■ Retarded growth ■ Testicular atrophy ■ Hyperpigmentation ■ Impaired wound healing ■ Diarrhea ■ Increased susceptibility to infection	*From ingestion:* ■ GI irritation with fever, cramps, diarrhea, nausea and vomiting ■ Metallic taste in mouth *From inhalation:* ■ Metal fume fever ■ Dry throat, cough, chest discomfort ■ Tachycardia, hypertension ■ Pulmonary edema due to inhalation

contamination of drinking water and of edible plants by industrial wastes dispersed in the soil can also cause overexposure to trace elements. The trace elements discussed in detail in this chapter are manganese and zinc.

VITAMIN ASSAYS

Vitamin A and carotene

The vitamin A and carotene test measures serum levels of vitamin A (retinol) and its precursor, carotene. A fat-soluble vitamin normally supplied by diet, vitamin A is important for reproduction, vision (especially night vision), and epithelial tissue and bone growth. Vitamin A is found mostly in fruits, vegetables, eggs, poultry, meat, and fish. Carotene is present in leafy green vegetables and in yellow fruits and vegetables.

In this serum test, the color reactions produced by vitamin A and related compounds with various reagents provide quantitative and qualitative information.

Purpose
- To investigate suspected vitamin A deficiency or toxicity
- To aid in the diagnosis of visual disturbances, especially night blindness and xerophthalmia
- To aid in the diagnosis of skin diseases, such as keratosis follicularis or ichthyosis
- To screen for malabsorption

Patient preparation
- Explain to the patient that this test measures the vitamin A level in the blood.
- Instruct the patient to fast overnight, but that he need not restrict water intake.

- Tell the patient that the test requires a blood sample. Explain who will perform the venipuncture and when.
- Explain to the patient that he may experience slight discomfort from the needle puncture and the tourniquet.

Procedure and posttest care
- Perform a venipuncture and collect the sample in a chilled 7-ml siliconized tube.
- Apply direct pressure to the venipuncture site until bleeding stops.
- If a hematoma develops at the venipuncture site, apply warm soaks.
- Instruct the patient that he may resume his usual diet discontinued before the test.

Precautions
- Protect the sample from light because vitamin A characteristically absorbs light.
- Handle the sample gently and send it to the laboratory immediately.
- Keep the specimen on ice.

Reference values
Normal serum levels for carotene are 10 to 85 µg/dl (SI, 0.19 to 1.58 µmol/L) and vitamin A are 30 to 80 µg/dl (SI, 1.05 to 2.8 µmol/L).

Abnormal findings
Low serum levels of vitamin A (hypovitaminosis A) may indicate impaired fat absorption, as in celiac disease, infectious hepatitis, cystic fibrosis of the pancreas, or obstructive jaundice. Low levels are also associated with protein-calorie malnutrition (marasmic kwashiorkor). Similar decreases in vitamin A levels may also result from chronic nephritis.

Elevated vitamin A levels (hypervitaminosis A) usually indicate chronically excessive intake of vitamin A supplements or of foods high in vitamin A. Increased levels are also associated with hyper-lipemia and hypercholesterolemia of uncontrolled diabetes mellitus.

Decreased serum carotene levels may indicate impaired fat absorption or, rarely, insufficient dietary intake of carotene. Carotene levels may also be suppressed during pregnancy. Elevated carotene levels indicate grossly excessive dietary intake.

Interfering factors
- Failure to observe overnight fast
- Hemolysis due to rough handling of the sample
- Mineral oil, neomycin, and cholestyramine (possible decrease)
- Glucocorticoids and hormonal contraceptives (possible increase)

Vitamin B$_2$

The serum vitamin B$_2$ test evaluates serum levels of vitamin B$_2$ (riboflavin), a vitamin essential for growth and tissue function. The serum test is considered more reliable than the urine test, which can produce artificially high values in patients after surgery or prolonged fasting.

Purpose
- To detect vitamin B$_2$ deficiency

Patient preparation
- Explain to the patient that this test evaluates vitamin B$_2$ levels.
- Instruct the patient to maintain a normal diet before the test.
- Tell the patient that the test requires a blood sample. Explain who will perform the venipuncture and when.
- Explain to the patient that he may experience slight discomfort from the needle puncture and the tourniquet.

Procedure and posttest care
- Perform a venipuncture and collect the sample in a 4.5-ml siliconized tube.
- Apply direct pressure to the venipuncture site until bleeding stops.
- If a hematoma develops at the venipuncture site, apply warm soaks.
- Inform the patient with vitamin B$_2$ deficiency that good dietary sources of vitamin B$_2$ are milk products, organ meats (liver and kidneys), fish, green leafy vegetables, legumes, and fortified breads and cereals.

Precautions
- Handle the sample gently to prevent hemolysis.
- Send the sample to the laboratory immediately.
- Don't refrigerate or freeze the sample.

Reference values
Normal test results are 3 to 15 µg/dl; 2 to 3 µg/dl is considered marginally low, and less than 2 µg/dl is considered significantly diminished.

Abnormal findings
Marginally low test results (< 3 µg/dl) indicate vitamin B$_2$ deficiency. Such deficiency can result from insufficient dietary intake of vitamin B$_2$, malabsorption syndrome, or conditions that increase metabolic demands such as stress.

Interfering factors
- Hemolysis due to rough handling of the sample

Vitamin B$_{12}$

The vitamin B$_{12}$ radioisotope assay of competitive binding is a quantitative analysis of serum levels of vitamin B$_{12}$ (also called cyanocobalamin, antiperni-

COBALT: CRITICAL TRACE ELEMENT

A trace element found mainly in the liver, cobalt is an essential component of vitamin B_{12} and therefore is a critical factor in hematopoiesis. A balanced diet supplies sufficient cobalt to maintain hematopoiesis, primarily through foods containing vitamin B_{12}.

However, excessive ingestion of cobalt may have toxic effects. Toxicity has occurred, for example, in individuals who consumed large quantities of beer containing cobalt as a stabilizer, resulting in heart failure from cardiomyopathy. Because quantitative analysis of cobalt alone is difficult because of the minute amount found in the body, cobalt is commonly measured by bioassay as part of vitamin B_{12} testing.

Normal cobalt concentration in human plasma is 60 to 80 pg/ml.

cious anemia factor, or extrinsic factor). This test is usually performed concurrently with measurement of serum folic acid levels.

A water-soluble vitamin containing cobalt, vitamin B_{12} is essential to hematopoiesis, deoxyribonucleic acid synthesis and growth, myelin synthesis, and central nervous system (CNS) integrity. This vitamin is found almost exclusively in animal products, such as meat, shellfish, milk, and eggs. (See *Cobalt: Critical trace element.*)

Purpose
- To aid in the differential diagnosis of megaloblastic anemia, which may be due to a vitamin B_{12} or folic acid deficiency
- To aid in the differential diagnosis of CNS disorders that are affecting peripheral and spinal myelinated nerves

Patient preparation
- Explain to the patient that this test determines the amount of vitamin B_{12} in the blood.
- Instruct the patient to fast overnight before the test.
- Tell the patient that the test requires a blood sample. Explain who will perform the venipuncture and when.
- Explain to the patient that he may experience slight discomfort from the needle puncture and the tourniquet.
- Check the patient's history for drugs that may alter test results, and note these on the laboratory request.

Procedure and posttest care
- Perform a venipuncture and collect the sample in a 4.5-ml siliconized tube.
- Apply direct pressure to the venipuncture site until bleeding stops.
- If a hematoma develops at the venipuncture site, apply warm soaks.
- Instruct the patient that he may resume his usual diet discontinued before the test.

Precautions
- Handle the sample gently to prevent hemolysis.
- Send the sample to the laboratory immediately.

Reference values
Normally, serum vitamin B_{12} values range from 200 to 900 pg/ml (SI, 148 to 664 pmol/L).

Abnormal findings
Decreased serum levels may indicate inadequate dietary intake, especially if the

patient is a strict vegetarian. Low levels are also associated with malabsorption syndromes, such as celiac disease; isolated malabsorption of vitamin B_{12}; hypermetabolic states, such as hyperthyroidism; pregnancy; and CNS damage (for example, posterolateral sclerosis or funicular degeneration).

Elevated levels of serum vitamin B_{12} may result from excessive dietary intake; hepatic disease, such as cirrhosis or acute or chronic hepatitis; and myeloproliferative disorders such as myelocytic leukemia.

Interfering factors
- Failure to fast overnight and administration of substances that decrease vitamin B_{12} absorption
- Neomycin, metformin, anticonvulsants, and ethanol (possible decrease)
- Hormonal contraceptives (increase)

Vitamin C

Vitamin C chemical assay measures plasma levels of vitamin C (ascorbic acid), a water-soluble vitamin required for collagen synthesis and cartilage and bone maintenance. Vitamin C also promotes iron absorption, influences folic acid metabolism, and may be necessary for withstanding the stresses of injury and infection.

This vitamin is present in generous amounts in citrus fruits, berries, tomatoes, raw cabbage, green peppers, green leafy vegetables, and fortified juices. Severe vitamin C deficiency, or scurvy, causes capillary fragility, joint abnormalities, and multisystemic symptoms.

Purpose
- To aid in the diagnosis of scurvy, scurvylike conditions, and metabolic disorders, such as malnutrition and malabsorption syndromes

Patient preparation
- Explain to the patient that this test detects the amount of vitamin C in the blood.
- Instruct the patient to fast overnight before the test.
- Tell the patient that the test requires a blood sample. Explain who will perform the venipuncture and when.
- Explain to the patient that he may experience slight discomfort from the needle puncture and the tourniquet.

Procedure and posttest care
- Perform a venipuncture and collect the sample in a 4.5-ml heparinized tube.
- Apply direct pressure to the venipuncture site until bleeding stops.
- If a hematoma develops at the venipuncture site, apply warm soaks.
- Instruct the patient that he may resume his usual diet discontinued before the test.

Precautions
- Avoid rough handling or excessive agitation of the sample to prevent hemolysis.
- Send the sample to the laboratory immediately.

Reference values
Normal plasma vitamin C levels range from 0.2 to 2 mg/dl (SI, 11 to 114 µmol/L).

Abnormal findings
Values less than 0.3 mg/dl (< 16.5 µmol/L) indicate significant deficiency. Vitamin C levels diminish during pregnancy to a low point immediately postpartum. Depressed levels occur with infection, fever, and anemia. Severe deficiencies result in scurvy.

High plasma levels can indicate increased ingestion of vitamin C. Excess vitamin C is converted to oxalate, which is excreted in the urine. Excessive concentration of oxalate can produce urinary calculi.

Interfering factors
- Failure to observe pretest restrictions
- Hemolysis due to rough handling of the sample
- Failure to promptly send the sample to the laboratory

Vitamin D₃

Vitamin D_3 (cholecalciferol), the major form of vitamin D, is endogenously produced in the skin by the sun's ultraviolet rays and occurs naturally in fish liver oils, egg yolks, liver, and butter.

This competitive protein-binding assay determines serum levels of 25-hydroxycholecalciferol after chromatography has separated it from other vitamin D metabolites and contaminants. It's commonly combined with measurement of serum calcium and alkaline phosphatase levels.

Purpose
- To evaluate skeletal disease, such as rickets and osteomalacia
- To aid in the diagnosis of hypercalcemia
- To detect vitamin D toxicity
- To monitor therapy with vitamin D_3

Patient preparation
- Explain to the patient that this test measures vitamin D in the body.
- Tell the patient to restrict food and fluids for 8 to 12 hours before the test.
- Tell the patient that the test requires a blood sample. Explain who will perform the venipuncture and when.

- Explain to the patient that he may experience slight discomfort from the needle puncture and the tourniquet.
- Check for drugs that alter test results (corticosteroids or anticonvulsants). If they must be continued, note this on the laboratory request.

Procedure and posttest care
- Perform a venipuncture and collect the sample in a 4.5-ml siliconized tube.
- Apply direct pressure to the venipuncture site until bleeding stops.
- If a hematoma develops at the venipuncture site, apply warm soaks.
- Inform the patient that he may resume his usual medications discontinued before the test, as ordered.

Precautions
- Handle the sample carefully to prevent hemolysis.

Reference values
The range for serum 25-hydroxycholecalciferol values is from 10 to 60 ng/ml (SI, 25 to 150 nmol/L).

Abnormal findings
Low or undetectable levels may result from vitamin D deficiency, which can cause rickets or osteomalacia. Such deficiency may stem from poor diet, decreased exposure to the sun, or impaired absorption of vitamin D (secondary to hepatobiliary disease, pancreatitis, celiac disease, cystic fibrosis, or gastric or small-bowel resection). Low levels may also be related to various hepatic, parathyroid, and renal diseases that directly affect vitamin D metabolism.

Elevated levels (over 100 ng/ml [SI, >250 nmol/L]) may indicate toxicity due to excessive self-medication or prolonged therapy. Elevated levels associated with hypercalcemia may be due to hypersensitivity to vitamin D, as in sarcoidosis.

Interfering factors
- Hemolysis due to rough handling of the sample
- Anticonvulsants, isoniazid, mineral oil, corticosteroids, aluminum hydroxide, cholestyramine, and colestipol (possible decrease)

Folic acid

The folic acid test is a quantitative analysis of serum folic acid levels (also called pteroylglutamic acid, folacin, or folate) by radioisotope assay of competitive binding. It's commonly performed concomitantly with measurement of serum vitamin B_{12} levels. Like vitamin B_{12}, folic acid is a water-soluble vitamin that influences hematopoiesis, deoxyribonucleic acid synthesis, and overall body growth.

Normally, diet supplies folic acid in organ meats, such as liver or kidneys, yeast, fruits, leafy vegetables, fortified breads and cereals, eggs, and milk. Inadequate dietary intake may cause a deficiency, especially during pregnancy. Because of folic acid's vital role in hematopoiesis, the usual indication for this test is a suspected hematologic abnormality.

Purpose
- To aid in the differential diagnosis of megaloblastic anemia, which may result from folic acid or vitamin B_{12} deficiency
- To assess folate stores in pregnancy

Patient preparation
- Explain to the patient that this test determines the folic acid level in the blood.
- Instruct the patient to fast overnight before the test.

- Tell the patient that the test requires a blood sample. Explain who will perform the venipuncture and when.
- Explain to the patient that he may experience slight discomfort from the needle puncture and the tourniquet.
- Check the patient's history for drugs that may affect test results, such as phenytoin or pyrimethamine.

Procedure and posttest care
- Perform a venipuncture and collect the sample in a 4.5-ml tube without additives.
- Apply direct pressure to the venipuncture site until bleeding stops.
- If a hematoma develops at the venipuncture site, apply warm soaks.
- Instruct the patient that he may resume his usual diet.

Precautions
- Handle the sample gently to prevent hemolysis.
- Protect the sample from light.
- Send the sample to the laboratory immediately.

Reference values
Normally, serum folic acid values are 1.8 to 9 ng/ml (SI, 4 to 20 nmol/L).

Abnormal findings
Low serum levels may indicate hematologic abnormalities, such as anemia (especially megaloblastic anemia), leukopenia, and thrombocytopenia. The Schilling test is usually performed to rule out vitamin B_{12} deficiency, which also causes megaloblastic anemia. Decreased folic acid levels can also result from hypermetabolic states (such as hyperthyroidism), inadequate dietary intake, small-bowel malabsorption syndrome, hepatic or re-

nal diseases, chronic alcoholism, or pregnancy.

Serum levels greater than normal may indicate excessive dietary intake of folic acid or folic acid supplements. Even when taken in large doses, this vitamin is nontoxic.

Interfering factors
■ Hemolysis due to rough handling of the sample
■ Alcohol; phenytoin; pyrimethamine; anticonvulsants, such as primidone; antineoplastics; antimalarials; and hormonal contraceptives (possible decrease)

TRACE ELEMENT ASSAYS

Manganese

The manganese test, an analysis by atomic absorption spectroscopy, measures serum levels of manganese, a trace element. Although its function is only partially understood, manganese is known to activate several enzymes — including cholinesterase and arginase — that are essential to metabolism. Dietary sources of manganese include unrefined cereals, green leafy vegetables, and nuts.

Manganese toxicity may result from the inhalation of manganese dust or fumes — a hazard in the steel and dry-cell battery industries — or from ingestion of contaminated water.

Purpose
■ To detect manganese toxicity

Patient preparation
■ Explain to the patient that this test determines the level of manganese in the blood.
■ Inform the patient that he need not restrict food and fluids.
■ Tell the patient that the test requires a blood sample. Explain who will perform the venipuncture and when.
■ Explain to the patient that he may experience slight discomfort from the needle puncture and the tourniquet.
■ Check the patient's history for medications that may influence serum manganese levels, such as estrogens and glucocorticoids.

Procedure and posttest care
■ Perform a venipuncture and collect the sample in a metal-free collection tube. Laboratories will supply a special kit for this test on request.
■ Apply direct pressure to the venipuncture site until bleeding stops.
■ If a hematoma develops at the venipuncture site, apply warm soaks.

Precautions
■ Handle the sample gently to prevent hemolysis.
■ Send the sample to the laboratory immediately.

Reference values
Normally, serum manganese values range from 0.4 to 1.4 μg/ml.

Abnormal findings
Significantly elevated serum levels indicate manganese toxicity, which requires prompt medical attention to prevent central nervous system deterioration. Depressed serum manganese levels may indicate deficient dietary intake, although deficiency hasn't been linked to disease.

Interfering factors

- Failure to use a metal-free collection tube
- Hemolysis due to rough handling of the sample
- High dietary intake of calcium and phosphorus (possible decrease due to interference with intestinal absorption of manganese)
- Estrogen (increase)
- Glucocorticoids (increase or decrease due to altered distribution of manganese in the body)

Zinc

The zinc test, an analysis by atomic absorption spectroscopy, measures serum zinc levels. An important trace element, zinc is an integral component of more than 80 enzymes and proteins and plays a critical role in enzyme catalytic reactions.

Zinc occurs naturally in water and in most foods; high concentrations are found in meat, seafood, dairy products, whole grains, nuts, and legumes. Zinc deficiency can seriously impair body metabolism, growth, and development.

Purpose

- To detect zinc deficiency or toxicity

Patient preparation

- Explain to the patient that this test determines the concentration of zinc in the blood.
- Inform the patient that he need not restrict food and fluids.
- Tell the patient that the test requires a blood sample. Explain who will perform the venipuncture and when.
- Explain to the patient that he may experience slight discomfort from the needle puncture and the tourniquet.

Procedure and posttest care

- Perform a venipuncture and collect a 7- to 10-ml sample in a zinc-free collection tube.
- Apply direct pressure to the venipuncture site until bleeding stops.
- If a hematoma develops at the venipuncture site, apply warm soaks.

Precautions

- Handle the sample gently to prevent hemolysis.
- Send the sample to the laboratory immediately. Reliable analysis must begin before platelet disintegration can alter test results.

Reference values

Normally, plasma zinc values range from 70 to 120 µg/dl (SI, 10.7 to 18.4 µmol/L).

Abnormal findings

Decreased serum zinc levels may indicate an acquired deficiency (from insufficient dietary intake or due to an underlying disease) or a hereditary deficiency. Markedly depressed levels are common in leukemia and may be related to impaired zinc-dependent enzyme systems. Low serum zinc levels are commonly associated with alcoholic cirrhosis of the liver, myocardial infarction, ileitis, chronic renal failure, rheumatoid arthritis, and anemia (such as hemolytic or sickle cell anemia).

Elevated and potentially toxic serum zinc levels may result from accidental ingestion or industrial exposure.

Interfering factors

- Failure to use a metal-free collection tube
- Hemolysis due to rough handling of the sample
- Delayed transport to the laboratory

■ Time of day and time of last meal (possible increase or decrease)

■ Zinc-chelating agents, such as penicillinase, and corticosteroids (decrease)

■ Estrogens; penicillamine; antineoplastics, such as cisplatin; antimetabolites; and diuretics (possible decrease)

Selected readings

Anderson, S.C., and Poulsen, K.B. *Anderson's Atlas of Hematology.* Philadelphia: Lippincott Williams & Wilkins, 2003.

Cavanaugh, B.M. *Nurse's Manual of Laboratory and Diagnostic Tests,* 4th ed. Philadelphia: F.A. Davis Co., 2003.

Goldman, L., and Ausiello, D., eds. *Cecil Textbook of Medicine,* 22nd ed. Philadelphia: W.B. Saunders Co., 2004.

Guyton, A.C., and Hall, J.E. *Textbook of Medical Physiology,* 10th ed. Philadelphia: W.B. Saunders Co., 2001.

Henry, J.B., et al. *Clinical Diagnosis and Management by Laboratory Methods,* 20th ed. Philadelphia: W.B. Saunders Co., 2001.

McClatchey, K.D. *Clinical Laboratory Medicine,* 2nd ed. Philadelphia: Lippincott Williams & Wilkins, 2002.

Pagana, K.D., and Pagana, T.J. *Mosby's Diagnostic and Laboratory Test Reference,* 6th ed. St. Louis: Mosby Year–Book, Inc., 2003.

Schnell, Z., et al. *Davis's Comprehensive Handbook of Laboratory and Diagnostic Tests with Nursing Implications.* Philadelphia: F.A. Davis Co., 2003.

10

Immuno-hematology

Introduction

Immunohematology refers to the theory and techniques of blood banking. Included is the study of antigen-antibody reactions and their effects on blood. An *antigen* is a substance that can initiate an immune response and induce the formation of a corresponding antibody. Established antigens found in blood are inherited. Others can be introduced into the body from exogenous sources, such as blood transfusions or drugs. An *antibody* is an immunoglobulin molecule synthesized in response to a specific antigen.

Successful blood transfusions require tests that identify these naturally occurring or acquired antigens and antibodies to make possible correct matching of donor and recipient blood. The major blood group systems are the ABO and Rh-Hr systems. Among the most important of these tests are ABO blood typing, Rh typing, crossmatching, direct antiglobulin, and antibody screening. If a transfusion reaction occurs despite correct transfusion of compatible blood, tests for other antibodies (such as leuko-

247

agglutinins) help identify the cause and prevent further reactions.

ABO blood group system

All blood group classifications are based on the types of antigens present or absent on the surfaces of red blood cells (RBCs). Persons with group A blood have RBCs with A antigens; those with group B blood have B antigens. AB blood contains A and B antigens; group O blood contains neither.

In the ABO system, one or both of two naturally occurring antibodies, anti-A and anti-B, are found in the serum. Thus, a person with group A blood has anti-B antibodies, rather than anti-A antibodies, because the latter would destroy his RBCs. Similarly, a person with group B blood has anti-A antibodies. A person with group O blood has anti-A and anti-B antibodies; a person with AB blood has neither type of antibody.

Because group O blood lacks A and B antigens, it can be transfused in limited amounts to any recipient in an emergency, regardless of his blood type, with little risk of agglutination. For this reason, a person with group O blood is called a *universal donor*. However, transfusions of universal donor blood should be given as packed RBCs, from which the plasma has been removed. A person with AB blood, who has neither anti-A nor anti-B antibodies, can receive A, B, or O blood (packed cells) and is called a *universal recipient*.

Typing and crossmatching of donor and recipient blood are required before a transfusion to establish compatibility. These tests minimize the risk of a hemolytic reaction, an immune reaction that occurs when the donor's and recipient's blood types are mismatched—for example, when blood containing anti-A antibodies is mixed with blood containing A antigens or when blood containing anti-B antibodies is mixed with blood containing B antigens.

When mismatching occurs, two types of reactions are possible. One is agglutination where the antibodies attach to the surface of the foreign RBCs, causing the cells to clump together. This clumping can eventually plug small blood vessels and arterioles. The second type is hemolysis, which occurs when an antibody-antigen reaction activates the body's complement system—a group of enzymatic proteins—and promotes and accelerates RBC hemolysis and phagocytosis by the reticuloendothelial cells. RBC hemolysis releases free hemoglobin into the bloodstream, which can damage the renal tubules and lead to renal failure and death.

Rh blood group system

In 1940, the Rh blood group system was developed after discovery of a certain antigen on the surface of RBCs in virtually all rhesus monkeys. Among humans, about 85% of Whites and an even higher percentage of Blacks, Native Americans, and Asians carry the Rh antigen—known as $Rh_o(D)$ factor—on their RBCs. Such blood is therefore classified as *Rh-positive*. The remaining 15% or less of the population lack this factor, and their blood is typed *Rh-negative*. The Rh antigen is highly immunogenic—that is, it's more likely to stimulate formation of an antibody than other known antigens.

Consequently, a person with Rh-positive blood doesn't carry anti-Rh antibodies in his serum because they would destroy his RBCs. However, a person with Rh-negative blood develops anti-Rh antibodies following exposure to Rh-positive blood (by transfusion or pregnancy). A transfusion reaction usually doesn't occur after the initial exposure to Rh-positive blood. Rather, anti-Rh antibodies generally develop slowly, over several weeks, causing the transfusion recipient to become sensitized to the Rh antigen. Subsequent exposure to Rh-positive blood then provokes a transfusion reaction and hemolysis, as in hemolytic disease of the neonate.

An important variation in the Rh system is the weak D antigen (formerly known as D^u variant). This antigen, considered Rh-positive, is somewhat less immunogenic than $Rh_o(D)$ and may not provoke antibody production in persons who lack it. Thus, all prospective donors must be screened for the weak D antigen, which is more common in Blacks than in Whites.

Other clinically significant Rh antigens also have been discovered; these additional antigens, such as rh′ (C), rh″ (F), hr′ (c) and hr″ (e) are much less immunogenic and not as likely to provoke an antibody reaction as $Rh_o(D)$. Tests for these antigens are done only in special cases, as for establishing paternity, determining family studies, or distinguishing between heterozygous and homozygous Rh-positive factors.

Screening blood donors

To qualify for selection, prospective blood donors must meet strict criteria established by the Scientific Committee of the Joint Blood Council and the Standards Committee of the American Association of Blood Banks. The purpose of these guidelines is to protect the donor and the recipient and to ensure a safe, therapeutic blood transfusion.

Before donation, a detailed medical history must be obtained from the prospective donor to detect disorders or conditions that could exclude or defer the donation. Such conditions include any disease that can be transmitted by blood transfusion (such as viral hepatitis, malaria, Creutzfeldt-Jakob disease, babesiosis, Chagas' disease, or acquired immunodeficiency syndrome [AIDS]), active tuberculosis, alcoholism, drug addiction or drug therapy, pregnancy, cancer, and recent immunizations or dental surgery.

A physical examination and laboratory tests must then be done to determine if the prospective donor meets the following minimum health standards:

- *age:* between 17 and 65 (if the donor is younger than 17, he or she can donate blood with parental consent; if older than age 65, he or she can donate blood with a physician's consent).
- *weight:* should weigh at least 110 lb (50 kg)
- *blood pressure:* systolic pressure no higher than 180 mm Hg; diastolic pressure no higher than 100 mm Hg
- *pulse:* between 50 and 100 beats/minute and regular
- *oral temperature:* shouldn't exceed 99.5° (37.5° C)
- *skin:* should be free from all lesions at the venipuncture site; should show no evidence of I.V. drug abuse
- *hemoglobin:* no less than 12.5 g/dl
- *hematocrit:* no less than 38%.

The prospective donor also is required to give informed consent to allow donation to proceed.

Testing donor blood

Except in the case of identical twins or autologous transfusion (in which a person receives his own blood), testing for blood compatibility between donor and recipient can never be foolproof. Howev-

er, the following tests on donor blood can improve selection for the recipient:
- determining ABO and Rh blood groups
- detecting unexpected antibodies that can coat, hemolyze, or agglutinate RBCs
- crossmatching of donor blood and recipient blood (before transfusion)
- detecting hepatitis B surface antigen (HBsAg) as well as antibodies to hepatitis B core antigen (anti-HB$_c$); to hepatitis C virus (anti-HCV); to human T-cell lymphotropic virus, type I (anti-HTLV-I); to human immunodeficiency viruses (anti-HIV-1 and anti-HIV-2); and to syphilis.

Special considerations

After the compatibility of donor and recipient blood has been established, the most important consideration is to ensure matching of the *right* blood with the *right* patient. Hemolytic reactions are most commonly caused by giving blood to the wrong person and mislabeling the sample.

Double-check the patient's name, medical record number, and ABO and Rh status, preferably with another health care professional or a physician. If there's a discrepancy—no matter how slight—*don't* administer the blood. Instead, notify the blood bank immediately so a substitution can be made without delay. Preventing potentially fatal hemolytic reactions from mismatched blood transfusions ranks among the most critical of professional responsibilities. Uncompromising thoroughness and strict adherence to protocol ensures your patients' safety.

After blood is administered, watch for signs and symptoms of a transfusion reaction. Check the patient's vital signs before and during the blood transfusion. For the first 15 minutes, transfuse the

blood slowly to lessen the severity of any reaction that may occur, and stay with the patient. Notify the physician immediately at the first signs of a transfusion reaction.

AGGLUTINATION TESTS

ABO blood typing

ABO blood typing classifies blood according to the presence of major antigens A and B on red blood cell (RBC) surfaces and according to serum antibodies anti-A and anti-B. ABO blood typing using forward and reverse methods is required before transfusion to prevent a lethal reaction.

In forward typing, the patient's RBCs are mixed with anti-A serum, then with anti-B serum; the presence or absence of agglutination determines the blood group. In reverse typing, the results of the forward method are verified by mixing the patient's serum with known group A and group B cells. Blood group determination is confirmed when the results of forward and reverse typing match perfectly.

Purpose
- To establish blood group according to the ABO system
- To check compatibility of donor and recipient blood before transfusion

Patient preparation
- Tell the patient that this test determines his blood group.
- If the patient is scheduled for a transfusion, explain that after his blood group is

known, it can be matched with the right donor blood.

■ Inform the patient that he need not restrict food and fluids.

■ Tell the patient that the test requires a blood sample. Explain who will perform the venipuncture and when.

■ Explain to the patient that he may experience slight discomfort from the needle puncture and the tourniquet.

■ Check the patient's history for recent administration of blood, dextran, or I.V. contrast media.

Procedure and posttest care

■ Perform a venipuncture and collect the sample in a 10-ml tube without additives.

■ Apply direct pressure to the venipuncture site until bleeding stops.

■ If a hematoma develops at the venipuncture site, apply warm soaks.

Precautions

■ Label the sample with the patient's name, the hospital or blood bank number, the date, and the phlebotomist's initials.

■ Handle the sample gently to prevent hemolysis and send it to the laboratory immediately with a properly completed laboratory request.

■ Follow standard precautions with collection of sample.

Findings

In forward typing, if agglutination occurs when the patient's RBCs are mixed with anti-A serum, the A antigen is present and the blood is typed A. If agglutination occurs when the patient's RBCs are mixed with anti-B serum, the B antigen is present and the blood is typed B. If agglutination occurs in both mixes, A and B antigens are present and the blood is

typed AB. If it doesn't occur in either mix, no antigens are present and the blood is typed O.

In reverse typing, if agglutination occurs when B cells are mixed with the patient's serum, anti-B is present and the blood is typed A. If agglutination occurs when A cells are mixed, anti-A is present and the blood is typed B. If agglutination occurs when A and B cells are mixed, anti-A and anti-B are present and the blood is typed O. If agglutination doesn't occur when A and B cells are mixed, neither anti-A nor anti-B is present and the blood is typed AB.

▶ **CLINICAL ALERT** *Donor blood may be transfused only when ABO compatibility has been confirmed with the recipient's blood. The transfusion of blood containing either A or B antigens to a recipient whose RBCs lack these antigens can cause a potentially fatal reaction.*

Interfering factors

■ Recent administration of dextran or I.V. contrast media, causing cellular aggregation resembling antibody-mediated agglutination

■ Hemolysis due to rough handling of the sample

■ Blood transfusion or pregnancy in the past 3 months (possibility of lingering antibodies)

Rh typing

The Rhesus (Rh) system classifies blood by the presence or absence of Rh antigen, called $Rh_o(D)$ factor, on the surface of red blood cells (RBCs). In Rh typing, a patient's RBCs are mixed with serum containing anti-$Rh_o(D)$ antibodies and are observed for agglutination. If agglutination occurs, the $Rh_o(D)$ antigen is present, and the patient's blood is typed Rh-positive; if agglutination doesn't occur, the antigen is absent, and the patient's blood is typed Rh-negative.

Prospective blood donors are fully tested to exclude the D^u variant, a weak variant of the D antigen, before being classified as having Rh-negative blood. People who have this antigen are considered Rh-positive donors, but are generally transfused as Rh-negative recipients.

Purpose
■ To establish blood type according to the Rh system
■ To help determine the donor's compatibility before transfusion
■ To determine if the patient will require an $Rh_o(D)$ immune globulin injection

Patient preparation
■ Explain to the patient that the test determines or verifies blood group to ensure safe transfusion.
■ Inform the patient that he need not restrict food and fluids.
■ Tell the patient that the test requires a blood sample. Explain who will perform the venipuncture and when.
■ Explain to the patient that he may experience slight discomfort from the needle puncture and the tourniquet.
■ Check the patient's history for recent administration of dextran, I.V. contrast media, or drugs that may alter results.

Procedure and posttest care
■ Perform a venipuncture and collect the sample in a 7-ml EDTA tube.
■ Apply direct pressure to the venipuncture site until bleeding stops.
■ If a hematoma develops at the venipuncture site, apply warm soaks.

■ If necessary, give the pregnant patient a card identifying that she may need to receive $Rh_o(D)$ injection.

Precautions
■ Label the sample with the patient's name, the hospital or blood bank number, the date, and the phlebotomist's initials.
■ Handle the sample gently and send it to the laboratory immediately.
■ If a transfusion is ordered, be sure a transfusion request form accompanies the sample to the laboratory.

Findings
Classified as Rh-positive or Rh-negative, donor blood may be transfused only if it's compatible with the recipient's blood.

If an Rh-negative woman delivers an Rh-positive neonate or aborts a fetus whose Rh type is unknown, she should receive an $Rh_o(D)$ injection within 72 hours to prevent hemolytic disease of the neonate in future births.

Interfering factors
■ Recent administration of dextran or I.V. contrast media (cellular aggregation resembling antibody-mediated agglutination)
■ Methyldopa, cephalosporins, and levodopa (possible false-positive for the D^u antigen due to positive direct antiglobulin [Coombs'] test)

Fetal-maternal erythrocyte distribution

Some transfer of red blood cells (RBCs) from the fetal to the maternal circulation occurs during most spontaneous or elective abortions and most normal deliveries. Usually, the amount of blood transferred is minimal and has no clinical significance. However, transfer of significant amounts of blood from an Rh-positive fetus to an Rh-negative mother can result in maternal immunization to the D antigen and the development of anti-D antibodies in the maternal circulation.

During a subsequent pregnancy, the maternal immunization subjects an Rh-positive fetus to potentially fatal hemolysis and erythroblastosis. This test measures the number of fetal RBCs in the maternal circulation.

Purpose
- To detect and measure fetal-maternal blood transfer
- To determine the amount of $Rh_o(D)$ immune globulin needed to prevent maternal immunization to the D antigen

Patient preparation
- Explain to the patient that this test determines the amount of fetal blood transferred to the maternal circulation and helps determine the appropriate treatment, if necessary.
- Inform the patient that she need not restrict food and fluids.
- Tell the patient that the test requires a blood sample. Explain who will perform the venipuncture and when.
- Explain to the patient that she may experience slight discomfort from the needle puncture and the tourniquet.
- Check the patient's history for recent administration of dextran, I.V. contrast media, or drugs that may alter results.

Procedure and posttest care
- Perform a venipuncture and collect the sample in a 7-ml EDTA tube.
- Apply direct pressure to the venipuncture site until bleeding stops.
- If a hematoma develops at the venipuncture site, apply warm soaks.

Precautions
- Label the sample with the patient's name, the hospital or blood bank number, the date, and the phlebotomist's initials.
- Send the sample to the laboratory immediately with a properly completed laboratory request.

Normal findings
Normal maternal whole blood contains no fetal RBCs.

Abnormal findings
An elevated fetal RBC volume in the maternal circulation necessitates administration of more than one dose of $Rh_o(D)$ immune globulin. The number of vials needed is determined by dividing the calculated fetomaternal hemorrhage by 30. (A single vial of $Rh_o(D)$ immune globulin provides protection against a 30-ml fetomaternal hemorrhage.)

Administration of $Rh_o(D)$ immune globulin to an unsensitized Rh-negative mother as soon as possible (no later than 72 hours) after the birth of an Rh-positive infant or after a spontaneous or elective abortion prevents complications in subsequent pregnancies. Most clinicians are now administering $Rh_o(D)$ immune globulin prophylactically at 28 weeks' gestation to women who are Rh-negative but have no detectable Rh antibodies.

The following patients should be screened for Rh isoimmunization or irregular antibodies: all Rh-negative mothers during their first prenatal visit and at 28 weeks' gestation and all Rh-positive mothers with histories of transfusion, a jaundiced infant, stillbirth, cesarean delivery, or induced or spontaneous abortion.

Interfering factors
- Delay of testing for more than 72 hours after sample collection

Crossmatching

Crossmatching (also known as compatibility testing) establishes compatibility or incompatibility of a donor's and a recipient's blood. It's the best antibody detection test available for avoiding lethal transfusion reactions. After the donor's and the recipient's ABO and Rh-factor type are determined, major crossmatching determines compatibility between the donor's red blood cells (RBCs) and the recipient's serum. Minor crossmatching determines compatibility between the donor's serum and the recipient's RBCs. Because the antibody-screening test is routinely performed on all blood donors, minor crossmatching is commonly omitted.

Because a complete crossmatch may take from 45 minutes to 2 hours, an incomplete (10-minute) crossmatch may be performed in an emergency such as severe blood loss due to trauma. In an emergency, transfusion can begin with limited amounts of group O packed RBCs while crossmatching is completed. Incomplete typing and crossmatching increase the risk of complications. After crossmatching, compatible units of blood are labeled and a compatibility record is completed.

◆ **CLINICAL ALERT** *The most carefully performed crossmatch may not detect all the possible sources of patient-donor incompatibility.*

Purpose
- To serve as the final check for compatibility between a donor's and a recipient's blood

Patient preparation
- Explain to the patient that this test ensures that the blood he receives matches his own to prevent a transfusion reaction.
- Inform the patient that he need not restrict food and fluids.
- Tell the patient that the test requires a blood sample. Explain who will perform the venipuncture and when.
- Explain to the patient that he may experience slight discomfort from the needle puncture and the tourniquet.
- Check the patient's history for recent administration of blood, dextran, or I.V. contrast media.

Procedure and posttest care
- Perform a venipuncture and collect the sample in a 10-ml tube without additives or EDTA. ABO typing, Rh typing, and crossmatching are all done together.
- Apply direct pressure to the venipuncture site until bleeding stops.
- If a hematoma develops at the venipuncture site, apply warm soaks.

Precautions
- Handle the sample gently to prevent hemolysis, which can mask hemolysis of the donor's RBCs.
- Label the sample with the patient's name, the hospital or blood bank number, the date, and the phlebotomist's initials.
- Indicate on the laboratory request the amount and type of blood component needed.
- Send the sample to the laboratory immediately.
- If more than 72 hours have elapsed since an earlier transfusion, previously crossmatched donor blood must be recrossmatched with a new recipient serum sample to detect newly acquired incompatibilities before transfusion.

- If the patient is scheduled for surgery and has received blood during the past 3 months, be aware that his blood needs to be crossmatched again if his surgery is rescheduled to detect recently acquired incompatibilities.

Normal findings

Absence of agglutination indicates compatibility between the donor's and the recipient's blood, which means that the transfusion of donor blood can proceed. Note that this doesn't guarantee a safe transfusion.

Abnormal findings

A positive crossmatch indicates incompatibility between the donor's blood and the recipient's blood, which means that the donor's blood can't be transfused to the recipient. The sign of a positive crossmatch is agglutination, or clumping, when the donor's RBCs and the recipient's serum are correctly mixed and incubated. Agglutination indicates an undesirable antigen-antibody reaction. The donor's blood must be withheld and the crossmatch continued to determine the cause of the incompatibility and identify the antibody.

Interfering factors

- Recent administration of dextran or I.V. contrast media (causing cellular aggregation resembling antibody-mediated agglutination)
- Previous blood transfusion (possibility of new antibodies to donor blood)
- Hemolysis due to rough handling of the sample
- Delay of testing for more than 72 hours after sample collection

Direct antiglobulin

The direct antiglobulin test (or direct Coombs' test) detects immunoglobulins (antibodies) on the surface of red blood cells (RBCs). These immunoglobulins coat RBCs when they become sensitized to an antigen such as the Rh factor.

In this test, antiglobulin (Coombs') serum added to saline-washed RBCs results in agglutination if immunoglobulins or complement is present. This test is "direct" because it requires only one step — the addition of Coombs' serum to washed cells.

Purpose

- To diagnose hemolytic disease of the neonate (HDN)
- To investigate hemolytic transfusion reactions
- To aid in the differential diagnosis of hemolytic anemias, which may be congenital or may result from an autoimmune reaction or use of certain drugs

Patient preparation

AGE ISSUE *If the patient is a neonate, explain to the parents that this test helps diagnose HDN.*

- If the patient is suspected of having hemolytic anemia, explain that the test determines whether the condition results from an abnormality in the body's immune system, the use of certain drugs, or some unknown cause.
- Inform the adult patient that he need not restrict food and fluids.

AGE ISSUE *Tell the patient (or a neonate's parents) that the test requires a blood sample. Explain who will perform the venipuncture and when.*

- Explain to the patient that he may experience slight discomfort from the needle puncture and the tourniquet.

- Withhold medications that may interfere with test results, including quinidine, methyldopa, cephalosporins, sulfonamides, chlorpromazine, diphenylhydantoin, ethosuximide, hydralazine, levodopa, mefenamic acid, melphalan, penicillin, procainamide, rifampin, streptomycin, tetracyclines, and isoniazid, as ordered.

Procedure and posttest care
- For an adult, perform a venipuncture and collect the sample in two 5-ml EDTA tubes.

  ⊛ **AGE ISSUE** *For a neonate, draw 5 ml of cord blood into a tube with EDTA or additives, as ordered, after the cord is clamped and cut.*
- Apply direct pressure to the venipuncture site until bleeding stops.
- If a hematoma develops at the venipuncture site, apply warm soaks.
- Instruct the patient that he may resume medications discontinued before the test, as ordered.

  ⊛ **AGE ISSUE** *Tell the patient or the parents of the neonate with HDN that further tests will be necessary to monitor anemia.*

Precautions
- Handle the sample gently to prevent hemolysis.
- Label the sample with the patient's full name, the facility or blood bank number, the date, and the phlebotomist's initials.
- Send the sample to the laboratory immediately.

Normal findings
A negative test, in which neither antibodies nor complement appears on the RBCs, is normal.

Abnormal findings
A positive test on umbilical cord blood indicates that maternal antibodies have crossed the placenta and coated fetal RBCs, causing HDN. Transfusion of compatible blood lacking the antigens to these maternal antibodies may be necessary to prevent anemia.

In other patients, a positive test result may indicate hemolytic anemia and help differentiate between autoimmune and secondary hemolytic anemia, which can be drug-induced or associated with an underlying disease. A positive test can also indicate sepsis.

A weakly positive test may suggest a transfusion reaction in which the patient's antibodies react with transfused RBCs containing the corresponding antigen.

Interfering factors
- Hemolysis due to rough handling of the sample
- Quinidine, methyldopa, cephalosporins, sulfonamides, chlorpromazine, diphenylhydantoin, ethosuximide, hydralazine, levodopa, mefenamic acid, melphalan, penicillin, procainamide, rifampin, streptomycin, tetracyclines, and isoniazid (positive test results, possibly due to immune hemolysis)

Antibody screening

Also called the indirect Coombs' test, the antibody screening test detects unexpected circulating antibodies in the patient's serum. After incubating the serum with group O red blood cells (RBCs), which are unaffected by anti-A or anti-B antibodies, an antiglobulin (Coombs') serum is added. Agglutination occurs if the patient's serum contains an antibody to one or more antigens on the red cells.

The antibody screening test detects 95% to 99% of the circulating antibodies. After this screening procedure detects them, the antibody identification test can determine the specific identity of the antibodies present.

Purpose
- To detect unexpected circulating antibodies to RBC antigens in the recipient's or donor's serum before transfusion
- To determine the presence of anti-D antibody in maternal blood
- To evaluate the need for $Rh_O(D)$ immune globulin
- To aid in the diagnosis of acquired hemolytic anemia

Patient preparation
- Explain to the prospective blood recipient that the antibody screening test helps evaluate the possibility of a transfusion reaction or to determine if fetal antibodies are in the patient's blood and if treatment is needed, as appropriate.
- If the test is being performed because the patient is anemic, explain to him that it helps identify the specific type of anemia.
- Inform the patient that he need not restrict food and fluids.
- Tell the patient that the test requires a blood sample. Explain who will perform the venipuncture and when.
- Explain to the patient that he may experience slight discomfort from the needle puncture and the tourniquet.
- Check the patient's history for recent administration of blood, dextran, or I.V. contrast media.

Procedure and posttest care
- Perform a venipuncture and collect the sample in two 10-ml tubes. If the anti-

body screen is positive, antibody identification is performed on the blood.
- Apply direct pressure to the venipuncture site until bleeding stops.
- If a hematoma develops at the venipuncture site, apply warm soaks.

Precautions
- Handle the sample gently to prevent hemolysis.
- Label the sample with the patient's name, the hospital or blood bank number, the date, and the phlebotomist's initials. Be sure to include on the laboratory request the patient's diagnosis and pregnancy status, history of transfusions, and current drug therapy.
- Send the sample to the laboratory immediately.

Normal findings
Normally, agglutination doesn't occur, indicating that the patient's serum contains no circulating antibodies other than anti-A or anti-B.

Abnormal findings
A positive result indicates the presence of unexpected circulating antibodies to RBC antigens. Such a reaction demonstrates donor and recipient incompatibility.

A positive result in a pregnant patient with Rh-negative blood may indicate the presence of antibodies to the Rh factor from an earlier transfusion with incompatible blood or from a previous pregnancy with an Rh-positive fetus.

AGE ISSUE *A positive result indicates that the fetus may develop hemolytic disease of the neonate. As a result, repeated testing throughout the pregnancy is necessary to evaluate progressive development of circulating antibody levels.*

Interfering factors

- Previous administration of dextran or I.V. contrast media (causing aggregation resembling agglutination)
- Hemolysis due to rough handling of the sample
- Blood transfusion or pregnancy within the past 3 months (possible presence of antibodies)

Leukoagglutinins

This test detects leukoagglutinins (also known as white blood cell [WBC] antibodies or human leukocyte antigen [HLA] antibodies)—antibodies that react with WBCs and may cause a transfusion reaction. These antibodies usually develop after exposure to foreign WBCs through transfusions, pregnancies, and allografts.

If a blood recipient has these antibodies, a febrile nonhemolytic reaction may occur 1 to 4 hours after the start of whole blood, red blood cell, platelet, or granulocyte transfusion. This nonhemolytic reaction (marked by fever and severe chills, sometimes with nausea, headache, and transient hypertension) must be distinguished from a true hemolytic reaction before further transfusion can proceed.

The technique used to detect leukoagglutinins is the microlymphocytotoxicity test. In this test, the recipient serum is tested against donor lymphocytes or against a panel of lymphocytes of known HLA phenotype. The antibodies in the recipient serum bind to the corresponding antigen present in the lymphocytes and cause cell membrane injury when the complement is added to the test system. Cell injury is detected by examining the lymphocytes under a microscope. If the lymphocytes don't absorb the added dye,

the test is negative. If the lymphocytes show dye uptake, the test is positive.

Purpose

- To detect leukoagglutinins in blood recipients who develop transfusion reactions, thus differentiating between hemolytic and febrile nonhemolytic transfusion reactions
- To detect leukoagglutinins in blood donors after transfusion of donor blood causes a reaction

Patient preparation

- Explain to the patient that this test helps determine the cause of his transfusion reaction.
- Tell the patient that the test requires a blood sample. Explain who will perform the venipuncture and when.
- Explain to the patient that he may experience slight discomfort from the needle puncture and the tourniquet.
- Check the patient's history for recent administration of blood, dextran, or I.V. contrast media and note this on the laboratory request.

Procedure and posttest care

- Perform a venipuncture and collect a sample in a 10-ml clot-activator tube. The laboratory requires 3 to 4 ml of serum for testing.
- Apply direct pressure to the venipuncture site until bleeding stops.
- If a hematoma develops at the venipuncture site, apply warm soaks.
- If a transfusion recipient has a positive leukoagglutinin test, know that continued transfusions require premedication with acetaminophen 1 to 2 hours before the transfusion, specially prepared leukocyte-poor blood, or use of leukocyte-removal blood filters to prevent further reactions.

Precautions

- Label the sample with the patient's name, the hospital or blood bank number, the date, and the phlebotomist's initials.
- Be sure to include on the laboratory request the patient's suspected diagnosis and history of blood transfusions, pregnancies, and drug therapy.
- Note that tests for these antibodies aren't useful in deciding which patient should receive leukocyte-poor blood components; the decision must be based on clinical experience.

Normal findings

Normally, test results are negative. Agglutination doesn't occur because the serum contains no antibodies.

Abnormal findings

A positive result in a transfusion recipient indicates the presence of leukoagglutinins in his blood, identifying his transfusion reaction as a febrile nonhemolytic reaction to these antibodies.

Recipients who test positive for HLA antibodies may need HLA-matched platelets to control bleeding episodes caused by thrombocytopenia.

Interfering factors

None known

Selected readings

Anderson, S.C., and Poulsen, K.B. *Anderson's Atlas of Hematology.* Philadelphia: Lippincott Williams & Wilkins, 2003.

Cavanaugh, B.M. *Nurse's Manual of Laboratory and Diagnostic Tests,* 4th ed. Philadelphia: F.A. Davis Co., 2003.

Goldman, L., and Ausiello, D., eds. *Cecil Textbook of Medicine,* 22nd ed. Philadelphia: W.B. Saunders Co., 2004.

Guyton, A.C., and Hall, J.E. *Textbook of Medical Physiology,* 10th ed. Philadelphia: W.B. Saunders Co., 2001.

Henry, J.B., et al. *Clinical Diagnosis and Management by Laboratory Methods,* 20th ed. Philadelphia: W.B. Saunders Co., 2001.

McClatchey, K.D. *Clinical Laboratory Medicine,* 2nd ed. Philadelphia: Lippincott Williams & Wilkins, 2002.

Pagana, K.D., and Pagana, T.J. *Mosby's Diagnostic and Laboratory Test Reference,* 6th ed. St. Louis: Mosby Year–Book, Inc., 2003.

Pillitteri, A. *Maternal and Child Health Nursing,* 4th ed. Philadelphia: Lippincott Williams & Wilkins, 2003.

Schnell, Z., et al. *Davis's Comprehensive Handbook of Laboratory and Diagnostic Tests with Nursing Implications,* Philadelphia: F.A. Davis Co., 2003.

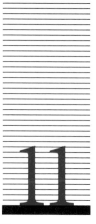

11

Immune response

Introduction

A normally functioning immune system provides continuous physiologic surveillance. It protects the body from the effects of invasion by microorganisms and maintains homeostasis by governing the degradation and removal of damaged cells. It also discovers and disposes of abnormal cells that continually arise within the body. Abnormal immune function causes serious physiologic disruptions. For example, immune hyperreactivity leads to allergic symptoms, immunodeficiency may lead to exaggerated vulnerability to infection, a misdirected immune response leads to autoimmune disorders, and failure of surveillance may allow uncontrolled growth of tumor cells. Thus, tests for immune dysfunction have great clinical significance.

The range of immunologic tests to study antigen-antibody reactions has expanded rapidly since the mid-1970s. Existing tests have been modified or replaced to reflect new data and technology. New tests of the cell-mediated immune response and of its components have been developed from the application of immunopotentiation, immunosuppression, and immunomodulation to clinical therapeutic medicine. New tests of the autoimmune response and of tumors have been developed using cell sorter technology and monoclonal antibodies.

Nonspecific and specific defense mechanisms protect the body against "nonself" attack. Nonspecific mechanisms — such as skin, mucous membranes and their secretions, and various enzymes, secretions, and cellular activities — protect the body from foreign invasion. However, when a foreign agent penetrates the body, a specific immune mechanism takes over, destroying the invading organism through the specialized activity of lymphocytes and macrophages. This response is the focus of the tests described in this chapter.

Lymphoreticular system

The lymphoreticular system — which consists of primary and secondary lymphoid organs (thymus, spleen, and lymph nodes and related areas in the liver, bone marrow, and respiratory and GI tracts) — is responsible for specific immune reactions to foreign substances. This system includes macrophages and T and B lymphocytes. To become properly differentiated, *T lymphocytes* need an intact, functioning thymus during their development. *B lymphocytes* mature through action of an unknown primary lymphoid organ, thought to be the bone marrow.

Macrophages recognize and phagocytize an antigen that enters the body, making it recognizable to lymphocytes as foreign. The lymphocytes then divide rapidly, forming a clone of cells that attempt (sometimes with the aid of complement) to destroy the antigen.

Antigenicity

Antigenicity is the very root of the immune response. A molecule or substance must be recognized as foreign and must provoke a specific immune response to be considered an *antigen*. Generally, antigens are proteins, polysaccharides, or lipoproteins of high molecular weight (10,000 daltons or more). The more complex the molecular configuration of the immunogenic substance, the more antigenic determinants it contains. The amount of antigen that penetrates the body and the route of invasion are also significant. An antigen must be presented in a unique manner to be optimally antigenic.

A *hapten* — a substance of lower molecular weight than an antigen — isn't antigenic by itself but can combine with a carrier protein to form a complete antigen that's recognized as such and is dealt with by antibodies specific for the hapten alone, the carrier protein, or the hapten-protein complex. Certain drugs may be haptens and can cause an allergic response if they combine with body proteins.

Immune response

Three sequentially dependent mechanisms, referred to as limbs, make up the immune response:

- The *afferent limb* recognizes and processes antigens and involves macrophages as well as T and B lymphocytes. (See *T and B cells: Their origin and role in the immune response,* pages 264 and 265.)
- The *central limb* makes possible an efferent immune response and includes cell cooperation, clonal expansion, and production of effectors and memory cells.
- The *efferent limb* involves destruction of specific antigens by sensitized T and B lymphocytes and their products. This destruction results from a system of humoral and cell-mediated mechanisms; although humoral and cell-mediated responses are present in most immune reactions, one response typically dominates. (See *Types of immune response,* page 266.)

Classification of the immune response into three functional limbs has practical application in diagnosis and treatment. When the immune response is evaluated, testing for defects in one or more limbs is common. Many drugs and therapies are directed primarily at particular activities or cell types within one limb.

Humoral immunity

Humoral immunity results from a clone of activated B lymphocytes that differentiates into plasma cells and synthesizes antibodies (immunoglobulins). These an-

tibodies bind to specific antigens on cell surfaces or circulate unattached body fluids. Specific binding of an antibody to an antigen typically leads to the destruction and removal of the complex. B lymphocytes usually require the cooperation of T lymphocytes and macrophages to initiate the production of antibodies.

Immunoglobulins, secreted by plasma cells as the effector agents of humoral immunity, circulate in the vascular system and in the intercellular fluids. Each immunoglobulin molecule is made up of two light and two heavy polypeptide chains attached by disulfide bridges. All four chains have a constant portion and a variable portion. The constant (Fc) portions of the heavy chains have certain regions that are of an unchanging amino acid sequence and can bind to any cell with an Fc receptor. The variable antibody portion (Fab) has a changing amino acid sequence and can lock onto the specific antigen that originally provoked its production. Thus, the Fab portion of immunoglobulin includes the antigen-binding variable portions of the heavy and light chains, whereas the Fc portion is associated with secondary biological activities, such as complement fixation and the release of histamine from mast cells.

Immunoglobulins

The known classes of immunoglobulins— IgG, IgM, IgA, IgE, and IgD — are distinguished by the constant portions of their heavy chains. However, each class has a kappa or a lambda light chain, which gives rise to many subtypes and provides almost limitless combinations of light and heavy chains that give immunoglobulins their specificity. The five classes of immunoglobulins are described below:

- *IgG,* the smallest immunoglobulin, appears in all body fluids because of its ability to move across membranes as a single structural unit (a monomer). It accounts for 75% of total immunoglobulins and is the major antibacterial and antiviral antibody.

- *IgM,* the largest immunoglobulin, appears as a pentamer (five monomers joined by a J-chain). Unlike IgG — which is produced mainly in the secondary, or recall, immune response — IgM dominates in the primary, or initial immune response. But like IgG, IgM is involved in classic antibody reactions, including precipitation, agglutination, neutralization, and complement fixation. Because of its size, IgM can't readily cross membrane barriers and is usually present only in the vascular system. IgM constitutes 5% of total serum immunoglobulins.
- *IgA* exists in serum primarily as a monomer; in secretory form, IgA exists almost exclusively as a dimer (two monomer molecules joined by a J-chain and a secretory component chain). As a secretory immunoglobulin, IgA defends external body surfaces and is present in colostrum, saliva, tears, nasal fluids, and respiratory, GI, and genitourinary secretions. This antibody is considered important in preventing antigenic agents from attaching to epithelial surfaces. IgA makes up 20% of total immunoglobulins.
- *IgE,* present in trace amounts in serum, is involved in the release of vasoactive amines stored in basophils and tissue mast cell granules. When released, these bioamines cause the allergic effects characteristic of this type of hypersensitivity (erythema, itching, smooth-muscle contraction, secretions, and swelling). (See *Four types of hypersensitivity,* page 266.)
- *IgD,* present as a monomer in serum in minute amounts, is the predominant antibody found on the surface of B lymphocytes and serves mainly as an antigen re-

ceptor. It may also help control lymphocyte activation or suppression.

Complement system
Complement is the collective term for a system of plasma proteins — labeled C1 through C9 — circulating in the blood as inactive enzyme precursors. The complement system is activated by the coupling of antigen and antibody on the surface of a cell, with a subsequent bonding of C1 to the Fc portion of the immunoglobulin heavy chain. The complement cascade that follows this activation causes cell membranes to undergo lysis. Activated complement fragments also cause chemotaxis of neutrophils and macrophages, initiate release of histamine from mast cells, neutralize viruses, and enhance phagocytosis and other nonspecific inflammatory effects. Alternately, the complement system can be activated by foreign polysaccharides and bacterial endotoxins.

Cell-mediated immune response
In the cell-mediated immune response, macrophages present antigens to T lymphocytes and activate them. Once activated, these T lymphocytes destroy the presenting antigen, either directly by cytotoxicity or indirectly by secreting lymphokines — soluble substances that stimulate proliferation of lymphocytes and cytotoxic macrophages. Thus, T lymphocytes respond differently than B lymphocytes. For example, B lymphocytes aren't required to be present at the antigen site, whereas T lymphocytes must be present and must actively participate in destroying the offending antigen.

Two subsets of regulatory T lymphocytes — *T-helper cells* and *T-suppressor cells* — function in humoral and cell-

(Text continues on page 266.)

T AND B CELLS: THEIR ORIGIN AND ROLE IN THE IMMUNE RESPONSE

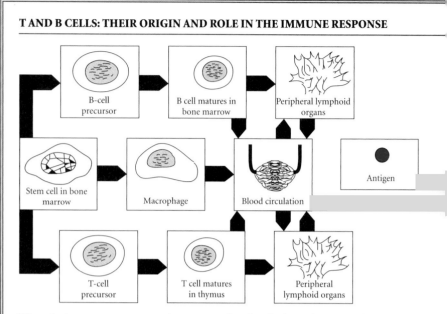

When the immune system recognizes an antigen as nonself, two distinct types of immune responses cooperate to protect the body. Both involve lymphocytes that share a common origin in stem cells. However, these lymphocytes differentiate and mature in different microenvironments, producing two populations: B cells and T cells.

In humoral immunity, antigen-stimulated B cells produce immunoglobulins (antibodies) to destroy antigens before they reach host cells. In cell-mediated immunity, antigen-activated T cells destroy antigens by direct cell-to-cell interaction. Macrophages, phagocytic cells of the reticuloendothelial system, affect both types of immune response by presenting antigens in the proper orientation to B cells and T cells for recognition and destruction.

Two groups of activated T cells trigger overlapping humoral and cell-mediated immune responses. T-regulatory cells (consisting of T-helper and T-suppressor cells) are influenced by interleukin-1 (IL-1), a monokine produced by antigen-stimulated macrophages. IL-1 activates T-helper cells and induces them to produce interleukin-2 (IL-2), B-cell growth factor (BCGF), and B-cell differentiating factor (BCDF); activated B cells then respond to these lymphokines by proliferating into clones of B cells, which differentiate into antibody-secreting plasma cells. The antibodies circulate through the body, find the antigen and bind to it, and assist in its destruction. IL-2 also stimulates effector-T-cell (natural killer and cytotoxic-T-cell) function and induces immune interferon production by T cells. Interferon suppresses B cells and enhances the cell-mediated immune response by effector T cells, which destroy antigenic substances. These effector T cells can also play a role in graft tissue rejection, delayed hypersensitivity, and graft-versus-host disease.

Macrophages activated by macrophage activating factor (MAF), a T-helper lymphokine, regulate the response by producing prostaglandin E2, which suppresses T-helper lymphokine activity and activates T-suppressor function. They also produce a tumor necrosis factor, which assists in destroying foreign antigens.

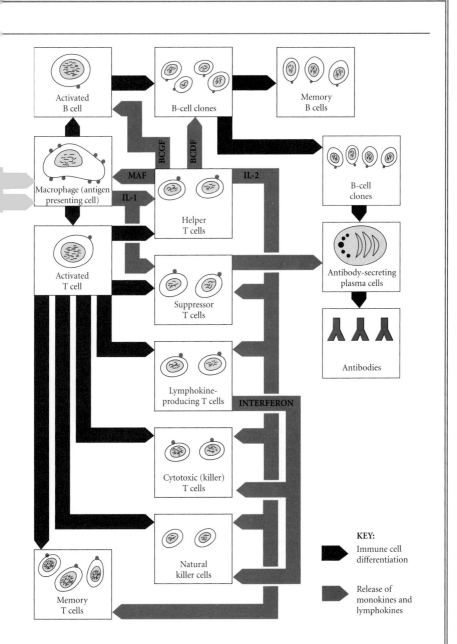

Humoral and cell-mediated immune responses record the battle by producing B- and T-memory cells. These memory cells can respond again to the same antigen, providing long-term immunity.

TYPES OF IMMUNE RESPONSE

Immune responses can be either cell-mediated or humoral. Here's a list of some of the common immune responses of each type.

Cell-mediated responses
- Transplant rejection
- Delayed hypersensitivity-tuberculin reaction, contact dermatitis
- Graft-versus-host reactions
- Tumor surveillance or destruction
- Intracellular infections

Humoral responses
- Bacterial phagocytosis and lysis
- Viral and toxin neutralization
- Anaphylaxis
- Allergic hay fever and asthma
- Immune complex disease

FOUR TYPES OF HYPERSENSITIVITY

Hypersensitivity states have been grouped into four major types:

- *Type I* (immediate hypersensitivity): an antigen reacts with an antibody (IgE) fixed on the surfaces of mast cells or basophils, causing release of vasoactive amines and histamine. These amines produce allergic symptoms, such as hives, secretions, erythema, itching, smooth-muscle contraction and, possibly, shock.

- *Type II* (cytotoxic): Antibody reacts with an antigenic component of a cell or with an antigen or a hapten associated with a cell. Complement or mononuclear cells (lymphocytes and macrophages) cause actual cellular destruction, resulting in lysis of the target cell. Thus, if erythrocytes are the target, such destruction causes hemolytic anemia; if platelets are the target, thrombocytopenia; and if white cells are the target, leukopenia.

- *Type III* (immune-complex mediated): Complexes of antigen-antibody and complement, forming in the blood, may precipitate onto "innocent bystander" cells and tissues, which are damaged by local inflammation. Type III hypersensitivity reactions include glomerulonephritis, arteritis, and rheumatoid arthritis.

- *Type IV* (delayed hypersensitivity): Sensitized T cells respond to antigens by excessive release of lymphokines or by direct cytotoxic injury. Type IV reactions are a delayed type of sensitivity, requiring 48 to 72 hours to occur. This form of hypersensitivity includes allergic contact dermatitis due to exposure to poison ivy as well as skin reactions to cosmetics, drugs, and industrial chemicals.

mediated immune responses and regulate the magnitude, intensity, and duration of the immune response. An equal number of helper and suppressor lymphocytes is required for a normally functioning immune response. An excess of either type can change the intensity and outcome of the immune response. T-helper cells appear to enhance the immune response, whereas T-suppressor cells seem to prevent an excessive immune response.

Activated by interleukin-1 (a soluble monokine produced by macrophages), T-helper cells secrete the lymphokine interleukin-2, which induces the growth and differentiation of B lymphocytes into antibody-secreting plasma cells and potentiates T-cell proliferation with subsequent cytotoxicity of effector cells. T-suppressor cells are also activated by interleukin-1 to produce interferon, a soluble protein that suppresses the growth and differentiation of B lymphocytes.

T-cell interferon enhances cell-mediated immune destruction by activating effector T cells — cytotoxic T lymphocytes and natural killer cells. Interferon can also promote the production of natural killer cells. These cells have the capacity to respond to an antigen immediately and without differentiation when they're targeting tumor cells, certain microbially infected cells, and perhaps other cells.

Misdirected response

Autoimmunity is the one form of hypersensitivity in which the immune response is misdirected against the body's own tissues. Disorders thought to result from autoimmunity include rheumatoid arthritis, systemic lupus erythematosus, scleroderma, Sjögren's syndrome, and hemolytic anemia. Autoantibodies usually attack intracellular "self-antigens" that aren't normally exposed to the lymphoreticular system, including inner layers of cell membranes, nucleoprotein, nucleic acids, and cytoplasmic structures such as mitochondria.

Viruses or haptens attached to the body's own cells also provoke autoimmune cell and tissue destruction. In many instances, tissue destruction results when intracellular antigens escape to form immune complexes, which are then deposited in the kidneys or blood vessels, activat-

ing complement and causing cytotoxic damage (type III hypersensitivity). Depletion of T-suppressor cells is believed to cause autoimmune disease by allowing unregulated function of T-helper cells.

In other hypersensitivity states, excessive amounts of immunoglobulins, T-helper cells, T-suppressor cells, B lymphocytes, or complement — or a combination of any of these — are present. In such conditions, overproduction of one immune response component retards the production of others. In multiple myeloma, for example, the excessive production of a single clone of plasma cells can result in a single type of immunoglobulin that completely inhibits the production of other types. In this respect, hypersensitivity reactions can lead to immunodeficiency.

Immunodeficiency is a congenital or acquired deficiency of the immune response. Congenital deficiencies include Bruton's agammaglobulinemia (B-cell deficiency) and DiGeorge syndrome (thymic parathyroid aplasia). Acquired immunodeficiency disorders can result from chemotherapy or from radiation or corticosteroid therapy. They're related to a change in the ratio of T-helper to T-suppressor cells or macrophages. An imbalance of these regulatory cells may also result from infection, stress, drug use, old age, malnutrition, and cancer.

Immunologic test methods

Most immunologic tests use a combination of techniques to evaluate humoral and cell-mediated immune responses or their individual components. The most commonly used laboratory methods include precipitation, immunodiffusion, agglutination, histochemical techniques (such as immunofluorescence), radioimmunoassay, enzyme-linked immunosorbent assay (ELISA), complement fixation and, most recently, monoclonal antibody assays. The ELISA test is used to screen blood for contamination with human immunodeficiency virus antibodies.

Precipitation

When a soluble antibody reacts with a soluble antigen, cross-linking occurs between the antibody and the antigen. This phenomenon, known as the *lattice hypothesis,* results from the presence of multiple receptor sites on the surfaces of the antibody and the antigen, allowing cross-linkage between them. As more antigens and antibodies cross-link, they create an insoluble lattice structure and precipitate out of solution.

The quantity of antibody and antigen in solution determines the precipitation reaction. When a small amount of antigen is added to a large amount of antibody, all antigen sites are satisfied, and the resultant complexes contain much antibody and little antigen. Optimal cross-linking occurs when antigen and antibody are present in equal proportions; this point of optimal proportion is called the *zone of equivalence.* An excess of antigen or antibody may produce false-negative test results.

Immunodiffusion

Immunodiffusion relies on the tendency of antigen and antibody particles to diffuse in an agar matrix and to form a precipitin line where they meet. This test may be performed using one of three methods:

- *Single diffusion* (radial immunodiffusion) uses an agar slide containing antibody specific to a certain antigen. A well is punched in the agar and is filled with the specific antigen. After 24 hours, a precipitation ring forms around the well.

The distance between the precipitation line and the well is proportional to the antigen concentration. Clinically, single diffusion is used to measure serum immunoglobulin concentrations. However, interference with diffusion (molecular size or weight) or precipitation (excess antigen or antibody) affects accurate determination of findings.

- *Double diffusion,* a similar method, uses an agar-filled slide or a Petri dish with small wells. After the addition of antigen to one well and antibody to the other, precipitin lines form where optimal proportions of antigen and antibody meet. The number of precipitin lines indicates the number of different antigen-antibody complexes present. Formation of a single precipitin line provides a rough quantitative estimate of antigen or antibody purity. Although double diffusion is a simple, useful method for detecting unknown antigens or antibodies, it lacks sensitivity and thus has limited practical application.

- *Immunoelectrophoresis* combines electrophoresis and immunodiffusion to identify and measure serum immunoglobulins and other proteins. A direct electric current is applied to an agar slide, causing each protein to migrate at a different speed, according to its size and net electrical charge. After the proteins are separated, addition of antigen to each one results in diffusion and the formation of precipitin lines; these lines may be photographed or stained for a permanent record. Clinically, immunoelectrophoresis aids in the diagnosis of monoclonal and polyclonal gammopathies as well as immunodeficiency diseases.

Agglutination

Agglutination occurs when large, insoluble particles, such as bacteria or red blood cells (RBCs), are clumped together by antibodies to the particles or to the antigens attached to the particles. Unlike precipitation, agglutination uses high-molecular-weight antigens for rough quantitation of antibody levels.

Direct agglutination results from the addition of antibody to a cell or to an insoluble particulate native antigen. If the antigen is added to increasing dilutions of antiserum in tubes or wells with rounded bottoms, the reciprocal of the dilution of antiserum in the last tube to show visible agglutination is the titer (relative concentration) of antibody.

Indirect or passive agglutination refers to the agglutination of soluble antigen attached to blood cells, bacteria, or latex particles, which are inert carrier particles.

Agglutination is clinically useful to detect specific antibodies, such as those that cause rheumatoid arthritis, syphilis, or salmonella infections.

Immunofluorescence

In this histochemical technique, fluorescent dyes are attached to antibody molecules. When complexed with antigen and viewed under an ultraviolet microscope, the antibody appears as a colored fluorescence. Direct and indirect immunofluorescence allow precise detection and demonstration of human tissue antigens and of bacterial, viral, and protozoan antigens. In the *direct* method, the fluorescein-labeled antibody reacts with an antigen specific to it. In the *indirect* method, a fluorescein-labeled antiglobulin reacts with an unlabeled antigen-antibody complex; the antiglobulin then binds to the unlabeled antibody.

Both methods are widely used to detect autoantibodies, immunoglobulins of cell surfaces, components of complement, T and B lymphocytes, tumor-specific antigens, and microorganisms.

Radioimmunoassay

This technique measures small quantities of a substance by combining a radiolabeled antigen with a particular antibody. Radiolabeled antigen is added to the sample, and binds with about 70% of antibody. Various amounts of unlabeled antibody are then added to the mixture, and the radiolabeled and unlabeled antigens compete for binding sites on the antibody. A curve is then constructed from the amount of radiolabeled antigen at various unlabeled antigen concentrations to determine the amount of antigen already present in the serum sample.

Enzyme-linked immunosorbent assay

Commonly known as ELISA, this technique can identify antibodies or antigens and is replacing or supplementing radioimmunoassay and immunofluorescence. ELISA is safe, sensitive, and simple to perform and provides reproducible results at a low cost. To measure a specific antibody, antigen is fixed to a solid-phase medium, incubated with a serum sample, and then incubated with an anti-immunoglobulin-tagged enzyme. Excess unbound enzyme is washed from the system and a substrate is added. To measure a specific antigen, antibody instead of antigen is fixed to a solid-phase medium. Hydrolysis of the substrate produces a color change that's quantified by a spectrophotometer. The amount of substrate hydrolyzed is directly proportional to the amount of antigen or antibody in the serum sample.

Complement fixation

Used to determine the presence and extent of an antigen-antibody reaction, complement fixation is performed by adding a known antigen or antibody, directed against an unknown antibody or antigen, to a patient's serum and then incubating the sample. Then, RBCs coated with the same known antigen or antibody are added. If hemolysis doesn't occur, complement must have been depleted in the original reaction; that is, the unknown antibody or antigen was present in the sample. The unknown antibody or antigen is then assayed.

Monoclonal antibody assays

B lymphocytes respond to antigen stimulation by rapidly proliferating and producing antibodies against the antigen. Laboratory production of monoclonal antibodies takes advantage of the B-lymphocyte reaction to an antigen to create unlimited numbers of completely homogenous antibodies.

Typically, a selected antigen is injected into a mouse, stimulating its immune response to develop antibody-secreting plasma cells. These cells are then harvested from the mouse's spleen and fused with myeloma cells — malignant cells that secrete an infinite amount of the single antibody specific to the antigen that's been injected. The resulting hybridomas are grown in culture, cloned, and tested for the desired antibody. Finally, selected hybridomas are grown in culture or injected into a mouse to produce monoclonal antibodies, which are purified for future use.

Monoclonal antibodies have been used extensively for typing cells and cell subsets, detecting specific antigens, and differentiating malignant from nonmalignant cells.

GENERAL CELLULAR TESTS

T- and B-lymphocyte assays

Lymphocytes — key cells in the immune system — have the capacity to recognize antigens through special receptors found on their surfaces. The two primary kinds of lymphocytes, T and B cells, originate in the bone marrow. T cells mature under the influence of the thymus gland; B cells evolve without thymic influence.

Cell separation is used to isolate lymphocytes from other cellular blood elements. In this method, a whole blood sample is layered on Ficoll-Hypaque in a narrow tube, which is then centrifuged. Granulocytes and erythrocytes form a sediment at the bottom of the tube, and lymphocytes, monocytes, and platelets form a distinct band at the Ficoll-Hypaque-plasma interface.

This procedure recovers approximately 80% of the lymphocytes, but doesn't differentiate between T and B cells. The percentage of T and B cells is determined by attaching a label or marker and by using different identification techniques. The E rosette test identifies T cells, which tend to form unstable clusterlike shapes (or rosettes) after exposure to sheep red blood cells at 39.2° F (4° C). Direct immunofluorescence detects B cells, which have monoclonal immunoglobulin on their surfaces; unlike T cells, B cells present receptors for complement as well as for Fc portions of immunoglobulin.

Null cells, which make up the remainder of the lymphocytes, possess Fc receptors but no other detectable surface markers, and presently have no diagnostic significance. Null cells are usually determined by subtracting the sum of T and B cells from total lymphocytes.

Purpose
- To aid in the diagnosis of primary and secondary immunodeficiency diseases
- To distinguish between benign and malignant lymphocytic proliferative diseases
- To monitor the patient's response to therapy

Patient preparation
- Explain to the patient that this test measures certain white blood cells.
- Tell the patient that this test requires a blood sample. Explain who will perform the venipuncture and when.
- Explain to the patient that he may experience slight discomfort from the needle puncture and the tourniquet.

Procedure and posttest care
- Perform a venipuncture and collect the sample in a 7 ml green-top tube.
- Apply direct pressure to the venipuncture site until bleeding stops.
- Because the patient with T- and B-cell changes may have a compromised immune system, keep the venipuncture site clean and dry. If a hematoma develops at the venipuncture site, apply warm soaks.

Precautions
- Fill the collection tube completely and invert it gently several times to mix the sample and the anticoagulant adequately.
- Send the sample to the laboratory immediately to ensure viable lymphocytes.
- If antilymphocyte antibodies are suspected, as in autoimmune disease, notify the laboratory.

Reference values
T-cell and B-cell values may differ from one laboratory to another, depending on test technique. Generally, T cells constitute 68% to 75% of total lymphocytes; B cells, 10% to 20%; and null cells, 5% to 20%. The total lymphocyte count ranges from 1,500 to 3,000/µl, the T-cell count varies from 1,400 to 2,700/µl, and the B-cell count ranges from 270 to 640/µl. These counts are higher in children.

Implications of results
An abnormal T-cell or B-cell count suggests but doesn't confirm specific diseases. The B-cell count is elevated in chronic lymphocytic leukemia (thought to be a B-cell malignancy), multiple myeloma, Waldenström's macroglobulinemia, and DiGeorge syndrome (a congenital T-cell deficiency). The B-cell count decreases in acute lymphocytic leukemia and in certain congenital or acquired immunoglobulin deficiency diseases. In other immunoglobulin deficiency diseases, especially if only one immunoglobulin class is deficient, the B-cell count remains normal.

The T-cell count rises occasionally in infectious mononucleosis; it's more common in multiple myeloma and acute lymphocytic leukemia. T cells decrease in congenital T-cell deficiency diseases, such as DiGeorge, Nezelof, and Wiskott-Aldrich syndromes, and in certain B-cell proliferative disorders, such as chronic lymphocytic leukemia, Waldenström's macroglobulinemia, and acquired immunodeficiency syndrome.

Normal T-cell and B-cell counts don't necessarily ensure a competent immune system. In autoimmune diseases, such as systemic lupus erythematosus and rheumatoid arthritis, T and B cells may be present in normal numbers but may not be functionally competent.

Interfering factors

- Exposing the sample to temperature extremes or failure to use the proper collection tube, to mix the sample adequately, or to send the sample to the laboratory
- Changes in health status, from the effects of stress, surgery, chemotherapy, steroid or immunosuppressive therapy, or radiography (possible rapid change in T- and B-cell counts)
- Immunoglobulins such as autologous antilymphocyte antibodies that sometimes occur in autoimmune disease (possible change in results)

Lymphocyte transformation

Transformation tests evaluate lymphocyte competency without injection of antigens into the patient's skin. These in vitro tests eliminate the risk of adverse effects, but can still accurately assess the ability of lymphocytes to proliferate and to recognize and respond to antigens.

The mitogen assay evaluates the mitotic response of T and B lymphocytes to a foreign antigen. The antigen assay uses specific substances, such as purified protein derivative, Candida, mumps, tetanus toxoid, and streptokinase, to stimulate lymphocyte transformation. The mixed lymphocyte culture (MLC) assay is useful in matching transplant recipients and donors and in testing immunocompetence. (See Lymphocyte marker assays.)

The neutrophils' ability to engulf and destroy bacteria and foreign particles can also be determined. (See Neutrophil function tests, page 274.)

Purpose

- To assess and monitor genetic and acquired immunodeficiency states

- To provide histocompatibility typing of tissue transplant recipients and donors
- To detect if a patient has been exposed to various pathogens such as those that cause malaria, hepatitis, and mycoplasmal pneumonia

Patient preparation

- Explain to the patient that this test evaluates lymphocyte function, which is crucial to the immune system.
- Inform the patient that the test monitors his response to therapy, if appropriate.
- For histocompatibility typing, explain that this test helps determine the best match for a transplant.
- Inform the patient that he need not restrict food and fluids.
- Tell the patient that the test requires a blood sample. Explain who will perform the venipuncture and when.
- Explain to the patient that he may experience slight discomfort from the needle puncture and the tourniquet.
- If a radioisotope scan is scheduled, make sure the serum sample for this test is drawn first.

Procedure and posttest care

- Perform a venipuncture. If the patient is an adult, collect the sample in a 7-ml heparinized tube; for a child, use a 5-ml heparinized tube.
- Because the patient may have a compromised immune system, take special care to keep the venipuncture site clean and dry.
- Apply direct pressure to the venipuncture site until bleeding stops.
- If a hematoma develops at the venipuncture site, apply warm soaks.

LYMPHOCYTE MARKER ASSAYS

A normal immune response requires a balance between the regulatory activities of several interacting cell types, most notably T-helper and T-suppressor cells. By using highly specific monoclonal antibodies, levels of lymphocyte differentiation can be defined, and normal and malignant cell populations can be analyzed. Direct and indirect immunofluorescence, microcytotoxicity, and immunoperoxidase immunoassay techniques are used most frequently: They use an anticoagulated blood sample combined with monoclonal antibodies that react with specific T- and B-cell markers. The chart below lists some commonly ordered lymphocyte marker assays and their indications.

Lymphocyte marker	Purpose
Pan T-cell marker (CD3)	■ To measure mature T cells in immune dysfunction
T-helper/inducer subset marker (CD4)	■ To identify and characterize the proportion of T-helper cells in autoimmune or immunoregulatory disorders ■ To detect immunodeficiency disorders such as acquired immunodeficiency syndrome ■ To differentiate T-cell acute lymphoblastic leukemia from T-cell lymphomas and other lymphoproliferative disorders
T-suppressor/cytotoxic subset marker (CD8)	■ To identify and characterize the proportion of T-suppressor cells in autoimmune and immunoregulatory disorders ■ To characterize lymphoproliferative disorders
T-cell/E-Rosette receptor (CD2)	■ To differentiate lymphoproliferative disorders of T-cell origin, such as T-cell lymphocytic leukemia and lymphoblastic lymphoma, from those of non-T-cell origin
Pan-B (B-1) marker (CD20)	■ To differentiate lymphoproliferative disorders of B-cell origin, such as B-cell chronic lymphocytic leukemia, from those of T-cell origin
Pan-B (BA-1) marker (CD19)	■ To identify B-cell lymphoproliferative disorders such as B-cell chronic lymphocytic leukemia
CALLA (common acute lymphocytic leukemia antigen) marker, CD10	■ To identify bone marrow regeneration ■ To identify non-T-cell acute lymphocytic leukemia
Lymphocyte subset panel (CD3/CD4/CD8/CD19)	■ To evaluate immunodeficiencies ■ To identify immunoregulation associated with autoimmune disorders ■ To characterize lymphoid neoplasms
Lymphocytic leukemia marker panel (CD3/CD4/CD8/CD19/CD10)	■ To characterize lymphocytic leukemias as T, B, non-T, or non-B, regardless of the stage of differentiation of the malignant cells

NEUTROPHIL FUNCTION TESTS

Neutrophil function tests may reveal the inability of neutrophils to kill a target bacteria or to migrate to the bacterial site (chemotaxis). The killing ability can be evaluated by the nitroblue tetrazolium (NBT) test, which relies on neutrophil generation of bactericidal enzymes and toxins during killing. This action results in increased oxygen consumption and glucose metabolism, which reduces colorless NBT to blue formazan. The reduced dye is then extracted with pyridine and measured photometrically; the level of reduction indicates phagocytic activity.

Neutrophil killing activity can also be evaluated by noting the neutrophil's chemiluminescence, its ability to emit light. After a neutrophil phagocytizes a microorganism, oxygen-containing substances form within phagocytic vacuoles. As the cell is stimulated, it emits light in proportion to the amount of oxygen-containing substances that are formed, providing an indirect measurement of phagocytosis.

Chemotaxis can be assessed in vitro by placing bacteria in the lower half of a two-part chamber and phagocytic neutrophils in the upper half. After incubation, migrating cells are counted microscopically and compared with standard values.

Precautions
■ Completely fill the collection tube and invert it gently several times to mix the sample and the anticoagulant.
■ Send the sample to the laboratory immediately.
■ Don't refrigerate or freeze the specimen.

Reference values
Results depend on the mitogens used. Reference ranges accompany test results. In general, a positive test is normal; a negative test indicates a deficiency.

Abnormal findings
In the mitogen and antigen assays, a low stimulation index or unresponsiveness indicates a depressed or defective immune system. Serial testing can be performed to monitor the effectiveness of therapy in a patient with an immunodeficiency disease.

In the MLC test, the stimulation index is a measure of compatibility. A high index indicates poor compatibility. Conversely, a low stimulation index indicates good compatibility.

A high stimulation index, in response to the relevant pathogen, can also demonstrate exposure to malaria, hepatitis, mycoplasmal pneumonia, periodontal disease, and certain viral infections in a patient who no longer has detectable serum antibodies.

Interfering factors
■ Pregnancy or use of hormonal contraceptives, depressing lymphocyte response to phytohemagglutinin (low stimulation index)
■ Chemotherapy (unless pretherapy baseline values are available for comparison)
■ Radioisotope scan within 1 week before the test
■ Failure to send the sample to the laboratory immediately

Terminal deoxynucleotidyl transferase

Using indirect immunofluorescence, the terminal deoxynucleotidyl transferase (TdT) test measures levels of TdT. The test differentiates certain types of leukemias and lymphomas marked by primitive cells that can't be identified by histology alone. Measurement of TdT may also help determine the prognosis for these diseases and may provide early diagnosis of a relapse.

Purpose

- To help differentiate acute lymphocytic leukemia (ALL) from acute nonlymphocytic leukemia
- To help differentiate lymphoblastic lymphomas from malignant lymphomas
- To monitor the patient's response to therapy, help determine his prognosis, or obtain early diagnosis of a relapse

Patient preparation

- Explain to the patient that this test detects an enzyme that can help classify tissue origin.

Blood test

- Tell the patient to fast for 12 to 14 hours before the test.
- Tell the patient that the test requires a blood sample. Explain who will perform the venipuncture and when.
- Explain to the patient that he may experience slight discomfort from the needle puncture and the tourniquet.

Bone marrow aspiration

- Describe the procedure to the patient and answer his questions.
- Inform the patient that he need not restrict food and fluids.

- Tell the patient who will perform the biopsy and where and that it usually takes 5 to 10 minutes.
- Make sure the patient or a responsible family member has signed an informed consent form.
- Administer a mild sedative 1 hour before the test, as ordered.
- Check the patient's history for hypersensitivity to the local anesthetic.
- After checking with the physician, tell the patient which bone will be the biopsy site.
- Inform the patient that he'll receive a local anesthetic, but will feel pressure on insertion of the biopsy needle and a brief, pulling pain when the marrow is withdrawn.

Procedure and posttest care

- If a blood test is scheduled, perform a venipuncture and collect the sample in one 10-ml heparinized blood tube and one EDTA tube.
- If assisting with bone marrow aspiration, inject 1 ml of bone marrow into a 7-ml heparinized tube and dilute it with 5 ml of normal saline solution, or submit four air-dried marrow smears.
- Send the sample to the laboratory immediately.
- Because the patient may have a compromised immune system, take special care to keep the venipuncture site clean and dry.
- Because a patient with leukemia may bleed excessively, apply pressure to the venipuncture site until bleeding stops.
- If a hematoma develops at the venipuncture site, apply warm soaks.
- Check the bone marrow aspiration site for bleeding and inflammation, and observe the patient for signs of hemorrhage and infection.

Precautions

■ Before performing the venipuncture, contact the laboratory to ensure that it can process the sample and to confirm how much blood to draw.

■ Because the patient with leukemia is more susceptible to infection, clean the skin thoroughly before performing the venipuncture.

■ Send the sample to the laboratory immediately.

Reference values

TdT is present in less than 2% of marrow cells and is undetectable in normal peripheral blood.

Abnormal findings

Positive cells are present in more than 90% of patients with ALL, in 33% of patients with chronic myelogenous leukemia in blast crisis, and in 5% of patients with nonlymphocytic leukemias. TdT-positive cells are absent in patients with ALL who are in remission.

Interfering factors

■ Failure to obtain a representative sample during bone marrow aspiration

■ Performing bone marrow aspiration on a child because of presence of TdT-positive bone marrow during proliferation of prelymphocytes (possible false-positive)

■ Bone marrow regeneration, idiopathic thrombocytopenic purpura, and neuroblastoma, causing TdT-positive bone marrow (possible false-positive)

■ Failure to send the sample to the laboratory immediately

GENERAL HUMORAL TESTS

Quantitative immunoglobulins G, A, and M

Immunoglobulins, proteins that can function as specific antibodies in response to antigen stimulation, are responsible for the humoral aspects of immunity. They are classified into five groups — immunoglobulin (Ig) G, IgA, IgM, IgD, and IgE — that are normally present in serum in predictable percentages.

IgG constitutes about 75% of serum immunoglobulins and includes the warm-temperature type; IgA, about 15% of the total; IgM, 5% to 7%, including cold agglutinins, rheumatoid factor, and ABO blood group isoagglutinins; and IgD and allergen-specific IgE, less than 2%. Deviations from normal immunoglobulin percentages are characteristic in many immune disorders, including cancer, hepatic disorders, rheumatoid arthritis, and systemic lupus erythematosus.

Immunoelectrophoresis identifies IgG, IgA, and IgM in a serum sample; the level of each is measured by radial immunodiffusion or nephelometry. Some laboratories detect immunoglobulin by indirect immunofluorescence and radioimmunoassay.

Purpose

■ To diagnose paraproteinemias, such as multiple myeloma and Waldenström's macroglobulinemia

■ To detect hypogammaglobulinemia and hypergammaglobulinemia as well as nonimmunologic diseases, such as cirrhosis and hepatitis, that are associated

with abnormally high immunoglobulin levels
- To assess the effectiveness of chemotherapy and radiation therapy

Patient preparation
- Explain to the patient that this test measures antibody levels.
- If appropriate, tell the patient that the test evaluates the effectiveness of treatment.
- Instruct the patient to restrict food and fluids, except for water, for 12 to 14 hours before the test.
- Tell the patient that the test requires a blood sample. Explain who will perform the venipuncture and when.
- Explain to the patient that he may experience slight discomfort from the needle puncture and the tourniquet.
- Check the patient's history for drugs that may affect test results.
- Be aware that alcohol or narcotic abuse may affect results.

Procedure and posttest care
- Perform a venipuncture and collect the sample in a 7-ml clot-activator tube.
- Advise the patient with abnormally low immunoglobulin levels (especially IgG or IgM) to protect himself against bacterial infection. When caring for such a patient, watch for signs of infection, such as fever, chills, rash, and skin ulcers.
- Instruct the patient with abnormally high immunoglobulin levels and symptoms of monoclonal gammopathies to report bone pain and tenderness. Such a patient has numerous antibody-producing malignant plasma cells in bone marrow, which hamper production of other blood components. Watch for signs of hypercalcemia, renal failure, and spontaneous pathologic fractures.

- Apply direct pressure to the venipuncture site until bleeding stops.
- If a hematoma develops at the venipuncture site, apply warm soaks.
- Instruct the patient that he may resume his usual diet and medications discontinued before the test, as ordered.

Precautions
- Send the sample to the laboratory immediately to prevent immunoglobulin deterioration.

Reference values
When using nephelometry, serum immunoglobulin levels for adults range as follows:
- IgG: 800 to 1,800 mg/dl (SI, 8 to 18 g/L)
- IgA: 100 to 400 mg/dl (SI, 1 to 4 g/L)
- IgM: 55 to 150 mg/dl (SI, 0.55 to 1.5 g/L).

Abnormal findings
The accompanying chart shows IgG, IgA, and IgM levels in various disorders. (See *Serum immunoglobulin levels in various disorders*, page 278) In congenital and acquired hypogammaglobulinemias, myelomas, and macroglobulinemia, the findings confirm the diagnosis. In hepatic and autoimmune diseases, leukemias, and lymphomas, such findings are less important, but they can support the diagnosis based on other tests, such as biopsies and white blood cell differential, and on the physical examination.

Interfering factors
- Radiation therapy or chemotherapy (possible decrease due to suppressive effects on bone marrow)
- Aminophenazone, anticonvulsants, asparaginase, hydralazine, hydantoin derivatives, hormonal contraceptives, and phenylbutazone (possible increase)

SERUM IMMUNOGLOBULIN LEVELS IN VARIOUS DISORDERS

Disorder	IgG	IgA	IgM
Immunoglobulin disorders			
Lymphoid aplasia	D	D	D
Agammaglobulinemia	D	D	D
Type I dysgammaglobulinemia (selective immunoglobulin [Ig] G and IgA deficiency)	D	D	N or I
Type II dysgammaglobulinemia (absent IgA and IgM)	N	D	D
IgA globulinemia	N	D	N
Ataxia-telangiectasia	N	D	N
Multiple myeloma, macroglobulinemia, lymphomas			
Heavy chain disease (Franklin's disease)	D	D	D
IgG myeloma	I	D	D
IgA myeloma	D	I	D
Macroglobulinemia	D	D	I
Acute lymphocytic leukemia	N	D	N
Chronic lymphocytic leukemia	D	D	D
Acute myelocytic leukemia	N	N	N
Chronic myelocytic leukemia	N	D	N
Hodgkin's disease	N	N	N
Hepatic disorders			
Hepatitis	I	I	I
Laënnec's cirrhosis	I	I	N
Biliary cirrhosis	N	N	I
Hepatoma	N	N	D
Other disorders			
Rheumatoid arthritis	I	I	I
Systemic lupus erythematosus	I	I	I
Nephrotic syndrome	D	D	N
Trypanosomiasis	N	N	I
Pulmonary tuberculosis	I	N	N

KEY:
N = normal; I = increased; D = decreased

- Methotrexate and severe hypersensitivity to bacille Calmette-Guérin vaccine (possible decrease)
- Dextrans and methylprednisolone (decrease in IgM levels)
- Dextrans and high doses of methylprednisolone and phenytoin (decrease in IgG and IgA levels)
- Methadone (increase in IgA levels)

Immune complex assays

When immune complexes are produced faster than they can be cleared by the lymphoreticular system, immune complex disease, such as postinfectious syndromes, serum sickness, drug sensitivity, rheumatoid arthritis, and systemic lupus erythematosus (SLE), may occur. Immune complexes can develop when a certain ratio of antigen reacts with antibody of isotopes immunoglobulin (Ig) G 1, 2, 3, or IgM in tissues. These complexes can fix the first component of complement (C1) and activate the complement cascade. Subsequent complement-mediated activity leads to inflammation and local tissue necrosis. In the blood, soluble circulating immune complexes may also activate complement and eventually cause damage, usually in the renal glomeruli, the aorta, and other large blood vessels.

Histologic examination of tissue obtained by biopsy and the use of fluorescence or peroxidase staining with antibodies specific for immunologic types generally detect immune complexes. However, tissue biopsies can't provide information about titers of complexes still in circulation; therefore, serum assays, which detect circulating immune complexes indirectly, may be required. Because of the inherent variability of these complexes, several serum test methods may be appropriate using C1, rheumatoid factor (RF), or cellular substrates, such as Raji cells, as reagents.

Most immune complex assays haven't been standardized, so more than one test may be required to achieve accurate results.

Purpose
- To demonstrate circulating immune complexes in serum
- To monitor the patient's response to therapy
- To estimate disease severity

Patient preparation
- Explain to the patient that these tests help evaluate his immune system.
- Inform the patient that the test will be repeated to monitor his response to therapy, if appropriate.
- Inform the patient that he need not restrict food and fluids.
- Tell the patient that the test requires a blood sample. Explain who will perform the venipuncture and when.
- Explain to the patient that he may experience slight discomfort from the needle puncture and the tourniquet.
- If the patient is scheduled for C1q assay (a component of C1), check his history for recent heparin therapy and report such therapy to the laboratory.

Procedure and posttest care
- Perform a venipuncture and collect the sample in a 7-ml clot-activator tube.
- Because many patients with immune complexes have a compromised immune system, keep the venipuncture site clean and dry.
- Apply direct pressure to the venipuncture site until bleeding stops.
- If a hematoma develops at the venipuncture site, apply warm soaks.

Precautions

- Send the sample to the laboratory immediately to prevent deterioration of immune complexes.

Normal findings

Normally, immune complexes aren't detectable in serum.

Abnormal findings

The presence of detectable immune complexes in serum has etiologic importance in many autoimmune diseases, such as SLE and rheumatoid arthritis. For definitive diagnosis, the presence of these complexes must be considered with the results of other studies. For example, in SLE, immune complexes are associated with high titers of antinuclear antibodies and circulating antinative deoxyribonucleic acid antibodies.

Because of their filtering function, renal glomeruli seem vulnerable to immune complex deposition, although blood vessel walls and choroid plexuses (vascular folds in the ventricles of the brain) can be affected. Renal biopsy to detect immune complexes can provide conclusive evidence for immune complex (type III) glomerulonephritis, differentiating it from other types of glomerulonephritis.

Interfering factors

- Failure to send the sample to the laboratory immediately
- Presence of cryoglobulins in the serum
- Inability to standardize RF inhibition tests and platelet aggregation assays

Raji cell assay

Raji cell assay, which is performed to detect the presence of circulating immune complexes, studies the Raji lymphoblastoid cell line. Identifying these cells, which have receptors for immunoglobulin G complement, helps to evaluate autoimmune disease.

Purpose

- To detect circulating immune complexes
- To aid in the study of autoimmune disease

Patient preparation

- Explain to the patient the purpose of the test, as appropriate.
- Tell the patient that the test requires a blood sample. Explain who will perform the venipuncture and when.
- Explain to the patient that he may experience slight discomfort from the needle puncture and the tourniquet.

Procedure and posttest care

- Perform a venipuncture, collect a sample in a clot-activator tube, and promptly send it to the laboratory.
- Apply direct pressure to the venipuncture site until bleeding stops.
- If a hematoma develops at the venipuncture site, apply warm soaks.

Precautions

- Handle the sample gently to prevent hemolysis.

Reference values

Normally, Raji cells aren't present.

Abnormal findings

A positive Raji cell assay can detect immune complexes, including those found in viral, microbial, and parasitic infections; metastasis; autoimmune disorders; and drug reactions. This test may also detect immune complexes associated with celiac disease, cirrhosis of the liver, Crohn's disease, cryoglobulinemia, dermatitis herpetiformis, sickle cell anemia, and ulcerative colitis.

Interfering factors
- Hemolysis due to rough handling of the sample

Complement assays

Complement is a collective term for a system of at least 20 serum proteins designed to destroy foreign cells and help remove foreign materials. The system may be triggered by contact with antigen-antibody complexes or by clotting factor XIIa. A cascade of events follows, resulting in the formation of a complex that ruptures cell membranes.

Complement components are numerically designated as C1 through C9, with C1 having three subcomponents: C1q, C1r, and C1s. These components constitute 3% to 4% of total serum globulins and play a key role in antibody-mediated immune reactions.

Complement can function as a defense by promoting the removal of infectious agents or as a threat by triggering destructive reactions in host tissues. Therefore, complement deficiency can increase susceptibility to infection and can predispose a person to other diseases. Complement assays are thus indicated in patients with known or suspected immunomediated disease or a repeatedly abnormal response to infection.

Normally, complement is present in serum in an inactive state until "fixed," or activated, in the classic pathway by binding to an antibody-coated surface. In the classic pathway, a specific antibody identifies and coats an antigen that enters the body. C1 then recognizes and binds with this specific antibody, activating the complement cascade—a series of enzymatic reactions involving all complement components—and producing a coordinated inflammatory response, which usually results in cell lysis or some other damaging outcome.

In the alternate pathway, substances, such as polysaccharides, bacterial endotoxins, and aggregated immunoglobulins, react with properdin and factors B, D, H, and I, producing an enzyme that activates C3. In turn, C3 activates the remainder of the complement cascade.

In both pathways, specific inhibitors regulate the sequential activation of complement components. The C1 esterase inhibitor, the most commonly studied inhibitor, regulates the classic pathway; the C3b inhibitor can regulate either pathway because C3 is a pivotal component of both.

Various laboratory methods are used to evaluate and measure total complement and its components; hemolytic assay, laser nephelometry, and radial immunodiffusion are the most common.

Although complement assays provide valuable information about the patient's immune system, the results must be considered in light of serum immunoglobulin and autoantibody tests for a definitive diagnosis of immunomediated disease or an abnormal response to infection.

Purpose
- To help detect immunomediated disease and genetic complement deficiency
- To monitor the effectiveness of therapy

Patient preparation
- Explain to the patient that this test measures a group of proteins that fight infection.
- Inform the patient that he need not restrict food and fluids.

- Tell the patient that the test requires a blood sample. Explain who will perform the venipuncture and when.
- Explain to the patient that he may experience slight discomfort from the needle puncture and the tourniquet.
- If the patient is scheduled for C1q assay, check his history for recent heparin therapy. Report such therapy to the laboratory.

Procedure and posttest care
- Perform a venipuncture and collect the sample in a 7-ml tube without additives.
- Because many patients with complement defects have a compromised immune system, keep the venipuncture site clean and dry.
- Apply direct pressure to the venipuncture site until bleeding stops.
- If a hematoma develops at the venipuncture site, apply warm soaks.

Precautions
- Handle the sample gently to prevent hemolysis.
- Send the sample to the laboratory immediately because complement is heat labile and deteriorates rapidly.

Reference values
Normal values for complement range as follows:
- total complement: 25 to 110 U/ml (SI, 0.25 to 1.1 g/L)
- C3: 70 to 150 mg/dl (SI, 0.7 to 1.5 g/L)
- C4: 15 to 45 mg/dl (SI, 0.15 to 0.45 g/L).

Abnormal findings
Complement abnormalities may be genetic or acquired; acquired abnormalities are most common. Depressed total complement levels (which are clinically more significant than elevations) may result from excessive formation of antigen-antibody complexes, insufficient complement synthesis, inhibitor formation, or increased complement catabolism and are characteristic in such conditions as systemic lupus erythematosus (SLE), acute poststreptococcal glomerulonephritis, and acute serum sickness. Low levels may also occur in some patients with advanced cirrhosis of the liver, multiple myeloma, hypogammaglobulinemia, or rapidly rejecting allografts.

Elevated total complement may occur in obstructive jaundice, thyroiditis, acute rheumatic fever, rheumatoid arthritis, acute myocardial infarction, ulcerative colitis, and diabetes.

C1 esterase inhibitor deficiency is characteristic in hereditary angioedema, the most common genetic abnormality associated with complement; C3 deficiency is characteristic in recurrent pyogenic infection and disease activation in SLE; C4 deficiency is characteristic in SLE and rheumatoid arthritis. C4 is increased in autoimmune hemolytic anemia.

Interfering factors
- Hemolysis due to rough handling of the sample
- Failure to send the sample to the laboratory immediately
- Recent heparin therapy

Radioallergosorbent test

The radioallergosorbent test (RAST) measures immunoglobulin (Ig) E antibodies in serum by radioimmunoassay and identifies specific allergens that cause rash, asthma, hay fever, drug reactions, and other atopic complaints. The RAST is easier to perform and more specific than skin testing; it's also less painful for and less dangerous to the patient. Careful selection of specific allergens, based on the patient's history, is crucial for effective testing.

Although skin testing is still the preferred means of diagnosing IgE-mediated hypersensitivities, the RAST may be more useful when a skin disorder makes accurate reading of skin tests difficult, when a patient requires continual antihistamine therapy, or when skin tests are negative but the patient's history supports IgE-mediated hypersensitivity.

In the RAST, a sample of the patient's serum is exposed to a panel of allergen particle complexes (APCs) on cellulose disks. The patient's IgE complexes with those APCs to which it's sensitive. Radiolabeled anti-IgE antibody is then added, and this binds to the IgE-APC complexes. After centrifugation, the amount of radioactivity in the particulate material is directly proportional to the amount of IgE antibodies present. Test results are compared with control values and represent the patient's reactivity to a specific allergen.

Purpose
■ To identify allergens to which the patient has an immediate (IgE-mediated) hypersensitivity
■ To monitor the patient's response to therapy

Patient preparation
■ Explain to the patient that this test may detect the cause of allergy or monitor the effectiveness of allergy treatment.
■ Inform the patient that he need not restrict food and fluids.
■ Tell the patient that the test requires a blood sample. Explain who will perform the venipuncture and when.
■ Explain to the patient that he may experience slight discomfort from the needle puncture and the tourniquet.

■ If the patient is scheduled for a radioactive scan, make sure the blood sample is collected before the scan.

Procedure and posttest care
■ Perform a venipuncture and collect the sample in a 7-ml clot-activator tube. Generally, 1 ml of serum is sufficient for five allergen assays.
■ Note on the laboratory request the specific allergens to be tested.
■ Apply direct pressure to the venipuncture site until bleeding stops.
■ If a hematoma develops at the venipuncture site, apply warm soaks.

Reference values
RAST results are interpreted in relation to a control or reference serum that differs among laboratories.

Abnormal findings
Elevated serum IgE levels suggest hypersensitivity to the specific allergen or allergens used.

Interfering factors
■ Radioactive scan within 1 week before sample collection

Ham test

The Ham test, or acidified serum lysis test, is performed to determine the cause of undiagnosed hemolytic anemia, hemoglobinuria, and bone marrow aplasia. This test determines the stability of the red blood cell (RBC) membrane. It helps establish a diagnosis of paroxysmal nocturnal hemoglobinuria (PNH), a rare hematologic disease.

The Ham test relies on the susceptibility of RBCs to lysis — RBCs from patients with PNH are unusually susceptible to lysis by complement. To perform the test, washed RBCs are mixed with ABO-compatible normal serum and acid. After incubation at 98.6° F (37° C), the cells are examined for hemolysis. In the presence of acidified human serum, a substantial portion of PNH cells are lysed, whereas normal RBCs show no hemolysis.

Purpose
- To aid in the diagnosis of PNH

Patient preparation
- Explain to the patient that this test helps determine the cause of his anemia or other signs.
- Inform the patient that he need not restrict food and fluids.
- Tell the patient that the test requires a blood sample. Explain who will perform the venipuncture and when.
- Explain to the patient that he may experience slight discomfort from the needle puncture and the tourniquet.

Procedure and posttest care
- Because the blood sample must be defibrinated immediately, laboratory personnel perform the venipuncture and collect the sample.
- Apply direct pressure to the venipuncture site until bleeding stops.
- If a hematoma develops at the venipuncture site, apply warm soaks.

Normal findings
Normally, RBCs don't undergo hemolysis. Test results should be negative.

Abnormal findings
Hemolysis of RBCs indicates PNH.

Interfering factors
- Blood containing large numbers of spherocytes (possible false-positive)

- Blood from patients with congenital dyserythropoietic anemia (false-positive)

Human leukocyte antigens

The human leukocyte antigen (HLA) test identifies a group of antigens present on the surface of all nucleated cells, but are most easily detected on lymphocytes. The four types of HLA are HLA-A, HLA-B, HLA-C, and HLA-D. These antigens are essential to immunity and determine the degree of histocompatibility between transplant recipients and donors. Numerous antigenic determinants (more than 60, for instance, at the HLA-B locus) are present for each site; one set of each antigen is inherited from each parent.

A high incidence of specific HLA types has been linked to specific diseases, such as rheumatoid arthritis and multiple sclerosis, but these findings have little diagnostic significance.

Purpose
- To provide histocompatibility typing of transplant recipients and donors
- To aid in genetic counseling
- To aid in paternity testing

Patient preparation
- Explain to the patient that this test detects antigens on white blood cells.
- Inform the patient that he need not restrict food and fluids.
- Tell the patient that the test requires a blood sample. Explain who will perform the venipuncture and when.
- Explain to the patient that he may experience slight discomfort from the needle puncture and the tourniquet.
- Check the patient's history for recent blood transfusions. HLA testing may

need to be postponed if he has recently undergone a transfusion.

Procedure and posttest care
- Perform a venipuncture and collect the sample in a tube containing anticoagulant acid citrate dextrose solution.
- Apply direct pressure to the venipuncture site until bleeding stops.
- If a hematoma develops at the venipuncture site, apply warm soaks.

Precautions
- Handle the sample gently to prevent hemolysis.

Normal findings
In HLA-A, HLA-B, and HLA-C testing, lymphocytes that react with the test antiserum undergo lysis; they're detected by phase microscopy. In HLA-D testing, leukocyte incompatibility is marked by blast formation, deoxyribonucleic acid synthesis, and proliferation.

Abnormal findings
Incompatible HLA-A, HLA-B, HLA-C, and HLA-D groups may cause unsuccessful tissue transplantation.

Many diseases have a strong association with certain types of HLAs. For example, HLA-DR5 is associated with Hashimoto's thyroiditis. B8 and Dw3 are associated with Graves' disease, whereas B8 alone is associated with chronic autoimmune hepatitis, celiac disease, and myasthenia gravis. Dw3 alone is associated with Addison's disease, Sjögren's syndrome, dermatitis herpetiformis, and systemic lupus erythematosus.

In paternity testing, a putative father who presents a phenotype (two haplotypes: one from the father and one from the mother) with no haplotype or antigen pair identical to one of the child's is ex-

cluded as the father. A putative father with one haplotype identical to one of the child's may be the father; the probability varies with the incidence of the haplotype in the population.

Interfering factors
- Hemolysis due to rough handling of the sample
- HLA from blood transfusion within 72 hours before sample collection

AUTOANTIBODY TESTS

Antinuclear antibodies

In such conditions as systemic lupus erythematosus (SLE), scleroderma, and certain infections, the body's immune system may perceive portions of its own cell nuclei as foreign and may produce antinuclear antibodies (ANAs). Specific ANAs include antibodies to deoxyribonucleic acid (DNA), nucleoprotein, histones, nuclear ribonucleoprotein, and other nuclear constituents.

Because they don't penetrate living cells, ANAs are harmless, but sometimes form antigen-antibody complexes that cause tissue damage (as in SLE). Because of multiorgan involvement, test results aren't diagnostic and can only partially confirm clinical evidence. (See *Comparative incidence of antinuclear antibodies,* page 286.)

This test measures the relative concentration of ANAs in a serum sample through indirect immunofluorescence. Serial dilutions of serum are mixed with either Hep-2 or mouse kidney substrate. If the serum contains ANAs, it forms antigen-antibody complexes with the substrate. After the preparation is mixed

COMPARATIVE INCIDENCE OF ANTINUCLEAR ANTIBODIES

Condition	Incidence of positive antinuclear antibodies
Systemic lupus erythematosus (SLE)	95% to 100%
Lupoid hepatitis	95% to 100%
Felty's syndrome	95% to 100%
Progressive systemic sclerosis (scleroderma)	75% to 80%
Drugs associated with SLE-like syndrome (hydralazine, procainamide, isoniazid)	Approximately 50%
Sjögren's syndrome	40% to 75%
Rheumatoid arthritis	25% to 60%
Healthy family member of patient with SLE	Approximately 25%
Chronic discoid lupus erythematosus	15% to 50%
Juvenile rheumatoid arthritis	15% to 30%
Polyarteritis nodosa	15% to 25%
Miscellaneous disorders	10% to 50%
Dermatomyositis, polymyositis	10% to 30%
Rheumatic fever	Approximately 5%

with fluorescein-labeled antihuman serum, it's examined under an ultraviolet microscope. If ANAs are present, the complex fluoresces. Titer is taken as the greatest dilution that shows the reaction.

About 99% of patients with SLE exhibit ANAs; a large percentage of these patients do so at high titers. Although this test isn't specific for SLE, it's a useful screening tool. Failure to detect ANAs essentially rules out active SLE.

Purpose
■ To screen for SLE (failure to detect ANAs essentially rules out active SLE)
■ To monitor the effectiveness of immunosuppressive therapy for SLE

Patient preparation
■ Explain to the patient that this test evaluates the immune system and that

further testing is usually required for diagnosis.
■ Inform the patient that the test will be repeated to monitor his response to therapy, if appropriate.
■ Inform the patient that he need not restrict food and fluids.
■ Tell the patient that the test requires a blood sample. Explain who will perform the venipuncture and when.
■ Explain to the patient that he may experience slight discomfort from the needle puncture and the tourniquet.
■ Check the patient's history for drugs that may affect test results, such as isoniazid and procainamide. Note findings on the laboratory request.

Procedure and posttest care
■ Perform a venipuncture and collect the sample in a 7-ml tube without additives.

- Because a patient with an autoimmune disease has a compromised immune system, observe the venipuncture site for signs of infection, and report changes to the physician immediately.
- Keep a clean, dry bandage over the site for at least 24 hours.
- Apply direct pressure to the venipuncture site until bleeding stops.
- If a hematoma develops at the venipuncture site, apply warm soaks.

Normal findings

Test results are reported as positive (with pattern and serum titer noted) or negative.

Abnormal findings

Although this test is a sensitive indicator of ANAs, it isn't specific for SLE. Low titers may occur in patients with viral diseases, chronic hepatic disease, collagen vascular disease, and autoimmune diseases and in some healthy adults; the incidence increases with age. The higher the titer, the more specific the test is for SLE (titer typically exceeds 1:256).

The pattern of nuclear fluorescence helps identify the type of immune disease present. A peripheral pattern is almost exclusively associated with SLE because it indicates the presence of anti-DNA antibodies; sometimes anti-DNA antibodies are measured by radioimmunoassay if ANA titers are high or if a peripheral pattern is observed. A homogeneous, or diffuse, pattern is also associated with SLE as well as with related connective tissue disorders; a nucleolar pattern, with scleroderma; and a speckled, irregular pattern, with infectious mononucleosis and mixed connective tissue disorders (for example, SLE and scleroderma).

A single serum sample, especially one collected from a patient with collagen vascular disease, may contain antibodies to several parts of the cell's nucleus. In addition, as serum dilution increases, the fluorescent pattern may change because different antibodies are reactive at different titers.

Interfering factors

- Most commonly isoniazid, hydralazine, and procainamide, but also para-aminosalicylic acid, chlorpromazine, clofibrate, phenytoin, griseofulvin, ethosuximide, gold salts, methyldopa, hormonal contraceptives, penicillin, propylthiouracil, phenylbutazone, methysergide, streptomycin, sulfonamides, tetracyclines, mephenytoin, quinidine, primidone, reserpine, and trimethadione (possible production of a syndrome resembling SLE)

Anti-deoxyribonucleic acid antibodies

About two-thirds of patients with active systemic lupus erythematosus (SLE) have measurable levels of autoantibodies to double-stranded (native) deoxyribonucleic acid (known as anti-ds-DNA). These antibodies are rarely detected in patients with other connective tissue diseases.

In autoimmune diseases, such as SLE, native DNA is thought to be the antigen that complexes with antibody and complement, causing local tissue damage where these complexes are deposited. Serum anti-ds-DNA levels are directly related to the extent of renal or vascular damage caused by the disease.

The anti-ds-DNA antibody test measures and differentiates these antibody levels in a serum sample, using radioimmunoassay, agglutination, complement fixation, or immunoelectrophoresis. If anti-ds-DNA antibodies are present, they combine with native DNA and form complexes that are too large to pass through a membrane filter. The test counts these oversized complexes.

Purpose
- To confirm a diagnosis of SLE
- To monitor the SLE patient's response to therapy and determine his prognosis

Patient preparation
- Explain to the patient that this test helps diagnose and determine the appropriate therapy for SLE.
- Inform the patient that he need not restrict food and fluids.
- Tell the patient that the test requires a blood sample. Explain who will perform the venipuncture and when.
- Explain to the patient that he may experience slight discomfort from the needle puncture and the tourniquet.
- Ask the patient if he has had a recent radioactive test; if so, note this on the laboratory request.

Procedure and posttest care
- Perform a venipuncture and collect the sample in a 7-ml tube without additives. (Some laboratories may specify a tube with either EDTA or sodium fluoride and potassium oxalate added.)
- Apply direct pressure to the venipuncture site until bleeding stops.
- If a hematoma develops at the venipuncture site, apply warm soaks.

Precautions
- Handle the sample gently to prevent hemolysis.

Reference values
An anti-ds-DNA antibody level less than 25 IU/ml (SI, < 25 kIU/L) is considered negative for SLE.

Abnormal findings
Elevated anti-ds-DNA antibody levels may indicate SLE. Values of 25 to 30 IU/ml (SI, 25 to 30 kIU/L) are considered borderline positive. Values of 31 to 200 IU/ml (SI, 31 to 200 kIU/L) are positive, and those greater than 200 IU/ml (SI, > 200 kIU/L) are strongly positive.

Depressed anti-ds-DNA antibody levels may follow immunosuppressive therapy, demonstrating effective treatment of SLE.

Interfering factors
- A radioactive scan performed within 1 week before sample collection
- Hemolysis due to rough handling of the sample

Extractable nuclear antigen antibodies

Extractable nuclear antigen (ENA) is a complex of at least four antigens. One of them — ribonucleoprotein (RNP) — is susceptible to degradation by ribonuclease. The second — Smith (Sm) antigen — is an acidic nuclear protein that resists ribonuclease degradation. The third and fourth antigens that are sometimes included in this group — Sjögren's syndrome A (SS-A) antigen and Sjögren's syndrome B (SS-B) antigen — form a precipitate when an antibody is present.

Antibodies to these antigens are associated with certain autoimmune disorders. Tests to detect ENA antibodies help differentiate autoimmune disorders with similar signs and symptoms.

The *RNP antibody test* detects RNP autoantibodies, which are associated with systemic lupus erythematosus (SLE), progressive systemic sclerosis, and other rheumatic disorders. This test aids in the differential diagnosis of systemic rheumatic disease and is a useful follow-up test for collagen vascular autoimmune disease.

The *anti-Sm antibody test* detects Sm autoantibodies, which are a specific marker for SLE; thus, positive results strongly suggest a diagnosis of SLE. This test, too, helps monitor collagen vascular autoimmune disease. The *Sjögren's antibody test* detects the SS-B autoantibodies produced by Sjögren's syndrome, an immunologic abnormality sometimes associated with rheumatic arthritis and SLE. However, this test doesn't confirm a diagnosis of Sjögren's syndrome.

Purpose
- To aid in the differential diagnosis of autoimmune disease
- To distinguish between anti-RNP and anti-Sm antibodies
- To screen for anti-RNP antibodies (common in mixed connective tissue disease)
- To screen for anti-Sm antibodies (common in SLE)
- To support the diagnosis of collagen vascular autoimmune diseases
- To monitor the patient's response to therapy

Patient preparation
- Explain to the patient that this test detects certain antibodies and that test results help determine diagnosis and treatment.
- Explain that the test assesses the effectiveness of treatment, when appropriate.
- Inform the patient that he need not restrict food and fluids.
- Tell the patient that the test requires a blood sample. Explain who will perform the venipuncture and when.
- Explain to the patient that he may experience slight discomfort from the needle puncture and the tourniquet.

Procedure and posttest care
- Perform a venipuncture and collect the sample in a 7-ml tube without additives.
- Because a patient with an autoimmune disease has a compromised immune system, check the venipuncture site for infection, and report changes promptly.
- Keep a clean, dry bandage over the site for at least 24 hours.
- Apply direct pressure to the venipuncture site until bleeding stops.
- If a hematoma develops at the venipuncture site, apply warm soaks.

Precautions
- Send the sample to the laboratory immediately.

Reference values
Serum should be negative for anti-RNP, anti-Sm, and SS-B antibodies.

Abnormal findings
Anti-RNP antibodies are elevated in SLE (35% to 40% of cases) and in mixed connective tissue disease. Anti-Sm antibodies are specific for SLE. Anti-SS-A and anti-SS-B antibodies are elevated in Sjögren's syndrome (40% to 45% of cases). Anti-SS-B antibodies are also elevated in SLE.

Interfering factors
- Failure to send the sample to the laboratory immediately

Antimitochondrial antibodies

Usually performed with the test for anti-smooth-muscle antibodies, the antimitochondrial antibodies test detects antimitochondrial antibodies in serum by indirect immunofluorescence. These autoantibodies are present in several hepatic diseases. Their role in disease pathogene-

INCIDENCE OF SERUM ANTIBODIES IN VARIOUS DISORDERS

The chart below shows the percentage of patients with certain disorders who have antimitochondrial or anti-smooth-muscle antibodies in the serum. The presence of these antibodies requires further testing to confirm the diagnosis. (Up to 1% of healthy people also show antimitochondrial antibodies.)

Disorder	Antimitochondrial antibodies	Anti-smooth-muscle antibodies
Primary biliary cirrhosis	75% to 95%	0% to 50%[a]
Chronic active hepatitis	0% to 30%	50% to 80%
Extrahepatic biliary obstruction	0% to 5%	0%
Cryptogenic cirrhosis	0% to 25%	0% to 1%
Viral (infectious) hepatitis	0%	1% to 2%[b]
Drug-induced jaundice	50% to 80%	
Intrinsic asthma		20%
Rheumatoid arthritis and other collagen diseases	1% to 2%	
Systemic lupus erythematosus	3% to 5%[c]	0%

[a] In chronic disease, values fall at upper end of range.
[b] Much higher incidence occurs with hepatic damage.
[c] Much higher incidence occurs with renal involvement.

sis is unknown, and there's no evidence that they cause hepatic damage. Most commonly, they're associated with primary biliary cirrhosis and, sometimes, chronic active hepatitis and drug-induced jaundice. Antimitochondrial antibodies are also associated with autoimmune diseases, such as systemic lupus erythematosus, rheumatoid arthritis, pernicious anemia, and idiopathic Addison's disease.

Purpose
- To aid in the diagnosis of primary biliary cirrhosis
- To distinguish between extrahepatic jaundice and biliary cirrhosis

Patient preparation
- Explain to the patient that this test evaluates liver function.
- Inform the patient that he need not restrict food and fluids.
- Tell the patient that the test requires a blood sample. Explain who will perform the venipuncture and when.
- Explain to the patient that he may experience slight discomfort from the needle puncture and the tourniquet.
- Check the patient's medication history for oxyphenisatin use and report it to the laboratory because it may produce antimitochondrial antibodies.

Procedure and posttest care
- Perform a venipuncture and collect the sample in a 7-ml tube with no additives.

- Because the patient with hepatic disease may bleed excessively, apply pressure to the venipuncture site until bleeding stops.
- If a hematoma develops at the venipuncture site, apply warm soaks.

Normal findings
Serum is normally negative for antimitochondrial antibodies. Positive results are titered.

Abnormal findings
Although antimitochondrial antibodies appear in 79% to 94% of patients with primary biliary cirrhosis, this test alone doesn't confirm the diagnosis. Further tests, such as serum alkaline phosphatase, serum bilirubin, aspartate aminotransferase, alanine aminotransferase and, possibly, liver biopsy or cholangiography, may also be necessary. The autoantibodies also appear in some patients with chronic active hepatitis, drug-induced jaundice, and cryptogenic cirrhosis. (See *Incidence of serum antibodies in various disorders.*) Antimitochondrial antibodies seldom appear in patients with extrahepatic biliary obstruction, and a positive test helps rule out this condition.

Interfering factors
- Confusion of antimitochondrial antibodies with heterophil antibodies, cardiolipin antibodies to syphilis, ribosomal antibodies, and microsomal hepatic or renal autoantibodies
- Oxyphenisatin (possible false-positive results)

Anti-smooth-muscle antibodies

Using indirect immunofluorescence, the anti-smooth-muscle antibodies test measures the relative concentration of anti-smooth-muscle antibodies in serum; it's usually performed with the test for antimitochondrial antibodies. The serum sample is exposed to a thin section of smooth muscle and incubated; then a fluorescent-labeled antiglobulin is added. This antiglobulin binds only to antibodies that have complexed with smooth muscle and appears fluorescent when viewed through the microscope under ultraviolet light.

Anti-smooth-muscle antibodies appear in several hepatic diseases, especially chronic active hepatitis and, less commonly, primary biliary cirrhosis. Although anti-smooth-muscle antibodies are usually associated with hepatic diseases, their etiologic role is unknown, and there's no evidence that they cause hepatic damage.

Purpose
- To aid in the diagnosis of active chronic hepatitis and primary biliary cirrhosis

Patient preparation
- Explain to the patient that this test helps evaluate liver function.
- Inform the patient that he need not restrict food and fluids.
- Tell the patient that the test requires a blood sample. Explain who will perform the venipuncture and when.
- Explain to the patient that he may experience slight discomfort from the needle puncture and the tourniquet.

Procedure and posttest care
- Perform a venipuncture and collect the sample in a 7-ml tube without additives.
- Because the patient with hepatic disease may bleed excessively, apply direct pressure to the venipuncture site until bleeding stops.

- If a hematoma develops at the venipuncture site, apply warm soaks.

Reference values
A normal titer of anti-smooth-muscle antibodies is negative. Positive results are titered.

Abnormal findings
The test for anti-smooth-muscle antibodies isn't specific; these antibodies appear in many patients with chronic active hepatitis and in fewer patients with primary biliary cirrhosis.

Anti-smooth-muscle antibodies may also be present in patients with infectious mononucleosis, acute viral hepatitis, a malignant tumor of the liver, and intrinsic asthma.

Interfering factors
- None significant

Antithyroid antibodies

In autoimmune disorders — such as Hashimoto's thyroiditis and Graves' disease (hyperthyroidism) — thyroglobulin, the major colloidal storage compound, is released into the blood. Because thyroxine usually separates from thyroglobulin before its release into the blood, thyroglobulin doesn't normally enter the circulation. When it does, antithyroglobulin antibodies are formed to attack this foreign substance; the ensuing autoimmune response damages the thyroid gland. The serum of a patient whose autoimmune system produces antithyroglobulin antibodies usually contains antimicrosomal antibodies, which react with the microsomes of the thyroid epithelial cells.

The tanned red cell hemagglutination test detects antithyroglobulin and antimicrosomal antibodies. Another laboratory technique, indirect immunofluorescence, can detect antimicrosomal antibodies.

Purpose
- To detect circulating antithyroglobulin antibodies when clinical evidence indicates Hashimoto's thyroiditis, Graves' disease, or other thyroid diseases

Patient preparation
- Explain to the patient that this test evaluates thyroid function.
- Inform the patient that he need not restrict food and fluids.
- Tell the patient that the test requires a blood sample. Explain who will perform the venipuncture and when.
- Explain to the patient that he may experience slight discomfort from the needle puncture and the tourniquet.

Procedure and posttest care
- Perform a venipuncture and collect the sample in a 7-ml tube without additives.
- Apply direct pressure to the venipuncture site until bleeding stops.
- If a hematoma develops at the venipuncture site, apply warm soaks.

Reference values
The normal titer is less than 1:100 for antithyroglobulin and antimicrosomal antibodies.

Abnormal findings
The presence of antithyroglobulin or antimicrosomal antibodies in serum can indicate subclinical autoimmune thyroid disease, Graves' disease, or idiopathic myxedema. Titers of 1:400 or greater strongly suggest Hashimoto's thyroiditis. Antithyroglobulin antibodies may also occur in some patients with other autoimmune disorders, such as systemic lupus

erythematosus, rheumatoid arthritis, and autoimmune hemolytic anemia.

Interfering factors
- None significant

Thyroid-stimulating immunoglobulin

Thyroid-stimulating immunoglobulin (TSI), formerly called long-acting thyroid stimulator, appears in the blood of most patients with Graves' disease. This auto-antibody reacts with the cell-surface receptors that usually combine with thyroid-stimulating hormone (TSH). TSI reacts with these receptors, activates intracellular enzymes, and promotes epithelial cell activity that functions outside the normal feedback regulation mechanism for TSH. It stimulates the thyroid gland to produce and excrete excessive amounts of thyroid hormone.

Reportedly, 90% of people with Graves' disease have elevated TSI levels. Positive results of this test strongly suggest Graves' disease, despite normal routine thyroid tests in patients still suspected of having Graves' disease or progressive exophthalmos.

Purpose
- To aid in the evaluation of suspected thyroid disease
- To aid in the diagnosis of suspected thyrotoxicosis, especially in patients with exophthalmos
- To monitor treatment of thyrotoxicosis

Patient preparation
- Explain to the patient that this test evaluates thyroid function, as appropriate.

- Tell the patient that the test requires a blood sample. Explain who will perform the venipuncture and when.
- Explain to the patient that he may experience slight discomfort from the needle puncture and the tourniquet.

Procedure and posttest care
- Perform a venipuncture and collect the sample in a 5-ml clot-activator tube.
- Apply direct pressure to the venipuncture site until bleeding stops.
- If a hematoma develops at the venipuncture site, apply warm soaks.
- If the patient had a radioactive iodine scan within 48 hours of the test, note this on the laboratory request.

Precautions
- Handle the sample gently to prevent hemolysis and send it to the laboratory immediately.

Reference values
TSI doesn't normally appear in serum. However, it's considered normal at levels equal to or greater than 1.3 index.

Abnormal findings
Increased TSI levels are associated with exophthalmos, Graves' disease (thyrotoxicosis), and recurrence of hyperthyroidism.

Interfering factors
- Hemolysis due to rough handling of the sample
- Administration of radioactive iodine within 48 hours of the test

Lupus erythematosus cell preparation

Lupus erythematosus (LE) cell preparation is an in vitro procedure used in diagnosing systemic lupus erythematosus (SLE). Although this test is less sensitive and reliable than either the antinuclear antibody (ANA) or the antideoxyribonucleic acid (DNA) antibody test, it's commonly used because it requires minimal equipment and reagents.

In this test, a blood sample is mixed with laboratory-treated nucleoprotein (the antigen). If the sample contains ANAs, they react with the nucleoprotein, causing swelling and rupture. Phagocytes from the serum then engulf the extruded nuclei, forming LE cells, which are then detected by microscopic examination of the sample.

Purpose
- To aid in the diagnosis of SLE
- To monitor treatment of SLE (About 60% of successfully treated patients fail to show LE cells after 4 to 6 weeks of therapy.)

Patient preparation
- Explain to the patient that this test helps detect antibodies to his own tissue. (See *Understanding autoantibodies in autoimmune disease.*)
- If appropriate, inform the patient that the test will be repeated to monitor his response to therapy.
- Inform the patient that he need not restrict food and fluids.
- Tell the patient that the test requires a blood sample. Explain who will perform the venipuncture and when.
- Explain to the patient that he may experience slight discomfort from the needle puncture and the tourniquet.
- Check the patient's medication history for drugs that may affect test results, such as isoniazid, hydralazine, and procainamide. If such drugs must be continued,

be sure to note this on the laboratory request.

Procedure and posttest care
- Perform a venipuncture and collect the sample in a 7-ml red-top tube.
- Because the patient with SLE may have a compromised immune system, keep a clean, dry bandage over the venipuncture site for at least 24 hours and check for infection.
- Apply direct pressure to the venipuncture site until bleeding stops.
- If a hematoma develops at the venipuncture site, apply warm soaks.
- If test results indicate SLE, tell the patient further tests may be required to monitor treatment.

Precautions
- Handle the sample gently to prevent hemolysis.

Normal findings
No LE cells are normally present in serum.

Abnormal findings
The presence of at least two LE cells may indicate SLE. Although these cells occur primarily in SLE, they may also appear in chronic active hepatitis, rheumatoid arthritis, scleroderma, and certain drug reactions. Also, up to 25% of patients with SLE demonstrate no LE cells.

Apart from supportive clinical signs, a definitive diagnosis of SLE may require a confirming ANA or anti-DNA test. The ANA test detects autoantibodies in the serum of many patients with SLE who have negative LE cell tests. Anti-DNA antibodies appear in two-thirds of all patients with SLE, but are rare in other conditions; thus, the presence of these antibodies is strong evidence of SLE.

UNDERSTANDING AUTOANTIBODIES IN AUTOIMMUNE DISEASE

When the immune system produces autoantibodies against the antigenic determinants on and in cells, two types of autoimmune disease can result. *Organ-specific diseases,* such as pernicious anemia, occur when the targeted antigenic determinants are specific to an organ or tissue or to certain cells or cell types. Lymphocytes invade the target organ, tissue, or cell and destroy targeted cells. *Non–organ-specific diseases,* such as myasthenia gravis, occur when the targeted antigenic determinants are shared with other cells (self-antigens). This causes deposition of immune complexes (type III hypersensitity) with subsequent lesions anywhere in the body.

Various diagnostic techniques are used to detect antibodies in autoimmune disease, including radioimmunoassay, hemagglutination, complement fixation, and immunofluorescence. The chart below lists common test methods and findings in various autoimmune diseases.

Disease	Affected area	Antigen	Antibody	Diagnostic technique
Hashimoto's thyroiditis	Thyroid gland	Thyroglobulin, second colloid antigen, cytoplasmic microsomes, cell-surface antigens	Antibodies to thyroglobulin and to microsomal antigens	Radioimmunoassay, hemagglutination, complement fixation, immunofluorescence
Pernicious anemia	Hematopoietic system	Intrinsic factor	Antibodies to gastric parietal cells and vitamin B_{12} binding site of intrinsic factor	Immunofluorecence, radioimmunoassay
Pemphigus vulgaris	Skin	Desmosomes between prickle cells in the epidermis	Antibodies to intercellular substances of the skin and mucous membranes	Immunofluorescence
Myasthenia gravis	Neuromuscular system	Acetylcholine receptors of skeletal and heart muscle	Antiacetylcholine antibodies	Immunoprecipitation radioimmunoassay
Autoimmune hemolytic anemia	Hematopoietic system	Red blood cells (RBCs)	Anti-RBC antibodies	Direct and indirect Coombs' test
Primary biliary cirrhosis	Small bile ducts in liver	Mitochondria	Antimitochondrial antibodies	Immunofluorescence of mitochondrial-rich cells (kidney biopsy)

(continued)

UNDERSTANDING AUTOANTIBODIES IN AUTOIMMUNE DISEASE
(continued)

Disease	Affected area	Antigen	Antibody	Diagnostic technique
Rheumatoid arthritis	Joints, blood vessels, skin, muscles, lymph nodes	Immunoglobu-lin (Ig) G	Antigamma-globulin antibodies	Sheep RBC agglutination, latex immuno-globulin agglu-tination, radi-oimmunoas-say, immuno-fluorescence, immuno-diffusion
Goodpasture's syndrome	Lungs and kidneys	Glomerular and lung basement membranes	Anti-basement membrane antibodies	Immunofluo-rescence of kidney biopsy sample, radio-immunoassay
Systemic lupus erythematosis	Skin, joints, muscles, lungs, heart, kidneys, brain, eyes	Deoxyribonu-cleic acid (DNA), nucleo-protein, blood cells, clotting factors, IgG, Wasserman antigen	Antinuclear antibodies, anti-DNA antibodies, Anti-ds-DNA antibodies, anti-SS-DNA antibodies, anti-ribonu-cleoprotein antibodies, antigamma-globulin anti-bodies, anti-RBC anti-bodies, anti-lymphocyte antibodies, antiplatelet antibodies, antineuronal cell antibodies, anti-Sm anti-bodies	Counterelec-trophoresis, hemagglutina-tion, radioim-munoassay, immunofluo-rescence, Coombs' test

Interfering factors
- Hemolysis due to rough handling of the sample

- Isoniazid, hydralazine, and procaina-mide (may produce a syndrome resem-bling SLE)

- Para-aminosalicylic acid, chlorpromazine, clofibrate, phenytoin, griseofulvin, ethosuximide, gold salts, methyldopa, hormonal contraceptives, penicillin, propylthiouracil, phenylbutazone, methysergide, streptomycin, sulfonamides, tetracyclines, mephenytoin, quinidine, primidone, reserpine, and trimethadione

Cardiolipin antibodies

The cardiolipin antibodies test measures serum concentrations of immunoglobulin (Ig) G and IgM antibodies in relation to the phospholipid cardiolipin. These antibodies appear in some patients with lupus erythematosus (LE) whose serum also contains a coagulation inhibitor (lupus anticoagulant). They also appear in some patients who don't fulfill all the diagnostic criteria for LE, but who experience recurrent episodes of spontaneous thrombosis, fetal loss, or thrombocytopenia. Serum concentrations of cardiolipin antibodies are measured by enzyme-linked immunosorbent assay.

Purpose
- To aid in the diagnosis of cardiolipin antibody syndrome in the patient with or without LE who experiences recurrent episodes of spontaneous thrombosis, fetal loss, or thrombocytopenia

Patient preparation
- Tell the patient that this test helps diagnose cardiolipin antibody syndrome and LE.
- Inform the patient that he need not restrict food and fluids.
- Tell the patient that the test requires a blood sample. Explain who will perform the venipuncture and when.

- Explain to the patient that he may experience slight discomfort from the needle puncture and the tourniquet.

Procedure and posttest care
- Perform a venipuncture and collect the sample in a 5-ml tube without additives.
- Apply direct pressure to the venipuncture site until bleeding stops.
- If a hematoma develops at the venipuncture site, apply warm soaks.

Precautions
- Handle the sample gently to prevent hemolysis and send it to the laboratory immediately.

Reference values
Cardiolipin antibody results are reported as negative or positive. A positive result is titered.

Abnormal findings
A positive result along with a history of recurrent spontaneous thrombosis, fetal loss, or thrombocytopenia suggests cardiolipin antibody syndrome. Treatment may involve anticoagulant or platelet inhibitor therapy.

Interfering factors
- Hemolysis due to rough handling of the sample
- Failure to send the sample to the laboratory immediately

Rheumatoid factor

The rheumatoid factor (RF) test is the most useful immunologic test for confirming rheumatoid arthritis (RA). In this disease, "renegade" immunoglobulin (Ig) G antibodies, produced by lymphocytes in the synovial joints, react with IgM antibody to produce immune complexes, complement activation, and tissue destruction. How IgG molecules become antigenic is still unknown, but they may be altered by aggregating with viruses or other antigens. Techniques for detecting RF include the sheep cell agglutination test and the latex fixation test. Although the presence of this autoantibody is diagnostically useful, it may not be etiologically related to RA.

Purpose
■ To confirm RA, especially when clinical diagnosis is doubtful

Patient preparation
■ Explain to the patient that this test helps confirm RA.
■ Inform the patient that he need not restrict food and fluids.
■ Tell the patient that the test requires a blood sample. Explain who will perform the venipuncture and when.
■ Explain to the patient that he may experience slight discomfort from the needle puncture and the tourniquet.

Procedure and posttest care
■ Perform a venipuncture and collect the sample in a 7-ml clot-activator tube.
■ Because a patient with RA may be immunologically compromised, keep the venipuncture site clean and dry for 24 hours.
■ Check regularly for signs of infection.
■ Apply direct pressure to the venipuncture site until bleeding stops.
■ If a hematoma develops at the venipuncture site, apply warm soaks.

Reference values
The normal RF titer is less than 1:20; a normal rheumatoid screening test is nonreactive.

Abnormal findings
Non-RA and RA populations aren't clearly separated with regard to the presence of RF: 25% of patients with RA have a nonreactive titer; 8% of non-RA patients are reactive at greater than 39 IU/ml, and only 3% of non-RA patients are reactive at greater than 80 IU/ml.

Patients with various non-RA diseases characterized by chronic inflammation may test positive for RF. These diseases include systemic lupus erythematosus, polymyositis, tuberculosis, infectious mononucleosis, syphilis, viral hepatic disease, and influenza.

Interfering factors
■ Inadequately activated complement (possible false-positive)
■ Serum with high lipid or cryoglobulin levels (possible false-positive, requiring a repeat test after restricting fat intake)
■ Serum with high IgG levels (possible false-negative due to competition with IgG on the surface of latex particles or sheep red blood cells used as substrate)

Cold agglutinins

Cold agglutinins are antibodies, usually of the immunoglobulin M type, that cause red blood cells (RBCs) to aggregate at low temperatures. They may occur in small amounts in healthy people. Transient elevations of these antibodies develop during certain infectious diseases, notably primary atypical pneumonia. This test reliably detects such pneumonia within 1 to 2 weeks after its onset.

Patients with high cold agglutinin titers, such as those with primary atypical pneumonia, may develop acute transient hemolytic anemia after repeated exposure to cold; patients with persistently high titers may develop chronic hemolytic anemia.

Purpose

■ To help confirm primary atypical pneumonia
■ To provide additional diagnostic evidence for cold agglutinin disease associated with many viral infections and lymphoreticular cancer
■ To detect cold agglutinins in the patient with suspected cold agglutinin disease

Patient preparation

■ Explain to the patient that this test detects antibodies in the blood that attack RBCs after exposure to low temperatures.
■ Tell the patient that the test will be repeated to monitor his response to therapy, if appropriate.
■ Tell the patient that he need not restrict food and fluids.
■ Tell the patient that the test requires a blood sample. Explain who will perform the venipuncture and when.
■ Explain to the patient that he may experience slight discomfort from the needle puncture and the tourniquet.
■ If the patient is receiving antimicrobial drugs, note this on the laboratory request because the use of such drugs may interfere with the development of cold agglutinins.

Procedure and posttest care

■ Perform a venipuncture and collect the sample in a 7-ml tube without additives that has been prewarmed to 98.6° F (37° C).
■ If cold agglutinin disease is suspected, keep the patient warm. If he's exposed to low temperatures, agglutination may occur within peripheral vessels, possibly leading to frostbite, anemia, Raynaud's phenomenon and, rarely, focal gangrene.
■ Watch for signs of vascular abnormalities, such as mottled skin, purpura, jaundice, pallor, pain or swelling of extremities, and cramping of fingers and toes. Hemoglobinuria may result from severe intravascular hemolysis on exposure to severe cold.
■ Apply direct pressure to the venipuncture site until bleeding stops.
■ If a hematoma develops at the venipuncture site, apply warm soaks.

Precautions

■ Handle the sample gently to prevent hemolysis and send it to the laboratory immediately.

▶ **CLINICAL ALERT** *Don't refrigerate the sample; cold agglutinins will coat the RBCs, leaving none in the serum for testing.*

Reference values

Cold agglutinin screening results are reported as negative or positive. A positive result, indicating the presence of cold agglutinin, is titered. A normal titer is less than 1:64.

Abnormal findings

High titers may occur as primary phenomena or secondary to infections or lymphoreticular cancer. They may be present in infectious mononucleosis, cytomegalovirus infection, hemolytic anemia, multiple myeloma, scleroderma, malaria, cirrhosis of the liver, congenital syphilis, peripheral vascular disease, pulmonary embolism, trypanosomiasis, tonsillitis, staphylococcemia, scarlatina, influenza and, occasionally, pregnancy. Chronically elevated titers are most commonly associated with pneumonia and lymphoreticular cancer; an acute transient elevation typically accompanies many viral infections.

In primary atypical pneumonia, cold agglutinins appear in serum in one-half to two-thirds of all patients during the first week of acute infection, even before antimycoplasmal antibodies can be detected by complement fixation or metabolic inhibition tests. Thus, titers usually become positive at 7 days, peak above 1:32 in 4 weeks, and disappear rapidly after 6 weeks. When sequential titers verify this pattern and clinical evidence of pneumonia exists, the diagnosis is confirmed.

Extremely high titers (> 1:2,000) can occur with idiopathic cold agglutinin disease that precedes lymphoma development. Patients with titers this high are susceptible to intravascular agglutination, which causes significant clinical problems.

Interfering factors
■ Hemolysis due to rough handling of the sample (possible false-low titer)
■ Refrigeration of the sample before serum is separated from RBCs (possible false-low titer)
■ Antimicrobial drugs

Cryoglobulins

Cryoglobulins are abnormal serum proteins that precipitate at low laboratory temperatures (39.2° F [4° C]) and redissolve after being warmed. Their presence in the blood (cryoglobulinemia) is usually associated with immunologic disease, but can also occur without known immunopathology. (See *Diseases associated with cryoglobulinemia.*) If patients with cryoglobulinemia are subjected to cold, they may experience Raynaud-like symptoms (pain, cyanosis, and cold fingers and toes), which generally result from cryoglobulin precipitation in cooler parts of the body. In some patients, for example, cryoglobulins may precipitate at tempera-

tures as high as 86° F (30° C); such temperatures are possible in some peripheral blood vessels.

The cryoglobulin test involves refrigerating a serum sample at 33.8° F (1° C) for 24 hours and observing for formation of a heat-reversible precipitate. Such a precipitate requires further study by immunoelectrophoresis or double diffusion to identify cryoglobulin components.

Purpose
■ To detect cryoglobulinemia in the patient with Raynaud-like vascular symptoms

Patient preparation
■ Explain to the patient that this test detects antibodies in blood that may cause sensitivity to low temperatures.
■ Instruct the patient to fast for 4 to 6 hours before the test.
■ Tell the patient that the test requires a blood sample. Explain who will perform the venipuncture and when.
■ Explain to the patient that he may experience slight discomfort from the needle puncture and the tourniquet.

Procedure and posttest care
■ Perform a venipuncture and collect the sample in a prewarmed 10-ml tube without additives.
■ Instruct the patient that he may resume his usual diet.
■ Tell the patient to avoid cold temperatures or contact with cold objects if the test is positive for cryoglobulins, as ordered.
■ Apply direct pressure to the venipuncture site until bleeding stops.
■ If a hematoma develops at the venipuncture site, apply warm soaks.
■ Observe for signs of intravascular coagulation, such as decreased color and

DISEASES ASSOCIATED WITH CRYOGLOBULINEMIA

The chart below indicates typical serum levels and diseases associated with the three types of cryoglobulins.

Type of cryoglobulin	Serum level	Associated diseases
Type I		
Monoclonal cryoglobulin	> 5 mg/ml	■ Myeloma ■ Waldenström's macroglobulinemia ■ Chronic lymphocytic leukemia
Type II		
Mixed cryoglobulin	> 1 mg/ml	■ Rheumatoid arthritis ■ Sjögren's syndrome ■ Mixed essential cryoglobulinemia
Type III		
Mixed polyclonal cryoglobulin	< 1 mg/ml (50% below 80 mcg/ml)	■ Systemic lupus erythematosus ■ Rheumatoid arthritis ■ Sjögren's syndrome ■ Infectious mononucleosis ■ Cytomegalovirus infection ■ Acute viral hepatitis ■ Chronic active hepatitis ■ Primary biliary cirrhosis ■ Poststreptococcal glomerulonephritis ■ Infective endocarditis ■ Leprosy ■ Kala-azar ■ Tropical splenomegaly syndrome

temperature in distal extremities, and increased pain.

Precautions
■ Warm the syringe and collection tube to 98.6° F (37° C) before venipuncture and keep the tube at that temperature to prevent cryoglobulin loss.
■ Send the sample to the laboratory immediately.

Normal findings
Normally, serum is negative for cryoglobulins. Positive results are reported as a percentage based on the amount of sample cryoprecipitation.

Abnormal findings
The presence of cryoglobulins in the blood confirms cryoglobulinemia. This finding doesn't always indicate the presence of clinical disease.

Interfering factors
■ Failure to adhere to dietary restrictions
■ Failure to keep the sample at 98.6° F (37° C) before centrifugation (possible loss of cryoglobulins)
■ Reading the sample before the 72-hour precipitation period ends (possible incorrect analysis of results because some cryoglobulins take several days to precipitate)

Acetylcholine receptor antibodies

The acetylcholine receptor (AChR) antibodies test is the most useful immunologic test for confirming acquired (autoimmune) myasthenia gravis (MG), a disorder of neuromuscular transmission. In MG, antibodies block and destroy AChR sites, causing muscle weakness that can be either generalized or localized to the ocular muscles.

Two test methods — a binding assay and a blocking assay — are now available to determine the relative concentration of AChR antibodies in serum. The blocking assay is relatively new, and its clinical significance isn't fully known. However, it's specific for the autoimmune form of MG and useful for research. Determination of AChR antibodies by either method also helps monitor immunosuppressive therapy for MG, although antibody levels don't usually parallel the severity of disease.

Purpose
- To confirm the diagnosis of MG
- To monitor the effectiveness of immunosuppressive therapy for MG

Patient preparation
- Explain to the patient that this test helps confirm the diagnosis of MG.
- Tell the patient that the test assesses the effectiveness of treatment, if appropriate.
- Inform the patient that he need not restrict food and fluids.
- Tell the patient that the test requires a blood sample. Explain who will perform the venipuncture and when.
- Explain to the patient that he may experience slight discomfort from the needle puncture and the tourniquet.
- Check the patient's history for immunosuppressive drugs that may affect test results and note such use on the laboratory request.

Procedure and posttest care
- Perform a venipuncture and collect the sample in a 7-ml tube without additives.
- Because a patient with an autoimmune disease has a compromised immune system, check the venipuncture site for infection and promptly report changes.
- Keep a clean, dry bandage over the site for at least 24 hours.
- Apply direct pressure to the venipuncture site until bleeding stops.
- If a hematoma develops at the venipuncture site, apply warm soaks.

Precautions
- Keep the sample at room temperature and send it to the laboratory immediately.

Normal findings
Normal serum is negative for AChR-binding antibodies and AChR-blocking antibodies.

Abnormal findings
Positive AChR antibodies in symptomatic adults confirm the diagnosis of MG. Patients who have only ocular symptoms have lower antibody titers than those who have generalized symptoms.

Interfering factors
- Failure to maintain the sample at room temperature and to send the sample to the laboratory immediately
- Thymectomy, thoracic duct drainage, immunosuppressive therapy, and plasmapheresis (possible decrease)
- Amyotrophic lateral sclerosis (possible false-positive)

Anti-insulin antibodies

Some patients with diabetes form antibodies to the insulin they take. These antibodies bind with some of the insulin, making less insulin available for glucose metabolism and necessitating increased insulin dosages. This phenomenon is known as insulin resistance.

Performed on the blood of a patient with diabetes who takes insulin, the anti-insulin antibody test detects insulin antibodies. Insulin antibodies are immunoglobulins, called anti-insulin Ab. The most common type of anti-insulin Ab is immunoglobulin (Ig) G, but anti-insulin Ab is also found in the other four classes of immunoglobulins — IgA, IgD, IgE, and IgM. IgM may cause insulin resistance, and IgE has been associated with allergic reactions.

Purpose
- To determine insulin allergy
- To confirm insulin resistance
- To determine if hypoglycemia is caused by insulin overuse

Patient preparation
- Explain to the patient that this test is used to determine the most appropriate treatment for his diabetes and to determine if he has insulin resistance or an allergy to insulin.
- Tell the patient that the test requires a blood sample. Explain who will perform the venipuncture and when.
- Explain to the patient that he may experience slight discomfort from the needle puncture and the tourniquet.
- Inform the patient that he need not restrict food and fluids.
- Ask the patient if he has had a radioactive test recently; if so, note this on the laboratory request.

Procedure and posttest care
- Perform a venipuncture and collect the sample in a 7-ml tube without additives.
- Apply direct pressure to the venipuncture site until bleeding stops.
- If a hematoma develops at the venipuncture site, apply warm soaks.

Precautions
- Handle the sample gently to prevent hemolysis.

Normal findings
There should be less than 3% binding of the patient's serum with labeled beef, human, and pork insulin.

Abnormal findings
Elevated levels may occur in insulin allergy or resistance and in factitious hypoglycemia.

Interfering factors
- Radioactive test performed within 1 week before the test

VIRAL TESTS

Rubella antibodies

Although rubella (German measles) is generally a mild viral infection in children and young adults, it can produce severe infection in the fetus, resulting in spontaneous abortion, stillbirth, or congenital rubella syndrome. Because rubella infection normally induces immunoglobulin (Ig) G and IgM antibody production, measuring rubella antibodies can determine present infection as well as immunity resulting from past infection. The hemagglutination inhibition test is the most commonly used serologic test for rubella antibodies.

Suspected cases of congenital rubella may be confirmed if rubella-specific IgM antibodies are present in the infant's serum. Immune status in adults can be confirmed by an existing IgG-specific titer.

Exposure risk (when the immunity status is unknown) may be evaluated using two serum samples. The first sample should be drawn in the acute phase of clinical symptoms. If clinical symptoms aren't apparent, the sample should be drawn as soon as possible after the suspected exposure. The second sample should be drawn 3 to 4 weeks later during the convalescent phase.

Purpose
- To diagnose rubella infection, especially congenital infection
- To determine susceptibility to rubella in children and in women of childbearing age

Patient preparation
- Explain to the patient that this test diagnoses or evaluates susceptibility to rubella.
- Inform the patient that she need not restrict food and fluids.
- Tell the patient that this test requires a blood sample and that if a current infection is suspected, a second blood sample will be needed in 2 to 3 weeks to identify a rise in the titer.
- Explain who will perform the venipuncture and when.
- Explain to the patient that she may experience slight discomfort from the needle puncture and the tourniquet.

Procedure and posttest care
- Perform a venipuncture and collect the sample in a 7-ml clot-activator tube.
- Apply direct pressure to the venipuncture site until bleeding stops.
- If a hematoma develops at the venipuncture site, apply warm soaks.
- Instruct the patient to return for an additional blood test, when appropriate.
- If a woman of childbearing age is found to be susceptible to rubella, explain that vaccination can prevent rubella and that she must wait at least 3 months after the vaccination to become pregnant or risk permanent damage or death to the fetus.
- If the pregnant patient is found to be susceptible to rubella, instruct her to return for follow-up rubella antibody tests to detect possible subsequent infection.
- If the test confirms rubella in a pregnant patient, provide emotional support. As needed, refer her for appropriate counseling.

Precautions
- Handle the specimen gently to prevent hemolysis.

Reference values
A titer of 1:8 or less indicates little or no immunity against rubella; titer more than 1:10 indicates adequate protection against rubella.

IgM results are reported as positive or negative.

Abnormal findings
Hemagglutination inhibition antibodies normally appear 2 to 4 days after the onset of the rash, peak in 3 to 4 weeks, and then slowly decline but remain detectable for life. A fourfold or greater rise from the acute to the convalescent titer indicates a recent rubella infection.

VIRAL HEPATITIS TEST PANEL

The six types of viral hepatitis produce similar symptoms, but differ in transmission mode, course of treatment, prognosis, and carrier status. When the clinical history is insufficient for differentiation, serologic tests can aid in diagnosis. Testing helps to identify antibodies specific to the causative virus and establish the type of hepatitis:

■ Type A: Detection of an antibody to hepatitis A, confirming the diagnosis
■ Type B: The presence of hepatitis B surface antigens and hepatitis B antibodies, confirming the diagnosis
■ Type C: Diagnosis depends on serologic testing for the specific antibody one or more months after the onset of acute illness: until then, diagnosis principally established by obtaining negative test results for hepatitis A, B, and D
■ Type D: Detection of intrahepatic delta antigens or immunoglobulin (Ig) M antidelta antigens in acute disease (or IgM and IgG in chronic disease), establishing the diagnosis

■ Type E: Detection of hepatitis E antigens supports the diagnosis; however, possibly ruling out hepatitis C
■ Type G: Detection of hepatitis G ribonucleic acid supporting the diagnosis (serologic assays are being developed).

Additional findings from liver function studies supporting the diagnosis include:

■ Serum aspartate aminotransferase and serum alanine aminotransferase levels increased in the prodromal stage of acute viral hepatitis
■ Serum alkaline phosphatase levels slightly increased
■ Serum bilirubin levels elevated; levels possibly remaining elevated late in the disease, especially with severe disease
■ Prothrombin time (PT) prolonged (PT of more than 3 seconds longer than normal, indicating severe liver damage)
■ White blood cell counts commonly revealing transient neutropenia and lymphopenia followed by lymphocytosis.

AGE ISSUE *The presence of rubella-specific IgM antibodies indicates recent infection in an adult and congenital rubella in an infant.*

Interfering factors

■ Hemolysis due to rough handling of the sample

Hepatitis B surface antigen

Hepatitis B surface antigen (HBsAg), also called hepatitis-associated antigen or Australia antigen, appears in the serum of the patient with hepatitis B virus. It can be detected by radioimmunoassay or, less commonly, reverse passive hemagglutination during the extended incubation period and usually during the first 3 weeks of acute infection or if the patient is a carrier.

Because hepatitis transmission is one of the gravest complications associated with blood transfusion, all donors must be screened for hepatitis B before their blood is stored. This screening, required by the Food and Drug Administration's Bureau of Biologics, has helped reduce the incidence of hepatitis. This test doesn't screen for hepatitis A virus (infectious hepatitis).

For information on related tests, see *Viral hepatitis test panel.* See also *Serodiagnosis of acute viral hepatitis,* page 306.

SERODIAGNOSIS OF ACUTE VIRAL HEPATITIS

The chart below helps evaluate positive test results in acute viral hepatitis.

Test results			Interpretation
HBsAg	*Anti-HBC IgM*	*Anti-HAV IgM*	
−	−	+	Recent acute hepatitis A infection
+	+	−	Acute hepatitis B infection
+	−	−	Early acute hepatitis B infection or chronic hepatitis B
−	+	−	Confirms acute or recent infection with hepatitis B virus
−	−	−	Possible hepatitis C infection, other viral infection, or liver toxin
+	+	+	Recent probable hepatitis A infection and superimposed acute hepatitis B infection; uncommon profile

KEY: + = positive   − = negative

Reprinted with permission of Abbott Laboratories, Abbott Park, Ill.

Purpose
- To screen blood donors for hepatitis B
- To screen people at high risk for contracting hepatitis B such as hemodialysis health care workers
- To aid in the differential diagnosis of viral hepatitis

Patient preparation
- Explain to the patient that this test helps identify a type of viral hepatitis.
- Inform the patient that he need not restrict food and fluids.
- Tell the patient that the test requires a blood sample. Explain who will perform the venipuncture and when.
- Explain to the patient that he may experience slight discomfort from the needle puncture and the tourniquet.
- Check the patient's history for administration of hepatitis B vaccine.
- If the patient is giving blood, explain the donation procedure to him.

Procedure and posttest care
- Perform a venipuncture and collect the sample in a 10-ml clot-activator tube.

- Apply direct pressure to the venipuncture site until bleeding stops.
- If a hematoma develops at the venipuncture site, apply warm soaks.
- Report confirmed viral hepatitis to public health authorities. This is a reportable disease in most states.

Precautions
- Wash your hands carefully after the procedure.
- Remember to wear gloves when drawing blood and dispose of the needle properly.

Normal findings
Normal serum is negative for HBsAg.

Abnormal findings
The presence of HBsAg in patients with hepatitis confirms hepatitis B. In chronic carriers and in people with chronic active hepatitis, HBsAg may be present in the serum several months after the onset of acute infection. It may also occur in more than 5% of patients with certain diseases other than hepatitis, such as hemophilia, Hodgkin's disease, and leukemia. If HbsAg is found in donor blood, that blood must be discarded because it carries a risk of transmitting hepatitis. Blood samples that test positive should be retested because inaccurate results do occur.

Interfering factors
- Hepatitis B vaccine (possible positive)

Heterophil antibodies

Heterophil antibody tests detect and identify two immunoglobulin (Ig) M antibodies in human serum that react against foreign red blood cells (RBCs): Epstein-Barr virus (EBV) antibodies and Forssman antibodies.

In the Paul-Bunnell test — also called the presumptive test — EBV antibodies, found in the sera of patients with infectious mononucleosis, agglutinate with sheep RBCs in a test tube. Forssman antibodies, present in the sera of some normal persons as well as in the sera of patients with such conditions as serum sickness, also agglutinate with sheep RBCs, thus rendering test results inconclusive for infectious mononucleosis.

If the Paul-Bunnell test establishes a presumptive titer, the Davidsohn differential absorption test can then distinguish between EBV and Forssman antibodies. (See *Monospot test for infectious mononucleosis*, page 308.)

Purpose
- To aid in the differential diagnosis of infectious mononucleosis

Patient preparation
- Explain to the patient that this test helps detect infectious mononucleosis.
- Tell the patient that the test requires a blood sample. Explain who will perform the venipuncture and when.
- Explain to the patient that he may experience slight discomfort from the needle puncture and the tourniquet.

Procedure and posttest care
- Perform a venipuncture and collect the sample in a 7-ml clot-activator tube.
- Apply direct pressure to the venipuncture site until bleeding stops.
- If a hematoma develops at the venipuncture site, apply warm soaks.
- If the titer is positive and infectious mononucleosis is confirmed, instruct the patient in the treatment plan.
- If the titer is positive but infectious mononucleosis isn't confirmed, or if the titer is negative but symptoms persist, ex-

MONOSPOT TEST FOR INFECTIOUS MONONUCLEOSIS

Several screening tests can detect the heterophil infectious mononucleosis (IM) antibody. One of these tests — the monospot — converts the Paul-Bunnell and the Davidsohn differential absorption tests into one rapid slide test without titration. Monospot relies on agglutination of horse red blood cells (RBCs) by heterophil antibodies.

Distinguishing antibodies

Because horse RBCs contain Forssman and IM antigens, differential absorption of the patient's serum is necessary to distinguish between them. This is done by mixing the serum sample with guinea pig kidney antigen (containing only Forssman antigen) on one end of a slide and with beef RBC stroma (containing only IM antigen) on the other end of the slide. Each absorbs only the heterophil antibody specific to it. After addition of horse RBCs to each spot, agglutination on the beef cell end of the slide indicates the presence of the IM heterophil antibody and confirms IM.

Monospot rivals the classic heterophil agglutination test for sensitivity. False-positives may occur in the presence of lymphoma, hepatitis A and B, leukemia, and pancreatic cancer.

Reference values

Normally, the titer is less than 1:56, but it may be higher in elderly people. Some laboratories refer to a normal titer as "negative" or as having "no reaction."

Abnormal findings

Although heterophil antibodies are present in the sera of about 80% of patients with infectious mononucleosis 1 month after its onset, a positive finding — a titer higher than 1:56 — doesn't confirm this disorder; a high titer can also result from systemic lupus erythematosus, syphilis, cryoglobulinemia, or the presence of antibodies to nonsyphilitic treponemata (yaws, pinta, bejel). A gradual increase in the titer during week 3 or 4 followed by a gradual decrease during weeks 4 to 8 proves most conclusive for infectious mononucleosis. A negative titer doesn't always rule out this disorder; occasionally, the titer becomes reactive 2 weeks later. Therefore, if symptoms persist, the test should be repeated in 2 weeks.

Confirming infectious mononucleosis depends on heterophil agglutination and hematologic tests that show absolute lymphocytosis, with 10% or more atypical lymphocytes.

Interfering factors
- Hemolysis due to rough handling of the sample
- Narcotic use, lymphomas, hepatitis, leukemia, and phenytoin therapy (false-positive)

plain that additional testing will be necessary in a few days or weeks to confirm the diagnosis and plan effective treatment.

Precautions
- Handle the sample gently to prevent hemolysis.

Epstein-Barr virus antibodies

Epstein-Barr virus (EBV), a member of the herpesvirus group, is the causative agent of heterophil-positive infectious mononucleosis, Burkitt's lymphoma, and nasopharyngeal carcinoma. Although the virus doesn't replicate in standard cell cultures, most EBV infections can be recognized by testing the patient's serum for heterophil antibodies (monospot test), which usually appear within the first 3 weeks of illness and then decline rapidly within a few weeks.

In about 10% of adults and a larger percentage of children, the monospot test is negative despite primary infection with EBV. Further, EBV has been associated with lymphoproliferative processes in immunosuppressed patients. These disorders occur with reactivated, rather than primary, EBV infections and therefore are also monospot-negative.

Alternatively, EBV-specific antibodies, which develop to several antigens of the virus during active infection, can be measured with a high level of sensitivity and specificity by indirect immunofluorescence.

Purpose

- To provide a laboratory diagnosis of heterophil- (or monospot-) negative cases of infectious mononucleosis
- To determine the antibody status to EBV of immunosuppressed patients with lymphoproliferative processes

Patient preparation

- Explain the purpose of the test to the patient.
- Tell the patient that the test requires a blood sample. Explain who will perform the venipuncture and when.
- Explain to the patient that he may experience slight discomfort from the needle puncture and the tourniquet.

Procedure and posttest care

- Perform a venipuncture and collect 5 ml of sterile blood in a clot-activator tube.
- Allow the blood to clot for at least 1 hour at room temperature.
- Apply direct pressure to the venipuncture site until bleeding stops.
- If a hematoma develops at the venipuncture site, apply warm soaks.

Precautions

- Handle the sample gently to prevent hemolysis.
- Transfer the serum to a sterile tube or vial and send it to the laboratory immediately.
- If transfer must be delayed, store the serum at 39.2° F (4° C) for 1 to 2 days or at −4° F (−20° C) for longer periods to prevent contamination.

Normal findings

Sera from patients who have never been infected with EBV have no detectable antibodies to the virus as measured by either the monospot test or the indirect immunofluorescence test. The monospot test is positive only during the acute phase of infection with EBV; the indirect immunofluorescence test detects and discriminates between acute and past infection with the virus.

Abnormal findings

EBV infection can be ruled out if no antibodies to EBV antigens are detected in the indirect immunofluorescence test. A positive monospot test or an indirect immunofluorescence test that's either immunoglobulin M (IgM)-positive or Epstein-Barr nuclear antigen (EBNA)-negative indicates acute EBV infection.

A monospot-negative result doesn't necessarily rule out acute or past infection with EBV. Conversely, IgG class antibody to viral capsid antigen and EBNA antigens (IgM-negative) indicates remote (more than 2 months) infection with EBV. Recognize that most cases of monospot-negative infectious mononucleosis are caused by cytomegalovirus infections.

Interfering factors
■ Hemolysis due to rough handling of the sample

Respiratory syncytial virus antibodies

Respiratory syncytial virus (RSV), a member of the paramyxovirus group, is the major viral cause of severe lower respiratory tract disease in infants, but may cause infections in people of any age. RSV infections are most common and produce the most severe disease during the first 6 months of life. Initial infection involves viral replication in epithelial cells of the upper respiratory tract, but in younger children especially, the infection spreads to the bronchi, the bronchioles, and even the parenchyma of the lungs.

In this test, immunoglobulin (Ig) G and IgM class antibodies are quantified using indirect immunofluorescence.

Purpose
■ To diagnose infections caused by RSV

Patient preparation
■ Explain the purpose of the test to the patient (or, to the patient's parents).
■ Tell the patient or parents that the test requires a blood sample. Explain who will perform the venipuncture and when.
■ Tell the patient he may experience slight discomfort from the needle puncture and the tourniquet.

Procedure and posttest care
■ Perform a venipuncture and collect 5 ml of sterile blood in a clot-activator tube.
■ Allow the blood to clot for at least 1 hour at room temperature.
■ Apply direct pressure to the venipuncture site until bleeding stops.
■ If a hematoma develops at the venipuncture site, apply warm soaks.

Precautions
■ Handle the sample gently to prevent hemolysis.
■ Transfer the serum to a sterile tube or vial and send it to the laboratory promptly.
■ If transfer must be delayed, store the serum at 39.2° F (4° C) for 1 to 2 days or at –4° F (–20° C) for longer periods to avoid contamination.

Reference values
Sera from patients who have never been infected with RSV have no detectable antibodies to the virus (less than 1:5).

Abnormal findings
The qualitative presence of IgM or a fourfold or greater increase in IgG antibodies indicates active RSV infection. Note that, in infants, serologic diagnosis of RSV infections is difficult because of the presence of maternal IgG antibodies. Thus, the presence of IgM antibodies is most significant.

Interfering factors
■ Hemolysis due to rough handling of the sample

Herpes simplex antibodies

Herpes simplex virus (HSV), a member of the herpesvirus group, causes various clinically severe manifestations, including genital lesions, keratitis or conjunctivitis, generalized dermal lesions, and pneumonia. Severe involvement is associated with intrauterine or neonatal infections and encephalitis; such infections are most severe in immunosuppressed patients. Of the two closely related antigenic types, type 1 usually causes infections above the waistline; type 2 infections predominantly involve the external genitalia. Primary contact with this virus occurs in early childhood as acute stomatitis or, more commonly, as an inapparent infection. More than 50% of adults have antibodies to HSV.

Sensitive assays, such as indirect immunofluorescence and enzyme immunoassay, are used to demonstrate immunoglobulin (Ig) M class antibodies to HSV or to detect a fourfold or greater increase in IgG class antibodies between acute- and convalescent-phase sera.

Purpose
- To confirm infections caused by HSV
- To detect recent or past HSV infection

Patient preparation
- Explain the purpose of the test to the patient.
- Tell the patient that the test requires a blood sample. Explain who will perform the venipuncture and when.
- Explain to the patient that he may experience slight discomfort from the needle puncture and the tourniquet.

Procedure and posttest care
- Perform a venipuncture and collect 5 ml of sterile blood in a tube designated by the laboratory.
- Allow the blood to clot for at least 1 hour at room temperature.
- Apply direct pressure to the venipuncture site until bleeding stops.
- If a hematoma develops at the venipuncture site, apply warm soaks.
- If the patient's immune system is compromised, check the venipuncture site for changes and report them promptly.

Precautions
- Handle the sample gently to prevent hemolysis.
- Transfer the serum to a sterile tube or vial and send it to the laboratory promptly.
- If transfer must be delayed, store the serum at 39.2° F (4° C) for 1 to 2 days or at −4° F (−20° C) for longer periods to avoid contamination.
- Because the patient may have a compromised immune system, keep the venipuncture site clean and dry.

Reference values
Sera from patients who have never been infected with HSV have no detectable antibodies (less than 1:5).

Abnormal findings
HSV infection can be ruled out in patients whose serum shows no detectable antibodies to the virus. The presence of IgM or a fourfold or greater increase in IgG antibodies indicates active HSV infection.

Interfering factors
- Hemolysis due to rough handling of the sample

Cytomegalovirus antibodies

After primary infection, cytomegalovirus (CMV) remains latent in white blood cells (WBCs). The presence of CMV antibodies indicates past infection with this virus. In an immunocompromised patient, CMV can be reactivated to cause active infection. Administration of blood or tissue from a seropositive donor may cause active CMV infection in a CMV-seronegative organ transplant recipient or neonate, especially one born prematurely.

Antibodies to CMV can be detected by several methods, including passive hemagglutination, latex agglutination, enzyme immunoassay, and indirect immunofluorescence. The complement fixation test is only 60% sensitive compared with other assays and shouldn't be used to screen for CMV antibodies. Screening tests for CMV antibodies are qualitative; they detect the presence of antibody at a single low dilution. In quantitative methods, several dilutions of the serum sample are tested to indicate acute CMV infection.

Purpose
- To detect CMV infection in donors and recipients of organs and blood and in immunocompromised patients
- To screen for CMV infection in infants who require blood transfusions or tissue transplants

Patient preparation
🟢 AGE ISSUE *Explain the purpose of the test to the patient or the parents of an infant, as appropriate.*
- Tell the patient that the test requires a blood sample. Explain who will perform the venipuncture and when.

- Explain to the patient that he may experience slight discomfort from the needle puncture and the tourniquet.

Procedure and posttest care
- Perform a venipuncture and collect the sample in a 5-ml tube designated by the laboratory.
- Allow the blood to clot for at least 1 hour at room temperature.
- Apply direct pressure to the venipuncture site until bleeding stops.
- If a hematoma develops at the venipuncture site, apply warm soaks.

Precautions
- Handle the sample gently to prevent hemolysis.
- Transfer the serum to a sterile tube or vial and send it to the laboratory.
- If transfer must be delayed, store the serum at 39.2° F (4° C) for 1 to 2 days or at −4° F (−20° C) for longer periods to avoid contamination.
- Because the patient may have a compromised immune system, keep the venipuncture site clean and dry.

Reference values
The patient who has never been infected with CMV has no detectable antibodies to the virus. Immunoglobulin (Ig) G and IgM are normally negative.

Abnormal findings
A serum sample collected early during the acute phase or late in the convalescent stage may not contain detectable IgG or IgM antibodies to CMV. Therefore, a negative result doesn't preclude recent infection. More than a single sample is needed to ensure accurate results.

A serum sample that tests positive for antibodies at this single dilution indicates that the patient has been infected with

CMV and that his WBCs contain latent virus capable of being reactivated in an immunocompromised host. An immunosuppressed patient who lacks antibodies to CMV should receive blood products or organ transplants from a donor who's also seronegative. The patient with CMV antibodies doesn't require seronegative blood products.

Interfering factors
- Hemolysis due to rough handling of the sample

Human immunodeficiency virus antibodies

The human immunodeficiency virus (HIV) antibodies test detects antibodies to HIV in serum. HIV is the virus that causes acquired immunodeficiency syndrome (AIDS). Transmission occurs by direct exposure of a person's blood to body fluids containing the virus. The virus may be transmitted from one person to another through exchange of contaminated blood and blood products, during sexual intercourse with an infected partner, when I.V. drugs are shared, and from an infected mother to her child during pregnancy or breast-feeding.

Initial identification of HIV is usually achieved through enzyme-linked immunosorbent assay. Positive findings are confirmed by Western blot test and immunofluorescence. There are also other tests available, which may be performed to detect antibodies. (See *Testing for HIV*.)

Purpose
- To screen for HIV in the high-risk patient
- To screen donated blood for HIV

TESTING FOR HIV

Newer tests are available to help identify human immunodeficiency virus (HIV)-infected antibodies quicker and more conveniently, including a test to identify genetic changes that may alter the patient's course of treatment.

OraQuick rapid HIV-1 antibody test
For the many people per year who don't check back for test results, rapid HIV testing may be done in any outpatient setting. The Ora-Quick rapid HIV-1 antibody test, approved by the Food and Drug Administration (FDA), allows results to be obtained in less than 20 minutes using 1 drop of blood. A color indicator similar to a home pregnancy test is used. If it's positive, another test must be done to confirm the results.

Nucleic acid test
The FDA has also approved a nucleic acid test to screen plasma donation for HIV and hepatitis C. This test has been shown to dramatically reduce the waiting time involved until blood and blood products may be used.

Gene-based test
Spikes of HIV virus in the bloodstream commonly mean that the individual being treated for HIV is growing resistant to the drug treatment being used. The government has approved the first gene-based test to help determine if an HIV-infected person's virus is mutating, making therapy fail. This test can help the physician to select more appropriate treatment.

Patient preparation

- Explain to the patient that this test detects HIV infection.
- Provide adequate counseling about the reasons for performing the test, which is usually requested by the patient's physician.
- If the patient has questions about his condition, be sure to provide full and accurate information.
- Tell the patient that the test requires a blood sample. Explain who will perform the venipuncture and when.
- Explain to the patient that he may experience slight discomfort from the needle puncture and the tourniquet.

Procedure and posttest care

- Perform a venipuncture and collect the sample in a 10-ml barrier tube. Barrier tubes help prevent contamination when pouring the serum in the laboratory.
- Apply direct pressure to the venipuncture site until bleeding stops.
- If a hematoma develops at the venipuncture site, apply warm soaks.
- Keep test results confidential.
- When the patient receives the results, give him another opportunity to ask questions.
- Encourage the patient with positive screening tests to seek medical follow-up care, even if he's asymptomatic.
- Tell the patient to report early signs of AIDS, such as fever, weight loss, axillary or inguinal lymphadenopathy, rash, and persistent cough or diarrhea. Women should also report gynecologic symptoms.
- Tell the patient to assume that he can transmit HIV to others until conclusively proved otherwise. To prevent possible virus transmission, advise him about safer sex practices.
- Instruct the patient not to share razors, toothbrushes, or utensils (which may be contaminated with blood) and to clean such items with household bleach diluted 1:10 in water.
- Advise the patient against donating blood, tissues, or an organ.
- Warn the patient to inform his physician and dentist about his condition so that they can take proper precautions.

Precautions

- Observe standard precautions when drawing a blood sample.
- Use gloves, properly dispose of needles, and use blood-fluid precaution labels on tubes, as necessary.
- Because the patient may have a compromised immune system, keep the venipuncture site clean and dry.

Normal findings

Test results are normally negative.

Abnormal findings

The test detects previous exposure to HIV. However, it doesn't identify a patient who has been exposed to the virus but hasn't yet made antibodies. In most cases, the patient with AIDS has antibodies to HIV. A positive test for the HIV antibody can't determine whether a patient harbors actively replicating virus or when the patient will manifest signs and symptoms of AIDS.

Many apparently healthy people have been exposed to HIV and have circulating antibodies. The test results for such people aren't false-positives. Furthermore, patients in the later stages of AIDS may exhibit no detectable antibody in their sera because they can no longer mount an antibody response.

Interfering factors

- None known

Parvovirus B-19 antibodies

Parvovirus B-19, a small, single-stranded deoxyribonucleic acid virus belonging to the family Parvoviridae, destroys red blood cell (RBC) precursors and interferes with normal RBC production. It's also associated with erythema infectiosum (a self-limiting, low-grade fever and rash in young children) and aplastic crisis (in patients with chronic hemolytic anemia and immunodeficient patients with bone marrow failure). Immunoglobulin (Ig) G and IgM antibodies can be detected by enzyme-linked immunosorbent assay and immunofluorescence.

Purpose
- To detect parvovirus B-19 antibody, especially in prospective organ donors
- To diagnose erythema infectiosum, parvovirus B-19 aplastic crisis, and related parvovirus B-19 diseases

Patient preparation
- Explain the test purpose and procedure to the patient. To a potential organ donor, explain that the test is part of a panel of tests performed before organ donation to protect the organ recipient from potential infection.
- Tell the patient that the test requires a blood sample. Explain who will perform the venipuncture and when.
- Explain to the patient that he may experience slight discomfort from the needle puncture and the tourniquet.

Procedure and posttest care
- Perform a venipuncture, collect the blood sample in a 5-ml clot-activator tube, and store it on ice.
- Apply direct pressure to the venipuncture site until bleeding stops.

- If a hematoma develops at the venipuncture site, apply warm soaks.

Precautions
- Handle the sample gently to prevent hemolysis.

Normal findings
Normally, results are negative for IgM- and IgG-specific antibodies to parvovirus B-19.

Abnormal findings
About 50% of all adults lack immunity to parvovirus B-19, with as many as 20% of susceptible adults becoming infected after exposure. Positive results have been associated with joint arthralgia, hydrops fetalis, fetal loss, transient aplastic anemia, chronic anemia in immunocompromised patients, and bone marrow failure.

Abnormal findings for parvovirus B-19 should be confirmed using the Western blot test.

Interfering factors
- Failure to put the sample on ice
- Hemolysis due to rough handling of the sample

BACTERIAL AND FUNGAL TESTS

Antistreptolysin-O

The antistreptolysin-O test measures the relative serum concentrations of the antibody to streptolysin-O (known as ASO). A serum sample is diluted with a commercial preparation of streptolysin-O and incubated. After the addition of human red blood cells, the tube is reincubated and examined visually. Failure of hemoly-

---

TEST FOR ANTI-DNASE B

The antideoxyribonuclease B (anti-DNase B) test, a process similar to the antistreptolysin-O (ASO) test, detects antibodies to DNase B, a potent antigen produced by all group A streptococci.

For adults, normal anti-DNase B titer is less than 85 Todd units/ml; for school-age children, it's less than 170 Todd units/ml; and for preschoolers, it's less than 60 Todd units/ml.

Elevated anti-DNase B titers appear in 80% of patients with acute rheumatic fever, in 75% of those with poststreptococcal glomerulonephritis (following streptococcal pharyngitis), and in 60% of those with glomerulonephritis (following group A streptococcal pyoderma). This is a much higher percentage than those with ASO titer elevations (25%), making the test for anti-DNase B especially valuable in detecting a reaction to group A streptococcal pyoderma.

Other streptococcal antigens are of limited diagnostic value, or their use is controversial.

---

sis to develop indicates recent streptococcal infection. The end point is read in Todd units, the reciprocal of the highest dilution (titer) that inhibits hemolysis.

Purpose
- To confirm recent or ongoing streptococcal infection
- To help diagnose rheumatic fever and poststreptococcal glomerulonephritis in the presence of clinical symptoms (See *Test for anti-DNase B*, for information about another method of diagnosing these two diseases.)
- To distinguish between rheumatic fever and rheumatoid arthritis when joint pains are present

Patient preparation
- Explain to the patient that this test detects an immunologic response to certain bacteria (streptococci).
- Inform the patient that he need not restrict food and fluids.
- Tell the patient that the test requires a blood sample. Explain who will perform the venipuncture and when.
- Explain to the patient that he may experience slight discomfort from the needle puncture and the tourniquet.
- If the test is to be repeated at regular intervals to identify active and inactive states of rheumatic fever or to confirm acute glomerulonephritis, tell the patient that measuring changes in antibody levels helps determine the effectiveness of therapy.
- Check the patient's history for drugs that may suppress the streptococcal antibody responses. If such drugs must be continued, note this on the laboratory request.

Procedure and posttest care
- Perform a venipuncture and collect the sample in a 7-ml tube without additives.
- Apply direct pressure to the venipuncture site until bleeding stops.
- If a hematoma develops at the venipuncture site, apply warm soaks.

Precautions
- Handle the sample gently to prevent hemolysis.

Reference values
 AGE ISSUE *Even healthy people have some detectable ASO titers from pre-*

vious minor streptococcal infections. Normal ASO titers range as follows:
- school-age children: 170 Todd units/ml
- preschoolers and adults: 85 Todd units/ml.

Abnormal findings

High ASO titers usually occur only after prolonged or recurrent infections. Generally, a titer higher than 166 Todd units/ml is considered a definite elevation. A low titer is good evidence of the absence of active rheumatic fever. A higher titer doesn't necessarily mean that rheumatic fever or glomerulonephritis is present; however, it does indicate the presence of a streptococcal infection.

Serial titers, determined at 10- to 14-day intervals, provide more reliable information than a single titer. An increase in titer 2 to 5 weeks after the acute infection, which peaks 4 to 6 weeks after the initial increase, confirms poststreptococcal disease.

Interfering factors

- Streptococcal skin infections, seldom producing abnormal ASO titers even with poststreptococcal disease (probable false-negative)
- Antibiotic or corticosteroid therapy (possible suppression of the streptococcal antibody response)
- Hemolysis due to rough handling of the sample

Febrile agglutination

Sometimes bacterial infections (such as tularemia, brucellosis, and the disorders caused by *Salmonella*) and rickettsial infections (such as Rocky Mountain spotted fever and typhus) cause puzzling fevers, called fevers of undetermined origin (FUO). In these infections and others in which microorganisms are difficult to isolate from blood or excreta, febrile agglutination tests can provide important diagnostic information.

The Weil-Felix test for rickettsial disease, Widal's test for *Salmonella,* and tests for brucellosis and tularemia are essentially the same. In these tests, a serum sample is mixed with a few drops of prepared antigens in normal saline solution on a slide and the reaction is observed.

The Weil-Felix test establishes rickettsial antibody titers. It uses three forms of *Proteus* antigens (OX-19, OX-2, and OX-K) that cross-react with the various strains of rickettsiae. Antibodies to certain rickettsial strains react with more than one *Proteus* antigen, whereas antibodies to other strains fail to react with any *Proteus* antigens.

Widal's test establishes the titers for flagellar (H) and somatic (O) antigens, which may indicate *Salmonella* gastroenteritis and extraintestinal focal infections, caused by *S. enteritidis,* or enteric (typhoid) fever, caused by *S. typhosa.* A third antigen, the Vi or envelope antigen, may indicate typhoid carrier status, which commonly tests negative for H and O antigens. Widal's test isn't recommended for diagnosing *Salmonella* gastroenteritis.

Slide agglutination and tube dilution tests, using killed suspensions of the disease organisms as antigens, establish titers for the gram-negative coccobacilli *Brucella* and *Francisella tularensis,* which cause brucellosis and tularemia, respectively.

Purpose

- To support clinical findings in diagnosis of disorders caused by *Salmonella, Rickettsia, F. tularensis,* and *Brucella* organisms
- To identify the cause of FUO

Patient preparation

- Explain to the patient that this test detects and quantifies microorganisms that may cause fever and other symptoms.
- Inform the patient that he need not restrict food and fluids.
- Tell the patient that the test requires a blood sample. Explain who will perform the venipuncture and when.
- Explain to the patient that he may experience slight discomfort from the needle puncture and the tourniquet.
- Explain to the patient that this test requires a series of blood samples to detect a pattern of titers characteristic of the suspected disorder, if appropriate. Reassure him that a positive titer only suggests a disorder.
- Note on the laboratory request when antimicrobial therapy began, if appropriate.

Procedure and posttest care

- Perform a venipuncture and collect the sample in a 7-ml clot-activator tube.
- Apply direct pressure to the venipuncture site until bleeding stops.
- If a hematoma develops at the venipuncture site, apply warm soaks.
- In FUO and suspected infection, contact the facility's infection control department. Isolation may be necessary.

Precautions

- Use standard isolation procedures when collecting and handling samples.
- Send samples to the laboratory immediately.

Reference values

Results are reported as negative or positive, and positive results are titered. Normal dilutions are:

- *Salmonella* antibody: < 1:80
- Brucellosis antibody: < 1:80

- Tularemia antibody: < 1:40
- Rickettsial antibody: < 1:40.

Abnormal findings

Observed rise and fall of titers is crucial for detecting active infection. If this isn't possible, certain titer levels can suggest the disorder. For all febrile agglutinins, a fourfold increase in titers is strong evidence of infection.

The Weil-Felix test is positive for rickettsiae with antibodies to *Proteus* 6 to 12 days after infection; titers peak in 1 month and usually drop to negative in 5 to 6 months. This test can't be used to diagnose rickettsialpox or Q fever because the antibodies of these diseases don't cross-react with *Proteus* antigens; the test shows positive titers in *Proteus* infections and, in such cases, is nonspecific for rickettsiae.

In *Salmonella* infection, H and O agglutinins usually appear in serum after 1 week, and titers rise for 3 to 6 weeks. O agglutinins usually fall to insignificant levels in 6 to 12 months. Agglutinin titers may remain elevated for years.

In brucellosis, titers usually rise after 2 to 3 weeks and reach their highest levels between 4 and 8 weeks. The absence of *Brucella* agglutinins doesn't rule out brucellosis. In tularemia, titers usually become positive during the second week of infection, exceed 1:320 by the third week, peak within 4 to 7 weeks, and usually decline gradually 1 year after recovery.

Interfering factors

- Failure to send the sample to the laboratory immediately
- Vaccination or continuous exposure to bacterial or rickettsial infection, resulting in immunity (high titers)
- Antibody cross-reaction with bacteria causing other infectious diseases such as

tularemia antibodies cross-reacting with *Brucella* antigens
- Immunodeficiency (negative titers even during symptomatic infection due to inability to form antibodies)
- Antibiotics (low titers early in the course of infection)
- Elevated immunoglobulin levels due to hepatic disease or excessive drug use (high *Salmonella* titers)
- Skin tests with *Brucella* antigen (possible high *Brucella* titers)
- *Proteus* infections (possible positive Weil-Felix titers for rickettsial disease)

Fungal serology

Most fungal organisms enter the body as spores inhaled into the lungs or infiltrated through wounds in the skin or mucosa. If the body's defenses can't destroy the organisms initially, the fungi multiply to form lesions; blood and lymph vessels may then spread the mycoses throughout the body. Most healthy people easily overcome initial mycotic infection, but elderly people and others with a deficient immune system are more susceptible to acute or chronic mycotic infection and to disorders secondary to such infection. Mycosis may be deep-seated or superficial. Deep-seated mycosis occurs primarily in the lungs; superficial mycosis, in the skin or mucosal linings.

Although cultures are usually performed to diagnose mycoses by identifying the causative organism, serologic tests occasionally provide the sole evidence for mycosis. Such serologic tests use immunodiffusion, complement fixation, precipitin, latex agglutination, or agglutination methods to demonstrate the presence of specific mycotic antibodies. (See *Serum test methods for fungal infections*, pages 320 and 321.)

Purpose
- To rapidly detect the presence of antifungal antibodies, aiding in the diagnosis of mycoses
- To monitor the effectiveness of therapy for mycoses

Patient preparation
- Explain to the patient that this test aids in the diagnosis of certain fungal infections. If appropriate, tell him that this test monitors his response to antimycotic therapy and that it may be necessary to repeat the test.
- Instruct him to restrict food and fluids for 12 to 24 hours before the test.
- Tell the patient that the test requires a blood sample. Explain who will perform the venipuncture and when.
- Explain to the patient that he may experience slight discomfort from the needle puncture and the tourniquet.

Procedure and posttest care
- Perform a venipuncture and collect the sample in a 10-ml sterile clot-activator tube.
- Apply direct pressure to the venipuncture site until bleeding stops.
- If a hematoma develops at the venipuncture site, apply warm soaks.

Precautions
- Send the sample to the laboratory immediately.
- If transport to the laboratory is delayed, store the sample at 39.2° F (4° C).

Normal findings
Depending on the test method, a negative finding, or normal titer, usually indicates the absence of mycosis.

SERUM TEST METHODS FOR FUNGAL INFECTIONS

Disease and normal values	Clinical significance of abnormal results
Blastomycosis	
Complement fixation: titers < 1:8	Titers ranging from 1:8 to 1:16 suggest infection; titers > 1:32 denote active disease. A rising titer in serial samples taken every 3 to 4 weeks indicates disease progression; a falling titer indicates regression. This test has limited diagnostic value because of a high percentage of false-negatives.
Immunodiffusion: negative	A more sensitive test for blastomycosis; detects 80% of infected people.
Coccidioidomycosis	
Complement fixation: titers < 1:2	Most sensitive test for this fungus. Titers ranging from 1:2 to 1:4 suggest active infection; titers > 1:16 usually denote active disease. Test may remain active in mild infections.
Immunodiffusion: negative	Most useful for screening, followed by complement fixation test for confirmation.
Precipitin: titers < 1:16	Good screening test; titers >1:16 usually indicate infection. About 80% of infected people show positive titers by 2 weeks; most revert to negative by 6 months. Early primary disease is shown by positive precipitin and negative complement fixation test. A positive complement fixation and negative precipitin test indicate chronic disease.
Histoplasmosis	
Complement fixation (histoplasmin): titers < 1:8	Titers ranging from 1:8 to 1:16 suggest infection; titers > 1:32 indicate active disease. Antibodies generally appear 10 to 21 days after initial infection. Test is positive in 10% to 15% of cases.
Complement fixation: titers < 1:18	Titers ranging from 1:8 to 1:16 suggest infection; titers > 1:32 indicate active disease. More sensitive than histoplasmin complement fixation test; gives positive results in 75% to 80% of cases. (Histoplasmin and yeast antigens are positive in 10% of cases.) A rising titer in serial samples taken every 2 to 3 weeks indicates progressive infection; a decreasing titer indicates regression.
Immunodiffusion (histoplasmin): negative	Appearance of H and M bands indicates active infection. If the M band appears first and lasts longer than the H band, the infection may be regressing. The M band alone may indicate early infection, chronic disease, or a recent skin test.

SERUM TEST METHODS FOR FUNGAL INFECTIONS *(continued)*

Disease and normal values	Clinical significance of abnormal results
Aspergillosis	
Complement fixation: titers < 1:8	Titers > 1:8 suggest infection; 70% to 90% of patients with known pulmonary aspergillosis or aspergillus allergy present antibodies. This test can't detect invasive aspergillosis because patients with this disease don't have antibodies; biopsy is required.
Immunodiffusion: negative	One or more precipitin bands suggests infection. The number of bands is related to complement fixation titers; the more precipitin bands, the higher the titer.
Sporotrichosis	
Agglutination: titers < 1:40	Titers >1:80 usually indicate active infection. The test usually is negative in cutaneous infections and positive in extracutaneous infections.
Cryptococcosis	
Latex agglutination for cryptococcal antigen: negative	About 90% of patients with cryptococcal meningitis exhibit positive latex agglutination in cerebrospinal fluid (CSF). (Serum is less frequently positive than CSF.) Culturing is definitive because false-positives do occur. (Presence of rheumatoid factor may cause a positive reaction.) Serum antigen tests are positive in 33% of patients with pulmonary cryptococcosis; biopsy is usually required.

Abnormal findings

The chart on pages 320 and 321 explains the significance of findings for specific organisms.

Interfering factors

- Failure to observe dietary restrictions
- Failure to send a sterile sample to the laboratory immediately or to properly store the sample in case of delay in transportation
- Cross-reaction of antibodies with other antigens, such as blastomycosis and histoplasmosis antigens (possible false-positive or high titers)
- Recent skin testing with fungal antigens (possible high titers)
- Mycosis-caused immunosuppression (low titers or false-negative)

Candida antibodies

Commonly present in the body, *Candida albicans* is a saprophytic yeast that can become pathogenic when the environment favors proliferation or the host's defenses have been significantly weakened.

Candidiasis is usually limited to the skin and mucous membranes, but may cause life-threatening systemic infection. Susceptibility to candidiasis is associated with antibacterial, antimetabolic, and corticosteroid therapy as well as with immunologic defects, pregnancy, obesity, diabetes, and debilitating diseases. Oral candidiasis is common and benign in children; in adults, it may be an early indication of acquired immunodeficiency syndrome.

Diagnosis of candidiasis is usually made by culture or histologic study. When such diagnosis can't be made, identifying *Candida* antibodies may be helpful in diagnosing systemic candidiasis. Be aware that serologic testing to detect antibodies in candidiasis isn't reliable, and investigators continue to disagree about its usefulness.

Purpose
■ To aid in the diagnosis of candidiasis when culture or histologic study can't confirm the diagnosis

Patient preparation
■ Explain the purpose of the test to the patient, as appropriate.
■ Inform the patient that he need not restrict food and fluids.
■ Tell the patient that the test requires a blood sample. Explain who will perform the venipuncture and when.
■ Explain to the patient that he may experience slight discomfort from the needle puncture and the tourniquet.

Procedure and posttest care
■ Perform a venipuncture and collect the sample in a 5-ml sterile collection tube without additives.
■ Apply direct pressure to the venipuncture site until bleeding stops.
■ If a hematoma develops at the venipuncture site, apply warm soaks.

Precautions
■ Handle the sample gently to prevent hemolysis.
■ Send the sample to the laboratory immediately.
■ Note recent antimicrobial therapy on the laboratory request form.
■ Because the patient's immune system may be compromised, keep the venipuncture site clean and dry.

Normal findings
A normal test result is negative for *Candida* antibodies.

Abnormal findings
A positive test for *C. albicans* antibodies is common in patients with disseminated candidiasis. However, this test yields a significant percentage of false-positive results.

Interfering factors
■ Hemolysis due to rough handling of the sample

Bacterial meningitis antigen

The bacterial meningitis antigen test can detect specific antigens of *Streptococcus pneumoniae*, *Neisseria meningitidis*, and *Haemophilus influenzae* type B, the principal etiologic agents in meningitis. It can be performed on samples of serum, cerebrospinal fluid (CSF), urine, pleural fluid, and joint fluid, but CSF and urine are preferred.

Purpose
■ To identify the etiologic agent in meningitis
■ To aid in the diagnosis of bacterial meningitis

- To aid in the diagnosis of meningitis when the Gram stain smear and culture are negative

Patient preparation
- Explain the purpose of the test to the patient, as appropriate.
- Inform the patient that this test requires a specimen of urine or CSF. Explain who will perform the procedure and when.
- If a CSF specimen is required, describe how it will be obtained.
- Explain to the patient that he may experience discomfort from the needle puncture.
- Advise the patient that a headache is the most common complication of lumbar puncture, but that his cooperation during the test minimizes such an effect.
- Make sure the patient or a family member has signed an informed consent form.

Procedure and posttest care
- Collect a 10-ml urine specimen or a 1-ml CSF specimen in a sterile container.

Precautions
- Maintain specimen sterility during collection.
- Wear gloves when obtaining or handling the specimen.
- Make sure the cap is tightly fastened on the specimen container.
- Place the specimen on a refrigerated coolant and send it to the laboratory immediately.

Normal findings
Normally, results are negative for bacterial antigens.

Abnormal findings
Positive results identify the specific bacterial antigen: *S. pneumoniae, N. meningitidis, H. influenzae* type B, or group B streptococci.

Interfering factors
- Previous antimicrobial therapy
- Failure to maintain sterility during specimen collection

Lyme disease serology

Lyme disease is a multisystem disorder characterized by dermatologic, neurologic, cardiac, and rheumatic manifestations in various stages. Epidemiologic and serologic studies implicate a common tickborne spirochete, *Borrelia burgdorferi,* as the causative agent. Serologic tests for Lyme disease, both indirect immunofluorescent and enzyme-linked immunosorbent assays, measure antibody response to this spirochete and indicate current infection or past exposure. Serologic tests can identify 50% of patients with early-stage Lyme disease and all patients with later complications of carditis, neuritis, and arthritis or patients in remission.

   In an indirect immunofluorescent assay, *B. burgdorferi* is grown in culture, fixed to a microscope slide, and then incubated with a human serum sample. A fluorescein-labeled antiglobulin is then introduced into the antigen-antibody complex. Any human antibody that binds to the spirochete is detected by viewing (under an ultraviolet microscope) the fluorescent antiglobulin that attaches to it.

Purpose
- To confirm a diagnosis of Lyme disease

Patient preparation

- Explain to the patient that this test helps determine whether his symptoms are caused by Lyme disease.
- Instruct the patient to fast for 12 hours before the sample is drawn, but to drink fluids as usual.
- Tell the patient that the test requires a blood sample. Explain who will perform the venipuncture and when.
- Explain to the patient that he may experience slight discomfort from the needle puncture and the tourniquet.

Procedure and posttest care

- Perform a venipuncture and collect the sample in a 7-ml clot-activator tube.
- Apply direct pressure to the venipuncture site until bleeding stops.
- If a hematoma develops at the venipuncture site, apply warm soaks.

Precautions

- Handle the specimen carefully to prevent hemolysis.
- Send the specimen to the laboratory immediately.

Reference values

Normal serum values are nonreactive.

Abnormal findings

A positive result can help confirm the diagnosis, but it isn't definitive. Other treponemal diseases and high rheumatoid factor titers can cause false-positive results. More than 15% of patients with Lyme disease fail to develop antibodies.

Interfering factors

- High serum lipid levels (possible inaccurate results, requiring a repeat test after a period of restricted fat intake)
- Samples contaminated with other bacteria (possible false-positive)

- Hemolysis due to rough handling of the sample

Helicobacter pylori antibodies

Helicobacter pylori is a spiral, gram-negative bacterium associated with chronic gastritis and idiopathic chronic duodenal ulceration. Although a gastric specimen can be obtained by endoscopy and cultured for *H. pylori*, the *H. pylori* antibody blood test is a more useful noninvasive screening procedure and may be performed using the enzyme-linked immunosorbent assay. (See *Additional tests for* Helicobacter pylori.)

Purpose

- To help diagnose *H. pylori* infection in the patient with GI symptoms

Patient preparation

- Inform the patient that this test is used to diagnose the infection that may cause ulcers.
- Inform the patient that he need not restrict food and fluids.
- Tell the patient that the test requires a blood sample. Explain who will perform the venipuncture and when.
- Explain to the patient that he may experience slight discomfort from the needle puncture and the tourniquet.

Procedure and posttest care

- Perform a venipuncture and collect the sample in a 7-ml clot-activator tube.
- Send the sample to the laboratory immediately.
- Apply direct pressure to the venipuncture site until bleeding stops.
- If a hematoma develops at the venipuncture site, apply warm soaks.

Precautions

- This test should be performed only on a patient with GI symptoms because of the large number of healthy people who have *H. pylori* antibodies.

Normal findings

Normally, no antibodies to *H. pylori* are revealed. Test results are reported as negative or positive.

Abnormal findings

A positive *H. pylori* test result indicates that the patient has antibodies to the bacterium. The serologic results should be interpreted in light of the clinical findings.

Interfering factors

- None significant

SYPHILIS TESTS

VDRL test

The Venereal Disease Research Laboratory (VDRL) test, a flocculation test, is widely used to screen for primary and secondary syphilis. Although the test has diagnostic significance during the first two stages of syphilis, transient or permanent biologic false-positive reactions can make accurate interpretation difficult. A biologic false-positive reaction can result from viral or bacterial infection, chronic systemic illness, or nonsyphilitic treponemal disease. Usually, a serum sample is used in the VDRL test, but this test may also be performed on a cerebrospinal fluid (CSF) specimen obtained by lumbar puncture to test for tertiary syphilis. The VDRL test of CSF is less sensitive than the

---

ADDITIONAL TESTS FOR *HELICOBACTER PYLORI*

Helicobacter pylori is diagnosed through blood, breath, stool, and tissue tests. Blood tests are the most common. They detect antibodies to *H. pylori* bacteria.

Urea breath tests are an effective diagnostic tool for *H. pylori*. They are also used after treatment to see whether it has been effective. In the physician's office, the patient drinks a urea solution that contains a special carbon atom. If *H. pylori* is present, it breaks down the urea, releasing the carbon. The blood carries the carbon to the lungs, where the patient exhales it. The breath test is 96% to 98% accurate.

Stool tests may be used to detect *H. pylori* infection in the patient's stool. Studies have shown that this test, called the *Helicobacter pylori* stool antigen (HpSA) test is accurate for diagnosing *H. pylori*.

Tissue tests are usually done using the biopsy sample taken with the endoscope. There are three types:
- The rapid urease detects the enzyme disease produced by *H. pylori*.
- A histology test allows the physician to find and examine the actual bacteria.
- A culture test involves allowing *H. pylori* to grow in the tissue sample.

In diagnosing *H. pylori*, blood, breath, and stool tests are commonly done before tissue tests because they are less invasive. However, blood tests aren't used to detect *H. pylori* following treatment because a patient's blood can show positive results even after *H. pylori* has been eliminated.

Source: U.S. National Institute of Diabetes & Digestive & Kidney Diseases of the National Institutes of Health, 2003.

RAPID PLASMA REAGIN TEST

The rapid plasma reagin (RPR) test is a rapid, macroscopic serologic test that's an acceptable substitute for the VDRL test in diagnosing syphilis. The RPR test, available as a kit, uses a cardiolipin antigen to detect reagin, the antibody relatively specific for *Treponema pallidum,* the causative agent of syphilis.

In the RPR test, the patient's serum is mixed with cardiolipin on a plastic-coated card, rotated mechanically, and then examined with the unaided eye. If flocculation occurs, the test sample is diluted until no visible reaction occurs. The last dilution to show visible flocculation is the titer of the reagin antibody.

In the RPR test, like the VDRL test, normal serum shows no flocculation.

---

fluorescent treponemal antibody absorption test.

The rapid plasma reagin test can also be used to diagnose syphilis. (See *Rapid plasma reagin test.*)

Purpose

■ To screen for primary and secondary syphilis

■ To confirm primary or secondary syphilis in the presence of syphilitic lesions

■ To monitor the patient's response to treatment

Patient preparation

■ Explain to the patient that this test detects syphilis.

■ Inform the patient that the disease usually goes undetected in the general population because infected people remain untreated.

■ Tell the patient that he need not restrict food, fluids, or medications, but should abstain from alcohol for 24 hours before the test.

■ Tell the patient that the test requires a blood sample. Explain who will perform the venipuncture and when.

■ Explain to the patient that he may experience slight discomfort from the needle puncture and the tourniquet.

Procedure and posttest care

■ Perform a venipuncture and collect the sample in a 7-ml clot-activator tube.

■ Apply direct pressure to the venipuncture site until bleeding stops.

■ If a hematoma develops at the venipuncture site, apply warm soaks.

■ If the test is nonreactive or borderline, but syphilis hasn't been ruled out, instruct the patient to return for follow-up testing. Explain that borderline test results don't necessarily mean that he's free from the disease.

■ If the test is reactive, explain the importance of proper treatment. Provide the patient with further information about sexually transmitted diseases and how they're spread and stress the need for antibiotic therapy. Report the results to state public health authorities and prepare the patient for mandatory inquiries.

■ If the test is reactive, but the patient shows no clinical signs of syphilis, explain that many uninfected people show false-positive reactions. Stress the need for further specific tests to rule out syphilis.

Precautions

■ Handle the specimen carefully to prevent hemolysis.

Normal findings

Normal serum shows no flocculation and is reported as a nonreactive test.

Abnormal findings

Definite flocculation is reported as a reactive test; slight flocculation is reported as a weakly reactive test. A reactive VDRL test occurs in about 50% of patients with primary syphilis and in nearly all patients with secondary syphilis. If syphilitic lesions exist, a reactive VDRL test is diagnostic. If no lesions are evident, a reactive VDRL test necessitates repeated testing. Biologic false-positive reactions can be caused by conditions unrelated to syphilis; for example, infectious mononucleosis, malaria, leprosy, hepatitis, systemic lupus erythematosus, rheumatoid arthritis, and nonsyphilitic treponemal diseases, such as pinta and yaws.

A nonreactive test doesn't rule out syphilis because *Treponema pallidum* causes no detectable immunologic changes in the serum for 14 to 21 days after infection. Darkfield microscopy of exudate from suspicious lesions can provide early diagnosis by identifying the causative spirochetes.

A reactive VDRL test using a CSF specimen indicates neurosyphilis, which can follow the primary and secondary stages in patients who remain untreated.

Interfering factors

■ Ingestion of alcohol within 24 hours of the test (possible transient nonreactive results)
■ Immunosuppression (possible nonreactive results)
■ Hemolysis due to rough handling of the sample

Fluorescent treponemal antibody absorption

The fluorescent treponemal antibody absorption (FTA-ABS or simply FTA) test uses indirect immunofluorescence to detect antibodies to the spirochete *Treponema pallidum* in serum. This spirochete causes syphilis.

In this test, prepared *T. pallidum* is fixed on a slide, and the patient's serum is added after the addition of an absorbed preparation of Reiter treponema. This addition to the test serum prevents interference by antibodies from nonsyphilitic treponemas; Reiter treponema combines with most nonsyphilitic antibodies, making the FTA-ABS test specific for *T. pallidum*

If syphilitic antibodies are present in the test serum, they will coat the treponemal organisms. The slide is then stained with fluorescein-labeled antiglobulin. This antiglobulin attaches to the coated spirochetes, which fluoresce when viewed under an ultraviolet microscope.

Although the FTA-ABS test is generally performed on a serum sample to detect primary or secondary syphilis, a cerebrospinal fluid (CSF) specimen is required to detect tertiary syphilis. Because antibody levels remain constant for long periods, the FTA-ABS test isn't recommended for monitoring the patient's response to therapy. (See *Two tests for* Treponema pallidum, page 328.)

Purpose

■ To confirm primary and secondary syphilis
■ To screen for suspected false-positive results of Venereal Disease Research Laboratories tests

Patient preparation

■ Explain to the patient that this test can confirm or rule out syphilis.
■ Inform the patient that he need not restrict food and fluids.

TWO TESTS FOR *TREPONEMA PALLIDUM*

The microhemagglutination assay for the *Treponema pallidum* antibody increases the specificity of syphilis testing by eliminating methodologic interference. In this assay, tanned sheep red blood cells are coated with *T. pallidum* antigen and combined with absorbed test serum. Hemagglutination occurs in the presence of specific anti-*T. pallidum* antibodies in the serum.

In the enzyme-linked immunosorbent assay, tubes coated with *T. pallidum* are washed and then treated with enzyme-labeled antihuman globulin. After the substrate for the enzymes is added to the tubes, the enzymatic activity is measured by quantitating the reaction product formed.

■ Tell the patient that the test requires a blood sample. Explain who will perform the venipuncture and when.
■ Explain to the patient that he may experience slight discomfort from the needle puncture and the tourniquet.

Procedure and posttest care

■ Perform a venipuncture and collect the sample in a 7-ml clot-activator tube.
■ Apply direct pressure to the venipuncture site until bleeding stops.
■ If a hematoma develops at the venipuncture site, apply warm soaks.
■ If the test is reactive, explain the nature of syphilis and stress the importance of proper treatment and the need to find and treat the patient's sexual contacts.
■ Provide the patient with additional information about syphilis and how it's spread; emphasize the need for antibiotic therapy, if appropriate. Report positive results to state public health authorities and prepare the patient for mandatory inquiries.
■ If the test is nonreactive or findings are borderline, but syphilis hasn't been ruled out, instruct the patient to return for follow-up testing; explain that inconclusive results don't necessarily indicate that he's free from the disease.

Precautions
■ Handle the sample gently to prevent hemolysis.

Normal findings
Normally, results of the FTA-ABS test are nonreactive.

Abnormal findings
The presence of treponemal antibodies in the serum — a reactive test result — doesn't indicate the stage or severity of infection. (The presence of these antibodies in CSF is strong evidence of tertiary neurosyphilis.) Elevated antibody levels appear in most patients with primary syphilis and in almost all patients with secondary syphilis. Higher antibody levels persist for several years, with or without treatment.

The absence of treponemal antibodies — a nonreactive test result — doesn't necessarily rule out syphilis. *T. pallidum* causes no detectable immunologic changes in the blood for 14 to 21 days after initial infection. Organisms may be detected earlier by examining suspicious lesions with a darkfield microscope. Low antibody levels and other nonspecific factors produce borderline findings. In such cases, repeated testing and a thorough review of the patient's history may be productive.

Although the FTA-ABS test is specific, some patients with nonsyphilitic conditions, such as systemic lupus erythematosus, genital herpes, and increased or abnormal globulins, or those who are pregnant may show minimally reactive levels. In addition, the FTA-ABS test doesn't always distinguish between *T. pallidum* and certain other treponemas, such as those that cause pinta, yaws, and bejel.

Interfering factors
- Hemolysis due to rough handling of the sample

FETAL ANTIGEN TESTS

Carcinoembryonic antigen

Carcinoembryonic antigen (CEA) is a protein normally found in embryonic entodermal epithelium and fetal GI tissue. Production of CEA stops before birth, but it may begin again later if a neoplasm develops. Because CEA levels are also raised by biliary obstruction, alcoholic hepatitis, chronic heavy smoking, and other conditions, this test can't be used as a general indicator of cancer. The measurement of enzyme CEA levels by immunoassay is useful for staging and monitoring treatment of certain cancers. (See *Using CEA to monitor cancer treatment,* pages 330 and 331.)

Purpose
- To monitor the effectiveness of cancer therapy
- To assist in preoperative staging of colorectal cancers, assess the adequacy of surgical resection, and test for the recurrence of colorectal cancers

Patient preparation
- Explain to the patient that this test detects and measures a special protein that isn't normally present in adults.
- Inform the patient that the test will be repeated to monitor the effectiveness of therapy, if appropriate.
- Inform the patient that he need not restrict food, fluids, or medications.
- Tell the patient that the test requires a blood sample. Explain who will perform the venipuncture and when.
- Explain to the patient that he may experience slight discomfort from the needle puncture and the tourniquet.

Procedure and posttest care
- Perform a venipuncture and collect the sample in a 7-ml tube without additives.
- Apply direct pressure to the venipuncture site until bleeding stops.
- If a hematoma develops at the venipuncture site, apply warm soaks.

Precautions
- Handle the sample gently to prevent hemolysis.
- Send the sample to the laboratory immediately.

Reference values
Normal serum CEA values are less than 5 ng/ml (SI, < 5 mg/L).

Abnormal findings
Persistent elevation of CEA levels suggests residual or recurrent tumor. If levels exceed normal before surgical resection, chemotherapy, or radiation therapy, their return to normal within 6 weeks suggests successful treatment.

High CEA levels are characteristic in various malignant conditions, particularly entodermally derived neoplasms of the GI organs and lungs, and in certain non-

USING CEA TO MONITOR CANCER TREATMENT

Because many patients in the early stages of colorectal cancer have normal or low levels of carcinoembryonic antigen (CEA), the CEA test doesn't screen successfully for early malignancy. It's a good tool, however, for monitoring response to cancer therapy.

After a patient's serum CEA level has dropped following surgery, chemotherapy, or other treatment, an increase suggests recurrence of cancer or diminished effectiveness of treatment.

Both charts to the right illustrate CEA levels in patients during and after treatment for colorectal cancer. In the near right chart, initial results show the usual dramatic drop in response to treatment; the subsequent rise in CEA indicates a diminishing response to chemotherapy. In the far right chart, the progressive rise in CEA signals a recurrence of cancer 8 months before clinical symptoms or radiologic evidence.

CEA LEVELS

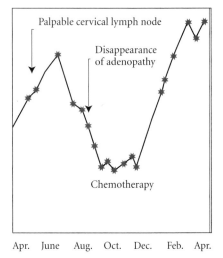

Apr.   June   Aug.   Oct.   Dec.   Feb.   Apr.

---

malignant conditions, such as benign hepatic disease, hepatic cirrhosis, alcoholic pancreatitis, and inflammatory bowel disease.

Elevated CEA concentrations may occur in nonendodermal carcinomas, such as breast and ovarian cancers.

Interfering factors
- Chronic cigarette smoking (possible increase)
- Hemolysis due to rough handling of the sample

Alpha-fetoprotein

Alpha-fetoprotein (AFP) is a glycoprotein produced by fetal tissue and tumors that differentiate from midline embryonic structures. During fetal development,

AFP levels in serum and amniotic fluid rise. AFP crosses the placenta and appears in maternal serum.

High maternal serum AFP levels may suggest fetal neural tube defects, such as spina bifida and anencephaly, but positive confirmation requires amniocentesis and ultrasonography. Other congenital anomalies, such as Down syndrome and other chromosomal disorders, may be associated with low maternal serum AFP concentrations.

Elevated AFP levels in the patient who isn't pregnant may occur in cancers, such as hepatocellular carcinoma, or certain nonmalignant conditions such as ataxia-telangiectasia. In these conditions, AFP assays are more useful for monitoring the patient's response to therapy than for diagnosis. AFP levels are best determined by

CEA LEVELS

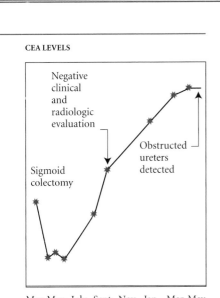

Mar. May July Sept. Nov. Jan. Mar. May

enzyme immunoassay on amniotic fluid or serum.

Purpose
- To monitor the effectiveness of therapy in malignant conditions, such as hepatomas and germ cell tumors, and certain nonmalignant conditions such as ataxiatelangiectasia
- To screen for the need for amniocentesis or high-resolution ultrasonography in a pregnant woman

Patient preparation
- Explain that this test helps in monitoring fetal development, screens for a need for further testing, helps detect possible congenital defects in the fetus, and monitors her response to therapy by measuring a specific blood protein, as appropriate.
- Inform the patient that she need not restrict food, fluids, or medications.
- Tell the patient that the test requires a blood sample. Explain who will perform the venipuncture and when.
- Explain to the patient that she may experience slight discomfort from the needle puncture and the tourniquet.

Procedure and posttest care
- Perform a venipuncture and collect the sample in a 7-ml clot-activator tube.
- Record the patient's age, race, weight, and gestational period on the laboratory request.
- Apply direct pressure to the venipuncture site until bleeding stops.
- If a hematoma develops at the venipuncture site, apply warm soaks.

Precautions
- Handle the sample gently to prevent hemolysis.

Reference values
When testing by immunoassay, AFP values are less than 15 ng/ml (SI, < 15 mg/L) in men and nonpregnant women. Values in maternal serum are less than 2.5 multiples of median for fetal gestational age.

Abnormal findings
Elevated maternal serum AFP levels may suggest neural tube defects or other tube anomalies. Maternal AFP levels rise sharply in the maternal blood of about 90% of women carrying a fetus with anencephaly and in 50% of those carrying a fetus with spina bifida. Definitive diagnosis requires ultrasonography and amniocentesis. High AFP levels may indicate intrauterine death. Sometimes high levels indicate other anomalies, such as duodenal atresia, omphalocele, tetralogy of Fallot, and Turner's syndrome.

Elevated serum AFP levels occur in 70% of nonpregnant patients with hepatocellular carcinoma. Elevated levels are also related to germ cell tumor of gonadal, retroperitoneal, or mediastinal origin. Serum AFP levels rise in ataxia-telangiectasia and sometimes in cancer of the pancreas, stomach, or biliary system and in nonseminiferous testicular tumors. Transient modest elevations can occur in nonneoplastic hepatocellular disease, such as alcoholic cirrhosis and acute or chronic hepatitis. Elevation of AFP levels after remission suggests tumor recurrence.

In hepatocellular carcinoma, a gradual decrease in serum AFP levels indicates a favorable response to therapy. In germ cell tumors, serum AFP levels and serum human chorionic gonadotropin levels should be measured concurrently.

Interfering factors
- Hemolysis due to rough handling of the sample
- Multiple pregnancies (possible false-positive)

MISCELLANEOUS TESTS

TORCH test

The TORCH test helps detect exposure to pathogens involved in congenital and neonatal infections. TORCH is an acronym for **TO**xoplasmosis, **R**ubella, **C**ytomegalovirus, and **H**erpes simplex antibodies. These pathogens are commonly associated with congenital and neonatal infections that aren't clinically apparent and may cause severe central nervous system impairment. This test detects specific

immunoglobulin M-associated antibodies in infant blood.

Purpose
- To aid in the diagnosis of acute, congenital, and intrapartum infections

Patient preparation
- Explain to the infant's parents the purpose of the test and mention that the test requires a blood sample.
- Tell the parents who will perform the venipuncture and when.
- Explain that the infant may experience slight discomfort from the needle puncture and the tourniquet.

Procedure and posttest care
- Obtain a 3-ml sample of venous or cord blood.
- Apply direct pressure to the venipuncture site until bleeding stops.
- If a hematoma develops at the venipuncture site, apply warm soaks.

Precautions
- Handle the sample gently to prevent hemolysis.
- Send the sample to the laboratory immediately.
- Don't freeze the sample.

Normal findings
Normal test results are negative for TORCH agents.

Abnormal findings
Toxoplasmosis is diagnosed by sequential examination that shows rising antibody titers, changing titers, and serologic conversion from negative to positive; a titer of 1:256 suggests recent *Toxoplasma* infection.

In infants less than 6 months old, rubella infection is associated with a marked and persistent rise in complement-fixing antibody titer over time. Persistence of rubella antibody in an infant after age 6 months strongly suggests congenital infection. Congenital rubella is associated with cardiac anomalies, neurosensory deafness, growth retardation, and encephalitic symptoms.

Detection of herpes antibodies in cerebrospinal fluid with signs of herpetic encephalitis and persistent herpes simplex virus type 2 antibody levels confirms herpes simplex infection in a neonate without obvious herpetic lesions.

Interfering factors
- Hemolysis due to rough handling of the sample

Tuberculin skin tests

Tuberculin skin tests are used to screen for previous infection by the tubercle bacillus. They're routinely performed in children, young adults, and patients with radiographic findings that suggest this infection. In the old tuberculin (OT) and purified protein derivative (PPD) tests, intradermal injection of the tuberculin antigen causes a delayed hypersensitivity reaction in patients with active or dormant tuberculosis (TB).

The Mantoux test uses a single-needle intradermal injection of PPD, permitting precise measurement of the dose. Multipuncture tests, such as the tine test, MonoVacc tests, and Aplitest, use intradermal injections with tines impregnated with OT or PPD. Because they require less skill and are more rapidly administered, multipuncture tests are generally used for screening. A positive multipuncture test usually requires a Mantoux test for confirmation.

Purpose
- To distinguish TB from blastomycosis, coccidioidomycosis, and histoplasmosis
- To identify people who need diagnostic investigation for TB because of possible exposure

Patient preparation
- Explain to the patient that this test helps detect TB.
- Tell the patient that the test requires an intradermal injection, which may cause him discomfort.
- Check the patient's history for active TB, the results of previous skin tests, and hypersensitivities.
- If the patient has had TB, don't perform a skin test.
- If the patient has had a positive reaction to previous skin tests, consult the physician or follow facility policy.
- If the patient has had an allergic reaction to acacia, don't perform an OT test because this product contains acacia.
- If you're performing a tuberculin test on an outpatient, instruct him to return at the specified time so that test results can be read.
- Inform the patient that a positive reaction to a skin test appears as a red, hard, raised area at the injection site. Although the area may itch, instruct him not to scratch it.
- Stress that a positive reaction doesn't always indicate active TB.

Procedure and posttest care
- Ask the patient to sit and support his extended arm on a flat surface.
- Clean the volar surface of the upper forearm with alcohol and allow the area to dry completely.

Mantoux test
- Perform an intradermal injection.

Multipuncture test

- Remove the protective cap on the injection device to expose the four tines.
- Hold the patient's forearm in one hand, stretching the skin of the forearm tightly. Then, with your other hand, firmly depress the device into the patient's skin without twisting it.
- Hold the device in place for at least 1 second before removing it.
- If you've applied sufficient pressure, you'll see four puncture sites and a circular depression made by the device on the patient's skin.

Both tests

- Record where the test was given, the date and time, and when the results are to be read. Tuberculin skin tests are generally read 48 to 72 hours after injection; the MonoVacc test can be read 48 to 96 hours after the test.
- If ulceration or necrosis develops at the injection site, apply cold soaks or a topical steroid.

Precautions

- Tuberculin skin tests are contraindicated in the patient with current reactions to smallpox vaccinations, a rash, a skin disorder, or active TB.
- Don't perform a skin test in areas with excessive hair, acne, or insufficient subcutaneous tissue, such as over a tendon or bone.
- If the patient is known to be hypersensitive to skin tests, use a first-strength dose in the Mantoux test to avoid necrosis at the puncture site.
- Have epinephrine available to treat a possible anaphylactic or acute hypersensitivity reaction.

Normal findings

In tuberculin skin tests, normal findings show negative or minimal reactions. In the Mantoux test, no induration may appear or the patient may develop induration less than 5 mm in diameter.

In the tine and Aplitest tests, no vesiculation or induration may appear or the patient may develop induration less than 2 mm in diameter. In the MonoVacc tests, no induration appears.

Abnormal findings

A positive tuberculin reaction indicates previous infection by tubercle bacilli. It doesn't distinguish between an active and a dormant infection or provide a definitive diagnosis. If a positive reaction occurs, sputum smear and culture and chest radiography are necessary for further information.

In the Mantoux test, induration 5 to 9 mm in diameter indicates a borderline reaction; larger induration, a positive reaction. Because patients infected with atypical mycobacteria other than tubercle bacilli may have borderline reactions, repeat testing is necessary.

In the tine or Aplitest tests, vesiculation indicates a positive reaction; induration 2 mm in diameter without vesiculation requires confirmation by the Mantoux test. Any induration in the MonoVacc test indicates a positive reaction; however, it requires confirmation by the Mantoux test.

Interfering factors

- Subcutaneous injection, usually indicated by erythema greater than 10 mm in diameter without induration
- Corticosteroids, other immunosuppressants, and live vaccine viruses, such as measles, mumps, rubella, and polio, with-

in 4 to 6 weeks before the test (possible suppression of skin reaction)

AGE ISSUE *In elderly people and patients with viral infection, malnutrition, febrile illness, uremia, immunosuppressive disorders, or miliary TB (possible suppression of skin reaction)*

- Less than 10-week period since infection (possible suppression of skin reaction)
- Improper dilution, dosage, or storage of the tuberculin

Tumor markers (CA 15-3 [27, 29]; CA 19-9; CA-125; and CA-50)

Tumor markers are substances produced and secreted by tumor cells to help determine tumor activity. They can be found in the serum of the cancer patient. Specific tests are ordered depending on the type of cancer the patient has. The CA 15-3 antigen (breast-cystic fluid protein or BCFP) may be used in conjunction with CEA and is helpful particularly in the breast cancer patient (CA 27, metastatic breast cancer, breast-cystic fluid protein 29, BCFP). CA 19-9 carbohydrate antigen may be ordered in the patient with pancreas, hepatobiliary, or lung cancer. The CA-125 glycoprotein antigen and serum carbohydrate antigen is commonly associated with types of ovarian cancers. The CA-50 may be ordered in the patient with GI or pancreatic cancer.

A combination of markers may be used due to low sensitivity and specificity of the markers. Few tumor markers meet Food and Drug Administration approval due to their controversy of their role in cancer diagnosis and treatment.

Purpose
- To assist tumor staging and identify possible metastasis
- To monitor and detect disease recurrence
- To assess the patient's response to therapy

Patient preparation
- Explain the purpose of the particular test ordered and that it may be helpful in the patient's disorder, as appropriate.
- Specific directions from the laboratory or cancer center should be followed for the particular test ordered. Fasting may be involved and factors may be identified that may interfere with test results. Note interfering factors on the appropriate laboratory requests.
- Tell the patient that the test requires a blood sample. Explain who will perform the venipuncture and when.
- Explain to the patient that he may experience slight discomfort from the needle puncture and the tourniquet.

Procedure and posttest care
- Obtain a 10-ml venous sample, as ordered, in the tube specified by the laboratory or cancer center and transport the sample as directed.
- Apply direct pressure to the venipuncture site until bleeding stops.
- If a hematoma develops at the venipuncture site, apply warm soaks.

Precautions
- Consult the laboratory or cancer center as to specific patient preparation required (fasting, identifying interfering factors).
- Transport the specimen as directed.
- Handle the sample gently to prevent hemolysis.

Reference values

Normal values for these tumor markers are:

- CA 15-3 (27, 29): < 30 U/ml
- CA 19-9: < 70 U/ml
- CA-125: < 34 U/ml
- CA-50: < 17 U/ml.

Abnormal findings

CA 15-3 (27, 29) is greatly increased in metastatic breast cancer; it's also increased in pancreas, lung, colorectal, ovarian, and liver cancers. It decreases with therapy; an increase after therapy suggests progressive disease.

CA 19-9 is increased in pancreas, hepatobiliary, and lung cancers. It may be mildly increased in gastric and colorectal cancers.

CA-125 is increased in epithelial ovary, fallopian tube, endometrial, endocervix, pancreas, and liver cancers. It's less increased in colon, breast, lung, and GI cancers.

CA-50 is increased in GI and pancreatic cancers.

Interfering factors

- CA 15-3 (27, 29) increased in benign breast or ovarian disease
- CA 19-9 increased in pancreatitis, cholecystitis, cirrhosis, gallstones, and cystic fibrosis (minimal elevations)
- CA-125 increased in pregnancy, endometriosis, pelvic inflammatory disease, menstruation, acute and chronic hepatitis, ascites, peritonitis, pancreatitis, GI disease, Meig's syndrome, pleural effusion, and pulmonary disease

Selected readings

Braunwald, E., et al., eds. *Harrison's Principles of Internal Medicine,* 15th ed. New York: McGraw-Hill Book Co., 2002.

Diseases, 3rd ed. Springhouse, Pa.: Lippincott Williams & Wilkins, 2002.

Fischbach, F. *A Manual of Laboratory and Diagnostic Tests,* 7th ed. Philadelphia: Lippincott Williams & Wilkins, 2004.

Guyton, A.C., and Hall, J.E. *Textbook of Medical Physiology,* 10th ed. Philadelphia: W.B. Saunders Co., 2001.

Henry, J.B., ed. *Clinical Diagnosis and Management of Laboratory Methods,* 20th ed. Philadelphia: W.B. Saunders Co., 2001.

Nursing2004 Drug Handbook, 24th ed. Philadelphia: Lippincott Williams & Wilkins, 2004.

SECTION II.
URINE TESTS

Urinalysis

Introduction

Routine urinalysis and special studies of renal function provide valuable information about the integrity of renal and urinary function and also serve as sensitive indicators of overall health. To understand the significance of such tests and their clinical applications, you need to know how urine is normally formed, what elements it contains, and the mechanisms that regulate urine volume.

Urine formation

The kidneys, through the activity of the nephrons, continuously remove metabolic wastes, drugs and other foreign substances, excess fluids, inorganic salts, and acid and base substances from the blood for eventual excretion in the urine. Each kidney has approximately 1 million *nephrons;* each nephron consists of a vascular ultrafilter called a *glomerulus* and a *renal tubule,* an epithelial-lined conduit for reabsorption of recyclable matter and secretion of foreign and waste substances. (See *Components of the nephron.*) The nephrons form urine through three mechanisms — *glomerular filtration,*

COMPONENTS OF THE NEPHRON

Each kidney has about 1 million functional units called nephrons. In turn, each nephron contains a vascular ultrafilter called a glomerulus and a renal tubule, an epithelial-lined conduit made up of four sections (proximal convoluted tubule, loop of Henle, distal convoluted tubule, and collecting tubule). As the filtrate from the glomerulus travels through the renal tubules, reabsorption and secretion modify it to meet the body's needs. The end result is urine.

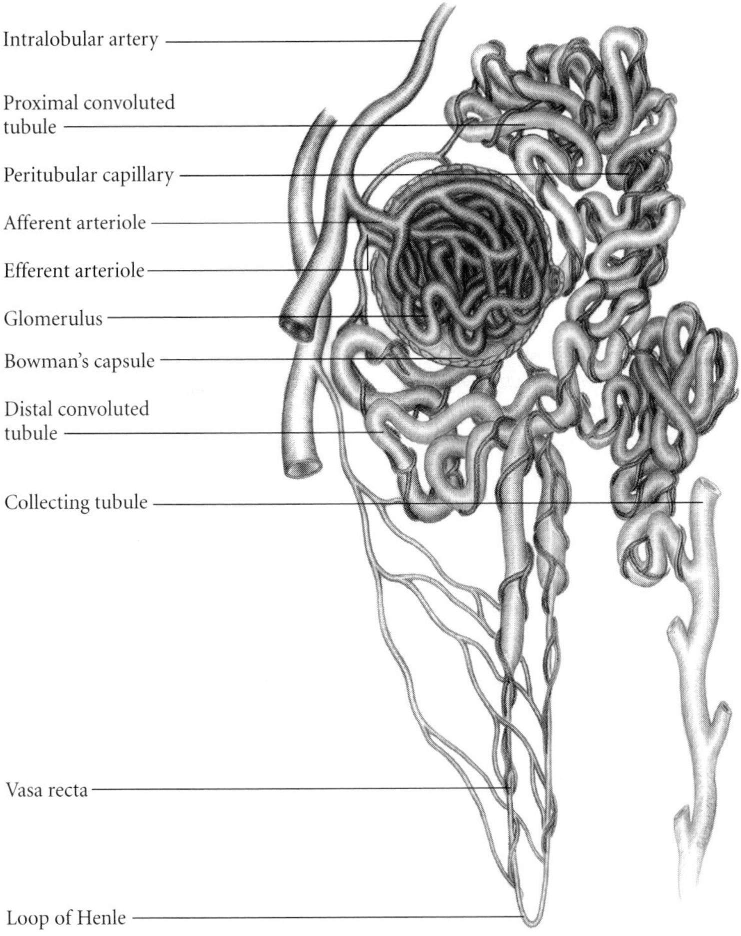

Intralobular artery

Proximal convoluted tubule

Peritubular capillary

Afferent arteriole

Efferent arteriole

Glomerulus

Bowman's capsule

Distal convoluted tubule

Collecting tubule

Vasa recta

Loop of Henle

tubular reabsorption, and *tubular secretion.*

Blood enters each kidney through the renal artery, passing through progressively smaller vascular channels and eventually entering the glomeruli through the afferent glomerular arterioles. These arterioles subdivide into clusters of capillary loops, each of which is partly enclosed in a membranous covering called Bowman's capsule. The walls of the capillaries are semipermeable so dissolved substances can pass by simple filtration from the plasma through the glomerular capillaries and into the capsule space.

Blood leaves the glomeruli through the efferent glomerular arterioles and travels to a network of peritubular capillaries, which encircle the renal tubules. Glomerular filtrate leaves the Bowman's capsule and enters the proximal convoluted tubules, where approximately 65% is selectively reabsorbed by the peritubular capillaries. (Reabsorbed substances include water, glucose, some proteins, amino acids, acetoacetate ions, vitamins, and hormones.) The remaining 35% of the filtrate proceeds through the loops of Henle and the distal convoluted tubules, where sodium and water are reabsorbed as needed.

During secretion, fluid, solutes (such as potassium), uric acid, exogenous substances (such as drugs), and other waste materials move from the peritubular capillaries back into the glomerular filtrate. As the liquid filtrate evolves, it's continuously modified by filtration, reabsorption, and secretion. The end product is urine.

Urine composition

Although the actual composition of normal urine changes — depending on diet, physical activity, and emotional stress — it always includes water, urea, uric acid, and sodium chloride. Urine also usually contains other nonprotein nitrogen compounds, citric acid, other organic acids, catecholamines, sulfur-containing compounds, phosphate, potassium, calcium, magnesium, reducing substances, mucoproteins, vitamins, and hormones.

In the presence of disease, urine may contain protein, glucose, ketone bodies, hemoglobin, lipids, bacteria, pus, urobilinogen, bilirubin, or calculi. Microscopic examination of centrifuged urine sediment can detect cells, casts, crystals, bacteria, yeasts, parasites, spermatozoa, contaminants, and artifacts.

Urine volume

Urine volume, closely regulated by the kidneys, reflects overall fluid homeostasis. The volume depends on fluid intake, the concentration of solutes in the filtrate, cardiac output, hormonal influences, physical activity, and fluid loss through the lungs, large intestine, and skin. In an adult, urine volume normally ranges from 800 to 2,000 ml/day and averages 1,200 to 1,500 ml/day. In a child, volume ranges from 300 to 1,500 ml/day; however, a child's urine output is three to four times greater per kilogram of body weight than an adult's.

Polyuria, urine volume that exceeds 2,000 ml/day, is typical of many abnormal conditions. For example, it's a common effect of osmotic diuresis in diabetes mellitus, hyperparathyroidism, and infections. Polyuria can also result from insufficient secretion of antidiuretic hormone (ADH), as in pituitary diabetes insipidus, or from an inability to respond to ADH, as in nephrogenic diabetes insipidus. Urine volume also increases from a lack of aldosterone, as in Addison's disease, which decreases renal reabsorption of sodium and water and decreases plasma volume. Polyuria follows the shift of interstitial fluid to plasma after burns or excessive intake or infusion of fluid. It also results from renal diseases in which the kidneys fail to concentrate urine and from the use of diuretics, alcohol, and caffeine.

Oliguria, excretion of less than 500 ml of urine per day, can result from depressed sodium concentration in the filtrate because sodium normally promotes water excretion. It also follows any condition that decreases plasma volume — for example, when fluid shifts from plasma to the interstitial spaces, as in heart failure; when fluid intake decreases; and when excess fluid escapes through extrarenal routes. Falling plasma volume and oliguria can follow dehydration due to prolonged vomiting, diarrhea, or profuse diaphoresis. Transfusion reactions, acute glomerulonephritis or pyelonephritis, and terminal chronic nephritis may cause oliguria and impair renal plasma flow and nephron function.

Anuria is the excretion of less than 100 ml of urine per day for 2 to 3 days despite high fluid intake. Anuria can follow oliguria in shock. It can also result from acute tubular necrosis caused by exposure to toxic agents, such as mercury bichloride, sulfonamides, and carbon tetrachloride, and from obstruction in bilateral hydronephrosis.

Nocturia, urine volume greater than 500 ml at night, with a specific gravity of less than 1.018, is characteristic of chronic glomerulonephritis and of heart or liver failure.

PHYSICAL AND CHEMICAL TESTS

Routine urinalysis

A routine urinalysis tests for urinary and systemic disorders. This test evaluates physical characteristics (color, odor, turbidity, and opacity) of urine; determines specific gravity and pH; detects and measures protein, glucose, and ketone bodies; and examines sediment for blood cells, casts, and crystals.

Diagnostic laboratory methods include visual examination, reagent strip screening, refractometry for specific gravity, and microscopic inspection of centrifuged sediment.

Purpose
■ To screen the patient's urine for renal or urinary tract disease (See *Urine cytology,* page 342.)
■ To help detect metabolic or systemic disease unrelated to renal disorders
■ To detect substances (drugs)

Patient preparation
■ Explain to the patient that this test aids in the diagnosis of renal or urinary tract disease and helps evaluate overall body function.
■ Inform the patient that he need not restrict food and fluids.
■ Notify the laboratory and physician of medications the patient is taking that may affect laboratory results; they may need to be restricted.

Procedure and posttest care
■ Collect a random urine specimen of at least 15 ml.
■ Obtain a first-voided morning specimen if possible.

URINE CYTOLOGY

Epithelial cells line the urinary tract and exfoliate easily into the urine, so a simple cytologic examination of these cells can aid diagnosis of urinary tract disease. Although urine cytology isn't performed routinely, it's useful for detecting cancer and inflammatory diseases of the renal pelvis, ureters, bladder, and urethra. It's especially useful for detecting bladder cancer in high-risk groups, such as smokers, people who work with aniline dyes (such as leather workers), and patients who have already received treatment for bladder cancer. Urine cytology can also determine whether bladder lesions that appear on X-rays are benign or malignant. This test can also detect cytomegalovirus infection and other viral disease.

To perform the test, the patient must collect a 100- to 300-ml clean-catch urine specimen 3 hours after his last voiding. (He should not use the first-voided specimen of the morning.) The urine specimen is sent to the cytology laboratory immediately so that it can be examined before the cells begin to degenerate.

Preparing the specimen

The specimen is prepared in one of the following ways and stained with Papanicolaou stain:

■ *Centrifuge:* After the urine is spun down, the sediment is smeared on a glass slide and stained for examination.

■ *Filter:* Urine is poured through a filter, which traps the cells so that they can be stained and examined directly.

■ *Cytocentrifuge:* After the urine is centrifuged, the sediment is resuspended and placed on slides, which are spun in a cytocentrifuge and stained for examination.

Implications of results

Normal urine is relatively free from cellular debris, but should have some epithelial and squamous cells that appear normal under a microscope. Identification of malignant cells or other signs of malignancy may indicate cancer of the kidney, renal pelvis, ureters, bladder, or urethra. It could also indicate a metastatic tumor.

An overgrowth of epithelial cells, an excess of red blood cells, or the presence of leukocytes or atypical cells may indicate a lower urinary tract inflammation, which can result from prostatic hyperplasia, urinary calculi, bladder diverticula, strictures, or malformation.

Large intranuclear inclusions may indicate a cytomegalovirus infection, which usually affects the renal tubular epithelium. This type of viral infection commonly occurs in cancer patients undergoing chemotherapy and transplant patients receiving immunosuppressant drugs. Cytoplasmic inclusion bodies may also indicate measles and may precede the characteristic Koplik's spots.

■ Inform the patient that he may resume his usual diet and medications, as ordered.

Precautions

■ Strain the specimen to catch stones or stone fragments if the patient is being evaluated for renal colic.

■ Carefully pour the urine through an unfolded 4″ × 4″ gauze pad or a fine-mesh sieve placed over the specimen container.

■ Send the specimen to the laboratory immediately.

■ Refrigerate the specimen if analysis will be delayed longer than 1 hour.

NORMAL FINDINGS IN ROUTINE URINALYSIS

Element	Findings
Macroscopic	
Color	▪ Straw to dark yellow
Odor	▪ Slightly aromatic
Appearance	▪ Clear
Specific gravity	▪ 1.005 to 1.035
pH	▪ 4.5 to 8
Protein	▪ None
Glucose	▪ None
Ketone bodies	▪ None
Bilirubin	▪ None
Urobilinogen	▪ Normal
Hemoglobin	▪ None
Erythrocytes (red blood cells [RBCs])	▪ None
Nitrites (bacteria)	▪ None
Leukocytes (white blood cells [WBCs])	▪ None
Microscopic	
RBCs	▪ 0 to 2/high-power field
WBCs	▪ 0 to 5/high-power field
Epithelial cells	▪ 0 to 5/high-power field
Casts	▪ None, except 1 to 2 hyaline casts/low-power field
Crystals	▪ Present
Bacteria	▪ None
Yeast cells	▪ None
Parasites	▪ None

Normal findings

See *Normal findings in routine urinalysis.*

Abnormal findings

Nonpathologic variations in normal values may result from diet, nonpathologic conditions, specimen collection time, and other factors. (See *Drugs that influence routine urinalysis results,* pages 344 and 345.) For example, specific gravity influences urine color and odor. As specific gravity increases, urine becomes darker and its odor becomes stronger.

Urine pH, which is greatly affected by diet and medications, influences the appearance of urine and the composition of crystals. An alkaline pH (above 7.0) — characteristic of a vegetarian diet —

DRUGS THAT INFLUENCE ROUTINE URINALYSIS RESULTS

Drugs that change urine color
Chlorzoxazone (orange to purple-red)
Deferoxamine mesylate (red)
Fluorescein sodium I.V. (yellow-orange)
Furazolidone (brown)
Iron salts (black)
Levodopa (dark)
Methylene blue (blue-green)
Metronidazole (dark)
Nitrofurantoin (brown)
Oral anticoagulants, indandione derivatives (orange)
Phenazopyridine (orange, red, or orange-brown)
Phenolphthalein (red to purple-red)
Phenolsulfonphthalein (pink or red)
Phenothiazines (dark)
Quinacrine (deep yellow)
Riboflavin (yellow)
Rifabutin (red-orange)
Rifampin (red-orange)
Sulfasalazine (orange-yellow)
Sulfobromophthalein (red)

Drugs that cause urine odor
Antibiotics
Paraldehyde
Vitamins

Drugs that increase specific gravity
Albumin
Dextran
Glucose

Radiopaque contrast media

Drugs that decrease pH
Ammonium chloride
Ascorbic acid
Diazoxide
Methenamine
Metolazone

Drugs that increase pH
Amphotericin B
Carbonic anhydrase inhibitors
Mafenide
Potassium citrate
Sodium bicarbonate

Drugs that cause false-positive results for proteinuria
Acetazolamide (Combistix)
Aminosalicylic acid (sulfosalicylic acid or Extons method)
Cephalothin in large doses (sulfosalicylic acid method)
Dichlorphenamide
Methazolamide
Nafcillin (sulfosalicylic acid method)
Sodium bicarbonate
Tolbutamide (sulfosalicylic acid method)
Tolmetin (sulfosalicylic acid method)

Drugs that cause true proteinuria
Aminoglycosides
Amphotericin B
Bacitracin
Cephalosporins
Cisplatin
Etretinate

Gold preparations
Isotretinoin
Nonsteroidal anti-inflammatory drugs
Phenylbutazone
Polymyxin B
Sulfonamides
Trimethadione

Drugs that can cause either true proteinuria or false-positive results
Penicillin in large doses (except with Ames reagent strips); however, some penicillins cause true proteinuria
Sulfonamides (sulfosalicylic acid method)

Drugs that cause false-positive results for glycosuria
Aminosalicylic acid (Benedict's test)
Ascorbic acid (Clinistix, Diastix, Tes-Tape)
Ascorbic acid in large doses (Clinitest tablets)
Cephalosporins (Clinitest tablets)
Chloral hydrate (Benedict's test)
Chloramphenicol (Clinitest tablets)
Isoniazid (Benedict's test)
Levodopa (Clinistix, Diastix, Tes-Tape)
Levodopa in large doses (Clinitest tablets)
Methyldopa (Tes-Tape)
Nalidixic acid (Benedict's test or Clinitest tablets)
Nitrofurantoin (Benedict's test)

DRUGS THAT INFLUENCE ROUTINE URINALYSIS RESULTS

Penicillin G in large doses (Benedict's test)
Phenazopyridine (Clinistix, Diastix, Tes-Tape)
Probenecid (Benedict's test, Clinitest tablets)
Salicylates in large doses (Clinitest tablets, Clinistix, Diastix, Tes-Tape)
Streptomycin (Benedict's test)
Tetracycline (Clinistix, Diastix, Tes-Tape)
Tetracyclines, due to ascorbic acid buffer (Benedict's test, Clinitest tablets)

Drugs that cause true glycosuria
Ammonium chloride
Asparaginase
Carbamazepine
Corticosteroids
Dextrothyroxine
Lithium carbonate
Nicotinic acid (large doses)
Phenothiazines (long-term)
Thiazide diuretics

Drugs that cause false-positive results for ketonuria
Levodopa (Ketostix, Labstix)
Phenazopyridine (Ketostix or Gerhardt's reagent strip shows atypical color)
Phenolsulfonphthalein (Rothera's test)
Phenothiazines (Gerhardt's reagent strip shows atypical color)
Salicylates (Gerhardt's reagent strip shows reddish color)
Sulfobromophthalein (Bili-Labstix)

Drugs that cause true ketonuria
Ether (anesthesia)
Insulin (excessive doses)
Isoniazid (intoxication)
Isopropyl alcohol (intoxication)

Drugs that increase white blood cell count
Allopurinol
Ampicillin
Aspirin (toxicity)
Kanamycin
Methicillin

Drugs that cause hematuria
Amphotericin B
Coumarin derivatives
Methenamine in large doses
Methicillin
Para-aminosalicylic acid
Phenylbutazone
Sulfonamides

Drugs that cause casts
Amphotericin B
Aspirin (toxicity)
Bacitracin
Ethacrynic acid
Furosemide
Gentamicin
Isoniazid
Kanamycin
Neomycin
Penicillin
Radiographic agents
Streptomycin
Sulfonamides

Drugs that cause crystals (if urine is acidic)
Acetazolamide
Aminosalicylic acid
Ascorbic acid
Nitrofurantoin
Theophylline
Thiazide diuretics

causes turbidity and the formation of phosphate, carbonate, and amorphous crystals. An acid pH (below 7.0) — typical of a high-protein diet — produces turbidity and the formation of oxalate, cystine, leucine, tyrosine, amorphous urate, and uric acid crystals.

Protein, normally absent from the urine, may be present in a benign condition known as orthostatic (postural) pro-teinuria. Most common in patients ages 10 to 20, this condition is intermittent, appears after prolonged standing, and disappears after recumbency. Transient benign proteinuria can also occur with fever, exposure to cold, emotional stress, or strenuous exercise. Systemic diseases that may cause proteinuria include lymphoma, hepatitis, diabetes mellitus, toxemia, hypertension, lupus erythematosus, and febrile illnesses.

Sugars, usually absent from the urine, may appear under normal conditions. The most common sugar in urine is glucose. Transient nonpathologic glycosuria may result from emotional stress or pregnancy and may follow ingestion of a high-carbohydrate meal.

Centrifuged urine sediment contains cells, casts, crystals, bacteria, yeast, and parasites. Red blood cells (RBCs) commonly don't appear in urine without pathologic significance; however, strenuous exercise can cause hematuria.

The following abnormal findings generally suggest pathologic conditions:
- *Color* — Color change can result from diet, drugs, and many diseases.
- *Odor* — In diabetes mellitus, starvation, and dehydration, a fruity odor accompanies formation of ketone bodies. In urinary tract infections (UTIs), a fetid odor commonly is associated with *Escherichia coli*. Maple syrup urine disease and phenylketonuria also cause distinctive odors. Other abnormal odors include those similar to a brewery, sweaty feet, cabbage, fish, and sulfur.
- *Turbidity* — Turbid urine may contain red or white cells, bacteria, fat, or chyle and may reflect renal infection.
- *Specific gravity* — Low specific gravity (< 1.005) is characteristic of diabetes insipidus, nephrogenic diabetes insipidus, acute tubular necrosis, and pyelonephritis. Fixed specific gravity, in which values remain 1.010 regardless of fluid intake, occurs in chronic glomerulonephritis with severe renal damage. High specific gravity (>1.035) occurs in nephrotic syndrome, dehydration, acute glomerulonephritis, heart failure, liver failure, and shock.

- *pH* — Alkaline urine pH may result from Fanconi's syndrome, UTI caused by urea-splitting bacteria (*Proteus* and *Pseudomonas*), and metabolic or respiratory alkalosis. Acid urine pH is associated with renal tuberculosis, pyrexia, phenylketonuria, alkaptonuria, and acidosis.
- *Protein* — Proteinuria suggests renal failure or disease (including nephrosis, glomerulosclerosis, glomerulonephritis, nephrolithiasis, nephrotic syndrome, and polycystic kidney disease) or, possibly, multiple myeloma.
- *Sugars* — Glycosuria usually indicates diabetes mellitus, but may result from pheochromocytoma, Cushing's syndrome, impaired tubular reabsorption, advanced renal disease, and increased intracranial pressure. I.V. solutions containing glucose and total parenteral nutrition containing from 10% to 50% glucose can cause glucose to spill over the renal threshold, leading to glycosuria. Fructosuria, galactosuria, and pentosuria generally suggest rare hereditary metabolic disorders (except for lactosuria during pregnancy and breast-feeding). However, an alimentary form of pentosuria and fructosuria may follow excessive ingestion of pentose or fructose. When the liver fails to metabolize these sugars, they spill into the urine because the renal tubules don't reabsorb them.
- *Ketone bodies* — Ketonuria occurs in diabetes mellitus when cellular energy needs exceed available cellular glucose. In the absence of glucose, cells metabolize fat for energy. Ketone bodies — the end products of incomplete fat metabolism — accumulate in plasma and are excreted in the urine. Ketonuria may also occur in starvation states, low- or no-carbohydrate diets, and following diarrhea or vomiting.
- *Bilirubin* — Bilirubin in urine may occur in liver disease resulting from ob-

structive jaundice or hepatotoxic drugs or toxins or from fibrosis of the biliary canaliculi (which may occur in cirrhosis).

■ *Urobilinogen* — Intestinal bacteria in the duodenum change bilirubin into urobilinogen. The liver reprocesses the remainder into bile. Increased urobilinogen in the urine may indicate liver damage, hemolytic disease, or severe infection. Decreased levels may occur with biliary obstruction, inflammatory disease, antimicrobial therapy, severe diarrhea, or renal insufficiency.

■ *Cells* — Hematuria indicates bleeding within the genitourinary tract and may result from infection, obstruction, inflammation, trauma, tumors, glomerulonephritis, renal hypertension, lupus nephritis, renal tuberculosis, renal vein thrombosis, renal calculi, hydronephrosis, pyelonephritis, scurvy, malaria, parasitic infection of the bladder, subacute bacterial endocarditis, polyarteritis nodosa, and hemorrhagic disorders. Strenuous exercise or exposure to toxic chemicals may also cause hematuria. An excess of white blood cells (WBCs) in urine usually implies urinary tract inflammation, especially cystitis or pyelonephritis. WBC and WBC casts in urine suggest renal infection or noninfective inflammatory disease. Numerous epithelial cells suggest renal tubular degeneration, such as heavy metal poisoning, eclampsia, and kidney transplant rejection.

■ *Casts (plugs of gelled proteinaceous material [high-molecular-weight mucoprotein])* — Casts form in the renal tubules and collecting ducts by agglutination of protein cells or cellular debris and are flushed loose by urine flow. Excessive numbers of casts indicate renal disease. Hyaline casts are associated with renal parenchymal disease, inflammation, trauma to the glomerular capillary membrane, and some physiologic states (such as after exercise); epithelial casts, with renal tubular damage, nephrosis, eclampsia, amyloidosis, and heavy metal poisoning; coarse and fine granular casts, with acute or chronic renal failure, pyelonephritis, and chronic lead intoxication; fatty and waxy casts, with nephrotic syndrome, chronic renal disease, and diabetes mellitus; RBC casts, with renal parenchymal disease (especially glomerulonephritis), renal infarction, subacute bacterial endocarditis, vascular disorders, sickle cell anemia, scurvy, blood dyscrasias, malignant hypertension, collagen disease, and acute inflammation; and WBC casts, with acute pyelonephritis and glomerulonephritis, nephrotic syndrome, pyogenic infection, and lupus nephritis.

■ *Crystals* — Some crystals normally appear in urine, but numerous calcium oxalate crystals suggest hypercalcemia or ethylene glycol ingestion. Cystine crystals (cystinuria) reflect an inborn error of metabolism.

■ *Other components* — Bacteria, yeast cells, and parasites in urine sediment reflect genitourinary tract infection or contamination of external genitalia. Yeast cells, which may be mistaken for RBCs, are identifiable by their ovoid shape, lack of color, variable size and, frequently, signs of budding. The most common parasite in sediment is *Trichomonas vaginalis,* which causes vaginitis, urethritis, and prostatovesiculitis.

Interfering factors

■ Strenuous exercise before routine urinalysis (may cause transient myoglobulinuria)

■ Insufficient urinary volume, less than 2 ml (possible limitation of the range of procedures)

■ Failure to send specimen to the laboratory immediately after the collection is completed or to refrigerate the specimen (false-low urobilinogen)
■ Foods, such as beets, berries, and rhubarb (false change in color)
■ Certain drugs
■ Highly dilute urine such as in diabetes insipidus

Urinary calculi

Urinary calculi (urolithiasis or, more commonly, urinary stones) are insoluble substances most commonly formed of the mineral salts — calcium oxalate, calcium phosphate, magnesium ammonium phosphate, urate, or cystine. They may appear anywhere in the urinary tract and range in size from microscopic to several centimeters. Calculi usually possess well-defined nuclei composed of bacteria, fibrin, blood clots, or epithelial cells that are enclosed in a protein matrix. Mineral salts accumulate around this matrix in layers, causing progressive enlargement.

Formation of calculi can result from reduced urinary volume, increased excretion of mineral salts, urinary stasis, pH changes, and decreased protective substances. Calculi commonly form in the kidney, pass into the ureter, and are excreted in the urine. Because not all calculi pass spontaneously, they may require surgical extraction or pulverization using extracorporeal shock-wave lithotripsy. Calculi don't always cause symptoms, but when they do, hematuria is most common. If calculi obstruct the ureter, they may cause severe flank pain, dysuria, and urinary retention, frequency, and urgency.

To test for urinary calculi, the patient must have all his urine carefully strained to remove any calculi. Qualitative chemical analysis then reveals the calculi's composition, which helps to identify their causes.

Purpose
■ To detect and analyze calculi in the urine

Patient preparation
■ Explain to the patient that this test detects urinary calculi and that laboratory analysis will reveal their composition.
■ Tell the patient that his urine will be collected and strained.
■ Advise the patient that he need not restrict food and fluids.
■ Inform the patient that medication to control pain will be administered.

Equipment
Strainer (an unfolded 4″ × 4″ gauze dressing or a fine-mesh sieve), specimen container

Procedure and posttest care
■ Have the patient void into the strainer.
■ Inspect the strainer carefully because calculi may be minute, looking like gravel or sand.
■ Document the appearance of the calculi and the number, if possible.
■ Place the calculi in a properly labeled container.
■ Send the container to the laboratory immediately for prompt analysis.
■ Observe the patient for severe flank pain, dysuria, and urinary retention, frequency, or urgency. Hematuria should subside.

Precautions
■ Keep the strainer and urinal or bedpan within the patient's reach if he has received analgesics because he may be drowsy and unable to get out of bed to void.

TYPES AND CAUSES OF CALCULI

A
Calcium oxalate calculi usually result from idiopathic hypercalciuria, a condition that reflects absorption of calcium from the bowel.

B
Calcium phosphate calculi usually result from primary hyperparathyroidism, which causes excessive reabsorption of calcium from bone.

C
Cystine calculi result from primary cystinuria, an inborn error of metabolism that prevents renal tubular reabsorption of cystine.

D
Urate calculi result from gout, dehydration (causing elevated uric acid levels), acidic urine, or hepatic dysfunction.

E
Magnesium ammonium phosphate calculi result from the presence of urea-splitting organisms, such as *Proteus,* which raises ammonia concentration and makes urine alkaline.

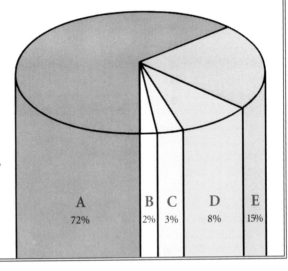

| A 72% | B 2% | C 3% | D 8% | E 15% |

Normal findings
Normally, calculi aren't present in urine.

Abnormal findings
More than one-half of all calculi in urine are of mixed composition, containing two or more mineral salts; calcium oxalate is the most common component. Determining the calculi's composition helps identify various metabolic disorders, guiding proper treatment and prevention measures. (See *Types and causes of calculi.*)

Interfering factors
■ Improper collection technique

TUBULAR FUNCTION TESTS

Urine osmolality

The kidneys normally concentrate or dilute urine according to fluid intake. When intake is excessive, the kidneys excrete more water in the urine; when intake is limited, they excrete less. To make such variation possible, the distal segment of the tubule varies its permeability to water in response to antidiuretic hormone, which, with renal blood flow, determines urine concentration or dilution.

This test measures the concentrating ability of the kidneys in acute and chronic renal failure. Osmolality is a more sensitive index of renal function than dilution techniques that measure specific gravity. It measures the number of osmotically active ions or particles present per kilogram of water. Osmolality is high in concentrated urine and low in dilute urine. It's determined by the effect of solute particles on the freezing point of the fluid.

Purpose
- To evaluate renal tubular function
- To detect renal impairment

Patient preparation
- Explain to the patient that this test evaluates kidney function.
- Tell the patient that the test requires a urine specimen and collection of blood within 1 hour before or after the urine is collected. Withhold diuretics, as ordered.
- Emphasize to the patient that his cooperation is necessary to obtain accurate results.

Procedure and posttest care
- Collect a random urine specimen and draw a blood sample within 1 hour of urine collection.
- If a 24-hour urine collection is ordered, record the total urine volume on the laboratory request. (Preservatives aren't required for a 24-hour container.)
- After collecting the final specimen, provide the patient with a balanced meal or snack.

- Make sure the patient voids within 8 to 10 hours after the catheter has been removed.

Precautions
- Send each specimen to the laboratory immediately after collection.
- If the patient is unable to urinate into the specimen containers, provide him with a clean bedpan, urinal, or toilet specimen pan. Rinse the collection device after each use.
- If the patient is catheterized, empty the drainage bag before the test. Obtain the specimen from the catheter.

Reference values
For a random urine specimen, osmolality normally ranges from 50 to 1,400 mOsm/kg; for a 24-hour urine specimen, osmolality ranges from 300 to 900 mOsm/kg.

Abnormal findings
Decreased renal capacity to concentrate urine in response to fluid deprivation, or to dilute urine in response to fluid overload, may indicate tubular epithelial damage, decreased renal blood flow, loss of functional nephrons, or pituitary or cardiac dysfunction.

Interfering factors
- Diuretics (increase urine volume and dilution, thereby lowering specific gravity)
- Nephrotoxic drugs (cause tubular epithelial damage, thereby decreasing renal concentrating ability)
- Patients who have been markedly overhydrated for several days before the test (may have depressed concentration values)
- Patients who are dehydrated or have electrolyte imbalances (may retain fluids, leading to inaccurate results)

Phenolsulfonphthalein excretion

The phenolsulfonphthalein (PSP) excretion test evaluates kidney function. This test is indicated in the patient with abnormal results in the urine concentration test, one of the earliest signs of renal dysfunction.

Purpose
- To determine renal plasma flow
- To evaluate tubular function

Patient preparation
- Explain to the patient that this test evaluates kidney function.
- Inform the patient that he need not restrict food before the test. Encourage him to drink fluids before and during the test to maintain adequate urine flow.
- Tell the patient the test requires an I.V. injection and collection of urine specimens 15 minutes, 30 minutes, 1 hour and, if ordered, 2 hours after the I.V. injection.
- Inform the patient who will administer the I.V. injection and when.
- Explain to the patient that he may experience slight discomfort from the needle puncture and the tourniquet and that the dye temporarily turns the urine red.
- If the patient can't void and requires catheterization, tell him that he may have the urge to void when the catheter is in place.
- Notify the laboratory and physician of medications the patient is taking that may affect test results; they may need to be restricted. If they must be continued, however, note this on the laboratory request.

Equipment
PSP dye (6 mg in 1 ml of solution), equipment for indwelling urinary catheterization, four urine specimen containers

Procedure and posttest care
- Instruct the patient to empty his bladder and discard the urine.
- The physician will administer 1 ml of PSP, which equals 6 mg of dye, I.V.
- Collect a urine specimen at 15 minutes, 30 minutes, 1 hour and, if ordered, 2 hours after the injection.
- Encourage fluid intake because 40 ml of urine is required for each specimen.
- If the patient is catheterized, be sure to clamp the catheter between collections.
- Record the PSP dosage on the laboratory request.
- Properly label each specimen and include the collection time.
- Elevate the arm and apply warm soaks if phlebitis develops at the I.V. site.
- If the patient is catheterized, make sure he voids within 8 hours after the catheter is removed.
- Inform the patient that he may resume his usual medications, as ordered.

Precautions
- Use this test cautiously in a patient with cardiac dysfunction or renal insufficiency because the increased fluid intake necessary for proper hydration may precipitate heart failure.
- Keep epinephrine, histamine-1 receptor antagonists (diphenhydramine), and a glucocorticoid (methylprednisolone) available because allergic reactions to PSP occasionally occur.
- Don't use the urine in the drainage bag if the patient already has a catheter in place.
- Empty the bag and clamp the catheter for 1 hour before the test.
- Send the specimen to the laboratory immediately after each collection.

- Refrigerate the specimen if more than 10 minutes will elapse before transport.

Normal findings

Normally, 25% of the PSP dose is excreted in 15 minutes, 50% to 60% in 30 minutes, 60% to 70% in 1 hour, and 70% to 80% in 2 hours. Normal excretion for children (excluding infants) is 5% to 10% higher than for adults.

Abnormal findings

The 15-minute value is the most sensitive indicator of tubular function and renal plasma flow because depressed excretion at this interval, with normal excretion later, suggests relatively mild or early-stage bilateral renal disease. However, a depressed 2-hour value may reveal moderate to severe renal impairment. Depressed PSP excretion is also characteristic in renal vascular disease, urinary tract obstruction, heart failure, and gout.

Elevated PSP excretion is characteristic in hypoalbuminemia, hepatic disease, and multiple myeloma.

Interfering factors

- Failure to collect an adequate specimen at required times
- Radiographic contrast agents, aspirin, chlorothiazide, salicylates, sulfonamides, penicillin, cascara sagrada, ethanol, indomethacin, nitrofurantoin, phenylbutazone, probenecid, and vitamins (possible increase or decrease)
- Beets, carrots, and rhubarb (possible increase or decrease)
- Incorrect PSP dosage (possible increase or decrease)
- High serum protein levels (decrease)
- Severe hypoalbuminemia, excessive albuminuria, or severe liver disease (possible effect on excretion)

Concentration and dilution

The kidneys normally concentrate or dilute urine according to fluid intake. When such intake is excessive, the kidneys excrete more water in the urine; when intake is limited, they excrete less. The concentration and dilution test evaluates renal capacity to concentrate urine in response to fluid deprivation or to dilute it in response to fluid overload. This test may also be referred to as the water loading or water deprivation test.

Purpose

- To evaluate renal tubular function
- To detect renal impairment
- To diagnose disorders such as diabetes insipidus

Patient preparation

- Explain to the patient that this test evaluates kidney function.
- Tell him the test requires multiple urine specimens. Explain how many specimens will be collected and at what intervals.
- Instruct him to discard urine voided for a specific time, as per laboratory protocol such as all urine collected during the night.
- Withhold diuretics as needed.

Concentration test

- Provide a high-protein meal and only 200 ml of fluid the night before the test.
- Instruct the patient to restrict food and fluids for at least 14 hours before the test. (Some concentration tests require that water be withheld for 24 hours, but permit relatively normal food intake.)
- Limit salt intake at the evening meal to prevent excessive thirst.

- Emphasize to the patient that his cooperation is necessary to obtain accurate results.

Dilution test
- Generally, this test directly follows the concentration test and necessitates no additional patient preparation. If it's performed alone, simply withhold breakfast.

Procedure and posttest care
Concentration test
- Collect urine specimens at 6 a.m., 8 a.m., and 10 a.m.

Dilution test
- Instruct the patient to void and discard the first urine sample.
- Give the patient 1,500 ml of water to drink within a 30-minute period.
- Collect urine specimens every half hour or every hour for 4 hours thereafter.

Both tests
- Provide a balanced meal or a snack after collecting the final specimen.
- Make sure the patient voids within 8 hours after the catheter is removed.

Precautions
- Testing may be contraindicated in the patient with advanced renal disease or cardiac dysfunction because fluid overload can precipitate water intoxication, sodium diuresis, or heart failure.
- Send each specimen to the laboratory immediately after collection.
- Provide the patient with a clean bedpan, urinal, or toilet specimen pan if he's unable to urinate into the specimen containers.
- Rinse the collection device after each use.
- If the patient is catheterized, empty the drainage bag before the test. Obtain the specimens from the catheter and clamp the catheter between collections.

Reference values
Normal specific gravity ranges from 1.005 to 1.035; osmolality normally ranges from 300 to 900 mOsm/kg.

Concentration test
Specific gravity ranges from 1.025 to 1.032, and osmolality rises above 800 mOsm/kg of water (SI, > 800 mmol/kg) in the patient with normal renal function.

Dilution test
Normally, specific gravity falls below 1.003 and osmolality below 100 mOsm/kg for at least one specimen; 80% or more of the ingested water is eliminated in 4 hours.

Abnormal findings
Decreased renal capacity to concentrate urine in response to fluid deprivation, or to dilute urine in response to fluid overload, may indicate tubular epithelial damage, decreased renal blood flow, loss of functional nephrons, or pituitary or cardiac dysfunction.

AGE ISSUE *In an elderly person, depressed values can be associated with normal renal function.*

Interfering factors
- Failure to observe pretest restrictions
- Use of radiographic contrast agents within 7 days of test (possible increase in osmolality)
- Diuretics and nephrotoxic drugs (possible increase or decrease in specific gravity and osmolality)
- Glycosuria

Tubular reabsorption of phosphate

The test for tubular reabsorption of phosphate is an indirect measure of parathyroid hormone (PTH) levels. PTH helps maintain optimum blood levels of ionized calcium and controls renal excretion of calcium and phosphate. Specifically, PTH stimulates reabsorption of calcium and inhibits reabsorption of phosphate from the glomerular filtrate. A regulatory feedback mechanism results in diminished PTH secretion as ionized calcium levels return to normal. In primary hyperparathyroidism, excessive secretion of PTH disrupts this calcium-phosphate balance. This test measures urine and serum phosphate and creatinine levels. These values are then used to calculate the tubular reabsorption of phosphate.

Purpose
- To evaluate parathyroid gland function
- To aid in the diagnosis of primary hyperparathyroidism
- To aid in the differential diagnosis of hypercalcemia

Patient preparation
- Explain to the patient that this test evaluates parathyroid gland function.
- Advise the patient that the test requires a blood sample and urine collection over a 24-hour period.
- Tell the patient who will perform the venipuncture and when.
- Advise the patient that he may experience slight discomfort from the needle puncture and the tourniquet.
- Instruct the patient to maintain a normal phosphate diet for 3 days before the test because low phosphate intake (< 500 mg/day) may elevate tubular reabsorption values and a high-phosphate

diet (3,000 mg/day) may lower them. Common nutritional sources of phosphorus include legumes, nuts, milk, egg yolks, meat, poultry, fish, cereals, and cheese. These foods should be eaten in moderate amounts.
- Instruct the patient to fast after midnight the night before the test.
- Notify the laboratory and physician of medications the patient is taking that may affect test results; they may need to be restricted. If they must be continued, however, note this on the laboratory request.

Procedure and posttest care
- Perform a venipuncture and collect the blood sample in a 10-ml clot-activator tube.
- Instruct the patient to empty his bladder and discard the urine; record this as time zero.
- Collect the patient's urine over a 24-hour period with the first sample discarded and the last sample retained; occasionally, a 4-hour collection or a random collection is ordered instead.
- Allow the patient to eat and encourage fluid intake to maintain adequate urine flow after the venipuncture.
- Apply direct pressure to the venipuncture site until bleeding stops. Apply warm soaks if a hematoma develops at the venipuncture site.
- Inform the patient that he may resume his usual diet and medications, as ordered.

Precautions
- Handle the blood collection tube gently to prevent hemolysis.
- Keep the urine specimen container refrigerated or on ice during the collection period.
- Tell the patient to avoid contaminating the specimen with toilet paper or stool.

- Label the specimen and send it to the laboratory as soon as the collection period has ended.

Normal findings

Renal tubules normally reabsorb 80% or more of phosphate.

Abnormal findings

Reabsorption of less than 74% of phosphate strongly suggests primary hyperparathyroidism. Hypercalcemia is the most common manifestation of primary hyperparathyroidism. However, a patient with hypercalcemia may still require additional testing to confirm primary hyperparathyroidism as the cause.

Interfering factors

- Uremia, renal tubular disease, osteomalacia, myeloma, and sarcoidosis (possible increase)
- Furosemide and gentamicin (possible increase)
- Renal calculi in the patient without a parathyroid tumor, amphotericin B, and thiazide diuretics (possible decrease)
- Contamination of the specimen with toilet tissue or stool
- Hemolysis due to rough handling of the sample
- Failure to keep the specimen on ice or to send it to the laboratory immediately after the collection is completed
- Failure to follow dietary restrictions

Selected readings

Black, J.M. *Medical-Surgical Nursing,* 6th ed. Philadelphia: W.B. Saunders Co., 2001.

Fischbach, F. *A Manual of Laboratory and Diagnostic Tests,* 7th ed. Philadelphia: Lippincott Williams & Wilkins, 2004.

Guyton, A.C., and Hall, J.E. *Textbook of Medical Physiology,* 10th ed. Philadelphia: W.B. Saunders Co., 2001.

Henry, J.B., ed. *Clinical Diagnosis and Management by Laboratory Methods,* 20th ed. Philadelphia: W.B. Saunders Co., 2001.

Malarkey, L.M., and McMorrow, M.E. *Nurse's Manual of Laboratory Tests and Diagnostic Procedures,* 2nd ed. Philadelphia: W.B. Saunders Co., 2000.

Phipps, W.J., et al. *Medical-Surgical Nursing: Health and Illness Perspectives,* 7th ed. St. Louis: Mosby–Year Book, Inc., 2003.

Urine enzymes

Introduction

Enzymes, protein molecules that promote chemical reactions in the body without being destroyed or permanently changed themselves, are present in all body tissues and fluids: tears, saliva, sweat, blood, urine, and digestive juices. Because enzyme actions are quite specific to tissue sites, abnormal enzyme levels typically can identify and locate tissue damage or disease. Cellular damage or necrosis is likely to cause the release of a large aggregation of enzymes into the blood. When such enzymes saturate the serum, they exceed the renal threshold and a significant quantity spill over into the urine. Because enzymes that circulate in the blood are normally reabsorbed by the renal tubules, with only small amounts excreted in the urine, increased enzyme levels in the urine may also signal renal dysfunction, especially impaired tubular reabsorption.

Because elevated urine levels may persist longer than serum levels (for example, of amylase), urine enzyme measurements can provide delayed or retrospective diagnosis. They also help monitor the progression of illness and the effectiveness of treatment in patients with confirmed disease.

Urine amylase, the most frequently performed urine enzyme test, can confirm acute pancreatitis and can aid diagnosis of chronic pancreatitis and salivary gland disorders. *Arylsulfatase A,* a rarely requested test, aids in the diagnosis of colorectal or bladder cancer, myeloid leukemia, and metachromatic leukodystrophy. *Lysozyme* (also known as *muramidase*), another rarely requested test, evaluates renal function, helps detect rejection or infarction of kidney transplants, and aids in the diagnosis of acute monocytic and granulocytic leukemia. *Cyclic adenosine monophosphate,* another enzyme detectable in urine, is measured after injection of parathyroid hormone to aid differential diagnosis of pseudohypoparathyroidism.

Enzymes are especially affected by pH, specific gravity, and bacteria. Thus, reliable enzyme measurement requires certain precautions during urine collection. Such testing requires an uncontaminated timed urine specimen and an adequate patient intake of fluid. For a valid specimen, the collection container must contain the proper preservative, if one is designated by the laboratory, to maintain the required pH. Finally, the specimen must be refrigerated or packed in ice throughout the collection period to inhibit bacterial growth. Failure to meet these requirements may invalidate the test results.

GENERAL TESTS

Urine amylase

Amylase is a starch-splitting enzyme produced primarily in the pancreas and sali-vary glands, which is usually secreted into the alimentary tract and absorbed into the blood; small amounts of amylase are also absorbed into the blood directly from these organs. Following glomerular filtration, amylase is excreted in the urine.

In the presence of adequate renal function, serum and urine levels usually rise in tandem. However, within 2 to 3 days of the onset of acute pancreatitis, serum amylase levels fall to normal, but elevated urine amylase persists for 7 to 10 days. One method for determining urine amylase levels is the dye-coupled starch method.

Purpose
■ To diagnose acute pancreatitis when serum amylase levels are normal or borderline
■ To aid in the diagnosis of chronic pancreatitis and salivary gland disorders

Patient preparation
■ Explain to the patient that this test evaluates the function of the pancreas and the salivary glands.
■ Inform the patient that he need not restrict food and fluids.
■ Tell the patient that the test requires urine collection for 2, 6, 8, or 24 hours, and teach him how to collect a timed specimen.
■ Instruct the patient to empty his bladder and then begin timing the collection.
■ Notify the laboratory and physician of medications the patient is taking that may affect test results; they may need to be restricted.

Procedure and posttest care
■ Collect the patient's urine over a 2-, 6-, 8-, or 24-hour period.
■ A 2-hour test is usually performed because collecting urine for a 2-hour period

produces fewer errors than a more diagnostic 24-hour collection.

Precautions
■ Cover and refrigerate the specimen during the collection period.
■ If the patient is catheterized, keep the collection bag on ice.
■ Instruct the patient not to contaminate the specimen with toilet tissue or stool.
■ Send the specimen on ice to the laboratory as soon as the test is complete.

Normal findings
Urine amylase is reported in various units of measure; therefore, values differ from laboratory to laboratory. The Mayo Clinic reports normal urinary excretion of 1 to 17 U/hour (SI, 0.017 to 0.29 µkat/h).

Abnormal findings
Elevated amylase levels occur in acute pancreatitis; obstruction of the pancreatic duct, intestines, or salivary duct; carcinoma of the head of the pancreas; mumps; acute injury of the spleen; renal disease, with impaired absorption; perforated peptic or duodenal ulcers; and gallbladder disease.

Depressed levels occur in pancreatitis, cachexia, alcoholism, cancer of the liver, cirrhosis, hepatitis, and hepatic abscess.

Interfering factors
■ Salivary amylase in the urine due to coughing or talking over the sample (possible increase)
■ Failure to collect all urine during the test period, to properly store the specimen, or to send the specimen to the laboratory immediately after the collection is completed
■ High levels of bacterial contamination of the specimen or blood in the urine

■ Morphine, meperidine, codeine, pentazocine, bethanechol, thiazide diuretics, indomethacin, or alcohol within 24 hours of the test (possible increase)
■ Fluorides (possible decrease)

Arylsulfatase A

Arylsulfatase A (ARSA), a lysosomal enzyme found in every cell except the mature erythrocyte, is principally active in the liver, pancreas, and kidneys, where exogenous substances are detoxified into ester sulfates.

Urine ARSA levels rise in transitional bladder cancer, colorectal cancer, and leukemia. However, research hasn't resolved whether elevated ARSA levels provoke malignant growths or are simply an enzymatic response to them. This test measures urine ARSA levels by colorimetric or kinetic techniques.

Purpose
■ To aid in the diagnosis of bladder, colon, or rectal cancer; myeloid (granulocytic) leukemia; and metachromatic leukodystrophy (an inherited lipid storage disease)

Patient preparation
■ Tell the patient that this test measures an enzyme that's present throughout the body.
■ Advise the patient that he need not restrict food and fluids.
■ Tell the patient that the test requires urine collection over a 24-hour period, and teach him how to collect a timed specimen.

Procedure and posttest care
■ Collect the patient's urine over a 24-hour period, discarding the first sample

and retaining the last sample in the appropriate container.

Precautions
- If a female patient is menstruating, anticipate possible test rescheduling.
- Tell the patient not to contaminate the urine specimen with toilet tissue or stool.
- Keep the collection container refrigerated or on ice during the collection period.
- Send the specimen to the laboratory as soon as the collection period has ended.
- If the patient has an indwelling urinary catheter in place, keep the collection bag on ice for the duration of the test.
- Begin the test period with a new, unused continuous urinary drainage apparatus.

Reference values
Normally, random values are 1.6 to 42 U/g creatinine; 24-hour urine values are 0.37 to 3.60 U/day creatinine; 1-hour test values are 2 to 19 U/1 hour (SI, 2 to 19 U/h); 2-hour test values are 4 to 37 U/2 hours (SI, 4 to 37 U/2 hours); 24-hour test values are 170 to 2,000 U/24 hours (SI, 2.89 to 34.0 μkat/ L).

Abnormal findings
Elevated ARSA levels may result from cancer of the bladder, colon, or rectum or from myeloid leukemia.

Depressed ARSA levels can result from metachromatic leukodystrophy. In a patient with this condition, urine studies show metachromatic granules in the urinary sediment.

Interfering factors
- Failure to collect all urine during the test period, to properly store the specimen, or to send the specimen to the laboratory immediately after the collection is completed
- Contamination of the specimen with toilet tissue, stool, or menstrual blood
- Surgery within 1 week before the test (possible increase)

Lysozyme

Lysozyme (also known as *muramidase*), a low-molecular-weight enzyme, is present in mucus, saliva, tears, skin secretions, and various internal body cells and fluids. This enzyme splits, or lyses, the cell walls of gram-positive bacteria and, with complement and other blood factors, acts to destroy them. Lysozyme seems to be synthesized in granulocytes and monocytes, first appearing in serum after the destruction of such cells. When the serum lysozyme level exceeds three times the normal level, the enzyme appears in the urine. However, because renal tissue also contains lysozyme, renal injury alone can cause measurable excretion of this enzyme.

This test measures urine lysozyme levels with a turbidimeter. Serum lysozyme determinations, using the same method, confirm the results of urine testing.

Purpose
- To aid in the diagnosis of acute monocytic or granulocytic leukemia and to monitor the progression of these diseases
- To evaluate proximal tubular function and to diagnose renal impairment
- To detect rejection or infarction of kidney transplantation

Patient preparation
- Explain to the patient that this test evaluates renal function and the immune system.

■ Advise the patient that he need not restrict food and fluids.
■ Tell the patient that the test requires collection of urine over a 24-hour period, and teach him how to collect the specimen correctly.

Procedure and posttest care
■ Collect the patient's urine over a 24-hour period, discarding the first specimen and retaining the last specimen in the appropriate container.

Precautions
■ If a female patient is menstruating, anticipate possible test rescheduling.
■ Tell the patient to avoid contaminating the urine specimen with toilet tissue or stool.
■ Cover and refrigerate the specimen throughout the collection period.
■ Keep the collection bag on ice if the patient has an indwelling urinary catheter in place.
■ Send the specimen to the laboratory as soon as the test is complete.

Reference values
Normally, urine lysozyme values are 0 to 3 mg/24 hours.

Abnormal findings
Elevated urine lysozyme levels are characteristic of impaired renal proximal tubular reabsorption, acute pyelonephritis, nephrotic syndrome, tuberculosis of the kidney, severe extrarenal infection, rejection or infarction of kidney transplantation (levels normally increase during the first few days after transplantation), and polycythemia vera.

Urine levels rise markedly after the acute onset or relapse of monocytic or myelomonocytic leukemia and rise moderately after acute onset or relapse of granulocytic (myeloid) leukemia.

Urine lysozyme levels remain normal or decrease in lymphocytic leukemia and remain normal in myeloblastic and myelocytic leukemias.

Interfering factors
■ Failure to collect all urine
■ Bacteriuria (decrease)
■ Blood or saliva in the specimen (increase)

STIMULATION TEST

Cyclic adenosine monophosphate

Formed from adenosine triphosphate by the action of the enzyme adenylate cyclase, the nucleotide cyclic adenosine monophosphate (cAMP) influences the protein synthesis rate within cells. Measurement of the urinary excretion of cAMP after an I.V. infusion of a standard dose of parathyroid hormone (PTH) can show renal tubular resistance in a patient with hypoparathyroid symptoms and high levels of PTH. Such findings suggest type I pseudohypoparathyroidism, a rare inherited disorder. (Urinary cAMP levels respond normally with type II pseudohypoparathyroidism because the defect is beyond the level of cAMP generation.)

Purpose
■ To aid in the differential diagnosis of hypoparathyroidism and pseudohypoparathyroidism

Patient preparation
■ Explain to the patient that this test evaluates parathyroid function.

- Tell the patient that the test requires a 15-minute I.V. infusion of PTH and a 3- to 4-hour urine specimen collection.

▶ **CLINICAL ALERT** *Perform a skin test to detect an allergy to PTH; keep epinephrine or a histamine-1-receptor antagonist, such as diphenhydramine or glucocorticoids (methylprednisolone), readily available in case of an adverse reaction.*

- Just before the procedure is performed, instruct the patient not to touch the I.V. line or exert pressure on the arm receiving the infusion.
- Tell the patient that he may experience discomfort from the needle puncture. Ask him to notify you if he feels severe burning or if the site becomes inflamed or swollen.

Equipment

PTH (300 units, in refrigerated ampules), vial of sterile water (saline solution causes precipitate to form), urine collection container with hydrochloric acid added as a preservative

Procedure and posttest care

- Instruct the patient to empty his bladder.
- If the patient has an indwelling urinary catheter in place, replace the collection apparatus with an unused one.
- Send this specimen to the laboratory, if ordered; otherwise, discard it.
- Prepare the PTH for infusion, as directed, using sterile water for dilution.
- Start the infusion with dextrose 5% in water, and infuse the PTH over 15 minutes. Record the start of the infusion as time zero.
- Collect a urine specimen 3 to 4 hours after the infusion.
- Discontinue the I.V. infusion, as ordered.

- Observe the patient for symptoms of hypercalcemia, including lethargy, anorexia, nausea, vomiting, vertigo, and abdominal cramps.
- Apply warm soaks if a hematoma or irritation develops at the venipuncture site.

Precautions

- The cAMP test is contraindicated in the patient with a positive PTH test as well as one with high calcium levels because PTH further raises calcium levels. It should be performed cautiously in the patient receiving a cardiac glycoside and in the patient with sarcoidosis or renal or cardiac disease.
- Tell the patient to avoid contaminating the urine specimen with toilet tissue or stool.
- Send the specimen to the laboratory immediately after the collection is completed; if transport is delayed, refrigerate the specimen.
- Keep the collection bag on ice if the patient has a catheter in place.

Reference values

Levels of cAMP are normally 0.3 to 3.6 mg/day (SI, 100 to 723 nmol/d) or 0.29 to 2.1 mg/g creatinine (SI, 100 to 723 nmol/d creatinine).

Abnormal findings

Failure to respond to PTH, indicated by normal urinary excretion of cAMP, suggests type I pseudohypoparathyroidism.

Interfering factors

- Contamination or improper storage of the specimen or failure to acidify the urine with hydrochloric acid

Selected readings

Anderson, S.C., and Poulsen, K.B. *Anderson's Atlas of Hematology.* Philadelphia: Lippincott Williams & Wilkins, 2003.

Cavanaugh, B.M. *Nurse's Manual of Laboratory and Diagnostic Tests,* 4th ed. Philadelphia: F.A. Davis Co., 2003.

Goldman, L., and Ausiello, D., eds. *Cecil Textbook of Medicine,* 22nd ed. Philadelphia: W.B. Saunders Co., 2004.

Guyton, A.C., and Hall, J.E. *Textbook of Medical Physiology,* 10th ed. Philadelphia: W.B. Saunders Co., 2001.

Henry, J.B., et al. *Clinical Diagnosis and Management by Laboratory Methods,* 20th ed. Philadelphia: W.B. Saunders Co., 2001.

McClatchey, K.D. *Clinical Laboratory Medicine,* 2nd ed. Philadelphia: Lippincott Williams & Wilkins, 2002.

Pagana, K.D., and Pagana, T.J. *Mosby's Diagnostic and Laboratory Test Reference,* 6th ed. St. Louis: Mosby Year–Book, Inc, 2003.

Schnell, Z., et al. *Davis's Comprehensive Handbook of Laboratory and Diagnostic Tests with Nursing Implications.* Philadelphia: F.A. Davis Co., 2003.

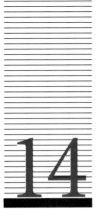

14
Urine hormones and metabolites

Introduction

Hormones are potent, complex chemicals produced and secreted primarily by the endocrine glands to promote and regulate the activity of target organs and tissues. To directly determine circulating hormone levels, laboratory methods commonly measure hormone concentrations in blood. But many hormones and their metabolites are also conveniently studied in urine.

Measuring urine hormone and metabolite levels provides a reliable estimate of the amount of circulating hormone. Moreover, timed, long-term urine measurements offer an advantage. Unlike a blood sample, which determines hormone levels only at the time of venipuncture, a 24-hour urine specimen reflects total daily secretion, offsets diurnal variations, and masks temporary fluctuations. (See *Key facts about urine hormones*, pages 364 and 365.)

Chemical classes
Chemically, hormones can be classified into three groups, each with a marked

363

KEY FACTS ABOUT URINE HORMONES

The chart below lists the secretion sites and methods of measuring the major hormones and their metabolites.

Hormone or metabolite	Principal secretion site	Laboratory tests
Aldosterone	Adrenal cortex	24-hour urine hormone analysis, urinary androgen evaluation, urinary thyroid panel
Free cortisol	Adrenal cortex	24-hour urine hormone analysis, urinary adrenal steroid evaluation, urinary cortisol or thyroid analysis
Catecholamines	Adrenal medulla	Urine catecholamines, HVA, VMA, adrenalin urine test, dopamine urine test
Total estrogens	Gonads, placenta, adrenal glands	24-hour urine steroid hormone panel
Estriol	Placenta, gonads, adrenal cortex	24-hour urine steroid hormone panel
Human chorionic gonadotropin (hCG)	Placenta	Urine hCG
Pregnanetriol	Adrenal cortex	24-hour urine hormone analysis
17-hydroxycorticosteroids	Adrenal cortex	24-hour urine hormone and steroid analysis
17-ketosteroids	Adrenal glands, testes	24-hour urine hormone and steroid analysis
17-ketogenic steroids	Adrenal cortex	24-hour urine hormone and steroid analysis
Vanillylmandelic acid (VMA)	Adrenal medulla	Urine VMA
Homovanillic acid (HVA)	Liver	Urine HVA
5-hydroxyindoleacetic acid	Intestinal wall, stomach	Urine 5-hydroxyindoleacetic acid
Pregnanediol	Corpus luteum, adrenal cortex	24-hour urine hormone analysis

Method of principal quantitation
Radioimmunoassay
Radioimmunoassay
Spectrophotofluorometry
Spectrophotofluorometry
Radioimmunoassay
Hemagglutination inhibition (antigen-antibody reaction)
Spectrophotofluorometry
Chromatography, spectrophotofluorometry
Spectrophotofluorometry
Spectrophotofluorometry
Spectrophotofluorometry
Chromatography
Colorimetry
Gas-liquid chromatography

structural specificity: *steroids* (such as estrogens and androgens), *amines* (such as dopamine and epinephrine), and *proteins* (such as human chorionic gonadotropin [hCG]). Steroid hormones are most commonly tested in urine. A single structural change in the composition of a steroid hormone can dramatically alter its physiologic activity. For example, the introduction of a new hydroxyl group is responsible for the conversion of estradiol to estriol.

Hormone metabolites

Although hormones have specific and characteristic functions, they rarely act independently. Quite the contrary, hormones are linked in an intricate series of complex interactions, including positive and negative feedback mechanisms that enable them to function efficiently and maintain homeostasis. Perhaps most important of these interactions is the formation of hormone metabolites. These metabolites can be degradation products or essential precursors with individual hormonal effects.

Urine levels of hormone metabolites reflect the secretory rates of the hormones from which these metabolites are derived and serve as valuable diagnostic indicators when the hormones themselves aren't excreted in measurable quantities. Metabolite levels also provide important information about the integrity of degradation pathways. A case in point is the conversion of 17-hydroxycorticosteroid progesterone to cortisol; when this metabolic process is blocked, as in adrenogenital syndrome (congenital adrenal hyperplasia), excessive amounts of pregnanetriol appear in the urine.

The hormones produced by the endocrine glands and their metabolites that are commonly measured in urine include:

■ *Adrenocortical hormones:* These hormones and metabolites are steroids that are synthesized and secreted primarily by the adrenal cortex. Formed from acetyl coenzyme A, cholesterol, and many other precursors, adrenocortical hormones and metabolites fall into three major groups:
– *glucocorticoids* (17-hydroxycorticosteroids, particularly cortisol), which maintain carbohydrate, protein, and fat metabolism
– *mineralocorticoids,* principally aldosterone, which help regulate blood pressure and fluid and electrolyte balance
– *adrenal androgens* (sex hormones), the most potent of which is dehydroepiandrosterone, which aid development of male secondary sex characteristics.

Androgens are secreted in minute amounts and are usually measured as part of the 17-ketosteroids. The most inclusive test of adrenocortical hormones, however, measures urine levels of 17-ketogenic steroids.

■ *Adrenal medullary hormones:* The adrenal medullae synthesize and secrete the catecholamines *norepinephrine* and *epinephrine,* which help mediate stress. Although these hormones are less vital to life than the adrenocortical hormones, measuring them and their principal metabolite, *vanillylmandelic acid,* in urine can be extremely useful in detecting catecholamine-producing tumors.

■ *Dopamine and other amines:* a catecholamine secreted primarily by the basal ganglia of the brain, dopamine is the precursor of norepinephrine and epinephrine. When a pheochromocytoma — a catecholamine-secreting tumor — is suspected, measuring urine levels of dopamine and its major metabolite, *homovanillic acid,* can aid in the diagnosis. Urine levels of *serotonin,* an indole amine synthesized by the argentaffin cells of the intestinal mucosa, are reflected by the excretion of *5-hydroxyindoleacetic acid,* its primary metabolite, and aid in the diagnosis of certain carcinoid tumors.

■ *Gonadal and placental hormones:* Urine levels of gonadal and placental hormones, which are principally steroids, are clinically useful for detecting hormone-secreting tumors and pregnancy. Early in pregnancy, the corpus luteum secretes greater amounts of progesterone and estrogen to maintain the pregnancy until the placenta can produce these hormones. Thus, urine levels of total estrogens, estriol, and pregnanediol help evaluate placental status and fetal well-being.

HCG may also be measured in the urine to detect pregnancy early. Soon after conception, the trophoblastic cells that develop into the chorionic villi of the placenta secrete hCG; thus, the presence of hCG in urine indicates pregnancy.

Four useful test methods

Quantitative assays of urine hormone levels are usually performed by using one or more of these methods:

■ *Colorimetry* is based on the principle that some groups of hormones, when combined with certain chemical reagents, take on individual colors; the intensity of color indicates the degree of hormone concentration. A colorimeter or spectrophotometer measures the wavelength of maximum absorption.

■ *Fluorometry* reveals the characteristic fluorescence of hormones on placement in specific media. Under certain laboratory conditions, the wavelengths activated and emitted are specific for a given hormone and can be measured.

■ *Chromatography* determines the adsorption or fractionation of a hormone to a specific medium (solid or liquid). In *gas chromatography,* a urine specimen is mixed with an inert gas to create vapors that are passed over in the medium. Adsorption of the hormone to the medium is measured. In *paper* chromatography, blotting or filter paper replaces the solid or liquid medium.

■ *Radioimmunoassay* involves combining a urine specimen with a radioactively tagged antigen (hormone) and its antibody. The unlabeled hormone being measured displaces the radioactively tagged hormone, which is then measured to determine the urine concentration of the hormone.

Special considerations

When measuring urine hormone levels, 24-hour urine specimens provide more accurate information than random urine specimens by compensating for diurnal variations in hormonal secretion. For the same reason, urine assays from a 24-hour specimen are typically more accurate than serum hormone determinations. However, accurate results require strict adherence to collection procedures and precautions:

■ Before beginning a 24-hour urine collection, confer with the laboratory to determine if the test requires special collection procedures or precautions. In many cases, enforce medication and diet restrictions to ensure accurate results. Many of these tests require dark collection containers and the addition of a preservative to the specimen. The specimen may have to be refrigerated or kept on ice during the collection period.

■ Make sure all urine voided during the 24-hour test period is collected. If a voiding is discarded accidentally, make sure that this is noted on the laboratory request so the laboratory can take this lost specimen into consideration when determining test results.

■ Because strenuous physical exercise and emotional stress can significantly alter the patient's hormone levels, encourage him to rest and relax before the test.

URINE HORMONE TESTS

Urine aldosterone

The urine aldosterone test measures urine levels of aldosterone, the principal mineralocorticoid secreted by the adrenal cortex. Aldosterone promotes sodium retention and potassium excretion by the renal tubules, thereby helping to regulate blood pressure and fluid and electrolyte balance. In turn, aldosterone secretion is controlled by the renin-angiotensin system. This feedback mechanism is vital to maintaining fluid and electrolyte balance. If, for instance, sodium intake is low, aldosterone production increases considerably. If, on the other hand, sodium consumption is high, aldosterone is less necessary and production decreases.

Urine aldosterone levels, measured through radioimmunoassay, are usually evaluated after measurement of serum electrolyte and renin levels.

Purpose

■ To aid in the diagnosis of primary and secondary aldosteronism

Patient preparation

■ Explain to the patient that the urine aldosterone test evaluates hormonal balance.

■ Instruct the patient to maintain a normal sodium diet (3 g/day) before the test and to avoid sodium-rich foods, such as bacon, barbecue sauce, corned beef, bouillon cubes or powder, pickles, snack foods (potato chips), and olives.

■ Advise the patient to avoid strenuous physical exercise and stressful situations during the collection period.

■ Tell the patient that the test requires collection of urine during a 24-hour period, and teach him the proper collection technique.

■ Notify the laboratory and physician of medications the patient is taking that may affect test results; they may need to be restricted.

Procedure and posttest care

■ Collect the patient's urine over a 24-hour period, discarding the first specimen and retaining the last. Use a bottle containing a preservative, such as boric acid, to keep the specimen at a pH of 4.0 to 4.5.

■ Instruct the patient that he may resume his usual activities, diet, and medications, as ordered.

Precautions

■ Refrigerate the specimen or place it on ice during the collection period.

■ Send the specimen to the laboratory as soon as the collection is completed.

Reference values

Normally, urine aldosterone levels range from 3 to 19 µg/24 hours (SI, 8 to 51 nmol/d).

Abnormal findings

Elevated urine aldosterone levels suggest primary or secondary aldosteronism. The primary form usually arises from an aldosterone-secreting adenoma of the adrenal cortex, but may also result from adrenocortical hyperplasia. Secondary aldosteronism, the more common form, results from external stimulation of the adrenal cortex such as that produced

when the renin-angiotensin system is activated by hypertensive and edematous disorders.

Disorders that may result in secondary aldosteronism are malignant hypertension, heart failure, cirrhosis of the liver, nephrotic syndrome, and idiopathic cyclic edema.

Low urine aldosterone levels may result from Addison's disease, salt-losing syndrome, and toxemia of pregnancy. These levels normally rise during pregnancy, but rapidly decline following parturition.

Interfering factors

■ Failure to maintain normal dietary sodium intake as well as excess intake of licorice or glucose

■ Failure to avoid strenuous physical exercise and emotional stress before the test (possible increase due to stimulation of adrenocortical secretions)

■ Radioactive scan performed within 1 week before the test

■ Failure to collect all urine during the collection period, to properly store the specimen, or to send it to the laboratory immediately after the collection is completed

■ Antihypertensive drugs (possible decrease due to sodium and water retention)

■ Diuretics and most steroids (possible increase due to sodium excretion)

■ Some corticosteroids, such as fludrocortisone, which mimic mineralocorticoid activity (possible decrease)

Urine free cortisol

Used as a screen for adrenocortical hyperfunction, the free cortisol test measures urine levels of the portion of cortisol not bound to the corticosteroid-binding globulin transcortin. It's one of the best diagnostic tools for detecting Cushing's syndrome.

Unlike a single measurement of plasma cortisol, radioimmunoassay determinations of free cortisol levels in a 24-hour urine specimen reflect overall secretion levels instead of diurnal variations. Concurrent measurements of plasma cortisol and corticotropin, with urine 17-hydroxycorticosteroids and the dexamethasone suppression test, may be used to confirm the diagnosis.

Purpose
- To aid in the diagnosis of Cushing's syndrome
- To evaluate adrenocortical function

Patient preparation
- Explain to the patient that the urine free cortisol test helps evaluate adrenal gland function.
- Inform the patient that he need not restrict food and fluids, but should avoid stressful situations and excessive physical exercise during the collection period.
- Tell the patient that the test requires collection of urine over a 24-hour period.
- Teach the patient the proper collection technique for a 24-hour urine specimen.
- Notify the laboratory and physician of medications the patient is taking that may affect test results; they may need to be restricted.

Procedure and posttest care
- Collect the patient's urine over a 24-hour period, discarding the first specimen and retaining the last specimen. Use a bottle containing a preservative to keep the specimen at a pH of 4.0 to 4.5.
- Instruct the patient that he may resume his usual activities and medications, as ordered.

Precautions
- Refrigerate the specimen or place it on ice during the collection period.

Reference values
Normal free cortisol values are less than 50 µg/24 hours (SI, < 138 mmol/24 hours).

Abnormal findings
Elevated free cortisol levels may indicate Cushing's syndrome resulting from adrenal hyperplasia, adrenal or pituitary tumor, or ectopic corticotropin production. Hepatic disease and obesity, which can raise plasma cortisol levels, generally don't appreciably raise urine levels of free cortisol. Low levels have little diagnostic significance and don't necessarily indicate adrenocortical hypofunction.

Interfering factors
- Failure to collect all urine during the test period or to properly store the specimen
- Pregnancy (possible increase)
- Reserpine, phenothiazines, morphine, amphetamines, hormonal contraceptives, danazol, aldactone, and prolonged steroid therapy (possible increase)
- Dexamethasone, ethacrynic acid, thiazides, and ketoconazole (decrease)

Urine catecholamines

The test for catecholamines uses spectrophotofluorometry to measure urine levels of the major catecholamines — epinephrine, norepinephrine, and dopamine. Epinephrine is secreted by the adrenal medulla; dopamine, by the central nervous system; and norepinephrine, by both. Catecholamines help regulate metabolism and prepare the body for the fight-or-flight response to stress. Certain tumors can also secrete catecholamines.

A 24-hour urine specimen is preferred because catecholamine secretion fluctuates diurnally and in response to pain, heat, cold, emotional stress, physical exercise, hypoglycemia, injury, hemorrhage, asphyxia, and drugs. However, a random specimen may be useful for evaluating catecholamine levels after a hypertensive episode.

For a complete diagnostic workup of catecholamine secretion, urine levels of catecholamine metabolites are also measured. These metabolites — metanephrine, normetanephrine, homovanillic acid (HVA), and vanillylmandelic acid (VMA) — normally appear in the urine in greater quantities than the catecholamines.

Purpose
- To aid in the diagnosis of pheochromocytoma in a patient with unexplained hypertension
- To aid in the diagnosis of neuroblastoma, ganglioneuroma, and dysautonomia

Patient preparation
- Explain to the patient that the urine catecholamine test evaluates adrenal function.
- Inform the patient that he should avoid chocolate, coffee, and bananas for 7 hours before the test and should avoid stressful situations and excessive physical activity during the collection period.
- Tell the patient that the test requires either the collection of urine over 24 hours or a random specimen, and explain the collection procedure.
- Notify the laboratory and physician of medications the patient is taking that may affect test results; they may need to be restricted.

Procedure and posttest care
- Collect the patient's urine over a 24-hour period. Use a bottle containing a preservative to keep the specimen acidified to a pH of 3.0 or less. (If a random specimen is ordered, collect it immediately after a hypertensive episode.)
- Instruct the patient that he may resume his usual activities, diet, and medications, as ordered.

Precautions
- Refrigerate a 24-hour specimen or place it on ice during the collection period.
- Send the specimen to the laboratory as soon as the collection is complete.

Reference values
Values for catecholamine fractionalization range as follows:
- *Epinephrine:* 0 to 20 µg/24 hours (SI, 0 to 109 nmol/24 hours)
- *Norepinephrine:* 15 to 80 µg/24 hours (SI, 89 to 473 nmol/24 hours)
- *Dopamine:* 65 to 400 µg/24 hours (SI, 425 to 2,610 nmol/24 hours)

Abnormal findings
In a patient with undiagnosed hypertension, elevated urine catecholamine levels following a hypertensive episode usually indicate a pheochromocytoma. If tests indicate a pheochromocytoma, the patient may also be tested for multiple endocrine neoplasia. With the exception of HVA — a dopamine metabolite — catecholamine metabolites may also be elevated. Abnormally high HVA levels rule out a pheochromocytoma because this tumor mainly secretes epinephrine, whose primary metabolite is VMA, not HVA.

Elevated catecholamine levels, without marked hypertension, may be due to a neuroblastoma or a ganglioneuroma, although HVA levels reflect these conditions more accurately. Elevated levels are also seen in severe systemic situations (burns, peritonitis, shock, and septicemia), cor pulmonale, manic depressive disorders, or depressive neurosis. Myasthenia gravis and progressive muscular dystrophy commonly cause urine catecholamine levels to rise above normal, but this test is rarely performed to diagnose these disorders. Consistently low-normal catecholamine levels may indicate dysautonomia marked by orthostatic hypotension.

Interfering factors
■ Failure to comply with drug restrictions, to collect all urine during the collection period, or to properly store the specimen
■ Excessive physical exercise or emotional stress (increase)
■ Caffeine, insulin, nitroglycerin, aminophylline, sympathomimetics, methyldopa, tricyclic antidepressants, chloral hydrate, quinidine, quinine, tetracycline, B-complex vitamins, isoproterenol, levodopa, and monoamine oxidase inhibitors (possible increase)
■ Clonidine, guanethidine, reserpine, and iodine-containing contrast media (possible decrease)
■ Phenothiazines, erythromycin, and methenamine compounds (possible increase or decrease)

Total urine estrogens

The total urine estrogens test is a quantitative analysis of total urine levels of estradiol, estrone, and estriol — the major estrogens present in significant amounts in urine. A common method for measuring total urine estrogen levels involves purification by gel filtration, followed by spectrophotofluorometry. Supplementary tests that may provide further information about ovarian function include cytologic examination of vaginal smears, measurement of urine levels of pregnanediol and follicle-stimulating hormone, and evaluation of response to a progesterone injection.

Purpose
■ To evaluate ovarian activity and to help determine the cause of amenorrhea and female hyperestrogenism
■ To aid in the diagnosis of tumors of ovarian, adrenocortical, or testicular origin
■ To assess fetoplacental status

Patient preparation
■ Explain to the female patient that the total urine estrogens test helps evaluate ovarian function; to the pregnant patient that this test helps evaluate fetal development and placental function; and to the male patient that this test helps evaluate testicular function.
■ Inform the patient that the test requires collection of urine over a 24-hour period.
■ Advise the patient that he need not restrict food and fluids.
■ If the 24-hour specimen is to be collected at home, teach the patient the proper collection technique.
■ Notify the laboratory and physician of medications the patient is taking that may affect test results; they may need to be restricted.

Procedure and posttest care
■ Collect the patient's urine over a 24-hour period, discarding the first specimen and retaining the last. Use a bottle containing a preservative to keep the specimen at a pH of 3 to 5.

- If the patient is pregnant, note the approximate week of gestation on the laboratory request.
- If the patient isn't pregnant, note the stage of her menstrual cycle.
- Instruct the patient that she may resume her usual medications, as ordered.

Precautions
- Refrigerate the specimen or keep it on ice during the collection period.

Normal findings
In nonpregnant females, total urine estrogen levels rise and fall during the menstrual cycle, peaking shortly before midcycle, decreasing immediately after ovulation, increasing through the life of the corpus luteum, and decreasing greatly as the corpus luteum degenerates and menstruation begins.

Total estrogen levels range as follows:
Nonpregnant females
- 4 to 60 μg/24 hours
Pregnant females
- First trimester: 0 to 800 μg/24 hours
- Second trimester: 800 to 5,000 μg/24 hours
- Third trimester: 5,000 to 50,000 μg/24 hours

In postmenopausal females, values are less than 10 μg/24 hours. In males, total estrogen levels range from 4 to 25 μg/24 hours.

Abnormal findings
Decreased total urine estrogen levels may reflect ovarian agenesis, primary ovarian insufficiency (due to Stein-Leventhal syndrome, for example), or secondary ovarian insufficiency (due to pituitary or adrenal hypofunction or metabolic disturbances).

Elevated total estrogen levels in the nonpregnant female may indicate tumors of ovarian or adrenocortical origin, adrenocortical hyperplasia, or a metabolic or hepatic disorder. In a male, elevated total estrogen levels are associated with testicular tumors.

Elevated total urine estrogen levels are normal during pregnancy; serial determinations should show a rising titer.

Interfering factors
- Steroid hormones, methenamine mandelate, phenazopyridine hydrochloride, phenothiazines, tetracyclines, phenolphthalein, ampicillin, meprobamate, senna, cascara sagrada, and hydrochlorothiazide (possible increase or decrease)

Urine placental estriol

The urine placental estriol test, also referred to as maternal urine estriol, monitors fetal viability by measuring urine levels of placental estriol, the predominant estrogen excreted in urine during pregnancy. A steady rise in estriol reflects a properly functioning placenta and, in most cases, a healthy, growing fetus. Normally, estriol is secreted in much smaller amounts by the ovaries in the nonpregnant female, by the testes in the male, and by the adrenal cortex in both sexes.

The usual clinical indication for this test is high-risk pregnancy. Serial testing is necessary to plot the expected rise in estriol levels or to show the absence of such a rise. A 24-hour urine specimen is recommended because estriol levels fluctuate diurnally. Radioimmunoassay is the usual test method. Generally, serum estriol levels are considered more reliable than urine levels.

Purpose
- To assess fetoplacental status, especially in high-risk pregnancy

Patient preparation
- Explain to the patient that the urine placental estriol test helps determine if the placenta is functioning properly, which is essential to the health of the fetus.
- Tell the patient that she need not restrict food and fluids.
- Advise the patient that this test requires urine collection over a 24-hour period, and instruct her how to collect the specimen. Emphasize that proper collection technique is necessary for the results to be valid.
- Notify the laboratory and physician of medications the patient is taking that may affect test results; they may need to be restricted.

Procedure and posttest care
- Collect the patient's urine over a 24-hour period, discarding the first specimen and retaining the last. Use a bottle containing a preservative to keep the specimen at a pH of 3 to 5. The test may also be done serially, requiring collection twice per week.
- Send the specimen to the laboratory. If the patient is pregnant, note the week of gestation on the laboratory request.
- Instruct the patient that she may resume her usual medications, as ordered.

Precautions
- Refrigerate the specimen or keep it on ice during the collection period.
- Some physicians may use an average of 3 previous values as a control because levels vary daily and false-positive and false-negative results are possible.

Normal findings
Normal urine estriol values vary considerably, but serial measures of urine estriol levels, when plotted on a graph, should share a steadily rising curve. (See *Urine estriol levels,* page 374.)

Abnormal findings
A 40% drop from baseline values that occurs on 2 consecutive days strongly suggests placental insufficiency and impending fetal distress. A 20% drop over 2 weeks or failure of consecutive estriol levels to rise in a normal curve similarly indicates inadequate placental function and undesirable fetal status. These developments may necessitate cesarean section, depending on the patient's condition and other apparent signs of fetal distress.

A chronically low urine estriol curve may result from fetal adrenal insufficiency, congenital anomalies (such as anencephaly), Rh isoimmunization, or placental sulfatase deficiency.

A high-risk pregnancy in which the maternal glomerular filtration rate decreases may cause a low-normal estriol curve. Such a pregnancy may occur in a patient with hypertension or diabetes mellitus, for example. The pregnancy may continue, as long as no complications develop and estriol levels continue to rise. However, falling estriol levels or a sudden drop from baseline values indicates severe fetal distress.

High urine estriol levels may occur in a multiple pregnancy.

Interfering factors
- Failure to collect all urine during the 24-hour period and properly store the specimen during the collection period
- Failure to refrigerate the specimen or keep it on ice

URINE ESTRIOL LEVELS

Because urine estriol levels rise as normal gestation proceeds (as shown below), any significant changes in serial urine determinations suggest abnormal conditions that require prompt medical interventions.

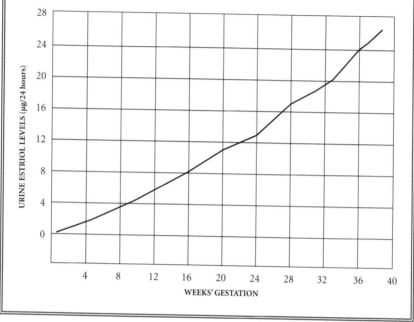

- Failure to maintain the prescribed pH level of the specimen
- Steroid hormones, methenamine mandelate, phenothiazines, phenazopyridine, tetracyclines, phenolphthalein, ampicillin, meprobamate, senna, cascara sagrada, and hydrochlorothiazide
- Maternal hemoglobinopathy, anemia, malnutrition, and hepatic or intestinal diseases (decrease)

Urine human chorionic gonadotropin

Qualitative analysis of urine levels of human chorionic gonadotropin (hCG) allows for the detection of pregnancy as early as 14 days after ovulation. Production of hCG, a glycoprotein, which prevents degeneration of the corpus luteum at the end of the normal menstrual cycle, begins after conception. During the first trimester, hCG levels rise steadily and rapidly, peaking around 10 weeks' gestation, subsequently tapering off to less than 10% of peak levels.

The most common method of evaluating hCG in urine is hemagglutination inhibition. This laboratory procedure can provide qualitative and quantitative information. The qualitative urine test is easier and less expensive than the serum hCG test (beta-subunit assay); therefore, it's used more commonly to detect pregnancy.

Purpose

- To detect and confirm pregnancy
- To aid in the diagnosis of hydatidiform mole or hCG-secreting tumors, threatened abortion, or dead fetus

Patient preparation

- If appropriate, explain to the patient that the urine hCG test determines whether she's pregnant or the status of her pregnancy. Alternatively, explain how the test functions as a screen for some types of cancer.
- Tell the patient that she need not restrict food, but should restrict fluids for 8 hours before the test.
- Inform the patient that the test requires a first-voided morning specimen or urine collection over a 24-hour period, depending on whether the test is qualitative or quantitative.
- Notify the laboratory and physician of medications the patient is taking that may affect test results; they may need to be restricted.

Procedure and posttest care

- For verification of pregnancy (qualitative analysis), collect a first-voided morning specimen. If this isn't possible, collect a random specimen.
- For quantitative analysis of hCG, collect the patient's urine over a 24-hour period in the appropriate container, discarding the first specimen and retaining the last.
- Specify the date of the patient's last menstrual period on the laboratory request.
- Instruct the patient that she may resume her usual diet and medications, as ordered.

Precautions

- Refrigerate the 24-hour specimen or keep it on ice during the collection period.
- Be sure the test is performed at least 5 days after a missed period to avoid a false-negative result.

Normal findings

In a qualitative immunoassay analysis, results are reported as negative (nonpregnant) or positive (pregnant) for hCG. In quantitative analysis, urine hCG levels in the first trimester of a normal pregnancy may be as high as 500,000 IU/24 hours; in the second trimester, they range from 10,000 to 25,000 IU/24 hours; and in the third trimester, from 5,000 to 15,000 IU/24 hours.

Measurable hCG levels don't normally appear in the urine of men or nonpregnant women.

Abnormal findings

During pregnancy, elevated urine hCG levels may indicate multiple pregnancy or erythroblastosis fetalis; depressed urine hCG levels may indicate threatened abortion or ectopic pregnancy.

Measurable levels of hCG in males and nonpregnant females may indicate choriocarcinoma, ovarian or testicular tumors, melanoma, multiple myeloma, or gastric, hepatic, pancreatic, or breast cancer.

Interfering factors

- Gross proteinuria (> 1 g/24 hours), hematuria, or an elevated erythrocyte sedimentation rate (possible false-positive, depending on the laboratory method)
- Early pregnancy, ectopic pregnancy, or threatened abortion (possible false-negative)

- Phenothiazine (possible false-negative or false-positive)

URINE METABOLITE TESTS

Urine pregnanetriol

Using spectrophotometry, the pregnanetriol test determines urine levels of pregnanetriol, the metabolite of the cortisol precursor 17-hydroxyprogesterone. Pregnanetriol is normally excreted in the urine in minute amounts. However, when cortisol biosynthesis is impaired at the point of 17-hydroxyprogesterone conversion, urinary excretion of pregnanetriol rises significantly.

Elevated urine pregnanetriol levels suggest adrenogenital syndrome. Urine 17-ketosteroids and urine 17-ketogenic steroids may be measured concurrently to assess androgen levels. Elevated androgen levels are characteristic of adrenogenital syndrome (congenital adrenal hyperplasia).

Purpose
- To aid in the diagnosis of adrenogenital syndrome
- To monitor cortisol replacement
- To detect anterior pituitary hypofunction or adrenocortical hyperfunction

Patient preparation
- Explain to the patient (or to the parents if the patient is a child) that the urine pregnanetriol test evaluates hormonal secretion.
- Inform the patient that he need not restrict food and fluids.
- Tell the patient that the test requires collection of urine over a 24-hour period, and teach him the proper collection technique.
- Notify the laboratory and physician of medications the patient is taking that may affect test results; they may need to be restricted.

Procedure and posttest care
- Collect the patient's urine over a 24-hour period, discarding the first specimen and retaining the last. Use a bottle containing a preservative to keep the specimen at a pH of 4.0 to 4.5.
- Instruct the patient that he may resume his usual medications, as ordered.

Precautions
- Refrigerate the specimen or keep it on ice during the collection period.
- Send the specimen to the laboratory as soon as the collection is complete.

Reference values
The normal value of pregnanetriol excretion for males age 16 and older are 0.4 to 2.5 mg/24 hours (SI, 1.2 to 7.5 µmol/d). For females age 16 and older, normal values are 0.1 to 1.8 mg/24 hours (SI, 0.3 to 5.3 µmol/d).

Abnormal findings
Elevated urine pregnanetriol levels suggest adrenogenital syndrome: excessive adrenal androgen secretion and resulting virilization.

AGE ISSUE *Females with adrenogenital syndrome fail to develop normal secondary sex characteristics and show marked masculinization of external genitalia at birth. Males usually appear normal at birth, but later develop signs of somatic and sexual precocity.*

In monitoring treatment with cortisol replacement, elevated urine pregnanetriol levels indicate an insufficient cortisol dosage. When cortisol replacement adequately inhibits hypersecretion of corticotropin and subsequent overproduction of 17-hydroxyprogesterone, pregnanetriol levels fall within the normal range.

Interfering factors
- Corticotropin (increase)
- Hormonal contraceptives and progesterone (decrease)
- Failure to store the specimen properly during the collection period or to send the sample to the laboratory immediately after the collection is completed

Urine 17-hydroxycorticosteroids

The 17-hydroxycorticosteroid (17-OHCS) test measures urine levels of 17-OHCS — metabolites of the hormones that regulate glyconeogenesis. More than 80% of all urinary 17-OHCS are metabolites of cortisol, the primary adrenocortical steroid. Test findings thus reflect cortisol secretion and, indirectly, adrenocortical function.

Urine 17-OHCS levels are most accurately determined from a 24-hour specimen because cortisol secretion varies diurnally and in response to stress and many other factors. Column chromatography and spectrophotofluorometry with the Porter-Silber reagent are used to measure 17-OHCS levels.

Levels of plasma cortisol, urine free cortisol, and urine 17-ketosteroids may be measured and corticotropin stimulation and suppression testing performed to confirm test results. Of these, urine free cortisol is a more sensitive and specific test for hypercortisolism.

Purpose
- To assess adrenocortical function

Patient preparation
- Explain to the patient that this test evaluates how his adrenal glands are functioning.
- Inform the patient that he should restrict food and fluids that will alter test results (coffee, tea) and avoid excessive physical exercise and stressful situations during the collection period.
- Tell the patient that the test requires collection of urine over a 24-hour period, and instruct him in the proper collection technique.
- Notify the laboratory and physician of medications the patient is taking that may affect test results; they may need to be restricted.

Procedure and posttest care
- Collect the patient's urine over a 24-hour period, discarding the first specimen and retaining the last. Use a bottle containing a preservative to prevent deterioration of the specimen. Label the specimen appropriately, including the patient's gender on the request forms.
- Instruct the patient that he may resume his usual activities, diet, and medications, as ordered.

Precautions
- Refrigerate the specimen or place it on ice during the collection period.

Reference values
Normally, urine 17-OHCS values range from 4.5 to 12 mg/24 hours in males (SI, 12.4 to 33.1 µmol/d) and from 2.5 to 10 mg/24 hours in females (SI, 6.9 to 27.6 µmol/d). In children ages 8 to 12, levels are less than 4.5 mg/24 hours (SI, < 12.4 µmol/d); in children younger than age 8, levels are normally less than 1.5 mg/24 hours (SI, < 4.14 µmol/d).

Abnormal findings

Elevated urine 17-OHCS levels may indicate Cushing's syndrome, an adrenal carcinoma or adenoma, or a pituitary tumor. Increased levels may also occur in the patient with virilism, hyperthyroidism, or severe hypertension. Extreme stress induced by such conditions as acute pancreatitis and eclampsia also causes urine 17-OHCS levels to rise above normal.

Low urine 17-OHCS levels may indicate Addison's disease, hypopituitarism, or myxedema.

Interfering factors

■ Failure to observe restrictions, to collect all urine during the test period, or to properly store the specimen
■ Meprobamate, phenothiazines, spironolactone, ascorbic acid, chloral hydrate, glutethimide, chlordiazepoxide, penicillin G, hydroxyzine, quinidine, quinine, iodides, and methenamine (possible increase)
■ Hydralazine, phenytoin, thiazide diuretics, estrogens, hormonal contraceptives, phenothiazines, nalidixic acid, and reserpine (possible decrease)

Urine 17-ketosteroids

The 17-ketosteroids (17-KS) is a fractionation test that uses the spectrophotofluorometric technique to measure urine levels of 17-KS. Steroids and steroid metabolites characterized by a ketone group on carbon 17 in the steroid nucleus, 17-KS originate primarily in the adrenal glands, but also in the testes and ovaries.

Although not all 17-KS are androgens, they cause androgenic effects. For example, excessive secretion of 17-KS may result in hirsutism and may increase clitoral or phallic size; in utero, elevated 17-KS

levels may cause a female fetus to develop a male urogenital tract. Because 17-KS don't include all the androgens (testosterone, for example, the most potent androgen), these levels provide only a rough estimate of androgenic activity. To provide additional information about androgen secretion, plasma testosterone levels may be measured concurrently.

Purpose

■ To aid in the diagnosis of adrenal and gonadal dysfunction
■ To aid in the diagnosis of adrenogenital syndrome (congenital adrenal hyperplasia)
■ To monitor cortisol therapy in the treatment of adrenogenital syndrome

Patient preparation

■ Explain to the patient that the urine 17-KS test evaluates hormonal balance.
■ Inform the patient that he need not restrict food and fluids, but should avoid excessive physical exercise and stressful situations during the collection period.
■ Tell the patient that the test requires urine collection over a 24-hour period, and instruct him in the proper collection technique.
■ Notify the laboratory and physician of medications the patient is taking that may affect test results; they may need to be restricted.

Procedure and posttest care

■ Collect the patient's urine over a 24-hour period, discarding the first sample and retaining the last. Use a bottle containing a preservative to keep the specimen at a pH of 4.0 to 4.5. Appropriately label the specimen and laboratory requisition requests with the patient's gender.

- Instruct the patient that he may resume his usual activities and medications, as ordered.

Precautions

- Refrigerate the specimen or place it on ice during the collection period.
- Send the specimen to the laboratory immediately after the collection is completed.

Reference values

Normally, urine 17-KS values range from 10 to 25 mg/24 hours (SI, 35 to 87 µmol/d) in men and from 4 to 6 mg/24 hours (SI, 4 to 21 µmol/d) in women. Children between ages 10 and 14 excrete 1 to 6 mg/24 hours (SI, 2 to 21 µmol/d); children younger than age 10 excrete less than 3 mg/24 hours (SI, <10 µmol/d).

For more information about specific steroids in the 17-KS group, the 17-KS fractionation test may be performed. (See *Normal values for the 17-ketosteroid fractionation test,* pages 380 and 381.)

Abnormal findings

Elevated urine 17-KS levels may result from adrenal hyperplasia, carcinoma or adenoma, or adrenogenital syndrome. In women, elevated levels may also indicate ovarian dysfunction, such as polycystic ovary disease (Stein-Leventhal syndrome), lutein cell tumor of the ovary, or androgenic arrhenoblastoma. In men, elevated 17-KS levels may indicate interstitial cell tumor of the testis. Characteristically, 17-KS levels also rise during pregnancy, severe stress, chronic illness, or debilitating disease.

Depressed urine 17-KS levels may result from Addison's disease, panhypopituitarism, eunuchoidism, or castration and may occur in cretinism, myxedema, and nephrosis. When this test is used to monitor cortisol therapy for adrenogenital syndrome, 17-KS levels typically return to normal with adequate cortisol administration.

Interfering factors

- Failure to observe restrictions, to collect all urine during the collection period, to properly store the specimen, or to send it to the laboratory immediately after the collection is completed
- Presence of menstrual blood in the specimen
- Meprobamate, phenothiazines, corticotropin, antibiotics, dexamethasone, spironolactone, and oleandomycin (possible increase)
- Estrogens, penicillin, ethacrynic acid, and phenytoin (possible decrease)
- Nalidixic acid and quinine (possible increase or decrease)

Urine 17-ketogenic steroids

Using spectrophotofluorometry, the 17-ketogenic steroids (17-KGS) test determines urine levels of 17-KGS, which consist of the 17-hydroxycorticosteroids — cortisol and its metabolites, for example — and other adrenocortical steroids, such as pregnanetriol, that can be oxidized in the laboratory to 17-ketosteroids. Because 17-KGS represent such a large group of steroids, this test provides an excellent overall assessment of adrenocortical function. For accurate diagnosis of a specific disease, 17-KGS levels must be compared with results of other tests, including plasma corticotropin, plasma cortisol, corticotropin stimulation, single-dose metyrapone, and dexamethasone suppression.

NORMAL VALUES FOR THE 17-KETOSTEROID FRACTIONATION TEST

Through gas-liquid chromatography, the 17-ketosteroid (17-KS) fractionation test shows which specific steroids in the 17-KS group are elevated or suppressed and thus aids differential diagnosis of conditions suggested by abnormal 17-KS levels. Note that 17-KS levels are measured in milligrams per 24 hours.

Steroid	Adult male	Adult female	Male ages 10 to 15	Female ages 10 to 15
Androsterone	0.9 to 6.1	0 to 3.1	0.2 to 2	0.5 to 2.5
Dehydroepiandrosterone	0 to 3.1	0 to 1.5	< 0.4	< 0.4
Etiocholanolone	0.9 to 5.2	0.1 to 3.5	0.1 to 1.6	0.7 to 3.1
11-hydroxyandrosterone	0.2 to 1.6	0 to 1.1	0.1 to 1.1	0.2 to 1
11-hydroxyetiocholanolone	0.1 to 0.9	0.1 to 0.8	< 0.3	0.1 to 0.5
11-ketoandrosterone	0 to 0.5	0 to 0.3	< 0.1	< 0.1
11-ketoetiocholanolone	0 to 1.6	0 to 1	< 0.3	0.1 to 0.5
Pregnanetriol	0.2 to 2	0 to 1.4	0.2 to 0.6	0.1 to 0.6

Purpose
- To evaluate adrenocortical and testicular function
- To aid in the diagnosis of Cushing's syndrome and Addison's disease

Patient preparation
- Explain to the patient that the urine 17-KGS test evaluates adrenal function.
- Inform the patient that he need not restrict food and fluids, but should avoid excessive physical exercise and stressful situations during the collection period.
- Tell the patient that the test requires urine collection over a 24-hour period, and teach him how to collect the specimen correctly.
- Notify the laboratory and physician of medications the patient is taking that may affect test results; they may need to be restricted.

Procedure and posttest care
- Collect the patient's urine over a 24-hour period, discarding the first specimen and retaining the last. Use a bottle containing a preservative to keep the specimen at a pH of 4.0 to 4.5. Appropriately label the specimen and laboratory requisition requests with the patient's gender.
- Instruct the patient that he may resume his usual activities and medications, as ordered.

Both sexes ages 6 to 9	Both sexes ages 3 to 5	Both sexes ages 1 to 2	Both sexes birth to age 1
0.1 to 1	< 0.3	< 0.3	< 0.1
< 0.2	< 0.1	< 0.1	< 0.1
0.3 to 1	< 0.7	< 0.4	< 0.1
0.4 to 1	< 0.4	< 0.3	< 0.3
0.1 to 0.5	< 0.4	< 0.1	< 0.1
< 0.1	< 0.1	< 0.1	< 0.1
0.1 to 0.5	< 0.4	< 0.1	< 0.1
< 0.3	< 0.1	< 0.1	< 0.1

Precautions

■ Refrigerate the specimen or keep it on ice during the collection period.

■ Send the specimen to the laboratory as soon as the collection is complete.

Reference values

Normally, urine 17-KGS levels range from 4 to 14 mg/24 hours (SI, 13 to 49 µmol/d) in men and from 2 to 12 mg/24 hours (SI, 7 to 42 µmol/d) in females. Children ages 11 to 14 excrete 2 to 9 mg/24 hours (SI, 7 to 31 µmol/d); younger children and infants excrete 0.1 to 4 mg/24 hours (SI, 0.3 to 14 µmol/d).

Abnormal findings

Elevated urine 17-KGS levels indicate hyperadrenalism, which may occur in Cushing's syndrome, adrenogenital syndrome (congenital adrenal hyperplasia), and adrenal carcinoma or adenoma. Levels also rise with severe physical stress (burns, infections, or surgery, for example) or emotional stress.

Low levels may reflect hypoadrenalism, which may occur in Addison's disease and may also be associated with panhypopituitarism, cretinism, and general wasting.

Interfering factors

■ Failure to observe restrictions, to collect all urine during the collection period, to properly store the specimen, or to send it to the laboratory immediately after the collection is completed

■ Corticotropin, meprobamate, phenothiazines, spironolactone, penicillin, oleandomycin, and hydralazine (possible increase)

■ Estrogens, quinine, reserpine, thiazide diuretics, and long-term corticosteroid therapy (possible decrease)

■ Nalidixic acid, dexamethasone, carbamazepine, cephalothin, and tiaprofenic acid (possible increase or decrease)

Urine vanillylmandelic acid

Using spectrophotofluorometry, the vanillylmandelic acid (VMA) test determines urine levels of VMA, a phenolic acid. VMA is the catecholamine metabolite that's normally most prevalent in the urine and is the product of hepatic conversion of epinephrine and norepinephrine; urine VMA levels reflect endogenous production of these major catecholamines. Like the test for urine total catecholamines, this test helps to detect catecholamine-secreting tumors — especially pheochromocytoma — and helps evaluate adrenal medulla function, the primary site of catecholamine production.

The VMA test ideally should be performed on a 24-hour urine specimen (not a random specimen) to overcome the effects of diurnal variations in catecholamine secretion. Other catecholamine metabolites — metanephrine, normetanephrine, and homovanillic acid (HVA) — may be measured at the same time. If evaluating hypertension, specimen collection may be of greatest value during the hypertensive episode.

Purpose
- To help detect pheochromocytoma, neuroblastoma, and ganglioneuroma
- To evaluate the function of the adrenal medulla

Patient preparation
- Explain to the patient that the urine VMA test evaluates hormonal secretion.
- Instruct the patient to restrict foods and beverages containing phenolic acid, such as coffee, tea, bananas, citrus fruits, chocolate, and vanilla, and carbonated beverages for 3 days before the test.
- Advise the patient to avoid stressful situations and excessive physical activity during the urine collection period.
- Tell the patient that the test requires collection of urine over a 24-hour period, and teach him the proper collection technique.
- Notify the laboratory and physician of medications the patient is taking that may affect test results; they may need to be restricted.

Procedure and posttest care
- Collect the patient's urine over a 24-hour period, discarding the first specimen and retaining the last. Use a bottle containing a preservative to keep the specimen at a pH of 3.
- Instruct the patient that he may resume his usual activities, diet, and medications, as ordered.

Precautions
- Refrigerate the specimen or keep it on ice during the collection period.
- Send the specimen to the laboratory immediately after the collection is completed.

Reference values
Normally, VMA levels in adults are 1.4 to 6.5 mg/24 hours (SI, 7 to 33 μmol/d).

Abnormal findings
Elevated urine VMA levels may result from a catecholamine-secreting tumor. Further testing, such as measurement of urine HVA levels to rule out pheochromocytoma, is necessary for precise diagnosis. If pheochromocytoma is confirmed, the patient may be tested for multiple endocrine neoplasia, an inherited condition commonly associated with pheochromocytoma. (Family members of a patient with confirmed pheochromocytoma should also be carefully evaluated for multiple endocrine neoplasia.)

Interfering factors
- Excessive exercise or emotional stress (increase)
- Failure to observe restrictions, to properly store the specimen during the collection period, or to send the sample to the laboratory immediately after the collection is completed

- Epinephrine, norepinephrine, lithium carbonate, and methocarbamol (increase); chlorpromazine, guanethidine, reserpine, monoamine oxidase inhibitors, and clonidine (decrease); levodopa and salicylates (increase or decrease)

Urine homovanillic acid

The urine homovanillic acid (HVA) test is a quantitative analysis of urine HVA levels, which is a metabolite of dopamine, one of the three major catecholamines. Synthesized primarily in the brain, dopamine is a precursor to epinephrine and norepinephrine, the other principal catecholamines. The liver breaks down most dopamine into HVA for eventual excretion; a minimal amount of dopamine appears in the urine.

Using two-dimensional chromatography, urine HVA levels are usually measured simultaneously with the major catecholamines and other catecholamine metabolites — metanephrine, normetanephrine, and vanillylmandelic acid (VMA).

Purpose
- To aid in the diagnosis of neuroblastoma and ganglioneuroma
- To rule out pheochromocytoma

Patient preparation
- Explain to the patient that the urine HVA test assesses hormone secretion.
- Inform the patient that he need not restrict food and fluids, but should avoid stressful situations and excessive physical exercise during the collection period.
- Tell the patient that the test requires collection of urine over a 24-hour period, and teach him the proper collection technique.

- Notify the laboratory and physician of medications the patient is taking that may affect test results; they may need to be restricted.

Procedure and posttest care
- Collect the patient's urine over a 24-hour period, discarding the first specimen and retaining the last. Use a bottle containing a preservative to keep the specimen at a pH of 2 to 4.
- Instruct the patient that he may resume his usual activities and medications, as ordered.

Precautions
- Refrigerate the specimen or keep it on ice during the collection period.
- Send the specimen to the laboratory immediately after the collection is completed.

Reference values
The normal urine HVA value for adults is less than 10 mg/24 hours (SI, < 55 µmol/d).

Abnormal findings
Elevated urine HVA levels suggest neuroblastoma, a malignant soft-tissue tumor that develops in infants and young children, or ganglioneuroma, a tumor of the sympathetic nervous system that develops in older children and adolescents and rarely metastasizes. HVA levels don't usually rise in patients with pheochromocytoma because this tumor secretes mainly epinephrine, which metabolizes primarily into VMA. Thus, an abnormally high urine HVA level generally rules out pheochromocytoma.

Interfering factors
- Failure to observe restrictions, to collect all urine during the test period, to

store the specimen properly, or to send the sample to the laboratory immediately after the collection is completed
- Excessive physical exercise or emotional stress during the collection period (possible increase)
- Monoamine oxidase inhibitors (decrease due to inhibition of dopamine metabolism)
- Aspirin, methocarbamol, and levodopa (possible increase or decrease)

Urine 5-hydroxyindoleacetic acid

The quantitative analysis of urine levels of 5-hydroxyindoleacetic acid (5-HIAA) is used mainly to screen for carcinoid tumors (argentaffinomas). Such tumors, found generally in the intestine or appendix, secrete an excessive amount of serotonin, which is reflected by high 5-HIAA levels. This test measures 5-HIAA levels by the colorimetric technique and is most accurate when performed with a 24-hour urine specimen, which can detect small or intermittently secreting carcinoid tumors.

Purpose
- To aid in the diagnosis of carcinoid tumors (argentaffinomas)

Patient preparation
- Explain to the patient what serotonin is and why the urine 5-HIAA test is important.
- Instruct the patient not to eat foods containing serotonin, such as bananas, plums, pineapples, avocados, eggplants, tomatoes, and walnuts, for 4 days before the test.
- Tell the patient that the test requires collection of urine over a 24-hour period,

and teach him the proper collection technique.
- Notify the laboratory and physician of medications the patient is taking that may affect test results; they may need to be restricted.

Procedure and posttest care
- Collect the patient's urine over a 24-hour period, discarding the first specimen and retaining the last. Use a bottle containing a preservative to keep the specimen at a pH of 2 to 4.
- Instruct the patient that he may resume his usual diet and medications, as ordered.

Precautions
- Refrigerate the specimen or keep it on ice during the collection period.
- Send the specimen to the laboratory as soon as the collection is complete.

Reference values
Normally, urine 5-HIAA values are qualitatively reported as negative; quantitative results are 2 to 7 mg/24 hours (SI, 10.4 to 36.6 µmol/d).

Abnormal findings
Marked elevation of urine 5-HIAA levels, possibly as high as 200 to 600 mg/24 hours (SI, 1,040 to 3,120 µmol/d), indicates a carcinoid tumor. However, because these tumors vary in their capacity to store and secrete serotonin, some patients with carcinoid syndrome (metastatic carcinoid tumors) may not show elevated levels. Repeated testing is usually necessary.

Interfering factors
- Failure to observe pretest restrictions, to collect all urine during the test period,

to properly store the specimen, or to send the sample to the laboratory immediately after the collection is completed

- Severe GI disturbance or diarrhea
- Melphalan, reserpine, methamphetamine, and fluorouracil (increase)
- Ethanol, tricyclic antidepressants, monoamine oxidase inhibitors, methyldopa, and isoniazid (decrease in most cases)
- Methenamine compounds, phenothiazines, salicylates, guaifenesin, methocarbamol, and acetaminophen (possible increase or decrease)

Urine pregnanediol

Using gas chromatography or radioimmunoassay, this test measures urine levels of pregnanediol, the chief metabolite of progesterone. Although biologically inert, pregnanediol has diagnostic significance because it reflects about 10% of the endogenous production of its parent hormone.

Progesterone is produced in nonpregnant females by the corpus luteum during the latter half of each menstrual cycle, preparing the uterus for implantation of a fertilized ovum. If implantation doesn't occur, progesterone secretion drops sharply; if implantation does occur, the corpus luteum secretes more progesterone to further prepare the uterus for pregnancy and to begin development of the placenta. Toward the end of the first trimester, the placenta becomes the primary source of progesterone secretion, producing the progressively larger amounts needed to maintain pregnancy.

Normally, urine levels of pregnanediol reflect variations in progesterone secretion during the menstrual cycle and during pregnancy. Direct measurement of plasma progesterone levels by radioimmunoassay may also be done.

Purpose

- To evaluate placental function in pregnant females
- To evaluate ovarian function in nonpregnant females
- To aid in the diagnosis of menstrual disorders

Patient preparation

- Explain to the patient that the urine pregnanediol test evaluates placental or ovarian function.
- Inform the patient that she need not restrict food and fluids.
- Tell the patient that the test requires collection of urine over a 24-hour period, and teach her the proper collection technique.
- Advise the pregnant patient that this test may be repeated several times to obtain serial measurements.
- Notify the laboratory and physician of medications the patient is taking that may affect test results; they may need to be restricted.

Procedure and posttest care

- Collect the patient's urine over a 24-hour period, discarding the first specimen and retaining the last.
- Instruct the patient that she may resume her usual medications, as ordered.

Precautions

- Refrigerate the specimen or keep it on ice during the collection period.
- If the patient is pregnant, note the approximate week of gestation on the laboratory request.
- For premenopausal women who aren't pregnant, note the stage of the menstrual cycle on the laboratory request.

Normal findings

In nonpregnant females, urine pregnanediol values normally range from 0.5 to 1.5 mg/24 hours during the follicular phase of the menstrual cycle. In pregnant females, the values are:

- *first trimester:* 10 to 30 mg/24 hours
- *second trimester:* 35 to 70 mg/24 hours
- *third trimester:* 70 to 100 mg/24 hours.

Normal postmenopausal values range from 0.2 to 1 mg/24 hours. In males, urine pregnanediol levels are 0 to 1 mg/24 hours.

Abnormal findings

During pregnancy, a marked decrease in urine pregnanediol levels based on a single 24-hour urine specimen or a steady decrease in pregnanediol levels in serial measurements may indicate placental insufficiency and requires immediate investigation. A precipitous drop in pregnanediol values may suggest fetal distress — for example, threatened abortion or preeclampsia — or fetal death. However, pregnanediol measurements aren't reliable indicators of fetal viability because levels can remain normal even after fetal death, as long as maternal circulation to the placenta remains adequate.

In nonpregnant females, abnormally low urine pregnanediol levels may occur with anovulation, amenorrhea, or other menstrual abnormalities. Low to normal pregnanediol levels may be associated with hydatidiform mole. Elevations may indicate luteinized granulosa or theca cell tumors, diffuse thecal luteinization, or metastatic ovarian cancer.

Adrenal hyperplasia or biliary tract obstruction may elevate urine pregnanediol values in males or females. Some forms of primary hepatic disease produce abnormally low levels in both sexes.

Interfering factors

- Failure to properly store the specimen during the collection period
- Methenamine mandelate, methenamine hippurate, progestogens, combination hormonal contraceptives, and drugs containing corticotropin (possible increase or decrease)

Selected readings

Anderson, S.C., and Poulsen, K.B. *Anderson's Atlas of Hematology.* Philadelphia: Lippincott Williams & Wilkins, 2003.

Cavanaugh, B.M. *Nurse's Manual of Laboratory and Diagnostic Tests,* 4th ed. Philadelphia: F.A. Davis Co., 2003.

DeGroot, L., and Jameson, J.L., eds. *Endocrinology,* 4th ed. Philadelphia: W.B. Saunders Co., 2001.

Goldman, L., and Ausiello, D., eds. *Cecil Textbook of Medicine,* 22nd ed. Philadelphia: W.B. Saunders Co., 2004.

Guyton, A.C., and Hall, J.E. *Textbook of Medical Physiology,* 10th ed. Philadelphia: W.B. Saunders Co., 2001.

Henry, J.B., et al. *Clinical Diagnosis and Management by Laboratory Methods,* 20th ed. Philadelphia: W.B. Saunders Co., 2001.

McClatchey, K.D. *Clinical Laboratory Medicine,* 2nd ed. Philadelphia: Lippincott Williams & Wilkins, 2002.

Monsaingeon, M., et al. "Comparative Values of Catecholamines and Metabolites for the Diagnosis of Neuroblastoma," *European Journal of Pediatrics* 162(6):397-402, June 2003.

Pagana, K.D., and Pagana, T.J. *Mosby's Diagnostic and Laboratory Test Reference,* 6th ed. St. Louis: Mosby Year–Book, Inc. 2003.

Schnell, Z., et al. *Davis's Comprehensive Handbook of Laboratory and Diagnostic Tests with Nursing Implications.* Philadelphia: F.A. Davis Co., 2003.

Scott, J., et al., eds. *Danforth's Obstetrics and Gynecology,* 9th ed. Philadelphia: Lippincott Williams & Wilkins, 2003.

15

Urine protein, protein metabolites, and pigments

Introduction

Laboratory analysis of urine specimens for abnormal levels of proteins, protein metabolites, and pigments is a significant factor in the detection and management of renal disorders and in the diagnosis of certain extrarenal or systemic diseases. Abnormalities that can be easily detected by analytical techniques include proteinuria and the presence of the pigments hemoglobin, bilirubin, urobilinogen, and the porphyrins. Examination of urine for protein metabolites is especially useful in evaluating renal function because healthy kidneys excrete these nonprotein nitrogenous (NPN) end products of protein metabolism.

Proteins
Normally, the protein content of urine is too small to be detected by routine screening procedures. Urine contains minute amounts of plasma proteins of

387

low molecular weight or renal mucoproteins derived from the tubular cells. Benign proteinuria can result from changes in body position, as occurs in orthostatic proteinuria, or it can be associated with stress, exposure to cold, or fever.

More than trace amounts of proteins in urine, which are detectable by screening tests, nearly always indicate renal disease. Pathologic proteinuria can result from increased glomerular permeability due to many causes, including glomerulonephritis, heart failure, or renal tubular damage with defective reabsorption of protein. Infections of the lower urinary tract (cystitis, for example) can also cause proteinuria.

In most forms of renal disease marked by proteinuria, the predominant protein found in the urine is albumin because it's the smallest, the most easily filterable, and the most prevalent of all proteins. As kidney damage progresses, however, proteins of higher molecular weight — including the larger globulins — escape into the urine. The presence of certain abnormal proteins in the urine has special diagnostic significance; for example, Bence Jones protein greater than 60 mg/L in urine strongly suggests multiple myeloma.

Protein metabolites
Plasma contains more than 15 different NPN compounds, primarily urea, amino acids, creatine, creatinine, and uric acid. The kidneys normally excrete these nitrogenous waste products of protein metabolism, but diminished renal function causes these substances (including urea, uric acid, and creatinine) to accumulate in plasma. Consequently, renal dysfunction lowers the urine levels of these substances.

However, urine levels of urea and uric acid may change as a result of conditions other than renal disease — an important diagnostic consideration. Excessive purine catabolism, for example — which may be caused by a pathologic condition, such as leukemia, or simply by a high-purine diet — can raise serum and urine uric acid levels because uric acid is a product of purine metabolism. Several factors, including dehydration, dietary ingestion of protein, and hepatic disease, can cause alteration in the levels of blood urea nitrogen and urine urea.

Because formation and urinary excretion of creatinine are more constant than urea and uric acid levels, serum and urine creatinine values provide a more reliable index of renal function. By comparing serum creatinine concentration with the total amount of creatinine excreted within a specified period, the creatinine clearance test shows how efficiently the kidneys are removing this substance from the blood. Values for this extremely important diagnostic test typically decrease when renal function is impaired.

Urinary excretion of amino acids is fairly constant in a healthy adult. However, metabolic disturbances can cause amino acids to accumulate in plasma and — when they exceed the renal threshold — to appear in the urine in excessive amounts. Urine amino acid screening can detect these overflow amino acids. Testing for the amino acid hydroxyproline helps detect disorders that affect bone metabolism.

Urine pigments
Pigments are involved in the biosynthesis of hemoglobin and its subsequent breakdown. A conjugated protein consisting of an iron-containing pigment (heme) and a protein (globin), *hemoglobin* normally appears in red blood cells, where its primary function is to carry oxygen from the

lungs to body tissues. Hemoglobin is *not* a normal component of urine. However, when the amount of free hemoglobin in plasma exceeds the binding capacity of haptoglobin, as in severe intravascular hemolysis, hemoglobinuria results.

Myoglobin, which is closely related to hemoglobin in chemical composition, usually appears in cardiac and skeletal muscle; like hemoglobin, it doesn't usually appear in urine. Consequently, the presence of myoglobin in urine may indicate extensive muscle damage such as rhabdomyolysis.

Porphyrins may be considered metabolic intermediates in heme synthesis, which takes place mainly in the marrow of the long bones and in the liver. Biosynthesis of heme begins with formation of delta-aminolevulinic acid and progresses through porphobilinogen to the precursors uroporphyrinogen, coproporphyrinogen, protoporphyrinogen and, finally, protoporphyrin, which chelates iron to form heme. Porphyrinogens are hematologically active. The inactive end products are normally excreted in small quantities: Protoporphyrin is excreted exclusively in stool; coproporphyrin and uroporphyrin, in stool or urine.

Metabolic defects in heme biosynthesis may cause inherited or acquired porphyrin disorders. Increased urinary excretion of specific porphyrins may aid in the diagnosis of a particular porphyrin disorder, perhaps in combination with results of fecal and erythrocyte porphyrin testing.

The breakdown of the heme fraction of hemoglobin results in the formation of *bilirubin.* In the liver, free bilirubin conjugates with glucuronic acid, which allows bilirubin to be filtered by the glomeruli (unconjugated bilirubin isn't filterable). Bilirubin is normally excreted in bile as its principal pigment, but it's an abnormal element of urine. Conjugated bilirubin is present in urine when serum levels are elevated, as in biliary tract obstruction or hepatocellular damage, and is accompanied by jaundice.

Urobilinogen, formed in the intestine by bacterial action on conjugated bilirubin, is eventually excreted in stool, producing its characteristic color. A small amount of urobilinogen is reabsorbed by the portal system and is excreted mainly in bile, although the kidneys do excrete some. Therefore, elevated urine urobilinogen levels may be an early indication of hepatic damage. Urine urobilinogen levels decrease in biliary obstruction because bilirubin doesn't reach the intestine.

Melanin, the main pigment of hair, skin, and the choroid of the eye, is formed from the metabolism of tyrosine. This pigment isn't normally present in urine, but melanin-producing tumors (melanomas) may produce sufficient amounts of it to be detected in urine. In live metastasis, melanins and their precursors — melanogens — commonly appear in urine.

PROTEIN TESTS

Urine protein

A urine protein test is a quantitative test for proteinuria. Normally, the glomerular membrane allows only proteins of low molecular weight to enter the filtrate. The renal tubules then reabsorb most of these proteins, normally excreting a small amount that's undetectable by a screening test. A damaged glomerular capillary membrane and impaired tubular reabsorption allow excretion of proteins in the urine.

A qualitative screening commonly precedes this test. A positive result requires quantitative analysis of a 24-hour urine specimen by acid precipitation tests. Electrophoresis can detect Bence Jones proteins, hemoglobins, myoglobins, or albumin.

Purpose

- To aid in the diagnosis of pathologic states characterized by proteinuria, primarily renal disease

Patient preparation

- Explain to the patient that the urine protein test detects proteins in the urine.
- Inform the patient that he need not restrict food and fluids.
- Tell the patient that the test usually requires urine collection over a 24-hour period; random collection can be done.
- Notify the laboratory and physician of medications the patient is taking that may affect test results; they may need to be restricted.

Procedure and posttest care

- Collect the patient's urine over a 24-hour period, discarding the first specimen and retaining the last. A special specimen container can be obtained from the laboratory.
- Instruct the patient that he may resume his usual medications, as ordered.

Precautions

- Tell the patient not to contaminate the urine with toilet tissue or stool.
- Refrigerate the specimen or place it on ice during the collection period.

Normal findings

At rest, normal urine protein values range from 50 to 80 mg/24 hours (SI, 50 to 80 mg/d).

Abnormal findings

Proteinuria is a chief characteristic of renal disease. When proteinuria is present in a single specimen, a 24-hour urine collection is required to identify specific renal abnormalities.

Proteinuria can result from glomerular leakage of plasma proteins (a major cause of protein excretion), from overflow of filtered proteins of low molecular weight (when these are present in excessive concentrations), from impaired tubular reabsorption of filtered proteins, and from the presence of renal proteins derived from the breakdown of kidney tissue.

Persistent proteinuria indicates renal disease resulting from increased glomerular permeability. *Minimal proteinuria* (< 0.5 g/24 hours), however, is commonly associated with renal diseases in which glomerular involvement isn't a major factor, as in chronic pyelonephritis.

Moderate proteinuria (0.5 to 4 g/24 hours) occurs in several types of renal disease — acute or chronic glomerulonephritis, amyloidosis, or toxic nephropathies — or in diseases in which renal failure typically develops as a late complication (diabetes or heart failure, for example). *Heavy proteinuria* (> 4 g/24 hours) is commonly associated with nephrotic syndrome.

When accompanied by an elevated white blood cell count, proteinuria indicates urinary tract infection. When accompanied by hematuria, proteinuria indicates local or diffuse urinary tract disorders. Other pathologic states (infections and lesions of the central nervous system, for example) can also result in detectable amounts of proteins in the urine.

Many drugs (such as amphotericin B, gold preparations, aminoglycosides, polymyxins, and trimethadione) inflict renal damage, causing true proteinuria. This makes the routine evaluation of urine proteins essential during such treatment. In all forms of proteinuria, fractionation results obtained by electrophoresis provide more precise information than the screening test. For example, excessive hemoglobin in the urine indicates intravascular hemolysis; elevated myoglobin suggests muscle damage; albumin, increased glomerular permeability; and Bence Jones protein, multiple myeloma.

Not all forms of proteinuria have pathologic significance. *Benign proteinuria* can result from changes in body position. *Functional proteinuria* is associated with exercise as well as emotional or physiologic stress and is usually transient.

Interfering factors
■ Contamination of the specimen with toilet tissue or stool
■ Tolbutamide, para-aminosalicylic acid, acetazolamide, sodium bicarbonate, penicillin, sulfonamides, cephalosporins, and iodine-containing contrast media (possible false-positive or false-negative)
■ Very dilute urine, such as from forcing fluids, possibly depressing protein values and causing false-negative results

Bence Jones protein

Bence Jones proteins are abnormal light-chain immunoglobulins of low molecular weight that are derived from the clone of a single plasma cell. This globulin appears in the urine of 50% to 80% of patients with multiple myeloma and in most patients with Waldenström's macroglobulinemia.

Screening tests, such as thermal coagulation and Bradshaw's test, can detect Bence Jones proteins, but urine immunoelectrophoresis is usually the method of choice for quantitative studies. Serum immunoelectrophoresis, which is sometimes used, is less sensitive than other tests. Nevertheless, urine and serum studies are usually used when multiple myeloma is suspected.

Purpose
■ To confirm the presence of multiple myeloma in the patient with characteristic clinical signs, such as bone pain (especially in the back and the thorax) and persistent anemia and fatigue

Patient preparation
■ Tell the patient that the Bence Jones protein test can detect an abnormal protein in the urine.
■ Tell the patient that the test requires an early-morning urine specimen; teach him how to collect a midstream clean-catch specimen.

Procedure and posttest care
■ Collect an early-morning urine specimen of at least 50 ml.

Precautions
■ Instruct the patient not to contaminate the urine specimen with toilet tissue or stool.
■ Send the specimen to the laboratory immediately after collection, or refrigerate it if transport is delayed. A refrigerated specimen must be analyzed within 24 hours, or it should be discarded.

Normal findings

Normal urine should contain no Bence Jones proteins.

Abnormal findings

The presence of Bence Jones proteins in urine suggests multiple myeloma or Waldenström's macroglobulinemia. Very low levels in the absence of other symptoms may result from benign monoclonal gammopathy. However, clinical evidence figures prominently in the diagnosis of multiple myeloma.

Interfering factors

- Connective tissue disease, renal insufficiency, and certain cancers (possible false-positive)
- Contamination of the specimen with menstrual blood, prostatic secretions, or semen (possible false-positive)
- Contamination of the specimen with toilet tissue or stool
- Failure to properly store the specimen during the collection period or to send the sample to the laboratory immediately after the collection is completed (possible false-positive from protein deterioration)

PROTEIN METABOLITE TESTS

Urine amino acid screening

Urine amino acid screening tests screen for aminoaciduria — elevated urine amino acid levels — a condition that may result from inborn errors of metabolism due to the absence of specific enzymatic activities. Abnormal metabolism causes an excess of one or more amino acids to appear in plasma and, as the renal thresh-

old is exceeded, in urine. (See *Chromatographic identification of amino acid disorders,* pages 394 and 395.)

Aminoacidurias may be classified as either primary (overflow) aminoacidopathies or as secondary (renal) aminoacidopathies. The latter type is associated with conditions marked by defective tubular reabsorption from congenital disorders. A more specific defect, such as cystinuria, may cause one or more amino acids to appear in urine.

To screen neonates, children, and adults for congenital aminoacidurias, plasma or urine specimens may be used. The plasma test is the better indicator of overflow aminoacidurias; urine testing is used to confirm or monitor certain amino acid disorders and to screen for renal aminoacidurias.

Various laboratory techniques are available to screen for aminoacidurias, but chromatography is the preferred method. Positive findings on chromatography can be elaborated by fractionation, showing specific amino acid levels. Testing for specific amino acid levels is also necessary for infants or young children with acidosis, severe vomiting and diarrhea, and abnormal urine odor. Such testing is especially important in neonates because early diagnosis and prompt treatment of aminoacidurias may prevent mental retardation.

Purpose

- To screen for renal aminoacidurias
- To follow up on plasma test findings when results of these tests suggest overflow aminoacidurias

Patient preparation

- Explain to the patient (or the parents if the patient is an infant or a child) that the urine amino acid screening test helps de-

tect amino acid disorders. Advise him that additional tests may be necessary.
■ Inform the patient that he need not restrict food and fluids.
■ Tell the patient that the test requires a urine specimen.
■ Notify the laboratory and physician of medications the patient is taking that may affect test results; they may need to be restricted. If such drugs must be continued, however, note this on the laboratory request. (If the patient is a breast-fed infant, record any drugs the mother is receiving.)

Procedure and posttest care

⬦ AGE ISSUE *If the patient is an infant, clean and dry the genital area, attach the collection device, and observe for voiding. Transfer urine—at least 20 ml— to a specimen container. Remove the collection device carefully to prevent skin irritation, and make sure to remove all adhesive residues.*
■ If the patient is an adult or a child, collect a fresh random specimen.

Precautions

⬦ AGE ISSUE *For an infant, apply the adhesive flanges of the collection device securely to the skin to prevent leakage.*
■ Send the specimen to the laboratory immediately after collection.

Normal findings

Reported values are age-dependent and are indicated as normal or abnormal.

Abnormal findings

If thin-layer chromatography shows gross changes or abnormal patterns, blood and 24-hour urine quantitative column chromatography are performed to identify specific amino acid abnormalities and to differentiate overflow and renal aminoacidurias.

Interfering factors

■ Failure to send the urine specimen to the laboratory immediately after collection

⬦ AGE ISSUE *In the neonate, failure to ingest dietary protein during the 48 hours preceding the test*

Urine hydroxyproline

Total urine levels of hydroxyproline, an amino acid found mainly in collagen (a component of skin and bone), are a good index of bone matrix turnover because levels increase when collagen breaks down during bone resorption. Bone matrix turnover and hydroxyproline levels normally rise in children during periods of rapid skeletal growth. However, they also rise in disorders that increase bone resorption, such as Paget's disease, metastatic bone tumors, and certain endocrine disorders.

Hydroxyproline levels are typically determined colorimetrically on a timed urine sample; they may also be determined by ion-exchange or gas-liquid chromatography. A collagen-restricted diet is essential for this test because hydroxyproline levels reflect collagen intake. Free hydroxyproline, a small component of total hydroxyproline and a sensitive indicator of dietary collagen intake, may be measured to validate results.

Purpose

■ To monitor treatment for disorders characterized by bone resorption, including Paget's disease, metastatic bone tumors, certain endocrine disorders (hyperthyroidism), rheumatoid arthritis, and osteoporosis.
■ To aid in the diagnosis of disorders characterized by bone resorption

(Text continues on page 396.)

CHROMATOGRAPHIC IDENTIFICATION OF AMINO ACID DISORDERS

In chromatography — the preferred method for screening aminoacidurias — amino acids migrate into multicolored bands. The sequence of amino acids and their corresponding band numbers, as listed below, reflect these standard migratory patterns. When congeni-

Chromatographic band number	Amino acids	Phenylketonuria		Maple syrup urine disease		Cystinuria	
		Plasma	Urine	Plasma	Urine	Plasma	Urine
1	Leucine, isoleucine			+	+		
2	Phenylalanine	+	+				
3	Valine, methionine			+	+		
4	Tryptophan, beta-aminoisobutyric acid						
5	Tyrosine						
6	Proline			+			
7	Alanine, ethanolamine						
8	Threonine, glutamic acid						
9	Homocitrulline, glycine, serine, hydroxyproline, aspartic acid, glutamine, citrulline			+			
10	Homocystine, asparagine						
11	Argininosuccinic acid, histidine, arginine, lysine, ornithine, cystathionine, cystine, cysteine, hydroxylysine						+

tal enzyme deficiencies and subsequent metabolic disorders increase plasma and urine amino acid levels, these bands intensify.

Key: + = increased amino acids in plasma or urine

Metabolic amino acid disorders											
Homo-cystinuria		*Hartnup disease*		*Argininosuc-cinicaciduria*		*Histidinemia*		*Hyperprolin-emia type A*		*Citrullinuria*	
Plasma	Urine	Plasma	Urine	Plasma	Urine	Plasma	Urine	Plasma	Urine	Plasma	Urine
			+								
			+								
+			+							+	
			+								
			+								
								+	+		
			+				+				+
							+				+
			+		+				+	+	+
	+										
			+		+	+	+				+

Patient preparation

- Explain to the patient that the urine hydroxyproline test helps monitor treatment or detect an amino acid disorder related to bone formation.
- Inform the patient that he must follow a collagen-free diet and avoid eating ice cream, candy, meat, fish, poultry, jelly, and any foods containing gelatin for 24 hours before the test and during the test period itself.
- Tell the patient that the test requires urine collection over a 2-hour or 24-hour period, and teach him the correct collection technique.
- Note the patient's age and sex on the laboratory request.
- Notify the laboratory and physician of medications the patient is taking that may affect test results; they may need to be restricted.

Procedure and posttest care

- Collect the patient's urine over a 2-hour or 24-hour period. In a 24-hour collection, discard the first sample and retain the last. Use a container that has a preservative to prevent hydroxyproline degradation.
- Instruct the patient that he may resume his usual diet and medications, as ordered.

Precautions

- Refrigerate the specimen or keep it on ice during the collection period.
- Send the specimen to the laboratory immediately after the collection is completed.

Normal findings

Normal values typically range from 1 to 9 mg/24 hours (SI, 1.0 to 3.4 IU/d).

Abnormal findings

Hydroxyproline levels should decrease slowly during therapy for bone resorption disorders. Elevated levels may indicate bone disease, metastatic bone tumors, or endocrine disorders that stimulate hormonal secretion.

Interfering factors

- Failure to observe restrictions, to collect all urine during the collection period, to properly store the specimen, or to send the specimen to the laboratory immediately after the collection is completed
- Ascorbic acid, vitamin D, aspirin, glucocorticoids, antineoplastic agents, calcium gluconate, corticosteroids, estradiol, propranolol, calcitonin, and mithramycin (used to treat Paget's disease) (possible decrease)
- Psoriasis and burns (possible increase due to collagen turnover)
- Growth hormone, parathyroid hormone, phenobarbital, and sulfonylureas (increase)

Urine creatinine

The creatinine test measures urine levels of creatinine, the chief metabolite of creatine. Produced in amounts proportional to total body muscle mass, creatinine is removed from the plasma primarily by glomerular filtration and is excreted in the urine. Because the body doesn't recycle it, creatinine has a relatively high, constant clearance rate, making it an efficient indicator of renal function. However, the creatinine clearance test, which measures urine and plasma creatinine clearance, is a more precise index than this test. A standard method for determining urine creatinine levels is based on Jaffé's reaction, in which creatinine treated with an alkaline picrate solution yields a bright orange-red complex.

Purpose

- To help assess glomerular filtration
- To check the accuracy of 24-hour urine collection, based on the relatively constant levels of creatinine excretion

Patient preparation

- Explain to the patient that the urine creatinine test helps evaluate kidney function.
- Inform the patient that he need not restrict fluids, but that he shouldn't eat an excessive amount of meat before the test.
- Advise the patient that he should avoid strenuous physical exercise during the collection period.
- Tell the patient that the test usually requires urine collection over a 24-hour period, and teach him the proper collection technique.
- Notify the laboratory and physician of medications the patient is taking that may affect test results; they may need to be restricted.

Procedure and posttest care

- Collect the patient's urine over a 24-hour period, discarding the first specimen and retaining the last. Use a specimen bottle that contains a preservative to prevent creatinine degradation.
- Instruct the patient that he may resume his usual activities, diet, and medications, as ordered.

Precautions

- Refrigerate the specimen or keep it on ice during the collection period.
- Send the specimen to the laboratory immediately after the collection is completed.

Reference values

Normally, urine creatinine levels range from 14 to 26 mg/kg body weight/24 hours (SI, 124 to 230 μmol/kg body weight/d) in males and from 11 to 20 mg/kg body weight/24 hours (SI, 97 to 177 μmol/kg body weight/d) in females.

Abnormal findings

Decreased urine creatinine levels may result from impaired renal perfusion (associated with shock, for example) or from renal disease due to urinary tract obstruction. Chronic bilateral pyelonephritis, acute or chronic glomerulonephritis, and polycystic kidney disease may also depress creatinine levels. Increased levels generally have little diagnostic significance.

Interfering factors

- Failure to observe restrictions, to collect all urine during the test period, to properly store the specimen, or to send the specimen to the laboratory immediately after the collection is completed
- Corticosteroids, gentamicin, tetracyclines, diuretics, and amphotericin B (possible decrease)

Creatinine clearance

An anhydride of creatine, creatinine is formed and excreted in constant amounts by an irreversible reaction and functions solely as the main end product of creatine. Creatinine production is proportional to total muscle mass and is relatively unaffected by urine volume or normal physical activity or diet.

An excellent diagnostic indicator of renal function, the creatinine clearance test determines how efficiently the kidneys are clearing creatinine from the blood. The rate of clearance is expressed in terms of the volume of blood (in milliliters) that can be cleared of creatinine in 1 minute. Creatinine levels become abnormal when more than 50% of the nephrons have been damaged.

Purpose
■ To assess renal function (primarily glomerular filtration)
■ To monitor progression of renal insufficiency

Patient preparation
■ Explain to the patient that the creatinine clearance test assesses kidney function.
■ Inform the patient that he may need to avoid meat, poultry, fish, tea, or coffee for 6 hours before the test.
■ Advise the patient that he should avoid strenuous physical exercise during the collection period.
■ Tell the patient that the test requires a timed urine specimen and at least one blood sample.
■ Tell the patient how the urine specimen will be collected. Also inform him who will perform the venipuncture and when and that he may feel some discomfort from the needle puncture.
■ Explain that more than one venipuncture may be necessary.
■ Notify the laboratory and physician of medications the patient is taking that may affect test results; they may need to be restricted.

Procedure and posttest care
■ Collect a timed urine specimen at 2, 6, 12, or 24 hours in a bottle containing a preservative to prevent creatinine degradation.
■ Perform a venipuncture anytime during the collection period and collect the sample in a 7-ml tube without additives.

■ Apply direct pressure to the venipuncture site until bleeding stops.
■ If a hematoma develops at the venipuncture site, apply warm soaks.
■ Instruct the patient that he may resume his usual activities, diet, and medications, as ordered.

Precautions
■ Refrigerate the urine specimen or keep it on ice during the collection period.
■ Send the specimen to the laboratory as soon as the collection is completed.

Reference values
Normal creatinine clearance varies with age; in males, it ranges from 94 to 140 ml/min/1.73 m² (SI, 0.91 to 1.35 ml/s/m²); in females, 72 to 110 ml/min/1.73 m² (SI, 0.69 to 1.06 ml/s/m²).

Abnormal findings
Low creatinine clearance may result from reduced renal blood flow (associated with shock or renal artery obstruction), acute tubular necrosis, acute or chronic glomerulonephritis, advanced bilateral chronic pyelonephritis, advanced bilateral renal lesions (which may occur in polycystic kidney disease, renal tuberculosis, and cancer), nephrosclerosis, heart failure, or severe dehydration.

High creatinine clearance can suggest poor hydration.

Interfering factors
■ Failure to observe restrictions, to collect all urine during the test period, to properly store the specimen, or to send the sample to the laboratory immediately after the collection is completed
■ Amphotericin B, thiazide diuretics, furosemide, and aminoglycosides (possible decrease)

■ High-protein diet or strenuous exercise (increase)

Urea clearance

The urea clearance test is a quantitative analysis of urine levels of urea, the main nitrogenous component in urine and the end product of protein metabolism. (See *How urea is formed.*) After filtration by the glomeruli, roughly 40% of the urea is reabsorbed by the renal tubules. Because of this reabsorption, urea clearance was once considered a precise fraction (60%) of the glomerular filtration rate (GFR). However, because the reabsorption rate of urea varies with the amount of water reabsorbed, this test actually assesses overall renal function; the creatinine clearance test provides a more accurate evaluation of the GFR.

In urea clearance, blood urea content and the total amount of urea excreted in the urine are proportional only when the rate of urine flow is 2 ml/minute or higher (maximal clearance). At lower flow rates, the test's accuracy decreases. The equation for determining urea clearance is $C = (U \times V) \div P$; it's similar to the equation used for creatinine clearance.

Purpose
■ To assess overall renal function

Patient preparation
■ Explain to the patient that the urea clearance test evaluates kidney function.
■ Instruct the patient to fast from midnight before the test and to abstain from exercise before and during the test.
■ Tell the patient that the test requires two timed urine specimens and one blood sample.
■ Tell him how the urine specimens will be collected, who will perform the veni-

---

HOW UREA IS FORMED

Urea, the main nitrogenous component in urine, is the final product of protein metabolism. Amino acids absorbed by the intestinal villi pass from the portal vein into the liver. Because the liver stores only small amounts of amino acids — which are later returned to the blood for use in the synthesis of enzymes, hormones, or new protoplasm — the excess is converted into other substances, such as glucose, glycogen, and fat.

Before this conversion, the amino acids are deaminated — they lose their nitrogenous amino groups. These amino groups are then converted to ammonia. Because ammonia is very toxic, especially to the brain, it must be removed as quickly as it's formed. (Serious liver disease causes elevated blood ammonia levels and eventually leads to hepatic coma.)

In the liver, ammonia combines with carbon dioxide to form urea, which is released into the blood and ultimately secreted in urine.

---

puncture and when, and that he may experience slight discomfort from the needle puncture and the tourniquet.
■ Check the patient's medication history for drugs that may affect urea clearance.
■ Review your findings with the laboratory and then notify the physician; he may want to restrict these medications.

Procedure and posttest care
■ Instruct the patient to empty his bladder and discard the urine. Then give him water to drink to ensure adequate urine output.

■ Collect two specimens 1 hour apart, and mark the collection time on the laboratory request.
■ Perform a venipuncture anytime during the collection period and collect the sample in a 7-ml red-top tube.
■ If a hematoma develops at the venipuncture site, apply warm soaks.
■ Tell the patient that he may resume his usual diet, activities, and medications, as ordered.

Precautions
■ Because this is a clearance test, make sure the patient empties his bladder completely and that the total amount of urine is collected from each hour's specimen.
■ Send each specimen to the laboratory as soon as it's collected.
■ If the patient is catheterized, empty the drainage bag before beginning the specimen collection.
■ Handle the blood sample gently to prevent hemolysis, and send it to the laboratory immediately.

Reference values
Normally, urea clearance ranges from 64 to 99 ml/minute with maximal clearance. If the flow rate is less than 2 ml/minute, normal clearance is 41 to 68 ml/minute. (If the urine flow rate is less than 1 ml/minute, this test shouldn't be performed.)

Abnormal findings
Low urea clearance values may indicate decreased renal blood flow (due to shock or renal artery obstruction), acute or chronic glomerulonephritis, advanced bilateral chronic pyelonephritis, acute tubular necrosis, or nephrosclerosis. Low clearance rates may also result from advanced bilateral renal lesions (as in polycystic kidney disease, renal tuberculosis,

or cancer), bilateral ureteral obstruction, heart failure, or dehydration.

High urea clearance rates usually aren't diagnostically significant.

Interfering factors
■ The patient's failure to empty his bladder completely — the most common error in this test — or to observe pretest restrictions
■ Caffeine, milk, or small doses of epinephrine (increase)
■ Antidiuretic hormone or large doses of epinephrine (decrease)
■ Corticosteroids, amphotericin B, thiazide diuretics, and streptomycin
■ Hemolysis due to rough handling of the blood sample

Urine uric acid

A quantitative analysis of urine uric acid levels may supplement serum uric acid testing when seeking to identify disorders that alter production or excretion of uric acid (such as leukemia, gout, and renal dysfunction).

The most specific laboratory method for detecting uric acid is spectrophotometric absorption after treatment of the specimen with the enzyme uricase.

Purpose
■ To detect enzyme deficiencies and metabolic disturbances that affect uric acid production such as gout
■ To help measure the efficiency of renal clearance and to determine the risk of stone formation

Patient preparation
■ Explain to the patient that this test measures the body's production and excretion of a waste product known as uric acid.

■ Anticipate the need for a diet low or high in purines before or during urine collection.

■ Tell the patient that the test requires urine collection over a 24-hour period, and teach him the proper collection technique.

■ Notify the laboratory and physician of medications the patient is taking that may affect test results; they may need to be restricted.

Procedure and posttest care

■ Collect the patient's urine over a 24-hour period, discarding the first specimen and retaining the last.

■ Instruct the patient that he may resume his usual diet and medications, as ordered.

Precautions

■ Send the specimen to the laboratory immediately after the collection is completed.

Reference values

Normal urine uric acid values vary with diet, but generally are 250 to 750 mg/24 hours (SI, 1.48 to 4.43 mmol/d).

Abnormal findings

Elevated urine uric acid levels may result from chronic myeloid leukemia, polycythemia vera, multiple myeloma, early remission in pernicious anemia, lymphosarcoma and lymphatic leukemia during radiotherapy, or tubular reabsorption defects, such as Fanconi's syndrome and hepatolenticular degeneration (Wilson's disease).

Low urine uric acid levels occur in gout (when associated with normal uric acid production but inadequate excretion) and in severe renal damage such as that resulting from chronic glomerulonephritis, dia-

betic glomerulosclerosis, and collagen disorders.

Interfering factors

■ Failure to send the sample to the laboratory immediately after the collection is completed

■ Diuretics, such as benzthiazide, furosemide, and ethacrynic acid (decrease); pyrazinamide, salicylates, phenylbutazone, probenecid, and allopurinol (increase)

■ High-purine diet (increase)

■ Low-purine diet (decrease)

PIGMENT TESTS

Urine hemoglobin

An abnormal finding, free hemoglobin (Hb) in the urine may occur in hemolytic anemias, infection, strenuous exercise, or severe intravascular hemolysis from a transfusion reaction. Contained in red blood cells (RBCs), Hb consists of an iron-protoporphyrin complex (heme) and a polypeptide (globin). Usually, RBC destruction occurs within the reticuloendothelial system. However, when RBC destruction occurs within the circulation, free Hb enters the plasma and binds with haptoglobin. If the plasma level of Hb exceeds that of haptoglobin, the excess of unbound Hb is excreted in the urine (hemoglobinuria).

Heme proteins act like enzymes that catalyze oxidation of organic substances. This reaction produces a blue coloration; the intensity of color varies with the amount of Hb present. Microscopic examination is required to identify intact RBCs in urine (hematuria), which can occur in the presence of unbound Hb.

BEDSIDE TESTING FOR URINE BLOOD PIGMENTS

To test a patient's urine for blood pigments at the bedside, use one of these methods.

Dipstick, Multistix, or Chemstrip
- Collect a urine specimen.
- Dip the stick into the specimen and withdraw it.
- After 30 seconds, compare the stick to the color chart. Blue indicates a positive reaction; the intensity of color indicates pigment concentration.

Occult tablet
- Collect a urine specimen.
- Put one drop of urine on the filter paper. Place the tablet on the urine, and then put two drops of water on the tablet.
- After 2 minutes, inspect the filter paper around the tablet. Blue indicates a positive reaction; the intensity of color indicates pigment concentration.

Occult solution
- Collect a urine specimen.
- After placing one drop of urine on the filter paper, close the package and turn it over. Open the opposite ends, and place two drops of solution on the filter paper.
- After 30 seconds, inspect the filter paper. Blue indicates a positive reaction; the intensity of color indicates pigment concentration.

Distinguishing hemoglobin
Because these methods detect only blood pigments, immunochemical studies are necessary to differentiate hemoglobin from other blood pigments such as myoglobin.

Purpose
- To aid in the diagnosis of hemolytic anemias, infection, or severe intravascular hemolysis from a transfusion reaction

Patient preparation
- Explain to the patient that the urine hemoglobin test detects excessive RBC destruction.
- Inform the patient that he need not restrict food and fluids.
- Tell the patient that the test requires a random urine specimen, and teach him the proper collection technique.
- If the female patient is menstruating, reschedule the test, as results may be altered.
- Notify the laboratory and physician of medications the patient is taking that may affect test results; they may need to be restricted.

Procedure and posttest care
- Collect a random urine specimen. (See *Bedside testing for urine blood pigments.*)
- Instruct the patient that he may resume his usual medications, as ordered.

Precautions
- Have a female patient who's menstruating reschedule her test because contamination of the specimen with menstrual blood alters results.
- Send the specimen to the laboratory immediately after collection.

Normal findings
Normally, Hb isn't present in the urine.

Abnormal findings

Hemoglobinuria may result from severe intravascular hemolysis due to a blood transfusion reaction, burns, or a crush injury. It may result from acquired hemolytic anemias caused by chemical or drug intoxication or malaria; congenital hemolytic anemias, such as hemoglobinopathies or enzyme defects; or paroxysmal nocturnal hemoglobinuria (another type of hemolytic anemia). Less commonly, it may signal cystitis, ureteral calculi, or urethritis.

Hemoglobinuria and hematuria occur in renal epithelial damage (which may result from acute glomerulonephritis or pyelonephritis), renal tumor, and tuberculosis.

Interfering factors

- Failure to send the specimen to the laboratory immediately after collection
- Nephrotoxic drugs and anticoagulants (positive results)
- Large doses of vitamin C or drugs that contain vitamin C as a preservative (false-negative)
- Lysis of RBCs in stale or alkaline urine and contamination of the specimen by menstrual blood
- Bacterial peroxidases in highly infected specimens (false-positive)

Urine myoglobin

The myoglobin test detects the presence of myoglobin—a red pigment found in the cytoplasm of cardiac and skeletal muscle cells—in the urine. When muscle cells are extensively damaged, as by disease or severe crushing trauma, myoglobin is released into the blood, quickly cleared by renal glomerular filtration, and eliminated in the urine (myoglobinuria). For example, myoglobin appears in the urine within 24 hours after a myocardial infarction (MI).

Urine myoglobin must be differentiated from urine hemoglobin because of their marked structural similarities. The most commonly used test method is the differential precipitation test. Hemoglobin—bound to haptoglobin—precipitates when urine is mixed with ammonium sulfate. Myoglobin, however, remains soluble and can be measured.

Purpose

- To aid in the diagnosis of muscular disease of rhabdomyolysis
- To detect extensive infarction of muscle tissue
- To assess the extent of muscular damage from crushing trauma

Patient preparation

- Explain to the patient that the urine myoglobin test detects a red pigment found in muscle cells and helps evaluate muscle injury or disease.
- Inform the patient that he need not restrict food and fluids.
- Tell the patient that this test requires a random urine specimen, and teach him the proper collection technique.

Procedure and posttest care

- Collect a random urine specimen.

Precautions

- Send the specimen to the laboratory immediately after collection.

Normal findings

Normally, myoglobin doesn't appear in urine.

Abnormal findings

Myoglobinuria occurs in acute or chronic muscular disease, alcoholic polymyopathy, familial myoglobinuria, extensive MI, and in severe trauma to the skeletal muscles (which may result from a crush injury, extreme hyperthermia, or severe burns). It also occurs in strenuous or prolonged exercise, but disappears after rest.

Interfering factors
- Extremely dilute urine (reduces sensitivity)
- Contamination with iodine during surgery (positive results)
- Recent ingestion of large amounts of vitamin C (inhibits reaction if testing is performed with Chemstrip or other reagent strips)
- Failure to send the specimen to the laboratory immediately after collection

Urine porphyrins

The test for porphyrins is a quantitative analysis of urine porphyrins (most notably, uroporphyrins and coproporphyrins) and their precursors (porphyrinogens such as porphobilinogen [PBG]). Tests for porphyrins may include PBG and urine ∂-aminolevulinic acid. Porphyrins are red-orange fluorescent compounds consisting of four pyrrole rings that are produced during heme biosynthesis. They're present in all protoplasm, figure in energy storage and utilization, and are normally excreted in urine in small amounts. Elevated urine levels of porphyrins or porphyrinogens, therefore, reflect impaired heme biosynthesis. Such impairment may result from inherited enzyme deficiencies (congenital porphyrias) or from defects due to such disorders as hemolytic anemias and hepatic disease (acquired porphyrias).

Determination of the specific porphyrins and porphyrinogens found in a urine specimen can help identify the impaired metabolic step in heme biosynthesis. Occasionally, a preliminary qualitative screening is performed on a random specimen. However, a positive finding on the screening test must be confirmed by the quantitative analysis of a 24-hour specimen. For correct diagnosis of a specific porphyria, urine porphyrin levels should be correlated with plasma and fecal porphyrin levels.

Purpose
- To aid in the diagnosis of congenital or acquired porphyrias

Patient preparation
- Explain to the patient that the urine porphyrin test detects abnormal hemoglobin formation.
- Inform the patient that he need not restrict food and fluids.
- Tell the patient that the test requires urine collection over a 24-hour period, and teach him the proper collection technique.
- Notify the laboratory and physician of medications the patient is taking that may affect test results; they may need to be restricted.

Procedure and posttest care
- Collect the patient's urine over a 24-hour period, discarding the first specimen and retaining the last. Use a light-resistant specimen bottle containing a preservative to prevent degradation of the light-sensitive porphyrins and their precursors.
- Instruct the patient that he may resume his usual medications, as ordered.

Precautions
- Be aware that pregnancy or menstruation may affect the accuracy of test results.

URINE PORPHYRIN LEVELS IN PORPHYRIA

In porphyria, defective heme biosynthesis increases urinary porphyrins and their corresponding precursors.

Porphyria	Porphyrins		Porphyrin precursors	
	Uropor-phyrins	Capropor-phyrins	∂-amino levulinic acid	Porpho-bilinogens
Erythropoietic porphyria	Highly increased	Increased	Normal	Normal
Erythropoietic protoporphyria	Normal	Normal	Normal	Normal
Acute intermittent porphyria	Variable	Variable	Highly increased	Highly increased
Variegate porphyria	Normal or slightly increased; may be highly increased during acute attack	Normal or slightly increased; may be highly increased during acute attack	Highly increased during acute attack	Normal or slightly increased; highly increased during acute attack
Coproporphyria	Not applicable	May be highly increased during acute attack	Increased during acute attack	Increased during acute attack
Porphyria cutanea tarda	Highly increased	Increased	Variable	Variable

- Refrigerate the specimen or keep it on ice during the collection period.
- Send the specimen to the laboratory as soon as the collection is completed.
- Protect the specimen from light exposure if a light-resistant container isn't available.
- Put the collection bag in a dark plastic bag if an indwelling urinary catheter is in place.

Normal findings

Normal urine porphyrin and precursor values fall in the following ranges:

- *uroporphyrins:* 27 to 52 µg/24 hours (SI, 32 to 63 nmol/d)
- *coproporphyrins:* 34 to 230 µg/24 hours (SI, 52 to 351 nmol/d).

Abnormal findings

Increased urine levels of porphyrins and porphyrin precursors are characteristic of porphyria. (See *Urine porphyrin levels in porphyria.*) Infectious hepatitis, Hodgkin's disease, central nervous system disorders, cirrhosis, and heavy metal, benzene, or carbon tetrachloride toxicity may also increase porphyrin levels.

Interfering factors

- Failure to properly store the specimen during the collection period, to protect it from exposure to light, or to send the specimen to the laboratory immediately after the collection is completed
- Barbiturates, chloral hydrate, chlorpropamide, sulfonamides, meprobamate, and chlordiazepoxide (induce porphyria or porphyrinuria); discontinue 12 days before the test if possible (possible increase or decrease)
- Hormonal contraceptives and griseofulvin (increase)
- Pregnancy or menstruation (possible increase or decrease)
- Rifampin (elevated urine urobilinogen)

Urine delta-aminolevulinic acid

Using the colorimetric technique, the quantitative analysis of urine delta-aminolevulinic acid (ALA) levels helps diagnose porphyrias, hepatic disease, and lead poisoning. In an emergency, a simple qualitative screening test may be performed.

ALA, the basic precursor of the porphyrins, normally converts to porphobilinogen during heme synthesis. Impaired conversion, which occurs in porphyrias and lead poisoning, causes urine ALA levels to rise before other chemical or hematologic changes occur.

Purpose

- To screen for lead poisoning
- To aid in the diagnosis of porphyrias and certain hepatic disorders, such as hepatitis and hepatic carcinoma

Patient preparation

- Explain to the patient that the urine ALA test detects abnormal hemoglobin formation.
- If lead poisoning is suspected, tell the patient (or parents, because the patient is usually a child) that the test helps detect the presence of excessive lead in the body.
- Inform the patient or his parents that he need not restrict food and fluids.
- Tell the patient that the test requires urine collection over a 24-hour period, and teach him or his parents the proper collection technique.
- Notify the laboratory and physician of medications the patient is taking that may affect test results; they may need to be restricted.

Procedure and posttest care

- Collect the patient's urine over a 24-hour period, discarding the first specimen and retaining the last. Use a light-resistant bottle containing a preservative (usually glacial acetic acid) to prevent ALA degradation.
- Instruct the patient that he may resume his usual medications, as ordered.

Precautions

- Refrigerate the specimen or keep it on ice during the collection period.
- Send the specimen to the laboratory as soon as the collection is complete.

 ▶ **CLINICAL ALERT** *Protect the specimen from direct sunlight.*

- Insert the drainage bag in a dark plastic bag if the patient has an indwelling urinary catheter in place.
- Blood levels for lead aren't sensitive indicators of lead poisoning in a child.

Reference values

Normally, urine ALA values range from 1.3 to 7.0 mg/24 hours (SI, 10 to 53 μmol/d).

Abnormal findings

Elevated urine ALA levels may occur in lead poisoning, hereditary tyrosinemia, acute porphyria, hepatic carcinoma, or hepatitis.

Interfering factors

- Failure to collect all urine during the test period, to properly store the specimen and protect it from light, or to send the specimen to the laboratory immediately after the collection is completed
- Barbiturates and griseofulvin (increase due to accumulation of porphyrins in the liver)
- Vitamin E in pharmacologic doses (possible decrease)

Urine bilirubin

The bilirubin screening test, based on a color reaction with a specific reagent, detects water-soluble direct (conjugated) bilirubin in the urine. Detectable amounts of bilirubin in the urine may indicate liver disease caused by infections, biliary disease, or hepatotoxicity.

When combined with urobilinogen measurements, the bilirubin test helps identify disorders that can cause jaundice. The analysis can be performed at the bedside, using a bilirubin reagent strip, or in the laboratory.

Purpose

- To help identify the cause of jaundice
- To compare urine and serum bilirubin levels and other liver enzyme tests

Patient preparation

- Explain to the patient that the urine bilirubin test helps determine the cause of jaundice.
- Inform the patient that he need not restrict food and fluids.
- Tell the patient that the test requires a random urine specimen.
- Advise the patient that the specimen will be tested at the bedside or in the laboratory.
- Notify the laboratory and physician of medications the patient is taking that may affect test results; they may need to be restricted.

Procedure and posttest care

- Collect a random urine specimen in the container provided.

Bedside analysis using the dipstrip procedure

- Dip the reagent strip into the specimen and remove it immediately.
- Compare the strip color with the color standards after 20 seconds.
- Record the test results on the patient's chart.

Bedside analysis using the ictotest procedure

- Place five drops of urine on the asbestos-cellulose test mat. If bilirubin is present, it will be absorbed into the mat.
- Put a reagent tablet on the wet area of the mat, and place two drops of water on the tablet. If bilirubin is present, a blue to purple coloration will develop on the mat. Pink or red indicates absence of bilirubin.
- Instruct the patient that he may resume his usual medications, as ordered.

Precautions

■ Use only a freshly voided specimen. Bilirubin disintegrates after 30 minutes of exposure to room temperature or light.

■ If the specimen is to be analyzed in the laboratory, send it there at once.

■ If the specimen is tested at the bedside, make sure 20 seconds elapse before interpreting the color change on the dipstrip. Make sure lighting is adequate to make this color determination.

Normal findings

Normally, bilirubin isn't found in urine in a routine screening test.

Abnormal findings

High concentrations of direct bilirubin in urine may be evident from the specimen's appearance (dark, with a yellow foam). To diagnose jaundice, however, the presence or absence of direct bilirubin in urine must be correlated with serum test results and with urine and fecal urobilinogen levels. (See *Comparative values of bilirubin and urobilinogen.*)

Interfering factors

■ Failure to test the specimen promptly or to send it to the laboratory immediately after collection

■ Phenazopyridine and phenothiazine derivatives (chlorpromazine and acetophenazine maleate) (false-positive)

■ Large amounts of ascorbic acid and nitrite (false-negative if using dipstick testing, such as Chemstrip or N-multistix)

■ Exposure of specimen to room temperature or light (decrease due to bilirubin degradation)

Urine urobilinogen

The urobilinogen test detects impaired liver function by measuring urine levels of urobilinogen, the colorless, water-soluble product that results from the reduction of bilirubin by intestinal bacteria. Absent or altered urobilinogen levels can indicate hepatic damage or dysfunction. Increased urine urobilinogen levels may indicate hemolysis of red blood cells.

Quantitative analysis of urine urobilinogen involves the addition of a reagent to a 2-hour urine specimen. The resulting color reaction is read promptly by spectrophotometry.

Purpose

■ To aid in the diagnosis of extrahepatic obstruction such as blockage of the common bile duct

■ To aid in the differential diagnosis of hepatic and hematologic disorders

Patient preparation

■ Explain to the patient that the urine urobilinogen test helps assess liver and biliary tract function.

■ Inform the patient that he need not restrict food and fluids, except for bananas, which he should avoid for 48 hours before the test.

■ Tell the patient that the test requires a 2-hour urine specimen, and teach him how to collect it.

■ Notify the laboratory and physician of medications the patient is taking that may affect test results; they may need to be restricted.

Procedure and posttest care

■ Most laboratories request a random urine specimen; others prefer a 2-hour specimen, usually during the afternoon (ideally, between 1 p.m. and 3 p.m.), when urobilinogen levels peak.

■ Instruct the patient that he may resume his usual diet and medications, as ordered.

COMPARATIVE VALUES OF BILIRUBIN AND UROBILINOGEN

Causes of jaundice	Serum		Urine		Stool
	Indirect bilirubin	*Direct bilirubin*	*Bilirubin*	*Urobilinogen*	*Urobilinogen*
Unconjugated hyperbilirubinemia					
Hemolytic disorders: hemolytic anemia, erythroblastosis fetalis	↑	N	O	N↑	↑
Gilbert's syndrome: constitutional hepatic dysfunction	↑↑	N	O	N↓	N↓
Crigler-Najjar syndrome: congenital hyperbilirubinemia	↑↑↑	N	O	N↓	N↓
Conjugated hyperbilirubinemia					
Extrahepatic obstruction: calculi, tumor, scar tissue in common bile duct or hepatic excretory duct	N	↑	+	↓O	↓O
Hepatocellular disorders: viral, toxic, or alcoholic hepatitis; cirrhosis; parenchymal injury	↑	↑	+	↓N↑	N↑
Hepatocanalicular disorders or intrahepatic obstruction: drug-induced cholestasis; some familial defects, such as Dubin-Johnson and Rotor's syndromes; viral hepatitis; and primary biliary cirrhosis	↑	↑	+	↓N↑	N↑

Key:

↑	Increased	↑↑↑	Markedly increased	N↓	Normal or reduced
N↑	May be increased	N	Normal	↓O	Decreased or absent
↑↑	Moderately increased	O	Absent	↓N↑	Variable
		+	Present		

Precautions

- Send the specimen to the laboratory immediately after collection. This test must be performed within 30 minutes of collection because urobilinogen quickly oxidizes into an orange compound called urobilin.

Reference values

Normally, urine urobilinogen values are 0.1 to 0.8 EU/2 hours (SI, 0.1 to 0.8 EU/ 2 hours) or 0.5 to 4.0 EU/24 hours (SI, 0.5 to 4.0 EU/d).

Abnormal findings

Absence of urine urobilinogen may result from complete obstructive jaundice or treatment with broad-spectrum antibiotics, which destroy the intestinal bacterial flora. Low urine urobilinogen levels may result from congenital enzymatic jaundice (hyperbilirubinemia syndromes) or from treatment with drugs that acidify urine, such as ammonium chloride or ascorbic acid.

Elevated levels may indicate hemolytic jaundice, hepatitis, or cirrhosis.

Interfering factors

- Failure to observe pretest restrictions or to send the specimen to the laboratory immediately after collection
- Para-aminosalicylic acid, phenazopyridine, procaine, phenothiazines, and sulfonamides (possible decrease)
- Acetazolamide and sodium bicarbonate (increase)
- Bananas eaten up to 48 hours before the test (increase)

Urine melanin

This relatively rare test measures urine levels of melanin, the brown-black pigment that covers the skin, hair, and eyes.

An end product of tyrosine metabolism, melanin is normally produced by specialized cells and melanocytes.

Cutaneous melanomas — malignant tumors that produce excessive amounts of melanin — develop most commonly around the head and neck, but may also originate in mucous membranes (as in the rectum), the retinas, or the central nervous system, where melanocytes appear. Patients with these tumors may excrete melanin precursors — melanogens — in their urine. If the urine is left standing, exposure to air converts the melanogens to melanin in about 24 hours.

Tormählen's test uses sodium nitroprusside (nitrofericyanide) to detect melanogens or melanin in urine, based on characteristic color changes. More specific tests for melanin, such as chromatography, isolate and measure the pigment.

Purpose

- To aid in the diagnosis of malignant melanomas

Patient preparation

- Explain to the patient what melanin is, and tell him the urine melanin test detects its presence in urine.
- Inform the patient that he need not restrict food and fluids.
- Tell the patient that the test requires a random urine specimen, and teach him the correct collection technique.

Procedure and posttest care

- Collect a random urine specimen.

Precautions

- Send the specimen to the laboratory immediately.

Normal findings

Urine shouldn't contain melanogens or melanin.

Abnormal findings

In the presence of a visible skin tumor, melanin or melanogens in urine indicates advanced internal metastasis. Because malignant melanomas may also develop in internal organs, large quantities of melanin or melanogens in a urine specimen in the absence of a visible skin tumor indicate an internal melanoma.

Interfering factors

■ Failure to send the urine specimen to the laboratory immediately after collection

Selected readings

Anderson, S.C., and Poulsen, K.B. *Anderson's Atlas of Hematology.* Philadelphia: Lippincott Williams & Wilkins, 2003.

Bradwell, A.R., et al. "Serum Test for Assessment of Patients with Bence-Jones Myeloma," *Lancet* 361(9356):489-91, February 2003.

Cavanaugh, B.M. *Nurse's Manual of Laboratory and Diagnostic Tests,* 4th ed. Philadelphia: F.A. Davis Co., 2003.

Goldman, L., and Ausiello, D., eds. *Cecil Textbook of Medicine,* 22nd ed. Philadelphia: W.B. Saunders Co., 2004.

Gonzalez-Arriaza, H.L., and Bostwick, J.M. "Acute Porphyrias: A Case Report and Review," *American Journal of Psychiatry* 160(3):450-59, March 2003.

Guyton, A.C., and Hall, J.E. *Textbook of Medical Physiology,* 10th ed. Philadelphia: W.B. Saunders Co., 2001.

Henry, J.B., et al. *Clinical Diagnosis and Management by Laboratory Methods,* 20th ed. Philadelphia: W.B. Saunders Co., 2001.

McClatchey, K.D. *Clinical Laboratory Medicine,* 2nd ed. Philadelphia: Lippincott Williams & Wilkins, 2002.

Pagana, K.D., and Pagana, T.J. *Mosby's Diagnostic and Laboratory Test Reference,* 6th ed. St. Louis: Mosby Year–Book, Inc., 2003.

Schnell, Z., et al. *Davis's Comprehensive Handbook of Laboratory and Diagnostic Tests with Nursing Implications.* Philadelphia: F.A. Davis Co., 2003.

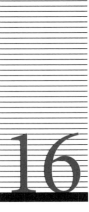

16

Urine sugars, ketones, and mucopoly-saccharides

Introduction

This group of tests is used to detect excessive urinary excretion of glucose, ketones, and mucopolysaccharides. Although plasma or serum glucose levels are typically used, several of these tests are sufficiently reliable and accessible to screen for diabetes.

Glycosuria significant
Because the renal tubules normally reabsorb glucose completely and return it to the blood, the presence of glucose in the urine (glycosuria) is abnormal and usually indicates a pathologic condition. Rarely, transient urinary traces of glucose and other reducing sugars (galactose, lactose, and pentose) reflect a benign state, such as the third trimester of pregnancy or lactation, or occur as a metabolic complication of total parenteral nutrition.

Characteristically, however, glycosuria reflects decreased glucose reabsorption in the renal tubules or increased amounts of glucose entering the renal tubules per minute — almost invariably the result of blood glucose concentration above the threshold level (180 mg/dl of venous blood). Such glycosuria with hyperglycemia suggests diabetes mellitus, one of the most common metabolic disorders.

The severity and prevalence of diabetes mandate routine screening of urine specimens for glucose in neonates. In some patients, urine levels of glucose don't reflect blood levels.

Ketone bodies

Substances designated ketone bodies (acetone bodies) include acetoacetic (diacetic) acid, acetone (formed by the spontaneous decarboxylation of acetoacetic acid), and beta-hydroxybutyric acid. Formed in the liver during fatty acid metabolism, ketone bodies circulate through the blood to the tissues for further oxidation. Normally, on the usual carbohydrate-protein-fat diet, less than 125 mg of such substances are excreted daily in the urine. Under conditions of absolute or relative carbohydrate deprivation, fat metabolism greatly accelerates. Such acceleration exceeds the liver's capacity to metabolize the fragments of acetyl coenzyme A derived from the fatty acid, causing the formation and release of significant quantities of ketone bodies into the blood.

The extrahepatic tissues (such as the kidneys) have a great capacity for utilizing ketone bodies (ketolysis). However, when the rate of ketogenesis by the liver exceeds the rate of ketolysis in peripheral tissues, the blood concentration of ketone bodies rises (ketonemia), causing these bodies to appear in the urine (ketonuria). Ketonuria is characteristic in starvation, fasting, uncontrolled diabetes mellitus,

and alcohol ingestion with poor dietary intake. It offers clues to various causes of metabolic acidosis; it's usually unrelated to intrinsic urinary system disease.

Screening for ketonuria

Ketonuria is commonly nonspecific, indicating urinary excretion of acetoacetic acid, acetone, or beta-hydroxybutyric acid. Consequently, a test that identifies any one of these three ketones generally confirms ketonuria. Commercially prepared *dip-and-read reagent strips* (such as Ketostix) are available as screening tools. These reagent strips, which are impregnated with sodium nitroprusside, are specific for acetoacetic acid and sensitive to 10 mg/dl. When the strip is dipped into the specimen, the presence of acetoacetic acid produces a color change that can be compared to a standard color block to determine approximate concentrations.

The *tablet test* (Acetest) is another convenient screening procedure sometimes used because it works equally well with plasma or urine and reacts to concentrations as low as 5 mg/dl of acetone. (It isn't specific for acetoacetic acid.) The Acetest tablet contains glycine, sodium nitroprusside, disodium phosphate, and lactose. Acetoacetic acid or acetone, in the presence of glycine, turns the tablet lavender-purple.

Mucopolysaccharides

These large polymer compounds are present in various body tissues and fluids, including connective tissue, fetal and adult mucous membranes, and blood group substances. Mucopolysaccharides occur in the free state or are bound to small quantities of proteins. The most important mucopolysaccharides include dermatan sulfate (also known as chondroitin sulfate B), derived from fibroblasts; heparan sulfate (heparitin sulfate), derived from mast cells; keratosulfate (keratan sulfate), distributed in costal cartilage and the cornea; and hyaluronic acid, present in synovial fluid, the umbilical cord, and vitreous humor.

Normally, the mucopolysaccharides contribute viscosity and permeability to the tissues, controlling the intercellular migration of small molecules. Hyaluronic acid, for example, decreases fluid viscosity and enhances the lubricating property of synovial fluid. Ordinarily, only minute quantities (10 to 15 mg/day) of these compounds are excreted in the urine. However, in certain hereditary disorders known as mucopolysaccharidosis, excessive quantities of these glycoproteins can accumulate in the tissues, eventually resulting in abnormal levels excreted in the urine (100 to 500 mg/day). In such patients, the primary defect seems to be the genetically determined absence of the target enzymes that catabolize the mucopolysaccharides.

These genetic disorders are marked by severe clinical abnormalities that usually become apparent during the first decade of life, including mental retardation, aortic insufficiency, and pronounced skeletal deformities. The most common types of mucopolysaccharidosis are Hurler's, Hunter's, and Sanfilippo's syndromes.

Screening for mucopolysaccharidosis

Screening tests for mucopolysaccharidosis use an organic dye (toluidine blue) that changes color in the presence of large amounts of acid mucopolysaccharides. One convenient method uses litmus paper impregnated with the dye: A drop of urine is placed on the paper and treated with acidified methyl alcohol. If a blue dye spot persists, acid mucopolysaccha-

rides are present. If the specimen is normal, no dye remains. However, up to 30% of spot tests produce false-negative results.

Another primarily qualitative test uses turbidimetry: Buffered urine is mixed with albumin at acid pH; if acid mucopolysaccharides are present, the solution grows uniformly turbid. (False-negative results occur in about 10% of these tests.) If spot or turbidity tests are positive, paper chromatography can identify the specific mucopolysaccharide. If the patient has Hurler's, Hunter's, or Sanfilippo's syndrome and his initial screening was negative, further tests are needed (paper or column chromatography, or electrophoresis).

CARBOHYDRATE AND FAT METABOLISM TESTS

Glucose oxidase

The glucose oxidase test—which involves the use of commercial, plastic-coated reagent strips (Clinistix, Diastix) or Tes-Tape—is a specific, qualitative test for glycosuria. The test is used primarily to monitor urine glucose in patients with diabetes. Patients can perform this test at home because of its simplicity and convenience.

Purpose
■ To detect glycosuria and determine the renal threshold for glucose
■ To monitor urine glucose levels during insulin therapy

Patient preparation

- Explain to the patient that the glucose oxidase test determines urine glucose concentration.
- If the patient is newly diagnosed with diabetes, teach him how to perform a reagent strip test.
- If the patient is taking levodopa, ascorbic acid, phenazopyridine, salicylates, peroxides, or hypochlorites, use Clinitest tablets instead.

Equipment

Specimen container, glucose test strips, reference color blocks

Procedure and posttest care

- Have the patient void; then give him a drink of water.
- Collect a second-voided specimen after 30 to 45 minutes.

Clinistix test

- Dip the test area of the reagent strip in the specimen for 2 seconds.
- Remove excess urine by tapping the strip against a clean surface or the side of the container and begin timing.
- Hold the strip in the air and "read" the color *exactly 10 seconds* after taking the strip out of the urine by comparing it with the reference color blocks on the label of the container.
- Record the results.
- Ignore color changes that develop after 10 seconds.

Diastix test

- Dip the reagent strip in the specimen for 2 seconds.
- Remove excess urine by tapping the strip against the container and begin timing.
- Hold the strip in the air and compare the color to the color chart *exactly 30 sec-*

onds after taking the strip out of the urine.
- Record the results.
- Ignore color changes that develop after 30 seconds.

Tes-Tape

- Withdraw about 1″ (2.5 cm) of the reagent tape from the dispenser; dip ¼″ (0.6 cm) in the specimen for 2 seconds.
- Remove excess urine by tapping the strip against the side of the container and begin timing.
- Hold the tape in the air and compare the color of the darkest part of the tape to the color chart *exactly 60 seconds* after taking the strip out of the urine.
- If the tape indicates 0.5% or higher, wait an additional 60 seconds to make the final color comparison.
- Record the results.

Precautions

- Instruct the patient not to contaminate the urine specimen with toilet tissue or stool.
- Keep the test strip container tightly closed to prevent deterioration of strips by exposure to light or moisture.
- Store the container in a cool place (under 86° F [30° C]) to avoid heat degradation.
- Don't use discolored or darkened Clinistix or Diastix or dark yellow or yellow-brown Tes-Tape.

Normal findings

Normally, no glucose is present in urine.

Abnormal findings

Glycosuria occurs in diabetes mellitus, adrenal and thyroid disorders, hepatic and central nervous system diseases, conditions involving low renal threshold (such as Fanconi's syndrome), toxic renal tubular disease, heavy metal poisoning, glomerulonephritis, and nephrosis; in pregnant women; and in those receiving total parenteral nutrition. It also occurs with the administration of large amounts of glucose and of certain drugs, such as asparaginase, corticosteroids, carbamazepine, ammonium chloride, thiazide diuretics, dextrothyroxine, large doses of nicotinic acid, lithium carbonate, and prolonged use of phenothiazines.

Interfering factors
- Dilute, stale urine or contamination of the specimen by toilet tissue, stool, or bacteria
- Use of reagent strips after the expiration date, failure to keep the reagent strip container tightly closed, or failure to record the reagent strip method used
- Presence of reducing substances, such as levodopa, ascorbic acid, phenazopyridine, methyldopa, and salicylates (possible false-negative)
- Tetracyclines (false-negative)

Ketones

In the ketone test, a routine, semiquantitative screening test, a commercially prepared product is used to measure the urine level of ketone bodies. Ketone bodies are the by-products of fat metabolism; they include acetoacetic acid, acetone, and beta-hydroxybutyric acid. Excessive amounts may appear in the patient with carbohydrate dehydration, which may occur in starvation or diabetic ketoacidosis (DKA).

Commercially available tests include the Acetest tablet, Chemstrip K, Ketostix, or Keto-Diastix. Each product measures a specific ketone body. For example, Acetest

measures acetone, and Ketostix measures acetoacetic acid.

Purpose
- To screen for ketonuria
- To identify DKA and carbohydrate deprivation
- To distinguish between a diabetic and a nondiabetic coma
- To monitor control of diabetes mellitus, ketogenic weight reduction, and treatment of DKA

Patient preparation
- Explain to the patient that the ketone test evaluates fat metabolism.
- If the patient is newly diagnosed with diabetes, tell him how to perform the test.

▶ **CLINICAL ALERT** *If the patient is taking levodopa or phenazopyridine or has recently received sulfobromophthalein, use Acetest tablets because reagent strips may produce inaccurate results.*

Procedure and posttest care
- Instruct the patient to void; then give him a drink of water.
- Collect a second-voided midstream specimen about 30 minutes later.

Acetest
- Lay the tablet on a piece of white paper, and place one drop of urine on the tablet.
- Compare the tablet color (white, lavender, or purple) with the color chart after 30 seconds.

Ketostix
- Dip the reagent stick into the specimen, and remove it immediately.
- Compare the stick color (buff or purple) with the color chart after 15 seconds.
- Record the results as negative, small, moderate, or large amounts of ketones.

Keto-Diastix

- Dip the reagent strip into the specimen, and remove it immediately.
- Tap the edge of the strip against the container or a clean, dry surface to remove excess urine.
- Hold the strip horizontally to prevent mixing the chemicals from the two areas.
- Interpret each area of the strip separately. Compare the color of the ketone section (buff or purple) with the appropriate color chart after exactly 15 seconds; compare the color of the glucose section after 30 seconds.
- Ignore color changes that occur after the specified waiting periods.
- Record the results as negative or positive for small, moderate, or large amounts of ketones.

Precautions

- Test the specimen within 60 minutes after it's obtained, or you must refrigerate it.
- Allow refrigerated specimens to return to room temperature before testing.
- Don't use tablets or strips that have become discolored or darkened.

Normal findings

Normally, no ketones are present in urine.

Abnormal findings

Ketonuria may occur in uncontrolled diabetes mellitus or starvation. It also occurs as a metabolic complication of total parenteral nutrition.

Interfering factors

- Failure to keep the reagent container tightly closed to prevent absorption of light or moisture or bacterial contamination of the specimen (false-negative)
- Failure to test the specimen within 1 hour or to refrigerate it

- Levodopa, phenazopyridine, and sulfobromophthalein (false-positive results when Ketostix or Keto-Diastix is used instead of Acetest)

Acid mucopolysaccharides

The acid mucopolysaccharides test is a quantitative test that helps detect mucopolysaccharidosis, a rare disorder that may affect the skeleton, joints, liver, spleen, eye, ear, skin, teeth, and the cardiovascular, respiratory, and central nervous systems. This test measures the urine level of acid mucopolysaccharides, a group of polysaccharides or carbohydrates.

Purpose

- To diagnose mucopolysaccharidosis in infants with a family history of the disease

Patient preparation

- Explain to the parents of the infant that the acid mucopolysaccharide test helps determine the efficiency of carbohydrate metabolism.
- Inform them that they need not restrict the child's food and fluids.
- Tell the parents that the test requires urine collection for 24 hours, and instruct them on the proper way to collect the specimen at home.
- If the child is receiving therapy with heparin and must continue it, note this on the laboratory request.

Equipment

Pediatric urine collectors, 24-hour collection container, 20 ml toluene (usually obtained from the laboratory)

Procedure and posttest care

■ Collect the patient's urine over a 24-hour period, discarding the first specimen and retaining the last.

■ Add 20 ml of toluene (as a preservative) to the collection container at the start of the collection.

■ Indicate the patient's age on the laboratory request.

■ Send the specimen to the laboratory immediately after the 24-hour collection period.

■ Make sure all adhesive from the urine collector is removed from the infant's perineum.

■ Wash the area gently with soap and water, and watch for irritation.

Precautions

■ Refrigerate the specimen or place it on ice during the collection period.

Normal findings

The acid mucopolysaccharide value is expressed as milligrams of glucuronic acid divided by the amount of creatinine in the same specimen (which reflects glomerular filtration rate) to overcome irregularities in the 24-hour urine collection.

Normal acid mucopolysaccharide values for adults are less than 13.3 µg glucuronic acid/mg/creatinine/24 hours. For children, values vary with age.

Abnormal findings

Elevated acid mucopolysaccharide levels reliably indicate mucopolysaccharidosis. Supplementary quantitative analysis and detailed blood studies can identify the defective enzyme.

Interfering factors

■ Failure to collect all urine during the test period, to properly store the specimen, or to send the specimen to the laboratory immediately after the collection is completed

■ Heparin (increase)

Selected readings

Anderson, S.C., and Poulsen, K.B. *Anderson's Atlas of Hematology.* Philadelphia: Lippincott Williams & Wilkins, 2003.

Bradwell, A.R., et al. "Serum Test for Assessment of Patients with Bence-Jones Myeloma," *Lancet* 361(9356):489-91, February 2003.

Cavanaugh, B.M. *Nurse's Manual of Laboratory and Diagnostic Tests,* 4th ed. Philadelphia: F.A. Davis Co., 2003.

Goldman, L., and Ausiello, D., eds. *Cecil Textbook of Medicine,* 22nd ed. Philadelphia: W.B. Saunders Co., 2004.

Gonzalez-Arriaza, H.L., and Bostwick, J.M. "Acute Porphyrias: A Case Report and Review," *American Journal of Psychiatry* 160(3):450-59, March 2003.

Guyton, A.C., and Hall, J.E. *Textbook of Medical Physiology,* 10th ed. Philadelphia: W.B. Saunders Co., 2001.

Henry, J.B., et al. *Clinical Diagnosis and Management by Laboratory Methods,* 20th ed. Philadelphia: W.B. Saunders Co., 2001.

McClatchey, K.D. *Clinical Laboratory Medicine,* 2nd ed. Philadelphia: Lippincott Williams & Wilkins, 2002.

Pagana, K.D., and Pagana, T.J. *Mosby's Diagnostic and Laboratory Test Reference,* 6th ed. St. Louis: Mosby Year–Book, Inc. 2003.

Schnell, Z., et al. *Davis's Comprehensive Handbook of Laboratory and Diagnostic Tests with Nursing Implications.* Philadelphia: F.A. Davis Co., 2003.

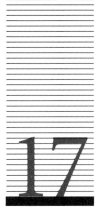

17

Urine vitamins and minerals

Introduction

Vitamins, a class of biochemical compounds essential for growth and metabolism, are classified into two groups according to their solubility. The *fat-soluble* vitamins include vitamins A, D, E, and K. The *water-soluble* group includes vitamins B$_1$ (thiamine) and B$_2$ (riboflavin), niacinamide (niacin or nicotinic acid), vitamin B$_6$ (pyroxidine), pantothenic acid, lipoic acid, folic acid, inositol, and vitamins B$_{12}$ (cyanocobalamin) and C (ascorbic acid).

Fat-soluble vitamins
Fat-soluble vitamins require bile salts and lipids for intestinal absorption; much of the amount absorbed is stored — mainly in the liver; the rest is excreted in stool. Storage of these vitamins promotes excessive accumulation; for this reason, toxicity is more common than deficiency. Because fat-soluble vitamins aren't readily excreted in the urine, serum assay is the preferred method of measuring their concentrations within the body.

419

Water-soluble vitamins

Water-soluble vitamins are present in all living cells and act primarily as coenzymes or their precursors. Because water-soluble vitamins are easily absorbed, readily excreted, and stored only briefly (or not at all), they are characteristically vulnerable to deficiency.

Deficiency may result from inadequate diet, malabsorption, chronic alcoholism, or increased metabolic demands, as occurs in stress, pregnancy, lactation, or chronic illness. When correlated with the patient's clinical features, water-soluble vitamin levels in urine help evaluate metabolic disorders, malabsorption, and nutritional deficiency. For example, the urine test for vitamin B helps detect neurologic disorders.

Minerals

Minerals are inorganic elements that are necessary for metabolism. Essential minerals — such as calcium, magnesium, and copper — participate in enzymatic catalysis directly and by binding with substrates to form metalloenzymes. Because minerals are stored in the body and tend to accumulate, toxicity is usually more common than deficiency. Minerals are classified according to their prevalence in the body: Major minerals are present in large amounts; trace elements are present in small amounts.

The following major minerals are commonly measured in the urine:

■ *Sodium* helps maintain osmotic pressure as well as water, electrolyte, and acid-base balance; with potassium, it also plays a part in transmission of nerve impulses and in muscle contractility. Sodium excretion is usually regulated by adrenocortical hormones, especially aldosterone.

■ *Chloride* helps control water, electrolyte, and acid-base balance and osmotic pressure; it's excreted mainly through the kidneys. Chloride levels usually parallel sodium levels.

■ *Potassium,* the major intracellular cation, helps maintain normal acid-base balance and neuromuscular function. Potassium excretion and concentration is regulated by the kidneys.

■ *Magnesium* activates several enzyme systems, aids cell metabolism, influences nucleic acid and protein metabolism, and enhances neuromuscular integration. Magnesium and calcium levels may be inversely related. Parathyroid hormone reduces magnesium excretion, but excessive secretion of aldosterone increases it.

■ *Calcium,* a vital component of bones and teeth, supports blood coagulation, muscle contractility, nerve impulse transmission, and cell wall permeability. It's excreted in urine as a result of excessive mobilization of bone calcium.

■ *Phosphorus* is necessary for mineralization of bones and teeth, energy metabolism, and fatty acid transport. Urine concentration of phosphorus is regulated by the renal tubules.

The following trace minerals may be measured in the urine:

■ *Iron* is needed for hemoglobin and myoglobin formation as well as cellular oxidation. It's stored in the body as hemosiderin and ferritin and is excreted in urine, stool, sweat, and menstrual flow.

■ *Copper* aids in the formation of hemoglobin and absorption of iron from the GI tract. It's a component of several enzymes for energy production and is excreted mainly in stool.

■ *Oxalate,* a salt of oxalic acid, combines with calcium in the digestive tract to form calcium oxalate, a component of urinary calculi.

DIETARY SOURCES OF VITAMINS AND MINERALS

Nutrient	Food sources
Thiamine (vitamin B₁)	Pork, liver, dried yeast, whole-grain cereals, enriched cereals, nuts, legumes, potatoes
Pyridoxine (vitamin B₆)	Dried yeast, liver, whole-grain cereals, fish, legumes
Ascorbic acid (vitamin C)	Citrus fruits, tomatoes, potatoes, cabbage, green peppers
Sodium	Table salt, beef, pork, sardines, cheese, milk, eggs
Chloride	Table salt, seafood, milk, meat, eggs
Potassium	Potatoes, dried beans, squash, scallops, veal, dried figs, cantaloupes, bananas
Calcium	Milk, milk products, meat, fish, eggs, cereals, beans, fruit, vegetables
Phosphorus	Milk, cheese, meat, poultry, fish, whole-grain cereals, nuts, legumes
Magnesium	Seafood, soybeans, nuts, cocoa, whole-grain cereals, peas, dried beans, meat, milk
Copper	Liver, shellfish, nuts, dried legumes, poultry, whole-grain cereals
Iron	Liver, meat, egg yolks, beans, clams, peaches, whole or enriched grains, legumes
Oxalic acid	Strawberries, tomatoes, rhubarb, spinach

These vitamins and minerals are found in many different foods (See *Dietary sources of vitamins and minerals.*)

Tests that determine serum or urine concentrations of vitamins and minerals help assess nutritional status and detect metabolic disorders that cause deficiency or toxicity. Less common uses include assessing the effects of I.V. therapy or therapy with megavitamins or hormonal contraceptives and monitoring the progression of debilitating diseases.

Serum analysis is generally preferred for determining mineral concentrations.

However, urine levels are more significant in some cases—for instance, in detecting primary oxalosis.

VITAMIN ASSAYS

Urine vitamin B₁

The vitamin B₁ test is used to detect a deficiency of vitamin B₁ (thiamine), a condition called beriberi. This water-soluble vitamin, which requires folic acid (folate) for effective uptake, is absorbed in the duodenum and excreted in the urine. Urine levels of vitamin B_1 reflect dietary intake and metabolic storage of thiamine. A coenzyme in decarboxylase reactions with citric acids, vitamin B_1 helps metabolize carbohydrates, fats, and proteins.

Rare in the United States, vitamin B_1 deficiency is most common in Asians because of their subsistence on polished rice. Vitamin B_1 deficiency may result from inadequate dietary intake (usually associated with alcoholism), impaired absorption (malabsorption syndrome), impaired utilization (hepatic disease), or conditions that increase metabolic demand (pregnancy, lactation, fever, exercise, hyperthyroidism, surgery, and high carbohydrate intake). High dietary intake of fats and proteins spares the vitamin B_1 necessary for tissue respiration.

The clinical effects of vitamin B_1 deficiency vary. Early deficiency produces nonspecific symptoms that may include fatigue, irritability, sleep disturbances, and abdominal and precordial discomfort. Severe deficiency states vary in several distinct patterns: Infantile beriberi produces abdominal pain, edema, irritability, vomiting, pallor and, possibly, seizures; wet, or edematous, beriberi (a complication of chronic alcoholism) produces severe neurologic symptoms — which may lead to Wernicke-Korsakoff's syndrome and Korsakoff's psychosis — emaciation, and edema that rises from the legs. Beriberi also causes arrhythmias, cardiomegaly, and circulatory collapse.

Purpose
- To help confirm vitamin B_1 deficiency (beriberi) and to distinguish it from other causes of polyneuritis

Patient preparation
- Explain to the patient that this test evaluates the body's stores of vitamin B_1.
- Tell the patient that the test requires a 24-hour urine specimen. If the patient is to collect the specimen, teach him the proper technique.
- Check the patient's diet history to rule out a deficiency due to inadequate intake.

Procedure and posttest care
- Collect a 24-hour urine specimen.
- Educate the patient who's deficient in vitamin B_1 about good dietary sources of this vitamin: beef, pork, organ meats, fresh vegetables (especially peas and beans), and wheat and other whole grains.

Precautions
- Tell the patient to save all urine voided in a 24-hour period and not to contaminate the urine specimen with toilet tissue or stool. If any urine is lost, discard the entire specimen and restart collecting with the next void.
- Refrigerate the specimen or place it on ice during the collection period.

Reference values
Normal urinary excretion ranges from 100 to 200 µg/24 hours.

Abnormal findings
Deficient urine levels of vitamin B_1 can result from inadequate dietary intake, hyperthyroidism, alcoholism, severe hepatic disease, chronic diarrhea, or prolonged diuretic therapy. Negative results indicate neuritis unrelated to deficiency.

Interfering factors
- Failure to collect all urine during the test period or to store the specimen properly

Tryptophan challenge

Measurement of urine xanthurenic acid after a challenge dose of tryptophan confirms vitamin B_6 deficiency long before symptoms appear.

Although vitamin B_6 isn't directly involved in energy metabolism, it's essential for reactions that occur in protein metabolism and for amino acid synthesis. Vitamin B_6 deficiency can cause hypochromic microcytic anemia without iron deficiency and central nervous system disturbances. When normal magnesium levels accompany a vitamin B_6 deficiency, urinary citrate and oxalate solubility may decrease, causing urinary calculi formation.

Purpose
- To detect vitamin B_6 deficiency

Patient preparation
- Explain to the patient that the tryptophan challenge test determines the body's stores of vitamin B_6.
- Tell the patient that he'll receive an oral dose of medication.
- Explain that this test requires urine collection over a 24-hour period.
- Notify the laboratory and physician of medications the patient is taking that may affect test results; they may need to be restricted.

Procedure and posttest care
- Administer L-tryptophan by mouth (usually, 50 mg/kg for children and up to 2 g/kg for adults).
- Have the patient void and discard the urine. Immediately begin collection of a 24-hour urine specimen.
- Inform the patient with vitamin B_6 deficiency that yeast, wheat, corn, liver, and kidneys are good sources of pyridoxine.
- Instruct the patient that he may resume his usual medications, as ordered.

Precautions
- Make sure the specimen bottle contains a crystal of thymol, a preservative.
- Tell the patient not to contaminate the urine specimen with toilet tissue or stool.
- Refrigerate the specimen or place it on ice during the collection period.

Normal findings
Normal excretion of xanthurenic acid after a tryptophan challenge dose is less than 50 mg/24 hours.

Abnormal findings
Urine levels of xanthurenic acid exceeding 100 mg/24 hours indicate vitamin B_6 deficiency. This rare disorder may result from malnutrition, malignancy, pregnancy, familial xanthurenic aciduria, or the use of hormonal contraceptives, hydralazine, D-penicillamine, or isoniazid.

Interfering factors
- Contamination of the specimen with toilet tissue or stool
- Failure to properly handle the specimen
- Hormonal contraceptives, hydralazine, D-penicillamine, and isoniazid (decrease)

Urine vitamin C

Through colorimetric measurement of urinary levels, the urine vitamin C test determines body stores of vitamin C (ascorbic acid). This water-soluble vitamin, which is easily absorbed by the intestine, acts as a reversible reducing agent in metabolic processes, aids collagen formation, and helps maintain connective and osteoid tissues.

This analysis is particularly useful in diagnosing scurvy, an extreme vitamin C deficiency characterized by the degeneration of connective and osteoid tissues, dentin, and endothelial membranes. Although now uncommon in North America, scurvy may occur in alcoholics, people on low-residue or low-citrus diets, and infants who have been weaned to cow's milk that doesn't contain a vitamin C supplement.

Purpose
■ To aid in the diagnosis of scurvy, scurvylike conditions, and metabolic disorders, such as malnutrition, that interfere with oxidative processes

Patient preparation
■ Explain to the patient that the urine vitamin C test detects vitamin C deficiency.
■ Inform the patient that he should maintain a normal diet.
■ Tell the patient that the test requires urine collection over a 24-hour period.
■ If the specimen is to be collected at home, instruct the patient on proper collection technique.

Procedure and posttest care
■ Collect the patient's urine over a 24-hour period, discarding the first specimen and retaining the last.
■ Advise the patient with vitamin C deficiency that citrus fruits, tomatoes, potatoes, cabbage, and strawberries are good dietary sources of vitamin C.

Precautions
■ Tell the patient not to contaminate the specimen with toilet tissue or stool.
■ Refrigerate the specimen, or place it on ice during the collection period.

Reference values
Normal urine vitamin C excretion is 30 mg/24 hours.

Abnormal findings
Depressed urine vitamin C levels are common in the patient with infection, cancer, burns, or other stress-producing conditions. Decreased vitamin C levels may also indicate malnutrition, malabsorption, renal deficiencies, or prolonged I.V. therapy without vitamin C replacement. Severe vitamin C deficiency causes scurvy.

Interfering factors
■ Improper specimen collection or storage or exposure to light
■ Contamination of the specimen with toilet tissue or stool

MINERAL ASSAYS

Urine sodium and chloride

The sodium and chloride test determines urine levels of sodium, the major extracellular cation, and of chloride, the major extracellular anion. Less significant than serum levels and, consequently, performed less frequently, the measurement of urine sodium and chloride concentrations is used to evaluate renal conservation of these two electrolytes and to confirm serum sodium and chloride values.

Normal ranges of sodium and chloride in the urine vary greatly with dietary salt intake and perspiration.

Purpose
■ To help evaluate fluid and electrolyte imbalance
■ To monitor the effects of a low-salt diet
■ To help evaluate renal and adrenal disorders

Patient preparation
- Explain to the patient that the urine sodium and chloride test helps determine the balance of salt and water in the body.
- Advise the patient that no special restrictions are necessary.
- Tell the patient that the test requires urine collection over a 24-hour period.
- If the specimen is to be collected at home, instruct the patient on proper collection technique.
- Notify the laboratory and physician of medications the patient is taking that may affect test results; they may need to be restricted.

Procedure and posttest care
- Collect the patient's urine over a 24-hour period, discarding the first specimen and retaining the last.
- Instruct the patient that he may resume his usual medications, as ordered.

Precautions
- Tell the patient not to contaminate the specimen with toilet tissue or stool.
- Tell the patient not to use a metallic bedpan for specimen collection.

Reference values
Normal urine sodium excretion in adults ranges from 40 to 220 mEq/L/24 hours (SI, 40 to 220 mmol/d); in children, it ranges from 41 to 115 mEq/L/24 hours (SI, 41 to 115 mmol/d). Normal urine chloride excretion in adults ranges from 110 to 250 nmol/24 hours (SI, 110 to 250 mmol/d); in children, from 15 to 40 nmol/24 hours (SI, 15 to 40 mmol/d); and in infants, from 2 to 10 mmol/24 hours (SI, 2 to 10 mmol/d).

Abnormal findings
Most commonly, urine sodium and urine chloride levels are parallel, rising and falling in tandem. Abnormal levels of both minerals may indicate the need for more specific testing.

Elevated urine sodium levels may reflect increased salt intake, adrenal failure, salicylate toxicity, diabetic acidosis, salt-losing nephritis, and water-deficient dehydration.

Decreased urine sodium levels suggest decreased salt intake, primary aldosteronism, acute renal failure, and heart failure.

Elevated urine chloride levels may result from water-deficient dehydration, salicylate toxicity, diabetic ketoacidosis, adrenocortical insufficiency (Addison's disease), or salt-losing renal disease. Decreased levels may result from excessive diaphoresis, heart failure, hypochloremic metabolic alkalosis, or prolonged vomiting or gastric suctioning.

To evaluate fluid-electrolyte imbalance, results must be correlated with findings of serum electrolyte studies.

Interfering factors
- Failure to collect all urine during the test period
- Sodium bicarbonate and thiazide diuretics (increase in sodium)
- Steroids (decrease in sodium)
- Ammonium chloride and potassium chloride (increase in chloride)

Urine potassium

The urine potassium test is a quantitative test that measures urine levels of potassium, a major intracellular cation that helps regulate acid-base balance and neuromuscular function. Potassium imbalance may cause such signs and symptoms as muscle weakness, nausea, diarrhea, confusion, hypotension, and electrocardiogram changes; severe imbalance may lead to cardiac arrest.

Most commonly, a serum potassium test is performed to detect hyperkalemia (abnormally high levels) or hypokalemia (abnormally low levels). A urine potassium test may be performed to evaluate hypokalemia when a history and physical examination fail to uncover the cause. If results suggest a renal disorder, additional renal function tests may be ordered.

Purpose
■ To determine whether hypokalemia is caused by renal or extrarenal disorders

Patient preparation
■ Explain to the patient that the urine potassium test evaluates his kidney function.
■ Advise the patient that no special dietary restrictions are necessary.
■ Tell the patient that the test requires urine collection over a 24-hour period.
■ If the specimen is to be collected at home, teach the patient the correct collection technique.
■ Notify the laboratory and physician of medications the patient is taking that may affect test results; they may need to be restricted.

Procedure and posttest care
■ Collect the patient's urine over a 24-hour period, discarding the first specimen and retaining the last.
■ Administer potassium supplements and monitor serum levels as appropriate.
■ Provide dietary supplements and nutritional counseling as necessary.
■ Replace fluid volume loss with I.V. or oral fluids as necessary.
■ Instruct the patient that he may resume his usual medications, as ordered.
■ Don't use a metallic bedpan for collection.

Precautions
■ Tell the patient not to contaminate the specimen with toilet tissue or stool.
■ Refrigerate the specimen, or place it on ice during the collection period.
■ Send the specimen to the laboratory immediately after the collection is completed, or refrigerate it.

Reference values
Normal potassium excretion in adults is 25 to 125 mmol/24 hours (SI, 25 to 125 mmol/d) and varies with diet. In children, normal excretion is 22 to 57 mmol/24 hours (SI, 22 to 57 mmol/d).

Abnormal findings
In a patient with hypokalemia, potassium concentration less than 10 mmol/24 hours (SI, <10 mmol/d) suggests normal renal function, indicating that potassium loss is most likely the result of a GI disorder such as malabsorption syndrome.

In a patient with hypokalemia lasting more than 3 days, urine potassium concentration above 10 mmol/24 hours (SI, >10 mmol/d) indicates renal loss of potassium. These losses may result from such disorders as aldosteronism, renal tubular acidosis, or chronic renal failure. However, extrarenal disorders, such as dehydration, starvation, Cushing's disease, or salicylate intoxication, may also elevate urine potassium levels.

Interfering factors
■ Excess dietary potassium (increase)
■ Contamination of the specimen with toilet tissue or stool
■ Failure to collect all urine and send the specimen to the laboratory immediately after collection or to refrigerate it

- Potassium-wasting medications, such as ammonium chloride, thiazide diuretics, and acetazolamide (increase)
- Excess vomiting or stomach suctioning

Urine calcium and phosphates

The calcium and phosphates test measures the urine levels of calcium and phosphates, elements essential for bone formation and resorption. Urine calcium and phosphate levels generally parallel serum levels.

Normally absorbed in the upper intestine and excreted in stool and urine, calcium and phosphates help maintain tissue and fluid pH, electrolyte balance in cells and extracellular fluids, and permeability of cell membranes. Calcium promotes enzymatic processes, aids blood coagulation, and lowers neuromuscular irritability; phosphates aid carbohydrate metabolism.

Purpose
- To evaluate calcium and phosphate metabolism and excretion
- To monitor treatment of calcium or phosphate deficiency

Patient preparation
- Explain to the patient that the urine calcium and phosphates test measures the amount of calcium and phosphates in the urine.
- Encourage the patient to be as active as possible before the test.
- Tell the patient that the test requires urine collection over a 24-hour period. If the patient is to collect the specimen, teach him the proper technique.
- Provide a diet that contains about 130 mg of calcium/24 hours for 3 days

before the test or provide a copy of the diet for the patient to follow at home.
- Notify the laboratory and physician of medications the patient is taking that may affect test results; they may need to be restricted.

Procedure and posttest care
- Collect the patient's urine over a 24-hour period, discarding the first specimen and retaining the last.
- Observe the patient with low urine calcium levels for tetany.
- Inform the patient that he may resume his usual diet, activities, and medications, as ordered.

Precautions
- Tell the patient not to contaminate the specimen with toilet tissue or stool.

Reference values
Normal values depend on dietary intake. For a normal diet, urine calcium levels for a 24-hour period range from 100 to 300 mg/24 hours (SI, 2.5 to 7.5 mmol/d). Normal excretion of phosphate is less than 1,000 mg/24 hours.

Abnormal findings
Many disorders may affect calcium and phosphorus levels. (See *Disorders that affect urine calcium and urine phosphorus levels,* page 428.)

Interfering factors
- Failure to collect all urine during the test period
- Parathyroid hormones (increase phosphates excretion and decrease calcium excretion)
- Thiazide diuretics (decreases calcium excretion)

DISORDERS THAT AFFECT URINE CALCIUM AND URINE PHOSPHORUS LEVELS

Disorder	Urine calcium level	Urine phosphate level
Hyperparathyroidism	Elevated	Elevated
Vitamin D intoxication	Elevated	Suppressed
Metastatic carcinoma	Elevated	Normal
Sarcoidosis	Elevated	Suppressed
Renal tubular acidosis	Elevated	Elevated
Multiple myeloma	Elevated or normal	Elevated or normal
Paget's disease	Normal	Normal
Milk-alkali syndrome	Suppressed or normal	Suppressed or normal
Hypoparathyroidism	Suppressed	Suppressed
Acute nephrosis	Suppressed	Suppressed or normal
Chronic nephrosis	Suppressed	Suppressed
Acute nephritis	Suppressed	Suppressed
Renal insufficiency	Suppressed	Suppressed
Osteomalacia	Suppressed	Suppressed
Steatorrhea	Suppressed	Suppressed

- Prolonged inactivity and ingestion of corticosteroids, sodium phosphate, calcitonin (increases calcium excretion)
- Vitamin D (increases phosphate absorption and excretion)

Urine magnesium

Measurement of urine magnesium is especially useful because magnesium deficiency is detectable in urine before it changes serum magnesium levels. This test may be used to rule out magnesium deficiency as the cause of neurologic symptoms and to help evaluate glomerular function in suspected renal disease.

Magnesium is a cation found primarily in the bones and in intracellular fluid; a small amount is present in extracellular fluid. This element activates many enzyme systems, helps transport sodium and potassium across cell membranes, affects nucleic acid and protein metabolism, and influences intracellular calcium levels through its effect on parathyroid hormone secretion.

Purpose
- To rule out magnesium deficiency in the patient with symptoms of central nervous system irritation
- To detect excessive urinary excretion of magnesium
- To help evaluate glomerular function in renal disease

Patient preparation
- Explain to the patient that the urine magnesium test determines urine magnesium levels.
- Tell the patient that this test requires urine collection over a 24-hour period.
- Notify the laboratory and physician of medications the patient is taking that may affect test results; they may need to be restricted.

Procedure and posttest care
- Collect the patient's urine over a 24-hour period, discarding the first specimen and retaining the last.
- Inform the patient that he may resume his usual medications, as ordered.

Precautions
- Tell the patient to be careful not to contaminate the urine specimen with toilet tissue or stool.
- Tell the patient not to use a metallic bedpan for collection.

Reference values
Normal urinary excretion of magnesium is 6 to 10 mEq/24 hours (SI, 3 to 5 mmol/d).

Abnormal findings
Low urine magnesium levels may result from malabsorption, acute or chronic diarrhea, diabetic ketoacidosis, dehydration, pancreatitis, advanced renal failure, and primary aldosteronism. They may

also result from decreased dietary intake of magnesium.

Elevated urine magnesium levels may result from early chronic renal disease, adrenocortical insufficiency (Addison's disease), chronic alcoholism, or chronic ingestion of magnesium-containing antacids.

Interfering factors
- Failure to collect all urine during the test period
- Spirolactone (decrease)
- Increased calcium intake (decrease)
- Magnesium-containing antacids, ethacrynic acid, thiazide diuretics, and aldosterone (possible increase)

Urine copper

The copper test measures the urine level of copper, an essential trace element and a component of several metalloenzymes and proteins necessary for hemoglobin synthesis and oxidation reduction. Most copper in plasma is bound to and transported by an $alpha_2$-globulin (plasma protein) called ceruloplasmin. When copper is unbound, the ions can inhibit many enzyme reactions, resulting in copper toxicity. Urine normally contains only a small amount of free copper.

Determination of urine copper levels is frequently used to detect Wilson's disease, a rare, inborn metabolic error most common among people of eastern European Jewish, southern Italian, or Sicilian ancestry.

Purpose
- To help detect Wilson's disease, chronic active hepatitis, or environmental exposure
- To screen infants with family histories of Wilson's disease

Patient preparation

■ Explain to the patient that the urine copper test determines the amount of copper in urine.
■ Inform the patient that no special restrictions are necessary.
■ Tell the patient that the test requires urine collection over a 24-hour period. If the specimen is to be collected at home, describe the proper collection technique.
■ Notify the laboratory and physician of medications the patient is taking that may affect test results; they may need to be restricted.

Procedure and posttest care

■ Collect the patient's urine over a 24-hour period, discarding the first specimen and retaining the last, using no preservatives.
■ Refrigerate the specimen during the collection period.
■ Instruct the patient that he may resume his usual medications, as ordered.

Precautions

■ Tell the patient not to contaminate the urine specimen with toilet tissue or stool.

Reference values

Normal urinary excretion of copper is 3 to 35 µg/24 hours (SI, 0.05 to 0.55 µmol/d).

Abnormal findings

Elevated urine copper levels usually indicate Wilson's disease (a liver biopsy helps establish this diagnosis), which is marked by decreased ceruloplasmin, increased urinary excretion of copper, and accumulation of copper in the interstitial tissues of the liver and brain. Early detection and treatment (low-copper diet and D-penicillamine) are vital to prevent irreversible changes, such as nerve tissue degeneration and cirrhosis of the liver.

Elevated copper levels may also occur in nephrotic syndromes, chronic active hepatitis, biliary cirrhosis, and rheumatoid arthritis.

Interfering factors

■ D-penicillamine (increase)
■ Failure to collect all urine during the test period and to refrigerate the specimen

Urine hemosiderin

The test for hemosiderin measures the urine level of hemosiderin — a colloidal iron oxide and one of the two forms of iron that are stored and deposited in body tissue.

When iron storage mechanisms fail to manage iron overload, excess iron may escape to cells unaccustomed to high iron concentrations and may produce toxic effects. Toxicity may affect the liver, myocardium, bone marrow, pancreas, kidneys, and skin. Subsequent tissue damage is referred to as hemochromatosis. Hemochromatosis may occur in a rare hereditary form (primary hemochromatosis) and in exogenous forms.

Purpose

■ To aid in the diagnosis of hemochromatosis, hemolytic anemia associated with intravascular hemolysis

Patient preparation

■ Explain to the patient that the urine hemosiderin test helps determine if the body is accumulating excessive amounts of iron.
■ Inform the patient that no restrictions are necessary and that the test requires a urine specimen.

Procedure and posttest care
■ Collect a random urine specimen of approximately 30 ml, preferably the first void of the morning.

Precautions
■ Seal the container securely, and send the specimen to the laboratory immediately after collection.

Normal findings
Normally, hemosiderin isn't found in urine.

Abnormal findings
The presence of hemosiderin, appearing as yellow-brown granules in urinary sediment, indicates hemochromatosis; liver or bone marrow biopsy is necessary to confirm primary hemochromatosis. Hemosiderin may also suggest pernicious anemia, chronic hemolytic anemia, multiple blood transfusions, and paroxysmal nocturnal hemoglobinuria, the result of excessive iron injections or dietary iron intake.

Interfering factors
■ Failure to send the specimen to the laboratory immediately after collection

Urine oxalate

Oxalate, a salt of oxalic acid, is an end product of metabolism and is excreted almost exclusively in the urine. Measuring urine levels of oxalate detects hyperoxaluria, a disorder in which oxalate accumulates in the soft and connective tissue, especially in the kidneys and bladder, causing chronic inflammation and fibrosis. Calcium oxalate deposits are the most common cause of renal calculi, which may produce kidney damage.

Purpose
■ To detect primary hyperoxaluria in infants
■ To rule out hyperoxaluria in renal insufficiency

Patient preparation
■ Explain to the patient (or to the parents if the patient is a child) that the urine oxalate test determines if the urine contains excess oxalate.
■ Tell the patient or parents that the test requires urine collection over a 24-hour period.
■ Tell the patient to avoid foods high in oxalate — such as tomatoes, strawberries, rhubarb, and spinach — for 1 week before the test.

Procedure and posttest care
■ Collect the patient's urine over a 24-hour period, discarding first specimen and retaining the last. Use a light-protected container with 30 ml of 6 N hydrochloric acid.
■ Inform the patient that he may resume his usual diet.

Precautions
■ Tell the patient not to urinate directly into the 24-hour specimen container, but to use an appropriate container.
■ Advise the patient not to contaminate the urine specimen with toilet tissue or stool.
■ Keep in mind that oxalate in acidified urine is stable for up to 7 days at room temperature or when refrigerated at 35.6° to 46.4° F (2° to 8° C)

Reference values
Normal urine oxalate levels are less than or equal to 40 mg/24 hours (SI, ≤ 456 μmol/d).

Abnormal findings

Elevated urine oxalate levels (hyperoxaluria) may result from excessive metabolic production of oxalate or increased oxalate intake. Levels as high as 400 mg/24 hours (SI, 4,560 μmol/d) can occur.

Primary hyperoxaluria, a rare inborn metabolic disorder, causes excessive production and urinary excretion of oxalate. In this type of hyperoxaluria, urine oxalate levels become elevated before serum levels become elevated.

Secondary hyperoxaluria can result from pancreatic insufficiency, diabetes mellitus, cirrhosis, pyridoxine deficiency, Crohn's disease, ileal resection, or ingestion of antifreeze (ethylene glycol) or stain remover or it can occur as a reaction to a methoxyflurane anesthetic.

Interfering factors

- Tomatoes, strawberries, rhubarb, and spinach (possible false increase)
- Vitamin C (increase in oxalate excretion, which may be a risk for calcium oxalate nephrolithiasis in individuals consuming megadoses of this vitamin)
- Failure to collect all urine during the test period or properly store the specimen

Selected readings

Anderson, S.C., and Poulsen, K.B. *Anderson's Atlas of Hematology.* Philadelphia: Lippincott Williams & Wilkins, 2003.

Cavanaugh, B.M. *Nurse's Manual of Laboratory and Diagnostic Tests,* 4th ed. Philadelphia: F.A. Davis Co., 2003.

Elisaf, M. "Effects of Fibrate on Serum Metabolic Parameters," *Current Medical Research and Opinion* 18(5):269-76, August 2002.

Goldman, L., and Ausiello, D., eds. *Cecil Textbook of Medicine,* 22nd ed. Philadelphia: W.B. Saunders Co., 2004.

Guyton, A.C., and Hall, J.E. *Textbook of Medical Physiology,* 10th ed. Philadelphia: W.B. Saunders Co., 2001.

Henry, J.B., et al. *Clinical Diagnosis and Management by Laboratory Methods,* 20th ed. Philadelphia: W.B. Saunders Co., 2001.

McClatchey, K.D. *Clinical Laboratory Medicine,* 2nd ed. Philadelphia: Lippincott Williams & Wilkins, 2002.

Pagana, K.D., and Pagana, T.J. *Mosby's Diagnostic and Laboratory Test Reference,* 6th ed. St. Louis: Mosby Year–Book, Inc., 2003.

Schnell, Z., et al. *Davis's Comprehensive Handbook of Laboratory and Diagnostic Tests with Nursing Implications.* Philadelphia: F.A. Davis Co., 2003.

SECTION III.
HISTOLOGIC
AND
MICROBIOLOGIC
TESTS

18

Histology

Introduction

Histology, the study of the microscopic structure of tissues and cells, is vital to confirm malignant disease and has made biopsy — extraction of a living tissue specimen — a common procedure. New tissue preparation techniques and needle designs have made biopsy more accessible — even allowing rapid specimen removal from deep tissues without surgery.

Accurate histologic diagnosis requires a representative or complete tissue specimen, procured with good technique to prevent damage; proper specimen handling and storage, usually in a fixative; and knowledge of the tissue's origin, the suspected diagnosis, previous biopsies at the site, and any current treatments.

Types of biopsy

In *incisional biopsy*, a scalpel, a cutting or aspiration needle, or a punch is used to remove a portion of tissue from large, multiple, hidden lesions. Fine-needle aspiration differs slightly from traditional needle biopsy. It provides a smaller specimen, requires cytologic (not histologic) studies, and is usually performed on outpatients for breast biopsies. Incision of a hidden lesion is called a closed, or blind, biopsy. In *excisional biopsy,* a scalpel is used to remove abnormal tissue from the skin or subcutaneous tissue. A brush biopsy is used to obtain tissue samples from the urinary system.

When such tissue can be easily and completely removed, excisional biopsy is preferred because it combines diagnosis and treatment. (For more information, see *Common types of tissue biopsy,* pages 436 and 437.)

A biopsy is commonly performed in a physician's office or an outpatient surgical clinic; when the patient is already hospitalized, it's performed at the bedside or in a treatment room. It can also be done in the operating room, using open technique. An open biopsy is usually performed if results of a closed biopsy or other tests suggest the need for complete excision of a tissue mass. During open biopsy, a tissue specimen is obtained (usually under general anesthesia) and sent immediately to the histology laboratory for rapid analysis. Test results are relayed to the operating room, and a decision is made about subsequent surgery.

Tissue preparation critical

Because a decomposed tissue specimen is diagnostically useless, fixation — a process that arrests cellular structures and prevents decomposition — is very important in slide preparation. Inadequately fixed tissue breaks down immediately after removal from the body, losing one or more components. To prevent this, biopsy specimens are placed immediately in fixing fluid to kill and harden the tissue and

make it resistant to damage by reagents used to process it for microscopic study. The most common fixative solution is 10% neutral buffered formaldehyde; however, some laboratories require different fixatives and procedures for specimen fixation.

Temperature also influences specimen preservation: Cold slows decomposition, and heat speeds it. If a fixative isn't immediately available, temporarily refrigerating the specimen prevents deterioration. However, even a refrigerated specimen deteriorates significantly after 24 hours.

When a tissue specimen arrives in the histology department, a histologist numbers and labels it and a pathologist examines it, recording its weight, length, width, color, contents, unusual markings, and hollowness. After sectioning, the pathologist selects representative cuts of tissue and places them in numbered capsules for processing. To prevent tissue loss in processing, small pieces of tissue, such as those obtained from needle biopsies or curettage, are placed in embedding bags, wrapped in lens paper, or placed between wet sponges before being inserted in the capsules. A histologist then places the capsules in an automatic processor that moves them through a fixing fluid, through ascending strengths of dehydrating fluids, through a clearing fluid, and finally, into melted paraffin, which infiltrates the tissue. This procedure generally takes place overnight.

After processing, the tissue, now embedded in paraffin, is ready for cutting and staining. Special stains color various cellular components and permit identification. One stain that's used routinely — hematoxylin-eosin stain — is an example of this: Hematoxylin stains the nucleus, while eosin stains the cytoplasm. After staining, the histologist seals the tissues

COMMON TYPES OF TISSUE BIOPSY

Biopsy type and target tissue	Equipment

Excision
Surgical removal of entire lesion from any tissue; may be excised under local anesthetic

Scalpel

Shaving
Tissue shaved from raised surface lesion on the skin

Scalpel

Needle
Removal of a core of tissue from bone, bone marrow, breast, lung, pleura, lymph node, liver, kidney, prostate, synovial membrane, or thyroid

Cutting needle (such as Cope's needle or Vim-Silverman needle)

Aspiration
Aspiration of tissue sample from bone marrow or breast

Flexible or fine aspiration needle, needle guide, and aspiration syringe

Punch incision
Removal of tissue specimen from core of lesion in skin or cervix

Punch (such as Tischler forceps)

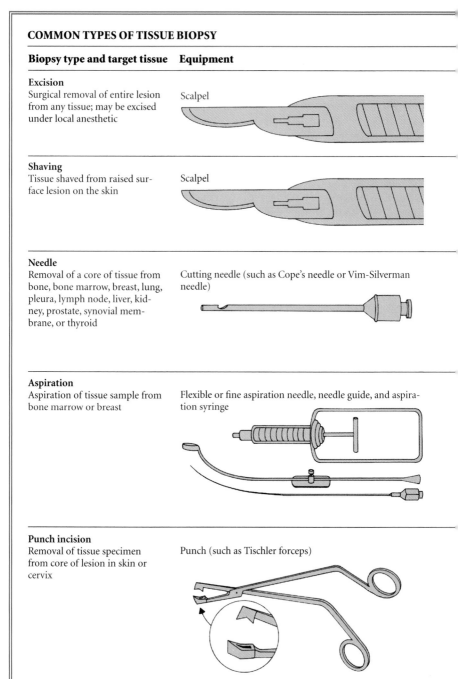

Advantages and disadvantages

- *Advantage:* combines diagnosis and treatment of lesion
- *Disadvantage:* may require major surgery under general anesthesia

---

- *Advantages:* generally safe; combines diagnosis and treatment of benign lesion; yields good cosmetic results
- *Disadvantages:* may require excision or other treatment if lesion is malignant; may cause seeding of malignant cells

---

- *Advantages:* avoids need for surgery; usually furnishes a representative specimen; preserves cell architecture
- *Disadvantages:* may require excision or other treatment based on histologic results; may be traumatic to surrounding tissues; may not furnish a representative specimen; may cause seeding of malignant cells

---

- *Advantages:* avoids need for surgery; aspiration of fluid from a breast cyst combines diagnosis and treatment; fine-needle aspiration causes less pain and can be done on outpatients
- *Disadvantages:* disturbs cell architecture; permits study of individual cells but not of intercellular structure; may not furnish a representative specimen; may cause seeding of malignant cells (less likely with fine-needle aspiration)

- *Advantages:* avoids need for surgery; furnishes a representative specimen
- *Disadvantages:* may cause seeding of malignant cells when part of mass is removed; may require excision or other treatment based on histologic results

---

under labeled coverslips and delivers them to the pathologist for diagnosis. Because of these preparations, a stat tissue report generally takes 24 hours.

Rapid analysis: Frozen sections

Frozen sections, an alternative method of preparing tissue for study, permit rapid, accurate analysis of potentially malignant tissue during surgery. In this method, an individual tissue specimen is sent directly from the operating room to the histology department, where a pathologist grossly examines the tissue, sections it, and selects a representative section for quick freezing. Freezing fixes the tissue, hardening it to allow cutting into microscopic sections. After rapid staining, the pathologist analyzes the tissue for malignant cells and tissue margins, which indicate adequate excision, and reports findings to the surgeon, who then closes the wound or further excises malignant tissue.

Generally, this technique allows pathologic diagnosis within 10 to 15 minutes after excision. Results from frozen section analysis are usually reliable, but standard analysis on tissue from the same specimen must verify the diagnosis. Frozen sections can eliminate the need for two separate surgical and anesthetic procedures (one for biopsy, the second for treatment) and spare the patient the anxiety of waiting for the biopsy report.

GLAND BIOPSIES

Breast biopsy

Breast biopsy is performed to confirm or rule out breast cancer after clinical examination, mammography, or thermography has identified a mass. Fine-needle or nee-

BRCA TESTING

Recently, genetic researchers located two genes, BRCA1 and BRCA2, that have been linked to certain forms of breast cancer. BRCA testing can detect the presence of BRCA gene mutations, which may increase an individual's susceptibility to some breast cancers.

The test, performed on a blood sample, is available for a woman with a family history of breast cancer. Controversy continues over whether BRCA testing should be made available to the general public.

Purpose
- To differentiate between benign and malignant breast tumors

Patient preparation
- Describe the procedure to the patient, and explain that this test permits microscopic examination of a breast tissue specimen. Offer her emotional support, and assure her that breast masses don't always indicate cancer.
- If the patient is to receive a local anesthetic, tell her that she need not restrict food, fluids, and medication.
- If the patient is to receive a general anesthetic, advise her to fast from midnight before the test until after the biopsy.
- Tell the patient who will perform the biopsy and where it will be done.
- Explain that pretest studies, such as blood tests, urine tests, and chest X-rays, may be required.
- Make sure the patient or a responsible family member has signed an informed consent form.
- Check the patient's history for hypersensitivity to anesthetics.

Procedure and posttest care
Needle biopsy
- Instruct the patient to undress to the waist, and guide her to a sitting or recumbent position with her hands at her sides, reminding her to remain still.
- The biopsy site is prepared, a local anesthetic is administered, and the syringe (luer-lock syringe for aspiration, Vim-Silverman needle for tissue specimen) is introduced into the lesion.
- Fluid aspirated from the breast is expelled into a properly labeled, heparinized tub; the tissue specimen is placed in a labeled specimen bottle containing normal saline solution or formalin.

dle biopsy is usually done on a mass that has been identified by ultrasonography as being fluid-filled. Both methods have limited diagnostic value because of the small and perhaps unrepresentative specimens they provide. Open biopsy provides complete tissue system, which can be sectioned to allow more accurate evaluation. Local anesthesia can usually be given to outpatients for these three techniques. Stereotactic breast biopsy immobilizes the breast and allows the computer to calculate the exact location of the mass based on X-rays from two angles.

An excisional biopsy may be done under general anesthesia. If sufficient tissue is obtained and the mass is found to be a malignant tumor, specimens are sent for estrogen and progesterone receptor assays to assist in determining future therapy and the prognosis.

Because breast cancer remains the most prevalent cancer in women, genetic researchers are continually working to identify women at risk. (See *BRCA testing.*)

- With fine-needle aspiration, a slide is made for cytology and viewed immediately under a microscope.
- Pressure is exerted on the biopsy site and, after bleeding stops, an adhesive bandage is applied. Because breast fluid aspiration isn't considered diagnostically accurate, some physicians aspirate fluid only from cysts. If such fluid is clear yellow and the mass disappears, the aspiration procedure is diagnostic and therapeutic, and the aspirate is discarded. If aspiration yields no fluid or if the lesion recurs two or three times, an open biopsy is then considered appropriate.

Open biopsy
- After the patient receives a general or local anesthetic, an incision is made in the breast to expose the mass.
- The examiner may then incise a portion of tissue or excise the entire mass. If the mass is smaller than ¾″ (2 cm) in diameter and appears benign, it's usually excised; if it's larger or appears malignant, a specimen is usually incised before the mass is excised. Incisional biopsy generally provides an adequate specimen for histologic analysis.
- The specimen is placed in a properly labeled specimen bottle containing 10% formalin solution. Tissue that appears malignant is sent for frozen section and receptor assays. Receptor assay specimens must not be placed in the formalin solution.
- The wound is sutured, and an adhesive bandage applied.

All procedures
- If the patient has received a general or local anesthetic, check the patient's vital signs, and provide medication for pain. If she has received a general anesthetic, check her vital signs every 15 minutes for

1 hour, every 30 minutes for 2 hours, every hour for the next 4 hours, and then every 4 hours.
- Administer an analgesic, as ordered. An ice bag may provide comfort. Instruct the patient to wear a support bra at all times until healing is complete.
- Watch for and report bleeding, tenderness, and redness at the biopsy site.
- Provide emotional support to the patient who's awaiting diagnosis.

Precautions
- Open breast biopsy is contraindicated in the patient with a condition that precludes surgery.
- Send the specimen to the laboratory immediately.

Normal findings
Normally, breast tissue consists of cellular and noncellular connective tissue, fat lobules, and various lactiferous ducts. It's pink, more fatty than fibrous, and shows no abnormal development of cells or tissue elements.

Abnormal findings
Abnormal breast tissue may exhibit a wide range of malignant or benign pathology. Breast tumors are common in women and account for 32% of female cancers; such tumors are rare in men (0.2% of male cancers). Benign tumors include fibrocystic disease, adenofibroma, intraductal papilloma, mammary fat necrosis, and plasma cell mastitis (mammary duct ectasia). Malignant tumors include adenocarcinoma, cystosarcoma, intraductal carcinoma, infiltrating carcinoma, inflammatory carcinoma, medullary or circumscribed carcinoma, colloid carcinoma, lobular carcinoma, sarcoma, and Paget's disease.

The receptor assays evaluate tumors for estrogen and progesterone protein and assign a positive or negative value to the estrogen and progesterone receptors. This positive or negative value assists in the prognosis and treatment of breast cancer.

Interfering factors
- Failure to obtain an adequate tissue specimen
- Failure to place the specimen in the proper solution and to send it to the laboratory immediately

Prostate gland biopsy

Prostate gland biopsy is the needle excision of a prostate tissue specimen for histologic examination. Indications include potentially malignant prostatic hypertrophy and prostatic nodules. A perineal, transrectal, or transurethral approach may be used — the transrectal approach is used for high prostatic lesions.

Purpose
- To confirm prostate cancer
- To determine the cause of prostatic hyperplasia

Patient preparation
- Describe the procedure to the patient, answer his questions, and tell him that the test provides a tissue specimen for microscopic study.
- Tell the patient who will perform the biopsy, where it will be done, and that he'll receive a local anesthetic.
- Make sure the patient or a responsible family member has signed an informed consent form.
- Check the patient's history for hypersensitivity to the anesthetic or other drugs.

- For a transrectal approach, administer enemas until the return is clear and administer an antibacterial agent to minimize the risk of infection. This approach may be performed on an outpatient without an anesthetic.
- Just before the biopsy, check the patient's vital signs and administer a sedative.
- Administer a prophylactic antibiotic, as ordered.
- Instruct the patient to remain still during the procedure and to follow instructions.

Procedure and posttest care
Perineal approach
- Place the patient in the proper position (left lateral, knee-chest, or lithotomy), and clean the perineal skin.
- After the local anesthetic is administered, a 2-mm incision may be made into the perineum.
- The examiner immobilizes the prostate by inserting a finger into the rectum and introduces the biopsy needle into a prostate lobe. The needle is rotated gently, pulled out about 5 mm, and reinserted at another angle. The procedure is repeated at several areas.
- Pressure is exerted on the puncture site, which is then bandaged.

Transrectal approach
- Place the patient in the left lateral position.
- A digital rectal examination is performed before an ultrasound probe is inserted. A curved needle guide is attached to the finger palpating the rectum. The biopsy needle is pushed along the guide into the prostate that was localized by ultrasonography.
- As the needle enters the prostate, the patient may experience pain. The needle

is rotated to cut off the tissue and is then withdrawn.

■ An alternative method of transrectal detection is the automated cone biopsy, in which the physician uses a spring-powered device with an inner trocar needle to cut through prostatic tissue. This technique is quick and reportedly painless.

Transurethral approach

■ An endoscopic instrument is passed through the urethra, permitting direct viewing of the prostate and passage of a cutting loop.
■ The loop is rotated to obtain tissue and then withdrawn.

All approaches

■ The specimen is placed immediately in a labeled specimen bottle containing 10% formalin solution and sent to the laboratory for analysis.
■ Check the patient's vital signs immediately after the procedure, every 2 hours for 4 hours, and then every 4 hours.
■ Observe the biopsy site for hematoma and for signs and symptoms of infection, such as redness, swelling, and pain. Watch for urine retention, urinary frequency, and hematuria.

Precautions

■ Complications may include transient, painless hematuria and bleeding into the prostatic urethra and bladder.

Normal findings

Normally, the prostate gland consists of a thin, fibrous capsule surrounding the stroma, which is made up of elastic and connective tissues and smooth-muscle fibers. The epithelial glands found in these tissues and muscle fibers drain into the chief excreting ducts.

Abnormal findings

Histologic examination can confirm cancer. Further tests — bone scans, bone marrow biopsy, tests for prostate-specific antigen, and serum acid phosphatase and prostatic acid phosphatase determinations — identify the extent of the cancer. Acid phosphatase levels usually rise in metastatic prostatic carcinoma; they tend to be low in carcinoma that's confined to the prostatic capsule.

Histologic examination can also be used to detect benign prostatic hyperplasia, prostatitis, tuberculosis, lymphomas, and rectal or bladder cancer.

Interfering factors

■ Failure to obtain an adequate tissue specimen
■ Failure to place the specimen in formalin

Thyroid biopsy

Thyroid biopsy is the excision of a thyroid tissue specimen for histologic examination. This procedure is indicated in patients with thyroid enlargement or nodules (even if serum triiodothyronine [T_3] and thyroxine [T_4] levels are normal), breathing and swallowing difficulties, vocal cord paralysis, weight loss, hemoptysis, and a sensation of fullness in the neck. It's commonly performed when noninvasive tests, such as thyroid ultrasonography and scans, are abnormal or inconclusive. Coagulation studies should always precede thyroid biopsy.

Thyroid tissue may be obtained with a hollow needle under local anesthesia or during open (surgical) biopsy under general anesthesia. Fine-needle aspiration with a cytologic smear examination can aid in diagnosis and replace an open biopsy. Open biopsy, performed in the operating room, provides more information than needle biopsy; it also permits direct examination and immediate excision of suspicious tissue.

Purpose

- To differentiate between benign and malignant thyroid disease
- To help diagnose Hashimoto's disease, hyperthyroidism, and nontoxic nodular goiter

Patient preparation

- Describe the procedure to the patient, and answer his questions.
- Explain that this test permits microscopic examination of a thyroid tissue specimen.
- Inform the patient that he need not restrict food and fluids (unless he receives a general anesthetic).
- Tell the patient who will perform the biopsy and where it will be done.
- Make sure the patient or a responsible family member has signed an informed consent form.
- Check the patient's history for hypersensitivity to anesthetics or analgesics.
- Tell the patient that he'll receive a local anesthetic to minimize pain during the procedure but may experience some pressure when the tissue specimen is procured.
- Check the results of the patient's coagulation studies, and make sure they're in his chart.
- Advise the patient that he may have a sore throat the day after the test.
- Administer a sedative to the patient 15 minutes before biopsy.

Procedure and posttest care

- For needle biopsy, place the patient in the supine position with a pillow under his shoulder blades. (This position pushes the trachea and thyroid forward and allows the neck veins to fall backward.)
- Prepare the skin over the biopsy site.
- As the examiner prepares to inject the local anesthetic, warn the patient not to swallow.
- After the anesthetic is injected, the carotid artery is palpated and the biopsy needle is inserted parallel to the thyroid cartilage to prevent damage to the deep structures and the larynx.
- When the specimen is obtained, the needle is removed and the specimen is placed in formalin immediately.
- Apply pressure to the biopsy site to stop bleeding. If bleeding continues for more than a few minutes, press on the site for up to an additional 15 minutes. Apply an adhesive bandage. (Bleeding may persist in a patient with a prolonged prothrombin time [PT] or partial thromboplastin time [PTT] or in a patient with a large, vascular thyroid with distended veins.)
- To make the patient more comfortable, place him in the semi-Fowler position; tell him to avoid straining the biopsy site by putting both hands behind his neck when he sits up.
- Watch for tenderness or redness, and report signs of bleeding at the biopsy site immediately. Check the back of the patient's neck and his pillow for bleeding every hour for 8 hours. Observe for difficult breathing due to edema or hematoma, with resultant tracheal collapse.
- Keep the biopsy site clean and dry.

Precautions

- Thyroid biopsy should be used cautiously in the patient with coagulation defects, as indicated by a prolonged PT or PTT.

- The specimen must be placed immediately in formalin solution because cell breakdown in the tissue specimen begins immediately after excision.

Normal findings

Histologic examination of normal tissue shows fibrous networks dividing the gland into pseudolobules that are made up of follicles and capillaries. Cuboidal epithelium lines the follicle walls and contains the protein thyroglobulin, which stores T_4 and T_3.

Abnormal findings

Malignant tumors appear as well-encapsulated, solitary nodules of uniform but abnormal structure. Papillary carcinoma is the most common thyroid cancer. Follicular carcinoma, a less common form, strongly resembles normal cells.

Benign tumors, such as nontoxic nodular goiter, demonstrate hypertrophy, hyperplasia, and hypervascularity. Distinct histologic patterns characterize subacute granulomatous thyroiditis, Hashimoto's thyroiditis, and hyperthyroidism.

Because thyroid tumors are usually multicentric and small, a negative histologic report doesn't rule out cancer.

Interfering factors

- Failure to obtain a representative tissue specimen
- Failure to place the specimen in formalin solution immediately

Lymph node biopsy

Lymph node biopsy is the surgical excision of an active lymph node or the needle aspiration of a nodal specimen for histologic examination. Both techniques usually use a local anesthetic and sample the superficial nodes in the cervical, supraclavicular, axillary, or inguinal region. Excision is preferred because it yields a larger specimen.

Although lymph nodes swell during infection, biopsy is indicated when nodal enlargement is prolonged and accompanied by backache, leg edema, breathing and swallowing difficulties and, later, weight loss, weakness, severe itching, fever, night sweats, cough, hemoptysis, and hoarseness. Generalized or localized lymph node enlargement is typical of such diseases as chronic lymphatic leukemia, Hodgkin's disease, infectious mononucleosis, and rheumatoid arthritis.

Complete blood count, liver function studies, liver and spleen scans, and X-rays should precede this test.

Purpose

- To determine the cause of lymph node enlargement
- To distinguish between benign and malignant lymph node processes
- To stage metastatic cancer

Patient preparation

- Explain to the patient that this test allows microscopic study of lymph node tissue.
- Describe the procedure to the patient, and answer his questions.
- For excisional biopsy, instruct the patient to restrict food after midnight and to drink only clear liquids on the morning of the test (if general anesthesia is needed for deeper nodes, he must also restrict fluids).
- For needle biopsy, inform him that he need not restrict food and fluids. Tell him who will perform the biopsy and where it will be done.
- Make sure the patient or a responsible family member has signed an informed consent form.

- Check the patient's history for hypersensitivity to the anesthetic.
- If the patient is to receive a local anesthetic, explain that he may experience slight discomfort during the injection.
- Record the patient's baseline vital signs just before the biopsy.

Procedure and posttest care
Excisional biopsy
- After the skin over the biopsy site is prepared and draped, the local anesthetic is administered.
- The examiner makes an incision, removes an entire node, and places it in a properly labeled bottle containing normal saline solution.
- The wound is sutured, and a sterile dressing is applied.

Needle biopsy
- After preparing the biopsy site and administering a local anesthetic, the examiner grasps the node between his thumb and forefinger, inserts the needle directly into the node, and obtains a small core specimen.
- The needle is removed, and the specimen is placed in a properly labeled bottle containing normal saline solution.
- Pressure is exerted at the biopsy site to control bleeding, and an adhesive bandage is applied.

Both procedures
- Check the patient's vital signs, and watch for bleeding, tenderness, and redness at the biopsy site.
- Inform the patient that he may resume his usual diet.

Precautions
- Storing the tissue specimen in normal saline solution instead of 10% formalin solution allows part of the specimen to be used for cytologic impression smears, which are studied along with the biopsy specimen.

Normal findings
The normal lymph node is encapsulated by collagenous connective tissue and divided into smaller lobes by tissue strands called *trabeculae*. It has an outer cortex, composed of lymphoid cells and nodules or follicles containing lymphocytes, and an inner medulla, composed of reticular phagocytic cells that collect and drain fluid.

Abnormal findings
Histologic examination of the tissue specimen distinguishes between malignant and nonmalignant causes of lymph node enlargement. Lymphatic cancer accounts for up to 5% of all cancers and is slightly more prevalent in males than in females. Hodgkin's disease, a lymphoma affecting the entire lymph system, is the leading cancer affecting adolescents and young adults. Lymph node cancer may also result from metastatic cancer.

When histologic results aren't clear or nodular material isn't involved, mediastinoscopy or laparotomy can provide another nodal specimen. Occasionally, lymphangiography can furnish additional diagnostic information.

Interfering factors
- Failure to obtain a representative tissue specimen
- Improper specimen storage
- Inability to differentiate nodal pathology

Sentinel lymph node biopsy

Sentinel lymph node biopsy is considered experimental for breast cancer patients but has become part of the standard of care for melanoma patients. A sentinel lymph node is defined as the first node in the lymphatic basin into which a primary tumor site drains. Hypothetically, the histology of the sentinel node will reflect the histology of the rest of the nodes in that basin. Hence, if that sentinel node is identified and found to be negative for tumor invasion, it's hypothesized that the rest of the nodes are also negative for tumor. In breast cancer, if the hypothesis is proven true, axillary lymph node dissections and their resulting morbidity could be avoided.

Sentinel lymph node biopsy is performed using one of two techniques; the techniques are usually combined to increase the likelihood of identifying the sentinel node. One technique is lymphoscintigraphy, performed in nuclear medicine using injected technetium-99m (^{99m}Tc), a radioactive isotope. The second technique uses the injection of blue dye.

Purpose
- To identify the sentinel lymph node and evaluate it for the presence or absence of tumor cells, indicating nodal metastasis

Patient preparation
- Explain to the patient that this test evaluates a particular lymph node to determine if cancer has spread into the lymph system. Tell her that it's usually done in conjunction with lumpectomy or mastectomy.

- Tell the patient that a radioactive substance will be injected under the skin. Assure her that she won't be radioactive and that the amount of radiation exposure will be less than that of a routine chest X-ray.

Procedure and posttest care
- The patient is positioned on the table in the nuclear medicine suite.
- A standard dose of ^{99m}Tc is injected circumferentially around the margins of a palpable mass using a 25G needle. For a nonpalpable mass, injections are guided with ultrasound or mammographic techniques. If the tumor has already been excised, the injections are made around the tumor bed.
- Images of the axilla are taken with a gamma camera. The location of the sentinel node is marked on the skin in indelible ink and noted on a data sheet.
- The patient is then transported to the operating room and placed under appropriate anesthesia.
- Blue dye is injected circumferentially in the tissue immediately surrounding the biopsy site using a 25G needle.
- Within 10 to 15 minutes of the dye injection, a small incision is made in the axilla over the suspected location of the sentinel lymph node. The surgeon follows the trail of stained lymphatics to the sentinel lymph node. The node is identified by the blue dye and by using an intraoperative gamma probe that measures radioactivity; the node having the highest radioactivity is deemed the sentinel node and removed.
- The axilla is then checked for remaining radioactivity; if none is noted, the surgical procedure concludes.
- Because of the radioactivity, the sentinel lymph node is maintained in forma-

lin for 24 to 48 hours before it can be processed.

■ Other than routine postoperative care, no special posttest care is required for this procedure.

Precautions

■ Because ^{99m}Tc is a radioactive substance, all radiation precautions must be implemented. Staff members need to be monitored for radiation exposure. Radiation levels need to be determined in the nuclear medicine suite and the operating room postsurgically.

■ Rare cases of allergy to the ^{99m}Tc or blue dye have been noted; the patient should be observed for signs of allergic reaction (skin changes and respiratory difficulties).

Normal findings

Normal findings are the same as for a normal lymph node biopsy.

Abnormal findings

Sentinel lymph node biopsy is performed only in breast cancer and melanoma, so abnormal findings mean the identification of melanoma or breast cancer cells. Their presence indicates lymph node metastasis and guides the prognosis and treatment.

Interfering factors

■ Allergy to a radioactive substance
■ Inability to raise arm to allow access to axilla
■ Inability to obtain an adequate specimen
■ Improper specimen storage

ORGAN BIOPSIES

Skin biopsy

Skin biopsy is the removal of a small piece of tissue under local anesthesia from a lesion suspected of being malignant or from other dermatoses. One of three techniques may be used: shave biopsy, punch biopsy, or excisional biopsy. Shave biopsy uses a scalpel to slice a superficial specimen from the site. Punch biopsy removes an oval core from the center of a lesion down to the dermis or subcutaneous tissue. Excisional biopsy removes the entire lesion with a small border of normal skin.

Lesions suspected of being malignant usually have changed color, size, or appearance or have failed to heal properly after injury. Fully developed lesions should be selected for biopsy whenever possible because they provide more diagnostic information than lesions that are resolving or in early developing stages.

Purpose

■ To provide differential diagnosis among basal cell carcinoma, squamous cell carcinoma, malignant melanoma, and benign growths
■ To diagnose chronic bacterial or fungal skin infections

Patient preparation

■ Explain to the patient that the biopsy provides a specimen for microscopic study.
■ Describe the procedure to the patient, and answer his questions.
■ Inform the patient that he need not restrict food and fluids.
■ Tell the patient who will perform the procedure and where it will be done.

- Tell the patient that he'll receive a local anesthetic to minimize pain during the procedure.
- Make sure the patient or a responsible family member has signed an informed consent form.
- Check the patient's history for hypersensitivity to the local anesthetic.

Procedure and posttest care
- Position the patient comfortably, and clean the biopsy site before the local anesthetic is administered.

Shave biopsy
- The protruding growth is cut off at the skin line with a #15 scalpel, and the tissue is placed immediately in a properly labeled specimen bottle containing 10% formalin solution.
- Apply pressure to the area to stop the bleeding.

Punch biopsy
- The skin surrounding the lesion is pulled taut, and the punch is firmly introduced into the lesion and rotated to obtain a tissue specimen. The plug is lifted with forceps or a needle and severed as deeply into the fat layer as possible.
- The specimen is placed in a properly labeled specimen bottle containing 10% formalin solution or in a sterile container, if indicated.
- Closing the wound depends on the size of the punch: A 3-mm punch requires only an adhesive bandage, a 4-mm punch requires one suture, and a 6-mm punch requires two sutures.

Excisional biopsy
- A #15 scalpel is used to excise the entire lesion; the elliptical incision is made as wide and as deep as necessary.

- The tissue specimen is removed and placed immediately in a properly labeled specimen bottle containing 10% formalin solution.
- Apply pressure to the site to stop bleeding.
- The wound is closed using 4-0 suture. If the incision is large, skin grafting may be required.

All procedures
- Check the biopsy site for bleeding.
- If the patient experiences pain, administer an analgesic, as ordered.
- Advise the patient with sutures to keep the area as clean and dry as possible. Facial sutures are removed in 3 to 5 days; trunk sutures, in 7 to 14 days. Tell the patient with adhesive strips to leave them in place for 14 to 21 days or until they fall off.

Precautions
- Send the specimen to the laboratory immediately.

Normal findings
Normal skin consists of squamous epithelium (epidermis) and fibrous connective tissue (dermis).

Abnormal findings
Histologic examination of the tissue specimen may reveal a benign or malignant lesion. Benign growths include cysts, seborrheic keratoses, warts, pigmented nevi (moles), keloids, dermatofibromas, and multiple neurofibromas.

Malignant tumors include basal cell carcinoma, squamous cell carcinoma, and malignant melanoma. Basal cell carcinoma occurs on hair-bearing skin; the most common location is the face, including the nose and its folds. Squamous cell carcinoma most commonly appears on the lips, mouth, and genitalia. Malignant melanoma, the deadliest skin cancer, can spread through the body by way of the lymphatic system and blood vessels.

Cultures can be used to detect chronic bacterial and fungal infections in which flora are relatively sparse.

Interfering factors
- Improper selection of the biopsy site
- Failure to use the appropriate fixative or a sterile container

Small bowel biopsy

Small-bowel biopsy is used to evaluate diseases of the intestinal mucosa, which may cause malabsorption or diarrhea. It produces larger specimens than those produced by endoscopic biopsy and allows removal of tissue from areas beyond an endoscope's reach. (See *Endoscopic biopsy of the GI tract.*)

Several similar types of capsules are available for tissue collection. In each, a mercury-weighted bag is attached to one end of the capsule; a thin polyethylene tube about 5′ (1.5 m) long is attached to the other end. When the bag, capsule, and tube are in place in the small bowel, suction on the tube draws the mucosa into the capsule and closes it, cutting off the piece of tissue within. Although this is an invasive procedure, it causes little pain and rarely causes complications.

Small-bowel biopsy verifies the diagnosis of some diseases, such as Whipple's disease, and may help confirm others, such as tropical sprue. Capsule biopsy is an invasive procedure, but it causes little pain and complications are rare.

Purpose
- To help diagnose diseases of the intestinal mucosa

Patient preparation
- Explain to the patient that this test is used to identify intestinal disorders.
- Describe the procedure to the patient, and answer his questions.
- Instruct the patient to restrict food and fluids for at least 8 hours before the test.
- Tell the patient who will perform the biopsy and where it will be done.
- Make sure the patient or a responsible family member has signed an informed consent form.
- Ensure that coagulation tests have been performed and that the results are recorded on the patient's chart.
- Withhold aspirin and anticoagulants, as ordered. If these drugs must be continued, note this on the laboratory request.

Procedure and posttest care
- Check the tubing and the mercury bag for leaks.
- Lightly lubricate the tube and capsule with a water-soluble lubricant, and moisten the mercury bag with water.
- Spray the back of the patient's throat with a local anesthetic to decrease gagging.
- Ask the patient to sit upright.
- The capsule is placed in the patient's pharynx, and he's asked to flex his neck and swallow as the tube is advanced.
- If a local anesthetic is used to control the gag reflex, the patient must not receive any fluids to help him swallow the capsule.
- Place the patient on his right side; the tube is then advanced another 20″ (50.8 cm). The tube's position is checked by fluoroscopy or by instilling air through the tube and listening with a stethoscope for air to enter the stomach.
- Next, the tube is advanced 2″ to 4″ (5 to 10 cm) at a time to pass the capsule through the pylorus. (Talk to the patient

ENDOSCOPIC BIOPSY OF THE GI TRACT

Endoscopy allows direct visualization of the GI tract and any site that requires biopsy of tissue specimens for histologic analysis. This relatively painless procedure helps detect, support diagnosis of, or monitor GI tract disorders. Its complications, notably hemorrhage, perforation, and aspiration, are rare.

Endoscopic biopsy of the GI tract can be used to diagnose cancer, lymphoma, amyloidosis, candidiasis, and gastric ulcers; to support a diagnosis of Crohn's disease, chronic ulcerative colitis, gastritis, esophagitis, and melanosis coli in laxative abuse; and to monitor progression of Barrett's esophagus, multiple gastric polyps, colon cancer and polyps, and chronic ulcerative colitis.

Preparing the patient

Careful patient preparation is vital for this procedure. Describe the procedure to the patient, and reassure him that he'll be able to breathe with the endoscope in place. Tell him to fast for at least 8 hours before the procedure. For lower GI biopsy, clean the bowel. Make sure the patient or a responsible family member has signed an informed consent form.

Just before the procedure, administer the prescribed sedative to the patient. He should be relaxed but not asleep because his cooperation is necessary to promote smooth passage of the endoscope. Spray the back of his throat with a local anesthetic to suppress his gag reflex. Have suction equipment and bipolar cauterizing electrodes available to prevent aspiration and excessive bleeding.

Obtaining the sample

After the endoscope is passed into the upper or lower GI tract and a lesion, node, or other abnormal area is visualized, a biopsy forceps is pushed through a channel in the endoscope until this, too, can be seen. The forceps are then opened, positioned at the biopsy site, and closed on the tissue. The closed forceps and tissue specimen are removed from the endoscope, and the tissue is taken from the forceps. Then the forceps may be used to cauterize any remaining abnormal tissue or stop bleeding.

The specimen is placed mucosal side up on fine-mesh gauze or filter paper and then placed in a labeled biopsy bottle containing fixative. When all specimens have been collected, the endoscope is removed. Specimens are sent to the laboratory immediately.

---

about food to stimulate the pylorus and help the capsule pass.)

■ When fluoroscopy confirms that the capsule has passed the pylorus, keep the patient on his right side to allow the capsule to move into the second and third portions of the small bowel.

■ Tell the patient that he may hold the tube loosely to one side of his mouth if it makes him more comfortable.

■ Capsule position is checked again by fluoroscopy. When the capsule is at or beyond the ligament of Treitz, the biopsy

sample can be taken. (The physician will determine the biopsy site.)

■ Place the patient in a supine position so that the capsule's position can be verified fluoroscopically. A 100-ml glass syringe is placed on the end of the tube, and steady suction is applied to close the capsule and cut off a tissue specimen. Suction is maintained on the syringe as the tube and capsule are removed; then the suction is released. This opens the capsule and exposes the specimen, mucosal side down.

USING A MENGHINI NEEDLE

In percutaneous liver biopsy, a Menghini needle attached to a 5-ml syringe containing normal saline solution is introduced through the chest wall and intercostal space (1). Negative pressure is created in the syringe. Then the needle is pushed rapidly into the liver (2) and pulled out of the body entirely (3) to obtain a tissue specimen.

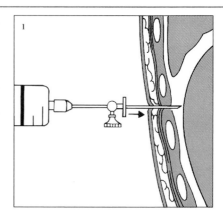

■ The specimen is gently removed with forceps, placed mucosal side up on a piece of mesh, and then placed in a biopsy bottle with required fixative.

■ As ordered, resume the patient's diet after confirming return of the gag reflex.

■ Although complications are rare, watch for signs of hemorrhage, bacteremia with transient fever and pain, and bowel perforation. Tell the patient to report abdominal pain or bleeding.

Precautions

■ Keep suction equipment nearby to prevent aspiration if the patient vomits.

■ Don't allow the patient to bite the tubing.

■ Handle the tissue carefully, and place it correctly on the slide.

■ Send the specimen to the laboratory immediately.

■ Biopsy is contraindicated in an uncooperative patient, one taking aspirin or anticoagulants, and the patient with uncontrolled coagulation disorders.

Normal findings

A normal small-bowel biopsy specimen consists of fingerlike villi, crypts, columnar epithelial cells, and round cells.

Abnormal findings

Small-bowel tissue that reveals histologic changes in cell structure may indicate Whipple's disease, abetalipoproteinemia, lymphoma, lymphangiectasia, eosinophilic enteritis, and such parasitic infections as giardiasis and coccidiosis. Abnormal specimens may also suggest celiac sprue, tropical sprue, infectious gastroenteritis, intraluminal bacterial overgrowth, folate and vitamin B_{12} deficiency, radiation enteritis, and malnutrition, but such disorders require further studies.

Interfering factors

■ Failure to fast before biopsy (possible poor specimen or vomiting and aspiration)

■ Mechanical failure of the biopsy capsule or hole in the tubing (possible difficulty in removing tissue specimen)

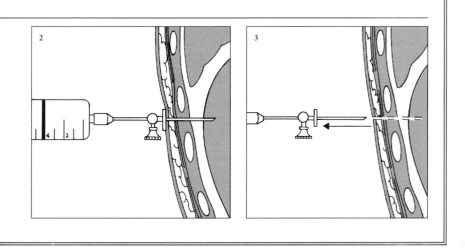

- The patient's inability to remain still or keep from coughing during the procedure
- Incorrect handling or positioning of the specimen or failure to place it in a fixative
- Delay in transporting the specimen to the laboratory

Percutaneous liver biopsy

Percutaneous biopsy of the liver is the needle aspiration of a core of liver tissue for histologic analysis. This procedure is performed under local or general anesthesia using a special needle. (See *Using a Menghini needle.*) Findings may help to identify hepatic disorders after ultrasonography, computed tomography scan, and radionuclide studies have failed to detect them. Because many patients with hepatic disorders have clotting defects, testing for hemostasis should precede liver biopsy.

Purpose

- To diagnose hepatic parenchymal disease, malignant tumors, and granulomatous infections

Patient preparation

- Explain to the patient that this test is used to diagnose liver disorders.
- Describe the procedure to the patient, and answer his questions.
- Instruct the patient to restrict food and fluids for 4 to 8 hours before the test.
- Tell the patient who will perform the biopsy and where it will be done.
- Make sure the patient or a responsible family member has signed an informed consent form.
- Check the patient's history for hypersensitivity to the local anesthetic.
- Make sure coagulation studies (prothrombin time [PT], partial thromboplastin time, and platelet counts) have been performed and that the results are recorded on the patient's chart.
- A blood sample is usually drawn for baseline hematocrit assessment.

- Just before the biopsy, tell the patient to void, and then record his vital signs.
- Inform the patient that he'll receive a local anesthetic but may experience pain similar to that of a punch in his right shoulder as the biopsy needle passes the phrenic nerve.

Procedure and posttest care
- For aspiration biopsy using the Menghini needle, place the patient in a supine position with his right hand under his head. Instruct him to maintain this position and remain as still as possible during the procedure.
- The liver is palpated, the biopsy site is selected and marked, and the local anesthetic is then injected.
- The needle flange is set to control the depth of penetration, and 2 ml of sterile normal saline solution are drawn into the syringe.
- The syringe is attached to the biopsy needle, and the needle is introduced into the subcutaneous tissue through the right eighth or ninth intercostal space at the midaxillary line and advanced up to the pleura.
- Next, 1 ml of normal saline solution is injected to clear the needle and the plunger, and then the plunger is drawn back to the 4-ml mark to create negative pressure.
- At this point in the procedure, ask the patient to take a deep breath, exhale, and hold his breath at the end of expiration to prevent movement of the chest wall.
- As the patient holds his breath, the biopsy needle is quickly inserted into the liver and withdrawn in 1 second.
- For the patient who can't hold his breath, the biopsy needle is quickly inserted and withdrawn at the end of expiration.

- After the needle is withdrawn, tell the patient to resume normal respirations.
- The tissue specimen is then placed in a properly labeled specimen cup containing 10% formalin solution. This is done by releasing negative pressure while the point of the needle is in the formalin solution. Send the specimen to the laboratory immediately.
- Again, 1 ml of normal saline solution is injected to clear the needle of the tissue specimen.
- Apply pressure to the biopsy site to stop bleeding.
- Position the patient on his right side for 2 to 4 hours, with a small pillow or sandbag under the costal margin to provide extra pressure. Advise bed rest for at least 24 hours.
- Check the patient's vital signs every 15 minutes for 1 hour, every 30 minutes for 4 hours, and every 4 hours thereafter for 24 hours. Throughout, observe him carefully for signs of shock.

CLINICAL ALERT *Immediately report bleeding or signs of bile peritonitis, such as tenderness and rigidity around the biopsy site. Be alert for symptoms of pneumothorax, such as rising respiratory rate, depressed breath sounds, dyspnea, persistent shoulder pain, and pleuritic chest pain. Report such complications promptly.*
- If the patient experiences pain, which may persist for several hours after the test, administer an analgesic.
- Inform the patient that he may resume his usual diet, as ordered.

Precautions
- Percutaneous liver biopsy is contraindicated in a patient with a platelet count below 100,000/µl; PT time longer than 15 seconds; empyema of the lungs, pleurae, peritoneum, biliary tract, or liver; vascular tumor; hepatic angiomas; hy-

datid cyst; or tense ascites. If extrahepatic obstruction is suspected, ultrasonography or subcutaneous transhepatic cholangiography should rule out this condition before the biopsy is considered.

■ Pain in the abdomen or dyspnea after the biopsy may indicate perforation of an abdominal organ or pneumothorax, respectively. In such cases, complete a thorough assessment and notify the physician at once.

■ Instruct the patient to hold his breath while the needle is in place.

Normal findings

The normal liver consists of sheets of hepatocytes supported by a reticulin framework.

Abnormal findings

Examination of the hepatic tissue may reveal diffuse hepatic disease, such as cirrhosis or hepatitis, or granulomatous infections such as tuberculosis. Primary malignant tumors include hepatocellular carcinoma, cholangiocellular carcinoma, and angiosarcoma, but hepatic metastasis is more common.

Nonmalignant findings with a known focal lesion require further studies, such as laparotomy or laparoscopy with biopsy.

Interfering factors

■ Failure to obtain a representative specimen

■ Failure to place the specimen in the proper preservative

■ Failure to send the specimen to the laboratory immediately

■ Hemorrhage caused by inadvertent puncture of a liver blood vessel

Percutaneous renal biopsy

Percutaneous renal biopsy is the needle excision of a core of kidney tissue for histologic examination. This biopsy may help assess histologic changes caused by acute or chronic glomerulonephritis, pyelonephritis, renal vein thrombosis, amyloid infiltration, and systemic lupus erythematosus. In the case of a mass, results can differentiate a primary renal cancer from a metastatic lesion.

Complications of percutaneous biopsy include bleeding, hematoma, arteriovenous fistula, and infection. This procedure is safer than open biopsy, which is the preferred method for sampling a solid lesion, but noninvasive procedures, especially renal ultrasonography and computed tomography, have replaced percutaneous renal biopsy in many facilities. (See *Urinary tract brush biopsy,* page 454.)

Purpose

■ To aid in the diagnosis of renal parenchymal disease

■ To monitor the progression of renal disease and assess the effectiveness of therapy

Patient preparation

■ Explain to the patient that this test is used to diagnose kidney disorders.

■ Describe the procedure to the patient, and answer his questions.

■ Instruct the patient to restrict food and fluids for 8 hours before the test.

■ Tell the patient who will perform the biopsy and where it will be done.

■ Ensure that blood samples and urine specimens are collected and tested before the biopsy and that results of other tests to determine the biopsy site, such as excretory urography, ultrasonography, and

URINARY TRACT BRUSH BIOPSY

Retrograde brush biopsy of the urinary tract may be used to obtain a renal tissue specimen when X-rays show a lesion in the renal pelvis or calyx. It can also be used to obtain specimens from other areas of the urinary tract. Retrograde brush biopsy is contraindicated in the patient with an acute urinary tract infection or an obstruction at or below the biopsy site.

Patient preparation

To prepare the patient for brush biopsy, describe the procedure, and tell him that he may experience some discomfort. Inform him who will perform the biopsy and when. Reassure the patient that the procedure will take only 30 to 60 minutes.

Make sure the patient or a responsible family member has signed an informed consent form. Because this procedure requires the use of a contrast medium and a general, local, or spinal anesthetic, check the patient's history for hypersensitivity to anesthetics, contrast media, or iodine-containing foods such as shellfish. Just before the biopsy procedure, administer a sedative to the patient.

Obtaining the biopsy

After the patient has received a sedative and an anesthetic, place him in the lithotomy position. Using a cystoscope, a guide wire is passed up the ureter and a urethral catheter is passed over the guide wire. Contrast medium is instilled through the catheter, which is positioned next to the lesion under fluoroscopic guidance. The contrast medium is washed out with normal saline solution to prevent cell distortions from the dye. A nylon or steel brush is passed up the catheter and the lesion is brushed. This procedure is repeated at least six times, using a new brush each time.

As each brush is removed from the catheter, a smear is made for Papanicolaou staining, and the brush tip is cut off and placed in formalin solution for 1 hour. The biopsy material is then removed from the brush tip for histologic examination. When the last brush is withdrawn, the catheter is irrigated with normal saline solution to remove additional cells. These cells are also sent for histologic examination.

Results differentiate between malignant and benign lesions, which may appear the same on X-rays.

Posttest care

Because brush biopsy may cause complications, such as perforation, hemorrhage, sepsis, and contrast medium extravasation, carefully monitor the patient's vital signs. Be sure to record the time, color, and amount of voiding, being alert for hematuria and abdominal or flank pain. Report abnormal findings immediately, and administer analgesics and antibiotics, as ordered.

an erect film of the abdomen, are available.
■ Make sure the patient or a responsible family member has signed an informed consent form.
■ Check the patient's history for hemorrhagic tendencies and hypersensitivity to the local anesthetic.

■ Administer a mild sedative 30 minutes to 1 hour before the biopsy to help the patient relax, as ordered.
■ Inform the patient that he'll receive a local anesthetic but may experience a pinching pain when the needle is inserted through the back into the kidney.
■ Check the patient's vital signs, and tell him to void just before the test.

Procedure and posttest care

- Place the patient in a prone position on a firm surface with a sandbag beneath his abdomen.
- Tell him to take a deep breath while his kidney is being palpated.
- A 7″ 20G needle is used to inject the local anesthetic into the skin at the biopsy site. Instruct the patient to hold his breath and remain still as the needle is inserted through the back muscles, the deep lumbar fascia, the perinephric fat, and the kidney capsule. After the needle is inserted, tell the patient to take several deep breaths. If the needle swings smoothly during deep breathing, it has penetrated the kidney capsule. After the penetration depth is marked on the needle shaft, instruct the patient to hold his breath and remain as still as possible while the needle is withdrawn.
- After a small incision is made in the anesthetized skin, instruct the patient to hold his breath and remain still while the Vim-Silverman needle with stylet is inserted to the measured depth.
- Tell the patient to breathe deeply. Then tell him to remain still while the tissue specimen is obtained.
- The tissue is examined immediately under a hand lens to ensure that the specimen contains tissue from the cortex and medulla. Then it's placed on a saline-soaked gauze pad and placed in a properly labeled container.
- If an adequate tissue specimen hasn't been obtained, the procedure is repeated immediately.
- After an adequate specimen is secured, apply pressure to the biopsy site for 3 to 5 minutes to stop superficial bleeding. Then apply a pressure dressing.
- Instruct the patient to lie flat on his back without moving for at least 12 hours to prevent bleeding. Check his vital signs every 15 minutes for 4 hours, every 30 minutes for 4 hours, every hour for 4 hours and, finally, every 4 hours. Report any changes.
- Examine the patient's urine for blood; small amounts may be present after the biopsy but should disappear within 8 hours. Hematocrit may be monitored after the procedure to screen for internal bleeding.
- Encourage fluid ingestion to minimize colic and obstruction from blood clotting within the renal pelvis.
- Inform the patient that he may resume his usual diet.
- Discourage the patient from engaging in strenuous activities for several days after the procedure to prevent possible bleeding.

Precautions

- Percutaneous renal biopsy is contraindicated in a patient with a severe bleeding disorder, markedly reduced plasma or blood volume, severe hypertension, hydronephrosis, perinephric abscess, advanced renal failure with uremia, or only one kidney.
- Instruct the patient to hold his breath and remain still whenever the needle or prongs are advanced into or retracted from the kidney.
- Send the specimen to the laboratory immediately.

Normal findings

Usually, a section of kidney tissue shows Bowman's capsule — the area between two layers of flat epithelial cells — the glomerular tuft, and the capillary lumen. The tubule sections differ, depending on the area of tubule involved. The proximal tubule is one layer of epithelial cells with microvilli that form a brush border. The descending loop of Henle has flat squamous epithelial cells. The ascending loop is convoluted distally, and collecting tubules are lined with squamous epithelial cells.

Abnormal findings

Histologic examination of renal tissue can reveal cancer or renal disease. Malignant tumors include Wilms' tumor, which is usually present in early childhood, and renal cell carcinoma, which is most prevalent in people over age 40. Diseases indicated by characteristic histologic changes include disseminated lupus erythematosus, amyloid infiltration, acute or chronic glomerulonephritis, renal vein thrombosis, and pyelonephritis.

Interfering factors

■ Failure to obtain an adequate tissue specimen
■ Failure to store the specimen properly
■ Failure to send the specimen to the laboratory immediately

Lung biopsy

In lung biopsy, a specimen of pulmonary tissue is excised by closed or open technique for histologic examination. Closed technique, performed under local anesthesia, includes needle and transbronchial biopsies, transcatheter bronchial brushing, and video-assisted thoracotomy. Open technique, performed under general anesthesia in the operating room, includes limited and standard thoracotomies. Needle biopsy is appropriate when the lesion is readily accessible, originates in the lung parenchyma and is confined to it, or is affixed to the chest wall; it provides a much smaller specimen than the open technique. Transbronchial biopsy, the removal of multiple tissue specimens through a fiber-optic broncho-

scope, may be used in patients with diffuse infiltrative pulmonary disease or tumors or when severe debilitation contraindicates open biopsy. Open biopsy is appropriate for the study of a well-circumscribed lesion that may require resection.

Generally, a lung biopsy is recommended after chest X-rays, computed tomography scan, and bronchoscopy have failed to identify the cause of diffuse parenchymal pulmonary disease or a pulmonary lesion. Complications of lung biopsy include bleeding, infection, and pneumothorax.

Purpose

■ To confirm a diagnosis of diffuse parenchymal pulmonary disease and pulmonary lesions

Patient preparation

■ Explain to the patient that this test is used to confirm or rule out a diagnostic finding in the lung.
■ Describe the procedure to the patient, and answer his questions.
■ Tell the patient that a chest X-ray and blood studies (prothrombin time, partial thromboplastin time, and platelet count) will be performed before the biopsy.
■ Tell the patient who will perform the biopsy and where it will be done.
■ Instruct the patient to fast after midnight before the procedure. (Sometimes the patient is permitted to have clear liquids the morning of the test.)
■ Make sure the patient or a responsible family member has signed an informed consent form.
■ Check the patient's history for hypersensitivity to the local anesthetic.
■ Administer a mild sedative, as ordered, 30 minutes before the biopsy to help the patient relax. Tell him that he'll receive a

local anesthetic, but he may experience a sharp, transient pain when the biopsy needle touches the lung.

■ Reinforce that the patient needs to lie still during the procedure because any movement or coughing can result in laceration of lung tissue by the biopsy needle.

Procedure and posttest care

■ After the biopsy site is selected, lead markers are placed on the patient's skin, and X-rays are ordered to verify their correct placement.

■ Position the patient in a sitting position with his arms folded on a table in front of him; instruct him to maintain this position, remaining as still as possible, and to refrain from coughing.

■ Prepare the skin over the biopsy site and drape the appropriate area.

■ With a 25G needle, the local anesthetic is injected just above the rib below the selected site to prevent damage to the intercostal nerves and vessels.

■ Using a 22G needle, the examiner anesthetizes the intercostal muscles and parietal pleura, makes a small incision (2 to 3 mm) with a scalpel, and introduces the biopsy needle through the incision, chest wall, and pleura into the tumor or pulmonary tissue.

■ If the intercostal space at the incision site is wide, the needle is inserted at a 90-degree angle; if the ribs overlap and the intercostal space is narrow, the needle is inserted at a 45-degree angle. When the needle is in the tumor or pulmonary tissue, the specimen is obtained and the needle is withdrawn.

■ The specimen is divided immediately: The tissue for histology is placed in a properly labeled bottle containing 10% neutral buffered formalin solution; the

tissue for microbiology is placed in a sterile container.

■ Immediately following the procedure, apply pressure on the biopsy site to stop bleeding and apply a small bandage.

▶ **CLINICAL ALERT** *Check the patient's vital signs every 15 minutes for 1 hour, every 30 minutes for 2 hours, every hour for 4 hours, and then every 4 hours. Watch for bleeding, dyspnea, elevated pulse rate, diminished breath sounds on the biopsy side and, eventually, cyanosis. Complications include pneumothorax and bleeding. Make sure the chest X-ray is repeated as soon as the biopsy has been completed.*

■ Inform the patient that he may resume his usual diet.

Precautions

■ Needle biopsy is contraindicated in the patient with a lesion that's separated from the chest wall or accompanied by emphysematous bullae, cysts, or gross emphysema and in the patient with coagulopathy, hypoxia, pulmonary hypertension, or cardiac disease with cor pulmonale.

■ During biopsy, observe for signs of respiratory distress — shortness of breath, elevated pulse rate, and cyanosis (late sign). If such signs develop, report them immediately.

■ Because coughing and movement during biopsy can cause lung tearing by the biopsy needle, keep the patient calm and still.

Normal findings

Normal pulmonary tissue shows uniform texture of the alveolar ducts, alveolar walls, bronchioles, and small vessels.

Abnormal findings

Histologic examination of a pulmonary tissue specimen can reveal squamous cell or oat cell carcinoma and adenocarcinoma and supplements the results of microbiologic cultures, deep-cough sputum specimens, chest X-rays, bronchoscopy, and the patient's physical history in confirming cancer or parenchymal pulmonary disease.

Interfering factors
- Failure to obtain a representative tissue specimen
- Failure to store the specimen in the appropriate containers

Pleural tissue biopsy

Pleural tissue biopsy is the removal of pleural tissue by needle biopsy or open biopsy for histologic examination. Needle pleural biopsy is performed under local anesthesia. It generally follows or is done in conjunction with thoracentesis (aspiration of pleural fluid), which is performed when the cause of an effusion is unknown, but it can be performed separately.

Open pleural biopsy, performed in the absence of pleural effusion, permits direct visualization of the pleura and the underlying lung. It's performed in the operating room.

Purpose
- To differentiate between nonmalignant and malignant disease
- To diagnose viral, fungal, or parasitic disease and collagen vascular disease of the pleura

Patient preparation
- Explain to the patient that this test permits microscopic examination of pleural tissue.
- Describe the procedure to the patient, and answer his questions.

- Tell the patient who will perform the biopsy, where it will be done, and that no fasting is required.
- Explain that blood studies will precede the biopsy, and chest X-rays will be taken before and after the biopsy.
- Make sure the patient or a responsible family member has signed an informed consent form.
- Check the patient's history for hypersensitivity to the local anesthetic.
- Tell the patient that he'll receive a local anesthetic and should experience little pain.
- Record the patient's vital signs just before the procedure.

Procedure and posttest care
- Seat the patient on the side of the bed, with his feet resting on a stool and his arms on the overbed table or supported by his upper body. Tell him to hold this position and remain still during the procedure.
- Prepare the skin and drape the area.
- The local anesthetic is then administered.
- In a *Vim-Silverman needle biopsy,* a needle is inserted through the appropriate intercostal space into the biopsy site, with the outer tip distal to the pleura and the central portion pushed in deeper and held in place. The outer case is inserted about ⅜" (1 cm), the entire assembly is rotated 360 degrees, and the needle and tissue specimen are withdrawn. In *Cope's needle biopsy,* a trocar is introduced through the appropriate intercostal space into the biopsy site. To obtain the specimen, a hooked stylet is inserted through the trocar. While the outer tube is held stationary, the inner tube is twisted to cut off the tissue specimen, and the assembly is withdrawn. (See *Using Cope's needle.*)

USING COPE'S NEEDLE

Cope's needle, which is used to obtain a pleural biopsy specimen, consists of three parts: a sharp obturator (A) and a cannula (B), which when fitted together are called a trocar, and a blunt-ended, hooked stylet (C). The trocar is used to gain access to the pleural cavity. Then the obturator is removed, leaving the cannula in place. The stylet is passed through the cannula to excise a tissue specimen, as shown below.

Lung

Fluid

Muscle

Parietal pleura

Rib

A

B

C

■ After the specimens are obtained, additional parietal fluid may be removed to treat the effusion.

■ Put the specimen immediately into a 10% neutral buffered formalin solution in a labeled specimen bottle, and send it to the laboratory immediately.

■ Clean the skin around the biopsy site, and apply an adhesive bandage.

■ Make sure the chest X-ray is repeated immediately after the biopsy.

■ Check the patient's vital signs every 15 minutes for 1 hour and then every hour for 4 hours or until stable.

CLINICAL ALERT *Watch for signs of respiratory distress (dyspnea), shoulder pain, and such complications as pneumothorax (immediate), pneumonia (delayed), and hemorrhage.*

■ Instruct the patient to lie on his unaffected side to promote healing of the biopsy site, as indicated.

Precautions
■ Pleural biopsy is contraindicated in the patient with a severe bleeding disorder.

Normal findings
The normal pleura consists primarily of mesothelial cells that are flattened in a uniform layer. Layers of areolar connective tissue that contain blood vessels, nerves, and lymphatics lie below.

Abnormal findings
Histologic examination of the tissue specimen can reveal malignant disease, tuberculosis, and viral, fungal, parasitic, or collagen vascular disease. Primary neo-

plasms of the pleura are generally fibrous and epithelial.

Interfering factors

- Failure to use the proper fixative or to obtain an adequate specimen
- The patient's inability to remain still, keep from coughing, or follow instructions, such as "Hold your breath," during the procedure

Cervical biopsy

Cervical biopsy (also known as *cervical punch biopsy*) is the excision by sharp forceps of a tissue specimen from the cervix for histologic examination. Generally, multiple biopsies are done to obtain specimens from all areas with abnormal tissue or from the squamocolumnar junction and other sites around the cervical circumference. The biopsy site is selected by direct visualization of the cervix with a colposcope or by Schiller's test, which stains normal squamous epithelium a dark mahogany, but fails to color abnormal tissue. Other biopsies are done to detect other gynecological disorders. (See *Endometrial and ovarian biopsies.*) The biopsy is performed when the cervix is least vascular, usually 1 week after menses.

Purpose

- To evaluate suspicious cervical lesions
- To diagnose cervical cancer

Patient preparation

- Describe the procedure to the patient, and explain that it provides a cervical tissue specimen for microscopic study.
- Tell the patient who will perform the biopsy and where it will be done.

- Tell the patient that she may experience mild discomfort during and after the biopsy.
- Advise the outpatient to have someone accompany her home after the biopsy.
- Make sure the patient or a responsible family member has signed an informed consent form.
- Ask the patient to void just before the biopsy.

Procedure and posttest care

- Place the patient in the lithotomy position, and tell her to relax as the unlubricated speculum is inserted.
- *For direct visualization,* the colposcope is inserted through the speculum, the biopsy site is located, and the cervix is cleaned with a swab soaked in 3% acetic acid solution. The biopsy forceps are then inserted through the speculum or the colposcope, and tissue is removed from any lesion or from selected sites, starting from the posterior lip to avoid obscuring other sites with blood. Each specimen is immediately put in 10% formalin solution in a labeled bottle. To control bleeding after biopsy, the cervix is swabbed with 5% silver nitrate solution (cautery or sutures may be used instead). If bleeding persists, the examiner may insert a tampon.
- *For Schiller's test,* an applicator stick saturated with iodine solution is inserted through the speculum. This stains the cervix to identify lesions for biopsy.
- Record the patient's and physician's names and the biopsy sites on the laboratory request.
- Instruct the patient to avoid strenuous exercise for 24 hours after the biopsy. Encourage the outpatient to rest briefly before leaving the office.
- If a tampon was inserted after the biopsy, tell the patient to leave it in place for 8 to 24 hours. Inform her that some bleed-

ENDOMETRIAL AND OVARIAN BIOPSIES

This list includes purposes and special considerations involved in endometrial and ovarian biopsies.

Method	Purpose	Special considerations
Endometrial biopsy		
■ Dilatation and curettage (D&C) ■ Endometrial washing (by jet irrigation, aspiration, or brushing)	■ To evaluate uterine bleeding ■ To diagnose suspected endometrial cancer	■ Time of menstrual cycle affects the accuracy of biopsy results. ■ The type of specimen obtained depends on the patient's age and the disorder. ■ D&C by endometrial washing may follow a negative biopsy. ■ Specimens obtained by D&C may be processed as frozen sections.
Ovarian biopsy		
■ Transrectal or transvaginal fine-needle biopsy ■ Aspiration biopsy during laparoscopy	■ To diagnose a missed abortion ■ To detect an ovarian tumor ■ To determine the spread of cancer	■ Fine-needle biopsy may follow palpation, laparoscopy, or computed tomography that detects an abnormal ovary. ■ Aspiration during laparoscopy is particularly useful for young women who are infertile or who have lesions that appear benign.

ing may occur, but tell her to report heavy bleeding (heavier than menses). Warn the patient to avoid using tampons, which can irritate the cervix and provoke bleeding.

■ Tell the patient to avoid douching and intercourse for 2 weeks, or as directed, if she has undergone such treatments as cryotherapy or laser treatment during the procedure.

■ Tell the patient that a foul-smelling, gray-green vaginal discharge is normal for several days after the biopsy and may persist for 3 weeks.

Precautions
■ Send the specimens to the laboratory immediately.

Normal findings
Normal cervical tissue is composed of columnar and squamous epithelial cells, loose connective tissue, and smooth-muscle fibers with no dysplasia or abnormal cell growth.

Abnormal findings
Histologic examination of a cervical tissue specimen is used to identify abnormal cells and to differentiate the tissue as in-

traepithelial neoplasia or invasive cancer. If the cause of an abnormal Papanicolaou test isn't demonstrated by cervical biopsy or if the specimen shows advanced dysplasia or carcinoma in situ, a cone biopsy is performed under general anesthesia to obtain a larger tissue specimen and to allow a more accurate evaluation of dysplasia.

Interfering factors

- Failure to obtain representative specimens
- Failure to place the specimens in the preservative immediately

SKELETAL BIOPSIES

Bone biopsy

Bone biopsy is the removal of a piece or a core of bone for histologic examination. It's performed either by using a special drill needle under local anesthesia or by surgical excision under general anesthesia.

Bone biopsy is indicated in patients with bone pain and tenderness after bone scan, computed tomography scan, X-ray, or arteriography reveals a mass or deformity. Excision provides a larger specimen than drill biopsy and permits immediate surgical treatment if quick histologic analysis of the specimen reveals cancer.

Possible complications include bone fracture, damage to surrounding tissue, infection (osteomyelitis) and, possibly, contamination of normal tissue with tumor cells.

Purpose

- To distinguish between benign and malignant bone tumors

Patient preparation

- Describe the procedure to the patient, and answer his questions.
- Explain that this test permits microscopic examination of a bone specimen.
- If the patient is to have a drill biopsy, he need not restrict food and fluids; if he's to have open biopsy, he must fast overnight before the test.
- Tell the patient who will perform the biopsy and where it will be done.
- Tell the patient that he'll receive a local anesthetic but will still experience discomfort and pressure when the biopsy needle enters the bone.
- Explain that a special drill forces the needle into the bone; if possible, show him a photograph of the bone drill. Stress the importance of his cooperation during the biopsy.
- Make sure the patient or a responsible family member has signed an informed consent form.
- Check the patient's history for hypersensitivity to the local anesthetic.

Procedure and posttest care
Drill biopsy

- The patient is properly positioned, and the biopsy site is shaved and prepared.
- After the local anesthetic is injected, a small incision (usually about 3 mm) is made and the biopsy needle is pushed with a pointed trocar into the bone, and then it's rotated about 180 degrees.
- When the bone core is obtained, the trocar is withdrawn and the specimen is placed in a properly labeled bottle containing 10% formalin solution. Then pressure is applied to the site with a sterile gauze pad.
- When bleeding stops, apply a topical antiseptic (povidone-iodine ointment) and an adhesive bandage or other sterile

covering to close the wound and prevent infection.

Open biopsy

- The patient is anesthetized, and the biopsy site is shaved, cleaned with surgical soap, and disinfected with an iodine wash and alcohol.
- An incision is made, and a piece of bone is removed and sent to the histology laboratory immediately for analysis. Further surgery can then be performed, depending on findings.

Both procedures

- Check the patient's vital signs and the dressing at the biopsy site. Determine how much drainage is expected and report excessive drainage.
- If the patient experiences pain, administer an analgesic.
- **CLINICAL ALERT** *For several days after the biopsy, watch for and report indications of bone infection: fever, headache, pain on movement, and redness or abscess near the biopsy site. Notify the physician if these symptoms develop.*
- Advise the patient that he may resume his usual diet.

Precautions

- Bone biopsy should be performed cautiously in the patient with coagulopathy.
- Send the specimen to the laboratory immediately.

Normal findings

Normal bone tissue consists of fibers of collagen, osteocytes, and osteoblasts. It may be compact or cancellous. Compact bone has dense, concentric layers of mineral deposits, or lamellae. Cancellous bone has widely spaced lamellae, with osteocytes and red and yellow marrow between them.

Abnormal findings

Histologic examination of a bone specimen can reveal benign or malignant tumors. Benign tumors, generally well circumscribed and nonmetastasizing, include osteoid osteoma, osteoblastoma, osteochondroma, unicameral bone cyst, benign giant-cell tumor, and fibroma. Malignant tumors, which spread irregularly and rapidly, most commonly include multiple myeloma and osteosarcoma; the most lethal is Ewing's sarcoma. Most malignant tumors spread to the bone through the blood and lymphatic system from the breasts, lungs, prostate, thyroid, or kidneys.

Interfering factors

- Failure to obtain a representative bone specimen
- Failure to use the proper fixative
- Failure to send the specimen to the laboratory immediately

Bone marrow aspiration and biopsy

Bone marrow, the soft tissue contained in the medullary canals of the long bone and in the interstices of cancellous bone, may be removed by aspiration or needle biopsy under local anesthesia. The histologic and hematologic examination of bone marrow provides reliable diagnostic information about blood disorders. Marrow may be removed by aspiration or needle biopsy under local anesthesia. In aspiration biopsy, a fluid specimen in which pustulae of marrow are suspended is removed from the bone marrow. In needle biopsy, a core of marrow cells (not fluid) is removed. These methods are typically used concurrently to obtain the best possible marrow specimens. Red marrow, which constitutes about 50% of an adult's

COMMON SITES OF BONE MARROW ASPIRATION AND BIOPSY

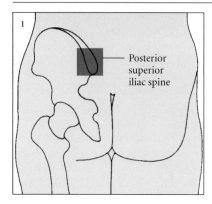

Posterior superior iliac spine

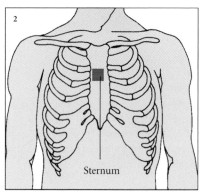

Sternum

The *posterior superior iliac spine* (1) is usually the preferred site for bone marrow aspiration and biopsy because no vital organs or vessels are located nearby. With the patient in a lateral position with one leg flexed, the health care provider inserts the needle several centimeters lateral to the iliosacral junction, entering the bone plane crest with the needle directed downward and toward the anterior inferior spine, or entering a few centimeters below the crest at a right angle to the surface of the bone.

The *sternum* (2) involves the greatest risks but is commonly used for marrow aspiration because it's near the surface, the cortical bone is thin, and the marrow cavity contains numerous cells and relatively little fat or supporting bone. For this procedure, the patient is supine on a firm bed or examining table with a small pillow beneath the shoulders to elevate the chest and lower the head. The health care provider secures the needle guard 3 to 4 mm from the tip of the needle to avoid accidental puncture of the heart or a major vessel. Then he inserts the needle at the midline of the sternum at the second intercostal space.

Preferred site

---

marrow, actively produces stem cells that ultimately evolve into red blood cells, white blood cells, and platelets. Yellow marrow contains fat cells and connective tissue and is inactive, but it can become active in response to the body's needs.

Bleeding and infection may result from bone marrow biopsy at any site, but the most serious complications occur at the sternum. Such complications are rare but

include puncture of the heart and major vessels, causing severe hemorrhage, and puncture of the mediastinum, causing mediastinitis or pneumomediastinum. (See *Common sites of bone marrow aspiration and biopsy*.)

Purpose

■ To diagnose thrombocytopenia, leukemias, and granulomas as well as

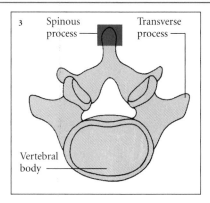

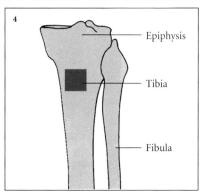

The *spinous process* (3) is the preferred site if multiple punctures are necessary, marrow is absent at other sites, or the patient objects to sternal puncture. For this procedure, the patient sits on the edge of the bed, leaning over the bedside stand; or, if he's uncooperative, he may be placed in the prone position with restraints. The health care provider selects the spinous process of the third or fourth lumbar vertebra and inserts the needle at the crest or slightly to one side, advancing the needle in the direction of the bone plane.

The *tibia* (4) is the site of choice for infants under age 1. The infant is placed in a prone position on a bed or examining table with a sandbag beneath the leg. The foot is taped to the surface of the table, or an assistant holds the leg stationary by placing a hand under it. The health care provider inserts the needle about ⅜″ (1 cm) below the tibial tuberosity and slightly toward the medial side, being careful to angle the needle point toward the foot to avoid epiphyseal injury.

aplastic, hypoplastic, and pernicious anemias
■ To diagnose primary and metastatic tumors
■ To determine the cause of infection
■ To aid in the staging of disease such as Hodgkin's disease
■ To evaluate the effectiveness of chemotherapy and monitor myelosuppression

Patient preparation
■ Explain to the patient that the test permits microscopic examination of a bone marrow specimen.
■ Describe the procedure to the patient, and answer his questions.
■ Inform the patient that he need not restrict food and fluids.
■ Tell the patient who will perform the biopsy and where it will be done.

PREPARING A CHILD FOR BONE MARROW BIOPSY

To prepare a child for a bone marrow biopsy, give him his own biopsy kit: a syringe without a needle, cotton balls, and adhesive bandages. Act out the procedure by using a doll or a stuffed animal as a model. This will help you gain the child's confidence and answer any questions he may have. Be sure to prepare him by describing the kinds of pressure and discomfort he will feel during the procedure.

Before the biopsy, explain the equipment on the tray to the child. Encourage the parents to get involved by helping you hold the child still and reassuring him. Tell the child that he'll feel some pain when the health care provider aspirates the bone marrow and that it's OK to cry or yell if he wants to, but the pain will go away quickly.

■ Inform the patient that more than one bone marrow specimen may be required and that a blood sample will be collected before biopsy for laboratory testing.

■ Make sure the patient or a responsible family member has signed an informed consent form.

■ Check the patient's history for hypersensitivity to the local anesthetic.

■ Tell the patient which bone—the sternum, anterior or posterior iliac crest, vertebral spinous process, rib, or tibia—will be the biopsy site.

■ Inform the patient that he'll receive a local anesthetic but will feel pressure on insertion of the biopsy needle and a brief, pulling pain on removal of the marrow.

Administer a mild sedative 1 hour before the test.

■ Preparation for children requires additional steps. (See *Preparing a child for bone marrow biopsy.*)

Procedure and posttest care

■ After positioning the patient, instruct him to remain as still as possible.

■ Offer emotional support during the biopsy by talking quietly to the patient, describing what's being done, and answering questions.

Aspiration biopsy

■ After the skin over the biopsy site is prepared and the area is draped, the local anesthetic is injected. With a twisting motion, the marrow aspiration needle is inserted through the skin, the subcutaneous tissue, and the cortex of the bone.

■ The stylet is removed from the needle, and a 10- to 20-ml syringe is attached. The examiner aspirates 0.2 to 0.5 ml of marrow and then withdraws the needle.

■ Apply pressure to the site for 5 minutes, while the marrow slides are being prepared. (If the patient has thrombocytopenia, apply pressure to the site for 10 to 15 minutes.)

■ The biopsy site is cleaned again, and a sterile adhesive bandage is applied.

■ If an adequate marrow specimen isn't obtained on the first attempt, the needle may be repositioned within the marrow cavity or removed and reinserted in another site within the anesthetized area. If the second attempt fails, a needle biopsy may be needed.

Needle biopsy

■ After preparing the biopsy site and draping the area, the examiner marks the skin at the site with an indelible pencil or marking pen.

■ A local anesthetic is then injected intradermally, subcutaneously, and at the bone's surface.

■ The biopsy needle is inserted into the periosteum, and the needle guard is set as indicated. The needle is advanced with a steady boring motion until the outer needle passes through the bone's cortex.

■ The inner needle with trephine tip is inserted into the outer needle. By alternately rotating the inner needle clockwise and counterclockwise, the examiner directs the needle into the marrow cavity and then removes a tissue plug.

■ The needle assembly is withdrawn, and the marrow is expelled into a labeled bottle containing Zenker's acetic acid solution.

■ After the biopsy site is cleaned, a sterile adhesive bandage or a pressure dressing is applied.

Both procedures
■ Check the biopsy site for bleeding and inflammation.

■ Observe the patient for signs of hemorrhage and infection, such as rapid pulse rate, low blood pressure, and fever.

Precautions
■ Bone marrow biopsy is contraindicated in the patient with a severe bleeding disorder.

■ Send the tissue specimen or slides to the laboratory immediately.

Normal findings
Yellow marrow contains fat cells and connective tissue; red marrow contains hematopoietic cells, fat cells, and connective tissue.

In addition, special stains that are used to detect hematologic disorders produce these normal findings: The iron stain, which is used to measure hemosiderin (storage iron), has a +2 level; the Sudan black B (SBB) fat stain, which shows granulocytes, is negative; and the periodic acid–Schiff (PAS) stain, which is used to detect glycogen reactions, is negative.

Abnormal findings
Histologic examination of a bone marrow specimen can be used to detect myelofibrosis, granulomas, lymphoma, and cancer. Hematologic analysis, including the differential count and myeloid-erythroid ratio, can implicate a wide range of disorders. (See *Bone marrow: Normal values and implications of abnormal findings*, pages 468 and 469.)

In an iron stain, decreased hemosiderin levels may indicate a true iron deficiency. Increased levels may accompany other types of anemias and blood disorders. A positive SBB stain can differentiate acute granulocytic leukemia from acute lymphocytic leukemia (SBB-negative) or may indicate granulation in myeloblasts. A positive PAS stain may indicate acute or chronic lymphocytic leukemia, amyloidosis, thalassemia, lymphomas, infectious mononucleosis, iron deficiency anemia, or sideroblastic anemia.

Interfering factors
■ Failure to obtain a representative specimen

■ Failure to use a fixative for histologic analysis

■ Failure to send the specimen to the laboratory immediately

(*Text continues on page 470.*)

BONE MARROW: NORMAL VALUES AND IMPLICATIONS OF ABNORMAL FINDINGS

Cell types	Normal mean values			Clinical implications
	Adults	*Children*	*Infants*	
Normoblasts, total	25.6%	23.1%	8%	*Elevated values:* polycythemia vera *Depressed values:* vitamin B_{12} or folic acid deficiency; hypoplastic or aplastic anemia
Pronormoblasts	0.2% to 1.3%	0.5%	0.1%	
Basophilic	0.5% to 2.4%	1.7%	0.34%	
Polychromatic	17.9% to 29.2%	18.2%	6.9%	
Orthochromatic	0.4% to 4.6%	2.7%	0.54%	
Neutrophils, total	56.5%	57.1%	32.4%	*Elevated values:* acute myeloblastic or chronic myeloid leukemia *Depressed values:* lymphoblastic, lymphatic, or monocytic leukemia; aplastic anemia
Myeloblasts	0.2% to 1.5%	1.2%	0.62%	
Promyelocytes	2.1% to 4.1%	1.4%	0.76%	
Myelocytes	8.2% to 15.7%	18.3%	2.5%	
Metamyelocytes	9.6% to 24.6%	23.3%	11.3%	
Bands	9.5% to 15.3%	0	14.1%	
Segmented	6% to 12%	12.9%	3.6%	
Eosinophils	3.1%	3.6%	2.6%	*Elevated values:* bone marrow carcinoma, lymphadenoma, myeloid leukemia, eosinophilic leukemia, pernicious anemia (in relapse)
Plasma cells	1.3%	0.4%	0.02%	*Elevated values:* myeloma, collagen disease, infection, antigen sensitivity, malignancy
Basophils	0.01%	0.06%	0.07%	*Elevated values:* no relation between basophil count and symptoms *Depressed values:* no relation between basophil count and symptoms

BONE MARROW: NORMAL VALUES AND IMPLICATIONS OF ABNORMAL FINDINGS (continued)

Cell types	Normal mean values			Clinical implications
	Adults	*Children*	*Infants*	
Lymphocytes	16.2%	16%	49.0%	*Elevated values:* B- and T-cell chronic lymphocytic leukemia, other lymphatic leukemias, lymphoma, mononucleosis, aplastic anemia, macroglobulinemia
Plasma cells	1.3%	0.4%	0.02%	*Elevated values:* myeloma, collagen disease, infection, antigen sensitivity, malignancy
Megakaryocytes	0.1%	0.1%	0.05%	*Elevated values:* advanced age, chronic myeloid leukemia, polycythemia vera, megakaryocytic myelosis, infection, idiopathic thrombocytopenic purpura, thrombocytopenia *Depressed values:* pernicious anemia
Myeloiderythroid ratio	2:1 to 4:1	2.9:1	4.4:1	*Elevated values:* myeloid leukemia, infection, leukemoid reactions, depressed hematopoiesis *Depressed values:* agranulocytosis, hematopoiesis after hemorrhage or hemolysis, iron deficiency anemia, polycythemia vera

Synovial membrane biopsy

Biopsy of the synovial membrane is needle excision of a tissue specimen for histologic examination of the thin epithelium lining the diarthrodial joint capsules. In a large joint, such as the knee, preliminary arthroscopy can aid selection of the biopsy site. Synovial membrane biopsy is performed when synovial fluid analysis — a viscous, lubricating fluid contained within the synovial membrane — proves nondiagnostic or when the fluid is absent.

Purpose
- To diagnose gout, pseudogout, bacterial infections and lesions, and granulomatous infections
- To aid in the diagnosis of systemic lupus erythematosus (SLE), rheumatoid arthritis, or Reiter's disease
- To monitor joint pathology

Patient preparation
- Explain to the patient that this test provides a tissue specimen from the membrane that lines the affected joint.
- Describe the procedure to the patient, and answer his questions.
- Advise the patient that he need not restrict food and fluids.
- Tell the patient who will perform the procedure and where it will be done.
- Inform the patient that complications include infection and bleeding into the joint, but they are rare.
- Advise the patient that he'll receive a local anesthetic to minimize discomfort but will experience pain when the needle enters the joint.
- Make sure the patient or a responsible family member has signed an informed consent form.
- Check the patient's history for hypersensitivity to the local anesthetic.
- Inform the patient which site — knee (most common), elbow, wrist, ankle, or shoulder — has been chosen for this biopsy (usually, the most symptomatic joint is selected).
- Administer a sedative to help the patient relax.

Procedure and posttest care
- Place the patient in the proper position, clean the biopsy site, and drape the area.
- The local anesthetic is injected into the joint space, and then the trocar is forcefully thrust into the joint space.
- The biopsy needle is inserted through the trocar. The hooked notch side of the biopsy needle is positioned against the synovium, and suction is applied with a 50-ml luer-lock syringe.
- While the trocar is held stationary, the biopsy needle is twisted to cut off a tissue segment.
- The biopsy needle is withdrawn, and the specimen is placed in a properly labeled sterile container or a specimen bottle containing absolute ethyl alcohol, as indicated.
- By changing the angle of the biopsy needle, several specimens can be obtained without reinserting the trocar.
- The trocar is then removed, the biopsy site is cleaned, and a pressure bandage is applied.
- Watch for signs of bleeding into the joint (swelling and tenderness) every hour for 4 hours and then every 4 hours for 12 hours.
- Administer an analgesic, as ordered, if the patient experiences pain.
- Tell the patient to rest the joint for 1 day before resuming normal activity.

Precautions

■ Send a specimen in a container with absolute ethyl alcohol to the histology laboratory immediately or send one in a sterile container to the microbiology laboratory.

Normal findings

The synovial membrane contains cells that are identical to those found in other connective tissue. The membrane surface is relatively smooth, except for villi, folds, and fat pads that project into the joint cavity. The membrane tissue produces synovial fluid and contains a capillary network, lymphatic vessels, and a few nerve fibers. A pathologic condition of the synovial membrane also affects the synovial fluid's cellular composition.

Abnormal findings

Histologic examination of synovial tissue can diagnose coccidioidomycosis, gout, pseudogout, hemochromatosis, tuberculosis, sarcoidosis, amyloidosis, pigmented villonodular synovitis, synovial tumors, and synovial cancer (rare). Such examination can also aid in the diagnosis of rheumatoid arthritis, SLE, and Reiter's disease.

Interfering factors

■ Failure to obtain several biopsy specimens
■ Failure to obtain the specimens away from the anesthetic's infiltration site
■ Failure to store the specimens in the appropriate solution or to send them to the laboratory immediately

Selected readings

Diseases, 3rd ed. Springhouse, Pa.: Springhouse Corp., 2001.

Guyton, A.C., and Hall, J.E. *Textbook of Medical Physiology,* 10th ed. Philadelphia: W.B. Saunders Co., 2001.

Pagana, K., and Pagana, T.J. *Diagnostic Testing and Nursing Implications: A Case Study Approach,* 5th ed. St. Louis: Mosby–Year Book, Inc., 1999.

Porth, C. *Pathophysiology: Concepts of Altered Health States,* 6th ed. Philadelphia: Lippincott Williams & Wilkins, 2002.

Yarbo, C.H., et al., eds. *Cancer Nursing: Principles and Practice,* 5th ed. Boston: Jones & Bartlett Pubs., Inc., 2000.

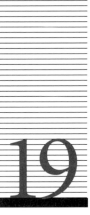

19

Microbes and parasites

Introduction

Microbiology is the study of microorganisms — bacteria, fungi, viruses, and protozoa — that are so small they require special techniques, such as staining or electron microscopy, to reveal their sizes, shapes, and cellular structures.

Gram stain

The Gram staining method, the most common and useful staining procedure, separates bacteria into two classifications, according to the composition of their cell walls: gram-positive organisms, which retain crystal violet stain after decolorization, and gram-negative organisms, which lose the purple stain but counterstain red with safranin.

Microscopic examination of a Gram-stained smear typically allows tentative identification of the suspected organism. Examining a direct Gram smear of the specimen for inflammatory cells, such as neutrophils and macrophages, can also provide clues about the type of infection present and consequent mobilization of the immune system. For example, many segmented neutrophils in a smear of cerebrospinal fluid suggests bacterial meningitis; many mononuclear cells suggests viral, fungal, or tubercular meningitis.

Acid-fast stain

Another staining procedure, the acid-fast method, helps identify organisms of the genus *Mycobacterium*. Since mycobacteria (including pathogens of tuberculosis and leprosy) are acid-fast, they retain carbolfuchsin stain after treatment with an acid-alcohol solution. This technique is particularly useful for identifying mycobacteria in sputum specimens, which may contain many different organisms.

Confirmation by culture

Although stained smears provide rapid, valuable diagnostic leads, they only tentatively identify a pathogen. For example, detection of acid-fast organisms in sputum doesn't conclusively diagnose tuberculosis; nor does a negative acid-fast smear preclude the possibility of tuberculosis. Generally, visualization of an acid-fast microorganism requires the presence of 10,000 to 100,000 microbes per gram of sputum or per milliliter of body fluid.

Confirmation requires culturing and identifying the microbes. Because this process depends on a particular organism's growth rate and nutritional requirements, growing microbes in culture takes longer than microscopic examination of a stained smear. For instance, slow-growing mycobacteria may need weeks of incubation before growth appears. Nevertheless, sufficient growth must take place before further microscopic and biochemical studies can identify the organism.

Sensitivity testing

After a microbe is isolated, its susceptibility to specific antimicrobials and the extent of infection must be determined before choosing antimicrobial therapy. Some pathogens, such as *Streptococcus pneumoniae* (pneumococci), *Streptococcus pyogenes,* and *Neisseria meningitidis,* usually have predictable sensitivity patterns; other pathogens, such as most gram-negative bacilli *(Escherichia coli, Enterobacter, Salmonella, Shigella, Klebsiella, Proteus,* and *Pseudomonas),* enterococci (such as *Streptococcus faecalis),* and *Staphylococcus* species, require testing to determine antimicrobial susceptibility.

These tests also help determine the dosage needed to inhibit or kill an organism in vivo. However, in vitro tests can't account for pharmacologic properties of the selected antimicrobial, such as toxicity, protein binding, absorption, and excretion; nor can they establish the immune status of the host or the nature of the underlying pathologic process. Thus, in vitro antimicrobial susceptibility studies provide only an approximate guide; the patient's clinical response determines the precise dosage.

In the Kirby-Bauer disk-diffusion method, the most widely used qualitative test, disks of filter paper are impregnated with exact amounts of different antimicrobial agents and are added to an agar plate seeded with the test organism. After overnight incubation, zones of inhibition around the disks demonstrate the sensitivity patterns of the organism. A *resistant* strain isn't inhibited by a therapeutic amount of an antimicrobial; a *moderately susceptible* strain may be inhibited by high doses of the antimicrobial; a *sensitive* strain is inhibited or killed by the recommended dosage of an antimicrobial; and an *intermediate* or *indeterminate* strain is equivocally susceptible.

Quantitative sensitivity testing may be necessary for the patient with bacterial endocarditis, bacteremia, or impaired renal function; for one who fails to respond to antimicrobial therapy; or for the patient who has a relapse during therapy. Quantitative sensitivity testing requires the dilution technique, in which serial dilutions of the antimicrobial are inoculated with the organism and incubated to determine the minimal inhibitory concentration and the minimum lethal concentration for the tested isolate.

The antibacterial serum level determination test can help evaluate the effectiveness of antimicrobial therapy. This test consists of titrating serum drawn at peak levels (when the antibacterial level is highest) or at trough levels (when the an-

tibacterial level is lowest, before the next antimicrobial dose) against dilutions of the infecting organism.

Parasitology

Transmission of parasites—organisms that live in or on other biological species to take nourishment from them—is affected by such factors as sanitation, diet, and climate. In countries with good sanitation and effective infection control, the incidence of parasitic disease is relatively low. The clinically important groups of parasites are protozoa (single-cell organisms), helminths (worms), and arthropods (insects and arachnids, such as spiders, mites, and ticks).

Protozoa

Protozoa are classified according to their means of locomotion:
- *Sarcodina* (amoebae) move on temporary cytoplasmic protrusions called pseudopodia. Most species of amoebae appear in humans in the motile, feeding stage (trophozoite form) and the infective stage (cyst form). Of these species, only *Entamoeba histolytica* causes significant disease.
- *Mastigophora* (flagellates) propel themselves by long filamentous appendages called flagella. The most common pathogenic species of flagellates in the United States are *Giardia lamblia,* which infests the intestinal tract, and *Trichomonas vaginalis,* which infests the genital tract. Hemoflagellates, an important subgroup, include the genera *Trypanosoma* and *Leishmania.*
- Ciliophora (ciliates and suctorians) move on hundreds of hairlike projections that cover their bodies. The only pathogenic ciliate is Balantidium coli, the largest protozoan parasite affecting hu-

mans and the cause of balantidial dysentery.

■ *Sporozoa,* which are immobile in the adult stages, include tissue and blood parasites, such as *Toxoplasma gondii, Pneumocystis carinii, Cryptosporidium,* and *Plasmodium* (the cause of malaria). (See *Four pathogenic protozoa,* page 476.)

Transmission of protozoa usually results from ingestion of parasitic cysts contained in fecally contaminated food, water, or soil; other modes of transmission include sexual intercourse *(Trichomonas vaginalis),* mechanical vectoring by flies and other insects *(E. histolytica, G. lamblia),* or the bites of blood-sucking insects *(Trypanosoma, Plasmodium,* and *Leishmania).*

Helminths

Both types of helminths — Platyhelminthes (flatworms) and Nemathelminthes (roundworms) — are usually visible to the naked eye, but confirming infestation requires microscopic examination of ova because the worms themselves are rarely passed. Flatworms include tapeworms, which inhabit the intestinal tract, and leaf-shaped flukes, which appear in the intestinal tract, bile ducts, and blood. Although some species of tapeworms, such as *Taenia saginata* and *Diphyllobothrium latum* are common in the United States, all fluke infections are rare.

Pathogenic species of the slender roundworms include blood and tissue parasites, such as *Wuchereria bancrofti* and *Onchocerca volvulus* (which rarely cause infection in the United States), and intestinal parasites, such as *Ascaris lumbricoides, Necator americanus, Enterobius vermicularis, Trichuris trichiura,* and *Strongyloides stercoralis* (which are indigenous to the United States).

Arthropods

Arthropods include flies, spiders, mites, ticks, crayfish, crabs, lice, fleas, beetles, gnats, and mosquitoes. Although some arthropods, such as lice and the itch mite *Sarcoptes scabiei,* are true parasites, most are vectors (carriers) of parasitic disease. Two kinds of vectors transmit such infections: A mechanical vector, such as an insect, simply carries parasites from one person or object to another; a biological vector, such as a mosquito, acts as a host, allowing parasites to develop and multiply before passing them to another host.

Testing procedures

All protozoan parasites, helminth eggs and larvae, and some arthropods require microscopic identification. Wet films of unstained material can detect various stages of intestinal parasites; the addition of iodine stains protozoan cysts. Permanent stains, such as Giemsa stain, help identify species of blood and tissue parasites and reveal the cytologic detail necessary to identify protozoan parasites. Preservation with formalin, followed by concentration procedures, can detect small numbers of ova, as in helminth infections.

Serologic tests are available for detecting at least 24 protozoan and helminth infections, especially those that cause high antibody levels (such as amebiasis, trichinosis, echinococcosis, and toxoplasmosis) and clinically occult infections (such as filariasis or cysticercosis). The degree of sensitivity and specificity of such testing varies with the disease and the serologic method.

Culturing is available for only a few protozoan parasites and larvae and is performed mainly for research purposes. A culture may be performed if infection with *E. histolytica, Trichomonas vaginalis,*

FOUR PATHOGENIC PROTOZOA

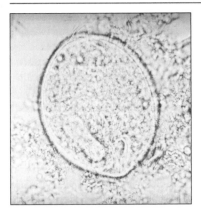

Balantidium coli: This is the largest intestinal protozoan found in humans and the only pathogenic ciliate. In this illustration of an unstained *B. coli* trophozoite taken from a stool specimen, food vacuoles and an anterior cytostome are visible.

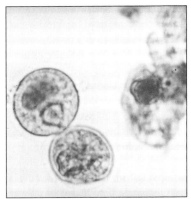

Entamoeba histolytica: This is the most common human pathogen of the six species of *Entamoeba* protozoa. Notice the large chromatoid bodies, diffused glycogen, and delicate chromatin beads on the inner surface of the nuclear membrane that distinguish these infective cysts from nonpathogenic amoebae.

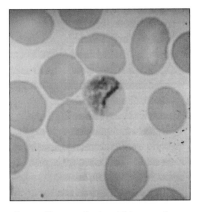

Plasmodium malariae: This organism attacks mature erythrocytes. The trophozoite shown in the illustration displays the granular band of dark brown or black pigment acquired during growth of this sporozoan.

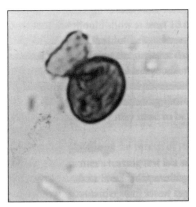

Giardia lamblia: These flagellates commonly infest the intestinal tract. The illustration shows an ellipsoid cyst with a smooth, well-defined wall and multiple nuclei. Notice the trophozoites—forms in the feeding stage—within the cyst.

Trypanosoma cruzi, Naegleria, Acan-thamoeba, or *Leishmania* is suspected and conventional methods fail to confirm it.

CULTURES FOR BACTERIA AND VIRUSES

Urine culture

Laboratory examination and culture of urine are used to evaluate urinary tract infections (UTIs), especially bladder infections. Urine in the kidneys and bladder is normally sterile, but a urine specimen may contain various organisms due to bacteria in the urethra and on external genitalia. Bacteriuria generally results from one prevalent bacteria type; the presence of more than two bacterial species in a specimen strongly suggests contamination during collection. A single negative culture doesn't always rule out infection; a quantitative examination of urine culture is needed.

Significant results of urine culture are possibly only after quantitative examination. To distinguish between true bacteriuria and contamination, it's necessary to know the number or organisms in a milliliter of urine, estimated by a culture technique known as "colony count." In addition, a quick centrifugation test can determine where a UTI originates. (See *Quick centrifugation test.*)

Clean-voided midstream collection, rather than suprapubic aspiration of catheterization, is now the method of choice for obtaining a urine specimen.

Purpose
- To diagnose UTI

QUICK CENTRIFUGATION TEST

The quick centrifugation test can determine whether the source of a urinary tract infection is in the lower tract (bladder) or the upper tract (kidneys). The test involves centrifugation of urine in a test tube, followed by staining of the sediment with fluorescein. If one-quarter of the bacteria fluoresce when viewed under a fluorescent microscope, an upper tract infection is present; if bacteria don't fluoresce, a lower tract infection is present.

- To monitor microorganism colonization after urinary catheter insertion

Patient preparation
- Explain to the patient that this test is used to detect UTIs.
- Inform the patient that the test requires a urine specimen and that no restriction of food and fluids is necessary.
- Instruct him how to collect a clean-voided midstream specimen; emphasize that external genitalia must be cleaned thoroughly.
- If appropriate, explain catheterization or suprapubic aspiration to the patient, and inform him that he may experience some discomfort during specimen collection.
- For the patient with suspected tuberculosis, specimen collection may be required on three consecutive mornings.
- Check the patient's history for current antimicrobial therapy.

Equipment
Gloves, sterile specimen cup, premoistened antiseptic towelettes (Commercial

clean-catch urine kits are available. Many include instructions in several languages.)

Procedure and posttest care

- Collect a urine specimen, as ordered.
- When obtaining a specimen from an indwelling urinary catheter, clamp the tubing below the collection port to collect a specimen in the tubing. Then use an alcohol pad to clean the port. Next, using a sterile needle and syringe, aspirate a 4-ml specimen from the port, and transfer it into a sterile specimen cup.
- Seal the cup with a sterile lid, and send it to the laboratory immediately. If transport is delayed longer than 30 minutes, store the specimen at 39.2° F (4° C) or place it on ice, unless a urine transport tube containing preservative is used.
- Instruct the patient to wash his hands, then clean the urethral area with antiseptic towelettes. Tell the patient to begin urinating in the toilet, then stop and continue to urinate into the sterile cup, without touching the inside of the cup.
- Record on the laboratory request the suspected diagnosis, the collection time and method, current antimicrobial therapy, and fluid- or drug-induced diuresis.

Precautions

- Wear gloves when performing the procedure and handling specimens.
- Collect at least 3 ml of urine, but don't fill the specimen cup more than halfway.

Normal findings

Culture results of sterile urine are usually reported as "no growth," which usually indicates the absence of a UTI.

Abnormal findings

Bacterial counts of 100,000/ml or more of a single microbe species indicate a probable UTI. Counts under 100,000/ml may

be significant, depending on the patient's age, sex, history, and other individual factors. Counts under 10,000/ml usually suggest that the organisms are contaminants, except in symptomatic patients, those with urologic disorders, and those whose urine specimens were collected by suprapubic aspiration. A special test for acid-fast bacteria isolates *Mycobacterium tuberculosis,* thus indicating tuberculosis of the urinary tract.

Isolation of more than two species of organisms or of vaginal or skin organisms usually suggests contamination and requires a repeat culture. Prolonged catheterization or urinary diversion may cause polymicrobial infection.

Interfering factors

- Failure to use the proper collection technique
- Failure to preserve the specimen properly or to send it to the laboratory immediately
- Fluid- or drug-induced diuresis and antimicrobial therapy (possible decrease)

Stool culture

Normal bacterial flora in stool include several potentially pathogenic organisms. Bacteriologic examination is valuable for identifying pathogens that cause overt GI disease — such as typhoid and dysentery — and carrier states. A sensitivity test may follow isolation of the pathogen. The most common pathogenic organisms of the GI tract are *Shigella, Salmonella,* and *Campylobacter jejuni.* Less common pathogenic organisms include *Vibrio cholerae, Clostridium botulinum, Clostridium difficile, Clostridium perfringens, Staphylococcus aureus,* enterotoxigenic *Escherichia coli, Bacillus cereus, Yersinia enterocolitica, Aeromonas hydrophila,* and *V.*

parahaemolyticus. (See *Pathogens of the GI tract.*) Identifying these organisms is vital to treat the patient, to prevent possibly fatal complications (especially in a debilitated patient), and to confine these severe infectious diseases. A sensitivity test may follow isolation of the pathogen.

Some viruses, such as rotavirus and parvovirus, may also cause GI symptoms. However, these viruses can be detected only by immunoassay or electron microscopy. Stool culture may detect other viruses, such as enterovirus, which can cause aseptic meningitis.

Purpose
- To identify pathogenic organisms caused by GI disease
- To identify carrier states

Patient preparation
- Explain to the patient that this test is used to determine the cause of GI distress or to determine if he's a carrier of infectious organisms.
- Advise the patient that he need not restrict food and fluids.
- Tell the patient that the test requires the collection of a stool specimen on 3 consecutive days.
- Check the patient's history for dietary patterns, recent antimicrobial therapy, and recent travel that might suggest endemic infections or infestations.

Equipment
Gloves, waterproof container with tight-fitting lid or sterile swab and commercial sterile collection and transport system, tongue blade, bedpan (if needed)

Procedure and posttest care
- Collect a stool specimen directly into the container. If the patient isn't ambulatory, collect the specimen in a clean, dry

---

PATHOGENS OF THE GI TRACT

The presence of the following pathogens in a stool culture may indicate certain disorders.

Aeromonas hydrophila: gastroenteritis, which causes diarrhea, especially in children

Bacillus cereus: food poisoning, acute gastroenteritis (rare)

Campylobacter jejuni: gastroenteritis

Clostridium botulinum: Food poisoning and infant botulism (a possible cause of sudden infant death syndrome)

Toxin-producing *Clostridium difficile:* pseudomembranous enterocolitis

Clostridium perfringens: food poisoning

Enterotoxigenic *Escherichia coli:* gastroenteritis (resembles cholera or shigellosis)

Salmonella: gastroenteritis, typhoid fever, nontyphoidal salmonellosis, paratyphoid fever

Shigella: shigellosis, bacillary dysentery

Staphylococcus aureus: food poisoning, suppression of normal bowel flora from antimicrobial therapy

Vibrio cholerae: cholera

Vibrio parahaemolyticus: food poisoning, especially seafood

Yersinia enterocolitica: gastroenteritis, enterocolitis (resembles appendicitis), mesenteric lymphadenitis, ileitis.

---

bedpan and, using a tongue blade, transfer the specimen to the container.

- If you must collect the specimen by rectal swab, insert the swab past the anal sphincter, rotate it gently, and withdraw it. Then place the swab in the appropriate container.
- Check with the laboratory for the proper collection procedure before obtaining a specimen for a virus test.
- Label the specimen with the patient's name, physician's name, facility number, and date and time of collection.
- Indicate the suspected cause of enteritis and current antimicrobial therapy on the laboratory request.

Precautions
- Wear gloves when performing the procedure and handling the specimen.
- If the patient uses a bedpan or a diaper, avoid contaminating the stool specimen with urine.
- The specimen must represent the first, middle, and last portion of the stool passed. Be sure to include mucoid and bloody portions.
- Put the specimen container in a leak-proof bag.
- Send the specimen to the laboratory immediately. Trophozoites and cysts may be destroyed if exposed to heat, cold, or a delay in delivery to the laboratory.
- Specimens should be collected before antimicrobial therapy is started.

Normal findings
A large percentage of normal fecal flora consists of anaerobes, including non-spore-forming bacilli, clostridia, and anaerobic streptococci. The remaining percentage consists of aerobes, including gram-negative bacilli (predominantly *E. coli* and other Enterobacteriaceae, plus small amounts of *Pseudomonas*), gram-positive cocci (mostly enterococci), and a few yeasts.

Abnormal findings
The most common pathogenic organisms of the GI tract are *Shigella*, *Salmonella*, and *Campylobacter jejuni*. Less common pathogenic organisms include *V. cholerae*, *V. parahaemolyticus*, *Clostridium botulinum*, *Clostridium difficile*, *Clostridium perfringens*, *S. aureus*, enterotoxigenic *E. coli*, and *Y. enterocolitica*. Isolation of some pathogens indicates bacterial infection in the patient with acute diarrhea and may require antimicrobial sensitivity tests. Normal fecal flora may include *Clostridium difficile*, *E. coli*, and other organisms. Therefore, isolation of these organisms may require further tests to demonstrate invasiveness or toxin production.

Isolation of pathogens such as *Clostridium botulinum* indicates food poisoning; the pathogens must also be isolated from the contaminated food. In a patient undergoing long-term antimicrobial therapy, isolation of large numbers of *S. aureus* or yeast may indicate infection. (Asymptomatic carrier states are also indicated by these enteric pathogens.) Isolation of enteroviruses may indicate aseptic meningitis.

If a stool culture shows no unusual growth, detection of viruses by immunoassay or electron microscopy may be used to diagnose nonbacterial gastroenteritis. Highly increased polymorphonuclear leukocytes in fecal material may indicate an invasive pathogen.

Interfering factors
- Failure to use proper collection technique
- Contamination of the specimen by urine (possible injury to or destruction of enteric pathogens)
- Antimicrobial therapy (possible decrease in bacterial growth)

■ Failure to transport the specimen promptly or, if delivery is delayed, to use a transport medium, such as buffered glycerol, that stabilizes pH (possible loss of enteric pathogens or overgrowth of nonpathogenic organisms)

Throat culture

A throat culture is used primarily to isolate and identify pathogens, thus allowing early treatment of pharyngitis and prevention of sequelae, such as rheumatic heart disease and glomerulonephritis. It's also used to screen for carriers of *Neisseria meningitidis*. In rare instances, a throat culture may be used to identify *Corynebacterium diphtheriae* or *Bordetella pertussis*. Although a throat culture may also be used to identify *Candida albicans,* direct potassium hydroxide preparation usually provides the same information faster.

A throat culture requires swabbing the throat, streaking a culture plate, and allowing the organisms to grow for isolation and identification of pathogens. A Gram-stained smear may provide preliminary identification, which may guide clinical management and determine the need for further tests. Culture results are considered in relation to the patient's clinical status, recent antimicrobial therapy, and amount of normal flora.

Purpose
■ To isolate and identify group A beta-hemolytic streptococci
■ To screen asymptomatic carriers of pathogens, especially *N. meningitidis*

Patient preparation
■ Explain to the patient that this test is used to identify microorganisms that may be causing his symptoms or to screen for asymptomatic carriers.
■ Inform the patient that he need not restrict food and fluids.
■ Tell the patient that a specimen will be collected from his throat and who will collect the specimen and when.
■ Describe the procedure, and warn the patient that he may gag during the swabbing.
■ Check the patient's history for recent antimicrobial therapy. Determine immunization history if it's pertinent to the preliminary diagnosis.

Equipment
Gloves, sterile swab and culture tube with transport medium or commercial collection and transport system

Procedure and posttest care
■ Tell the patient to tilt his head back and close his eyes.
■ With the throat well illuminated, check for inflamed areas using a tongue blade.
■ Swab the tonsillar areas from side to side; include inflamed or purulent sites.
■ *Don't* touch the tongue, cheeks, or teeth with the swab.
■ Immediately place the swab in the culture tube.
■ If a commercial sterile collection and transport system is used, crush the ampule and force the swab into the medium to keep the swab moist.
■ Note recent antimicrobial therapy on the laboratory request; label the specimen with the patient's name, the physician's name, the date and time of collection, and the origin of the specimen; indicate the suspected organism, especially *C. diphtheriae* (requires two swabs and a special growth medium), *B. pertussis* (requires a nasopharyngeal culture and a

special growth medium), and *N. meningitidis* (requires enriched selective media).
- Nonculture antigen testing methods can be used to detect group A streptococcal antigen in as few as 5 minutes. Cultures are then performed on negative specimens.

Precautions
- Procure the throat specimen before beginning antimicrobial therapy.
- Wear gloves when performing the procedure and handling specimens.
- Send the specimen to the laboratory immediately. Unless a commercial sterile collection and transport system is used, keep the container upright during transport.

▶ **CLINICAL ALERT** *Laryngospasm may occur after the culture is obtained if the patient has epiglottiditis or diphtheria. Keep resuscitation equipment nearby.*

Normal findings
Normal throat flora include nonhemolytic and alpha-hemolytic streptococci, *Neisseria* species, staphylococci, diphtheroids, some *Haemophilus* species, pneumococci, yeasts, enteric gram-negative rods, spirochetes, *Veillonella* species, and *Micrococcus* species.

Abnormal findings
Pathogens that may be cultured include group A beta-hemolytic streptococci (*Streptococcus pyogenes*), which can cause scarlet fever and pharyngitis; *Candida albicans*, which can cause thrush; *Corynebacterium diphtheriae*, which can cause diphtheria; and *B. pertussis*, which can cause whooping cough. The laboratory report should indicate the prevalent organisms and the quantity of pathogens cultured.

Interfering factors
- Failure to report recent or current antimicrobial therapy on the laboratory request (possible false-negative)
- Failure to use the proper transport medium
- More than a 15-minute delay in sending the specimen to the laboratory

Nasopharyngeal culture

A nasopharyngeal culture is used to evaluate nasopharyngeal secretions for the presence of pathogenic organisms. It requires direct microscopic examination of a Gram-stained smear of the specimen. Preliminary identification of organisms may be used to guide clinical management and determine the need for additional testing. Cultured pathogens may then require susceptibility testing to determine appropriate antimicrobial therapy.

Nasopharyngeal cultures are typically useful for identifying *Bordetella pertussis* and *Neisseria meningitidis,* especially in very young, elderly, or debilitated patients. They can also be used to isolate viruses, especially carriers of influenza virus A and B. However, because the laboratory procedure required for such testing is complex, time-consuming, and costly, this culture is performed infrequently.

Purpose
- To identify pathogens causing upper respiratory tract symptoms
- To identify proliferation of normal nasopharyngeal flora, which may be pathogenic in debilitated and other immunocompromised patients
- To identify *B. pertussis* and *N. meningitidis,* especially in very young, elderly, or debilitated patients and asymptomatic carriers

- Infrequently, to isolate viruses, especially to identify carriers of influenza virus A and B

Patient preparation
- Explain to the patient that this test is used to isolate the cause of nasopharyngeal infection.
- Describe the procedure to the patient; tell him that secretions will be obtained from the back of the nose and the throat, using a cotton-tipped swab, and who will collect the specimen.
- Warn the patient that he may experience slight discomfort and gagging, but reassure him that obtaining the specimen takes less than 15 seconds.

Equipment
Gloves; penlight; sterile, flexible wire swab; small, sterile, open-ended glass tube or sterile nasal speculum; tongue blade; culture tube; transport medium (broth), sterile water or saline

Procedure and posttest care
- Put on gloves.
- Moisten the swab with sterile water or saline.
- Ask the patient to cough before you begin collecting the specimen.
- Position the patient with his head tilted back.
- Using a penlight and a tongue blade, inspect the nasopharyngeal area.
- Gently pass the swab through the nostril and into the nasopharynx, keeping the swab near the septum and floor of the nose. Rotate the swab quickly and remove it.
- Alternatively, place the glass tube in the patient's nostril, and carefully pass the swab through the tube into the nasopharynx. (See *Obtaining a nasopharyngeal specimen.*) Rotate the swab for 5 seconds

> ### OBTAINING A NASOPHARYNGEAL SPECIMEN
>
> When the swab passes into the nasopharynx, gently but quickly rotate it to collect a specimen. Then remove the swab, taking care not to injure the nasal mucous membrane.
>
>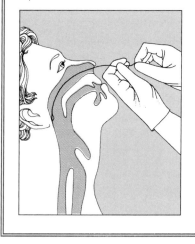

and then place it in the culture tube with transport medium. Remove the glass tube.
- Label the specimen with the patient's name, the physician's name, the date and time of collection, the origin of the material, and the suspected organism.
- Ideally, specimens for *B. pertussis* should be inoculated to fresh culture medium at the patient's bedside because of the organism's susceptibility to environmental changes.
- If the purpose of specimen collection is to isolate a virus, follow the laboratory's recommended collection technique.

Precautions
- Wear gloves when performing the procedure and handling the specimen.

■ *Don't* let the swab touch the sides of the patient's nostril or his tongue to prevent specimen contamination.

🔻 **CLINICAL ALERT** *Laryngospasm may occur after the culture is obtained if the patient has epiglottiditis or diphtheria. Keep resuscitation equipment nearby.*

■ Note antimicrobial therapy or chemotherapy on the laboratory request.

■ Keep the container upright.

■ Tell the laboratory if the suspected organism is *Corynebacterium diphtheriae* or *B. pertussis* because these need special growth media.

■ Refrigerate a viral specimen according to your laboratory's procedure.

■ If *B. pertussis* is suspected, Dacron or calcium alginate mini-tipped swabs should be used for collection.

■ When specimens can't be directly placed onto growth media, the best media-based transport is one supplemented with antibiotics to reduce the growth of normal flora.

Normal findings

Flora commonly found in the nasopharynx include nonhemolytic streptococci, alpha-hemolytic streptococci, *Neisseria* species (except *N. meningitidis* and *N. gonorrhoeae*), coagulase-negative staphylococci such as *Staphylococcus epidermidis* and, occasionally, the coagulase-positive *S. aureus.*

Abnormal findings

Pathogens include group A beta-hemolytic streptococci; occasionally groups B, C, and G beta-hemolytic streptococci; *B. pertussis, C. diphtheriae,* and *S. aureus;* large numbers of pneumococci; *Haemophilus influenzae;* Myxovirus influenzae; paramyxoviruses; *Candida albicans;* my-

coplasma species; and *Mycobacterium tuberculosis.*

Interfering factors

■ Recent antimicrobial therapy (decrease in bacterial growth)

■ Failure to use proper collection technique

■ Failure to place the specimen in transport medium

■ Failure to keep a viral specimen cold

■ Failure to send the specimen to the laboratory immediately

Sputum culture

Bacteriologic examination of sputum (material raised from the lungs and bronchi) is an important aid to the management of lung disease. During passage through the throat and oropharynx, sputum specimens are commonly contaminated with indigenous bacterial flora, such as alpha-hemolytic streptococci, *Neisseria* species, diptheroids, some *Haemophilus* species, pneumococci, staphylococci, and yeasts such as *Candida.*

Pathogenic organisms typically found in sputum include *Streptococcus pneumoniae, Mycobacterium tuberculosis, Klebsiella pneumoniae* (and other Enterobacteriaceae), *Haemophilus influenzae, Staphylococcus aureus,* and *Pseudomonas aeruginosa.* Other pathogens, such as *Pneumocystis carinii, Legionella* species, *Mycoplasma pneumoniae,* and respiratory viruses, may exist in the sputum and can cause lung disease, but they usually require serologic or histologic diagnosis rather than diagnosis by sputum culture.

The usual method of specimen collection is expectoration (which may require ultrasonic nebulization, hydration, physiotherapy, or postural drainage); other

USING AN IN-LINE TRAP

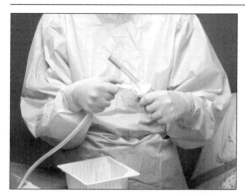

Push the suction tubing onto the male adapter of the in-line trap.

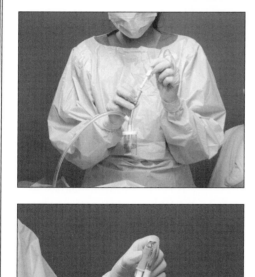

Put on sterile gloves; with one hand, insert the suction catheter into the rubber tubing of the trap. Then suction the patient.

After suctioning, disconnect the in-line trap from the suction tubing and catheter. To seal the container, connect the rubber tubing to the female adapter of the trap.

methods include tracheal suctioning and bronchoscopy. (See *Using an in-line trap*.)

A Gram stain of expectorated sputum must be examined to ensure that it's a representative specimen of secretions from the lower respiratory tract (many white blood cells [WBCs], few epithelial cells) rather than one contaminated by oral flora (few WBCs, many epithelial cells). Careful examination of an acid-fast smear of sputum may provide presumptive evidence of a mycobacterial infection such as tuberculosis.

Purpose
■ To isolate and identify the cause of pulmonary infection, thus aiding in the diagnosis of respiratory diseases (most commonly bronchitis, tuberculosis, lung abscess, and pneumonia)

Patient preparation
■ Explain to the patient that this test is used to identify the organism causing respiratory tract infection.
■ Tell the patient that the test requires a sputum specimen and who will collect the specimen.
■ If the suspected organism is *M. tuberculosis,* tell the patient that as many as three consecutive morning specimens may be required.
■ If testing is for tuberculosis, explain that cultures for tuberculosis may take some time to develop and that specimens may need to be collected on at least three consecutive mornings; therefore, diagnosis of this disorder generally depends on clinical symptoms, a smear for acid-fast bacilli, a chest X-ray, and response to a purified protein derivative skin test.
■ If the specimen will be collected by expectoration, encourage fluid intake the night before collection to help sputum production, unless contraindicated by a fluid restriction. Teach the patient how to expectorate by taking three deep breaths and forcing a deep cough; emphasize that sputum isn't the same as saliva, which is unacceptable for culturing. Tell him to brush his teeth and gargle with water before the specimen collection to reduce contaminating oropharyngeal bacteria.

■ If the specimen will be collected by tracheal suctioning, tell the patient that he'll experience discomfort as the catheter passes into the trachea.
■ If the specimen will be collected by bronchoscopy, instruct the patient to fast for 6 hours before the procedure.
■ Make sure the patient or a responsible family member has signed an informed consent form.
■ Tell the patient that he'll receive a local anesthetic just before the test to minimize discomfort during passage of the tube.

Equipment
For expectoration: clean gloves, sterile, disposable, impermeable container with a tight-fitting cap; normal saline solution, acetylcysteine, propylene glycol, or sterile or distilled water aerosols to induce cough as ordered; leakproof bag

For tracheal suctioning: #16 or #18 French suction catheter, water-soluble lubricant, sterile gloves, sterile specimen container or in-line specimen trap, normal saline solution

For bronchoscopy: bronchoscope, local anesthetic, sterile needle and syringe, sterile specimen container, normal saline solution, bronchial brush, sterile gloves

Procedure and posttest care
Expectoration
■ Put on gloves.
■ Instruct the patient to cough deeply and expectorate into the container. If the cough is nonproductive, use chest physiotherapy or a heated aerosol spray (nebulization) to induce sputum. Using sterile technique, close the container securely.
■ Dispose of equipment properly; seal the container in a leakproof bag before sending it to the laboratory.

Tracheal suctioning
- Administer oxygen to the patient before and after the procedure if necessary.
- Attach the sputum trap to the suction catheter. Using sterile gloves, lubricate the catheter with normal saline solution, and pass it through the patient's nostril without suction. (He'll cough when the catheter passes through the larynx.) Advance the catheter into the trachea. Apply suction for no longer than 15 seconds to obtain the specimen.
- Stop suction and gently remove the catheter. Discard the catheter and gloves in the proper receptacle. Then detach the in-line sputum trap from the suction apparatus, and cap the opening.

Bronchoscopy
- After a local anesthetic is sprayed into the patient's throat or after he gargles with a local anesthetic, the bronchoscope is inserted through the pharynx and trachea into the bronchus.
- Secretions are then collected with a bronchial brush or aspirated through the inner channel of the scope using an irrigating solution, such as normal saline solution, if necessary.
- After the specimen is obtained, the bronchoscope is removed.

CLINICAL ALERT *During and after bronchoscopy, observe the patient carefully for signs of hypoxemia (change in mental status), laryngospasm (laryngeal stridor), bronchospasm (paroxysms of coughing or wheezing), pneumothorax (dyspnea, cyanosis, pleural pain, tachycardia), perforation of the trachea or bronchus (subcutaneous crepitus), and trauma to respiratory structures (blood-tinged sputum, coughing up blood). Also, check for difficulty in breathing or swallowing. Don't give liquids until the gag reflex returns.*

All collection methods
- Provide good mouth care.
- Label the container with the patient's name. Include on the test request form the nature and origin of the specimen, the date and time of collection, the initial diagnosis, and any current antimicrobial therapy.

Precautions
- Tracheal suctioning is contraindicated in the patient with esophageal varices.

CLINICAL ALERT *In a patient with asthma or chronic bronchitis, watch for aggravated bronchospasms when using normal saline solution or acetylcysteine in an aerosol.*

- During tracheal suctioning, suction for only 5 to 10 seconds at a time. Never suction longer than 15 seconds. If the patient becomes hypoxic or cyanotic, remove the catheter immediately and administer oxygen.
- Wear gloves when performing the procedure and handling specimens.
- Because the patient may cough violently during suctioning, wear gloves, a mask and, if necessary, a gown to avoid exposure to pathogens.
- *Don't* use more than 20% propylene glycol with water as an inducer for a specimen scheduled for tuberculosis culturing because higher concentrations inhibit the growth of *M. tuberculosis*. (If propylene glycol isn't available, use 10% to 20% acetylcysteine with water or saline solution.)
- Send the specimen to the laboratory immediately after collection.

Normal findings
Flora commonly found in the respiratory tract include alpha-hemolytic streptococci, *Neisseria* species, and diphtheroids.

The presence of normal flora doesn't rule out infection.

Abnormal findings

Because sputum is invariably contaminated with normal oropharyngeal flora, a culture isolate must be interpreted in light of the patient's overall clinical condition. Isolation of *M. tuberculosis* is always a significant finding.

Interfering factors

- Failure to use the proper collection technique
- Failure to report current or recent antimicrobial therapy on the laboratory request (possible false-negative)
- Collection over an extended period, which may cause pathogens to deteriorate or become overgrown by commensals (not accepted as a valid specimen by laboratories)

Blood culture

A blood culture is performed to isolate and aid in the identification of the pathogens in bacteremia (bacterial invasion of the bloodstream) and septicemia (systemic spread of such infection). It requires inoculating a culture medium with a blood sample and incubating it.

Blood culture can identify about 67% of pathogens within 24 hours and up to 90% within 72 hours.

Bacteria from local tissue infection usually invade the bloodstream through the lymphatic system by way of the thoracic duct. (See *The lymphatic system*.) Occasionally, they enter the bloodstream directly through infusion lines, thrombophlebitis, or bacterial endocarditis from prosthetic heart valve replacements. Bacteremia may be transient, intermittent, or continuous. The timing of specimen collection for blood cultures varies;

THE LYMPHATIC SYSTEM

The lymphatic system—a network of capillary and venous channels—returns excess interstitial fluids and proteins to the blood. Materials flowing through these channels pass into the thoracic and right lymph ducts. The thoracic duct, the larger of the two, drains the lymphatic vessels from all but the upper right quadrant. This lymphatic drainage (commonly called *lymph*, the tissue fluid absorbed in the lymphatic vessels) then flows into the junction of the left internal jugular and left subclavian veins. The right lymph duct drains interstitial fluid from the upper right quadrant into the right subclavian vein.

Bacteria from local tissue infection usually enter the bloodstream through this system. When functioning properly, however, the lymphatic system provides a strong defense against bacteria and viruses. Before lymph reenters the bloodstream, afferent lymphatic vessels transport it to lymph nodes or glands—clusters of lymphatic tissues throughout the body—where numerous lymphocytes destroy microorganisms and foreign particles.

If the lymphatic system fails to destroy harmful particles before they enter the bloodstream, white blood cells (WBCs) in the spleen, liver, and bone marrow act as another defense mechanism. As blood circulates through the body, it flows into the spleen, where it's filtered. There, residing lymphocytes ingest abnormal or foreign cells while normal cells pass through. Bacteria that accompany digested food particles into the portal vein—which supplies the liver—are ingested by reticulum cells. Likewise,

---

it usually depends on the type of bacteremia (intermittent or continuous) suspected and on whether drug therapy needs to be started regardless of test results.

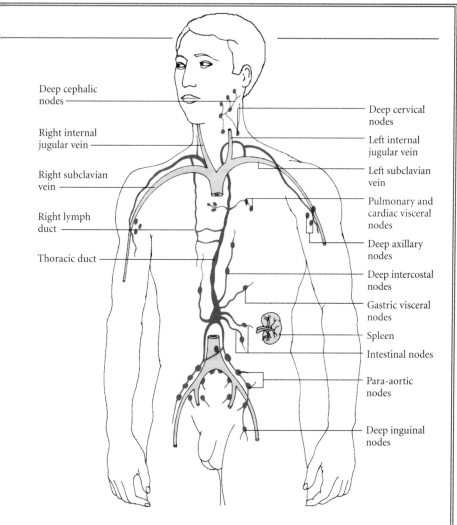

Deep cephalic nodes

Right internal jugular vein

Right subclavian vein

Right lymph duct

Thoracic duct

Deep cervical nodes

Left internal jugular vein

Left subclavian vein

Pulmonary and cardiac visceral nodes

Deep axillary nodes

Deep intercostal nodes

Gastric visceral nodes

Spleen

Intestinal nodes

Para-aortic nodes

Deep inguinal nodes

WBCs formed in the bone marrow protect the body from invading bacteria.

Macrophages constitute still another defense system. These WBCs in the tissues, lymph nodes, and red bone marrow are usually immobile, but they migrate to inflamed areas, where they ingest and destroy infective particles.

Purpose
- To confirm bacteremia
- To identify the causative organism in bacteremia and septicemia

Patient preparation
- Explain to the patient that this procedure is used to help identify the organism causing his symptoms.
- Inform the patient that he need not restrict food and fluids.

- Tell the patient how many samples the test will require and who will perform the venipunctures and when.
- Inform the patient that he may experience slight discomfort from the needle punctures and the tourniquet.

Equipment

Gloves; tourniquet; small adhesive bandages; alcohol swabs; povidone-iodine swabs; 10- to 20-ml syringe for an adult, 6-ml syringe for a child; three or four sterile needles; two blood culture bottles, one vented (aerobic) and one unvented (anaerobic), with nutritionally enriched broths and sodium polyethanol sulfonate added, or bottles with resin or a lysis-centrifugation tube

Procedure and posttest care

- Put on gloves.
- Clean the venipuncture site with an alcohol swab and then with an iodine swab, working in a circular motion from the site outward.
- Wait at least 1 minute for the skin to dry, and remove the residual iodine with an alcohol swab or remove the iodine after venipuncture.
- Apply the tourniquet.
- Perform a venipuncture; draw 10 to 20 ml of blood for an adult or 2 to 6 ml for a child.
- Clean the diaphragm tops of the culture bottles with alcohol or iodine, and change the needle on the syringe.
- If broth is used, add blood to each bottle until a 1:5 or 1:10 dilution is obtained. For example, add 10 ml of blood to a 100-ml bottle. (The size of the bottle varies, depending on facility procedure.)
- If a special resin is used, add blood to the resin in the bottles and invert them gently to mix.

- If you're using the lysis-centrifugation technique (Isolator), draw the blood directly into a special collection and processing tube.
- Indicate the tentative diagnosis on the laboratory request, and note current or recent antimicrobial therapy.
- Apply direct pressure to the venipuncture site until bleeding stops.
- If a hematoma develops at the venipuncture site, apply warm soaks.

Precautions

- Wear gloves when performing the procedure and handling specimens.
- Send each specimen to the laboratory immediately after collection.
- Don't draw blood from an existing I.V. catheter. Use a vein below an I.V. catheter or in the opposite arm.
- Whenever possible, blood cultures should be collected before administering antimicrobial agents.

Normal findings

Normally, blood cultures are negative for pathogens.

Abnormal findings

Positive blood cultures don't necessarily confirm pathologic septicemia. Mild, transient bacteremia may occur during the course of many infectious diseases or may complicate other disorders. Persistent, continuous, or recurrent bacteremia reliably confirms the presence of serious infection. To detect most causative agents, blood cultures are ideally drawn on 2 consecutive days.

Isolation of most organisms takes about 72 hours; negative cultures are held for 1 or more weeks before being reported negative.

Common blood pathogens include *Streptococcus pneumoniae* and other

Streptococcus species, *Haemophilus influenzae, Staphylococcus aureus, Pseudomonas aeruginosa, Bacteroides, Brucella,* Enterobacteriaceae, coliform bacilli, and *Candida albicans.* Although 2% to 3% of cultured blood samples are contaminated by skin bacteria, such as *Staphylococcus epidermidis,* diphtheroids, and *Propionibacterium,* these organisms may be clinically significant when isolated from multiple cultures or from immuno-compromised patients. Debilitated or im-munocompromised patients may have isolates of *C. albicans.* In patients with human immunodeficiency virus infec-tion, *Mycobacterium tuberculosis* and *M. avium* complex may be isolated as well as other *Mycobacterium* species on a less fre-quent basis.

Interfering factors
■ Previous or current antimicrobial ther-apy on the laboratory request (possible false-negative)
■ Failure to use the proper collection technique
■ Removal of culture bottle caps at the bedside (possible prevention of anaerobic growth)
■ Use of the incorrect bottle and media (possible prevention of aerobic growth)

Wound culture

Performed to confirm infection, a wound culture is a microscopic analysis of a specimen from a lesion. Wound cultures may be aerobic, for detection of organ-isms that usually appear in a superficial wound, or anaerobic, for organisms that need little or no oxygen and appear in ar-eas of poor tissue perfusion, such as post-operative wounds, ulcers, and compound fractures. Indications for wound culture

include fever as well as inflammation and drainage in damaged tissue.

Purpose
■ To identify an infectious microbe in a wound

Patient preparation
■ Explain to the patient that this test is used to identify infectious microbes.
■ Describe the procedure, informing the patient that a drainage specimen from the wound is withdrawn by a syringe or re-moved on sterile cotton swabs.
■ Tell the patient who will collect the specimen.

Equipment
Sterile cotton swabs and sterile culture tube or commercial sterile collection and transport system (for aerobic culture); sterile cotton swabs or sterile 10-ml sy-ringe with 21G needle, and special culture tube containing carbon dioxide or nitro-gen (for anaerobic culture); sterile gloves; alcohol pads; sterile gauze; povidone-iodine solution

Procedure and posttest care
■ Put on gloves, prepare a sterile field, and clean the area around the wound with antiseptic solution.
■ For an *aerobic culture,* express the wound and swab as much exudate as pos-sible, or insert the swab deeply into the wound and gently rotate. Immediately place the swab in the aerobic culture tube.
■ For an *anaerobic culture,* insert the swab deeply into the wound, gently ro-tate, and immediately place the swab in the anaerobic culture tube. (See *Anaerobic specimen collector,* page 492.) Or, insert the needle into the wound, aspirate 1 to 5 ml of exudate into the syringe, and im-mediately inject the exudate into the

ANAEROBIC SPECIMEN COLLECTOR

Some anaerobes die when exposed to oxygen. To facilitate anaerobic collection and culturing, tubes filled with carbon dioxide (CO_2) or nitrogen are used for oxygen-free transport.

The anaerobic specimen collector shown here consists of a rubber-stopper tube filled with CO_2, a small inner tube, and a swab attached to a plastic plunger. The drawing below left shows the tube before specimen collection. The small inner tube containing the swab is held in place by the rubber stopper.

After specimen collection (below right), the swab is quickly replaced in the inner tube, and the plunger is depressed. This separates the inner tube from the stopper, forcing it into the larger tube and exposing the specimen to the CO_2-rich environment.

The tube should be kept upright.

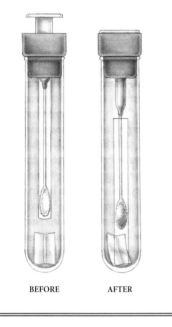

BEFORE   AFTER

anaerobic culture tube. If the needle is covered with a rubber stopper, the aspirate may be sent to the laboratory in the syringe.

■ Record on the laboratory request recent antimicrobial therapy, the source of the specimen, and the suspected organism. Label the specimen container with the patient's name, the physician's name, the facility number, the wound site, and the time of collection.

■ Dress the wound.

Precautions

■ Clean the area around the wound thoroughly to limit contamination of the culture by normal skin flora, such as diphtheroids, *Staphylococcus epidermidis,* and alpha-hemolytic streptococci. *Don't* clean the area around a perineal wound.

■ Make sure no antiseptic enters the wound.

■ Obtain exudate from the entire wound, using more than one swab if necessary.

■ Because some anaerobes die in the presence of even a small amount of oxygen, place the specimen in the culture tube quickly, take care that no air enters the tube, and check that double stoppers are secure.

■ Keep the specimen container upright, and send it to the laboratory within 15 minutes to prevent growth or deterioration of microbes.

■ Wear gloves during the procedure and when handling the specimen, and take necessary isolation precautions when sending the specimen to the laboratory.

Normal findings

Normally, no pathogenic organisms are present in a clean wound.

Abnormal findings

The most common aerobic pathogens for wound infection include *S. aureus*, group A beta-hemolytic streptococci, *Proteus*, *Escherichia coli* and other Enterobacteriaceae, and some *Pseudomonas* species; the most common anaerobic pathogens include some *Clostridium*, *Peptococcus*, *Bacteroides*, and *Streptococcus* species.

Interfering factors

■ Failure to report recent or current antimicrobial therapy (possible false-negative)
■ Failure to use the proper collection technique
■ Failure to use the proper transport medium, allowing the specimen to dry and the bacteria to deteriorate

Gastric culture

A gastric culture requires aspiration of gastric contents and cultivation of any microbes present. Performed in conjunction with a chest X-ray and a purified protein derivative skin test, it's especially useful when a sputum specimen can't be obtained by expectoration or nebulization. Gastric aspiration also provides a specimen for rapid presumptive identification of bacteria (by Gram stain) in neonatal septicemia.

Purpose

■ To aid in the diagnosis of mycobacterial infections
■ To identify the infectious bacteria in neonatal septicemia

Patient preparation

■ Explain to the patient (or parents if the patient is a child) that gastric culture helps diagnose tuberculosis.

■ Instruct the patient to fast for 8 hours before the test.
■ Tell the patient who will perform the procedure and that the same procedure may be performed on three consecutive mornings.
■ Instruct the patient to remain in bed each morning until specimen collection has been completed to prevent premature emptying of stomach contents.
■ Describe the procedure to the patient. Tell him that the nasogastric (NG) tube may make him gag but that it passes more easily if he relaxes and follows instructions about breathing and swallowing.
■ Just before the procedure, obtain baseline oxygen saturation and heart rate and rhythm, and place the patient in high Fowler's position.
■ Inform the patient (or his parents) that test results may be prolonged because acid-fast bacteria is slow-growing.
■ Check the patient's history for recent antimicrobial therapy. Inform the physician of your findings; he may want to discontinue medications before the test.

Equipment

Water-soluble lubricating jelly; sterile water; #16 or #18 French disposable, plastic NG tube; 50-ml sterile syringe; sterile specimen container; sterile gloves; emesis basin; stethoscope; clamp (if necessary)

Procedure and posttest care

■ As soon as the patient awakens in the morning, put on gloves, perform NG insertion, confirming position, and obtain gastric washings.
■ Clamp the tube before quickly removing it from the patient.
■ Note recent antimicrobial therapy on the laboratory request, along with the site and time of collection.

■ Label the specimen container with the patient's name, the physician's name, and the facility number.

■ Tell the patient that he may resume his usual diet and medications, as ordered.

■ Instruct the patient not to blow his nose for 4 hours to prevent bleeding.

Precautions

■ Gastric insertion is contraindicated in pregnancy, esophageal disorders (varices, stenosis, diverticula), malignant neoplasms, recent severe gastric hemorrhage, aortic aneurysm, heart failure, and myocardial infarction.

■ If possible, obtain the specimens before the start of antimicrobial therapy.

■ Watch for signs that the tube has entered the trachea, including coughing, cyanosis, decreasing oxygen saturation readings, and gasping.

▶ **CLINICAL ALERT** *Never inject water into an NG tube unless you're sure the tube is correctly placed in the patient's stomach. During lavage, use sterile distilled water to decrease the risk of contamination with saprophytic mycobacteria.*

■ Check the patient's pulse rate for irregularities during this procedure to detect arrhythmias and monitor for signs of hypoxia.

■ Wear gloves when performing the procedure and when handling specimens and the NG tube.

■ Put the specimen in a tightly capped container, wipe the outside of the container with disinfectant, and place it upright in a plastic bag.

■ Send the specimen to the laboratory immediately.

■ Dispose of all equipment carefully to prevent staff contamination.

Normal findings

Normally, the culture specimen is negative for pathogenic mycobacteria.

Abnormal findings

Isolation and identification of the organism *Mycobacterium tuberculosis* indicates the presence of active tuberculosis; other species, such as *M. bovis, M. kansasii, and M. avium,* may cause pulmonary disease that's clinically indistinguishable from tuberculosis. Treatment of these mycobacterial infections may be difficult and commonly requires susceptibility studies to determine the most effective antimicrobial therapy. Pathogenic bacteria causing neonatal septicemia may also be identified through culture.

Interfering factors

■ Failure to observe an 8-hour fast before the test (possible decrease)

■ Tetracycline and aminoglycosides (possible false-negative)

■ Presence of saprophytic mycobacteria in gastric contents because these mycobacteria can't be microscopically distinguished from pathogenic mycobacteria (possible false-positive acid-fast smears)

Duodenal contents culture

A duodenal contents culture requires duodenal tube insertion, aspiration of duodenal contents, and cultivation of microbes to isolate and identify pathogens that may cause duodenitis, cholecystitis, and cholangitis. Occasionally, a specimen may be obtained during surgery.

Duodenal contents (pancreatic and duodenal enzymes and bile) are normally almost sterile, but they're subject to infection by many pathogens, such as *Escherichia coli, Staphylococcus aureus,* and *Sal-*

monella. Such microbial infections of the biliary tract and duodenum can result in duodenitis, cholecystitis, or cholangitis.

Purpose
- To detect bacterial infection of the biliary tract and duodenum
- To differentiate between infection and gallstones
- To rule out bacterial infection as the cause of persistent GI symptoms (epigastric pain, nausea, vomiting, and diarrhea)

Patient preparation
- Explain to the patient that this test is used to determine the cause of his symptoms.
- Instruct the patient to restrict food and fluids for 12 hours before the test.
- Tell the patient who will perform the procedure and where it will be done.
- Describe the insertion procedure to the patient. Assure him that although this procedure is uncomfortable, it isn't dangerous; tell him that passage of the tube may cause gagging, but that following the examiner's instructions about proper positioning, breathing, swallowing, and relaxing will minimize his discomfort.
- Suggest that the patient empty his bladder before the procedure to increase his general comfort.

Equipment
Gloves, double-lumen nasoenteric tube with olive tip, water-soluble jelly, 30-ml sterile syringe, emesis basin, sterile specimen container, ½″ adhesive tape

Procedure and posttest care
- After the nasoenteric tube is inserted, place the patient in a left lateral decubitus position with his feet elevated to allow peristalsis to move the tube into the duodenum.

- Determine the pH of a small amount of aspirated fluid to ascertain tube position. If the tube is in the stomach, pH is lower than 7; if the tube is in the duodenum, pH is higher than 7. The position of the tube can also be confirmed by fluoroscopy.
- Aspirate duodenal contents.
- Occasionally, a specimen for culture of duodenal contents is obtained during duodenoscopy. (See "Esophagogastroduodenoscopy," page 764.)
- Transfer the specimen to a sterile container, and label it with the patient's name, the physician's name, the date and time of collection, and the collector's initials.
- After duodenal tube placement or duodenoscopy, observe the patient carefully for signs of perforation, such as dysphagia, epigastric or shoulder pain, dyspnea, and fever.
- After duodenoscopy, monitor the patient's vital signs until he's stable; keep the side rails up, and enforce bed rest until the he's fully alert.
- Tell the patient that he may resume his usual diet, as ordered.

Precautions
- Wear gloves when assisting with this procedure and handling the specimen.
- Duodenal tube insertion is contraindicated in pregnancy; acute pancreatitis or cholecystitis; esophageal varices, stenosis, and diverticular malignant neoplasms; recent severe gastric hemorrhage; aortic aneurysm; heart failure; and myocardial infarction.
- Collect the specimen for culture before antimicrobial therapy begins.
- Send the specimen to the laboratory immediately.
- Withdraw the tube slowly (6″ to 8″ [15 to 20 cm] every 10 minutes) until it

reaches the esophagus, and then clamp the tube and remove it quickly. If you can't withdraw the tube easily, report the problem; *never* force the tube.

Normal findings

Normally, a duodenal contents culture contains small amounts of polymorphonuclear leukocytes and epithelial cells with no pathogens. The bacterial count is usually less than 100,000/ml of body fluid.

Abnormal findings

Generally, bacterial counts of 100,000/ml or more or the presence of pathogens in any number indicates infection. Susceptibility testing may be required.

Numerous polymorphonuclear leukocytes, copious mucus, and bile-stained epithelial cells in the bile fluid suggest inflammation of the biliary tract; many segmented neutrophils and exfoliated epithelial cells suggest pancreas, duodenum, or bile duct inflammation. The presence of bile sand indicates cholelithiasis or calculi in the biliary tract. Differential diagnosis requires further testing.

Interfering factors

- Failure to observe a 12-hour fast before the test (possible decrease)
- Failure to use the proper collection technique

Culture for gonorrhea

Gonorrhea almost always results from sexual transmission of *Neisseria gonorrhoeae*. A stained smear of genital exudate can confirm gonorrhea in 90% of males with characteristic symptoms, but a culture is usually necessary, especially in asymptomatic females. Possible culture sites include the urethra (usual site in males), endocervix (usual site in females), anal canal, and oropharynx.

Purpose

- To confirm gonorrhea

Patient preparation

- Describe the procedure to the patient. Explain that this test is used to confirm gonorrhea.
- Inform the patient who will perform the test and when.
- Instruct the female patient not to douche for 24 hours before the test.
- Tell the male patient not to void during the hour preceding the test. Warn him that males sometimes experience nausea, sweating, weakness, and fainting due to stress or discomfort when the cotton swab or wire loop is introduced into the urethra.

Equipment

Sterile gloves, sterile cotton swabs, tongue blade, wire bacteriologic loop or thin urogenital alginate swabs (for male), vaginal speculum, modified Thayer-Martin medium in plates (or Transgrow medium in specimen bottles if laboratory isn't readily available), ring forceps, cotton balls

Procedure and posttest care
Endocervical culture

- Place the patient in the lithotomy position, drape her appropriately, and instruct her to take deep breaths.
- Using gloved hands, insert a vaginal speculum that has been lubricated only with warm water. Clean mucus from the cervix, using cotton balls in ring forceps.
- Insert a dry, sterile cotton swab into the endocervical canal and rotate it from side to side. Leave the swab in place for several seconds for optimum absorption of organisms.

- In cases of deep pelvic inflammatory disease, cultures of the endometrium or aspirations by laparoscopy or culdoscopy may be necessary. Endometrial specimens are obtained by inserting stents through a narrow-bore catheter introduced into the cervical canal.

Urethral culture

- Place the patient in a supine position, and drape him appropriately.
- Clean the urethral meatus with sterile gauze or a cotton swab, and then insert a thin urogenital alginate swab or a wire bacteriologic loop ⅜″ to ¾″ (1 to 2 cm) into the urethra, and rotate the swab or loop from side to side. Leave it in place for several seconds for optimum absorption of organisms. If permitted, the patient may milk the urethra, bringing urethral secretions to the meatus for collection on a cotton swab.

Rectal culture

- After obtaining an endocervical or a urethral specimen (while the patient is still on the examination table), insert a sterile cotton swab into the anal canal about 1″ (2.5 cm), move the swab from side to side, and leave it in place for several seconds for optimum absorption.
- If the swab is contaminated with stool, discard it and repeat the procedure with a clean swab.

Throat culture

- Position the patient with his head tilted back.
- Check his throat for inflamed areas using a tongue blade. Rub a sterile swab from side to side over the tonsillar areas, including inflamed or purulent sites. Be careful not to touch the teeth, cheeks, or tongue with the swab.

After specimen collection

- Roll the swab in a Z pattern in a plate containing modified Thayer-Martin medium. Then cross-streak the medium with a sterile wire loop or the tip of the swab and cover the plate. (See *Culturing for* Neisseria gonorrhoeae, page 498.)
- Label the specimen with the patient's name and room number (if applicable), the physician's name, and the date and time of collection.
- Direct smears of obtained material should be made immediately to prepare the Gram stain. Remaining material must be quickly inoculated into selective culture media or into a transport system. A culturette transport tube or a swab transport medium containing charcoal can be used. Charcoal helps neutralize toxic materials in the specimen.
- If laboratory facilities aren't readily available, do the following: Uncap the Transgrow medium specimen bottle just before inserting the swab of test material into the bottle. Keep the bottle upright to minimize loss of carbon dioxide. With the swab, absorb the excess moisture within the bottle, and then roll the swab across the Transgrow medium. Discard the swab. Place the lid on the bottle, and label it appropriately.
- Advise the patient to avoid all sexual contact until test results are available.
- Explain that treatment usually begins after confirming a positive culture, except in a person who has symptoms of gonorrhea or who has had intercourse with someone known to have gonorrhea.
- Advise the patient that a repeat culture is required 1 week after completion of treatment to evaluate the effectiveness of therapy.
- Inform the patient that positive culture findings must be reported to the local health department.

CULTURING FOR *NEISSERIA GONORRHOEAE*

Culturing for *Neisseria gonorrhoeae* requires use of a modified Thayer-Martin (MTM) medium. If a laboratory isn't readily available, you may use Transgrow medium.

Modified Thayer-Martin medium

MTM medium is a combination of hemoglobin, gonococcal growth-enhancing chemicals, and antimicrobial agents for culturing endocervical, urethral, and rectal specimens. To inoculate a culture plate treated with MTM medium and to spread organisms out of their associated mucus, take these steps:

■ Roll the swab in a Z pattern (illustration 1)

■ Using the swab or a sterile wire loop, immediately cross-streak the plate (illustration 2).

Incubate within 15 minutes of streaking.

TWO-STEP METHOD OF STREAKING THAYER-MARTIN MEDIUM

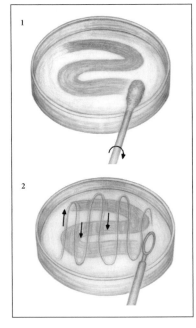

Transgrow medium

A modification of MTM medium, Transgrow is available in a screwcap bottle containing air and carbon dioxide. Transgrow bottles are used to transport suspect cultures when laboratory facilities aren't available at the site of specimen collection. Use this procedure:

■ To prevent loss of carbon dioxide, inoculate the specimen bottle while it's upright.

■ After uncapping the bottle, immediately insert the swab and soak up all excess moisture.

■ Starting at the bottom of the bottle, roll the swab from side to side across the medium.

■ Recap the bottle, and send it to the laboratory immediately. Subculturing should begin within 24 to 48 hours.

ONE-STEP METHOD OF STREAKING TRANSGROW MEDIUM

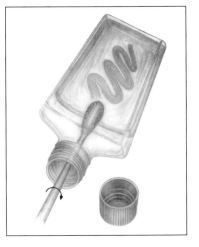

Precautions

- Wear gloves when performing the procedures and handling the specimens.
- Place the male patient in the supine position to prevent him from falling if vasovagal syncope occurs when the cotton swab or wire loop is introduced into the urethra. Observe for profound hypotension, bradycardia, pallor, and sweating.
- Collect a urethral specimen at least 1 hour after the patient has voided to prevent loss of urethral secretions.
- After collecting the specimens, carefully dispose of gloves, swabs, and speculum to prevent staff exposure.
- Send the specimens to the laboratory immediately, or arrange for transport of the Transgrow bottle because the specimen must be subcultured within 24 to 48 hours.

Normal findings

Normally, no *N. gonorrhoeae* appears in the culture.

Abnormal findings

A positive culture confirms gonorrhea.

Interfering factors

- Pretest antimicrobial therapy
- Contamination due to fecal material in a rectal culture
- Failure to use the collection technique (may provide a nonrepresentative or contaminated specimen)
- In males, voiding within 1 hour of specimen collection; in females, douching within 24 hours of specimen collection (fewer organisms available for culture)

Culture for herpes simplex virus

Herpes simplex virus (HSV) produces a wide spectrum of clinical manifestations, including keratitis, gingivostomatitis, and encephalitis. In the immunocompromised individual, it may lead to disseminated illness. The herpesvirus group includes Epstein-Barr virus, cytomegalovirus (CMV), varicella-zoster virus (VZV), human herpesvirus-6, herpesvirus-7, herpesvirus-8, and the two closely related serotypes of HSV — type 1 and type 2. Only CMV, VZV, and HSV replicate in the standard cell cultures used in diagnostic laboratories.

About 50% of HSV strains can be detected by characteristic cytopathic effects (CPE) within 24 hours after the laboratory receives the specimen; 5 to 7 days are required to detect the remaining HSV strains.

Alternatively, early HSV antigens can be detected by monoclonal antibodies in shell vial cell cultures within 16 hours after receipt of the specimen with the same sensitivity and specificity as standard tube cell cultures.

Purpose

- To confirm diagnosis of HSV infection by culturing the virus from specimens

Patient preparation

- Explain to the patient that this test is performed to detect HSV infection.
- Explain to the patient that specimens will be collected from suspected lesions during the prodromal and acute stages of clinical infection.

Procedure and posttest care

- Collect a specimen for culture in the appropriate collection device. Vesicle fluid can be obtained with a 27G needle or a tuberculin syringe. If the fluid is scant, the base of the ulcer can be scraped with a swab to remove cells.

- For the throat, skin, eye, or genital area, use a microbiologic transport swab.
- For body fluids or other respiratory specimens (washings, lavage), use a sterile screw-capped jar.
- Transport the specimen to the laboratory as soon as possible after collection. If the anticipated time between collection and inoculation of cell cultures is more than 3 hours, the specimen should be stored and transported at 39.2° F (4° C).

Precautions
- Wear gloves when obtaining and handling all specimens.
- Don't allow the specimen to dry up.

Normal findings
HSV is seldom recovered from an immunocompetent patient who shows no overt signs of disease.

Abnormal findings
HSV detected in specimens taken from dermal lesions, the eye, or cerebrospinal fluid is highly significant. Specimens from the upper respiratory tract may be associated with intermittent shedding of the virus, particularly in an immunocompromised patient.

Like other herpesviruses, HSV can be shed from the immunocompromised patient intermittently in the absence of apparent disease. For epidemiologic purposes, HSV detected by CPE in standard tube cell cultures is confirmed and identified as type 1 or 2.

Interfering factors
- Administration of antiviral drugs before specimen collection

Culture for chlamydia

The most common sexually transmitted disease in the United States, chlamydia is caused by the organism *Chlamydia trachomatis*. Identification of this parasite requires cultivation in the laboratory. After incubation, *Chlamydia*-infected cells can be detected by fluorescein isothiocyanate-conjugated monoclonal antibodies or by iodine stain. Detection in cell cultures of *C. psittaci* and *C. pneumoniae* requires specific technical manipulations and reagents; deoxyribonucleic acid detection may also be performed in women who may be susceptible to the infections, whether they have symptoms or not.

Culture is the detection method of choice, but rapid noncultural (antigen detection) procedures are also available.

Purpose
- To confirm infections caused by *C. trachomatis*

Patient preparation
- Explain the purpose of the test to the patient.
- Describe the procedure for collecting a specimen for culture.
- If the specimen will be collected from the patient's genital tract, instruct him not to urinate for 3 to 4 hours before the specimen is taken.
- Tell a female patient not to douche for 24 hours before the test.
- Tell a male patient that he may experience some burning and pressure as the culture is taken, but that the discomfort will subside after a few minutes.

Equipment
Gloves, sterile cotton swabs, wire bacteriologic loop or thin urogenital alginate swabs (for male), vaginal speculum, sucrose phosphate (2SP) transport medi-

um, microbiologic transport swab or cytobrush.

Procedure and posttest care

- Obtain a specimen of the epithelial cells from the infected site. In adults, these sites may include the eye, urethra (rather than from the purulent exudate that may be present), endocervix, and rectum.
- Obtain a urethral specimen by inserting a cotton-tipped applicator ¾″ to 2″ (2 to 5 cm) into the urethra.
- To collect a specimen from the endocervix, use a microbiologic transport swab or cytobrush.
- Extract the specimen into 2SP transport medium.
- Specimens collected from the throat, eye, or nasopharynx and aspirates from infants should be extracted into 2SP transport medium. The specimens are sent to the laboratory at 39.2° F (4° C).
- If the anticipated time between specimen collection and inoculation into cell culture is more than 24 hours, freeze the 2SP transport medium and send it to the laboratory with dry ice.

▶ **CLINICAL ALERT** *In the patient suspected of being sexually abused, be sure to process the specimen by culture rather than by antigen detection methods.*

- Advise the patient to avoid all sexual contact until after test results are available.
- If the culture confirms infection, provide counseling for the patient regarding treatment of sexual partners.

Precautions

- Place the male patient in the supine position to prevent him from falling if vasovagal syncope occurs when the cotton swab or wire loop is introduced into the urethra. Observe for profound hypotension, bradycardia, pallor, and sweating.
- Wear gloves when performing the procedures and handling the specimens.
- Collect a urethral specimen at least 1 hour after the patient has voided to prevent loss of urethral secretions.
- After collecting the specimens, carefully dispose of gloves, swabs, and speculum to prevent staff exposure.

Normal findings

Normally, no *C. trachomatis* appears in the culture.

Abnormal findings

A positive culture confirms *C. trachomatis* infection.

Interfering factors

- Using an antimicrobial drug within a few days before specimen collection (possible inability to recover *C. trachomatis*)
- In males, voiding within 1 hour of specimen collection; in females, douching within 24 hours of specimen collection (fewer organisms available for culture)
- Failure to use the proper collection technique
- Contamination of the specimen due to fecal material in a rectal culture

RAPID MONOCLONAL TESTS

Rapid monoclonal test for cytomegalovirus

Cytomegalovirus (CMV), a member of the herpesvirus group, can cause systemic infection in congenitally infected infants and in immunocompromised patients, such as transplant recipients, patients receiving chemotherapy for neoplastic disease, and those with acquired immunodeficiency syndrome (AIDS).

In the past, CMV infections were detected in the laboratory by recognizing the distinctive cytopathic effects (CPE) that the virus produced in conventional tube cell cultures. In this slow method of detecting CMV, CPE cultures grow in about 9 days. The faster shell vial assay (rapid monoclonal test) is based on the availability of a monoclonal antibody specific for the 72 kd protein of CMV synthesized during the immediate early stage of viral replication.

Through indirect immunofluorescence, CMV-infected fibroblasts are recognized by their dense, homogeneous staining confined to the nucleus. Because of the smooth, regular shape of the nucleus and the surrounding nuclear membrane, infected cells are readily differentiated from nonspecific background fluorescence that may be present in some specimens.

Purpose
■ To obtain rapid laboratory diagnosis of CMV infection, especially in the immunocompromised patient who currently has, or is at risk for developing, systemic infections caused by this virus

Patient preparation
■ Explain the purpose of the test, and describe the procedure for collecting the specimen, which will depend on the laboratory used.

Procedure and posttest care
■ Specimens should be collected during the prodromal and acute stages of clinical infection to maximize the chances of detecting CMV.
■ Each type of specimen requires a specific collection device, as listed below:

– *for throat:* microbiologic transport swab
– *for urine or cerebrospinal fluid:* sterile screw-capped tube or vial
– *for bronchoalveolar lavage tissue:* sterile screw-capped jar
– *for blood:* sterile tube with anticoagulant (heparin).

Precautions
■ Transport the specimen to the laboratory as soon as possible after the collection. If the anticipated time between collection and inoculation into shell vial cell cultures is longer than 3 hours, store the specimen at 39.2° F (4° C). Don't freeze the specimen or allow it to become dry.
■ Use gloves when obtaining and handling all specimens.

Normal findings
CMV shouldn't appear in a culture specimen.

Abnormal findings
CMV can be detected in urine and throat specimens from an asymptomatic patient. However, detection from these sites indicates active, asymptomatic infection, which may herald symptomatic involvement, especially in the immunocompromised patient. Detection of CMV in specimens of blood, tissue, and bronchoalveolar lavage generally indicates systemic infection and disease.

Interfering factors
■ Administration of antiviral drugs before collecting the specimen

Stool examination for rotavirus antigen

Rotaviruses are the most common cause of infectious diarrhea in infants and young children. They're most prevalent in children ages 3 months to 2 years during the winter months. Clinical features include diarrhea, vomiting, fever, and abdominal pain. Symptoms of infection may range from mild in adults to severe in young children, especially hospitalized infants.

Detection of human rotaviruses typically requires sensitive, specific enzyme immunoassays that provide results within minutes or hours (depending on the assay) because human rotaviruses don't replicate efficiently in laboratory cell cultures.

Purpose
■ To obtain a laboratory diagnosis of rotavirus gastroenteritis

Patient preparation
■ Explain the purpose of the test to the patient or his parents if the patient is a child.
■ Inform the patient that the test requires a stool specimen.
■ Collect the specimens during the prodromal and acute stages of clinical infection to ensure detection of the viral antigens by enzyme immunoassay.

Procedure and posttest care
■ Usually, a stool specimen (1 g in a screw-capped tube or vial) is used to detect rotaviruses. If a microbiological transport swab is used, it must be heavily stained with stool to be diagnostically productive for rotavirus.
■ Monitor the patient's intake and output and provide him with fluids to avoid dehydration caused by vomiting and diarrhea.

Precautions
■ Avoid using collection containers with preservatives, metal ions, detergents, and serum, which may interfere with the assay.
■ Store stool specimens for up to 24 hours at 35.6° to 46.4° F (2° to 8° C). If a longer period of storage or shipment is necessary, freeze specimens at –4° F (–20° C) or colder. Repeated freezing and thawing will cause the specimen to deteriorate and yield misleading results.
■ Don't store the specimen in a self-defrosting freezer.
■ Use gloves when obtaining or handling all specimens.

Normal findings
Rotavirus shouldn't appear in the specimen. Detection by enzyme immunoassay is laboratory evidence of current infection with the organism.

Abnormal findings
Rotavirus isn't normally detectable in the stool. It can infect all age-groups but is generally more severe in young children than in adults. Rotavirus infections are easily transmitted in group settings, such as nursing homes, preschools, and day-care centers. Transmission is presumed to occur from person to person by the fecal-oral route. In a facility setting, nosocomial spread of this viral infection can cause significant harm.

Interfering factors
■ Collection of a specimen in containers with preservatives, such as metal ions, detergents, or serum (decreased number of pathogens)

TESTS FOR OVA AND PARASITES

Stool examination

Examination of a stool specimen can detect several types of intestinal parasites. Some of these parasites live in nonpathogenic symbiosis; others cause intestinal disease. In the United States, the most common parasites include the roundworms *Ascaris lumbricoides* and *Necator americanus* (commonly called *hookworm*); the tapeworms *Diphyllobothrium latum, Taenia saginata* and, rarely, *T. solium;* the amoeba *Entamoeba histolytica;* and the flagellate *Giardia lamblia. Cyclospora* can also be detected in stool examination for ova and parasites.

Detection of pinworm requires a different collection method. (See *Collection procedure for pinworm.*)

Purpose
■ To confirm or rule out intestinal parasitic infection and disease

Patient preparation
■ Explain to the patient that this test detects intestinal parasitic infection.
■ Instruct the patient to avoid treatments with castor or mineral oil, bismuth, magnesium or antidiarrheal compounds, barium enemas, and antibiotics for 7 to 10 days before the test.
■ Tell the patient that the test requires three stool specimens—one every other day or every third day. Up to six specimens may be required to confirm the presence of *E. histolytica.*
■ If the patient has diarrhea, record recent dietary and travel history.
■ Check the patient's history for use of antiparasitic drugs, such as tetracycline,

paromomycin, metronidazole, and iodoquinol, within 2 weeks of the test.

Equipment
Gloves, waterproof container with tight-fitting lid, bedpan (if necessary), tongue blade

Procedure and posttest care
■ Put on gloves and collect a stool specimen directly in the container. If the patient is bedridden, collect the specimen in a clean, dry bedpan, and then, using a tongue blade, transfer it into a properly labeled container.
■ Note on the laboratory request the date and time of collection and the specimen consistency. Also record recent or current antimicrobial therapy and any pertinent travel or dietary history.
■ Tell the patient that he may resume his usual medications, as ordered.

Precautions
■ Don't contaminate the stool specimen with urine, which can destroy trophozoites.
■ Don't collect stool from a toilet bowl because water is toxic to trophozoites and may contain organisms that interfere with test results.
■ Send the specimen to the laboratory immediately. If a liquid or soft stool specimen can't be examined within 30 minutes of passage, place some of it in a preservative; if a formed stool specimen can't be examined immediately, refrigerate it or place it in preservative.
■ If the entire stool can't be sent to the laboratory, include macroscopic worms or worm segments as well as bloody and mucoid portions of the specimen.
■ Use gloves when performing the procedure and handling the specimen, disposing of equipment, sealing the container,

and transporting the specimen. Dispose of gloves after specimen collection and transport.

Normal findings

No parasites or ova should appear in stool.

Abnormal findings

The presence of *E. histolytica* confirms amebiasis; *G. lamblia*, giardiasis. However, the extent of infection depends on the degree of tissue invasion. If amebiasis is suspected, but stool examinations are negative, specimen collection after saline catharsis using buffered sodium biphosphate or during sigmoidoscopy may be necessary. If giardiasis is suspected, but stool examinations are negative, examination of duodenal contents may be necessary.

Because injury to the host is difficult to detect — even when helminth ova or larvae appear — the number of worms is usually correlated with the patient's clinical symptoms to distinguish between helminth infestation and helminth diseases. Eosinophilia may also indicate parasitic infection. Helminths may migrate from the intestinal tract, producing pathologic changes in other parts of the body. For example, the roundworm *Ascaris* may perforate the bowel wall, causing peritonitis, or may migrate to the lungs, causing pneumonitis. Hookworms can cause hypochromic microcytic anemia secondary to bloodsucking and hemorrhage, especially in the patient with an iron-deficient diet. The tapeworm *D. latum* may cause megaloblastic anemia by removing vitamin B_{12}.

COLLECTION PROCEDURE FOR PINWORM

The ova of the pinworm *Enterobius vermicularis* seldom appear in stool because the female migrates to the anus and deposits her ova there. To collect them, place a piece of cellophane tape, sticky side out, on the end of a tongue blade, and press it firmly on the anal area. Then transfer the tape, sticky side down, to a slide (kits with tape and a slide or a sticky paddle are available). Because the female usually deposits her ova at night, collect the specimen early in the morning, before the patient bathes or defecates.

Interfering factors

■ Improper collection technique, not enough specimens, or the presence of urine (false-negative results)
■ Failure to transport the specimen promptly or to refrigerate or preserve it if transport is delayed
■ Excessive heat or cold
■ Failure to observe pretest drug restrictions

Examination of urogenital secretions for trichomonads

Microscopic examination of urine or vaginal, urethral, or prostatic secretions can detect urogenital infection by *Trichomonas vaginalis*, a parasitic, flagellate protozoan that's usually transmitted sexually. This test is more commonly performed on women than on men because women are more likely to exhibit symptoms of trichomoniasis; men may exhibit symptoms of urethritis or prostatitis.

Purpose
- To confirm trichomoniasis

Patient preparation
- Explain to the patient that this test can identify the cause of urogenital infection.
- If the patient is a woman, tell her that the test requires a specimen of vaginal secretions or urethral discharge and ask her not to douche before the test.
- If the patient is a man, tell him the test requires a specimen of urethral or prostatic secretions.
- Inform the patient who will perform the procedure and when.

Equipment
Gloves, cotton swab, test tube containing small amount of normal saline solution, vaginal speculum, specimen cup (if a urine specimen is being collected)

Procedure and posttest care
Vaginal secretions
- With the patient in the lithotomy position, an unlubricated vaginal speculum is inserted, and discharge is collected with a cotton swab. The swab is then placed in a tube containing normal saline solution and the speculum is removed.
- Another method is to smear the specimen on a glass slide, allow it to air-dry, and then transport it to the laboratory.

Prostatic material
- After prostatic massage, collect secretions with a cotton swab, and place the swab in normal saline solution.

Urethral discharge
- Collect the discharge with a cotton swab, and place the swab in normal saline solution.

Urine
- Include the first portion of a voided random specimen (not midstream).

All procedures
- Label the specimen container appropriately, including the date and time of collection.
- Provide perineal care.

Precautions
- Remember to use gloves when performing procedures and handling specimens.
- If possible, obtain the urogenital specimen before treatment with a trichomonacide begins.
- Send the specimen to the laboratory immediately after collection because trichomonads can be identified only while they're still motile.

Normal findings
Trichomonads are normally absent from the urogenital tract.

Abnormal findings
Trichomonads confirm trichomoniasis. In approximately 25% of women and in most infected men, trichomonads may be present without associated pathology.

Interfering factors
- Improper collection technique
- Failure to send the specimen to the laboratory immediately after collection, causing trichomonads to lose motility
- Collection of the specimen after trichomonacide therapy begins (fewer trichomonads in the specimen)

Examination of duodenal contents

The test for duodenal parasites evaluates duodenal contents for the presence of parasites in a specimen obtained by duodenal intubation and aspiration or by the string test (Entero test). Such parasites include trophozoites of *Giardia lamblia* and *G. duodenalis,* the ova and larvae of *Strongyloides stercoralis,* and the ova of *Entamoeba histolytica, Necator americanus,* or *Ancylostoma duodenale* in various stages of cleavage. This test can also detect ova of the liver flukes *Clonorchis sinensis* and *Fasciola hepatica* in the biliary tract. However, liver fluke infestations are rare in North America.

Examination of duodenal contents for ova and parasites is performed only in a symptomatic patient with negative stool examinations.

Purpose
■ To detect parasitic infestation when stool examinations are negative

Patient preparation
■ Explain to the patient that this test detects parasitic infestation of the GI tract.
■ Instruct the patient to restrict food and fluids for 12 hours before the test.
■ Tell the patient who will perform the test and when.
■ If the test will be done with a nasoenteric tube, warn the patient that he may gag during the tube's passage, but assure him that following the examiner's instructions about positioning, breathing, and swallowing will minimize discomfort.
■ Instruct the patient to empty his bladder just before the procedure.

Equipment
Gloves, double-lumen tube with olive tip (or weighted gelatin capsule with string attached, for string test), water-soluble jelly, 30-ml sterile syringe, emesis basin, sterile specimen container, ½″ adhesive tape

Procedure and posttest care
Nasoenteric tube
■ After inserting the tube, place the patient in a left lateral decubitus position with his feet elevated to allow peristalsis to move the tube into the duodenum.
■ The pH of a small amount of aspirated fluid determines tube position: If the tube is in the stomach, the pH is lower than 7; if it's in the duodenum, the pH is higher than 7.
■ Fluoroscopy can also determine correct positioning. When position is confirmed, residual duodenal contents are aspirated.
■ Transfer the entire specimen to a sterile container, and label the container appropriately.

Entero test capsule with string
■ Tape the free end of the string to the patient's cheek.
■ Instruct him to swallow the capsule (on the other end of the string) with water.
■ As ordered, leave the string in place for 4 hours; then pull it out gently and place it in a sterile container.
■ Label the container appropriately.
■ Dispose of the equipment properly.
■ Provide oral hygiene and offer the patient water.
■ Observe carefully for signs of perforation, such as dysphagia or fever.
■ Tell the patient he can resume his usual diet.

Precautions

- Use gloves when performing the procedure and handling specimens.
- Duodenal intubation is contraindicated for the pregnant patient and for one with acute cholecystitis; acute pancreatitis; esophageal varices, stenosis, diverticula, or malignant neoplasms; recent severe gastric hemorrhage; aortic aneurysm; or heart failure.
- When possible, obtain the specimen before the start of drug therapy.
- Send the specimen to the laboratory immediately.
- As ordered, withdraw the tube slowly (about 6″ to 8″ [15 to 20 cm] every 10 minutes) to the esophagus, and then clamp the tube and remove it quickly. *Never* force the tube.

Normal findings

Normally, no ova or parasites appear in duodenal contents.

Abnormal findings

Finding *G. lamblia* or *G. duodenalis* indicates giardiasis, possibly causing malabsorption syndrome; *S. stercoralis* suggests strongyloidiasis; *A. duodenale* and *N. americanus* imply hookworm disease; and *C. sinensis* and *F. hepatica* signify histopathologic changes in the bile ducts.

Interfering factors

- Failure to observe pretest restrictions (possible dilution of the specimen)
- Previous drug therapy or delay in transporting the specimen to the laboratory

Sputum examination

Parasitic infestation is rare in North America, but may result from exposure to *Entamoeba histolytica, Ascaris lumbri-*coides, *Echinococcus granulosus, Strongyloides stercoralis, Paragonimus westermani,* or *Necator americanus.* A sputum specimen is obtained by expectoration or tracheal suctioning to evaluate for parasites.

Purpose

- To identify pulmonary parasites

Patient preparation

- Explain to the patient that this test helps identify parasitic pulmonary infection.
- Tell the patient that the test requires a sputum specimen or, if necessary, tracheal suctioning.
- Inform the patient that early morning collection is preferred because secretions accumulate overnight.
- Encourage the patient to help sputum production by drinking fluids the night before collection.
- Teach the patient how to expectorate by taking three deep breaths and forcing a deep cough.
- Tell the patient that he'll experience some discomfort from the catheter during tracheal suctioning.
- Notify the laboratory and physician of medications the patient is taking that may affect test results; they may need to be restricted.

Equipment

For expectoration: Sterile, disposable, impermeable container with screw cap or tight-fitting cap, nebulizer, intermittent positive-pressure breathing ventilator, and 10% sodium chloride, acetylcysteine, or sterile or distilled water aerosols, to induce cough

  For tracheal suctioning: #16 or #18 French suction catheter, sterile gloves, sterile specimen container or sputum trap, sterile normal saline solution, and protective eyewear

Procedure and posttest care
Expectoration
■ Instruct the patient to breathe deeply a few times and then to "deep cough" and expectorate into the container.

■ Use chest physiotherapy, or heated aerosol spray (nebulization), if the patient's cough is unproductive.

■ Take proper precautions in sending the specimen to the laboratory.

Tracheal suctioning
■ Administer oxygen before and after the procedure, if necessary.

■ Attach a sputum trap to the suction catheter.

■ Wearing a sterile glove, lubricate the tip of the catheter and then pass the catheter through the patient's nostril without suction. (He'll cough when the catheter passes into the larynx.)

■ Advance the catheter into the trachea.

■ Apply suction for no longer than 15 seconds to obtain the specimen.

■ Stop suctioning and gently remove the catheter.

■ Discard the catheter and glove in a proper receptacle.

■ Detach the sputum trap from the suction apparatus and cap the opening.

■ Label all specimens carefully.

■ Provide proper mouth care. After suctioning, offer the patient water.

■ Monitor the patient's vital signs every hour until he's stable.

Precautions
■ Be sure to wear gloves and protective eyewear when performing procedures and handling specimens.

▶ **CLINICAL ALERT** *Don't perform tracheal suctioning on the patient with esophageal varices.*

▶ **CLINICAL ALERT** *If the patient has asthma or chronic bronchitis, watch for aggravated bronchospasms with use of more than 10% concentration of sodium chloride or acetylcysteine in an aerosol.*

■ Suction for only 5 to 10 seconds at a time during tracheal suctioning. Never suction for longer than 15 seconds. If the patient shows signs of hypoxia or cyanosis, remove the suctioning catheter immediately and administer oxygen.

■ Send the specimen to the laboratory or place it in preservative immediately after collection.

Normal findings
Normally, no parasites or ova are present in sputum.

Abnormal findings
The parasite identified indicates the type of pulmonary infection as well as the presence and stage of intestinal infection.

■ *E. histolytica* trophozoites: pulmonary amebiasis

■ *A. lumbricoides* larvae and adults: pneumonitis

■ *E. granulosus* cysts of larval stage: hydatid disease

■ *P. westermani* ova: paragonimiasis

■ *S. stercoralis* larvae: strongyloidiasis

■ *N. americanus* larvae: hookworm disease

Interfering factors
■ Improper collection technique or failure to send the specimen to the laboratory immediately after collection

■ Recent therapy with antihelmintics or amebicides

Selected readings

Baron, E.J., et al. *Bailey and Scott's Diagnostic Microbiology,* 11th ed. St. Louis: Mosby–Year Book, Inc., 2002.

Diseases, 3rd ed. Springhouse, Pa.: Springhouse Corp., 2001.

Fischbach, F. *A Manual of Laboratory and Diagnostic Tests,* 7th ed. Philadelphia: Lippincott Williams & Wilkins, 2004.

Guyton, A.C., and Hall, J.E. *Textbook of Medical Physiology,* 10th ed. Philadelphia: W.B. Saunders Co., 2001.

Henry, J.B., ed. *Clinical Diagnosis and Management by Laboratory Methods,* 20th ed. Philadelphia: W.B. Saunders Co., 2001.

Nursing2004 Drug Handbook, 24th ed. Philadelphia: Lippincott Williams & Wilkins, 2004.

Ryan, K.J., ed. *Sherris Medical Microbiology: An Introduction to Infectious Diseases,* 3rd ed. Stamford, Conn.: Appleton & Lange, 2003.

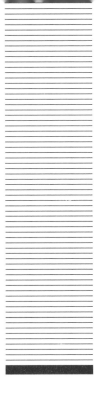

SECTION IV.
ORGAN TESTS

Thyroid

Introduction

A number of sensitive and specific laboratory tests are available to evaluate thyroid function and hormone use. These tests make diagnosis of thyroid dysfunction possible even in patients with marginal or obscure thyroid abnormalities. However, because no one test diagnoses all thyroid disorders and interpretation of test results may be complicated by many factors, a combination of laboratory tests is usually required to ensure accurate diagnosis.

Laboratory tests of thyroid function can be classified into the following categories:

■ *direct tests of thyroid function* that measure thyroid hormone synthesis and excretion such as the radioactive iodine uptake test

■ *tests that measure concentration and binding of the thyroid hormones* and other iodinated materials in the blood, such as serum free thyroxine, triiodothyronine (T_3) resin uptake (see chapter 5), and protein-binding iodine

■ *tests that assess the metabolic effects of thyroid hormones on the tissues,* such as serum cholesterol, basal metabolic rate (BMR), and Achilles reflex time (however, BMR and Achilles reflex time have largely been replaced by other tests)

■ *tests that evaluate hormonal regulating mechanisms,* such as the thyroid-stimulating hormone (TSH) test (see chapter 5) and the thyroid suppression and stimulation tests

■ *tests that evaluate anatomic detail of the thyroid gland* and aid in the evaluation of thyroid masses, such as radionuclide thyroid imaging and thyroid ultrasonography.

Thyroid disorders

Thyroid dysfunction can cause several disorders, most commonly hyperthyroidism, hypothyroidism, thyroiditis, and goiter.

Hyperthyroidism, which is four times more common in females than in males, results from excessive secretion of thyroid hormone. Conversely, *hypothyroidism* results from inadequate thyroid hormone production. *Thyroiditis* may occur as an acute inflammation, as a subacute viral inflammation that generally subsides spontaneously, or as a chronic disorder (Hashimoto's disease). *Simple goiter* results from inadequate iodine intake and tends to occur in certain geographic areas.

Benign adenomas and malignant tumors cause one-third of all thyroid enlargements. Well-encapsulated and non-invasive, a benign adenoma usually causes no symptoms until it grows large enough to cause respiratory distress by compressing the trachea. Malignant thyroid tumors are rare, accounting for fewer than 1% of all cancer deaths. However, large doses of radiation to the head and neck may predispose a person to develop thyroid nodules and cancer later in life, and prolonged TSH production may lead to malignant transformation of benign adenomas.

Testing procedures

Measurement of the ultrasensitive TSH is the first step in thyroid evaluation. If it's abnormal, then measuring serum thyroid hormone levels—T_3 and thyroxine (T_4)—is warranted. Abnormal hormone levels should be treated. If T_4 levels are elevated and TSH levels are suppressed, then visualization of the thyroid gland to assess function is needed. (See *Thyroid anatomy and physiology,* pages 514 and 515.)

Thyroid tests can determine the thyroid gland's size, identify tumors or cysts, and measure the thyroid's ability to retain iodine (essential for thyroid hormone synthesis). Such tests, which commonly include the radioactive iodine uptake test, T_3 resin uptake study, radionuclide thyroid imaging, and thyroid ultrasonography, are commonly performed as part of a series to provide a complete analysis.

Radioactive iodine tests

Measuring thyroid uptake of radioactive iodine reflects the gland's ability to handle stable dietary iodine and allows direct evaluation of thyroid function. This measurement is especially significant in assessing thyroid hyperfunction, thyrotoxicosis factitia, and subacute thyroiditis. In the radioactive iodine uptake test, the patient's thyroid is scanned at specific intervals after oral administration of a radioisotope of iodine (usually ^{131}I) to help determine the degree of iodine retention.

Three radioisotopes of iodine — [123]I, ^{125}I, and [131]I — are useful because they differ in terms of half-life and amount of radiation emitted. All are synthetic isotopes and are indistinguishable from the naturally occurring stable isotope, [127]I.

THYROID ANATOMY AND PHYSIOLOGY

The thyroid gland is located in the neck, just below the cricoid cartilage. Its two lateral lobes straddle the trachea, usually connected by an isthmus that crosses in front of the trachea. The right lobe is a bit larger and higher in the neck than the left lobe. About 50% of people have a third, pyramidal lobe rising from the isthmus. Occasionally, this lobe is the site of a malignant tumor.

Visualization of the thyroid can determine abnormalities in gland size and the ability to absorb iodine as well as the presence and quality of tumors and cysts. The parathyroid glands, two upper and two lower, sit behind the thyroid and are so closely involved in its tissue that they're usually inadvertently removed during thyroid surgery, causing hypoparathyroidism.

Thyroid tissue is composed of follicles filled with colloid, a substance consisting primarily of an iodine-containing pro-

tein known as *thyroglobulin*. Normally, the thyroid weighs about 20 g, but certain disorders, such as goiter, can grossly enlarge it to more than several hundred grams.

The thyroid controls the body's metabolism primarily through the secretion of two hormones, *thyroxine* (T_4) and *triiodothyronine* (T_3). T_4 regulates body metabolism and helps control physical and mental development, resistance to infection, and vitamin requirements. Its production is regulated by release of thyroid-stimulating hormone, a pituitary hormone, and the ingestion of iodine and protein. T_4 may also be converted to T_3, a more potent hormone, by deiodination. T_3 is essential for maintaining metabolic rates in all cells. A third thyroid hormone, *thyrocalcitonin*, is a polypeptide whose function is limited to lowering plasma phosphate and calcium levels.

All emit gamma radiation, which allows their external measurement in sites of concentration, such as the thyroid gland or aberrant thyroid tissue.

Radionuclide thyroid imaging

Thyroid imaging, which uses radionuclides to locate sites of radioactive iodine accumulation, is valuable in the diagnosis and management of thyroid disease. In this test, the patient is given a radiopharmaceutical and then a gamma camera is placed near the anterior portion of his neck, where it assesses and processes the radioactivity of the radionuclide, producing a precise image of the thyroid gland.

Radionuclide thyroid imaging provides information on overall thyroid size and shape. More important, it can define areas of hyperfunction (hot spots) or hypofunction (cold spots) and is especially valuable in detecting nodules that may harbor cancer. Palpable nodules shown to be nonfunctioning may be malignant. Conversely, functioning nodules, particularly if they're more active than surrounding tissue, are unlikely to be malignant. Radionuclide thyroid imaging may also reveal substernal goiters; the location of ectopic thyroid tissue in the tongue, chest, or ovary; and functioning metastasis of thyroid cancer. Accurate interpretation of

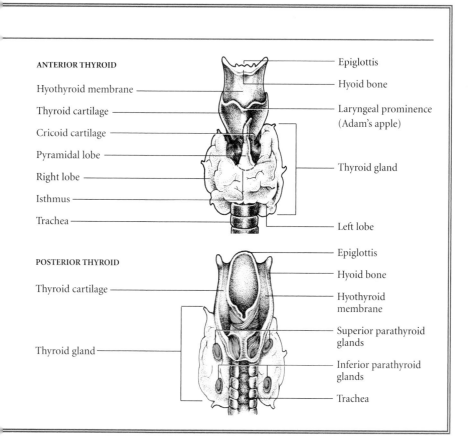

ANTERIOR THYROID

Hyothyroid membrane

Thyroid cartilage

Cricoid cartilage

Pyramidal lobe

Right lobe

Isthmus

Trachea

Epiglottis

Hyoid bone

Laryngeal prominence (Adam's apple)

Thyroid gland

Left lobe

POSTERIOR THYROID

Thyroid cartilage

Thyroid gland

Epiglottis

Hyoid bone

Hyothyroid membrane

Superior parathyroid glands

Inferior parathyroid glands

Trachea

thyroid imaging results requires careful correlation with findings on palpation.

Ultrasonography
Thyroid ultrasonography allows visualization of the thyroid gland through high-frequency sound waves that are converted to images on an oscilloscope screen. This test is especially useful for distinguishing cystic from solid thyroid nodules. When used during pregnancy, thyroid ultrasonography doesn't expose the fetus to radioactive materials.

Magnetic resonance imaging
A noninvasive procedure, magnetic resonance imaging (MRI) uses magnetic energy to obtain images of the posterior and substernal thyroid. This test helps to detect tumors or tissue abnormalities in these areas. Because the MRI scanner records magnetic signals and translates them into detailed pictures, this test involves no exposure to radiation.

SCANNING

Radioactive iodine uptake test

The radioactive iodine uptake (RAIU) test evaluates thyroid function by measuring the amount of orally ingested iodine 123 (^{123}I) or iodine 131 (^{131}I) that accumulates in the thyroid gland after 2, 6, and 24 hours. An external single counting probe measures the radioactivity in the thyroid as a percentage of the original dose, thus indicating its ability to trap and retain iodine. The RAIU test accurately diagnoses hyperthyroidism but is less accurate for hypothyroidism. When performed concurrently with radionuclide thyroid imaging and the T_3 resin uptake test, the RAIU test helps differentiate Grave's disease from hyperfunctioning toxic adenoma. Indications for this test include abnormal results of chemical tests used to evaluate thyroid function.

Patients with suspected Hashimoto's disease may undergo the perchlorate suppression test in addition to the RAIU test. (See *Perchlorate suppression test.*)

Purpose
■ To evaluate thyroid function
■ To help diagnose hyperthyroidism or hypothyroidism
■ To help distinguish between primary and secondary thyroid disorders (in combination with other tests)

Patient preparation
■ Tell the patient that the RAIU test assesses thyroid function.
■ Instruct the patient to begin fasting at midnight the night before the test.

■ Explain to the patient that he'll receive radioactive iodine (capsule or liquid) and that he'll then be scanned after 2 hours, 6 hours, and 24 hours.
■ Assure the patient that the test is painless and that the small amount of radioactivity used is harmless.
■ Check the patient's history for iodine exposure, which may interfere with test results. Note previous radiologic tests using contrast media, nuclear medicine procedures, or current use of iodine preparations or thyroid medications on the film request slip. Iodine hypersensitivity isn't considered a contraindication because the amount of iodine used is similar to the amount consumed in a normal diet.
■ Make sure the patient or a responsible family member has signed an informed consent form, if required.

Equipment
Oral dose of ^{123}I or ^{131}I (the radiologist determines the exact dosage), external single counting probe

Procedure and posttest care
■ After ingesting an oral dose of radioactive iodine, the patient's thyroid is scanned at 2 hours, 6 hours, and 24 hours by placing the anterior portion of his neck in front of an external single counting probe.
■ The amount of radioactivity detected by the probe is compared with the amount of radioactivity contained in the original dose to determine the percentage of radioactive iodine retained by the thyroid.
■ Instruct the patient to resume a light diet 2 hours after taking the oral dose of radioactive iodine. When the study is complete, the patient may resume his usual diet.

Precautions

■ RAIU testing is contraindicated during pregnancy and lactation because of possible teratogenic effects. It's also contraindicated in the patient who's allergic to iodine and shellfish.

Normal findings

After 2 hours, 4% to 12% of the radioactive iodine should have accumulated in the thyroid; after 6 hours, 5% to 20%; at 24 hours, accumulation should be 8% to 29%. The remaining radioactive iodine is excreted in the urine. Local variations in the normal range of iodine uptake may occur due to regional differences in dietary iodine intake and procedural differences among laboratories.

Abnormal findings

Below-normal iodine uptake may indicate hypothyroidism, subacute thyroiditis, or iodine overload. Above-normal uptake may indicate hyperthyroidism, early Hashimoto's thyroiditis, hypoalbuminemia, lithium ingestion, or iodine-deficient goiter. However, in hyperthyroidism, the rate of turnover may be so rapid that a false normal measurement occurs at 24 hours.

Interfering factors

■ Renal failure; diuresis; severe diarrhea; X-ray contrast media studies; ingestion of iodine preparations, including iodized salt, cough syrups, and some multivitamins (decrease)
■ Thyroid hormones, thyroid hormone antagonists, salicylates, penicillins, antihistamines, anticoagulants, corticosteroids, and phenylbutazone (decrease)
■ Phenothiazines or an iodine-deficient diet (increase)

PERCHLORATE SUPPRESSION TEST

The perchlorate suppression test is used to evaluate the patient with suspected Hashimoto's disease or to demonstrate an enzyme deficiency within the thyroid gland. Because potassium perchlorate competes with and displaces the iodide ions that aren't organified, this study can identify defects in the iodide organification process within the thyroid.

In this procedure, a small dose of radioactive iodine is administered orally. A radioactive iodine uptake (RAIU) test is performed 1 and 2 hours afterward. After the 2-hour RAIU test, the patient receives 400 mg to 1 g of potassium perchlorate orally. RAIU tests are performed every 15 minutes for the first hour after the dose and then every 30 minutes for the next 2 to 3 hours.

The results of the RAIU tests performed after administration of potassium perchlorate are compared with those of the 2-hour RAIU test performed before perchlorate was administered. In a normal person, the uptake of radioactive iodine won't change significantly after administration of perchlorate. The patient with either Hashimoto's disease or an enzyme deficiency will experience a decrease in uptake. The patient with an enzyme deficiency will experience a drop in his uptake of more than 15% after perchlorate administration.

Radionuclide thyroid imaging

In radionuclide thyroid imaging, the thyroid is studied by gamma camera after the patient receives a radioisotope (iodine 123 [^{123}I], technetium [^{99m}Tc] pertechnetate, or iodine 131 [^{131}I]). Thyroid imaging typically follows discovery of a palpable mass, an enlarged gland, or an asymmetrical goiter and is performed concurrently with thyroid uptake tests and measurements of serum triiodothyronine (T_3) and serum thyroxine (T_4) levels. Later, thyroid ultrasonography may be performed.

Purpose

- To assess the size, structure, and position of the thyroid gland
- To evaluate thyroid function (in conjunction with other thyroid tests)

Patient preparation

- Tell the patient that radionuclide thyroid imaging helps determine the cause of thyroid dysfunction.
- If ^{123}I or ^{131}I will be used, tell the patient to fast after midnight the night before the test. Fasting isn't required if an I.V. injection of ^{99m}Tc pertechnetate is used.
- Explain to the patient that after he receives the radiopharmaceutical, a gamma camera will be used to produce an image of his thyroid. Tell him that the imaging procedure will take about 30 minutes and assure him that his exposure to radiation is minimal.
- Ask the patient if he has undergone tests that used radiographic contrast media within the past 60 days. Note previous radiographic contrast media exposure on the X-ray request.

- Check the patient's diet and medication history. Medications, such as thyroid hormones, thyroid hormone antagonists, and iodine preparations (Lugol's solution, some multivitamins, and cough syrups) should be discontinued 2 to 3 weeks before the test, as ordered. Phenothiazines, corticosteroids, salicylates, anticoagulants, and antihistamines should be discontinued 1 week before the test, as ordered. Instruct the patient to stop consuming iodized salt, iodinated salt substitutes, and seafood for 14 to 21 days, as ordered. Liothyronine, propylthiouracil, and methimazole should be discontinued 3 days before the test, and T_4 should be discontinued 10 days before the test, as ordered.
- The patient receives ^{123}I or ^{131}I (oral) or ^{99m}Tc pertechnetate (I.V.). Record the date and the time of administration.
- The patient receiving an oral radioisotope should fast for another 2 hours after administration.
- Just before the test, tell the patient to remove dentures, jewelry, and other materials that may interfere with the imaging process.
- Make sure the patient or a responsible family member has signed an informed consent form, if required.

Procedure and posttest care

- The test is performed 24 hours after oral administration of ^{123}I or ^{131}I or 20 to 30 minutes after I.V. injection of ^{99m}Tc pertechnetate. Just before the test, tell the patient to remove his dentures and any jewelry that could interfere with visualization of the thyroid.
- The patient is placed in a supine position with his neck extended; the thyroid gland is palpated. The gamma camera is positioned above the anterior portion of his neck.

RESULTS OF THYROID IMAGING IN THYROID DISORDERS

This chart shows the characteristic findings in radionuclide imaging tests that are associated with various thyroid disorders as well as the possible causes of those disorders.

Condition	Findings	Causes
Hypothyroidism	■ Glandular damage or absent gland	■ Surgical removal of gland ■ Inflammation ■ Radiation ■ Neoplasm (rare)
Hypothyroid goiter	■ Enlarged gland ■ Decreased uptake (of radioactive iodine) if glandular destruction is present ■ Increased uptake possible from congenital error in thyroxine synthesis	■ Insufficient iodine intake ■ Hypersecretion of thyroid-stimulating hormone (TSH) caused by thyroid hormone deficiency
Myxedema (cretinism in children)	■ Normal or slightly reduced gland size ■ Uniform pattern ■ Decreased uptake	■ Defective embryonic development, resulting in congenital absence or underdevelopment of thyroid gland ■ Maternal iodine deficiency
Hyperthyroidism (Graves' disease)	■ Enlarged gland ■ Uniform pattern ■ Increased uptake	■ Unknown, but may be hereditary ■ Production of thyroid-stimulating immunoglobulins
Toxic nodular goiter	■ Multiple hot spots	■ Long-standing simple goiter
Hyperfunctioning adenomas	■ Solitary hot spot	■ Adenomatous production of triiodothyronine and thyroxine, suppressing TSH secretion and producing atrophy of other thyroid tissue
Hypofunctioning adenomas	■ Solitary cold spot	■ Cyst or nonfunctioning nodule
Benign multinodular goiter	■ Multiple nodules with variable or no function	■ Local inflammation ■ Degeneration
Thyroid carcinoma	■ Usually a solitary cold spot with occasional or no function	■ Neoplasm

■ Images of the patient's thyroid gland are projected on a monitor and are recorded on X-ray film. Three views of the thyroid are obtained: a straight-on anterior view and two bilateral oblique views.

■ Tell the patient that he may resume his usual diet and medications, as ordered.

Precautions

■ Radionuclide thyroid imaging is contraindicated during pregnancy and lactation and in the patient with a previous allergy to iodine, shellfish, or radioactive tracers.

Normal findings

Normally, radionuclide thyroid imaging reveals a thyroid gland that's about 2″ (5 cm) long and 1″(2.5 cm) wide, with a uniform uptake of the radioisotope and without tumors. The gland is butterfly-shaped, with the isthmus located at the midline. Occasionally, a third lobe called the *pyramidal lobe* may be present; this is a normal variant.

Abnormal findings

During radionuclide thyroid imaging, hyperfunctioning nodules (areas of excessive iodine uptake) appear as black regions called *hot spots*. The presence of hot spots requires a follow-up T_3 thyroid suppression test to determine if the hyperfunctioning areas are autonomous. Hypofunctioning nodules (areas of little or no iodine uptake) appear as white or light gray regions called *cold spots.* If a cold spot appears, subsequent thyroid ultrasonography may be performed to rule out cysts; in addition, fine-needle aspiration and biopsy of such nodules may be performed to rule out malignancy. (See *Results of thyroid imaging in thyroid disorders,* page 519.)

Interfering factors

■ An iodine-deficient diet and phenothiazines (increase)
■ Decreased uptake of radioactive iodine due to renal disease; ingestion of iodized salt, iodine preparations, iodinated salt substitutes, or seafood; and use of thyroid hormones, thyroid hormone antagonists, aminosalicylic acid, corticosteroids, multivitamins, or cough syrups containing inorganic iodine (decrease)
■ Severe diarrhea and vomiting, impairing GI absorption of radioiodine (decrease)

ULTRASONOGRAPHY

Thyroid ultrasonography

In thyroid ultrasonography, high-frequency sound waves emitted from a transducer are directed at the thyroid gland and reflected back to produce structural images on a monitor.

When a mass is located by palpation or by thyroid imaging, thyroid ultrasonography can differentiate between a cyst and a tumor larger than ¼″ (1 cm) with a high degree of accuracy. This test is also used to evaluate thyroid nodules during pregnancy because it doesn't require use of radioactive iodine.

Purpose

■ To evaluate thyroid structure
■ To differentiate between a cyst and a solid tumor
■ To monitor the size of the thyroid gland during suppressive therapy

Patient preparation

■ Describe the procedure to the patient, and explain that this test defines the size and shape of the thyroid gland.
■ Inform the patient that he need not restrict food and fluids.
■ Tell the patient who will perform the procedure, where it will take place, and that it's painless and safe.

Procedure and posttest care

- The patient is placed in a supine position with a pillow under his shoulder blades to hyperextend his neck.
- His neck is coated with water-soluble conductive gel.
- The transducer then scans the thyroid, projecting its echographic image on the oscilloscope screen.
- The image on the monitor is photographed for subsequent examination.
- Accurate visualization of the anterior portion of the thyroid requires use of a short-focused transducer.
- Thoroughly clean the patient's neck to remove the conductive gel.

Normal findings

Thyroid ultrasonography exhibits a uniform echo pattern throughout the gland.

Abnormal findings

Cysts appear as smooth-bordered, echo-free areas with enhanced sound transmission; adenomas and carcinomas appear either solid and well demarcated with identical echo patterns or, less commonly, solid with cystic areas. Carcinoma infiltrating the gland may not be well demarcated.

Identification of a tumor is generally followed up by fine needle aspiration or an excisional biopsy to determine malignancy.

Interfering factors

- None significant

Selected readings

Braunwald, E., et al., eds. *Harrison's Principles of Internal Medicine,* 15th ed. New York: McGraw-Hill Book Co., 2001.

Guyton, A.C., and Hall, J.E. *Textbook of Medical Physiology,* 10th ed. Philadelphia: W.B. Saunders Co., 2001.

Henry, J.B., ed. *Clinical Diagnosis and Management by Laboratory Methods,* 20th ed. Philadelphia: W.B. Saunders Co., 2001.

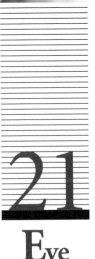

21

Eye

Introduction

Numerous disorders can affect the anatomical structures of the eye with outcomes ranging from moderate discomfort to vision loss.

Tests to diagnose eye disorders fall into three categories. *Subjective tests,* such as visual acuity tests and the tangent screen examination, require oral responses from the patient that must be interpreted by the examiner. These tests need to be correlated with *objective tests,* such as tonometry and ophthalmoscopy, in which the examiner obtains measurements or directly visualizes the eye's interior. When severe abnormalities result from ocular disease or trauma, the ophthalmologist can resort to *special procedures* such as computed tomography. Understanding the diagnostic application and significance of these tests begins by reviewing the eye's anatomic structure and physiology.

Outer layer
The cornea and sclera constitute the outermost portion of the eye's three layers. The *cornea,* a transparent structure com-

posed of avascular tissue, lies in the anterior portion of the eye. It bends light rays that enter the eye and helps to focus the images on the retina. Adjoining the cornea is the *sclera,* an opaque, white, fibrous coat covering the posterior five-sixths of the eye through which nerves and blood vessels pass to penetrate the eye's interior.

Middle layer

The middle vascular layer, known as the *uveal tract,* consists of the iris, ciliary body, and choroid. The *iris,* the colored part of the eye, is composed of muscle fibers that regulate the amount of light admitted to the eye's interior through the pupil, the circular opening in its center. Behind the iris lies the *lens,* a biconvex, transparent structure that can change its shape to focus light rays precisely on the retina. The *ciliary body* produces aqueous humor and permits flexibility of the lens for clearer vision. The highly vascular and pigmented *choroid* supplies blood to the retina and conducts blood and nerve impulses to the eye's anterior structures.

Inner layer

The third layer of the eye, the *retina,* consists of rods and cones. These photoreceptive cells translate light into nerve impulses. In the posterior portion of the retina lies the *fovea;* composed entirely of cones, it's the area of most acute vision. The *macula,* a spot on the retina, appears different in color (yellow) from the surrounding tissue. High-acuity vision occurs when an image is focused directly on the fovea centralis of the macula lutea.

Chambers and their fluids

The iris forms a curtain that divides the space between the cornea and the lens into the eye's anterior and posterior chambers. *Aqueous humor* secreted by the ciliary body processes in the posterior chamber flows through the pupil into the anterior chamber. This fluid nourishes the internal eye structures and maintains constant pressure within the eyeball. Defective drainage of aqueous humor can increase intraocular pressure (IOP) and eventually cause glaucoma.

The *vitreous body* is surrounded by the retina and the optic nerve and constitutes four-fifths of the back of the eye. It's filled with *vitreous humor*—a clear, avascular, gelatinous substance. Vitreous humor helps maintain the transparency and shape of the eye. (See *Cross section of the eye,* page 524.)

How the eye moves

The eye rests on a cushion of fat within its bony orbit, which also contains the eye's appendages—eyelids, lacrimal system, and conjunctiva. Six extraocular muscles attached to the sclera control the eyeball's movements. Although each has at least one specific action, these muscles never act independently. Complex muscular interactions allow the eyes to move in different directions and make possible coordinated use of both eyes.

Progressive change

The eye is a dynamic organ that changes progressively throughout life. Because the lens's elasticity greatly affects its ability to change its shape, alterations in visual acuity from adolescence to adulthood are quite common as the lens becomes increasingly less elastic.

Presbyopia, impaired near vision caused by the loss of the lens's natural elasticity, occurs commonly in middle age. This disorder typically requires the use of reading glasses. In older persons, eye tissue may degenerate and seriously affect vision, especially in those with

CROSS SECTION OF THE EYE

This illustration highlights the major anatomical structures of the eye.

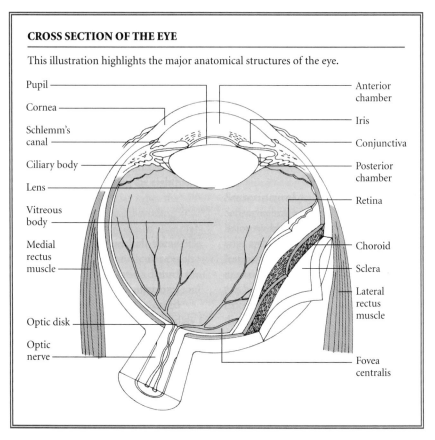

Pupil
Cornea
Schlemm's canal
Ciliary body
Lens
Vitreous body
Medial rectus muscle
Optic disk
Optic nerve

Anterior chamber
Iris
Conjunctiva
Posterior chamber
Retina
Choroid
Sclera
Lateral rectus muscle
Fovea centralis

chronic diseases, such as diabetes and macular degeneration. *Cataracts* — degenerative clouding of the lens — commonly afflict elderly patients.

Types of eye examinations

A thorough eye examination begins with a patient history, including documentation of medical conditions and past eye surgery. Identify the patient's reason for seeking care, such as discharge, pain, itching, blurred vision, blind spots, vertigo, photophobia, difficulty in distinguishing color, or poor visual acuity. Determine the location, duration, and intensity of the symptom. Ask the patient about his occupation and if there are any environ-

mental agents that might affect his eyes; ask whether he has had facial pain or headaches. In addition, ask about systemic diseases that may cause ocular changes, such as diabetes, thyroid problems, hypertension, and acquired immunodeficiency syndrome. Note the patient's current medication regimen because many drugs have ophthalmic effects. Tailor questions to the patient's age, ability, and cultural background.

The next step in the examination is visual acuity testing, using standardized vision charts such as the Snellen chart and the Jaeger card. After assessing acuity, look for clinical features, such as redness, excessive tearing or blinking, displacement of the eye within the orbit, and asymmetry of ocular and facial structures. External examination assesses pupillary light reflexes, inspects anterior segments, and evaluates extraocular muscle function and ocular alignment. The interior structures of the eye are inspected with an ophthalmoscope and a slit-lamp biomicroscope. Tonometry, which measures IOP, is done to assess for glaucoma. (See *Common ophthalmologic abbreviations and symbols.*)

Observe the patient's appearance and posture. Odd clothing combinations may indicate a color vision defect. Be alert to nonverbal behavior, such as squinting or abnormal eye movements. Head tilting may signal that the patient is compensating for a defect (for example, to focus double images into one image). Extend your hand as the patient approaches you to check depth perception.

Abnormalities detected by routine procedures may require more refined tests. Suspected abnormalities can commonly be located more precisely with orbital radiography, computed tomography, or ocular ultrasonography (or a combination of these tests).

Important considerations

In several routine tests, the physician may request ophthalmic drugs. *Cycloplegic agents* and *mydriatic agents* are the primary classes used to perform a dilated fundoscopic examination. Cycloplegics cause paralysis of accommodation and are commonly required before refraction. Mydriatics cause pupillary dilation and are commonly used to inspect intraocular structures. Generally, two instillations are required to induce maximum mydriasis. To help prevent contamination, avoid touching the eyedropper to the eye or eyelids during instillation.

COMMON OPHTHALMOLOGIC ABBREVIATIONS AND SYMBOLS

When recording the patient's responses during eye examinations, use these ophthalmic abbreviations.

AC	anterior chamber
$\overline{cc}$	with spectacles
CF	count fingers (visual acuity)
EOM	extraocular muscles
HM	hand motion (visual acuity)
IOP	intraocular pressure
LP	light perception
NLP	no light perception
NPC	near point of convergence
OD	right eye (oculus dexter)
OS	left eye (oculus sinister)
OU	both eyes (oculi uterque)
PERRLA	pupils equal, round, reactive to light, and accommodation
PH	pinhole
$\overline{sc}$	without spectacles
VF	visual field
Δ	prism diopters
D	lens diopters
(+)	convex lens
(−)	concave lens

◀ **CLINICAL ALERT** *Never instill dilating drops in a patient who has or is suspected of having angle-closure glaucoma. In such a patient, pupillary dilation* *could trigger an acute attack of angle closure.*

To ensure the patient's cooperation during an eye examination, provide a thorough explanation of each test and reassure him that the procedures are painless. These measures are essential with tests that require subjective responses from the patient.

The first section of this chapter deals with subjective tests; the second section focuses on objective tests. The final section covers special diagnostic procedures that are usually performed in a hospital or radiology department.

SUBJECTIVE TESTS
Visual acuity

The visual acuity test evaluates the patient's ability to distinguish the form and detail of an object. The patient is asked to read letters on a standardized visual chart, commonly called the *Snellen chart,* from a distance of 20′ (6.1 m). Charts showing the letter "E" in various positions and sizes are used for young children and other people who can't read. The smaller the symbol the patient can identify, the sharper his visual acuity. A patient's near (reading) vision may be tested as well, using a standardized chart such as the Jaeger card (a card with print in graded sizes).

The Snellen test should be performed on all patients with eye complaints.

AGE ISSUE *The near-vision test is routine for those complaining of eyestrain or reading difficulty and for everyone over age 40. Results serve as a baseline for treatments, follow-up examinations, and referrals.*

Purpose
- To test distance and near visual acuity
- To identify refractive errors in vision

Patient preparation
- Tell the patient that the tests evaluate distant and near vision.
- Tell the patient that the tests take only a few minutes. If he wears glasses, tell him to bring them to the examination.

Procedure and posttest care
Distance visual acuity
- Have the patient sit 20′ (6.1 m) away from the eye chart. If he's wearing glasses, tell him to remove them so his uncorrected vision can be tested first.
- Begin with the right eye unless vision in the left eye is known to be more acute. Have the patient occlude the left eye; then ask him to read the smallest line of letters he can see on the chart. Encourage him to try to read lines he can't see clearly because intelligent guesses usually indicate that the patient can recognize some of the symbols' details.

AGE ISSUE *If using the "E" chart with preschool children, have the child compare the letter to a table with three legs. Then ask the child to point to the direction in which the legs of the table are pointing.*
- Record the number of the smallest line the patient can read. This number is expressed as a fraction. The numerator is the distance between the patient and the chart; the denominator is the distance from which a patient with normal vision can read the line. The greater the denominator, the poorer the vision.
- If the patient makes an error on a line, record the results with a minus number. For example, if the patient reads the 20/40 line but makes one error, record his vision as 20/40 – 1. If the patient reads

sler's grid test can also detect microscopic areas of macular or perimacular edema that cause visual distortions. However, because this test is only a screening procedure, it must be supplemented with other tests, such as ophthalmoscopy, visual field testing, and fluorescein angiography, to determine the cause of abnormal vision.

Purpose
- To detect central scotomas
- To evaluate the stability or progression of macular disease

Patient preparation
- Explain to the patient that this test evaluates his central field of vision and takes 5 to 10 minutes to perform.
- If he normally wears corrective lenses, instruct him to keep them on during the test.

Procedure and posttest care
- Occlude one of the patient's eyes and hold Amsler's grid at his customary reading distance, approximately 11″ to 12″ (28 to 30 cm) in front of the unoccluded eye.
- Tell the patient to stare at the central dot on the grid, and then ask these questions:
– Can you see the black dot in the center?
– When you look directly at the dot, can you see all four sides of the grid? All of the little squares?
– Do all the lines appear ruler-straight?
– Is there any blurring, distortion, or movement?
– If the patient answers yes to any of these questions, ask him to elaborate.
– Give him a pencil and paper, and encourage him to outline and describe the specific areas that appear distorted.

– After recording the patient's observations, occlude the other eye and repeat the procedure.

Precautions
- Remind the patient to keep his unoccluded eye fixed on the central black dot on the grid.
- Perform this test before dilating the patient's pupils and performing fundoscopic examination or the refraction test.

Normal findings
The patient should be able to see the central black dot and, while staring at the dot, all four sides of the grid and all the little squares. All the lines should appear ruler-straight. He should not see any blurring, distortion, or missing squares. (See *Amsler's grid: Normal and abnormal views,* page 530.)

Abnormal findings
The inability to see the black dot in the center of the grid suggests a central scotoma. If any of the lines don't appear ruler-straight to the patient, metamorphopsia (distorted perception of objects) may be indicated. Blurring, distortion, or movement may signal an imminent scotoma. Abnormal findings indicate the need for further evaluation by ophthalmoscopy, visual field testing, and fluorescein angiography.

Interfering factors
- The patient's inability to see Amsler's grid because of poor eyesight or failure to cooperate or to keep his unoccluded eye fixed on the central dot
- Bleaching of the retina with the bright light of a retinoscope or an ophthalmoscope before the test, impairing the ability to see the grid

AMSLER'S GRID: NORMAL AND ABNORMAL VIEWS

The top illustration shows a normal view of Amsler's grid. The bottom illustration shows a grid as it might look to a patient with a central scotoma due to a macular hole. The center dot is entirely absent, as are the lines around it. The lines of the periphery of the scotoma appear bowed in an asymmetrical pattern.

NORMAL VIEW

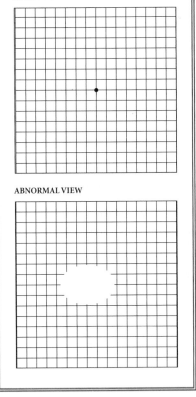

ABNORMAL VIEW

tral field—a 25-degree area surrounding the fixation point—and a peripheral field—the remainder of the area within which objects can be visualized. The tangent screen examination evaluates a patient's central visual field through systematic movement of a test object across a tangent screen, usually a piece of black felt with concentric circles and lines radiating from a central fixation point, much like a spider web.

Monocular visual field examinations are important in detecting and following the progression of ocular diseases, such as glaucoma and optic neuritis. They're also used to detect and evaluate neurologic disorders, such as brain tumors and strokes. Localization of a specific visual field defect commonly points to the underlying pathology. However, the tangent screen examination provides only a general evaluation of the patient's visual field. Abnormal findings warrant further examination with a perimeter to evaluate areas of the peripheral visual field. (Perimeters are used almost exclusively by ophthalmologists.) Another test that can assess the visual field is the confrontation test. (See *Confrontation test.*)

Purpose
■ To detect central visual field loss and evaluate its progression or regression

Patient preparation
■ Explain to the patient that the tangent screen examination evaluates his central field of vision and takes about 30 minutes to perform.
■ Reassure him that it causes no pain but requires his full cooperation.
■ If he normally wears corrective lenses, tell him to wear them during the test.

Tangent screen examination

The area within which objects can be seen as the eye fixates on a central point is called the *visual field*. It consists of a cen-

CONFRONTATION TEST

If a tangent screen or perimeter isn't available or if the patient can't cooperate for other tests, use the confrontation test to evaluate the visual field. Sit or stand about 2′ (0.6 m) directly in front of the patient and test his right eye first. Have him occlude his left eye, and tell him to look at your right eye and maintain fixation during the test. Explain that you'll hold up fingers or a fist in various positions. When he sees your hand, he should tell you what he can see — a fist or the number of fingers. Instruct him not to look for your hand, but to stare at your eye and say "now" when your hand appears.

Occlude your right eye, and in each quadrant, hold up your hand midway between yourself and the patient. Move it from nonseeing to seeing areas. Alternate between presenting fingers and a fist. You and the patient should see your hand at the same time, and the patient should correctly identify what you're presenting.

If the patient responds correctly in all quadrants, present fingers on both sides of fixation to test horizontal, vertical, and oblique meridians. If the patient re-sponds correctly, wiggle the index finger of each hand in the horizontal, vertical, and oblique meridians, and ask the patient if one finger is clearer than the other. If the patient reports that both fingers appear equally clear, occlude and fixate the opposite eyes, and repeat the procedure to test the left visual field.

However, if the patient reports that one finger is clearer than the other, you'll need to pinpoint the questionable area. To do this, simultaneously hold fingers above and below the area, and ask the patient which finger he sees better. Then proceed to test the other eye. If any areas of the visual field remain questionable, the patient should be tested with a tangent screen or a perimeter. A patient with "field cuts" may have a neurologic disorder such as multiple sclerosis.

Although the confrontation test is a simple means of screening a patient's visual field for gross abnormalities, it can't replace quantitative methods of evaluation. Also, the examiner's own visual field must be normal to produce valid test results.

Procedure and posttest care

■ Have the patient sit comfortably about 3′ (1 m) from the tangent screen so that the eye being tested is directly in line with the central fixation target on the screen.
■ Occlude the patient's left eye, and tell him that while he fixates on the central target, you'll move a test object into his visual field. The test object is white on one side and black on the other; its diameter varies in size from 1 to 10 mm, depending on the patient's visual acuity (for example, if he has 20/20 vision, the test object should have a diameter of 1 mm).

■ Tell the patient not to look for the test object, but to wait for it to appear and then to signal when he sees it. Stand to the side of the eye being tested.
■ Move the test object inward from the periphery of the screen at 30-degree intervals, as represented by the radiating lines on the screen.
■ Using black-tipped straight pins, plot the points on the screen at which the patient can see the object. When connected, these points define areas of equal visual acuity. The boundary of a visual field for a specific target size and distance is called an *isopter*. To guarantee the adequacy of

fixation, the blind spot (projection of optic nerve into the visual field) should be clearly identified.

- After the boundaries of the patient's central visual field have been plotted, test how well he can see within his visual field by turning the test object to the black side. Then turn it over within each 30-degree interval, and ask the patient to signal when he sees the test object.
- Plot suspicious areas — those in which the patient has failed to identify the test object — for size, shape, and density.
- Record the patient's visual field on the recording chart, marked in degrees, and note any abnormal areas within the field.
- Because isopters vary with the patient's age, visual acuity, and pupil size; the size and color of the test object; and the distance between the patient and the screen, carefully record all measurements.
- Occlude the patient's right eye and repeat the test.

Precautions

- Remind the patient that he must maintain fixation on the central target on the tangent screen.
- Watch the patient's eyes carefully to make sure he's following your instructions.

Normal findings

The central visual field normally forms a circle, extending 25 degrees superiorly, nasally, inferiorly, and temporally. The physiologic blind spot lies 12 to 15 degrees temporal to the central fixation point, approximately 1.5 degrees below the horizontal meridian. It extends approximately 7.5 degrees in height and 5.5 degrees in width. The test object should be visible throughout the patient's entire central visual field, except within the physiologic blind spot.

Abnormal findings

Visual field defects appear in several forms and may arise from many causes. For example, the inability to see the test object within the temporal half of the central visual field may indicate bitemporal hemianopia. Lesions of the optic chiasm (commonly caused by a pituitary tumor), craniopharyngiomas in the young, and meningiomas or an aneurysm of the circle of Willis in adults can cause bitemporal hemianopsia. (See *Complete bitemporal hemianopsia.*) Hemianopsia may also occur after a stroke. Although bilateral homonymous hemianopsia is uncommon, it may follow multiple thrombosis in the posterior cerebral circulation. Plotting visual fields after a stroke helps to locate cerebrovascular lesions.

When a disease, such as glaucoma, involves the optic nerve, an enlarged blind spot, a central scotoma, or a centrocecal scotoma may result. A ring scotoma (a scotoma 10 or more degrees away from the fixation point) is characteristic of retinitis pigmentosa, a slowly progressive disease that leads to night blindness. The peripheral area beyond this ring is usually spared. Retinal detachment (a separation of the retina from the retinal pigment epithelium in the posterior portion of the eye) can be outlined as well.

Repeat tangent screen examinations can help evaluate progression or regression of a diagnosed disorder.

Interfering factors

- An uncooperative patient or one who has severe vision loss that causes him to have difficulty seeing even the largest test object

COMPLETE BITEMPORAL HEMIANOPSIA

These illustrations show the results of an examination of the peripheral visual field with a perimeter. The heavy black line encloses the normal visual field. The white area within it represents the limited visual field in a person with complete bitemporal hemianopia, a serious eye disorder that's usually caused by lesions of the optic chiasm.

LEFT EYE

RIGHT EYE

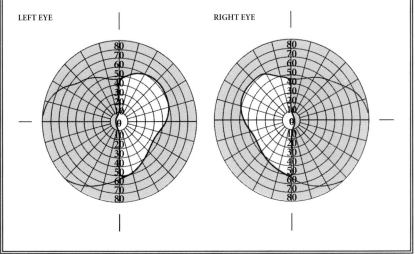

Color vision

The human eye perceives color through the cones of the retina, which are also responsible for central visual acuity. The most widely accepted theories of color vision propose that these retinal cones contain three different photosensitive pigments, each of which absorbs light of different wavelengths. Specifically, these pigments are sensitive to red, green, and blue—the primary colors of light. Mixtures of these three pigments allow perception of other colors.

Color vision tests assess the ability to recognize differences in color. They're commonly used to evaluate patients with suspected retinal disease or with a family history of color vision deficiency. A color vision deficiency may be inherited—a sex-linked recessive trait affecting approx-

imately 8% to 10% of males and less than 1% of females—or acquired as a result of disease. These tests are also used to screen applicants for jobs in which accurate color perception is vital, as in the military and electronics fields.

The most common color vision tests use pseudoisochromatic plates made up of dot patterns of the primary colors superimposed on backgrounds of randomly mixed colors. A patient with normal color vision can identify the dot pattern; a patient with a color vision deficiency can't distinguish between the pattern and the background. Basic color vision tests merely indicate the presence of a deficiency; more sophisticated tests can determine the degree of deficiency.

Purpose

■ To detect color vision deficiency

Patient preparation

- Explain to the patient that this test evaluates color perception, takes only a few minutes, and causes no pain.
- If the patient normally wears glasses or contact lenses, tell him to wear them during the test.

Procedure and posttest care

- After seating the patient comfortably, occlude one of his eyes.
- Hold the test book approximately 14″ (35.5 cm) in front of his unoccluded eye and give him the pointer.
- Explain to the patient what patterns or symbols he may see. Show him the sample plates — which can be deciphered in most cases — and tell him you'll ask him to identify the symbols and then to trace them with the pointer. Inform him that some symbols are more difficult to see than others.
- Conduct the test, eliciting immediate responses from the patient.
- Record the responses according to the instructions included with the test kit.
- When testing the other eye (or repeating the test, if necessary), rotate the plates 90 to 180 degrees to minimize recall.

Precautions

- To prevent discoloration of the plates, keep the test book closed when it isn't being used and turn the pages by their edges.

Normal findings

A person with normal color vision — a trichromat — can identify all the patterns or symbols.

Abnormal findings

A patient with deficit color vision — an anomalous trichromat — can't identify all the patterns or symbols. This deficiency may be diagnosed more precisely by noting the combinations of colors that elicit incorrect responses. For example, *protanopia* is a deficiency of the retinal cone pigment that is sensitive to red. A patient with protanopia has difficulty discriminating between red/green and blue/green. A patient with *deuteranopia,* a deficiency of the retinal pigment sensitive to green, can't distinguish between green/purple and red/purple. *Tritanopia,* a deficiency of the pigment sensitive to blue, causes the patient to have difficulty discriminating between blue/green and yellow/green.

Achromatopsia — true color blindness — is a rare disease inherited as a Mendelian autosomal dominant or autosomal recessive trait. Patients with achromatopsia, called *monochromats,* see all colors as shades of gray. These patients may also have impaired visual acuity, nystagmus, and photophobia due to reduced or absent cone function.

Inherited color deficiency affects both eyes; acquired deficiency may affect only one eye. The patient with an acquired deficiency may complain of an inability to recognize colors that were formerly recognizable.

Abnormalities of the ocular media, retina, or optic nerve can cause deficient color vision. For this reason, a patient with an acquired color vision deficiency or an inherited deficiency accompanied by a loss of visual acuity should be referred for a complete ophthalmologic examination to determine the source of the deficiency.

Interfering factors

- Failure to cooperate, an inability to see the plates because of reduced visual acuity or failure to wear glasses, or improper lighting

- Errors in the testing procedure, such as inaccurately recording the patient's responses or allowing too much time for a response

Refraction

Refraction — the bending of light rays by the cornea, aqueous humor, lens, and vitreous humor in the eye — enables images to focus on the retina and directly affects visual acuity. The refraction test, done routinely during a complete eye examination or whenever a patient complains of a change in vision, defines the refractive error and determines the degree of correction required to improve visual acuity with corrective lenses. The ophthalmologist generally performs a refraction objectively, by using a retinoscope, and subjectively, by asking the patient about his visual acuity while placing trial lenses before his eyes.

Purpose
- To diagnose refractive error and prescribe corrective lenses, if necessary

Patient preparation
- Explain to the patient that the refraction test helps determine whether he needs corrective lenses.
- Tell the patient that eyedrops may be instilled to dilate his pupils and that the test takes 10 to 20 minutes.
- Reassure the patient that the test is painless and safe.
- Check the patient's history for angle-closure glaucoma. Also check for previous use of and hypersensitivity to dilating eyedrops.

Procedure and posttest care
- After short-acting mydriatic eyedrops are administered (if ordered), the exam-

iner directs the light of the retinoscope at the pupillary opening.
- Through the aperture at the top of the instrument, the examiner looks for an orange glow — the retinoscopic, or red, reflex, which represents the reflection of light from the retinoscope — and notes its brightness, clarity, and uniformity.
- Moving the retinoscope's light across the pupil, the examiner observes the reflex for any movement.
- The examiner then places trial lenses before the patient's eyes and adjusts the lens power to make the reflex clear, bright, and uniform and to neutralize its motion. The lens power necessary to make this adjustment is recorded.
- Objective findings can be refined by altering the trial lenses and having the patient read lines on a standardized visual chart. This helps determine which lens or combination of lenses provides the best correction of his visual acuity.
- If corrective lenses are prescribed, the patient is advised that images may appear blurred the first time he wears the lenses; eventually his eyes will adjust to the prescription.
- If the patient has worn glasses or contact lenses previously, the patient should wear only his new prescription lenses because changing back and forth from the old prescription to the new one will prevent his eyes from making the required adjustment to the new lenses.
- Laser-assisted *In Situ* Keratomileusis (LASIK) or optic laser surgery also may be used to correct refractive errors.

Precautions
CLINICAL ALERT *Don't administer dilating eyedrops to a patient who has angle-closure glaucoma or to any patient who has had a hypersensitivity reaction to such drops. Instruct the patient to*

NORMAL AND ABNORMAL REFRACTION

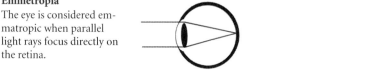

Emmetropia
The eye is considered emmatropic when parallel light rays focus directly on the retina.

Hyperopia
In hyperopia, parallel light rays focus behind the retina (left). This defect is corrected by placing a convex lens in front of the eye, which causes the rays to converge so they focus on the retina (right).

Myopia
In myopia, parallel light rays focus in front of the retina (left). A concave lens placed in front of the eye can correct this defect by diverging the rays so they focus on the retina (right).

report ocular discomfort or redness immediately.

Normal findings
Refractive power, measured in diopters, is greatest at the cornea (approximately 44 diopters) because of its curvature. The aqueous humor has the same refractive power as the cornea and is considered to be the same medium. The lens, normally a convex structure, has a refractive power of approximately 10 to 14 diopters, but can alter this power by changing its shape. This phenomenon is known as *accommodation* and occurs when the eye views objects closer than 20′(6.1 m).

The vitreous humor, a gelatinous medium, has little refractive power and mainly transmits light. In the absence of accommodation, the average refractive power of the human eye is 58 diopters.

Ideally, the eyes have no refractive error (emmetropia). Parallel light rays emanating from a point source can be focused directly on the retina to produce a clear image.

Abnormal findings
Most patients show some degree of refractive error (ametropia). *Hyperopia*, or farsightedness, occurs when the eyeball is too short and parallel light rays focus behind the retina. Examination with the

retinoscope shows a red reflex moving in the same direction as the retinoscope's light. A patient with hyperopia sees clearly at a distance, but experiences blurring of near objects.

Myopia, or nearsightedness, occurs when the eyeball is too long and parallel light rays focus in front of the retina. Retinoscopic examination reveals reflex motion opposite to movement of the retinoscope's light. A patient with myopia sees near objects clearly, but experiences blurring of distant images. (See *Normal and abnormal refraction.*)

When light rays entering the eye aren't refracted uniformly and a clear focal point on the retina isn't attained, the patient has *astigmatism.* This disorder is usually caused by unequal curvature of the cornea and is typically associated with some degree of hyperopia or myopia.

Interfering factors

■ Inadequate paralysis of accommodation or pupil dilation or the patient's failure to cooperate with the test

OBJECTIVE TESTS

Exophthalmometry

Exophthalmometry determines the relative forward protrusion of the eye from its orbit by using an exophthalmometer to measure the distance from the apex of the cornea to the lateral orbital margin. The exophthalmometer is a horizontal calibrated bar with movable carriers on both sides. These carriers hold mirrors inclined at a 45-degree angle that reflect the scale readings and the corneal apex in profile.

This test provides information that's useful in detecting and evaluating thyroid disease, eye tumors, and any condition that displaces the eye in the orbit.

Purpose

■ To measure the amount of forward eye protrusion
■ To evaluate the progression or regression of exophthalmos

Patient preparation

■ Explain to the patient that this test determines the degree of eye protrusion.

Procedure and posttest care

■ Ask the patient to sit upright facing you with his eyes on the same level as yours.
■ Hold the horizontal bar of the exophthalmometer in front of the patient's eyes, parallel to the floor.
■ Move the device's two small concave carriers against the lateral orbital margins and carefully record the calibrated bar reading. The baseline reading should be used during follow-up examinations.
■ If the patient has already been measured with an exophthalmometer, set the calibrated bar at the baseline reading. Tighten the locking screws on the mirrors to keep them properly positioned.
■ Measure each eye separately.
■ First, instruct the patient to fixate his right eye on your left eye. Using the inclined mirrors, superimpose the apex of the right cornea on the millimeter scale and record the reading, which represents the eye's relative forward displacement from its orbit.
■ Then instruct the patient to fixate his left eye on your right eye and repeat the procedure.
■ Refer the patient to an appropriate specialist, as needed.

Precautions
■ For follow-up examinations, set the calibrated bar at the baseline reading.

Normal findings
Normally, readings range from 12 to 20 mm. Measurements for each eye are similar, usually differing by 1.5 mm or less and rarely by more than 3 mm.

Abnormal findings
A difference between the eyes of more than 3 mm may indicate exophthalmos (outward displacement) or enophthalmos (inward displacement). A single reading that exceeds 20 mm may indicate exophthalmos; readings under 12 mm may indicate enophthalmos.

A patient with exophthalmos should receive a thorough ophthalmologic examination because the underlying cause may be local in origin. Any mass in the orbital cavity, edematous or hemorrhagic conditions, inflammatory diseases (such as periostitis or cellulitis), hyperostosis of the orbit, or other conditions causing a reduction in orbit size result in exophthalmos. However, it may also result from a systemic disorder, such as thyroid disease, as well as xanthomatosis or a blood dyscrasia, in which case a complete medical examination is indicated. In such cases, exophthalmos is usually bilateral.

Enophthalmos may result from traumatic injury, such as a fractured orbital floor. Less commonly, it may be a congenital or developmental defect.

Interfering factors
■ Failure to set the calibrated bar of the exophthalmometer at the baseline distance

Slit-lamp examination

The slit lamp is an instrument equipped with a special lighting system and a binocular microscope that allows an ophthalmologist to visualize in detail the anterior segment of the eye, including the eyelids, eyelashes, conjunctiva, sclera, cornea, tear film, anterior chamber, iris, crystalline lens, and vitreous face. To evaluate normally transparent or near-transparent ocular fluids and tissues, the size, shape, intensity, and depth of the light source as well as the magnification of the microscope may be altered. If abnormalities are noted, special devices are attached to the slit lamp to allow more detailed investigation.

Purpose
■ To detect and evaluate abnormalities of anterior segment tissues and structures

Patient preparation
■ Tell the patient that the slit-lamp examination evaluates the front portion of the eyes and that it requires that he remain still. Reassure him that the examination is painless.
■ If the patient wears contact lenses, tell him to remove them for the test, unless the test is being performed to evaluate the fit of the lens.
■ If the test calls for dilating eyedrops, check the patient's history for adverse reactions to mydriatics or for the presence of narrow-angle glaucoma before administering the drops. Dilating eyedrops aren't used in routine eye examinations; however, some diseases require pupillary dilation before slit-lamp examination.

Procedure and posttest care
■ Seat the patient in the examining chair. Have him place his feet on the floor and position his chin on the rest and his fore-

head against the bar. Dim the lights in the room.

■ The ophthalmologist examines the patient's eyes starting with the lids and lashes and progressing to the vitreous face, altering light and magnification as necessary. In some cases, a special camera can be attached to the slit lamp to photograph portions of the eye.

■ If dilating drops were instilled, tell the patient that his near vision will be blurred for up to 2 hours.

Precautions

■ Don't instill mydriatic drops into the eyes of a patient who has had a hypersensitivity reaction to them or who has angle-closure glaucoma.

Normal findings

Slit-lamp examination should reveal no abnormalities of anterior segment tissues and structures.

Abnormal findings

Slit-lamp examination may detect pathologic conditions, such as corneal abrasions and ulcers, lens opacities, iritis, and conjunctivitis as well as irregularly shaped corneas. A parchmentlike consistency of the lid skin, with redness, minor swelling, and moderate itching, may indicate a hypersensitivity reaction. If a corneal abrasion or ulcer is detected, a fluorescein stain may be applied to allow better viewing of the area. If a tearing deficiency is suspected, the ophthalmologist may examine the eye after applying a fluorescein or rose Bengal stain; he may also perform Schirmer's test. Some abnormal findings may indicate impending disorders. For example, early-stage lens opacities may signify cataract development.

PROPER FILTER PLACEMENT IN SCHIRMER'S TEST

This illustration shows the proper placement of the filter paper for Schirmer's test. The filter paper should be inserted into the inferior conjunctival sac of each eye.

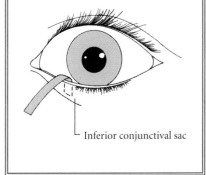

Inferior conjunctival sac

Interfering factors

■ The patient's inability to cooperate

Schirmer's tearing

Schirmer's test assesses the function of the major lacrimal glands, which are responsible for reflex tearing in response to stressful situations such as the presence of a foreign body. Reflex tearing is stimulated by inserting a strip of filter paper into the lower conjunctival sac, followed by measuring the amount of moisture absorbed by the paper. (See *Proper filter placement in Schirmer's test.*) Both eyes are tested simultaneously.

A variation of this test evaluates the function of the accessory lacrimal glands of Krause and Wolfring by instilling a topical anesthetic before inserting the filter papers. The anesthetic inhibits reflex tearing by the major lacrimal glands, ensuring measurement of only the basic tear film normally produced by the accessory glands. This tear film usually maintains adequate corneal moisture under normal circumstances.

Purpose
- To measure tear secretion in the patient with a suspected tearing deficiency

Patient preparation
- Explain to the patient that this test measures tear secretion.
- Tell the patient that the test requires that a strip of filter paper be placed in the lower part of each eye for 5 minutes.
- Reassure the patient that the procedure is painless.
- If the patient wears contact lenses, ask him to remove them before the test. If an anesthetic is instilled, he won't be able to reinsert the lenses for 2 hours after the test.

Procedure and posttest care
- Seat the patient in the examining chair with his head against the headrest.
- To remove the test strip from the wrapper, bend the rounded wick end at the indentation and cut open the envelope at the other end.
- Tell the patient to look up, and then gently lower the inferior eyelid.
- Hook the bent end of the strip over the inferior eyelid at the junction of the medial and nasal segments.
- Insert one strip in each eye and note the time of insertion. Tell the patient not to squeeze or rub his eyes, but to blink normally or to keep his eyes closed lightly.
- After 5 minutes, remove the strips from the patient's eyes and measure the length of the moistened area from the indentation, using the millimeter scale on the envelope.
- Report the results as a fraction: the numerator is the length of the moistened area, and the denominator is the time the

strips were left in place. Also note which eye was tested. Thus, if a strip inserted in the right conjunctival sac for 5 minutes shows 8 mm of moisture, the correct notation is OD (*oculus dexter,* or right eye), 8 mm/5 minutes.
- To measure the function of the accessory lacrimal glands of Krause and Wolfring, instill one drop of topical anesthetic into each conjunctival sac before inserting the test strips.
- If a topical anesthetic was instilled, advise the patient not to rub his eyes for at least 30 minutes after instillation because this can cause a corneal abrasion. The patient who wears contact lenses shouldn't reinsert them for at least 2 hours.

Precautions
- To prevent patient discomfort, be careful not to touch the cornea while inserting the test strip.

Normal findings
The test strip should show at least 15 mm of moisture after 5 minutes. Both eyes usually secrete the same amount of tears.

AGE ISSUE *Because tear production decreases with age, normal test results in a patient over age 40 may range from 10 to 15 mm.*

Abnormal findings
Although Schirmer's tearing test is a simple and efficient method of measuring the rate of tear secretion, up to 15% of the patients tested have false-positive or false-negative results. Because the test is rapid and simple, it may be repeated and findings compared. Additional testing, such as a slit-lamp examination with fluorescein or rose Bengal stain, is necessary to corroborate results.

A positive result confirmed by additional testing indicates a definite tearing deficiency, which may result from aging or, more seriously, from Sjögren's syndrome, a systemic disease of unknown origin most common among post-menopausal women. A tearing deficiency may also arise secondarily to systemic diseases, such as lymphoma, leukemia, and rheumatoid arthritis. Regardless of the cause, a tearing deficiency is a matter of clinical concern because it can lead to corneal erosions, scarring, and secondary infection.

Interfering factors
- The patient closing his eyes too tightly during the test
- Reflex tearing due to contact of the test strip with the cornea

Ophthalmoscopy

Ophthalmoscopy allows magnified examination of the vascular and nerve tissue of the fundus, including the optic disk, retinal vessels, macula, and retina. This test is conducted with either a direct or an indirect ophthalmoscope — one of the most important diagnostic tools in ophthalmology. Generally, examiners use the direct ophthalmoscope, a small, handheld instrument consisting of a light source, a viewing device, a reflecting device to channel light into the patient's eyes, and spherical lenses to correct refractive error of the patient or examiner. If a slit lamp isn't available, the examiner may also use the ophthalmoscope to examine the patient's cornea, iris, and lens.

If an abnormality of the retina is suspected, further testing, such as fluorescein angiography, may be necessary.

Purpose
- To detect and evaluate eye disorders as well as ocular manifestations of systemic disease

Patient preparation
- Explain to the patient that this test permits examination of the back of the eye.
- Describe the test, including who will perform it, where it will take place, and how long it will last.
- Advise the patient that eyedrops may be used to dilate the pupils for a clearer examination, but reassure him that he'll experience no discomfort during the test.
- When using eyedrops, check the patient's history for previous use of dilating eyedrops, indications of possible hypersensitivity, and angle-closure glaucoma.

Procedure and posttest care
- Routine examination of the ocular media and fundus is usually conducted without dilating the pupil if there's sufficient light in the ophthalmoscope and room lighting is subdued. If indicated, two instillations of mydriatic eyedrops are usually necessary to achieve maximum dilation.
- The patient sits upright in the examination chair, and the room lights are dimmed to keep irregular reflections from interfering with the examination.
- The examiner sits about 2′(0.6 m) away from the patient and slightly to his right. The examination begins with the patient's right eye. The ophthalmoscope is held in the right hand in front of the examiner's right eye. A small adjustment near the forefinger allows him to select different lenses quickly.
- The illuminated dial should be set to zero and the patient told to look straight ahead at a specific object 20′(6.1 m) away — for example, a large symbol on a

standardized vision chart — for the duration of the examination.

- Remaining on the patient's right side, the examiner moves forward until he's within 6″ (15 cm) of the patient. At this point, he directs the light beam into the pupil and looks for the red reflex (red reflection from the fundus), which is visible without magnification. Then he focuses on the optic disk, noting its size, shape, and color.
- Next, the examiner looks for a white central depression in the optic disk — the physiologic cup — and observes the retinal vessels that emerge from the disk.
- Finally, the examiner focuses on the macula — a yellowish depression slightly below the center of the optic disk — and its center, the fovea. The examiner tells the patient to look up, down, and to each side to examine the extreme periphery. The superior, inferior, temporal, and nasal portions of the retina are examined respectively.
- This procedure is then repeated for the left eye, with the examiner moving slightly to the patient's left side and holding the ophthalmoscope in the left hand and in front the examiner's left eye.

Precautions

- Don't administer dilating eyedrops to a patient who has a history of hypersensitivity reactions to them or who has angle-closure glaucoma.
- Make sure the patient maintains fixation throughout the procedure.

Normal findings

With the beam of light from the ophthalmoscope directed into the patient's pupil, the red reflex should be visible through the aperture. The slightly oval optic disk lies to the nasal side of the fundus center. Although its color varies widely, it's usually pink with darker edges at its nasal border. The physiologic cup, a pale depression in the center of the optic disk, varies widely in size; it tends to be larger in the patient with myopia and smaller in one with hyperopia.

The semitransparent retina surrounds the optic disk. Branching out from the disk are the retinal vessels, including the venules and the slightly smaller arterioles. Vessel diameter progressively decreases with distance from the optic disk. Retinal arterioles generally have a medium red color; venules appear dark red or blue.

The macula is the most darkly pigmented area of the retina. In its center lies a small, even darker spot — the fovea. A tiny light reflex can be seen at the center of the fovea, caused by reflection of the ophthalmoscopic light from the concave inner surface of the area.

Abnormal findings

An absent or a diminished red reflex may be due to gross corneal lesions, dense opacities of the aqueous or vitreous (such as from blood after hemorrhage), cataracts, or a detached retina. A cloudy vitreous that obscures the fundus may be caused by inflammatory disease of the optic disk, retina, or uvea. Fundal lesions should be sketched or photographed for further study.

Optic neuritis causes the optic disk to become elevated and more vascular; small hemorrhages may also occur. Optic nerve atrophy causes the disk to appear white. Papilledema, which may result from increased intracranial pressure, causes an abnormal elevation of the disk, blurring of disk margins, engorged vessels, and hemorrhages.

In glaucoma, the physiologic cup may appear enlarged and gray with white edges. A milky white retina characterizes the acute phase of a central retinal artery occlusion; the fovea, in contrast to the ischemic macula, appears as a bright red spot. Central retinal vein occlusion is marked by widespread retinal hemorrhaging, patches of white exudate, and disk elevation.

Retinal detachments appear as gray elevated areas, possibly with areas of red vascular choroid exposed by retinal tears. A choroidal tumor appears as a dark lesion.

The integrity of retinal vessels is commonly evaluated to aid in the diagnosis of systemic disease. Hypertension, for example, causes vasospasm, sclerosis, and eventual occlusion of retinal arterioles, leading to retinal edema and hemorrhage and papilledema. Diabetes mellitus may be complicated by retinal fibroses, patches of white exudate, and microaneurysms. Other systemic disorders present similar findings.

Interpretation of ophthalmoscopic findings depends largely on the examiner's knowledge and experience because an abnormality can arise from several sources. After an ophthalmoscopic evaluation, referral for a complete medical evaluation may be necessary.

Interfering factors
■ Room not sufficiently dark, inadequate light source, or other condition improper for examination
■ The patient's inability to cooperate
■ Conditions prohibiting a good view of the fundus, such as insufficient dilation, dense cataracts, cloudy media, and gross nystagmus

Corneal staining

Corneal staining with fluorescein dye allows a detailed view of the anterior part of the eye that can't ordinarily be seen during slit-lamp examination. A special attachment is used during the slit-lamp examination to enhance visualization.

Purpose
■ To detect the depth and pattern of injuries to the corneal surface of the eye
■ To diagnose corneal injuries

Patient preparation
■ Describe the procedure to the patient. Explain that corneal staining evaluates the eye surface and is painless.
■ Tell the patient who will perform the test and where it will take place.
■ Ask the patient for a detailed history of the eye injury and the symptoms associated with the injury.
■ Ask the patient to remove his glasses or contact lenses before the test.

Procedure and posttest care
■ Seat the patient in the examination chair.
■ Stain the patient's eye surface with the fluorescein dye by touching the tip of the fluorescein strip to the lower conjunctival sac.
■ Ask the patient to close his eye to help spread the dye over the corneal surface.
■ Have the patient sit properly in the examination chair with his forehead placed against the bar apparatus.
■ Instruct the patient to look straight ahead while his eyes are examined with the slit lamp.
■ Defects are recorded while the eye is being examined with a bright light.
■ Inform the patient that any blurring of vision will gradually disappear within 2 hours.

Precautions
■ Monitor the patient for allergic reaction to the fluorescein dye.

■ Because the dye used in this test causes blurred vision, ensure that the patient has a responsible person to take him home.

Normal findings

The normal cornea is convex in shape and has a smooth, shiny appearance. No scratches or indentations are noted.

Abnormal findings

Abnormal findings include corneal scratches, abrasions, ulcerations, and keratitis.

Interfering factors

■ The patient's inability to remain still during the examination
■ Allergy to the fluorescein dye

Tonometry

Tonometry allows indirect measurement of intraocular pressure (IOP) and serves as an effective screen for early detection of glaucoma, which occurs in 2% of people over age 40 and is a common cause of blindness. Indentation tonometry measures this resistance by observing how deeply a known weight depresses the cornea; applanation tonometry provides the same information by measuring the amount of force required to flatten a known area of the cornea. Both procedures necessitate corneal anesthetization and careful examination technique. Patients with IOP problems can now monitor their pressure at home with a portable tonometer. If the IOP is elevated, other tests, such as applanation tonometry, visual field testing, and ophthalmoscopy, must confirm the diagnosis.

Purpose

■ To measure IOP

■ To aid in the diagnosis and follow-up evaluation of glaucoma

Patient preparation

■ Explain to the patient that tonometry measures the pressure within his eyes.
■ Tell the patient that the test takes only a few minutes and requires that his eyes be anesthetized, but reassure him that the procedure is painless.
■ If the patient wears contact lenses, instruct him to remove them before the test or until the anesthetic wears off completely.
■ Ask the patient to assume a supine position. Make sure he's relaxed and have him loosen restrictive clothing around his neck. Instruct him not to cough or squeeze his eyelids together.

Procedure and posttest care

■ Ask the patient to look down. Raise his superior eyelid with your thumb, place one drop of the topical anesthetic at the top of the sclera, and have the patient blink.
■ Check the tonometer for a zero reading on the steel test block that comes with the instrument. Make sure the plunger moves freely. The first measurement on each eye is obtained with the 5.5-g weight.
■ Have the patient look up and stare at a spot on the ceiling. Then ask him to open his mouth, take a deep breath, and exhale slowly for distraction.
■ With the thumb and forefinger of one hand, hold the lids of his right eye open against the orbital rim.
■ Hold the tonometer vertically with the thumb and forefinger of the other hand, and rest the footplate on the apex of the cornea.
■ With the footplate in place, check the indicator needle for a rhythmic transmission caused by the ocular pulse, and then

record the calibrated scale reading that converts to a measurement of IOP. If the reading doesn't exceed 4, add an additional weight (7.5, 10, or 15 g) to obtain a reliable result.

- Repeat the procedure on the left eye and record the time the test is performed.
- Tell the patient not to rub his eyes for at least 20 minutes after the test to prevent corneal abrasion.
- If the patient wears contact lenses, tell him not to reinsert them for at least 2 hours.
- If the tonometer moved across the cornea during the test, tell the patient he may feel a slight scratching sensation in the eye when the anesthetic wears off. This sensation should disappear within 24 hours because most abrasions resulting from tonometry affect only the epithelium, which regenerates in 24 hours.

Precautions

⏵ **CLINICAL ALERT** *Tonometry should never be performed on a patient with a corneal ulcer or infection, except by a skilled examiner and only in an emergency such as suspected acute angle-closure glaucoma.*
- Avoid resting your fingers on the cornea or pressing on the cornea because this increases IOP.
- Don't touch the patient's lashes; this could trigger a blink response or Bell's phenomenon (upward movement of the eyes with forced closure of the lids), which can cause the footplate to move and scratch the cornea.

Normal findings

IOP normally ranges from 12 to 20 mm Hg, with diurnal variations. The highest point is reached at the time of waking; the lowest point, in the evening.

Abnormal findings

Elevated IOP requires further testing for glaucoma. Because IOP varies diurnally, findings must be supplemented with serial measurements obtained at different times on different days.

Interfering factors

- Poor patient cooperation
- Deformed corneal curvature that prevents proper placement of the footplate
- Corneoscleral rigidity or flaccidity, as determined by an ophthalmologist (falsely elevated or depressed readings)

Fluorescein angiography

In fluorescein angiography, a special camera takes rapid-sequence photographs of the fundus following I.V. injection of sodium fluorescein (a contrast medium), thereby recording the appearance of blood vessels within the eye. This technique provides enhanced visibility of the microvascular structures of the retina and choroid, which permits the evaluation of the entire retinal vascular bed, including retinal circulation.

Purpose

- To document retinal circulation when evaluating intraocular abnormalities, such as retinopathy, tumors, and circulatory or inflammatory disorders

Patient preparation

- Explain that fluorescein angiography takes about 30 minutes and evaluates the small blood vessels in the eyes.
- Make sure the patient or a responsible family member has signed an informed consent form.
- Check the patient's history for glaucoma and hypersensitivity reactions or allergies, especially to contrast media and

dilating eyedrops. If necessary, tell a patient with glaucoma not to use miotic eyedrops on the day of the test.

■ Explain that eyedrops will be instilled to dilate his pupils and that a dye will be injected into his arm. Tell him that his eyes will be photographed with a special camera before and after the injection. Stress that these are photographs, not X-rays.

■ Warn the patient that his skin may be discolored and his urine may appear orange for 24 to 48 hours after the procedure.

Procedure and posttest care

■ Administer mydriatic eyedrops. Usually, two instillations are necessary to achieve maximum mydriasis within 15 to 40 minutes.

■ Following mydriasis, seat the patient comfortably in the examining chair facing the camera.

■ Have the patient loosen or remove any restrictive clothing around his neck.

■ Tell the patient to place his chin in the chin rest and his forehead against the bar. Tell him to open his eyes wide and stare straight ahead, while keeping his teeth together and maintaining normal breathing and blinking.

■ The antecubital vein is prepared and punctured; however, dye isn't injected yet. At this time, a few photographs may be taken. Make sure the patient keeps his arm extended; if necessary, use an arm board.

■ Warn the patient that the dye will be injected rapidly. Remind him to maintain his position and to continue to stare straight ahead, and then inject the dye.

■ The patient may experience nausea and a feeling of warmth. Provide reassurance and observe him for hypersensitivity reactions, such as vomiting, dry mouth, metallic taste, suddenly increased salivation, sneezing, light-headedness, fainting, or hives. In rare instances, anaphylactic shock may occur.

■ As the dye is injected, 25 to 30 photographs are taken in rapid sequence. Each photograph is taken 1 second after the other.

■ The needle and syringe are removed carefully; pressure and a dressing are applied to the injection site.

■ If late-phase photographs are needed, tell the patient to sit and relax for 20 minutes, and then reposition him for 5 to 10 photographs. If necessary, photographs may be taken up to 1 hour after the injection.

■ Remind the patient that his skin and urine will be slightly discolored for 24 to 48 hours after the test. Encourage the patient to drink increased amounts of fluids to help excrete the dye.

■ Explain to the patient that his near vision will be blurred for up to 12 hours and that he should avoid direct sunlight and refrain from driving during this time.

Precautions

■ Don't leave the patient unattended because may experience mild adverse reactions, such as nausea, vomiting, sneezing, paresthesia of the tongue, and dizziness.

CLINICAL ALERT *Have emergency resuscitation equipment at hand. Serious adverse effects (laryngeal edema, bronchospasm, and respiratory arrest) are possible. If a reaction occurs, note it on the patient's allergy history.*

■ Keep in mind that the needle must be placed in the vein correctly; extravasation of dye around the injection site is painful.

Normal findings

After rapid injection into the antecubital vein, sodium fluorescein reaches the retina in 12 to 15 seconds (filling phase). As the choroidal vessels and choriocapillaries fill, the background of the retina fluoresces, taking on an evenly mottled appearance known as the *choroidal flush.* Then the dye fills the arteries (arterial phase). The arteriovenous (AV) phase lasts from the complete filling of the arteries and capillaries to the earliest evidence of dye in the veins. The time the arteries begin to empty to the time the veins fill and empty is known as the *venous phase.* Finally, the recirculation phase occurs 30 to 60 minutes after the injection, when the fluorescein — if at all present — is barely detectable in the retinal vessels. Normally, there's no leakage from the retinal vessels.

Abnormal findings

The varying and complex findings after fluorescein angiography require interpretation by a highly skilled ophthalmologist with extensive experience in diagnosing retinal disorders.

Abnormalities detected in the early filling phase may include microaneurysms, AV shunts, and neovascularization. The test may identify arterial occlusion by showing delayed or absent flow of the dye through the arteries, stenosis, and prolonged venous drainage. Venous occlusion may be associated with vessel dilation and fluorescein leakage. Chronic obstruction may produce recanalization and collateral circulation.

In hypertensive retinopathy, abnormalities may include areas of increased vascular tortuosity, microaneurysms around zones of capillary nonperfusion, and generalized suffusion of the dye in the retina. Aneurysms and capillary hemangiomas may leak fluorescein and are typically surrounded by hard yellow exudate. Tumors exhibit variable fluorescein patterns, de-

pending on the histologic type. Retinal edema or inflammation and fibrous tissue may show variable degrees of fluorescence. Papilledema produces vascular leakage in the disk area.

Interfering factors

- Inadequate view of the fundus due to insufficient pupillary dilation (possible poor imaging)
- Cataract, media opacity, or inability to keep eyes open and to maintain fixation (possible poor imaging)

SPECIAL PROCEDURES

Orbital radiography

Orbital radiography evaluates the orbit, the bony cavity that houses the eye and the lacrimal glands, as well as blood vessels, nerves, muscles, and fat. Because portions of the orbit are composed of thin bone that fractures easily, X-rays are commonly taken following facial trauma. They're also useful in diagnosing ocular and orbital pathologies. Special radiographic techniques can reveal foreign bodies in the orbit or eye that are invisible to an ophthalmoscope. In some cases, radiography is used in conjunction with computed tomography scans and ultrasonography to better define an abnormality.

Purpose

- To aid in the diagnosis of orbital fractures and pathologies
- To help locate intraorbital or intraocular foreign bodies

Patient preparation

■ Explain that orbital radiography involves taking several X-rays to assess the condition of the bones around the eye.

■ Describe the test, including who will perform it and where it will take place.

■ Reassure the patient that the procedure is usually painless unless he has suffered facial trauma, in which case positioning may cause some discomfort. Explain that he'll be asked to turn his head from side to side and to flex or extend his neck.

■ Instruct the patient to remove all jewelry and other metallic objects from the X-ray field.

Procedure and posttest care

■ Have the patient recline on the X-ray table or sit in a chair.

■ Instruct the patient to remain still while the X-rays are taken.

■ Remember that usually a series of orbital X-rays includes a lateral view, posteroanterior view, submentovertical (base) view, stereo Waters' views (views from both sides), Towne's (half-axial) projection, and optic canal projections. If enlargement of the superior orbital fissure is suspected, apical views are obtained.

■ The films are first developed and inspected by the radiography department before the patient is released.

Normal findings

Each orbit is composed of a roof, a floor, and medial and lateral walls. The bones of the roof and floor are very thin (the floor can be less than 1 mm thick). The medial walls, which parallel each other, are slightly thicker, except for the portion formed by the ethmoid bone. The lateral walls are the thickest part of the orbit and are strongest at the orbital rim.

The superior orbital fissure, at the back of the orbit between the lateral wall and the roof, is actually a gap between the greater and lesser wings of the sphenoid bone. The optic canal, which carries the optic nerve and ophthalmic artery, is an opening in the lesser wing of the sphenoid bone located at the apex of the orbit.

Abnormal findings

Orbital fractures associated with facial trauma are most common in the thin structures of the floor and ethmoid bone. Abnormalities are detected by comparing the size and shape of orbital structures on the affected side with those on the opposite side.

Generally, orbit enlargement indicates the presence of a lesion that has caused proptosis due to increased intraorbital pressure. Any growing tumor can produce these changes. Superior orbital fissure enlargement can result from orbital meningioma, from intracranial conditions such as pituitary tumors or, more characteristically, from vascular anomalies. Optic canal enlargement may result from extraocular extension of a retinoblastoma or, in children, from an optic nerve glioma. In adults, only prolonged pathology can increase orbital size; however, in children, even a rapidly growing lesion can cause orbital enlargement because orbital bones aren't fully developed. A decrease in the size of the orbit may follow childhood enucleation of the eye or conditions such as congenital microphthalmia.

Destruction of the orbital walls may indicate a malignant neoplasm or an infection. A benign tumor or cyst produces a clear-cut local indentation of the orbital wall. Lesions of adjacent structures may also produce radiographic changes due to enlargement and erosion of the orbit.

Increased bone density may be seen in such conditions as osteoblastic metastasis, sphenoid ridge meningioma, or Paget's disease. To confirm orbital pathology, however, radiographic findings must be supplemented with results from other appropriate tests and procedures.

Interfering factors
- None significant

Orbital computed tomography

Orbital computed tomography (CT) allows visualization of abnormalities not readily seen on standard radiographs, delineating their size, position, and relationship to adjoining structures. A series of tomograms reconstructed by a computer and displayed as anatomic slices on a monitor, the orbital CT scan identifies space-occupying lesions earlier and more accurately than other radiographic techniques and provides three-dimensional images of orbital structures, especially the ocular muscles and the optic nerve.

Purpose
- To evaluate pathologies of the orbit and eye — especially expanding lesions and bone destruction
- To evaluate fractures of the orbit and adjoining structures
- To determine the cause of unilateral exophthalmos

Patient preparation
- Describe the procedure to the patient, and explain that the orbital CT scan visualizes the anatomy of the eye and its surrounding structures.
- If contrast enhancement isn't scheduled, inform the patient that he need not restrict food and fluids. If contrast enhancement is scheduled, withhold food and fluids from the patient for 4 hours before the test.
- Tell the patient that a series of X-ray films will be taken of his eye and explain who will perform the test and where it will take place.
- Reassure the patient that the test will cause him no discomfort.
- Tell the patient that he'll be positioned on an X-ray table and that the head of the table will be moved into the scanner, which will rotate around his head and make loud clacking sounds.
- If a contrast medium will be used for the procedure, tell the patient that he may feel flushed and warm and may experience a transient headache, a salty or metallic taste, and nausea or vomiting after the contrast medium is injected. Reassure him that these reactions are normal.
- Ensure that the patient or a responsible family member has signed an informed consent form, if required.
- Check the patient's history for hypersensitivity reactions to iodine, shellfish, or contrast media, and notify the physician of the sensitivities.
- Instruct the patient to remove jewelry, hairpins, or other metal objects in the X-ray field to allow for precise imaging of the orbital structures.

Procedure and posttest care
- The patient is placed in a supine position on the X-ray table with his head immobilized by straps, if required. Ask him to lie still.
- The head of the table is moved into the scanner, which rotates around the patient's head, taking radiographs.
- Information obtained is stored on magnetic tapes, and the images are displayed on a monitor. Photographs may be made if a permanent record is desired.

■ When this series of radiographs has been taken, contrast enhancement is performed. The contrast medium is injected intravenously, and a second series of scans is recorded.

■ If a contrast medium was used, watch for its residual adverse effects, including headache, nausea, or vomiting. After the procedure, advise the patient that he may resume his usual diet.

Precautions

▶ **CLINICAL ALERT** *Use of contrast enhancement is contraindicated in the patient with known hypersensitivity reactions to iodine, shellfish, or contrast media used in other tests.*

Normal findings

Orbital structures are evaluated for size, shape, and position. Dense orbital bone provides a marked contrast to less dense periocular fat. The optic nerve and the medial and lateral rectus muscles are clearly defined. The rectus muscles appear as thin dense bands on each side, behind the eye. The optic canals should be equal in size.

Abnormal findings

Orbital CT scans can identify intraorbital and extraorbital space-occupying lesions that obscure the normal structures or cause orbital enlargement, indentation of the orbital walls, or bone destruction. This test can also help determine the type of lesion. For example, infiltrative lesions, such as lymphomas and metastatic carcinomas, appear as irregular areas of density. However, encapsulated tumors, such as benign hemangiomas and meningiomas, appear as clearly defined masses of consistent density. CT scans can also visualize intracranial tumors that invade the orbit, thickening of the optic nerve that may oc-

cur with gliomas, meningiomas, and secondary tumors that may cause enlargement of the optic canal.

In evaluating fractures, CT scans allow a complete three-dimensional view of the affected structures. In determining the cause of unilateral exophthalmos, CT scans can show early erosion or expansion of the medial orbital wall that may arise from lesions in the ethmoidal cells. It can also detect space-occupying lesions in the orbit or paranasal sinuses that cause exophthalmos. CT scans can also show thickening of the medial and lateral rectus muscles in proptosis resulting from Graves' disease.

Enhancement with a contrast medium may provide information about the circulation through abnormal ocular tissues.

Interfering factors

■ Head movement

■ Failure to remove metallic objects from examination field (possible poor imaging)

Ocular ultrasonography

Ocular ultrasonography involves the transmission of high-frequency sound waves through the eye and the measurement of their reflection from ocular structures. An A-scan converts the resulting echoes into waveforms whose crests represent the positions of different structures, providing a linear dimensional picture. The B-scan converts the echoes into patterns of dots that form a two-dimensional, cross-sectional image of the ocular structure.

Because the B-scan is easier to interpret than the A-scan, it's used more commonly to evaluate the structures of the eye and to diagnose abnormalities. However, the A-scan is more valuable in measuring the eye's axial length and characterizing the tissue texture of abnormal lesions. Thus, a combination of A- and B-scans produces the most useful test results.

Illustrating the eyes' structures through ultrasound is especially helpful in evaluating a fundus clouded by an opaque medium such as a cataract. In such a patient, this test can identify pathologies that are normally undetectable through ophthalmoscopy.

Ophthalmologists may also perform this test before surgery — for example, cataract removal — to ensure the integrity of the retina. If an intraocular lens is to be implanted, ultrasound may be used preoperatively to measure the length of the eye and the curvature of the cornea as a guide for the surgeon. Unlike computed tomography, ocular ultrasonography is readily available and provides information immediately.

In addition to its diagnostic capabilities, ocular ultrasonography can also identify intraocular foreign bodies and determine their position in relation to ocular structures as well as assess the severity of resulting ocular damage.

Purpose
■ To aid in evaluating the fundus in an eye with an opaque medium such as a cataract
■ To aid in the diagnosis of vitreous disorders and retinal detachment
■ To diagnose and differentiate between intraocular and orbital lesions and to follow their progression through serial examinations
■ To locate intraocular foreign bodies

Patient preparation
■ Describe the procedure to the patient and explain that ocular ultrasonography evaluates the eye's structures.

■ Inform the patient that he need not restrict food and fluids.
■ Tell the patient who will be performing the test and where it will be done.
■ Reassure the patient that it's safe and painless and takes about 5 minutes to perform.
■ Tell the patient that a small transducer will be placed on his closed eyelid and that the transducer transmits high-frequency sound waves that are reflected by the structures in the eye.
■ Inform the patient that he may be asked to move his eyes or change his gaze during the procedure and that his cooperation is required to ensure accurate test results.

Procedure and posttest care
■ The patient is placed in the supine position on an X-ray table.
■ For the *B-scan*, the patient is asked to close his eyes, and a water-soluble gel (such as Goniosol) is applied to his eyelid. The transducer is then placed on the eyelid.
■ For the *A-scan*, the patient's eye is numbed with anesthetizing drops and a clear plastic eye cup is placed directly on the eyeball. A water-soluble gel is then applied to the eye cup, and the transducer is positioned on the medium.
■ The transducer then transmits high-frequency sound waves into the patient's eye, and the resulting echoes are transformed into images or waveforms on the oscilloscope screen.
■ After the test, the water-soluble gel is removed from the patient's eyelid.

Precautions
■ None

NORMAL B-SCAN

This is a normal B-scan using the lid contact method. The posterior lens capsule is visible, but the cornea and iris aren't because of obscuring echoes from the eyelid.

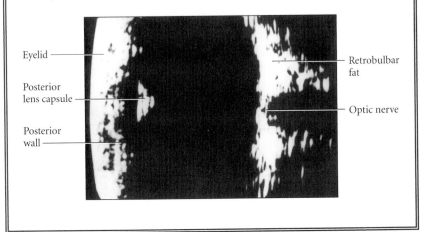

Eyelid

Posterior
lens capsule

Posterior
wall

Retrobulbar
fat

Optic nerve

Normal findings

The optic nerve and the posterior lens capsule produce echoes that take on characteristic forms on A- and B-scan images. The posterior wall of the eye appears as a smooth, concave curve; retrobulbar fat can also be identified. The lens and vitreous humor, which don't produce echoes, can also be identified. Normal orbital echo patterns depend on the position of the transducer and the position of the patient's gaze during the procedure. (See *Normal B-scan.*)

Abnormal findings

In eyes clouded by a vitreous hemorrhage, the organization of the hemorrhage can be identified by the degree of density that appears on the image. In some instances, the cause of the hemorrhage, the prognosis, and associated abnormalities can also be determined.

Other vitreous abnormalities, such as massive vitreous organization and vitreous bands, may also be detected by ultra-

sonography. Retinal detachment, commonly found in a patient with an opaque medium, characteristically produces a dense, sheetlike echo on a B-scan. The extent of retinal or choroidal detachment can be defined by transmitting ultrasound waves through the quadrants of the patient's eye.

Ocular ultrasonography can be used to diagnose and differentiate intraocular tumors according to size, shape, location, and texture. The most common tumors identified are melanomas, metastatic tumors, and hemangiomas. This test can also identify retinoblastomas and measure the dimensions of other tumors detectable by ophthalmoscopy.

Hemangiomas and cystic lesions produce characteristic ultrasound patterns. Other orbital lesions detectable by ultrasound include meningiomas, neurofibromas, gliomas, neurilemomas, and the inflammatory changes associated with Graves' disease.

Interfering factors
- None

Selected readings

Carlson, N., and Kurtz, D., eds. *Clinical Procedures for Ocular Examination,* 3rd ed. New York: McGraw-Hill Professional, 2004.

Cavanaugh, B.M. *Nurse's Manual of Laboratory and Diagnostic Tests,* 4th ed. Philadelphia: F.A. Davis Co., 2003.

McClatchey, K.D. *Clinical Laboratory Medicine,* 2nd ed. Philadelphia: Lippincott Williams & Wilkins, 2002.

Pagana, K.D., and Pagana, T.J. *Mosby's Diagnostic and Laboratory Test Reference,* 6th ed. St. Louis: Mosby Year–Book, Inc., 2003.

Roy, F.H. *Ocular Differential Diagnosis,* 7th ed. Philadelphia: Lippincott Williams & Wilkins, 2002.

Schnell, Z., et al. *Davis's Comprehensive Handbook of Laboratory and Diagnostic Tests with Nursing Implications.* Philadelphia: F.A. Davis Co., 2003.

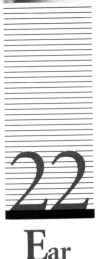

22
Ear

Introduction

Numerous disorders can affect the anatomical structures of the ear with outcomes ranging from moderate discomfort to hearing loss.

Tests that diagnose ear disorders fall into three categories. *Audiologic tests* can detect hearing impairment and reveal the presence of lesions or disorders requiring treatment. *Scanning tests*, or nonphysiologic tests, can determine the site of lesions and identify the type, such as a brain stem tumor or a brain abscess. *Vestibular tests*, which investigate the function of the labyrinth structures of the inner ear and the central nervous system coordination of balance, are used to evaluate equilibrium disorders and can locate a vestibular lesion. Understanding the diagnostic application and significance of these tests begins with a review of the ear's anatomic structure and physiology. The ear has three parts—the external, middle, and inner ear—and is innervated by several sensory nerves. (See *Evaluating ear structures.*)

EVALUATING EAR STRUCTURES

Because the ear is so complex, a thorough examination of all its structures requires a battery of diagnostic tests. For example, otoscopy provides direct visualization of the external ear canal and tympanic membrane, acoustic immittance tests evaluate middle ear and eustachian tube function, and electronystagmography and falling and past-pointing tests evaluate the vestibular system. Pure tone audiometry and tuning for tests evaluate conductive and sensorineural function and help determine the cause and extent of hearing loss.

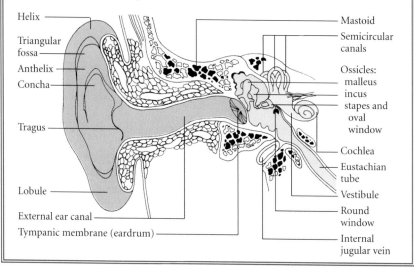

The external ear

The external ear consists of the auricle, or pinna (the visible flap), and the external ear canal. These structures direct and transmit sound waves toward the tympanic membrane (eardrum). The external ear canal also serves as a resonating tube, amplifying sound frequencies between 2,000 and 6,000 Hz. These frequencies are critical for perceiving consonants. Cerumen (earwax) results from the combined secretions of the canal's sebaceous and apocrine glands. The tympanic membrane separates the external and the middle ear; disease can significantly alter the concavity of the drumhead (umbo) and its position relative to the ear canal.

The middle ear

The middle ear, which lies directly behind the tympanic membrane, is a small air space in the tympanic region of the temporal bone. Three small bones — the malleus (hammer), incus (anvil), and stapes (stirrup) — make up the auditory ossicles. The vibrations of these bones transmit sound waves from the tympanic membrane to the inner ear through a membrane called the *oval window*. The eustachian tube's connection to the nasopharynx makes it a direct route for middle ear infection.

The inner ear

The inner ear contains the sensory end organs for hearing and balance. The temporal bone surrounds and protects these interconnected, fluid-filled membranous structures. The auditory end organ, or cochlea, is a coiled tube that is divided into three compartments; vibration of the ossicles sets the fluid in these compartments into motion. The middle compartment, or cochlear duct, contains the organ of Corti. Here, sensitive hair cells convert fluid disturbance into neural impulses, which travel along the eighth cranial nerve to the brain.

Vestibular organs

The vestibular organs include the utricle, the saccule, and the semicircular canals. Changes in body orientation disturb the fluid in the canals (the equilibrium) and stimulate vestibular hair cells, called *cristae* or *maculae*. These hair cells dispatch messages to the brain, enabling muscles to respond to position changes.

Types of hearing loss

Hearing loss can result from injury to or disease of any part of the auditory system. For example, foreign objects, impacted cerumen, or growths can obstruct the external ear canal; perforation may damage the tympanic membrane; and various diseases may affect the delicate parts of the middle and inner ear.

There are essentially three types of hearing loss: conductive hearing loss, sensorineural hearing loss, and mixed hearing loss.

Conductive

Conductive hearing loss results from a decrease in the strength of a sound and is caused by injury or disease of any part of the outer or middle ear. When a conductive hearing loss is present, the normal pathway for sound is blocked; therefore, the transmission of sound via air conduc-

tion will become diminished. Sound energy transferred to the inner ear via bone conduction bypasses the normal pathway of sound and is transferred directly to the sensorineural mechanisms of the inner ear. Examples of conductive hearing loss include cerumen impaction, otitis media or otitis externa, a perforated tympanic membrane, foreign objects, and otosclerosis.

Sensorineural

Sensorineural hearing loss is caused by a lesion within the inner ear and the nervous system structures of the retrocochlear pathways, which involve the sensorineural mechanism of hearing. The lesions can be either cochlear or retrocochlear. Cochlear lesions result from Ménière's disease, ototoxic agents, or viral labyrinthitis and retrocochlear lesions can be caused by tumors or multiple sclerosis. Distinguishing cochlear from retrocochlear types of lesions is essential because retrocochlear lesions are potentially life-threatening.

Mixed

Mixed hearing loss may occur due to a combination of conductive hearing loss and sensorineural hearing loss. The mechanism of hearing loss may work in conjunction with one another to produce this type of hearing loss. Further evaluation by an audiologist may help determine the underlying causes involved.

Types of ear examinations

A thorough otoscopic examination of the external ear, ear canal, and tympanic membrane should precede auditory and vestibular testing. After otoscopy, a basic audiologic examination includes puretone audiometry to measure thresholds for air- and bone-conducted sound, speech detection and understanding tests, measurement of otoacoustic emissions, and acoustic immittance measurements, such as tympanometry and acoustic reflex testing. Tuning fork tests are screening tests that also may be performed, but aren't typically included in an audiologic evaluation.

An audiologic examination reveals the degree and type of hearing loss. When the examination or the patient's history suggests that signs of retrocochlear involvement are present, radiographic testing may be ordered by the referring physician. Patients with dizziness may require vestibular testing, such as videonystagmography or electronystagmography. Nonphysiologic tests may also be useful in determining the site of a lesion. Numerous radiographic techniques, such as computed tomography (CT) scans and magnetic resonance imaging (MRI), may detect or confirm a lesion and identify its type. CT and MRI scans can also help to detect cranial nerve eight and brain stem tumors, neural degeneration, hydrocephalus, brain abscesses, and other tumors that may disrupt auditory and vestibular function.

Screening neonates and infants

Hearing loss in children is estimated to range from 1 to 6 children per 1,000. Therefore, screening infants and children is imperative. Because the first three years of life are the most important period for language and speech development, early detection in high-risk infants and continued monitoring throughout infancy is recommended. High-risk infants include those who are born prematurely; have a family history of hearing impairment; have congenital anomalies of the face and skull, low birth weight, or hyperbiliru-

binemia; and those whose mothers had an intrauterine infection.

The Joint Committee on Infant Hearing recommends that screening be conducted on all neonates at birth. Identifying hearing-impaired neonates early is important so that treatment can begin within the first 6 months. In the absence of neonatal screening and identification systems, parents are the ones who identify 70% of neonates and infants with hearing deficits.

Screening may include the auditory brain stem response, evoked otoacoustic emissions, and modified forms of audiometry if the child is older.

Screening school-aged children

Screening school-aged children helps to accurately identify those with hearing loss that can affect or interfere with their language development and general learning capabilities. School screening programs must provide proper medical and audiologic referrals, involve consultation with the parents, and provide information for the teachers.

For specific screening guidelines for children age 5 through 18, contact the American Speech-Language Hearing Association.

Screening adults

Aging can lead to gradual bilateral hearing loss. Approximately 25% of adults age 45 to 64 and 40% of those over age 65 experience presbycusis, which results from degeneration of the middle ear. This type of hearing loss is primarily sensorineural, bilateral, and irreversible and is commonly accompanied by tinnitus.

Noise-induced hearing loss in the workplace — from loud music, power tools, hunting, and other activities that involve loud noises — also requires evaluation in an adult. An accurate and thorough history of each patient is necessary. In most cases, an adult is reluctant to seek medical attention regarding his hearing loss. Therefore, vigilance on the part of the health care professional is essential to encourage proper management.

AUDIOLOGIC TESTS

Otoscopy

Otoscopy is the direct visualization of the external auditory canal and the tympanic membrane through an otoscope. It's a basic part of physical examination of the ear and should be performed before other auditory or vestibular tests. Otoscopy indirectly provides information about the eustachian tube and the middle ear cavity.

Purpose
- To visualize inner ear structures
- To detect foreign bodies, cerumen, or stenosis in the external canal
- To detect external or middle ear pathology, such as an infection or a tympanic membrane perforation

Patient preparation
- Describe the procedure to the patient and explain that this test permits visualization of the ear canal and eardrum.
- Reassure the patient that the examination is usually painless.
- Tell the patient that his ear will be pulled upward and backward to straighten the canal, to facilitate insertion of the otoscope.
- If the patient will undergo pneumatic otoscopy, tell him that he may experience dizziness with nystagmus, a positive fistula sign.

Procedure and posttest care
- When assembling the otoscope, test the lamp and make sure you attach the largest speculum that fits comfortably into the patient's ear.
- With the patient seated, tilt his head slightly away from you so that the ear to be examined is pointed upward.
- Pull the auricle up and back. Insert the otoscope gently into the ear canal with a downward and forward motion. If insertion is difficult, replace the speculum with a smaller one.

▶ **CLINICAL ALERT** *If the patient is under age 3, pull the auricle downward to insert the otoscope.*

- If you still feel resistance, withdraw the otoscope and tell the physician.
- Look through the lens and gently advance the speculum until you see the tympanic membrane. Obtain as full a view as possible and note redness, swelling, lesions, discharge, foreign bodies, and scaling in the canal. Check the tympanic membrane for color, scarring, contours, perforation, and a cone of light that appears at the 5 o'clock position in the right ear and at the 7 o'clock position in the left; this is a reflection of the otoscope lamp.
- Locate the malleus, partially visible through the translucent tympanic membrane. Examine the membrane itself and the surrounding fibrous rim (annulus).

Precautions
- The otoscope should be advanced slowly and gently through the medial portion of the ear canal to avoid irritation of the canal lining, especially if an infection is suspected.
- Continuing to insert an otoscope against resistance may cause the tympanic membrane to perforate.

COMMON ABNORMALITIES OF THE TYMPANIC MEMBRANE

Visual examination of the tympanic membrane may reveal abnormal findings. This chart lists some of the more common findings as well as their typical causes.

Abnormal findings	Usual cause
Bright red color	Inflammation (otitis media)
Yellowish color	Pus or serum behind the tympanic membrane (acute or chronic otitis media)
Bubble behind the tympanic membrane	Serous fluid in the middle ear (serous otitis media)
Absent light reflection	Bulging tympanic membrane (acute otitis media)
Absent or diminishing landmarks	Thickened tympanic membrane (chronic otitis media, otitis externa, or tympanosclerosis)
Oval dark areas	Perforated or scarred tympanic membrane (otitis media or trauma)
Prominent malleus	Retracted tympanic membrane (nonfunctional eustachian tube)
Reduced mobility	Stiffened middle ear system (serous otitis media or, less commonly, middle ear adhesions)

Normal findings

The normal tympanic membrane is thin, translucent, shiny, and slightly concave. It appears as a pearl gray or pale pink disk that reflects light in its inferior portion. The short process, manubrium mallei, and umbo should be visible but not prominent.

Abnormal findings

Scarring, discoloration, or retraction or bulging of the tympanic membrane indicates a pathologic condition. (See *Common abnormalities of the tympanic membrane.*) Movement of the tympanic membrane in tandem with respiration suggests abnormal patency of the eustachian tube.

Normal light reflex extends inferiorly and anteriorly from the umbo. However, an altered or absent light reflex isn't a reliable indicator of disease because there can be many normal variations of the tympanic membrane and posterior bony ear canal.

Interfering factors

- Obstruction of the ear canal by cerumen or foreign matter
- Recumbent position during otoscopy (possible masking of serous otitis media)

Tuning fork

The Weber, Rinne, and Schwabach tuning fork tests are quick, valuable screening tools for detecting hearing loss and obtaining preliminary information as to its type. The Weber test determines whether a patient lateralizes the tone of the tuning fork to one ear. The Rinne test compares air and bone conduction in both ears. The Schwabach test compares the patient's bone conduction response with that of the examiner, who's assumed to have normal hearing.

Test results are most reliable when a low-frequency tuning fork is used; results aren't definitive because they depend on subjective factors, such as the examiner's ability to strike the fork with equal force each time and the patient's ability to report audible tones correctly.

Results of the Weber test may be misleading, and the Rinne test commonly doesn't detect a mild conductive hearing loss (10 to 35 dB). Thus, abnormal test results require confirmation by pure tone audiometry.

Purpose
- To screen for or confirm hearing loss
- To help distinguish conductive from sensorineural hearing loss

Patient preparation
- Describe the procedure to the patient and explain that the tuning fork tests help detect and assess hearing loss. Tell him who will conduct the tests and reassure him that they're painless.
- Explain to the patient that concentration and prompt responses are essential for accurate testing. Have him use hand signals to indicate whether a tone is louder in his right ear or left ear and when he stops hearing the tone.
- Inform the patient that tuning fork tests aren't definitive and that further testing may be necessary to confirm abnormal results.

Procedure and posttest care
- Using a low-frequency tuning fork (256 or 512 Hz), practice achieving a consistent tone by gently striking a prong

against your elbow or the heel of your hand, by stroking the prongs upward, or by pinching them together.
- When performing each test, be careful to strike the tuning fork with equal force. Hold the fork at its base to allow the prongs to vibrate freely. Record the name of the test, the result, and the vibrating frequency of the tuning fork.

Weber test
- Vibrate the fork, and place its base on the midline of the patient's skull at the forehead.
- Ask the patient whether the tone is louder in his left ear or his right ear or is equally loud in both. Describe the results as Weber left, Weber right, or Weber midline, according to his response.

Rinne test
- Test bone conduction by holding the tuning fork between your thumb and index finger and placing the base of the vibrating fork against the patient's mastoid process.
- Test air conduction by moving the vibrating prongs next to (but not touching) the external ear. Ask the patient which location has the louder or longer sound. Repeat the procedure for the other ear.
- Record results as Rinne-positive, if the air-conducted sound is heard louder or longer, or Rinne-negative, if the bone-conducted sound is heard louder or longer.

Schwabach test
- Holding the tuning fork between your thumb and index finger, place the base of the vibrating tuning fork against the patient's left mastoid process, and ask whether he hears the tone. If he does, immediately place the tuning fork on your left mastoid process and listen for the tone.

- Alternate the tuning fork between the patient's left mastoid process and your own until one of you stops hearing the sound. Record the length of time the patient continues to hear it.
- Repeat the procedure on the right mastoid process.

All tests
- Refer the patient for further audiologic testing if the tuning fork tests suggest a hearing loss.

Precautions
- None

Normal findings
A patient with normal hearing will respond to the Weber test by hearing the same tone equally loudly in both ears (Weber midline result); to the Rinne test, by hearing the air-conducted tone louder or longer than the bone-conducted tone (Rinne-positive result); and to the Schwabach test, by hearing the tone for the same duration as the examiner.

Abnormal findings
In the Weber test, lateralization of the tone to one ear suggests a conductive loss on that side or a sensorineural loss on the other side. Lateralization results if the tone is louder in one ear (Stenger effect) or reaches one ear sooner (phase effect). If one ear has a sensorineural loss, the Stenger effect causes lateralization to the unaffected ear; if one ear has a conductive loss, either the Stenger or the phase effect produces lateralization to that ear. If a patient's hearing loss is unilateral, the Weber test may suggest the type of loss. If a patient's hearing loss is bilateral, this test may help to identify the ear with the better bone conduction.

In the Rinne test, hearing the bone-conducted tone louder or longer than the air-conducted tone indicates a conductive loss. In unilateral hearing loss, the tone may be heard louder when conducted by bone, but in the opposite ear; this is a false-negative Rinne test result. A sensorineural loss is indicated when the sound is heard louder by air conduction.

In the Schwabach test, hearing the tone longer than the examiner hears it suggests a conductive loss; conversely, a shorter duration indicates a sensorineural loss. A conductive loss attenuates (decreases the energy of) air-conducted sound in a room with ambient noise, enabling the patient with this type of loss to hear bone-conducted sound longer than the examiner can hear it.

If the patient has abnormal results on retesting, pure tone audiometry is indicated to confirm hearing loss and determine its type and severity.

Interfering factors
- Failure to strike the tuning fork with equal force or to hold it correctly during the procedure
- Striking the tuning fork on a hard surface rather than on the elbow or knee
- Failure to use either the 512-Hz frequency tuning fork or the more sensitive 256-Hz tuning fork
- Inaccurate patient response due to poor understanding of his task
- Undetected hearing loss in the examiner

Pure tone audiometry and pure tone screening

Pure tone audiometry, performed with an audiometer, provides a record of the thresholds (the lowest intensity levels) at which a patient can hear a set of test tones introduced through earphones or a bone conduction (sound) vibrator. The energy of these pure tones is concentrated at discrete frequencies. The octave fre-

PATIENTS WHO REQUIRE HEARING SCREENING

Listed here are various patient groups that require hearing screening and the risk factors that warrant the screening.

Neonates
In most of the United States, all neonates are screened using physiologic procedures before leaving the health care facility. Pure tone screening isn't possible in neonates.

Infants and toddlers (up to age 2)
Screening for this patient group is required if the child meets any of these risk criteria:
- parental or caregiver concern about hearing
- expressive or receptive language delay or disorder
- history of hyperbilirubinemia, which can cause progressive hearing loss
- use of ototoxic agents, including aminoglycoside or macrolide antibiotics, or ototoxic chemotherapy agents such as cisplatin
- bacterial meningitis
- family history of childhood hearing loss
- head trauma causing loss of consciousness and skull fracture
- exposure to potentially damaging noise levels.

Infants or toddlers up to age 2 who didn't receive hearing screening at birth will require screening by an audiologist if they have any of these characteristics:
- craniofacial anomalies, including of the pinna or ear canal, or stigmata of syndromes associated with sensorineural hearing loss
- birth weight less than 1,500 g
- Apgar scores of 0 to 4 at 1 minute or 0 to 6 at 5 minutes
- mechanical ventilation lasting 5 days or longer
- in utero infections of cytomegalovirus, rubella, syphilis, herpes, or toxoplasmosis
- recurrent or persistent otitis media with effusion for at least 3 months
- neurofibromatosis type II or neurodegenerative disease.

Children (age 3 to 18)
Children in this age-group require hearing screening if they have the same risk factors as those for younger children as well as:
- evidence of parental or caregiver concern
- concern about speech and language development.

Adults
Screening once per decade until age 50, then every 3 years is recommended for all adults. Also, screening is valid with any of these risk factors:
- any decrease in hearing
- report of decreased hearing by family members
- patients with mental health concerns.

quencies between 125 and 8,000 Hz are used to obtain air conduction thresholds; frequencies between 250 and 4,000 Hz are used to obtain bone conduction thresholds.

Comparison of air and bone conduction thresholds can suggest a conductive, sensorineural, or mixed hearing loss, but doesn't indicate the cause of the loss; further audiologic and vestibular tests and X-rays may be needed. Pure tone audiometry results may also suggest a need to consult an audiologist to evaluate communication difficulties. (See *Patients who require hearing screening.*)

Pure tone audiometry is indicated for any patient who requires a quantitative hearing assessment. There are no contraindications; however, results depend on the patient's cooperation. Acoustic immittance test results may provide additional information.

Purpose

- To determine the presence, type, and degree of hearing loss
- To assess communication abilities and rehabilitation needs
- To accurately determine pure tone and speech reception threshold

Patient preparation

- Describe the procedure to the patient and explain that this test determines the presence and degree of hearing loss. Explain who will perform the test and where it will take place.
- Tell the patient that each ear will be tested, beginning with the ear with the better hearing acuity. Explain that he'll hear tones at various intensities and that he should signal (or press the response button) each time he hears the tone. Emphasize that he should respond even if the tone is faint.
- Just before the test, ask the patient to remove jewelry or apparel that obstructs proper earphone placement.
- Postpone the test if the patient has been exposed to loud noises (loud enough to cause tinnitus or to make face-to-face communication difficult) within the past 16 hours.

Procedure and posttest care

- The patient's ear canal is checked with the otoscope for impacted cerumen.
- The examiner presses a finger on the auricle and then the tragus to rule out possible closure of the ear canal under pressure from the earphones. If the canal tends to close, a stiff-walled plastic tube is carefully inserted into the canal. This

modification is recorded on the audiogram.

- The earphones are positioned properly and the headband is tightened.
- A test tone is presented to the patient's better ear.

Air conduction testing

- A 1,000-Hz tone is presented to the patient's better ear. The intensity of the tone is decreased in 10-dB steps until the patient fails to respond. Then intensity is increased in 5-dB steps until he hears the tone again. Sequences of 10-dB decrements and 5-dB increments are repeated until the patient responds to at least two of three presentations at a single level. The threshold level is the lowest decibel level at which the response rate is at least 50%.
- Using this procedure, tones are presented to the better ear in this order: 1,000 Hz, 2,000 Hz, 4,000 Hz, 8,000 Hz, 1,000 Hz, 500 Hz, and 250 Hz.
- After testing the better ear, the other ear is tested. In each ear, test or retest differences may be + or −5 dB. If the difference between the first and second threshold at 1,000 Hz is greater than 10 dB, test results are unreliable; equipment should be checked for malfunction and the patient should be reinstructed and retested.
- Many audiologists sample hearing only at octave points. Others may prefer the detail resulting from testing the mid-octave frequencies. The American Speech-Language-Hearing Association recommends testing the better ear first and that mid-octave points be tested when a difference of 20 dB or greater is seen in the thresholds at adjacent octaves.

Bone conduction testing

- The earphones are removed and the vibrator is placed on the mastoid process of the better ear (the auricle shouldn't touch the vibrator).

- Ascending and descending tones are presented, as in air conduction testing, using 250, 500, 1,000, 2,000, and 4,000 Hz.

Both tests
- Refer the patient to an audiologist if test results are inconsistent or are confounded by possible crossover.

Precautions
- Any modifications of standard testing procedure—such as inserting a plastic tube to prevent ear canal collapse—must be recorded on the audiogram.
- Be on the alert for false responses; they can be misleading and influence interpretation of test results. False responses include failure to indicate when a tone has been heard or responding when no tone has been heard.

Normal findings
The normal range of hearing sensitivity is 0 to 25 dB for adults and 0 to 15 dB for children. Normal test results don't rule out a hearing disorder; a mild middle ear infection or other disorder may exist without interfering with auditory function.

Abnormal findings
The pure tone average—the average of pure tone air conduction thresholds obtained at 500, 1,000, and 2,000 Hz—quantifies the degree of hearing loss. When these three thresholds vary widely, the mean of the best two, known as the *Fletcher average*, indicates the degree of hearing loss.

The relation between threshold responses for air and bone conduction tones determines the type of hearing loss. In *sensorineural hearing loss*, both thresholds are depressed; in *conductive hearing loss*, air thresholds are depressed, but bone thresholds are unchanged; and in *mixed hearing loss*, both thresholds are abnormal, with air conduction more depressed than bone conduction.

Interfering factors
- Impacted cerumen or a closed ear canal (possible 35- to 40-dB artifactual conductive hearing loss)
- Patient's confusion of vibrotactile with auditory sensation or tinnitus with the signal (invalid results)
- Cracked or poorly fitting earphones (low-frequency leakage and false-high thresholds)
- Uncalibrated audiometer or background noise (possible invalidation)
- Presenting extraneous cues to the patient, such as a rhythmic pattern of test tones or hand movement near the attenuator dial (possible invalidation)
- Patient uncooperative or inattentive (possible invalidation)
- Ear infection

Acoustic immittance

Acoustic immittance tests evaluate middle ear function by measuring the flow of sound energy into the ear (admittance). Not all sound energy that impinges on the tympanic membrane reaches the inner ear; some reflects into the external ear canal. The relationship between incident and reflected sound energy determines the admittance, which depends on the resistance, stiffness, and mass of the auditory system. Normally, stiffness is the predominant factor in the middle ear.

Admittance is commonly measured by two tests: *tympanometry* and *acoustic reflex testing*. Each of these tests uses an electronic tone generator, an air pressure manometer, and a tone probe that delivers sound and air pressure stimuli to the ear canal and tympanic membrane through an airtight seal. Tympanometry measures middle ear admittance in response to changes in air pressure in the ear canal; the acoustic reflex test measures the change in admittance produced by contraction of the stapedius muscle in response to an intense sound. Stapedial contraction stiffens the tympanic membrane and ossicular chain, causing a measurable reduction in middle ear admittance. Reflex decay, part of the acoustic reflexes test, is a function of eighth cranial nerve adaptation or fatigue in response to a sustained reflex-eliciting stimulus.

Tympanometry helps diagnose middle ear pathology and assesses eustachian tube function. Acoustic reflex testing assesses the seventh (facial) and eighth cranial nerve function and helps establish the site of the lesion. Because admittance tests require little patient cooperation, they are reliable in testing young children and individuals with physical or mental challenges.

Purpose
Tympanometry
■ To assess the continuity and admittance of the middle ear
■ To evaluate the status of the tympanic membrane

Acoustic reflex testing
■ To distinguish between cochlear and retrocochlear lesions
■ To differentiate eighth nerve or peripheral brain stem lesions from intra-axial brain stem lesions
■ To locate seventh nerve lesions relative to stapedius muscle innervation
■ To confirm conductive hearing loss
■ To help confirm nonorganic loss (feigning or exaggerating hearing loss, also called *pseudohypoacusis*)

Patient preparation
■ Ensure that the patient's ear is free from significant cerumen accumulation.
■ Describe the procedure to the patient and explain that acoustic immittance tests evaluate the condition of the middle ear.
■ Tell the patient that he will feel pressure in the ear, but that the test isn't painful.
■ Ask the patient not to move during the test, which takes just a few seconds.

Procedure and posttest care
For tympanometry
■ Otoscopic examination is performed to verify that no impacted cerumen or other obstruction is present in the ear canal.
■ The size and shape of the canal are checked to select the appropriate-size probe tip, which is then attached to the probe.
■ The probe tip is inserted into the ear canal while pulling upward and backward on the auricle; a proper seal can maintain a negative pressure of +200 daPa. Once a hermetic seal is obtained, the pressure in the ear canal will automatically vary from +200 to –400 daPa.
■ A graphic display of the tympanogram is obtained. If the tympanogram has a clear peak, the pressure of the peak is noted and usually printed with the test results. This indicates the pressure within the middle ear cavity. The sound admittance through the middle ear system is noted by the height of the tympanogram, its peak compliance. This value is also typically printed.
■ If a flat tympanogram is obtained (no change in admittance), the possibility that the probe tip may have rested against the canal wall or that it was clogged with cerumen must be ruled out with ear canal volume measurements and repeated testing. Measurement error is more likely to be the cause of the flat tympanogram if

the ear canal volume is low (0.3 ml or less). The probe tip is removed, cleaned, reinserted, and the test is repeated.

For acoustic reflex testing

- The audiologist positions the immittance probe in the patient's ear the same as for tympanometry, but uses a device to fix the probe to the patient's head to reduce artifacts that can invalidate test results.
- For threshold testing, stimuli of progressively louder levels are presented until a reflex, if present, is noted.
- Acoustic reflex decay testing involves presentation of a tone, 10 dB above the reflex threshold, at one or more frequency 1,000 Hz and below, for a 10-second period. The time that the auditory system sustains the contraction at least half strength is measured. The patient must remain still and quiet during reflex testing.
- Reflexes and reflex decay may be measured ipsilaterally (in the same ear as the probe that measures the contraction) or contralaterally (the probe measuring the reflex is in the opposite ear from the ear presented with the loud tone.) Ipsilateral reflexes are also called *uncrossed reflexes;* contralateral can be called *crossed reflexes.*

Precautions

- Obtain medical clearance before performing admittance tests in the patient with head trauma or a possible labyrinthine fistula and on one who has recently had middle ear surgery.
- Check equipment carefully. If the probe tip is clogged with cerumen or debris, the measured admittance won't change, even when the probe isn't coupled to the ear. To clean the probe, carefully insert a wire through each bore, wipe the wire, and then withdraw it.

- If you can't obtain a seal even though the probe seems well seated, look for leakage elsewhere in the air system. Check the system by putting the probe in the supplied coupler. If it can't seal, then the tubing has a leak or the equipment is malfunctioning.
- While some screening systems permit acoustic reflex measurements, the results aren't reliable if the probe is handheld in the ear. Refer to an audiologist, as required.

Normal findings
Tympanometry

Four measurements are important on the tympanogram: the ear canal volume, the peak compliance reading, the peak pressure reading, and the slope gradient. These measures are interpreted along with the shape or "type" of the tympanogram and together determine the implication of the tympanometric results. A type A tympanogram is a normal finding.

Acoustic reflex testing

Acoustic reflexes are normally present at an intensity of 65 to 100 dB HL. The sensation level of the reflex is computed by subtracting the hearing threshold for the ear by the frequency receiving the tone. The sensation level of the reflex should also be 65 to 100 dB.

Abnormal findings
Tympanometry

Any evidence that doesn't reflect a type A tympanogram is considered abnormal. (See *Interpreting tympanograms.*)

Acoustic reflex testing

The patient with ears that have conductive involvement commonly have absent reflexes. If the conductive loss is unilater-

INTERPRETING TYMPANOGRAMS

Four measurements are important when interpreting tympanograms: static compliance, ear canal volume, peak pressure reading, and slope gradient.

Static compliance

Also called *static immittance, static admittance,* or *peak compliance,* this is a measurement of the relative ease of sound transmission through the middle ear. The unit of measurement is typically the "equivalent volume" of air, measured in cubic centimeters or milliliters.

Ear canal volume

Also called *base compliance* and *physical volume,* this is an estimate of the size of the space between the probe tip and the sound-reflecting surface. Like static compliance, it's measured in cubic centimeters or milliliters.

Peak pressure reading

This reading refers to the pressure reading reflecting the best sound transmission through the middle ear.

Slope gradient

This reading indicates whether the tympanogram is sharply peaking or whether the peak is more moundlike. For example, a nearly flat tympanogram would have a very large slope gradient. The term "tympanometric width" may also be used, as the test is based on the concept that the width of the tympanogram at the point half way to the peak is being measured. Slope gradient calculations permit prediction of the presence of effusion. The smaller the slope gradient, the more peaked the curve, and the lower the chance of an ear effusion. Slope gradients larger than 250 daPa or static compliance less than or equal to 0.2 cc is consistent with the clinical finding of otitis media.

Currently, the presence of a type B tympanogram or an abnormally wide slope gradient are the best predictors of effusion.

Type A tympanogram

■ Type A tympanograms include subtypes A_S and A_D that have peaks occurring near 0 daPa (pressure reading) indicating the best sound transmission through the eardrum when the pressure in the ear canal is near ambient and the air of the middle ear system is at or near ambient pressure.
■ Type A tympanograms and their subtypes indicate that the eustachian tube has recently opened, equalizing air pressure between the middle ear space and the nasopharynx.
■ The different subtypes of type A tympanograms are defined based on the height of the curve, or static compliance,

which measures the mobility of the middle ear system:
– Subtype A_S tympanograms show too little mobility of the middle ear system; generally static compliance is less than 0.25 cc. The stiffness may come from pathology, such as otosclerosis, or from benign sclerosis of the tympanic membrane, typically secondary to childhood tympanic membrane perforation.
– Subtype A_D tympanograms indicate that the middle ear system is inordinately flaccid. Peaks above 2 cc are typically classified as A_D. A break of the ossicular chain can create this condition; however, benign flaccidity of the tympanic mem-

(continued)

INTERPRETING TYMPANOGRAMS *(continued)*

brane can also create this tympanometric type.

– The presence of hearing loss along with an A_S or A_D tympanogram requires complete audiometric testing to determine if middle ear abnormality is contributing to the hearing loss.

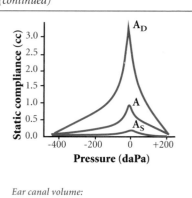

Peak pressure:

- + 100 to – 100 daPa

Static compliance:

- < 0.25 cc = Type A_S
- 0.25 to 2.0 cc = Type A
- > 2.0 = Type A_D

Ear canal volume:

- not a classification criterion

Type B tympanogram

- Type B tympanograms don't have a defined peak and have low static compliance at the highest point in the trace.
- A gentle mound shape may occur, or the trace may gradually rise toward the negative pressure side.
- Type B tympanograms indicate that the system being measured is abnormally stiff.
- The ear canal volume must be considered when evaluating type B tympanograms. If small, less than about 0.4 cc in a child or 0.6 cc in an adult, the probe tone from the tympanometer is likely reflected off an obstruction in the ear canal or the side of the ear canal; if ear canal volume is normal (nominally 0.4 to 1.0 cc in children or 0.6 to 2.0 cc in adults, although adults commonly have ear canal volumes as high as 2.8 cc), then the probe tone is being reflected off an abnormally stiff tympanic membrane/middle ear system, most likely fluid behind the tympanic membrane; if large, it's possible that the sound is passing through a hole in the tympanic membrane and is reflected off the back of the middle ear, such as when the patient has a pressure equalizing tube inserted through the tympanic membrane or a perforated tympanic membrane.

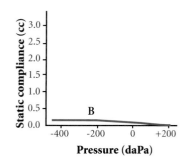

Peak pressure:

- no peak observed

Static compliance:

- < 0.25 cc

Ear canal volume:

- < 0.4 cc (children) or 0.6 cc (adults) suggests canal obstruction
- 0.4 to 1 cc (children) or 0.6 to 2 cc (adults) indicates middle ear pathology
- > 1 cc (children) or 2 cc (adults) may indicate the tympanic membrane isn't intact

INTERPRETING TYMPANOGRAMS *(continued)*

Type C tympanogram
- Type C tympanograms result when the peak is visible, but shifted to the left.
- Typically, peaks must be shifted beyond −100 daPa for this classification.
- Shifting occurs when the pressure in the middle ear system is negative due to the mucosa of the middle ear absorbing air and eustachian tube dysfunction that prevents the equalization of middle ear pressure.
- Forceful sniffling can also evacuate some air from the middle ear space, creating a type C tympanogram.
- Interpretation of type C tympanograms is somewhat controversial. Children commonly have type C tympanograms and the degree of hearing loss, if any, apparently is more important than the peak pressure itself.
- Negative pressure doesn't necessarily indicate that otitis media will develop.
- Adults typically don't have type C tympanograms.

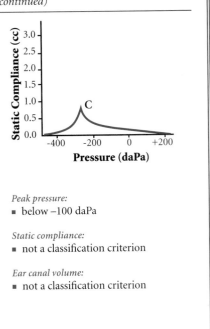

Peak pressure:
- below −100 daPa

Static compliance:
- not a classification criterion

Ear canal volume:
- not a classification criterion

al, presentation of the reflex tone to the involved ear, with measurement contralaterally, may reveal a reflex at an elevated hearing level. The calculated sensation level would be normal in this case. The finding of a reflex when the probe is in an affected ear is negative for conductive involvement.

If the cochlea is the site of the lesion, reflexes may be present at normal hearing levels, elevated, or absent. The more severe the loss, the more likely the finding of an absent reflex. Most mild to moderately severe hearing losses have present acoustic reflexes. When the audiologist computes the sensation level of the reflex, it's noted as being reduced if there's significant loss at that frequency.

Absent acoustic reflexes raise the possibility of a retrocochlear lesion if conduc-

tive involvement or severe cochlear loss isn't present. Acoustic reflex decay (failure to have a sustained reflex for 5 or more seconds) is also an indicator of possible retrocochlear involvement.

The patient with nonorganic loss (or pseudohypoacousis, a feigned hearing loss or exaggeration of hearing thresholds) may be discovered during immittance testing. Reflexes present below the admitted threshold are an indicator of a nonorganic problem.

Interfering factors
- Interpretation by audiologist of reflex findings in light of audiologic results
- Patient movement resulting in false readings

Speech

The audiologist administers tests that use speech signals to determine the lowest level that the patient is able to hear words and the ability to correctly recognize words presented above the threshold level. Auditory processing tests also involve speech materials, but an auditory processing evaluation may use tests with non-speech material. In auditory processing speech testing, the speech signal is degraded. Interfering speech may be present, the speech may be filtered to remove some frequencies, or the speed of the material is increased. These tests place greater stress on the auditory processing system to determine the patient's function in challenging conditions.

Purpose

■ To determine the degree of hearing loss for speech recognition

Patient preparation

■ Explain the procedure to the patient and what the speech test evaluates.
■ Review any materials given to the patient by the audiologist.
■ Remove any significant cerumen accumulation.

Procedure and posttest care

■ To obtain the threshold of speech reception, the audiologist presents two-syllable words (spondee words) to the patient, decreasing the intensity until the threshold is obtained. Threshold testing results are reported as spondee thresholds, which is synonymous with speech reception thresholds (SRTs).

AGE ISSUE *Children may be asked to point to pictures representing the words. Very young children who don't have the vocabulary to identify pictures are test-*ed by having them point to body parts, such as eyes, nose, and "Mommy's" mouth.

■ Occasionally, speech awareness thresholds are used in lieu of speech reception threshold testing to assess the lowest level at which a patient can detect speech (typically 10 dB below the speech reception threshold). The test may be used as a substitute for the SRT in a young child and for someone who speaks a foreign language.

■ To estimate the patient's ability to understand speech, lists of one-syllable words are presented, typically in quiet and at an intensity that's comfortable for the patient. Word understanding testing is referred to as *speech discrimination testing* or *word recognition testing.* This test can be administered at the level of typical conversational speech (40 to 50 dB HL) to estimate the impact of the hearing loss on communication in ideal environments. A percentage correct score is obtained. The test can alternatively be administered at an intensity level that's comfortable for the patient, which provides limited prognostic information about probable benefit from amplification.

■ When there's a suspicion of cranial nerve VIII or other retrocochlear involvement, the speech understanding testing may be repeated at a very high intensity. This form of testing is referred to as *rollover testing.*

Precautions

■ None

Normal findings

A normal speech threshold (spondee threshold, SRT) is in the range of –10 to 15 dB HL for children age 2 and over and –10 to 25 dB HL for adults.

Word recognition scores are normally 100%, though typically reduced in the presence of hearing loss. Speech tests for auditory processing are interpreted by comparing the patient's score to age-appropriate norms.

Abnormal findings

SRTs higher than 25 dB HL indicate that the patient can't hear a whispered sound. Thresholds that range up to 40 dB HL suggest that the patient has difficulty hearing faint or distant speech. If the person doesn't wear a hearing aid and has a SRT of 30 to 40 dB HL, make sure that you speak to the patient in a quiet environment from a distance of no more than 6′ (1.8 m). Speech reception thresholds above 40 dB HL indicate increasing difficulty understanding speech. Closer proximity to the patient, if unaided, is required. When thresholds exceed 50 dB HL, the patient can't be expected to understand you without amplification. Health care facilities can obtain portable personal amplification systems to aid in communicating with this patient.

The audiologist will compare the SRT with the pure tone average to cross-check test reliability. The patient who doesn't have agreement within 10 dB between the SRT and pure tone average may not have understood test instructions. The patient with nonorganic loss (exaggeration of hearing thresholds) commonly has a better SRT than pure tone testing would predict.

Word understanding scores below 90% indicate that the patient has some degree of communication difficulty. The audiologist uses the score, interpreted in conjunction with the presentation level and the audiometric configuration, as a prognostic indicator of potential for success with amplification. Amplification is most successful in the patient with higher word understanding scores, although a patient with limited word understanding ability may be a candidate for amplification. (See *Classifying word recognition ability,* page 572.)

The audiologist's finding of decreased word understanding at a high intensity level indicates "rollover," which, if significant, is an indicator of possible retrocochlear involvement. The significance of this finding is interpreted along with the results of immittance tests.

Abnormal auditory processing test results are those significantly below the expected level when compared to age-appropriate norms. This test finding indicates difficulty processing auditory information. Auditory processing disorders are specific to the auditory modality. For example, the patient with attention deficit hyperactivity disorder may function abnormally if he lacks motivation for completing the task. The patient with an auditory processing disorder may require language testing/treatment, specific treatments for auditory processing dysfunction, and may need modification of the classroom environment. Amplification, whether for the entire classroom or using a personal unit for that child, may be recommended by the audiologist to ensure that the child receives a signal of sufficient quality to permit speech understanding and learning.

Interfering factors

- Failure to consider receptive vocabulary when interpreting test results
- A speaker of a foreign language with biased estimates of speech understanding ability if the testing isn't conducted in the patient's native language, by a speaker who can accurately interpret the patient's responses

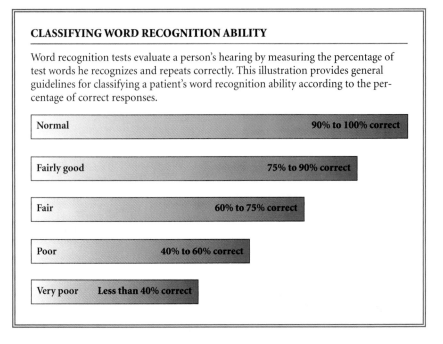

CLASSIFYING WORD RECOGNITION ABILITY

Word recognition tests evaluate a person's hearing by measuring the percentage of test words he recognizes and repeats correctly. This illustration provides general guidelines for classifying a patient's word recognition ability according to the percentage of correct responses.

Normal	90% to 100% correct
Fairly good	75% to 90% correct
Fair	60% to 75% correct
Poor	40% to 60% correct
Very poor	Less than 40% correct

Otoacoustic emissions

Otoacoustic emissions testing is a rapid method of screening that assesses the function of outer hair cells of the cochlea. Because outer hair cells almost invariably are lost before damage to inner hair cells, this technique screens for cochlear hearing loss. Otoacoustic emissions are absent when more than a slight to mild hearing loss is present. Subtle changes in otoacoustic emissions are sometimes present in normal hearing carriers of recessive hearing loss genes. Abnormalities of otoacoustic emissions may precede hearing loss.

Commercially available since 1988, this test has provided a cost-effective method of neonatal screening because patient participation isn't necessary. It provides a measure of outer hair cell function, assists in patient triage during diagnostic testing, and provides a rapid indication of whether the outer hair cells are intact. It can assist in detecting nonorganic hearing loss. However, hearing loss developing after birth, such as from maternal cytomegalovirus infection, and some genetic hearing losses may not be identified with neonatal screening. Moreover, slight (minimal) hearing loss may go undetected.

Purpose
■ To screen and assess the health of the outer hair cells of the cochlea
■ To screen hearing of neonates

Patient preparation
■ Remove significant cerumen accumulation from the patient's ear canals.
■ Inform the patient (if appropriate) that the test is rapidly administered, requiring approximately 1 minute per ear (if the patient is quiet and has normal hearing) or just slightly longer (if findings aren't immediately normal).

Procedure and posttest care

- In screening, the technician places the probe in the patient's ear after having cleared it of debris, such as vernix, which is present in the neonate's ear.
- The audiologist adjusts signal levels, and in the case of distortion-product otoacoustic emissions, the frequency characteristics.
- The emission level is monitored and compared to the background noise level.

Precautions

- None

Normal findings

Otoacoustic emissions are normally present at 500 to 6,000 Hz, with signal-to-noise ratios of at least 5 dB. Emissions sufficiently above the background physiologic and ambient noise provide evidence of functional outer hair cells in the cochlea, typically associated with normal or near-normal hearing. Results are frequency specific.

Abnormal findings

An absence of otoacoustic emissions at any test frequency suggests outer hair cell dysfunction and hearing loss of at least 25 dB HL. The presence of otoacoustic emissions at traditional screening levels indicates no more than a slight cochlear hearing disorder. Significant conductive hearing loss can reduce or eliminate the size of the otoacoustic emission.

Interfering factors

- Screening by inexperienced technicians in the technique, possibly leading to high false-positive rates (Retesting is typically incorporated into screening programs.)
- Significant conductive hearing loss, which can create a failure during diagnostic testing or a "refer to" during screening

(While this allows most congenital conductive losses to be discovered, it means that some children with transient conductive loss will fail to pass the screening or diagnostic version of otoacoustic emissions testing.)

- Presence of cerumen obstruction
- Auditory dysynchrony, sometimes called *auditory neuropathy,* such as from hyperbilirubinemia or kernicterus, undetected with this procedure (If outer hair cells function, but the disorder is such that a neural signal isn't transmitted to the brain, otoacoustic emissions will be normal and the hearing deficit won't be discovered.)

Auditory brain stem evoked-response testing

Auditory brain stem evoked-response (ABR, also called *brain stem auditory evoked response*) testing is the most common form of auditory evoked potentials testing. In ABR testing, electrodes are attached to the surface of the patient's scalp, following cleaning and mild abrasion of the electrode sites. The EEG activity, including the auditory evoked potential present in response to a signal, is amplified, filtered, digitized, and subjected to time-domain signal averaging to separate the response from the background EEG. The resulting traces are analyzed to determine if a response is present, and the characteristics of that response are noted. Various peaks are associated with the ABR (the most prominent are labeled I, III, and V). They occur at predictable times after signal presentation in the patient with normal hearing and normal neural synchronization.

The stimulus characteristics depend upon the type of evoked potential and its use. In threshold estimation and hearing screening, the signal may be tonal or may be a very short duration square wave, or click. The click contains energy throughout the frequency spectrum, but the evoked response generally comes from the high-frequency region of the cochlea.

Various forms of auditory evoked responses can be used to evaluate the function of the auditory pathways in a child or adult suspected of having auditory processing deficits.

Electrocochleography (ECoG or ECochG) can be used in the differential diagnosis of Ménière's disease (endolymphatic hydrops), although its diagnostic sensitivity and specificity is considered by some to be lacking, particularly in the early stages of the disease.

Purpose

- To screen neonatal hearing
- To estimate or confirm the extent of hearing loss in infants and toddlers
- To estimate threshold in other difficult-to-test patients, such as those with developmental disabilities and those suspected of nonorganic hearing loss
- To evaluate cranial nerve (CN) VIII and lower brain stem auditory synchronization, which is abnormal with lesions of this area and with auditory dysynchronization (auditory neuropathy)

Patient preparation

- Cerumen removal is required before referring the patient for this form of testing, which is conducted by an audiologist, and sometimes at a neurology facility. Clean ear canals are particularly important when referring for ECoG.

AGE ISSUE *Depending upon the age of the child, sedation may be required. Sedated ABR testing can only be conducted at health care facilities. In other facilities, sleep deprivation of the child may* *be required to ensure that the patient sleeps during testing.*

- The patient should be advised to dress comfortably and be aware that although the test is painless, electrodes will be applied to the skin and will require 1 to 1½ hours to complete. Therefore, a woman may wish to not use foundation make-up on the test day.

Procedure and posttest care

- Electrodes are connected to a physiologic amplifier that allows the minute voltages coming from the auditory system to be amplified enough to allow them to be read by the signal-averaging computer. The waveforms are displayed as the amplitude of the response across the time after the presentation of the signals.
- Threshold estimation is typically conducted by an audiologist. In this testing, he varies the intensity of the signal until the threshold of the response is obtained. The response threshold is typically slightly supra-threshold, but threshold estimation is possible if the patient has normal neural synchrony.
- In neurodiagnostic testing for CN VIII and auditory brain stem response, click signals are presented at intensities that are clearly audible and should elicit good synchronization of CN VIII. Typically, the click signals are presented at different presentation rates. More rapid presentations may reveal auditory pathology more readily. A click stimulus is presented at a supra-threshold level. The time at which wave V occurs in each ear, the time difference between the evoked waves I and V in each ear, and the time difference between both of these measures is used to indicate the probability of retrocochlear pathology. Assessment of central auditory processing ability typically involves assessing brain stem potentials and one or more of

the potentials generated by the neural structures superior to the brain stem.

- ECoG also involves the presentation of relatively intense signals. The recording electrodes are placed in the ear canal of the patient or on the tympanic membrane. Rarely, a physician places the electrode through the tympanic membrane and rests it on the promontory of the middle ear. The cochlear potentials and CN VIII response are recorded.
- If the patient required sedation, he must be medically supervised until he completely recovers.

Precautions

- Accurate test results require passive patient cooperation.
- Rarely, skin abrasion for electrode placement causes irritation and minor allergic reactions.
- ECoG using tympanic membrane electrodes requires skill on the part of the audiologist to place the electrode in contact with the tympanic membrane without creating patient discomfort.

Normal findings

The ABR wave latencies (time of the waveform occurrence after stimulus presentation) occur at predictable times for the patient with normal hearing or with cochlear loss who's hearing signals that are sufficiently above hearing threshold. The latency between wave I and V are approximately 4.0 ms (no longer than about 4.4 ms). The interaural latency difference of wave V and the I-V interaural latency differences are small, generally less than 0.3 or 0.4 ms. (See *Auditory brain evoked response,* page 576.)

The threshold of the ABR is typically about 10 to 20 dB nHL for click or high-frequency stimuli, and 20 or 30 dB nHL for lower-frequency stimuli.

ECoG reveals an amplitude ratio of the summating potential and action potential that's within normal limits for the type of electrode used.

Abnormal findings

Cochlear loss increases the threshold of the ABR response, but doesn't typically alter the wave V latency for stimuli that are well above the threshold. The time between waves I and V is unaffected or shortens with cochlear loss; however, establishing wave I may be more difficult. Prolongation of the I-V interpeak latency is an indicator of CN VIII or lower brain stem pathology. This requires confirmation with imaging studies. Asymmetry of the I-V interpeak interval between ears is also a strong sign of a retrocochlear disorder. Asymmetry of absolute latency of wave V, abnormal prolongation of V with an increase in the stimulus repetition rate, poor replicability or morphology, and atypical amplitude ratios of waves I to V fail to rule out a retrocochlear abnormality.

A normal supra-threshold response — for example, an ABR to a 80 dB nHL click — doesn't indicate normal hearing. Assessment of the threshold of the ABR must be conducted. The threshold of the ABR is slightly above the expected actual hearing threshold. The audiologist interprets the findings in terms of probable hearing loss type and degree. While ABR testing is subject to some level of imprecision, amplification shouldn't be delayed because of incomplete test results. Amplification should be provided using conservative gain levels and protection against high output levels that can damage hearing. Careful audiologic follow-up is required. The goals of neonatal hearing screening programs are to identify hear-

AUDITORY BRAIN EVOKED RESPONSE

These graphs are an example of an auditory brain stem evoked response elicited by 100 ms click stimuli. The patient's auditory neural activity is recorded using surface electrodes. The peaks on the graphs represent activity from cranial nerve VIII and brain stem structures. Traces are repeated for accuracy at each intensity. The morphology and time between labeled peaks is evaluated when assessing the patient's neural integrity. Additionally, the symmetry of left and right ear responses are evaluated (not illustrated). When used to estimate the hearing threshold, the stimuli's intensity is decreased. A prolonged wave V occurs. The lowest intensity eliciting an evoked potential is assumed to be slightly suprathreshold.

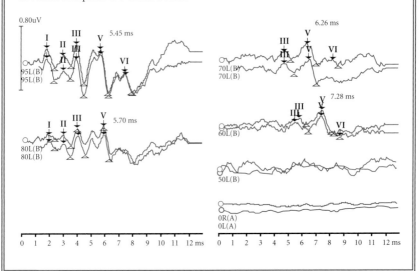

ing problems in children at birth and provide amplification by age 6 months.

ECoG that indicates abnormally large summating potential amplitude, compared to action potential amplitude, is a positive indicator of Ménière's disease.

Interfering factors

■ Hearing loss developed after birth, such as from some congenital diseases as maternal cytomegalovirus infection and some genetic hearing losses or progressive hearing loss

■ Patient moving leading to inaccurate results: if the young child isn't asleep or if the older child or adult is restless

■ Threshold testing with click stimuli, possibly creating false-negative results with normal hearing occurring due to a region of residual hearing

■ Some uncertainty of ABR threshold estimation

■ Auditory dyssynchronization, possibly eliminating an ABR even though cochlear function may be normal (The use of otoacoustic emissions testing in conjunction with ABR testing is recommended.)

■ Lack of use of age-specific norms (Neonates and infants have longer latency responses than adults.)

■ Asymptomatic Ménière's disease, leading to high false-negative results via ECoG (Normal ECoG findings don't rule out Ménière's disease.)

SCANNING

Computed tomography of the ear

Computed tomography (CT) scanning combines the use of a computer and X-rays passed through the body at different angles to produce clear cross-sectional images of body tissues. High-resolution computed tomography (HRCT) is the most commonly used radiographic diagnostic procedure since its invention in the early 1980s. The technique has been perfected over the last 2 decades, and it's used to evaluate patients for cochlear implants, differentiate osseous changes involving the external auditory canal and middle ear, differentiate the osseous structures of the temporal bone and petrous bone, and for providing differential diagnoses for middle ear and inner ear problems.

Purpose

■ To investigate the cause of bilateral hearing loss

■ To confirm cochlear abnormalities

■ To differentiae chronic inflammation from cholesteatoma

■ To evaluate ossification of the cochlea coils before cochlear implantation

■ To depict osseous changes involving the temporal and petrous bone contained in the inner ear

■ To accurately define appropriate surgical and therapeutic approaches for patients with middle ear and inner ear disorders

■ To assess postsurgical management for patients with middle ear and inner ear disorders

Patient preparation

■ Describe the procedure to the patient. Tell him to remove any metal objects, such as jewelry, before the procedure.

■ Explain to the patient that he will be secured to the scanner table to eliminate movement.

■ Check the patient for allergies to iodine products if a contrast medium is to be used (Contrast medium isn't required for evaluating ossification of the cochlea coils or studying the petrous portion of the temporal bone.) Tell him that a contrast medium will be given intravenously.

■ Inform the patient that his body and head will be moved into the scanner, which is an air-conditioned chamber that resembles a giant doughnut. The technician will be able to stay with and communicate with the patient throughout the test, which averages between 15 to 20 minutes.

■ Warn the patient that he will hear a humming sound while the machine records the appropriate images.

Procedure and posttest care

■ The protocol for each HRCT depends on the purpose of the test, with most HRCT studies done in the axial and coronal planes.

■ The patient is taken to the radiology department and placed on the scanner table with his head toward the machine. The mobile scanner table allows for easy transfer and accurate positioning in the machine.

- A trained technician conducts the study under the supervision of a radiologist.
- The technician explains the details of the procedure to the patient to reassure him and gain his cooperation.
- Numerous low-dosage X-ray beams pass through the patient's body at different angles for a fraction of a second as the scanner rotates around him.
- Detectors in the scanner record the number of X-rays absorbed by different tissues, and a computer transforms these data into an image, which is interpreted by the radiologist.
- The temporal bones are imaged separately in the axial and coronal planes. Because contrast already exists between bone, air and soft tissue, the use of a contrast medium isn't necessary in most cases.

Precautions

- If a contrast medium will be used, ask the patient if he has a history of iodine sensitivity.
- Ask the patient about feelings of claustrophobia, which can be an issue. He may require preprocedure medication to alleviate his fears and allow for an accurate study. The ordering physician will make this determination.

Normal findings

Normal anatomic structures should be readily identified in the patient without disease.

Abnormal findings

A CT scan can reveal such diagnoses as tympanosclerosis and the osseous changes of the external auditory canal and middle and inner ear structures, confirm cochlear abnormalities, evaluate cholesteatomas, establish surgical and other therapeutic approaches for the patient, and evaluate the postsurgical management of a patient with middle or inner ear disorder.

Interfering factors

- The patient's inability to lie still during the scan
- Failure to remove all metal objects
- Allergies to iodine if a contrast medium is needed

Magnetic resonance imaging of the ear

Magnetic resonance imaging (MRI) provides high-quality, cross-sectional images of the body. It's a noninvasive test that doesn't use ionizing radiation. MRI images are based upon the radio-frequency (RF) signal emitted by hydrogen nuclei of tissues after they have been perturbed by RF pulses in the presence of a strong magnetic field. MRI is used to assess soft tissues, the cranial nerves, and bone.

Because of improvements in equipment and more highly trained personnel, MRI of the ear is quicker and more economical to perform than it was in the past. Advances have also led to the use of fast-spin echo (FSE) MRIs and diffusion weighted images for otologic and neurologic assessment, especially when a retrocochlear lesion is suspected or other neurologic etiology is under investigation.

For studies of the inner ear and its connections, MRI complements high-resolution computed tomography by providing more accurate assessments of intracranial and infracranial extension as well as the patency of the jugular bulb.

Purpose

- To assess the cause of sudden unilateral sensorineural hearing loss
- To show early nonossified soft-tissue scarring in the membranous labyrinth
- To investigate lesions of the petrous apex
- To diagnose vestibular schwannomas as small as 2 mm
- To visualize cranial nerves VII and VIII, especially when anticipating excision of an auditory neuroma

Patient preparation

- Explain to the patient that MRI is valuable in studying the internal structures of the ear.
- Tell the patient that the MRI machine itself emits a loud, banging noise when it's operating.
- Advise the patient that the test may require the use of an I.V. contrast medium, which seldom causes adverse reactions.
- Inform the patient that the procedure takes about 15 minutes when contrast medium isn't used. (FSE MRI takes even less time.)
- Have the patient remove all jewelry (including watches and rings) and metal objects, such as hairpins and barrettes.
- Tell the patient to inform the physician if he has a pacemaker, hearing aid, or other electrical device because these items can interfere with the scanner.

Procedure and posttest care

- The protocol for each MRI depends on the purpose of the test.
- After the patient is prepared and placed on the MRI table, the technician, under the direction of the radiologist, sets the parameter that will provide optimum spatial resolution in a reasonable scan time.
- The patient's head is moved into a large, hollow, cylindrical magnet. The machine surrounds the patient with short bursts of powerful magnetic fields and radio waves.
- These bursts stimulate hydrogen atoms in the patient's system to emit signals, which are detected and analyzed by the computer to create images that resemble "slices" of the patient's body.

Precautions

- If a contrast medium will be used, ask the patient if he has a history of iodine sensitivity.
- Ask the patient about feelings of claustrophobia, which can be an issue. He may require preprocedure medication to alleviate his fears and allow for an accurate study. The ordering physician will make this determination.

Normal findings

Normal anatomic structures should be readily identified in the patient without disease.

Abnormal findings

MRI can detect viral labyrinthitis, increased intracranial pressure, paragangliomas, acoustic neuromas, vestibular schwannomas, and other disorders. If a large lesion is identified in a vascular or cranial nerve area, angiography may be necessary to prevent difficulties during surgery to remove the paraganglioma.

Interfering factors

- The patient's inability to lie still during the scan
- Failure to remove all metal objects

VESTIBULAR TESTS

Electronystagmography and videonystagmography

In electronystagmography (ENG) testing and videonystagmography (VNG) testing, eye movements in response to specific stimuli are recorded and used to evaluate the interactions of the vestibular system and the muscles controlling eye movement in what is known as the *vestibulo-ocular reflex*. Nystagmus, the involuntary back-and-forth eye movements caused by this reflex, results from the vestibular system's attempts to maintain visual function during head movement. When the patient turns his head in one direction, the eyes deviate slowly in the opposite direction; on reaching their deviation limit, they quickly return to the center. If the head continues to turn, the pattern of eye movement continues. (See *Understanding eye movement patterns.*)

The nystagmus cycle has two parts: Slow deviation against the direction of the turn (the slow phase) is controlled by the vestibular system; rapid return to center (the fast phase) is controlled by the central nervous system (CNS). Nystagmus is described as "beating" in the direction of the fast phase. Thus, a head turn to the right yields a right-beating nystagmus, with its slow phase to the left and its fast phase to the right.

Nystagmus accompanying a head turn is normal; prolonged nystagmus after a head turn or nystagmus when the patient isn't turning his head is abnormal. Because of the interaction of the vestibular and ocular systems, abnormal nystagmus can result from lesions of either system; such lesions can be peripheral (end organ or vestibular nerve involvement) or cen-

tral (cerebellar or brain stem involvement). Abnormal nystagmus is the main sign of vestibular disturbances, such as dizziness and vertigo.

Nystagmography is a technique for monitoring nystagmus and other eye movements. The eye movements can be monitored using electrodes placed near the eyes. Traditional ENG records the corneoretinal potential—the difference of 1 mV between the positive charge of the cornea and the negative charge of the retina—to record nystagmus through electrodes placed near the eyes. As the eyes move horizontally or vertically, the electrodes pick up the corneoretinal potential and chart it. This method permits the recordings of nystagmus in dimly lit surroundings, with the patient's eyes open or closed. (See *ENG eye movements,* page 582.) In VNG, goggles are placed over the patient's eyes, and eye movements are recorded with an infrared camera. The lenses of the goggles can be closed, excluding outside light and preventing the patient from visually fixating. Additional information about eye movement, such as torsion of the eyes, is also observable. Tracings representing eye movements are obtained.

The ENG/VNG test battery includes oculomotor and caloric tests. The tests seek to determine whether the disorder is peripheral (inner ear or related to cranial nerve VIII involvement) or central (originating from problems of the CNS, brain stem, cerebellum, or cerebrum).

Purpose
- To help identify the cause of dizziness and vertigo
- To confirm the presence and location (central or oculomotor, peripheral, or both) of a lesion
- To assess neurologic disorders

UNDERSTANDING EYE MOVEMENT PATTERNS

There are several types of eye movement patterns to look for during ENG testing. Here are some terms along with their definitions.

Bilateral weakness: reduced nystagmus slow-phase velocity for the caloric irrigation of both ears.

Conjugate deviation: drawing of the eyes to one side in unison.

Directional preponderance: difference in beat intensity in one direction as opposed to the other direction during caloric testing; commonly associated with existing spontaneous nystagmus.

Nystagmus: involuntary, rhythmic, back-and-forth movement of the eyes, usually composed of a slow deviation in one direction and a rapid return in the other. Types of nystagmus include:

■ *Fast phase of nystagmus:* quick, jerky component of nystagmus controlled by the central nervous system.

■ *Horizontal nystagmus:* nystagmus in the horizontal plane, either left- or right-beating.

■ *Inverted nystagmus:* nystagmus that beats in the direction opposite to that anticipated.

■ *Positional nystagmus:* a persistent nystagmus that appears while in a particular head position.

■ *Positioning nystagmus:* a transient nystagmus occurring immediately after a change in head position.

■ *Rotary nystagmus:* a nystagmus that rotates about the axis of the eye.

■ *Slow phase of nystagmus:* the vestibular phase of nystagmus or the slow deviation of the eyes from the midline.

■ *Spontaneous nystagmus:* a nystagmus occurring in the absence of stimuli.

■ *Vertical nystagmus:* nystagmus occurring in the vertical plane, either up- or down-beating.

Saccades: rapid, involuntary, jerky movements that occur simultaneously in both eyes when they change their fixation to a new point.

Unilateral weakness: reduced nystagmus (slow phase velocity) after one ear is exposed to cold and warm irrigations (averaged), and then those results are compared with the other ear's results.

Patient preparation

■ Make sure that the patient's ear canals are free from cerumen before referring him for ENG testing. The caloric testing portion of the ENG can't be conducted safely or accurately if he has cerumen accumulation or a tympanic membrane perforation.

■ Inform the patient that tympanometry will be conducted before caloric testing to ensure tympanic membrane integrity.

■ Tell the patient that his dizziness problems will be assessed by recording eye movements.

■ Inform the patient that the procedure will require approximately 1½ hours to complete.

■ Reassure the patient that the test isn't painful and someone will be present to ensure that he doesn't fall, but that some portions may briefly make him dizzy. Because of this, advise him not to eat or drink for 3 to 4 hours before the test.

■ Suggest that someone accompany the patient to the evaluation, as occasionally the patient doesn't feel well enough to drive after the appointment. Avoid overemphasizing the risk of discomfort because patient anxiety increases the risk of

ENG EYE MOVEMENTS

Traditional electronystagmography (ENG) involves electrodes that are placed above and below (vertical channel), and at the inner and outer canthi (horizontal channel) of one or both of the patient's eyes. Videonystagmography records the patient's eye movements optically. Both systems create traces of eye movement over time. The horizontal and vertical eye movements over time are shown separately here. The top illustration depicts a right beating nystagmus, and the bottom illustration shows an upbeating nystagmus. The direction of the more rapid portion of the nystagmus determines the labeled direction.

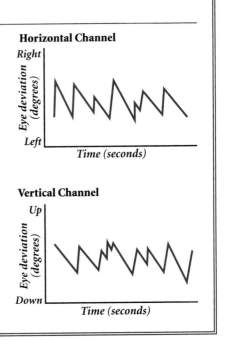

nausea and vomiting during the procedure.

■ Encourage the patient to wear comfortable clothing. A woman should wear pants.

■ If testing involves traditional ENG with attachment of recording electrodes, inform the patient that his skin will need to be cleaned, so ideally make-up or facial creams shouldn't be used on the day of the test. VNG testing is compromised by mascara, so a woman should refrain from wearing make-up on the day of the test.

■ Instruct the patient not to smoke or drink caffeinated beverages the day of the test. He should refrain from taking nonessential medication for 48 hours before the test.

■ Ask the patient to bring a list of his medications to the evaluation. He must not take these agents 48 hours before the test because they prevent accurate collection and interpretation of the results: alcoholic beverages, tranquilizers, sleeping pills, antihistamines, antivertigo agents, and opioids. Other medications can create dizziness, which include salicylates, antidepressants, diuretics, stimulants, and certain aminoglycoside antibiotics.

■ Alert the health care facility performing the test if the patient has a history of back or neck problems that would be exacerbated by head or neck movement.

■ If the patient wears glasses, tell him to bring them to the test. The patient who wears contact lenses should bring eyeglasses to the examination, if possible.

■ Tell the patient that the audiologist will ask for a description of the dizziness and to describe when it began. It's helpful if the patient thinks about what situations creates or makes the dizziness worse. Additionally, find out about the progression of the patient's symptoms by asking him to think about words that might describe the dizziness other than the word "dizzy."

Procedure and posttest care

■ After the device is set up, light bars are connected to the equipment.

■ The patient is positioned a calibrated distance from the light source and asked to follow the movement of the lights using eye movement only. The eye movements are recorded and graphed.

■ After testing is complete, the patient may resume his usual diet.

Oculomotor testing

Saccade testing

■ The patient is asked to watch the movement of a dot on the light bar. The dot position will move varying amounts, which correspond to eye deviations in degrees. The accuracy and velocity of the eye tracking of the rapidly moving light is measured. The traces are analyzed to determine if there's symmetrical (right versus left and up versus down) eye movement or dysmetria such as excessive overshoot or undershoot. Glissades, a slowing of the eye movement as it approaches a target, is also ruled out.

Gaze nystagmus testing

■ The patient is asked to look at the light on the light bar and hold the gaze steady. Gaze is directed left, right, up, and down.

■ The patient is also asked to close his eyes and retain the gaze direction in traditional ENG testing. When VNG recordings are made, the goggles exclude light and the recordings are made with the eyes open. Nystagmus shouldn't occur with the patient's eyes open while he fixates on the target and should be minimal with his eyes closed or when goggles exclude light.

Smooth pursuit (sinusoidal) tracking testing

■ The patient watches the dot on the light bar as it moves smoothly back and forth at varying rates.

■ The eye movement is observed to determine if the patient can track the target accurately.

■ Tracings are analyzed for left/right symmetry and "smoothness" of the eye's tracking (pursuit) of the target.

Optokinetics testing

■ The patient is instructed to look at the light bar as a series of dots moves across the screen, first in one direction (for example, right to left), and then in the other direction.

■ The patient's eyes rapidly move back to center and track another dot. This creates a tracing that looks like nystagmus: the patient follows a dot for a brief period; the eyes rapidly move back to center and track another moving dot. This test assesses the CNS's ability to control rapid eye movement and will be affected by an existing nystagmus.

Positional and positioning testing

■ The patient's eye movements are recorded as he's moved into various body positions and as he remains in these body positions. Recordings note whether nystagmus is present, and if so, the positions that elicit the nystagmus are noted and have diagnostic significance.

■ In the Dix-Hallpike test, diagnostic for benign paroxysmal positional vertigo (BPPV), the patient is initially seated. He's then rapidly moved into a supine, head hanging position, with the head deviated to the side and then returned to a sitting position.

■ If torsional eye movements are observed, time-locked to the subjective report of dizziness, the findings are positive for BPPV. The test is repeated to establish fatigability, also classic in BPPV. The direction of the rotational eye movement assists in diagnosing which semicircular canal is involved and helps to establish the appropriate BPPV repositioning treatment.

Caloric testing

■ The patient lies supine with his head elevated 30 degrees so that the horizontal semicircular canals are perpendicular to the floor.

■ The patient's ear is irrigated with water or air (depending upon the system used) for approximately 60 seconds per irrigation. Four irrigations are completed (both temperatures for each ear).

■ Heating and cooling the outer ear causes a change in temperature of the middle ear. The horizontal semicircular canal is located behind the medial wall of the middle ear. The fluid in the semicircular canal moves when the temperature of the fluid is changed, eliciting nystagmus. Thus, for caloric testing, nystagmus is normal.

■ The patient is instructed to open his eyes during one portion of each recording. Visual fixation reduces nystagmus if the CNS is normal.

■ The symmetry of the nystagmus elicited by irrigation of each ear is assessed. The different temperatures produce different directions of nystagmus. The symmetry of the left beating nystagmus and the right beating nystagmus is analyzed.

■ If the patient fails to respond to standard caloric stimulation, ice calorics may be used. A small quantity of ice water or very cold air is introduced into the ear canal to determine if there's residual functioning of that ear's vestibular system.

Precautions

■ If the patient has a back or neck condition that could be aggravated by rapid changes in position, check with the physician to determine if any of the positional tests should be omitted.

■ Water caloric testing can't be safely used if the patient has a perforated tympanic membrane. Air caloric test results won't be accurate.

■ After testing, the audiologist monitors the patient's status and advises him to remain in a position that reduces dizziness, if present after the procedure.

■ The patient is advised not to drive until all symptoms of imbalance have subsided.

Normal findings

See *Results of electronystagmography.*

Abnormal findings

ENG/VNG results are reported as normal, vestibular (peripheral), CNS, or multifactorial. A peripheral lesion may involve the end organ or the vestibular branch of the eighth cranial nerve and may result from conditions, such as Ménière's disease, multiple sclerosis, ischemic damage to the cochlea, autoimmune disease, and vestibular ototoxity and eighth nerve tumors. A central lesion may involve the brain stem, cerebellum, cerebrum, or any of the connecting structures and may result from demyelinating diseases, tumors, or circulatory disorders.

Interfering factors

■ Medication that suppresses or stimulates CNS function (See "Patient preparation," page 581.)

■ Poor eyesight or extraocular muscle weakness

■ Drowsiness and level of alertness

■ Poor patient cooperation

RESULTS OF ELECTRONYSTAGMOGRAPHY

Test and normal findings	Abnormal findings	Usual underlying conditions
Saccadic pursuit testing Square-wave patterns of differing amplitudes mimicking the target, minimal latency and good accuracy of eye movements	*Ocular dysmetria:* significant undershoots, overshoots, glissades, or pulsion; reduced eye velocity, accuracy, prolonged latency	Central nervous system (CNS) pathology: possible involvement of brain stem, cerebellum, or cortex. Nonlocalizing: spontaneous or gaze nystagmus may be the cause.
Gaze testing No nystagmus with eyes open, weak or no nystagmus with eyes closed	*Spontaneous nystagmus:* significant amount noted when eyes are closed or when tested in complete darkness under goggles while gazing forward	Nonlocalizing abnormality of the vestibular system: in acute peripheral disorders, is horizontal and initially beats away from the affected ear. If present with eyes open, viewing a target, or if the nystagmus changes direction, this is consistent with CNS involvement.
	Gaze nystagmus: presence of nystagmus only when the eyes are deviated from midline	Generally consistent with CNS involvement: the patient with spontaneous nystagmus due to peripheral lesions will have stronger nystagmus when looking in the direction of the nystagmus fast phase.
	Up-beating nystagmus: upward deviation of eye movement	Cerebellar or brain stem involvement
	Down-beating nystagmus: downward deviation of eye movement	Cerebellar or cervicomedullary junction involvement
	Rotary nystagmus: not classic benign paroxysmal positional vertigo (BPPV)	Brain stem or vestibular nuclei
Positional testing (head in position) Eyes open, no nystagmus; eyes closed or wearing light-excluding goggles, no more than weak nystagmus in one or more positions	*Nystagmus:* either changes direction across positions or positioning or remains in the same direction, but isn't spontaneous nystagmus	Nonlocalizing: suppression with visual fixation suggests peripheral involvement; enhancement of nystagmus or failure to suppress with visual fixation suggests central etiology.

(continued)

RESULTS OF ELECTRONYSTAGMOGRAPHY *(continued)*

Test and normal findings	Abnormal findings	Usual underlying conditions
Positioning testing (head in movement toward the position) Eyes open, no nystagmus; eyes closed or wearing light-excluding goggles, no more than weak nystagmus in one or more positions	*Transient, fatigable torsional eye movement*: during Dix-Hallpike procedure, occurring in concert with subjective dizziness	BPPV: responds well to repositioning maneuvers.
Smooth pursuit tracking Volitional smooth tracking of the target, accuracy within age norms	*Sinusoidal tracking*: with superimposed nystagmus	Nonlocalizing: spontaneous or gaze nystagmus may be the cause.
	Break-up in tracings or saccades: jerking, rather than smooth movements; reduced velocity, accuracy, prolonged latency that isn't accounted for by advanced age or poor cooperation	CNS involvement if peripheral visual problems are ruled out.
Optokinetic testing Eye movement follows stimulus at speeds to 30 degrees per second; clear triangular wave pattern; similar pattern for stimuli traveling in both directions	*Significant asymmetry*: not explained by spontaneous or gaze nystagmus	CNS involvement
	Reduced eye velocity: when compared to age-appropriate norms	CNS involvement if peripheral visual problems are ruled out.
Caloric testing Eyes closed, nystagmus occurring in all conditions; suppressed by visual fixation with cold stimuli, nystagmus beats to opposite ear; with warm stimuli, it beats to same ear (To help recall this phenomenon, use the acronym COWS — cold, opposite, warm, same.)	*Unilateral weakness*: over 20% to 30% difference in maximum slow phase velocities (averaged across temperatures) between ears	Peripheral lesion of weaker side
	Bilateral weakness: slow-phase velocity of the sum of the four caloric irrigations is reduced, typically below 20 degrees (average of each irrigation ≤ 5 degrees/second.)	Bilateral peripheral or CNS involvement
	Directional preponderance: more than 30% difference in maximum slow-phase velocities for right- versus left-beating nystagmus	Nonlocalizing, usually due to underlying spontaneous nystagmus.

RESULTS OF ELECTRONYSTAGMOGRAPHY (continued)		
Test and normal findings	**Abnormal findings**	**Usual underlying conditions**
Caloric testing (continued)	*Failure to suppress fixation:* visual fixation fails to reduce nystagmus by at least 40%	CNS involvement

Posturography

Balance involves the coordination of input from the vestibular system, from vision, and from proprioception. Posturography assesses the patient's ability to retain equilibrium when vision and proprioceptive input is removed.

Purpose

■ To objectively determine the functional impairment associated with dizziness
■ To determine the relative strengths and weaknesses of the vestibular system for establishing and monitoring the progress of a rehabilitation plan

Patient preparation

■ Advise the patient not to smoke or drink caffeinated beverages the day of the test.
■ Tell the patient to refrain from taking nonessential medication for 48 hours before the test.
■ Ask the patient to bring a list of his medications to the evaluation. He must not take these agents 48 hours before the test because they prevent accurate interpretation of the results: alcoholic beverages; tranquilizers; sleeping pills; antihistamines; antivertigo agents; opioids; and other medications that can create dizziness, including salicylates, antidepressants, diuretics, stimulants, and certain aminoglycoside antibiotics.

■ Inform the patient that during the test, he will stand on a platform. The platform can move, and the visual field in front will move.
■ Tell the patient that the test assesses how vision and motion affects his sense of balance. Assure him that he won't fall during the test.
■ Suggest that the patient wear comfortable, loose-fitting clothing; advise a woman to wear pants.

Procedure and posttest care

■ Procedures are somewhat specific to the equipment manufacturer. A battery of tests is typically administered.
■ After testing is complete, the patient may resume his usual diet and medications.

Sensory organization test

■ The patient is placed in a harness, standing on a platform, while looking forward toward a screen that encompasses the entire visual field.
■ The sensor on the platform measures the patient's sway and the strength and latency of leg movements that occur when the platform or visual field moves. Six test conditions include:
– The patient sees the screen in front and the platform is fixed. (Eyes open Rhomberg test)

– The patient closes his eyes. The platform remains fixed. (Eyes closed Rhomberg test)
– The visual field around the patient moves. The platform remains fixed. The visual system information conflicts with the vestibular and proprioceptive inputs. The patient with deficits in these areas experiences greater imbalance.
– The platform moves. The visual field remains fixed. The patient receives proprioceptive and vestibular input that differs from that of the visual system.
– The patient's eyes are closed. The platform moves. Proprioception and vestibular input are assessed.
– The platform and screen in front move in concert. The three sensory systems work together to maintain balance.
■ The test evaluates the person's ability to integrate information across the senses and to suppress information that results in sensory conflicts.

Motor control test
■ The platform makes a series of jerky motions, and the patient's responses are measured.

Adaptation test
■ The platform is tilted up or down, and the patient's ability to compensate for this movement during repetition of the platform tilt is analyzed.

Limit of stability test
■ The patient leans as far as possible in different directions and his responses are measured.

Precautions
■ The person conducting the posturography places the patient in a body harness to prevent falls.

Normal findings
Dynamic platform posturography sensory organization test results indicate whether the patient has a preference for visual, proprioceptive, or vestibular inputs. The analysis determines whether the patient is using ankle or hip strategies to compensate for platform or visual surround motion. This information can be used by the physical therapist in planning and monitoring treatment and can be used as a prognostic indicator.

Dynamic posturography provides age-norm scores to determine a patient's stability. A variety of information is available from the sensory organization test. A score of 100% indicates good stability; 0% indicates that the patient would have fallen had the patient not have been in the harness. Scores for the somatosensory, visual, and vestibular contributions to balance are also given. All tests are interpreted in light of age-appropriate norms.

Abnormal findings
Scores that don't meet age-appropriate norms are considered abnormal. For example, motor control test results assess whether there's normal or abnormal response to postural changes. Leg movements may either be too strong or too weak. Latency abnormalities are suggestive of extravestibular central nervous system lesions. Strength differences between legs may indicate long-loop autonomic nervous system disorders, and multiple sclerosis and spino-cerebellar problems yield specific types of abnormalities. The adaptation test reveals the patient's ability to compensate for movement change and can be compromised by range-of-motion limitations and ankle weakness or an inability to suppress automatic reactions.

The results of the limit of stability test have implications for analyzing the risk of a fall. The patient who can't voluntarily move from his center of gravity will have difficulty reaching for objects and moving his body in his home or work environment.

Interfering factors
- Failure to consider orthopedic and musculoskeletal problems in interpreting the results and recommending a treatment plan
- Medications, such as vestibular suppressants or centrally acting medicines

Selected readings

Cavanaugh, B.M. *Nurse's Manual of Laboratory and Diagnostic Tests,* 4th ed. Philadelphia: F.A. Davis Co., 2003.

McClatchey, K.D. *Clinical Laboratory Medicine,* 2nd ed. Philadelphia: Lippincott Williams & Wilkins, 2002.

Pagana, K.D., and Pagana, T.J. *Mosby's Diagnostic and Laboratory Test Reference,* 6th ed. St. Louis: Mosby Year–Book, Inc., 2003.

Roeser, R.J., et al., eds. *Audiology Diagnosis.* New York: Thieme, 2000.

Schnell, Z., et al. *Davis's Comprehensive Handbook of Laboratory and Diagnostic Tests with Nursing Implications.* Philadelphia: F.A. Davis Co., 2003.

Yueh, B., et al. "Screening and Management of Adult Hearing Loss in Primary Care," *JAMA* 289(15):1976-985, April 2003.

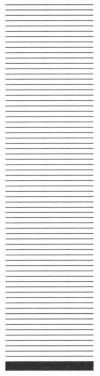

SECTION V.
BODY SYSTEM
TESTS

Respiratory system

Introduction

The pulmonary and circulatory systems are designed to provide the body with a continuous supply of oxygen and a quick, efficient removal of carbon dioxide. The pulmonary system controls the exchange of gases between the atmosphere and blood (known as external respiration), and the circulatory system transports these gases between the lungs and cells (known as internal respiration). A dysfunction in either system disrupts homeostasis and causes anoxia and even cell death. The tests described in this chapter are designed to identify and assess such dysfunction.

Pulmonary physiology

The organs and structures involved in the exchange of gases between the atmosphere and blood are the nose, pharynx, larynx, trachea, bronchi, and lungs. The trachea branches into primary bronchi, secondary bronchi, bronchioles, terminal bronchioles and, finally, alveolar sacs. The walls of the alveolar sacs are lined with

REVIEWING PULMONARY GAS EXCHANGE

Grapelike clusters of alveoli are the sites of gas exchange in the lungs. Each alveolus is served by two systems: the capillary network, which transports mixed venous blood to the alveolar membrane, and the tracheobronchial tree (trachea, bronchi, and bronchioles), which delivers air to the alveolar space. When venous blood passes through the alveolar membrane, it releases carbon dioxide and takes in oxygen. Then the oxygenated blood travels to the heart. From there, it circulates throughout the body, releasing oxygen and taking in carbon dioxide and cellular waste before returning to the lungs.

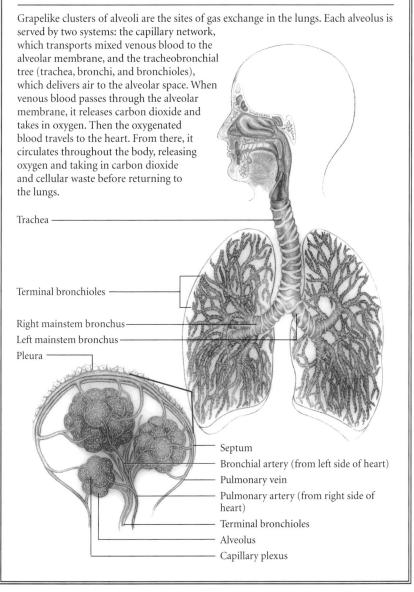

Trachea

Terminal bronchioles

Right mainstem bronchus
Left mainstem bronchus
Pleura

Septum
Bronchial artery (from left side of heart)
Pulmonary vein
Pulmonary artery (from right side of heart)
Terminal bronchioles
Alveolus
Capillary plexus

small outpouchings called *alveoli* and are covered by a capillary network of arterioles and venules. The alveoli, the functional units of the lungs, are responsible for gas exchange between the air and blood. (See *Reviewing pulmonary gas exchange.*)

Three concurrent processes permit gas exchange during respiration.

■ *Ventilation,* the movement of air between the atmosphere and the alveoli, is the result of the contraction and relaxation of the respiratory muscles (primarily the diaphragm), which alternately compress and distend the lungs, causing the decrease and increase of pressure within the alveoli. Inspiration occurs when the pressure in the alveoli is less than atmospheric pressure, and expiration occurs when the pressure in the alveoli is greater than atmospheric pressure.

■ *Diffusion* is the process by which oxygen and carbon dioxide cross the alveolar-capillary membrane. Oxygen (at a higher concentration in alveolar air than in blood) and carbon dioxide (at a higher concentration in blood than in alveolar air) move from their respective region of higher concentration to one of lower concentration.

■ *Perfusion* is the movement of blood through vessels that supply blood for an organ or tissue.

Primary controls

The primary controls of respiration include:

■ The *nervous system* adjusts the rate of respiration to satisfy physiologic demands. The respiratory center in the brain, located in the medulla oblongata and the pons, directs the contraction and relaxation of respiratory muscles.

■ The *Hering-Breuer reflex* controls the depth and rhythm of respiration and prevents overinflation of the lungs. This reflex occurs in response to nerve impulses transmitted from stretch receptors in the bronchi and bronchioles to the respiratory center in the brain.

■ *Carbon dioxide, oxygen,* and *hydrogen ion concentrations* determine the rate of respiration by acting directly on the respiratory center in the brain or on chemoreceptors located in the carotid arteries and the aorta.

Together, these control mechanisms keep blood oxygen and carbon dioxide levels remarkably stable.

Pulmonary assessment

Clinical evaluation of a patient with suspected pulmonary dysfunction begins with a physical examination and a thorough patient history. A *chest X-ray* usually is performed after initial assessment and, depending on its results, may be followed by a *sputum culture* (see chapter 19) or *arterial blood gas analysis* (see chapter 3).

Pulmonary function tests may then identify obstructive or restrictive ventilatory defects. Such tests measure lung capacity and volume and are useful in screening the patient preoperatively to evaluate surgical risk. (See *Evaluating pulmonary function and structure.*)

Endoscopic examinations permit direct observation of structures in the thorax. Such examinations may serve both diagnostic and therapeutic purposes. For example, they allow the removal of foreign bodies (with a rigid bronchoscope), secretions, and blood and aid in identifying abnormalities, such as tumors or strictures.

Finally, *radiographic* and *scanning tests* serve many purposes, from screening for asymptomatic cancer to determining perfusion and ventilation abnormalities. These tests visualize the entire pulmonary system or can provide a three-dimensional view of a specific area.

EVALUATING PULMONARY FUNCTION AND STRUCTURE

Test	Purpose
Volumetric tests	*Evaluate function*
Lung volumes and capacities Tidal volume Inspiratory reserve volume Expiratory reserve volume Residual volume Minute volume Vital capacity Inspiratory capacity Functional residual capacity Total lung capacity Forced vital capacity Flow-volume curve Forced expiratory volume Peak expiratory flow Forced expiratory flow Maximum voluntary ventilation	■ Differentiates between obstructive and restrictive disease patterns ■ Assesses response to therapeutic interventions ■ Aids in interpreting other function tests ■ Makes preoperative assessment in the patient with compromised lung function ■ Evaluates pulmonary disability ■ Quantifies the amount of nonventilated lung ■ Detects presence of lung dysfunction ■ Quantifies the severity of known lung disease ■ Assesses the change in lung function over time or after administration of or change in therapy ■ Assesses the potential effects or response to environmental or occupational exposure ■ Assesses the risk of surgical procedures known to affect lung function ■ Assesses impairment, disability, or both
Endoscopic tests	*Evaluate structure*
Bronchoscopy	■ Directly examines larger airways of tracheobronchial tree
Mediastinoscopy	■ Directly examines mediastinum for biopsy (usually supplements bronchoscopy)
Thoracoscopy	■ Directly examines pleural cavity
Radiographic and scanning tests	*Evaluate structure, function, and vascular status*
Chest radiography	■ Visualizes appearance and status of respiratory system
Paranasal sinus radiography	■ Visualizes appearance and status of paranasal sinus
Fluoroscopy	■ Visualizes thoracic organs in motion
Tomography	■ Supplements radiographs; visualizes target areas in a series of planes to reveal occult pathology
Bronchography	■ Visualizes size and appearance of tracheobronchial tree
Pulmonary angiography	■ Visualizes pulmonary vascular system
Lung perfusion scan	■ Visualizes distribution of blood flow patterns in lungs
Ventilation scan	■ Evaluates ventilatory function
Thoracic computed tomography	■ Locates suspected neoplasms, mediastinal nodes, and pleural involvement

FUNCTION TESTS

Pulmonary function

Pulmonary function tests (volume, capacity, and flow rate tests) are a series of measurements that evaluate ventilatory function through spirometric measurements; they're performed on patients with suspected pulmonary dysfunction.

Of the seven tests used to determine volume, tidal volume (V_T) and expiratory reserve volume (ERV) are direct spirographic measurements; minute volume, carbon dioxide response, inspiratory reserve volume, and residual volume are calculated from the results of other pulmonary function tests; and thoracic gas volume (TGV) is calculated from body plethysmography.

Of the pulmonary capacity tests, vital capacity (VC), inspiratory capacity (IC), functional residual capacity (FRC), total lung capacity, and forced expiratory flow may be measured directly or calculated from the results of other tests. Forced vital capacity (FVC), flow-volume curve, forced expiratory volume (FEV), peak expiratory flow rate, and maximal voluntary ventilation (MVV) are direct spirographic measurements. Diffusing capacity for carbon monoxide (DL_{CO}) is calculated from the amount of carbon monoxide exhaled. (See *Interpreting pulmonary function tests.*)

Purpose
- To determine the cause of dyspnea
- To assess the effectiveness of specific therapeutic regimens
- To determine whether a functional abnormality is obstructive or restrictive
- To measure pulmonary dysfunction
- To evaluate a patient before surgery
- To evaluate a person as part of a job screening (firefighting, for example)

Patient preparation
- Explain to the patient that pulmonary function tests evaluate pulmonary function. Instruct him to eat only a light meal and not to smoke for 12 hours before the tests.
- Describe the tests and equipment. Explain who will perform the tests, where they will take place, and how long they will last.
- Describe the operation of a spirometer.
- Advise the patient that the accuracy of the tests depends on his cooperation.
- Assure the patient that the procedures are painless and that he'll be able to rest between tests.
- Inform the laboratory if the patient is taking an analgesic that depresses respiration.
- As ordered, withhold bronchodilators for 8 hours.
- Just before the test, tell the patient to void and to loosen tight clothing. If he wears dentures, tell him to wear them during the test to help form a seal around the mouthpiece. Advise him to put on the noseclip so that he can adjust to it before the test.

Equipment
For direct spirography
Spirometer, noseclip, mouthpiece

For body plethysmography
Body plethysmograph, mouthpiece, transducer

Procedure and posttest care
- When measuring VT, tell the patient to breathe normally into the mouthpiece 10 times.

(Text continues on page 600.)

INTERPRETING PULMONARY FUNCTION TESTS

Pulmonary function tests are interpreted after data are collected and calculated. The implications are reviewed in the chart below.

Pulmonary function test	Method of calculation	Implications
Tidal volume (V_T): amount of air inhaled or exhaled during normal breathing	Determining the spirographic measurement for 10 breaths and then dividing by 10	Decreased V_T may indicate restrictive disease and requires further testing, such as full pulmonary function studies or chest X-rays.
Minute volume (MV): total amount of air expired per minute	Multiplying V_T by the respiratory rate	Normal MV can occur in emphysema; decreased MV may indicate other diseases such as pulmonary edema. Increased MV can occur with acidosis, increased carbon dioxide (CO_2), decreased partial pressure of arterial oxygen, exercise, and low compliance states.
Carbon dioxide (CO_2) response: increase or decrease in MV after breathing various CO_2 concentrations	Plotting changes in MV against increasing inspired CO_2 concentrations	Reduced CO_2 response may occur in emphysema, myxedema, obesity, hypoventilation syndrome, and sleep apnea.
Inspiratory reserve volume (IRV): amount of air inspired over above-normal inspiration	Subtracting V_T from inspiratory capacity (IC)	Abnormal IRV alone doesn't indicate respiratory dysfunction; IRV decreases during normal exercise.
Expiratory reserve volume (ERV): amount of air exhaled after normal expiration	Direct spirographic measurement	ERV varies, even in healthy people, but usually decreases in obese people.
Residual volume (RV): amount of air remaining in the lungs after forced expiration	Subtracting ERV from functional residual capacity (FRC)	RV > 35% of total lung capacity (TLC) after maximal expiratory effort may indicate obstructive disease.

(continued)

INTERPRETING PULMONARY FUNCTION TESTS *(continued)*

Pulmonary function test	Method of calculation	Implications
Vital capacity (VC): total volume of air that can be exhaled after maximum inspiration	Direct spirographic measurement or adding V_T, IRV, and ERV	Normal or increased VC with decreased flow rates may indicate any condition that causes a reduction in functional pulmonary tissue such as pulmonary edema. Decreased VC with normal or increased flow rates may indicate decreased respiratory effort resulting from neuromuscular disease, drug overdose, or head injury; decreased thoracic expansion; or limited diaphragm movement.
Inspiratory capacity (IC): amount of air that can be inhaled after normal expiration	Direct spirographic measurement or adding IRV and V_T	Decreased IC indicates restrictive disease.
Thoracic gas volume (TGV): total volume of gas in the lungs from ventilated and nonventilated airways	Body plethysmography	Increased TGV indicates air trapping, which may result from obstructive disease.
Functional residual capacity (FRC): amount of air remaining in the lungs after normal expiration	Nitrogen washout, helium dilution technique, or adding ERV and RV	Increased FRC indicates overdistention of the lungs, which may result from obstructive pulmonary disease.
Total lung capacity (TLC): total volume of the lungs when maximally inflated	Adding V_T, IRV, ERV, and RV; FRC and IC; or VC and RV	Low TLC indicates restrictive disease; high TLC indicates overdistended lungs caused by obstructive disease.
Forced vital capacity (FVC): amount of air exhaled forcefully and quickly after maximum inspiration	Direct spirographic measurement; expressed as a percentage of the total volume of gas exhaled	Decreased FVC indicates flow resistance in the respiratory system from obstructive disease such as chronic bronchitis, or from restrictive disease such as pulmonary fibrosis.

INTERPRETING PULMONARY FUNCTION TESTS *(continued)*

Pulmonary function test	Method of calculation	Implications
Flow-volume curve (also called flow-volume loop): greatest rate of flow (V_{max}) during FVC maneuvers versus lung volume change	Direct spirographic measurement at 1-second intervals; calculated from flow rates (expressed in L/second) and lung volume changes (expressed in liters) during maximal inspiratory and expiratory maneuvers	Decreased flow rates at all volumes during expiration indicate obstructive disease of the small airways such as emphysema. A plateau of expiratory flow near TLC, a plateau of inspiratory flow at mid-VC, and a square wave pattern through most of VC indicate obstructive disease of large airways. Normal or increased PEFR, decreased flow with decreasing lung volumes, and markedly decreased VC indicate restrictive disease.
Forced expiratory volume (FEV): volume of air expired in the 1st, 2nd, or 3rd second of an FVC maneuver	Direct spirographic measurement; expressed as a percentage of FVC	Decreased FEV_1 and increased FEV_2 and FEV_3 may indicate obstructive disease; decreased or normal FEV_1 may indicate restrictive disease.
Forced expiratory flow (FEF): average rate of flow during the middle half of FVC	Calculated from the flow rate and the time needed for expiration of the middle 50% of FVC	Low FEF (25% to 75%) indicates obstructive disease of the small and medium-sized airways.
Peak expiratory flow rate (PEFR): V_{max} during forced expiration	Calculated from the flow-volume curve or by direct spirographic measurement using a pneumotachometer or electronic tachometer with a transducer to convert flow to electrical output display	Decreased PEFR may indicate a mechanical problem, such as upper airway obstruction, or obstructive disease. PEFR is usually normal in restrictive disease but decreases in severe cases. Because PEFR is effort dependent, it's also low in a person who has poor expiratory effort or doesn't understand the procedure.

INTERPRETING PULMONARY FUNCTION TESTS *(continued)*

Pulmonary function test	Method of calculation	Implications
Maximal voluntary ventilation (MVV) (also called maximum breathing capacity): the greatest volume of air breathed per unit of time	Direct spirographic measurement	Decreased MVV may indicate obstructive disease; normal or decreased MVV may indicate restrictive disease such as myasthenia gravis.
Diffusing capacity for carbon monoxide (DL_{CO}): milliliters of carbon monoxide diffused per minute across the alveolocapillary membrane	Calculated from analysis of the amount of carbon monoxide exhaled compared with the amount inhaled	Decreased DL_{CO} due to a thickened alveolocapillary membrane occurs in interstitial pulmonary diseases, such as pulmonary fibrosis, asbestosis, and sarcoidosis; DL_{CO} is reduced in emphysema because of alveolocapillary membrane loss.

■ When measuring ERV, tell the patient to breathe normally for several breaths and then to exhale as completely as possible.

■ When measuring VC, tell the patient to inhale as deeply as possible and to exhale into the mouthpiece as completely as possible. This procedure is repeated three times, and the test result showing the largest volume is used.

■ When measuring IC, tell the patient to breathe normally for several breaths and then to inhale as deeply as possible.

■ When measuring FRC, tell the patient to breathe normally into a spirometer that contains a known concentration of an insoluble gas (usually helium or nitrogen) in a known volume of air. After a few breaths, the concentrations of gas in the spirometer and in the lungs reach equilibrium. Then the point of equilibrium and the concentration of gas in the spirometer are recorded.

■ When measuring TGV, be aware that the patient is put in an airtight box (or body plethysmograph) and told to breathe through a tube connected to a transducer. At end-expiration, the tube is occluded, the patient is told to pant, and changes in intrathoracic and plethysmographic pressures are measured. The results are used to calculate total TGV and FRC.

■ When measuring FVC and FEV, tell the patient to inhale as slowly and deeply as possible and then exhale into the mouthpiece as quickly and completely as possible. This procedure is repeated three times, and the largest volume is recorded. The volume of air expired at 1 second (FEV_1), at 2 seconds (FEV_2), and at 3 seconds (FEV_3) during all three repetitions is also recorded.

- When measuring MVV, tell the patient to breathe into the mouthpiece as quickly and deeply as possible for 15 seconds.
- When measuring DL_{CO}, the patient inhales a gas mixture with a low concentration of carbon monoxide and then holds his breath for 10 seconds before exhaling.
- After the tests, instruct the patient to resume his usual activities, diet, and medications, as ordered.

Precautions
- Know that pulmonary function tests are contraindicated in the patient with acute coronary insufficiency, angina, or recent myocardial infarction.
- Watch the patient for respiratory distress, changes in pulse rate and blood pressure, and coughing or bronchospasm.

Reference values
Normal values are predicted for each patient based on age, height, weight, and sex and are expressed as a percentage. Usually, results are considered abnormal if they're less than 80% of these values.

The following reference values can be calculated at bedside with a portable spirometer: VT, 5 to 7 ml/kg of body weight; ERV, 25% of VC; IC, 75% of VC; FEV_1, 83% of VC (after 1 second); FEV_2, 94% of VC (after 2 seconds); and FEV_3, 97% of VC (after 3 seconds).

Abnormal findings
See the accompanying chart.

Interfering factors
- Hypoxia, metabolic disturbances, or lack of patient cooperation
- Pregnancy or gastric distention (possible lung volume displacement)

- Narcotic analgesics or sedatives (possible decrease in inspiratory and expiratory forces)
- Bronchodilators (possible temporary improvement in pulmonary function)

FLUID ANALYSIS
Pleural fluid

The pleura, a two-layer membrane that covers the lungs and lines the thoracic cavity, maintains a small amount of lubricating fluid between its layers to minimize friction during respiration. Increased fluid in this space may result from such diseases as cancer or tuberculosis or from blood or lymphatic disorders and can cause respiratory difficulty.

In pleural fluid aspiration (thoracentesis), the thoracic wall is punctured to obtain a specimen of pleural fluid for analysis or to relieve pulmonary (and possibly cardiac) compression and resultant respiratory distress.

Purpose
- To determine the cause and nature of pleural effusion
- To permit better radiographic visualization of a lung with large effusions

Patient preparation
- Explain to the patient that pleural fluid analysis assesses the space around the lungs for fluid.
- Inform the patient that he need not restrict food and fluids.
- Tell the patient who will perform the test and where it will be done.
- Explain that chest X-rays or an ultrasound study may precede the test to help locate the fluid.

- Check the patient's history for hypersensitivity to local anesthetics.
- Warn the patient that he may feel a stinging sensation on injection of the anesthetic and some pressure during withdrawal of the fluid.
- Advise the patient not to cough, breathe deeply, or move during the test to minimize the risk of injury to the lung.

Equipment

Sterile collection bottles, sterile gloves, personal protective eyewear, adhesive tape, sterile thoracentesis tray (a prepackaged, disposable tray with the following: 70% alcohol or povidone-iodine solution for disinfection, drapes, local anesthetic [usually 1% lidocaine], 5-ml sterile syringe and 25G needle for local anesthetic, 50-ml syringe for removing fluid, 17G thoracentesis aspiration needle, sterile specimen bottle or tube, three-way stopcock or sterile tubing to prevent air from entering the pleural cavity, small sterile dressing)

Procedure and posttest care

- Record the patient's baseline vital signs.
- If necessary, shave the area around the needle insertion site.
- Position the patient to widen intercostal spaces and to allow easier access to the pleural cavity. He must be well-supported and comfortable, preferably seated at the edge of the bed with a chair or stool supporting his feet and his head and arms resting on a padded overbed table. If the patient can't sit up, he may be positioned on his unaffected side, with the arm on the affected side elevated above his head.
- Remind the patient not to cough, breathe deeply, or move suddenly during the procedure.

- After positioning, the physician disinfects the skin, drapes the area, injects a local anesthetic into the subcutaneous tissue, and inserts the thoracentesis needle above the rib to avoid lacerating intercostal vessels. When the needle reaches the pocket of fluid, the 50-ml syringe is attached and the stopcock and clamps are opened on the tubing to aspirate the fluid into the container.
- During aspiration, observe the patient for signs of respiratory distress, such as weakness, dyspnea, pallor, cyanosis, changes in heart rate, tachypnea, diaphoresis, blood-tinged frothy mucus, and hypotension.
- After the needle is withdrawn, apply slight pressure and a small adhesive bandage to the puncture site.
- Label the specimen container and record the date and time of the test and the amount, color, and character of the fluid (clear, frothy, purulent, bloody) on the laboratory request.
- Note any signs of distress exhibited during the procedure.
- Record the exact location from which the fluid was removed to aid diagnosis.
- Reposition the patient comfortably on the affected side. Tell him to remain on this side for at least 1 hour to seal the puncture site. Elevate the head of the bed to facilitate breathing.
- Monitor the patient's vital signs every 30 minutes for 2 hours and then every 4 hours until they're stable.
- Tell the patient to call a nurse immediately if he experiences difficulty breathing.

CLINICAL ALERT *Watch for signs of pneumothorax, tension pneumothorax, fluid reaccumulation and, if a large amount of fluid was withdrawn, pulmonary edema or cardiac distress due to mediastinal shift. Usually, a posttest X-ray is or-*

dered to detect these complications before clinical symptoms appear.

■ Check the puncture site for fluid leakage. A large amount of leakage is abnormal. Also check the site and surrounding area for subcutaneous emphysema.

Precautions

■ Keep in mind that thoracentesis is contraindicated in the patient who has a history of bleeding disorders or anticoagulant therapy.

■ Use strict aseptic technique.

■ Note the patient's temperature and whether he's receiving antimicrobial therapy on the laboratory request.

■ Send the specimen to the laboratory immediately after collection.

Normal findings

Normally, the pleural cavity maintains negative pressure and contains less than 20 ml of serous fluid.

Abnormal findings

Pleural effusion results from the abnormal formation or reabsorption of pleural fluid. Certain characteristics classify pleural fluid as either a transudate (a low-protein fluid leaked from normal blood vessels) or an exudate (a protein-rich fluid leaked from blood vessels with increased permeability).

Pleural fluid may contain blood (hemothorax), chyle (chylothorax), or pus (empyema) and necrotic tissue. Blood-tinged fluid may indicate a traumatic tap; if so, the fluid should clear as aspiration progresses.

Transudative effusion generally results from diminished colloidal pressure, increased negative pressure within the pleural cavity, ascites, systemic and pulmonary venous hypertension, heart failure, hepatic cirrhosis, and nephritis.

Exudative effusion results from disorders that increase pleural capillary permeability (possibly with changes in hydrostatic or colloid osmotic pressures), lymphatic drainage interference, infections, pulmonary infarctions, and neoplasms. Exudative effusion associated with depressed glucose levels, elevated lactate dehydrogenase (LD) isoenzymes, rheumatoid arthritis cells, and negative smears, cultures, and cytologic examination may indicate pleurisy associated with rheumatoid arthritis.

The most common pathogens that appear in pleural fluid culture studies are *Mycobacterium tuberculosis, Staphylococcus aureus, Streptococcus pneumoniae* and other streptococci, *Haemophilus influenzae* and, in the case of a ruptured pulmonary abscess, anaerobes such as *Bacteroides*. Cultures are usually positive during the early stages of infection; however, antibiotic therapy may produce a negative culture despite a positive Gram stain and grossly purulent fluid. Empyema may result from complications of pneumonia, pulmonary abscess, perforation of the esophagus, or penetration from mediastinitis. A high percentage of neutrophils suggests septic inflammation; predominating lymphocytes suggest tuberculosis or fungal or viral effusions.

Serosanguineous fluid may indicate pleural extension of a malignant tumor. Elevated LD in a nonpurulent, nonhemolyzed, nonbloody effusion may also suggest malignancy. Pleural fluid glucose levels 30 to 40 mg/dl lower than blood glucose levels may indicate a malignant tumor, a bacterial infection, nonseptic inflammation, or metastasis. Increased amylase levels occur in pleural effusions associated with pancreatitis.

Interfering factors

- Failure to use aseptic technique
- Failure to send the specimen to the laboratory immediately after collection
- Antimicrobial therapy before fluid aspiration for culture (possible decrease in numbers of bacteria, making it difficult to isolate the infecting organism)

Sweat

The sweat test is a quantitative measurement of electrolyte concentrations (primarily sodium and chloride) in sweat, usually performed using pilocarpine iontophoresis (pilocarpine is a sweat inducer). Although this test is primarily used to confirm cystic fibrosis (CF) in children, it's also performed in adults to determine if they're homozygous or heterozygous for CF.

Purpose

- To confirm CF
- To exclude the diagnosis in siblings of the patient with CF

Patient preparation

- Explain the sweat test to the child (if he's old enough to understand), using clear, simple terms.
- Inform the child and his parents that there are no restrictions on diet, medication, or activity before the test.
- Tell the child who will perform the test and where.
- Tell the child that he may feel a slight tickling sensation during the procedure, but won't feel any pain.
- Encourage the parents to assist with preparations and to stay with their child during the test. Their presence will minimize the child's anxiety.

Equipment

Analyzer, two skin chloride electrodes (positive and negative), distilled water, two standardizing solutions (chloride concentrations), $2'' \times 2''$ sterile gauze pads (kept in an airtight container), pilocarpine pads, forceps (for handling pads), straps (for securing electrodes), gram scale, normal saline solution

Procedure and posttest care

- Wash the area that will undergo iontophoresis with distilled water and dry it. (The flexor surface of the right forearm is commonly used or, when the patient's arm is too small to secure electrodes [as with an infant], the right thigh.)
- Place a gauze pad saturated with premeasured pilocarpine solution on the positive electrode; place the pad saturated with normal saline solution on the negative electrode.
- Apply both electrodes to the area to undergo iontophoresis and secure them with straps. Lead wires to the analyzer are given a current of 4 mA in 15 to 20 seconds. Iontophoresis will continue at 15- to 20-second intervals for 5 minutes.
- Try to distract the child with a book, television, toy, or another diversion if he becomes nervous or frightened during the test.
- Remove both electrodes after iontophoresis.
- Discard the pads, clean the skin with distilled water, and then dry it.
- Using forceps, place a dry gauze pad or filter paper (previously weighed on a gram scale) on the area that underwent iontophoresis.
- Cover the pad or filter paper with a slightly larger piece of plastic and seal the edges of the plastic with waterproof adhesive tape.

- Leave the gauze pad or filter paper in place for about 30 to 40 minutes. (The appearance of droplets on the plastic usually indicates induction of an adequate amount of sweat.)
- Remove the pad or filter paper with the forceps, place it immediately in the weighing bottle, and insert the stopper in the bottle. (The difference between the first and second weights indicates the weight of the sweat specimen collected.)
- Wash the area that underwent iontophoresis with soap and water and dry it thoroughly. If the area looks red, reassure the patient that this is normal and will disappear within a few hours.
- Tell the patient or his parents that he may resume his usual activities.

Precautions

- Always perform iontophoresis on the right arm (or right thigh) rather than on the left.
- Never perform iontophoresis on the chest, especially in a child, because the current can induce cardiac arrest.
- Use battery-powered equipment to prevent electric shock, if possible.
- Stop the test immediately if the patient complains of a burning sensation, which usually indicates that the positive electrode is exposed or positioned improperly. Adjust the electrode and continue the test.
- Make sure at least 100 mg of sweat is collected for analysis.
- Carefully seal the gauze pad or filter paper in the weighing bottle and immediately send the bottle to the laboratory.

Reference values

Normal sodium values in sweat range from 10 to 30 mEq/L (SI, 10 to 30 mmol/L). Normal chloride values range from 10 to 35 mEq/L (SI, 10 to 35 mmol/L).

Abnormal findings

Sodium concentrations of 50 to 60 mEq/L (SI, 50 to 60 mmol/L) strongly suggests CF. Concentrations above 60 mEq/L (SI, >60 mmol/L) with typical clinical features confirm the diagnosis.

Only a few conditions other than CF result in elevated sweat electrolyte levels—most notably, untreated adrenal insufficiency as well as type I glycogen storage disease, vasopressin-resistant diabetes insipidus, meconium ileus, and renal failure.

In women, sweat electrolyte levels fluctuate cyclically; chloride concentrations usually peak 5 to 10 days before onset of menses, and most women retain fluid before menses. Men also show fluctuations up to 70 mEq/L (SI, 70 mmol/L). However, CF is the only condition that raises sweat electrolyte levels above 80 mEq/L (SI, 80 mmol/L).

Interfering factors

- Dehydration or edema, especially in the collection area
- Failure to obtain an adequate amount of sweat, a common problem in neonates
- Presence of pure salt depletion, common during hot weather (possible false normal)
- Failure to clean the skin thoroughly or to use sterile gauze pads (possible false high)
- Failure to seal the gauze pad or filter paper carefully (possible false-high electrolyte levels due to evaporation)

ENDOSCOPY

Direct laryngoscopy

Direct laryngoscopy allows visualization of the larynx by the use of a fiber-optic endoscope or laryngoscope passed through the mouth and pharynx to the larynx. It's indicated for children, patients with strong gag reflexes due to anatomic abnormalities, and those who have had no response to short-term therapy for symptoms of pharyngeal or laryngeal disease, such as stridor and hemoptysis. Secretions or tissue may be removed during this procedure for further study. The test is usually contraindicated in patients with epiglottiditis, but may be performed on them in an operating room with resuscitative equipment available.

Purpose
■ To detect lesions, strictures, or foreign bodies
■ To remove benign lesions or foreign bodies from the larynx
■ To aid in the diagnosis of laryngeal cancer
■ To examine the larynx when indirect laryngoscopy is inadequate

Patient preparation
■ Explain to the patient that direct laryngoscopy is used to detect laryngeal abnormalities.
■ Instruct the patient to fast for 6 to 8 hours before the test.
■ Tell the patient who will perform the procedure and where it will be done.
■ Inform the patient that he'll receive a sedative to help him relax, medication to reduce secretions and, during the procedure, a general or local anesthetic. Reassure him that this procedure won't obstruct his airway.
■ Make sure that the patient or a responsible family member has signed an informed consent form.
■ Check the patient's history for hypersensitivity to the anesthetic.
■ Obtain the patient's baseline vital signs.

■ Administer the sedative and other medication (usually 30 minutes to 1 hour before the test), as ordered.
■ Instruct the patient to remove dentures, contact lenses, and jewelry and to void before giving him a sedative.

Equipment
Laryngoscope, sedative, atropine, local anesthetic (spray or jelly) or general anesthetic, sterile container for microbiology specimen, sterile gloves, Coplin jar with 95% ethyl alcohol for cytology smears, container with 10% formalin solution for histology specimen, forceps for biopsy, emesis basin, suction and resuscitation equipment

Procedure and posttest care
■ Place the patient in the supine position.
■ Encourage the patient to breathe through his nose and to relax with his arms at his sides.
■ Assist as appropriate when a general anesthetic is administered or when the patient's mouth and throat are sprayed with a local anesthetic.
■ A laryngoscope is introduced through the patient's mouth, the larynx is examined for abnormalities, and a specimen or secretions may be removed for further study; minor surgery, such as removal of polyps or nodules, may be performed at this time.
■ Place the specimens in their respective containers. Specimen collection should be done in accordance with laboratory and pathology guidelines.
■ Place the conscious patient in semi-Fowler's position; place the unconscious patient on his side with his head slightly elevated to prevent aspiration.
■ Check the patient's vital signs according to facility protocol, or every 15 minutes until the patient is stable and then

every 30 minutes for 2 hours, every hour for the next 4 hours, and then every 4 hours for 24 hours. Immediately report to the physician any adverse reaction to the anesthetic or sedative (tachycardia, palpitations, hypertension, euphoria, excitation, and rapid, deep respirations).

■ Apply an ice collar to minimize laryngeal edema.

■ Provide an emesis basin, and instruct the patient to spit out saliva rather than swallow it. Observe sputum for blood and report excessive bleeding immediately.

■ Instruct the patient to refrain from clearing his throat and coughing to prevent hemorrhaging at the biopsy site.

■ Advise the patient to avoid smoking until his vital signs are stable and there's no evidence of complications.

■ Immediately report subcutaneous crepitus around the patient's face and neck, which may indicate tracheal perforation.

■ Listen to the patient's neck with a stethoscope for signs of stridor and airway obstruction.

◣ **CLINICAL ALERT** *Observe the patient with epiglottiditis for signs of airway obstruction and immediately report signs of respiratory difficulty. Keep emergency resuscitation equipment available; keep a tracheotomy tray nearby for 24 hours.*

■ Restrict food and fluids to avoid aspiration until the gag reflex returns (usually within 2 hours). Then the patient may resume his usual diet, beginning with sips of water.

■ Reassure the patient that voice loss, hoarseness, and sore throat are temporary. Provide throat lozenges or a soothing liquid gargle when his gag reflex returns.

Precautions
■ Send the specimens to the laboratory immediately.

Normal findings
A normal larynx shows no evidence of inflammation, lesions, strictures, or foreign bodies.

Abnormal findings
The combined results of direct laryngoscopy, biopsy, and radiography may indicate laryngeal carcinoma. Direct laryngoscopy may also show benign lesions, strictures, or foreign bodies and, with a biopsy, may distinguish laryngeal edema from a radiation reaction or tumor. It can also determine vocal cord dysfunction.

Interfering factors
■ Failure to place the specimens in appropriate containers or to send them to the laboratory immediately

Bronchoscopy

Bronchoscopy allows direct visualization of the larynx, trachea, and bronchi through a flexible fiber-optic bronchoscope or a rigid metal bronchoscope. A more recent approach is the use of virtual bronchoscopy. (See *Virtual bronchoscopy*, page 608.) Although a flexible fiber-optic bronchoscope allows a wider view and is used more commonly, the rigid metal bronchoscope is required to remove foreign objects, excise endobronchial lesions, and control massive hemoptysis. A brush, biopsy forceps, or catheter may be passed through the bronchoscope to obtain specimens for cytologic examination.

VIRTUAL BRONCHOSCOPY

Using a computer and data from a spiral computed tomography (CT) scan, physicians can now examine the respiratory tract noninvasively with virtual bronchoscopy. Although still in its early stages, researchers believe that this test can enhance screening, diagnosis, preoperative planning, surgical technique, and postoperative follow-up.

Unlike its counterpart — conventional bronchoscopy — virtual bronchoscopy is noninvasive, doesn't require sedation, and provides images for examination beyond the segmental bronchi, thus allowing for possible diagnosis of areas that may be stenosed, obstructed, or compressed from an external source. The images obtained from the CT scan include views of the airways and lung parenchyma. Anatomic structures and abnormalities can be precisely identified and therefore can be helpful in locating potential biopsy sites to be obtained with conventional bronchoscopy and provide simulation for planning the optimal surgical approach.

Virtual bronchoscopy does have disadvantages. This technique doesn't allow for actual biopsies to be obtained from tissue sources. It also can't demonstrate details of the mucosal surface, such as color or texture. Moreover, if an area contains viscous secretions, such as mucus or blood, visualization becomes difficult.

More research on this technique is needed. However, researchers believe that virtual bronchoscopy may play a major role in the screening and early detection of certain cancers, thus allowing for treatment at an earlier, possibly curable stage.

Purpose
- To visually examine a tumor, an obstruction, secretions, bleeding, or a foreign body in the tracheobronchial tree
- To help diagnose bronchogenic carcinoma, tuberculosis, interstitial pulmonary disease, and fungal or parasitic pulmonary infection by obtaining a specimen for bacteriologic and cytologic examination
- To remove foreign bodies, malignant or benign tumors, mucus plugs, and excessive secretions from the tracheobronchial tree

Patient preparation
- Explain to the patient that bronchoscopy is used to examine the lower airways.
- Describe the procedure, and instruct the patient to fast for 6 to 12 hours before the test.
- Tell the patient who will perform the test, where it will be done, and that the room will be darkened.
- Tell the patient that a chest X-ray and blood studies will be performed before the bronchoscopy and afterward, if appropriate.
- Advise the patient that he may receive an I.V. sedative to help him relax.
- If the procedure isn't being performed under general anesthesia, inform the patient that a local anesthetic will be sprayed into his nose and mouth to suppress the gag reflex. Warn him that the spray has an unpleasant taste and that he may experience discomfort during the procedure.
- Reassure the patient that his airway won't be blocked during the procedure and that oxygen will be administered through the bronchoscope.

- Make sure that the patient or a responsible family member has signed an informed consent form.
- Check the patient's history for hypersensitivity to the anesthetic.
- Obtain the patient's baseline vital signs.
- Administer the preoperative sedative.
- Have the patient remove his dentures, if appropriate, before he receives a sedative.

Equipment

Flexible fiber-optic bronchoscope, sedative, local anesthetic (spray, jelly, or liquid), sterile gloves, sterile container for microbiology specimen, container with 10% formalin solution for histology specimen, Coplin jar with 95% ethyl alcohol for cytology smears, six glass slides (frosted, if possible, or with frosted tips), emesis basin, handheld resuscitation bag with face mask, oral and endotracheal airways, continuous suction equipment, laryngoscope, oxygen delivery equipment, ventilating bronchoscope for a patient requiring controlled mechanical ventilation

Procedure and posttest care

- Place the patient in the supine position or have him sit upright in a chair.
- Tell the patient to remain relaxed with his arms at his sides and to breathe through his nose.
- Provide supplemental oxygen by nasal cannula, if necessary.
- After the local anesthetic is sprayed into the patient's throat and it takes effect, assist as appropriate as a bronchoscope is introduced through the patient's mouth or nose. When the scope is just above the vocal cords, about 3 to 4 ml of 2% to 4% lidocaine is flushed through the inner channel of the scope to the vocal cords to anesthetize deeper areas. The physician inspects the anatomic structure of the trachea and bronchi, observes the color of the mucosal lining, and notes masses or inflamed areas.

- As indicated, provide biopsy forceps that may be used to remove a tissue specimen from a suspect area, a bronchial brush to obtain cells from the surface of a lesion, and a suction apparatus to remove foreign bodies or mucus plugs. Bronchoalveolar lavage may be performed to diagnose the infectious causes of infiltrates in an immunocompromised patient or to remove thickened secretions.
- After collection, place the specimens in their respective, properly labeled containers in accordance with laboratory and pathology guidelines and send them to the laboratory at once.
- Be aware that bronchoscopy may require fluoroscopic guidance for distal evaluation of lesions for a transbronchial biopsy in alveolar areas.
- Check the patient's vital signs per facility policy, or at least every 15 minutes until the patient is stable and then every 30 minutes for 4 hours, every hour for the next 4 hours, and then every 4 hours for 24 hours. Immediately notify the physician of adverse reactions to the anesthetic or sedative.
- Place the conscious patient in semi-Fowler's position; place the unconscious patient on his side with his head slightly elevated to prevent aspiration.
- Provide an emesis basin and instruct the patient to spit out saliva rather than swallow it. Observe sputum for blood and report excessive bleeding immediately.
- Tell the patient who has had a biopsy to refrain from clearing his throat and coughing, which may dislodge the clot at the biopsy site and cause hemorrhaging.
- Immediately report subcutaneous crepitus around the patient's face and

neck because this may indicate tracheal or bronchial perforation.

> **CLINICAL ALERT** *Watch for, listen for, and immediately report symptoms of respiratory difficulty resulting from laryngeal edema or laryngospasm, such as laryngeal stridor and dyspnea. Observe for signs of hypoxemia, pneumothorax, bronchospasm, and bleeding.*

- Restrict food and fluids to avoid aspiration until the gag reflex returns (usually in 1 to 2 hours). Then the patient may resume his usual diet, beginning with sips of clear liquid or ice chips.
- Reassure the patient that hoarseness, loss of voice, and sore throat are temporary. Provide lozenges or a soothing liquid gargle to ease discomfort when his gag reflex returns.

Precautions
- A patient with respiratory failure who can't breathe adequately by himself should be placed on a ventilator before bronchoscopy.
- Send the specimens to the laboratory immediately.

Normal findings
The trachea normally consists of smooth muscle containing C-shaped rings of cartilage at regular intervals, and it's lined with ciliated mucosa. The bronchi appear structurally similar to the trachea; the right bronchus is slightly larger and more vertical than the left. Smaller segmental bronchi branch off the main bronchi.

Abnormal findings
Bronchial wall abnormalities include inflammation, swelling, protruding cartilage, ulceration, enlargement of the mucous gland orifices or submucosal lymph nodes, and tumors. Endotracheal abnormalities include stenosis, compression,

ectasia (dilation of tubular vessel), irregular bronchial branching, and abnormal bifurcation due to diverticulum.

Abnormal substances in the trachea or bronchi include blood, secretions, calculi, and foreign bodies.

Results of tissue and cell studies may indicate interstitial pulmonary disease, bronchogenic carcinoma, tuberculosis, or other pulmonary infections. Correlation of radiographic, bronchoscopic, and cytologic findings with clinical signs and symptoms is essential.

Interfering factors
- Failure to observe pretest restrictions
- Failure to place specimens in the appropriate containers or to send them to the laboratory immediately

Mediastinoscopy

Using an exploring speculum with built-in fiber light and side slit, mediastinoscopy allows direct viewing of mediastinal structures. It also permits palpation and biopsy of paratracheal and carinal lymph nodes. This surgical procedure is indicated when other tests, such as sputum cytology, lung scans, radiography, and bronchoscopic biopsy, fail to confirm the diagnosis.

Scarring of the area from previous mediastinoscopy contraindicates this procedure.

Purpose
- To detect bronchogenic carcinoma, lymphoma (including Hodgkin's disease), and sarcoidosis
- To determine stages of lung cancer

Patient preparation
- Explain to the patient that mediastinoscopy is used to evaluate the lymph

nodes and other structures in the chest. Review his history for previous mediastinoscopy because scarring from a previous mediastinoscopy contraindicates the test.

- Describe the procedure to the patient and answer his questions.
- Instruct the patient to fast after midnight before the test.
- Tell the patient who will perform the procedure, where it will be done, that he'll be given general anesthesia, and that the procedure takes about 1 hour.
- Tell the patient that he may have temporary chest pain, tenderness at the incision site, or a sore throat (from intubation).
- Reassure the patient that complications are rare.
- Make sure that the patient or a responsible family member has signed an informed consent form.
- Check the patient's history for hypersensitivity to the anesthetic.
- Give a sedative the night before the test and again before the procedure, as ordered.

Procedure and posttest care
- After the endotracheal tube is in place, a small transverse suprasternal incision is made.
- Using finger dissection, the surgeon forms a channel and palpates the lymph nodes.
- The mediastinoscope is inserted, and tissue specimens are collected and sent to the laboratory for frozen section examination.
- If analysis confirms malignancy of a resectable tumor, thoracotomy and pneumonectomy may follow immediately.
- Monitor the patient's postoperative vital signs and check his dressings for bleeding and fluid drainage.

- Observe the patient for the following complications: fever (a sign of mediastinitis); crepitus (a sign of subcutaneous emphysema); dyspnea, cyanosis, and diminished breath sounds on the affected side (signs of pneumothorax); and tachycardia and hypotension (signs of hemorrhage).
- Administer the prescribed analgesic, as needed.

Precautions
- Immediately send collected specimens to the laboratory.

Normal findings
Lymph nodes appear as small, smooth, flat oval bodies of lymphoid tissue.

Abnormal findings
Malignant lymph nodes usually indicate inoperable, but not always untreatable, lung or esophageal cancer or lymphomas (such as Hodgkin's disease). Staging of lung cancer helps determine the therapeutic regimen. (For example, multiple nodular involvement can contraindicate surgery.)

Interfering factors
- Previous mediastinoscopy with scarring (makes lymph node dissection difficult or impossible)

Thoracoscopy

In thoracoscopy, an endoscope is inserted directly into the chest wall to view the pleural space, thoracic walls, mediastinum, and pericardium. It's used for diagnostic and therapeutic purposes and can sometimes replace traditional thoracotomy. Thoracoscopy reduces morbidity (by reducing the use of open chest surgery) and postoperative pain, decreases surgical and anesthesia time, and allows faster recovery.

Purpose

- To diagnose pleural disease
- To obtain biopsy specimens
- To treat pleural conditions, such as cysts, blebs, and effusions
- To perform wedge resections

Patient preparation

- Explain to the patient that thoracoscopy permits visual examination of the chest wall to view the pleural space, thoracic wall, mediastinum, and pericardium.
- Describe the procedure. Caution the patient that an open thoracotomy may still be needed for diagnosis or treatment and that general anesthesia may be required.
- Instruct the patient not to eat or drink for 10 to 12 hours before the procedure.
- Make sure that the appropriate preoperative tests (such as pulmonary function and coagulation tests, electrocardiography, and chest X-ray) have been performed and that an informed consent form has been signed.
- Tell the patient that he'll have a chest tube and drainage system in place after surgery. Reassure him that analgesics will be available and that complications are rare.

Equipment

Monitors, videocassette recorder, camera, light source, insufflator, cautery, suction and irrigation equipment, trocars, endostaplers, endosutures

Procedure and posttest care

- The patient is anesthetized, and a double-lumen endobronchial tube is inserted.

- The lung on the operative side is collapsed, and a small intercostal incision is made through which a trocar is inserted.
- A lens is then inserted to view the area and assess thoracoscopy access.
- Two or three more small incisions are made, and trocars are placed to insert suction and dissection instruments.
- The camera lens and instruments are moved from site to site as needed.
- After thoracoscopy, the lung is reexpanded, a chest tube is placed through one incision site, and a water-sealed drainage system is attached. The other incisions are closed with adhesive strips and dressed.
- Monitor the patient's postoperative vital signs as per facility policy or every 15 minutes for 1 hour, every 30 minutes for 2 hours, every hour for 2 hours, and then every 4 hours.
- Assess the patient's respiratory status and the patency of the chest drainage system.
- Give analgesics as needed for pain and monitor the patient for adverse effects.

Precautions

- Send specimens to the laboratory immediately.
- Know that thoracoscopy is contraindicated in the patient who has coagulopathies or lesions near major blood vessels, who has had previous thoracic surgery, or who can't be adequately oxygenated with one lung.
- Be alert for complications, although rare, including hemorrhage, nerve injury, perforation of the diaphragm, air emboli, and tension pneumothorax.

Normal findings

A normal pleural cavity contains a small amount of lubricating fluid that facilitates movement of the lung and chest wall. The parietal and visceral layers are lesion-free and can separate from each other.

Abnormal findings

Lesions—such as tumors, ulcers, and bleeding sites—adjacent to or involving the pleura or mediastinum can be seen and biopsies can be taken. Diagnosis may include carcinoma, empyema, pleural effusion, tuberculosis, or an inflammatory process. Areas of blebs can be removed by wedge resection to reduce the risk of repeat episodes of spontaneous pneumothorax.

Interfering factors

■ Extensive disease or inaccessibility (may prevent thoracoscopy)
■ Excessive bleeding during the procedure (may require open thoracotomy)

RADIOGRAPHY

Chest radiography

In chest radiography, X-rays or electromagnetic waves penetrate the chest and cause an image to form on specially sensitized film. Normal pulmonary tissue is radiolucent, whereas abnormalities—such as infiltrates, foreign bodies, fluids, and tumors—appear as densities on the film. A chest X-ray is most useful when compared with previous films to detect changes. (See *Selected clinical implications of chest X-ray films,* pages 614 and 615.)

Purpose

■ To detect pulmonary disorders, such as pneumonia, atelectasis, pneumothorax, pulmonary bullae, pleurisy, and tumors
■ To detect mediastinal abnormalities, such as tumors, and cardiac disease such as heart failure

■ To determine the correct placement of pulmonary catheters, endotracheal tubes, and other chest tubes
■ To determine the location and size of lesions or foreign bodies (coins, broken central lines) that were swallowed or aspirated
■ To help assess pulmonary status
■ To evaluate the patient's response to interventions

Patient preparation

■ Explain to the patient that chest radiography assesses respiratory status.
■ Tell the patient that he need not restrict food and fluids.
■ Describe the test, including who will perform it and when it will take place.
■ Provide a gown without snaps, and instruct the patient to remove jewelry and other metallic objects that may be in the X-ray field.
■ Explain to the patient that he'll be asked to take a deep breath and to hold it momentarily while the film is being taken to provide a clearer view of pulmonary structures.

Procedure and posttest care

■ If a stationary X-ray machine is used, the patient stands or sits in front of the machine so films can be taken of the posteroanterior and left lateral views.
■ If a portable X-ray machine is used at the patient's bedside, the patient is moved to the top of the bed, if his tolerance permits. The head of the bed is elevated for maximum upright positioning.
■ Place cardiac monitoring lead wires, I.V. tubing from central lines, pulmonary artery catheter lines, and safety pins as far from the X-ray field as possible.

SELECTED CLINICAL IMPLICATIONS OF CHEST X-RAY FILMS

Normal anatomic location and appearance	Possible abnormality	Implications
Trachea Visible midline in the anterior mediastinal cavity; translucent tubelike appearance	■ Deviation from midline	■ Tension pneumothorax, atelectasis, pleural effusion, consolidation, mediastinal nodes or, in children, enlarged thymus
	■ Narrowing with hourglass appearance and deviation to one side	■ Substernal thyroid or stenosis secondary to trauma
Heart Visible in the anterior left mediastinal cavity; solid appearance due to blood contents; edges may be clear in contrast with surrounding air density of the lung	■ Shift ■ Hypertrophy of right heart ■ Cardiac borders obscured by stringy densities ("shaggy heart")	■ Atelectasis, pneumothorax ■ Cor pulmonale, heart failure ■ Cystic fibrosis
Aortic knob Visible as water density; formed by the arch of the aorta	■ Solid densities, possibly indicating calcifications ■ Tortuous shape	■ Atherosclerosis ■ Atherosclerosis
Mediastinum (mediastinal shadow) Visible as the space between the lungs; shadowy appearance that widens at the hilum of the lungs	■ Deviation to nondiseased side; deviation to diseased side by traction ■ Gross widening	■ Pleural effusion or tumor, fibrosis or collapsed lung ■ Neoplasms of esophagus, bronchi, lungs, thyroid, thymus, peripheral nerves, lymphoid tissue; aortic aneurysm; mediastinitis; cor pulmonale
Ribs Visible as thoracic cavity encasement	■ Break or misalignment ■ Widening of intercostal spaces	■ Fractured sternum or ribs ■ Emphysema
Spine Visible midline in the posterior chest; straight bony structure	■ Spinal curvature ■ Break or misalignment	■ Scoliosis, kyphosis ■ Fractures
Clavicles Visible in upper thorax; intact and equidistant in properly centered X-ray films	■ Break or misalignment	■ Fractures

SELECTED CLINICAL IMPLICATIONS OF CHEST X-RAY FILMS *(continued)*

Normal anatomic location and appearance	Possible abnormality	Implications
Hila (lung roots) Visible above the heart, where pulmonary vessels, bronchi, and lymph nodes join the lungs; appear as small, white, bilateral densities	▪ Shift to one side ▪ Accentuated shadows	▪ Atelectasis ▪ Pneumothorax, emphysema, pulmonary abscess, tumor, enlarged lymph nodes
Mainstem bronchus Visible; part of the hila with translucent tubelike appearance	▪ Spherical or oval density	▪ Bronchogenic cyst
Bronchi Usually not visible	▪ Visible	▪ Bronchial pneumonia
Lung fields Usually not visible throughout, except for the blood vessels	▪ Visible ▪ Irregular	▪ Atelectasis ▪ Resolving pneumonia, infiltrates, silicosis, fibrosis, metastatic neoplasm
Hemidiaphragm Rounded, visible; right side $\frac{3}{8}''$ to $\frac{3}{4}''$ (1 to 2 cm)	▪ Elevation of diaphragm (difference in elevation can be measured on inspiration and expiration to detect movement) ▪ Flattening of diaphragm ▪ Unilateral elevation of either side ▪ Unilateral elevation of left side only	▪ Active tuberculosis, pneumonia, pleurisy, acute bronchitis, active disease of the abdominal viscera, bilateral phrenic nerve involvement, atelectasis ▪ Asthma, emphysema ▪ Possible unilateral phrenic nerve paresis ▪ Perforated ulcer (rare), gas distention of stomach or splenic flexure of colon, free air in abdomen

Precautions

▪ Know that chest radiography is usually contraindicated during the first trimester of pregnancy; however, when radiography is absolutely necessary, a lead apron placed over the patient's abdomen can shield the fetus.

▪ If the patient is intubated, check that no tubes have been dislodged during positioning.

▪ To avoid exposure to radiation, leave the room or the immediate area while the films are being taken. If you must stay in the area, wear a lead-lined apron or protective clothing.

Findings

For an overview of normal and abnormal chest radiography findings, see the accompanying chart. For an accurate diagnosis, radiography findings must be correlated with the results of additional radiologic and pulmonary tests as well as physical assessment findings. For example, pulmonary hyperinflation with a low diaphragm and generalized increased radiolucency may suggest emphysema, but may also occur in a healthy person.

Interfering factors

- Portable chest X-rays (possibly lower-quality image than stationary X-rays)
- Portable chest X-rays taken in the anteroposterior position (may show larger cardiac shadowing than other X-rays due to shorter distance between beam and anterior structures)
- Patient in a supine position (hides fluid levels that are visible in decubitus views)
- Age and sex of the patient (may influence findings)
- The patient's inability to take a full inspiration
- Underexposure or overexposure of films
- Incorrect view of the area (For example, lateral film views reveal infiltrates [pneumonia, atelectasis] that may not be seen in anteroposterior views or posteroanterior views because of heart obstruction.)

Paranasal sinus radiography

The paranasal sinuses—air-filled cavities lined with mucous membranes—lie within the maxillary, ethmoid, sphenoid, and frontal bones. Sinus abnormalities resulting from inflammation, trauma, cysts, mucoceles, granulomatosis, and other conditions may include distorted bony sinus walls, altered mucous membranes, and fluid or masses within the cavities. In paranasal sinus radiography, X-rays or electromagnetic waves penetrate the paranasal sinuses and react on specially sensitized film, forming a film image that differentiates sinus structures.

When surrounding facial structures that are superimposed on the paranasal sinuses interfere with visualization of relevant areas, computed tomography scanning may be performed to provide further information.

Purpose

- To detect unilateral or bilateral abnormalities, possibly indicating trauma or disease
- To confirm diagnosis of neoplastic or inflammatory paranasal sinus disease
- To determine the location and size of a malignant neoplasm

Patient preparation

- Explain to the patient that paranasal sinus radiography helps evaluate abnormalities of the paranasal sinuses.
- Describe the test, including who will perform it and where it will take place.
- Tell the patient that his head may be immobilized in a foam vise during the test to help him maintain the correct position, but that the vise doesn't hurt.
- Explain to the patient that he'll be asked to sit upright and avoid moving while the X-rays are being taken to prevent blurring of the image and to allow visualization of air-fluid levels, if present. Emphasize the importance of his cooperation.

ABNORMAL FINDINGS IN PARANASAL SINUS RADIOGRAPHY

Disorder	Abnormal findings
Paranasal sinus trauma or fracture	■ Edema or hemorrhage in mucous membrane lining or sinus cavity ■ Clouded sinus air cells ■ Air-fluid level ■ Radiolucent, linear bone defects ■ Irregular, overriding bone edges ■ Depression or displacement of bone fragments ■ Foreign bodies
Acute sinusitis	■ Swollen, inflamed mucous membrane ■ Inflammatory exudate ■ Hazy to opaque sinus air cells ■ Air-fluid level
Chronic sinusitis	■ Thickening or sclerosis of bony wall of affected sinus
Wegener's granulomatosis	■ Clouded to opaque sinus air cells ■ Destruction of bony sinus wall
Malignant neoplasm	■ Rounded or lobulated soft-tissue mass, projecting into sinus ■ Destruction of bony sinus wall
Benign bone tumor	■ Distortion of bony sinus wall in specific patterns
Cyst, polyp, or benign tumor	■ Rounded or lobulated soft-tissue mass, projecting into sinus
Mucocele	■ Clouded sinus air cells ■ Destruction of bony sinus wall resulting in various degrees of radiolucency

■ Instruct the patient to remove dentures, all jewelry, and metallic objects in the X-ray field.

Procedure and posttest care
■ Have the patient sit upright (his head may be placed in a foam vise) between the X-ray tube and a film cassette.
■ During the test, the X-ray tube is positioned at specific angles and the patient's head is placed in various standard positions while his paranasal sinuses are filmed from different angles. If necessary, assist with positioning the patient.

Precautions
■ Be aware that paranasal sinus radiography is usually contraindicated during pregnancy; however, when it's absolutely necessary, a lead-lined apron placed over the patient's abdomen can shield the fetus.
■ To avoid exposure to radiation, leave the room or the immediate area during the test; if you must stay in the area, wear a lead-lined apron.

Normal findings

Normal paranasal sinuses are radiolucent and filled with air, which appears black on films.

Abnormal findings

See *Abnormal findings in paranasal sinus radiography,* page 617.

Interfering factors

- The presence of dentures, jewelry, or other metallic objects in the X-ray field or the presence of numerous metallic foreign bodies around the paranasal sinuses (possible poor imaging)
- Patient movement (possible poor imaging)
- Patient unable to sit upright (may require supine position, reducing diagnostic value of test)
- Superimposition of the surrounding facial structures on the film (obscures paranasal sinuses)

Fluoroscopy

In fluoroscopy, a continuous stream of X-rays passes through the patient, casting shadows of the heart, lungs, and diaphragm on a fluorescent screen, which allows moving structures to be studied. Because fluoroscopy reveals less detail than standard chest radiography, it's indicated only when diagnosis requires visualization of physiologic or pathologic motion of thoracic contents — for example, to rule out paralysis in the patient with diaphragmatic elevation.

Purpose

- To assess lung expansion and contraction during quiet breathing, deep breathing, and coughing

- To assess movement and paralysis of the diaphragm (sniff test) or digestive tract
- To detect bronchial obstructions and pulmonary disease
- To assist with the placement of tubes or catheters, such as a pulmonary artery (PA) catheter or a central venous catheter

Patient preparation

- Explain to the patient that fluoroscopy assesses respiratory structures and their motion.
- Describe the test, including who will perform it and where it will take place.
- Tell the patient that he'll be asked to follow specific instructions — for example, to breathe deeply and cough — while X-ray images depict his breathing.
- Instruct the patient to remove all jewelry and other metallic objects within the X-ray field.

Procedure and posttest care

- If necessary, assist with positioning the patient.
- Move cardiac monitoring cables, I.V. tubing from subclavian lines, PA catheter lines, and safety pins as far from the X-ray field as possible.
- During the test, the patient's cardiopulmonary or digestive motion is observed on a screen. Special equipment may be used to intensify the images, or a videotape recording of the fluoroscopy may be made for later study.

Precautions

- Know that fluoroscopy is contraindicated during pregnancy.
- If the patient is intubated, check that no tubes have been dislodged during positioning.
- To avoid exposure to radiation, leave the room or the immediate area during

the test; if you must stay in the area, wear a lead-lined apron.

Normal findings

Normal diaphragmatic movement is synchronous and symmetrical. Normal diaphragmatic excursion ranges from ¾″ to 1⅝″ (2 to 4 cm).

Abnormal findings

Diminished diaphragmatic movement may indicate pulmonary disease. Increased lung translucency may indicate loss of elasticity or bronchial obstruction. In an elderly patient, the lowest part of the trachea may be displaced to the right by an elongated aorta.

Diminished or paradoxical diaphragmatic movement may indicate paralysis of the diaphragm; however, fluoroscopy may not detect such paralysis in the patient who compensates for diminished diaphragm function by forcefully contracting his abdominal muscles to aid expiration.

Gaps in the stomach or small intestine may indicate ulcers or poor peristalsis.

Interfering factors

■ Failure to remove all metallic objects within the X-ray field (possible poor imaging)

Chest tomography

Also called laminagraphy, planigraphy, stratigraphy, or body section roentgenography, chest tomography provides clearly focused radiographic images of selected body sections otherwise obscured by shadows of overlying or underlying structures. In this procedure, the X-ray tube and film move around the patient in opposite directions (a motion called the linear tube sweep), producing exposures in

---

SPIRAL CT

The spiral (helical) computed tomography (CT) scan is produced while the X-ray tube rotates continuously around the patient, forming a spiral path through the patient. This path represents a contiguous volumetric data set, covering a specific volume of the patient's anatomy with no spatial or temporal gaps. The patient continuously moves through the slip-ring gantry, and no two data points are taken in exactly the same plane.

Benefits include increased speed (spiral CT is typically 8 to 10 times faster than conventional CT), improved image quality and diagnostic accuracy, and reduced radiation exposure. The improved speed—the scan can usually be obtained during a single breath hold—is especially beneficial for elderly, pediatric, and critically ill populations, in which scanning commonly proves difficult.

There are disadvantages. Spiral CT delivers a limited amount of milliamperes, which can result in a grainier image than conventional CT (more common in larger patients). In addition, artifacts ("pseudothrombi") can be created in the infrahepatic inferior vena cava by the admixture of unopacified blood and contrast medium flowing in from the renal veins. These disadvantages are being resolved with improved equipment and technique.

---

which a selected body plane appears sharply defined and the areas above and below it are blurred. Some facilities have spiral computed tomography (CT) available. (See *Spiral CT.*) It's used to further evaluate chest lesions when other tests are inconclusive. In more modern facilities,

CT has superseded plain film tomography.

Purpose

■ To demonstrate pulmonary densities (for cavitation, calcification, and presence of fat), tumors (especially those obstructing the bronchial lumen), or lesions (especially those located deep within the mediastinum such as at lymph nodes at the hilum)
■ To evaluate severity of disease such as emphysema

Patient preparation

■ Explain to the patient that chest tomography helps evaluate lesions inside the chest.
■ Describe the test, including who will perform it and where it will take place.
■ Tell the patient that he need not restrict food and fluids.
■ Warn the patient that the equipment is noisy because of rapidly moving metal-on-metal parts and that the X-ray tube swings overhead.
■ Advise the patient to breathe normally during the test, but to remain immobile; tell him that foam wedges will be used to help him maintain a comfortable, motionless position.
■ Tell the patient to close his eyes to prevent involuntary movement.
■ Instruct the patient to remove all jewelry and metallic objects within the X-ray field.

Procedure and posttest care

■ The patient is placed in a supine position or in different degrees of lateral rotation on the X-ray table. The X-ray tube then swings over the patient, taking numerous films from different angles.
■ For lung tomography, the X-ray tube is usually moved in a linear direction, but

may be moved in a hypocycloid, circular, elliptic, trispiral, or figure-eight pattern. Multidirectional films aid in the diagnosis of mediastinal lesions or tumors.

Precautions

■ Know that tomography is contraindicated during pregnancy.
■ To avoid exposure to radiation, leave the room or the immediate area during the test; if you must stay in the area, wear a lead-lined apron.

Normal findings

A normal chest tomogram shows structures equivalent to those seen on a normal chest radiograph film.

Abnormal findings

Central calcification in a nodule suggests a benign lesion; an irregularly bordered tumor suggests malignancy; and a sharply defined tumor suggests granuloma or nonmalignancy. Evaluation of the hilum can help differentiate blood vessels from nodes, detect tumor extension into the hilar lung area, and identify bronchial dilation, stenosis, and endobronchial lesions. Tomography can also identify extension of a mediastinal lesion to the ribs or spine.

Interfering factors

■ Failure to remove all metallic objects within the X-ray field (possible poor imaging)
■ An uncooperative patient

Bronchography

Bronchography is X-ray examination of the tracheobronchial tree after instillation of a radiopaque iodine contrast agent through a catheter into the lumens of the trachea and bronchi. The contrast agent coats the bronchial tree, permitting visualization of any anatomic deviations. Bronchography of a localized lung area may be accomplished by instilling contrast dye through a fiber-optic bronchoscope placed in the area to be filmed.

Since the development of computed tomography scanning, bronchography is used less frequently. It may be performed using a local anesthetic instilled through the catheter or bronchoscope, although a general anesthetic may be necessary for children or during a concurrent bronchoscopy.

Purpose
- To help detect bronchiectasis and map its location for surgical resection
- To detect bronchial obstruction, pulmonary tumors, cysts, and cavities and, indirectly, to pinpoint the cause of hemoptysis
- To provide permanent films of pathologic findings
- To guide procedures such as bronchoscopy

Patient preparation
- Explain to the patient that bronchography helps evaluate abnormalities of the bronchial structures.
- Instruct the patient to fast for 12 hours before the test.
- Tell the patient to perform good oral hygiene the night before and the morning of the test.
- Explain who will perform the test and where and when it will take place.
- Make sure the patient or a responsible family member has signed an informed consent form.
- Check the patient's history for hypersensitivity to anesthetics, iodine, or contrast media.
- If the patient has a productive cough, administer a prescribed expectorant and perform postural drainage 1 to 3 days before the test.
- If the procedure is to be performed under a local anesthetic, tell the patient he'll receive a sedative to help him relax and to suppress the gag reflex. Prepare him for the unpleasant taste of the anesthetic spray. Warn him that he may experience some difficulty breathing during the procedure, but reassure him that his airway won't be blocked and that he'll receive enough oxygen. Tell him the catheter or bronchoscope will pass more easily if he relaxes.
- If bronchography is to be performed under a general anesthetic, inform the patient that he'll receive a sedative before the test to help him relax.
- Just before the test, instruct the patient to remove his dentures (if present) and to void.

Equipment
Radiograph machine, tilting table, sedative, anesthetic, catheter or bronchoscope, radiopaque oils or water-soluble contrast agent, emergency resuscitation equipment

Procedure and posttest care
- After a local anesthetic is sprayed into the patient's mouth and throat, a bronchoscope or catheter is passed into the trachea and the anesthetic and contrast medium are instilled.
- The patient is placed in various positions during the test to promote movement of the contrast medium into different areas of the bronchial tree. After X-rays are taken, the contrast medium is removed through postural drainage and by having the patient cough it up.

CLINICAL ALERT *Watch for signs of laryngeal spasms (dyspnea) or edema (hoarseness, dyspnea, laryngeal stridor) secondary to traumatic intubation. Also, immediately report signs of allergic reaction to the contrast medium or anesthetic, such as itching, dyspnea, tachycardia, palpitations, excitation, hypotension, hypertension, or euphoria.*

■ Withhold food, fluids, and oral medications until the gag reflex returns (usually in 2 hours). Fluid intake before the gag reflex returns may cause aspiration.

■ Encourage gentle coughing and postural drainage to facilitate clearing of the contrast medium. A postdrainage film is usually done in 24 to 48 hours.

■ Watch for signs of chemical or secondary bacterial pneumonia — fever, dyspnea, crackles, or rhonchi — the result of incomplete expectoration of the contrast medium.

■ If the patient has a sore throat, reassure him that it's only temporary and provide throat lozenges or a liquid gargle when his gag reflex returns.

■ Advise the outpatient not to resume his usual activities until the next day.

Precautions

■ Know that bronchography is contraindicated during pregnancy.

■ Keep in mind that the test is also contraindicated in people with hypersensitivity to iodine or contrast media, and usually in people with respiratory insufficiency.

■ Observe the patient with asthma for laryngeal spasm (such as dyspnea) secondary to the instillation of the contrast medium.

■ Observe the patient with chronic obstructive pulmonary disease for airway occlusion secondary to the instillation of the contrast medium.

Normal findings

The right mainstem bronchus is shorter, wider, and more vertical than the left bronchus. Successive branches of the bronchi become smaller in diameter and are free from obstruction or lesions.

Abnormal findings

Bronchography may demonstrate bronchiectasis or bronchial obstruction due to tumors, cysts, cavities, or foreign objects. Findings must be correlated with physical examination, patient history, and perhaps other pulmonary studies.

Interfering factors

■ Presence of secretions or improper patient positioning (possible poor imaging due to inadequate filling of bronchial tree)

■ Inability to suppress coughing (interferes with bronchial filling and retention of the contrast medium)

Pulmonary angiography

Also called *pulmonary arteriography,* pulmonary angiography is the radiographic examination of the pulmonary circulation following injection of a radiopaque iodine contrast agent into the pulmonary artery or one of its branches.

Possible complications include arterial occlusion, myocardial perforation or rupture, ventricular arrhythmias from myocardial irritation, and acute renal failure from hypersensitivity to the contrast agent.

Purpose

■ To detect pulmonary embolism in a patient who is equivocal

■ To evaluate pulmonary circulation abnormalities

- To evaluate pulmonary circulation preoperatively in the patient with congenital heart disease
- To locate a large embolus before surgical removal

Patient preparation
- Describe the pulmonary angiography procedure to the patient. Explain that this test permits evaluation of the blood vessels to help identify the cause of his symptoms.
- Instruct the patient to fast for 8 hours before the test or as prescribed. Tell him who will perform the test, where it will take place, and that laboratory work for kidney function and coagulation may precede the test.
- Tell the patient that a small puncture will be made in the blood vessel of his right arm where blood samples are usually drawn, or in the right groin at the femoral vein, and that a local anesthetic will be used to numb the area. Inform him that a small catheter will then be inserted into the blood vessel and passed into the right side of the heart to the pulmonary artery.
- Tell the patient the contrast medium will then be injected into this artery. Warn him that he may feel flushed, experience an urge to cough, or experience a salty taste for approximately 3 to 5 minutes after the injection.
- Inform the patient that his heart rate will be monitored continuously during the procedure and that he should tell the physician or nurse if he has concerns.
- Make sure that the patient or a responsible family member has signed an informed consent form. Check the patient's history for hypersensitivity to anesthetics, iodine, seafood, or radiographic contrast agents.

- Obtain or check laboratory tests (including prothrombin time, partial thromboplastin time, platelet count, and blood urea nitrogen [BUN] and serum creatinine levels), and notify the radiologist of any abnormal results. I.V. hydration may need to be considered depending on the patient's renal and cardiac status. The radiologist may want to discontinue a heparin drip 3 to 4 hours before the test.

Equipment
Angiography tray, 50 ml of contrast medium, imaging equipment, angiography catheters and guide wires, monitoring equipment (electrocardiogram, arterial oxygen saturation, blood pressure, pulmonary artery pressure), emergency resuscitation equipment

Procedure and posttest care
- After the patient is placed in a supine position, the local anesthetic is injected and the cardiac monitor is attached to the patient. Blood pressure and pulse oximeter are monitored as per facility protocol.
- A puncture is made at the procedure site, and a catheter is introduced into the antecubital or femoral vein. As the catheter passes through the right atrium, the right ventricle, and the pulmonary artery, pressures are measured and blood samples are drawn from various regions of the pulmonary circulation.
- The contrast medium is injected and circulates through the pulmonary artery and lung capillaries while X-rays are taken.
- Apply pressure over the catheter insertion site for 15 to 20 minutes or until bleeding stops.
- Maintain bed rest for about 6 hours.
- Observe the site for bleeding and swelling. If either occur, maintain pres-

sure at the insertion site for 10 minutes and notify the radiologist.

■ Check the patient's blood pressure and pulse rate and the catheter insertion site (arm or groin) every 15 minutes for 1 hour, every hour for 4 hours, and then every 4 hours for 16 hours.

■ Observe the patient for signs of myocardial perforation or rupture by monitoring vital signs.

■ Be alert for signs of acute renal failure, such as sudden onset of oliguria, nausea, and vomiting. Check BUN and serum creatinine levels.

■ Check the catheter insertion site for inflammation or hematoma formation and report symptoms of a delayed hypersensitivity response to the contrast agent or to the local anesthetic (dyspnea, itching, tachycardia, palpitations, hypotension or hypertension, excitation, or euphoria).

■ Advise the patient about any restriction of activity. Tell him that he may resume his usual diet after the test (encourage him to drink lots of fluids), or administer I.V. fluids, as ordered, to flush the contrast agent from his body.

Precautions

■ Pulmonary angiography is contraindicated during pregnancy.

■ Monitor the patient for ventricular arrhythmias due to myocardial irritation from passage of the catheter through the heart chambers.

■ Observe for signs of hypersensitivity to the contrast agent, such as dyspnea, nausea, vomiting, sweating, increased heart rate, and numbness of extremities.

■ Keep emergency equipment available in case of a hypersensitivity reaction to the contrast agent.

■ Measure pulmonary artery pressures. Right ventricular end-diastolic pressure is usually less than or equal to 20 mm Hg,

and pulmonary artery systolic pressure is usually less than or equal to 70 mm Hg. Pressures greater than this increase the risk of mortality associated with this procedure.

Normal findings

Normally, the contrast agent flows symmetrically and without interruption through the pulmonary circulatory system.

Abnormal findings

Interruption of blood flow may result from emboli and from other types of pulmonary vascular abnormalities or tumors.

Interfering factors

■ None significant

SCANNING

Lung perfusion scan

A lung perfusion scan produces an image of pulmonary blood flow after I.V. injection of a radiopharmaceutical, either human serum albumin microspheres or macroaggregated albumin bonded to technetium.

Purpose

■ To assess arterial perfusion of the lungs
■ To detect pulmonary emboli
■ To evaluate pulmonary function before lung resection

Patient preparation

■ Tell the patient that the lung perfusion scan helps evaluate respiratory function.
■ Explain to the patient that he need not restrict food and fluids.

■ Describe to the patient the test, including who will perform it and where it will take place.

■ Tell the patient that a radiopharmaceutical will be injected into a vein in his arm and that he'll then sit in front of a camera or lie under it. Explain that neither the camera nor the uptake probe emits radiation and that the amount of radioactivity in the radiopharmaceutical is minimal.

■ Assure the patient that he'll be comfortable during the test and that he doesn't have to remain perfectly still.

■ On the test request, note if the patient has conditions, such as chronic obstructive pulmonary disease (COPD), vasculitis, pulmonary edema, tumor, sickle cell disease, or parasitic disease.

■ Ensure that the patient or a responsible family member has signed an informed consent form, if required.

Equipment
Scanner; radiopharmaceutical agent for I.V. use; I.V. insertion equipment, if needed

Procedure and posttest care
■ With the patient supine and taking moderately deep breaths, the radiopharmaceutical is injected I.V. slowly over 5 to 10 seconds to allow more even distribution of pulmonary blood flow.

■ After the injection, the gamma camera takes a series of single stationary images in the anterior, posterior, oblique, and both lateral chest views.

■ Images, which are projected on an oscilloscope screen, show the distribution of radioactive particles.

■ If a hematoma develops at the injection site, apply warm soaks.

Precautions
■ A lung scan is contraindicated in the patient who's hypersensitive to the radiopharmaceutical.

Normal findings
Areas with normal blood perfusion, called hot spots, show a high uptake of the radioactive substance; a normal lung shows a uniform uptake pattern.

Abnormal findings
Areas of low radioactive uptake, called *cold spots,* indicate poor perfusion, suggesting an embolism; however, a ventilation scan is necessary to confirm diagnosis. Decreased regional blood flow that occurs without vessel obstruction may indicate pneumonitis.

Interfering factors
■ Scheduling more than one radionuclide test per day, especially if using different tracing substances (may hinder diffusion of tracer isotope in second test)

■ Administering all the radiopharmaceutical while the patient is sitting (possible poor imaging due to settling of tracer isotope in lung bases)

■ Conditions, such as COPD, vasculitis, pulmonary edema, tumor, sickle cell disease, and parasitic disease (possible poor imaging)

Lung ventilation scan

The lung ventilation scan is performed after the patient inhales a mixture of air and radioactive gas that delineates areas of the lung ventilated during respiration. The scan records gas distribution during three phases: the buildup of radioactive gas (wash-in phase), the time after rebreathing when radioactivity reaches a steady level (equilibrium phase), and after removal of the radioactive gas from the lungs (wash-out phase).

Purpose
- To help diagnose pulmonary emboli
- To identify areas of the lung capable of ventilation
- To help evaluate regional respiratory function
- To locate regional hypoventilation, which may indicate atelectasis, obstructing tumors, or chronic obstructive pulmonary disease

Patient preparation
- Describe the lung ventilation scan to the patient and explain that this test helps evaluate respiratory function.
- Tell the patient that he need not restrict food and fluids.
- Tell the patient who will perform the test and where it will take place.
- Ask the patient to remove all jewelry and metal objects from the scanning field.
- Explain to the patient that he'll be asked to hold his breath for a short time after inhaling a gas and to remain still while a machine scans his chest.
- Reassure the patient that a minimal amount of radioactive gas is used.
- Ensure that the patient or a responsible family member has signed an informed consent form, if required.

Equipment
Nuclear scanner, radioactive gas, mask

Procedure and posttest care
- After the patient inhales air mixed with a small amount of radioactive gas through a mask, its distribution in the lungs is monitored on a nuclear scanner.
- The patient's chest is scanned as he exhales.

Precautions
- Watch for leaks in the closed system of radioactive gas, such as through the mask, which can contaminate the surrounding atmosphere.

Normal findings
Normal findings include an equal distribution of gas in both lungs and normal wash-in and wash-out phases.

Abnormal findings
Unequal gas distribution in both lungs indicates poor ventilation or airway obstruction in areas with low radioactivity. When compared with a lung scan (perfusion scan), in vascular obstructions—such as pulmonary embolism—the perfusion to the embolized area is decreased, but the ventilation to this area is maintained; in parenchymal disease, such as pneumonia, ventilation is abnormal within the areas of consolidation.

Interfering factors
- Failure to remove jewelry and other metal objects from the scanning field (possible poor imaging)

Thoracic computed tomography

Thoracic computed tomography (CT) provides cross-sectional views of the chest by passing an X-ray beam from a computerized scanner through the body at different angles. CT scanning may be done with or without an injected contrast medium, which is primarily used to highlight blood vessels and to allow greater visual discrimination.

This test provides a three-dimensional image and is especially useful in detecting small differences in tissue density. The thoracic CT scan may replace mediastinoscopy in the diagnosis of mediastinal masses and Hodgkin's disease; its value in the evaluation of pulmonary pathology is proven.

Purpose

■ To locate suspected neoplasms (such as in Hodgkin's disease), especially with mediastinal involvement
■ To differentiate coin-sized calcified lesions (indicating tuberculosis) from tumors
■ To differentiate emphysema or bronchopleural fistula from lung abscess
■ To distinguish tumors adjacent to the aorta from aortic aneurysms
■ To detect the invasion of a neck mass in the thorax
■ To evaluate primary malignancy that may metastasize to the lungs, especially in the patient with a primary bone tumor, soft-tissue sarcoma, or melanoma
■ To evaluate the mediastinal lymph nodes
■ To evaluate the severity of lung disease such as emphysema
■ To detect a dissection or leak of an aortic aneurysm or aortic arch aneurysm
■ To plan radiation treatment

Patient preparation

■ Explain to the patient that the thoracic CT provides cross-sectional views of the chest and distinguishes small differences in tissue density.
■ If a contrast medium won't be used, inform the patient that he need not restrict food and fluids. If the test is to be performed with contrast enhancement, instruct him to fast for 4 hours before the test.
■ Tell the patient who will perform the test and where it will take place.
■ Inform the patient that he'll be positioned on an X-ray table that moves into

the center of a large ring-shaped piece of X-ray equipment and that the equipment may be noisy.
■ Inform the patient that a contrast medium may be injected into a vein in his arm. If so, he may experience nausea, warmth, flushing of the face, and a salty or metallic taste. Reassure him that these symptoms are normal and that radiation exposure is minimal.
■ Tell the patient not to move during the test, but to breathe normally until told to follow specific breathing instructions. Instruct him to remove all jewelry and metallic objects in the X-ray field.
■ Check the patient's history for hypersensitivity to iodine, shellfish, or contrast media.
■ Ensure that the patient or a responsible family member has signed an informed consent form, if required.

Equipment

CT scanner; contrast medium, if ordered; I.V. insertion equipment, if necessary

Procedure and posttest care

■ After the patient is placed in a supine position on the X-ray table and the contrast medium has been injected, the machine scans the patient at different angles while the computer calculates small differences in the densities of various tissues, water, fat, bone, and air.
■ This information is displayed as a printout of numerical values and as a projection on a monitor. Images may be recorded for further study.
■ Watch the patient for signs of delayed hypersensitivity to the contrast medium (itching, hypotension or hypertension, or respiratory distress).
■ After the test, encourage the patient to drink lots of fluids.

Precautions

- Know that thoracic CT scanning is contraindicated during pregnancy.
- Keep in mind that the test is also contraindicated—if a contrast medium is used—in a person who has a history of hypersensitivity reactions to iodine, shellfish, or contrast media.

Normal findings

Black and white areas on a thoracic CT scan refer, respectively, to air and bone densities. Shades of gray correspond to water, fat, and soft-tissue densities.

Abnormal findings

Abnormal thoracic CT findings include tumors, nodules, cysts, aortic aneurysms, enlarged lymph nodes, pleural effusion, and accumulations of blood, fluid, or fat.

Interfering factors

- Failure to remove all metallic objects from the scanning field (possible poor imaging)
- The patient's inability to remain still during the procedure
- An obese patient (may be too heavy for scanning table)

Selected readings

Cavanaugh, B.M. *Nurse's Manual of Laboratory and Diagnostic Tests*, 4th ed. Philadelphia: F.A. Davis Co., 2003.

Finkelstein, S.E., et al. "Virtual Bronchoscopy for Evaluation of Malignant Tumors of the Thorax," *Journal of Cardiovascular Surgery* 123(5):967-72, May 2002.

Gilkeson, R.C., and Ciancibello, L. "Virtual Bronchoscopy: Technical Features and Clinical Applications," *Applied Radiology* 32(4), May 2003. *www.medscape.com/viewarticle/452491*.

Goldman, L., and Ausiello, D., eds. *Cecil Textbook of Medicine*, 22nd ed. Philadelphia: W.B. Saunders Co., 2004.

Guyton, A.C., and Hall, J.E. *Textbook of Medical Physiology*, 10th ed. Philadelphia: W.B. Saunders Co., 2001.

Henry, J.B., et al. *Clinical Diagnosis and Management by Laboratory Methods*, 20th ed. Philadelphia: W.B. Saunders Co., 2001.

Hunter, C.J., et.al. "A Comparison of the Validity of Different Diagnostic Tests in Adults with Asthma," *Chest* 121(4):1051-57, April 2002.

McClatchey, K.D. *Clinical Laboratory Medicine*, 2nd ed. Philadelphia: Lippincott Williams & Wilkins, 2002.

Pagana, K.D., and Pagana, T.J. *Mosby's Diagnostic and Laboratory Test Reference*, 6th ed. St. Louis: Mosby Year–Book, Inc., 2003.

Schnell, Z., et al. *Davis's Comprehensive Handbook of Laboratory and Diagnostic Tests with Nursing Implications*. Philadelphia: F.A. Davis Co., 2003.

Wilkins, R.L., and Stoller, J.K. *Egan's Fundamentals of Respiratory Care*, 8th ed. St. Louis: Mosby Year–Book, Inc., 2003.

Wilkinson, T.M., et al. "Airway Bacterial Load and FEV_1 Decline in Patients with Chronic Obstructive Pulmonary Disease," *American Journal of Respiratory and Critical Care Medicine* 167(8):1090-95, April 2003.

Wood, B.J., and Razavi, P. "Virtual Endoscopy: A Promising New Technology," *American Family Physician* 66(1):107-12, July 2002.

Skeletal system

Introduction

Diagnostic tests of the skeletal system help evaluate bones and their inner structures as well as the joints and lubricating fluids within them. These tests include various radiographic, nuclear medicine, and endoscopic techniques as well as joint aspiration, computed tomography scans, and magnetic resonance imaging with or without a contrast agent.

Several skeletal tests combine diagnosis and treatment. For example, arthroscopy permits direct visualization of a joint as well as removal of loose bodies within the joint, meniscectomy, meniscal repair, rotator cuff repair, abrasion arthroplasty, and release of the vastus lateralis muscle. Arthrocentesis and synovial fluid analysis provide a fluid sample for laboratory analysis as well as an avenue for local drug therapy.

Structure of bone

Bones are complex structures composed of living cells and nonliving intercellular substances. The intercellular matrix consists of inorganic salts—mostly calcium and phosphate—embedded in collagen fibers. All bones have some basic structures in common. They are covered by the periosteum, which is a white membrane of connective tissue with two layers: a superficial layer of dense irregular connective tissue and a deep layer containing osteoblasts, osteoclasts, blood vessels, nerves, and lymphatics. All bones also have a thin connective tissue membrane called the *endostium*. Long bones have a medullary cavity in the center of the diaphysis filled with yellow bone marrow.

Histologically, bone is of two basic types. *Cancellous (spongy) bone* contains many open spaces, which are filled with red and yellow bone marrow, between thin strands of bone called *trabeculae,* which are oriented along lines of stress or pressure and give the bone extra structural strength. *Compact bone* is strong and dense with many networks of interconnecting canals, each of which is known as a *haversian system.* A haversian canal runs centrally through each system, parallel to the bone's long axis, and contains one or two blood vessels that provide much of the bone's blood supply. The haversian canals are surrounded by concentric cylindrical layers called *lamellae,* which are closely spaced in compact bone. Small cavities called *lacunae* appear between the lamellae; each lacuna contains *osteocytes,* mature bone-forming cells that are suspended in tissue fluid. The lacunae are joined by a network of tiny canals called *canaliculi,* each of which contains one or more capillaries and provides an additional route for tissue fluids.

Red marrow, which produces blood cells, occupies the spaces in cancellous bone. At birth, all marrow is red marrow. In adults, red marrow appears mainly in the spongy part of cranial bones, in the ribs and sternum, in the vertebrae, and in portions of the femur, humerus, and other long bones. In neonates and children, it appears in many other bones. *Yellow marrow* is present in the shafts of long bones and extends into the haversian system. It's composed of adipose cells and can change to red marrow, if necessary.

Types of bone
Bones classified by shape include:
- *long bones* that are found in the extremities and consist of a shaft *(diaphysis)* and two bulbous ends *(epiphyses).* The parts of the shaft that flare to join the epiphyses are called *metaphyses;* these contain the bone's growth zones and become continuous with the epiphyses at maturity. Long bones are composed primarily of compact bone and include the humerus, radius, ulna, femur, tibia, fibula, phalanges, metacarpals, and metatarsals.
- *short bones* that consist mainly of cancellous bone with a thin compact bone shell and include the tarsal and carpal bones.
- *flat bones* that have a large surface area and provide protection for soft body parts. They have an inner layer of cancellous bone surrounded by compact bone. Examples of flat bones are the frontal and parietal bones of the cranium and the ribs, sternum, scapulae, ilium, and pubis.
- *irregular bones* that are of various shapes and composition and include the spine (vertebrae, sacrum, coccyx) and certain skull bones (sphenoid, ethmoid, and mandible).

Bones not classified by shape include the sesamoid (free-floating) bones—such as the patella—and the wormian bones, small clusters of bones found between some cranial bones.

All bones are covered with a fibrous layer called the *periosteum*—except at joints, where they're covered by articular cartilage.

Types of joints

Joints consist of two bones joined in various ways; like bones, they have varying forms.

■ *Fibrous joints* (synarthroses) have only minute motion and provide stability when tight union is necessary, as in the sutures joining the cranial bones.

■ *Cartilaginous joints* (amphiarthroses) allow limited movement, as between vertebrae.

■ *Synovial joints* (diarthroses), the most common type, allow angular and circular movement. To achieve freedom of movement, synovial joints have special characteristics: The bones' two articulating surfaces have a smooth hyaline covering (articular cartilage) resilient to pressure, their opposing surfaces are congruous and glide smoothly on each other, and a fibrous capsule holds them together. Lining the joint cavity is the *synovial membrane,* which secretes a clear viscous fluid called synovial fluid. This fluid lubricates the two opposing surfaces during motion and nourishes the articular cartilage. Surrounding each synovial joint are ligaments, muscles, and tendons, which strengthen and stabilize the joint, but allow free movement.

In some synovial joints, the synovial membrane forms two additional structures — bursae and tendon sheaths — which reduce friction. *Bursae* are small cushionlike sacs that are lined with synovial membranes and filled with synovial fluid; most are located between tendons and bones, as in the shoulders, knees, and elbows, but others are found between muscles and bones, ligaments and bones, and skin and bones. *Tendon sheaths* are modified bursae that wrap around a ten-

don to cushion it as it stretches across a joint. (See *Types of bones and joints,* page 632.)

Evaluating skeletal disorders

When a patient's reason for seeking care involves the skeletal system, make sure to obtain an accurate history. Ask the patient about general activities that may be affected by skeletal disease or trauma, such as his job, diet, recreation, sexual activity, and elimination habits. Does he have difficulty getting around or performing normal daily activities? Has he recently experienced trauma or a change in physical activity?

Ask the patient to describe his symptoms. When did they begin? Have they lessened or worsened? Has he previously sought treatment for the problem? If so, what was the result? Did he comply with the prescribed treatment? Ask if he's in pain at the moment and have him rate his pain on a scale of 0 to 10 (with 10 being the greatest level of pain), at rest and with activity. Has he been able to get relief from the pain? Does he require medication? If so, what kind and how much does he take?

Because joint or bone pain symptoms may indicate a systemic disease, a complete physical examination is essential. Observe the patient's general appearance, checking for localized edema, reddening of pressure points, point tenderness, effusion, and other deformities. Check the joint's active and passive range of motion, which may be restricted or painful. Palpate swollen joints to determine the nature of the swelling, which may result from synovial thickening, bone enlargement, or simple fluid effusion.

Pain thought to originate in a major joint may actually come from a minor one. Check the patient's neurovascular

TYPES OF BONES AND JOINTS

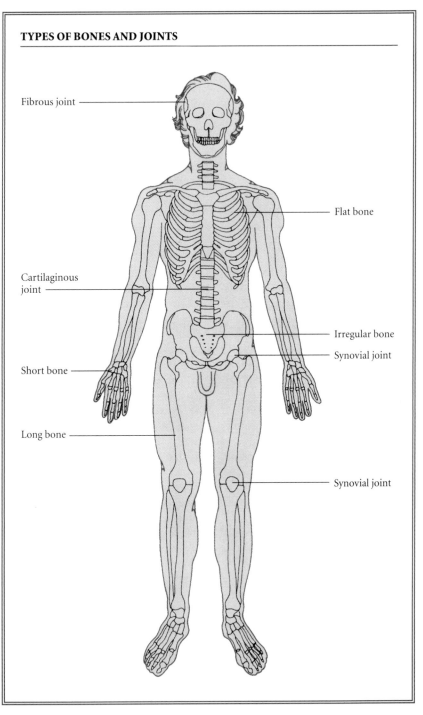

Fibrous joint

Flat bone

Cartilaginous joint

Irregular bone

Synovial joint

Short bone

Long bone

Synovial joint

status, including motion, sensation, and circulation. Measure and record dissimilarities in muscle circumference or limb length. Compare the size and shape of the affected joint with those of its unaffected opposite.

Types of diagnostic tests

Common diagnostic skeletal system tests include:

■ *Radiography* is probably the most widely used skeletal test. Because osseous tissue is quite dense, radiography readily demonstrates the skeletal system.

■ *Bone scan* is the examination of bone after I.V. injection of radioisotopes, which have an affinity for bone.

■ *Arthrography* is the radiographic examination of a joint after injection of air, a radiopaque dye, or both into the joint space.

■ *Arthrocentesis* is the aspiration of synovial fluid from a joint space (usually the knee) for diagnosis or to relieve pain caused by fluid accumulation.

■ *Arthroscopy,* the direct visualization of joint structures (usually the knee) using a fiber-optic endoscope, is particularly useful for detecting knee disorders (such as arthritis, a torn meniscus, cysts, and loose bodies) that aren't readily revealed by radiography or arthrography.

■ *Computed tomography scanning* provides cross-sectional images that can show successive layers or a specific plane of involved bone in detail.

■ *Magnetic resonance imaging,* a noninvasive imaging technique, uses magnetic fields, radio waves, and computers to show skeletal and soft-tissue abnormalities.

RADIOGRAPHY AND NUCLEAR MEDICINE

Vertebral radiography

Vertebral radiography visualizes all or part of the vertebral column. A commonly performed test, it's used to evaluate the vertebrae for deformities, fractures, dislocations, tumors, and other abnormalities. Bone films determine bone density, texture, erosion, and changes in bone relationships. X-rays of the cortex of the bone reveal the presence of any widening, narrowing, and signs of irregularity. Joint X-rays can reveal the presence of fluid, spur formation, narrowing, and changes in the joint structure.

The type and extent of vertebral radiography depends on the patient's clinical condition. For example, a patient with lower back pain requires only study of the lumbar and sacral segments.

Purpose

■ To detect vertebral fractures, dislocations, subluxations, and deformities

■ To detect vertebral degeneration, infection, and congenital disorders

■ To detect disorders of the intervertebral disks

■ To determine the vertebral effects of arthritic and metabolic disorders

Patient preparation

■ Explain to the patient that vertebral radiography permits examination of the spine.

■ Inform the patient that he need not restrict food and fluids.

■ Tell the patient the test requires X-ray films. Also tell him who will perform the test and where it will take place.

■ Advise the patient that he'll be placed in various positions for the X-ray films.

- Tell the patient that although some positions may cause slight discomfort, his cooperation is needed to ensure accurate results.
 - Stress to the patient that he must keep still and hold his breath during the procedure.

Procedure and posttest care
- The procedure varies considerably, depending on the vertebral segment being examined.
- Initially, the patient is placed in a supine position on the X-ray table for an anteroposterior view.
- The patient may be repositioned for lateral or right and left oblique views; specific positioning depends on the vertebral segment or adjacent structure of interest.
- Analgesics or local heat applications may relieve pain.

Precautions
- Vertebral radiography is contraindicated during the first trimester of pregnancy, unless the benefits outweigh the risk of fetal radiation exposure.
- Exercise extreme caution when handling a trauma patient with suspected spinal injuries, particularly of the cervical area. He should be filmed while on the stretcher to avoid further injury during transfer to the radiographic table.

Normal findings
Normal vertebrae show no fractures, subluxations, dislocations, curvatures, or other abnormalities. Specific positions and spacing of the vertebrae vary with the patient's age.

AGE ISSUE *In the lateral view, adult vertebrae are aligned to form four alternately concave and convex curves. The cervical and lumbar curves are convex an-teriorly; the thoracic and sacral curves are concave anteriorly. Although the structure of the coccyx varies, it usually points forward and downward. Neonatal vertebrae form only one curve, which is concave anteriorly.*

Abnormal findings
The vertebral radiograph readily shows spondylolisthesis, fractures, subluxations, dislocations, wedging, and such deformities as kyphosis, scoliosis, and lordosis.

To confirm other disorders, spinal structures and their spatial relationships on the radiograph must be examined, and the patient's history and clinical status must be considered. These disorders include congenital abnormalities, such as torticollis (wryneck), absence of sacral or lumbar vertebrae, hemivertebrae, and Klippel-Feil syndrome; degenerative processes, such as hypertrophic spurs, osteoarthritis, and narrowed disk spaces; tuberculosis (Pott's disease); benign or malignant intraspinal tumors; ruptured disk and cervical disk syndrome; and systemic disorders, such as rheumatoid arthritis, Charcot's disease, ankylosing spondylitis, osteoporosis, and Paget's disease.

Depending on radiographic results, definitive diagnosis may also require additional tests, such as myelography or computed tomography scanning.

Interfering factors
- Improper positioning of the patient or patient movement (possible poor imaging)

Arthrography

Arthrography allows radiographic examination of a joint after injection of a radiopaque dye, air, or both (double-contrast arthrogram) to outline soft-tissue structures and the contour of the joint. The joint is put through its range of motion while a series of radiographs are taken.

Indications for arthrography include persistent unexplained joint discomfort or pain. Complications may include persistent joint crepitus and allergic reactions to the contrast dye. Magnetic resonance imaging of the joint may be used in place of this test.

Purpose

■ To identify acute or chronic tears or other abnormalities of the joint capsule or supporting ligaments of the knee, shoulder, ankle, hips, or wrist
■ To detect internal joint derangements
■ To locate synovial cysts

Patient preparation

■ Describe arthrography to the patient and answer any questions he may have. Explain that this test permits examination of a joint.
■ Inform the patient that he need not restrict food and fluids.
■ Tell the patient who will perform the procedure and where it will take place.
■ Explain that the fluoroscope allows the physician to track the contrast medium as it fills the joint space.
■ Inform the patient that standard X-ray films will also be taken after diffusion of the contrast medium.
■ Tell the patient that, although the joint area will be anesthetized, he may experience a tingling sensation or pressure in the joint when the contrast medium is injected.
■ Instruct the patient to remain as still as possible during the procedure, except when following instructions to change position.
■ Stress to the patient the importance of his cooperation in assuming various posi-

tions because films must be taken as quickly as possible to ensure optimum quality.
■ Check the patient's history to determine if he's hypersensitive to local anesthetics, iodine, seafood, or dyes used for other diagnostic tests.

Equipment

Fluoroscope, skin-cleaning solution, local anesthetic, two 2″ 20G needles, two 24G needles, three 3-ml syringes, short lumbar puncture needle (3″ 22G needle for arthrography of the shoulder), water-soluble radiopaque dye (5 to 15 ml), four sterile sponges, elastic knee bandage, sterile towels, sterile specimen container for fluid, culture tube, sterile adhesive bandage, collodion (optional), shave preparation kit

Procedure and posttest care
Knee arthrography

■ The knee is cleaned with an antiseptic solution and the area around the puncture site is anesthetized. (It isn't usually necessary to anesthetize the joint space itself.)
■ A 2″ needle is then inserted into the joint space between the patella and femoral condyle and fluid is aspirated. The aspirated fluid is usually sent to the laboratory for analysis.
■ While the needle is still in place, the aspirating syringe is removed and replaced with a syringe containing dye.
■ If fluoroscopic examination demonstrates correct placement of the needle, the dye is injected into the joint space.
■ After the needle is removed, the site is rubbed with a sterile sponge and the wound may be sealed with collodion.
■ The patient is asked to walk a few steps or to move his knee through a range of motion to distribute the dye in the joint

space. A film series is quickly taken with the knee held in various positions.

■ If the films are clean and demonstrate proper dye placement, the knee is bandaged, possibly with an elastic bandage.

■ Tell the patient to keep the bandage in place for several days and teach him how to rewrap it.

Shoulder arthrography

■ The skin is prepared and a local anesthetic is injected subcutaneously just in front of the acromioclavicular joint.

■ Additional anesthetic is injected directly onto the head of the humerus.

■ The short lumbar puncture needle is inserted until the point is embedded in the joint cartilage.

■ The stylet is removed, a syringe of contrast medium is attached and, using fluoroscopic guidance, about 1 ml of dye is injected into the joint space, as the needle is withdrawn slightly.

■ If fluoroscopic examination demonstrates correct needle placement, the rest of the dye is injected while the needle is slowly withdrawn and the site is wiped with a sterile sponge.

■ A film series is taken quickly to achieve maximum contrast.

Both types

■ Tell the patient to rest the joint for at least 12 hours.

■ Inform the patient that he may experience some swelling or discomfort or may hear crepitant noises in the joint after the test, but that these symptoms usually disappear after 1 or 2 days; tell him to report persistent symptoms.

■ Advise the patient to apply ice to the joint if swelling occurs and to take a mild analgesic for pain.

■ Instruct the patient to report any signs of infection at the needle insertion site, such as warmth, redness, swelling, or foul-smelling drainage.

Precautions

■ Arthrography is contraindicated during pregnancy and in the patient with active arthritis, joint infection, or previous sensitivity to radiopaque media.

Normal findings

A normal knee arthrogram shows a characteristic wedge-shaped shadow, pointed toward the interior of the joint, which indicates a normal medial meniscus. A normal shoulder arthrogram shows the bicipital tendon sheath, redundant inferior joint capsule, and subscapular bursa intact.

Abnormal findings

Arthrography accurately detects medial meniscal tears and lacerations in 90% to 95% of cases. Because the entire joint lining is opacified, arthrography can demonstrate extrameniscal lesions, such as osteochondritis dissecans, chondromalacia patellae, osteochondral fractures, cartilaginous abnormalities, synovial abnormalities, tears of the cruciate ligaments, and disruption of the joint capsule and collateral ligaments.

Arthrography can reveal shoulder abnormalities, such as adhesive capsulitis, bicipital tenosynovitis or rupture, and rotator cuff tears. It can also evaluate damage from recurrent dislocations.

Interfering factors

■ Dilution of the contrast medium due to incomplete aspiration of joint effusion (possible poor imaging)

■ Improper injection technique (possible displacement of contrast medium)

Bone scan

A bone scan involves imaging the skeleton by a scanning camera after I.V. injection of a radioactive tracer compound. The tracer of choice, radioactive technetium diphosphonate, collects in bone tissue in increased concentrations at sites of abnormal metabolism. When scanned, these sites appear as hot spots that are typically detectable months before an X-ray can reveal a lesion. To promote early detection of lesions, this test may be performed with a gallium scan.

Purpose
- To detect or to rule out malignant bone lesions when radiographic findings are normal but cancer is confirmed or suspected
- To detect occult bone trauma due to pathologic fractures
- To monitor degenerative bone disorders
- To detect infection
- To evaluate unexplained bone pain
- To stage cancer

Patient preparation
- Describe the bone scan procedure to the patient. Explain that this test may detect skeletal abnormalities sooner than is possible with ordinary X-rays.
- Tell the patient who will perform the test, where it will take place, and that he may have to assume various positions on a scanner table. Emphasize that he must keep still for the scan.
- Assure the patient that the scan itself is painless and that the isotope, although radioactive, emits less radiation than a standard X-ray machine.
- Make sure that the patient or a responsible family member has signed an informed consent form, if required.

- If a bone scan is ordered to diagnose cancer, evaluate the patient's emotional state and offer support.
- Administer prescribed analgesics.
- After the patient receives an I.V. injection of the tracer and imaging agent, encourage him to increase his intake of fluids for the next 1 to 3 hours to facilitate renal clearance of the circulating free tracer.

Equipment
Bone mineral tracer; 3-ml syringe; 21G needle; I.V. insertion equipment, if needed; scanning camera

Procedure and posttest care
- Be aware that the patient receives an I.V. injection of tracer and imaging agent. Encourage increased fluids for the next 1 to 3 hours to facilitate renal clearance.
- Instruct the patient to void immediately before the procedure (otherwise, a urinary catheter may be inserted to empty the bladder), and then position him on the scanner table.
- As the scanner head moves back and forth over the patient's body, know that it detects low-level radiation emitted by the skeleton and translates this into a film, paper chart, or both to produce two-dimensional pictures of the area scanned.
- If appropriate, assist with repositioning the patient several times during the test to obtain adequate views. (The scanner takes as many views as needed to cover the specified area.)

⚙ **AGE ISSUE** *Anticipate the need to administer sedation to children who can't hold still for the scan.*
- Check the injection site for redness or swelling. If a hematoma develops, apply warm soaks.
- Don't schedule other radionuclide tests for 24 to 48 hours.

- Instruct the patient to drink lots of fluids and to empty his bladder frequently for the next 24 to 48 hours.
- Provide analgesics for pain resulting from positioning on the scanning table, as needed.

Precautions
- To avoid exposing the fetus or infant to radiation, a bone scan is contraindicated during pregnancy or lactation.
- Allergic reactions to radionuclides may occur.

Normal findings
The tracer concentrates in bone tissue at sites of new bone formation or increased metabolism. The epiphyses of growing bone are normal sites of high concentration, or hot spots.

Abnormal findings
Although a bone scan demonstrates hot spots that identify sites of bone formation, it doesn't distinguish between normal and abnormal bone formation. But scan results can identify all types of bone malignancy, infection, fracture, and other disorders if viewed in light of the patient's medical and surgical history, X-rays, and other laboratory tests.

Interfering factors
- Distended bladder (possible obscuring of pelvic detail)
- Improper injection technique (possible seepage of tracer into muscle tissue, creating false hot spots)
- Antihypertensives (invalidate test results)

Bone densitometry

Bone densitometry assesses bone mass quantitatively. This noninvasive technique, also known as dual energy X-ray absorptiometry, uses an X-ray tube to measure bone mineral density, but exposes the patient to only minimal radiation. The images detected are computer-analyzed to determine bone mineral status. The computer calculates the size and thickness of the bone as well as its volumetric density to determine its potential resistance to mechanical stress. It may be performed in the radiology department of a hospital, a physician's office, or a clinic.

Purpose
- To determine bone mineral density
- To identify the risk of osteoporosis
- To evaluate clinical response to therapy for reducing the rate of bone loss

Patient preparation
- Reassure the patient that the bone densitometry test is painless and that the exposure to radiation is minimal.
- Tell the patient that the test will take from 10 minutes to 1 hour, depending on the areas to be scanned.
- Tell the patient who will perform the test and where it will take place.

Procedure and posttest care
- Instruct the patient to remove all metallic objects from the area to be scanned.
- Know that the patient is positioned on a table under the scanning device, with the radiation source below and the detector above. The detector measures the bone's radiation absorption and produces a digital readout.

Precautions
- Bone densitometry is contraindicated during pregnancy.

Normal findings

Computer-analyzed results of the bone densitometry scan are within normal limits for the patient's age, sex, and height.

The patient's rate of bone loss can be treated over time.

Abnormal findings

The value and reliability of bone densitometry as a predictor of fractures are under investigation. Controversy exists regarding the scanning site and whether bone loss occurs as a general phenomenon or occurs first in the spine. Also, large-scale studies are being conducted to establish an "at-risk" level of bone density to help predict fractures.

Interfering factors

- Osteoarthritis (possible decrease)
- Fat tissue (poor visualization)
- Fractures
- Size of region to be scanned

SCANNING

Skeletal computed tomography

Skeletal computed tomography (CT) provides a series of tomograms, translated by a computer and displayed on a monitor, representing cross-sectional images of various layers (or slices) of bone. This technique can reconstruct cross-sectional, horizontal, sagittal, and coronal plane images.

Taking collimated (parallel) radiographs increases the number of radiation density calculations the computer makes, thereby improving the degree of resolution and thus specificity and accuracy. Hundreds of thousands of readings

of radiation levels absorbed by tissues may be combined to depict anatomic slices of varying thickness.

Purpose

- To determine the existence and extent of primary bone tumors, skeletal metastases, soft-tissue tumors, injuries to ligaments or tendons, and fractures
- To diagnose joint abnormalities difficult to detect by other methods

Patient preparation

- Explain to the patient that skeletal CT allows visualization of bones and joints. If contrast medium isn't ordered, tell him that he need not restrict food and fluids. If contrast medium is ordered, instruct him to fast for 4 hours before the test.
- Explain to the patient who will perform the procedure and where it will take place. Reassure him that the procedure is painless.
- Explain to the patient that he'll be positioned on an X-ray table inside a CT scanner and asked to lie still; the computer-controlled scanner will revolve around him taking multiple scans. Stress that he should lie as still as possible because movement may cause distorted images.
- If a contrast medium is used, tell the patient that he may feel flushed and warm and may experience a transient headache, a salty or metallic taste, and nausea or vomiting after its injection. Reassure him that these reactions are normal.
- Instruct the patient to wear a radiologic examining gown and remove all metal objects and jewelry in the X-ray field.

◆ **CLINICAL ALERT** *Check the patient's history for hypersensitivity reactions to iodine, shellfish, or contrast media. Mark such reactions in the chart and notify the physician, who may order pro-*

phylactic medications or choose not to use a contrast medium.

■ If the patient appears restless or apprehensive about the procedure, a mild sedative may be prescribed.

■ Ensure that the patient or a responsible family member has signed an informed consent form, if required.

Equipment

CT scanner; contrast medium; I.V. insertion equipment, if needed

Procedure and posttest care

■ Place the patient in a supine position on an X-ray table and tell him to lie as still as possible.

■ The table is slid into the circular opening of the CT scanner. The scanner revolves around the patient, taking radiographs at preselected intervals.

■ After the first set of scans is taken, the patient is removed from the scanner and a contrast medium is administered, if necessary.

■ Observe the patient for signs and symptoms of a hypersensitivity reaction, including pruritus, rash, and respiratory difficulty, for 30 minutes after the contrast medium has been injected.

■ After contrast medium I.V. injection, the patient is moved back into the scanner and another series of scans is taken. The images obtained from the scan are displayed on a monitor during the procedure and stored on magnetic tape to create a permanent record for subsequent study.

■ If contrast media is used, observe for a delayed allergic reaction and treat as necessary. (Diphenhydramine is the drug of choice.)

■ Encourage fluids to assist in eliminating the contrast medium.

■ Tell the patient that he may resume his usual diet and activities, if appropriate.

■ Provide comfort measures and pain medication, as ordered, because of prolonged positioning on the table.

Precautions

■ Know that this procedure is contraindicated during pregnancy.

■ Know that this test is contraindicated in a patient who's hypersensitive to iodine, shellfish, or contrast media, or in a patient with renal insufficiency (if he isn't on dialysis).

■ Be aware that the patient may experience strong feelings of claustrophobia or anxiety when inside the CT body scanner. In this case, a mild sedative may be ordered to help reduce anxiety.

■ For the patient with significant bone or joint pain, administer analgesics so that he can lie still comfortably during the scan.

Normal findings

The scan should reveal no pathology in the bones or joints. It produces crisp images of the structure while blurring or eliminating details of surrounding structures.

Abnormal findings

Because of its ability to display cross-sectional anatomy, CT scanning is useful for imaging the shoulder, spine, hip, and pelvis. The cross-sectional view eliminates the confusing shadows of superimposed structures that occur with conventional radiographs. The scan can reveal primary bone tumors and soft-tissue tumors as well as skeletal metastasis. It can also reveal joint abnormalities difficult to detect by other methods.

Interfering factors

■ Claustrophobia (possible interference with the patient's ability to lie in the scanner for long periods)

- Excessive patient movement
- Failure to remove metallic objects from the examination field (possible poor imaging)

Skeletal magnetic resonance imaging

A noninvasive technique, skeletal magnetic resonance imaging (MRI) produces clear and sensitive images of bone and soft tissue. The scan provides superior contrast of body tissues and allows imaging of multiple planes, including direct sagittal and coronal views in regions that can't be easily visualized with X-rays or computed tomography scans. MRI eliminates any risks associated with exposure to X-ray beams and causes no known harm to cells.

MRI is most easily generated from the proton of the hydrogen atom. Each water molecule has two hydrogen atoms, but the distribution of water molecules varies according to specific body tissue. For example, bone is considered "dry" because it doesn't contain much hydrogen. Consequently, bone produces a weak signal and can't be visualized. However, normal bone marrow has the brightest signal and can be seen well.

Purpose
- To evaluate bony and soft-tissue tumors
- To identify changes in bone marrow composition
- To identify spinal disorders

Patient preparation
- Make sure the scanner can accommodate the patient's weight and abdominal girth.
- Explain to the patient that skeletal MRI assesses bone and soft tissue. Tell him

who will perform the test and where it will take place.
- Explain to the patient that although MRI is painless and involves no exposure to radiation from the scanner, a contrast medium may be used, depending on the type of tissue being studied.
- If the patient is claustrophobic or if extensive time is required for scanning, explain to him that a mild sedative may be administered to reduce anxiety. Open scanners have been developed for use on the patient with extreme claustrophobia or morbid obesity, but tests using such machines take longer.
- Tell the patient that he must lie flat, and describe the test procedure.
- Explain to the patient that he'll hear the scanner clicking, whirring, and thumping as it moves inside its housing.
- Reassure the patient that he'll be able to communicate with the technician at all times.
- Instruct the patient to remove all metallic objects, including jewelry, hairpins, or watches.
- Ask whether the patient has any surgically implanted joints, pins, clips, valves, pumps, or pacemakers containing metal that could be attracted to the strong MRI magnet. If he does, he won't be able to have the test.
- Ensure that the patient or a responsible family member has signed an informed consent form, if required.

Procedure and posttest care
- At the scanner room door, check the patient one last time for metal objects.
- The patient is placed on a narrow, padded, nonmetallic table that moves into the scanner tunnel. Fans continuously circulate air in the tunnel, and a call bell or intercom is used to maintain verbal contact.

- Remind the patient to remain still throughout the procedure.
- While the patient lies within the strong magnetic field, the area to be studied is stimulated with radio-frequency waves.
- If the test is prolonged with the patient lying flat, monitor him for orthostatic hypotension.
- Provide comfort measures and pain medication as needed and ordered because of prolonged positioning in the scanner.
- After the test, tell the patient that he may resume his usual activity.
- Provide emotional support to the patient with claustrophobia or anxiety over his diagnosis.

Precautions
- Be aware that MRI can't be performed on a patient with a pacemaker, intracranial aneurysm clip, or other ferrous metal implants. Ventilators, I.V. infusion pumps, oxygen tanks, and other metallic or computer-based equipment must be kept out of the MRI area.
- If the patient is unstable, make sure an I.V. line without metal components is in place and that all equipment is compatible with MRI imaging. If necessary, monitor the patient's oxygen saturation, cardiac rhythm, and respiratory status during the test. An anesthesiologist may be needed to monitor a heavily sedated patient.
- Ensure that the technician maintains verbal contact with the conscious patient.

Normal findings
MRI should reveal no pathology in bone, muscles, and joints.

Abnormal findings
MRI is excellent for visualizing diseases of the spinal canal and cord and for identify-

ing primary and metastatic bone tumors. It's beneficial in anatomic delineation of muscles, ligaments, and bones. The images show superior contrast of body tissues and sharply define healthy, benign, and malignant tissues.

Interfering factors
- Excessive patient movement
- Patient unable to fit into scanner

ENDOSCOPY AND JOINT ASPIRATION

Arthroscopy

Arthroscopy is the visual examination of the interior of a joint (most commonly a major joint, such as a shoulder, hip, or knee) with a specially designed fiber-optic endoscope that's inserted through a cannula in the joint cavity. It usually follows and confirms a diagnosis made through physical examination, radiography, and arthrography.

Arthroscopy may be performed under local anesthesia, but it's usually performed under a spinal or general anesthesia, particularly when surgery is anticipated. A camera may be attached to the arthroscope to photograph areas for later study. (See *Arthroscopy of the knee.*)

Complications associated with arthroscopy are rare and may include infection, hemarthrosis, swelling, thrombophlebitis, and joint injury.

Purpose
- To detect and diagnose meniscal, patellar, condylar, extrasynovial, and synovial diseases
- To monitor disease progression
- To perform joint surgery

ARTHROSCOPY OF THE KNEE

With the patient's knee flexed about 40 degrees, the arthroscope is introduced into the joint. The examiner flexes, extends, and rotates the knee to view the joint space. Counterclockwise from the top right, these illustrations show a normal patello-femoral joint with smooth joint surfaces; the articular surface of the patella, showing chondromalacia; and a tear in the anterior cruciate ligament.

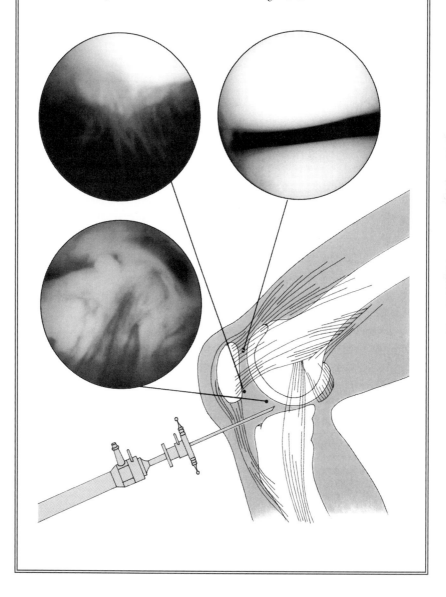

■ To monitor the effectiveness of therapy

Patient preparation

■ Explain to the patient that arthroscopy is used to examine the interior of the joint, to evaluate joint disease, or to monitor his response to therapy, as appropriate.

■ Describe the procedure to the patient and answer his questions.

■ If surgery or another treatment is anticipated, explain that this may be accomplished during arthroscopy.

■ Instruct the patient to fast after midnight before the procedure.

■ Tell the patient who will perform the procedure and where it will be done.

■ If local anesthesia is to be used, tell the patient that he may experience slight discomfort from the injection of the local anesthetic and the pressure of the tourniquet on his leg. The patient will also feel a thumping sensation as the cannula is inserted in the joint capsule.

■ Make sure that the patient or a responsible family member has signed an informed consent form.

■ Check the patient's history for hypersensitivity to the anesthetic.

■ Be aware that the surgical site is prepared by shaving the area 5″ (12.7 cm) above and below the joint and a sedative is administered, as ordered. The patient is positioned and draped according to facility policy.

Equipment

Skin antiseptic (povidone-iodine solution), arthroscope and accessory equipment, pointed scalpel, sterile gloves, local anesthetic, sterile needle, 12- and 60-ml syringes, waterproof stockinette, elastic bandages, pneumatic tourniquet, epinephrine (1:100,000 in 1% lidocaine solution), 500-ml sterile normal saline solution, continuous drainage system, sponges, 2″ × 2″ sterile gauze pads, sterile drapes, small adhesive bandages

Procedure and posttest care

■ Arthroscopic techniques vary depending on the surgeon and the type of arthroscope used.

■ The patient's leg is elevated and wrapped with an elastic bandage to drain as much blood from the leg as possible, or a mixture of lidocaine with epinephrine and normal saline is instilled into the patient's knee to distend the knee and help reduce bleeding.

■ The local anesthetic is administered, a small incision is made, and a cannula is passed through the incision and positioned in the joint cavity.

■ The arthroscope is then inserted, and the knee structures are visually examined and photographed for further study.

■ After visual examination, a synovial biopsy or appropriate surgery is performed as indicated.

■ When the examination is completed, the arthroscope is removed, the joint is irrigated, the cannula is removed, and an adhesive strip and compression dressing are applied over the incision site.

■ Watch the patient for fever, swelling, increased pain, and localized inflammation at the incision site. If the patient reports discomfort, provide an analgesic, as ordered.

■ Monitor the patient's circulation and sensation in his leg.

■ Advise the patient to elevate the leg and apply ice for the first 24 hours.

■ Instruct the patient to report fever, bleeding, drainage, or increased swelling or pain in the joint.

■ Advise the patient to bear only partial weight, using crutches, a walker, or a cane for 48 hours.

- If an immobilizer is ordered, teach the patient how to apply it.
- Tell the patient that showering is permitted after 48 hours, but a tub bath should be avoided until after the postoperative visit.
- Tell the patient that he may resume his usual diet, as ordered.

Precautions

- Arthroscopy is contraindicated in a patient with fibrous ankylosis with flexion of less than 50 degrees.
- The procedure is contraindicated when a patient with local skin or wound infections has a risk of subsequent joint involvement.

Normal findings

The knee is a typical diarthrodial joint surrounded by muscles, ligaments, cartilage, and tendons and lined with a synovial membrane. In children, the menisci are smooth and opaque, with their thick outer edges attached to the joint capsule and their inner edges lying snugly against the condylar surfaces, unattached. Articular cartilage appears smooth and white; ligaments and tendons appear cablelike and silvery. The synovium is smooth and marked by a fine vascular network. Degenerative changes begin during adolescence.

Abnormal findings

Arthroscopic examination can reveal meniscal disease, such as a torn medial or lateral meniscus or other meniscal injuries; patellar disease, such as chondromalacia, dislocation, subluxation, parapatellar synovitis or fracture; condylar disease, such as degenerative articular cartilage, osteochondritis dissecans, and loose bodies; extrasynovial disease, such as torn anterior cruciate or tibial collateral ligaments, Baker's cyst, and ganglionic cyst; and synovial disease, such as synovitis, rheumatoid and degenerative arthritis, and foreign bodies associated with gout, pseudogout, and osteochondromatosis.

Depending on test findings, appropriate treatment or surgery can follow arthroscopy. If arthroscopic surgery can't be performed, arthrotomy is the procedure of choice.

Interfering factors

- Failure to use the arthroscope properly

Synovial fluid analysis

In synovial fluid aspiration, or arthrocentesis, a sterile needle is inserted into a joint space — most commonly the knee — to obtain a fluid specimen for analysis. This procedure is indicated for the patient with undiagnosed articular disease and symptomatic joint effusion, a condition marked by the excessive accumulation of synovial fluid. Although rare, complications associated with synovial fluid aspiration include joint infection and hemorrhage leading to hemarthrosis (accumulation of blood within the joint).

Purpose

- To aid differential diagnosis of arthritis, particularly septic or crystal-induced arthritis
- To identify the cause and nature of joint effusion
- To relieve the pain and distention resulting from the accumulation of fluid within the joint
- To administer a drug locally (usually corticosteroids)

Patient preparation

- Describe synovial fluid analysis to the patient and answer his questions.
- Explain that this test helps determine the cause of joint inflammation and swelling and also helps relieve the associated pain.
- Instruct the patient to fast for 6 to 12 hours before the test if glucose testing of synovial fluid is ordered; otherwise, inform him that he need not restrict food and fluids.
- Tell the patient who will perform the test and where it will be done.
- Warn the patient that although he'll receive a local anesthetic, he may still feel slight pain when the needle penetrates the joint capsule.
- Make sure that the patient or a responsible family member has signed an informed consent form.
- Check the patient's history for hypersensitivity to iodine compounds (such as povidone-iodine), procaine, lidocaine, or other local anesthetics.
- Administer a sedative, as ordered.

Equipment

Surgical detergent; skin antiseptic (usually tincture of povidone-iodine); alcohol pads; local anesthetic (procaine or lidocaine, 1% or 2%); sterile, disposable 1½″ 25G needle; sterile, disposable 1½″ to 2½″ 20G needle; sterile 5-ml syringe for injecting anesthetic; sterile 20-ml syringe for aspiration; 3-ml syringe for administering sedative; sterile dressings; 2″ × 2″ sterile gauze pads; sterile drapes; elastic bandage; tubes for culture, cytologic, clot, and glucose analysis; anticoagulants (heparin, EDTA, and potassium oxalate); venipuncture equipment

For corticosteroid administration

Corticosteroid suspension such as hydrocortisone, 2-ml and 5-ml syringes (or one 10-ml syringe if procaine and steroid are to be injected simultaneously)

Procedure and posttest care

- Position the patient and explain that he'll need to maintain this position throughout the procedure.
- Clean the skin over the puncture site with surgical detergent and alcohol.
- Paint the site with tincture of povidone-iodine and allow it to air-dry for 2 minutes.
- Know that after the local anesthetic is administered, the aspirating needle is quickly inserted through the skin, subcutaneous tissue, and synovial membrane into the joint space.
- Be aware that as much fluid as possible is aspirated into the syringe; at least 15 ml should be obtained, although a smaller amount is usually adequate for analysis.
- Assist as appropriate to maintain the joint (except for the area around the puncture site) wrapped with an elastic bandage to compress the free fluid into this portion of the sac, ensuring maximal fluid collection.
- If a corticosteroid is being injected, prepare the dose as necessary. For instillation, the syringe is detached, leaving the needle in the joint, and the syringe containing the steroid is attached to the needle instead.
- After the steroid is injected and the needle withdrawn, wipe the puncture site with an alcohol pad.
- Apply pressure to the puncture site for about 2 minutes to prevent bleeding, and then apply a sterile dressing.
- If synovial fluid glucose levels are being measured, perform a venipuncture to ob-

tain a specimen for blood glucose analysis.

■ Apply ice or cold packs to the affected joint for 24 to 36 hours after aspiration to decrease pain and swelling. Use pillows for support. If a large quantity of fluid was aspirated, apply an elastic bandage to stabilize the joint.

■ If the patient's condition permits, tell him that he may resume his usual activity immediately after the procedure. However, warn him to avoid excessive use of the affected joint for a few days even if pain and swelling subside.

■ Watch for increased pain or fever; these symptoms may indicate joint infection.

■ Be careful when handling the dressings and linens of the patient with drainage from the joint space, especially if septic arthritis is confirmed or suspected.

■ Tell the patient that he may resume his usual diet, as ordered.

Precautions
■ Wear gloves when handling all specimens.

■ Don't perform the test in areas of skin or wound infections.

■ Use strict sterile technique throughout aspiration to prevent contamination of the joint space or the synovial fluid specimen.

■ Add an anticoagulant to the specimen, according to the laboratory tests requested. Gently invert the tube several times to mix the specimen and anticoagulant adequately.

For cultures
■ Obtain 2 to 5 ml of synovial fluid and, if possible, inoculate the medium immediately. Otherwise, add one or two drops of heparin to the specimen.

For cytologic analysis
■ Add 5 mg of EDTA or one or two drops of heparin to 2 to 5 ml of synovial fluid.

For glucose analysis
■ Add potassium oxalate, as specified by the laboratory, to 3 to 5 ml of fluid.

For crystal examination
■ Add heparin if specified by the laboratory.

For other studies
■ For general appearance and clot evaluation, obtain 2 to 5 ml of synovial fluid, but don't add an anticoagulant.

■ Send the properly labeled specimens to the laboratory immediately after collection — gonococci are particularly labile. If a white blood cell (WBC) count is being obtained as well, clearly label the specimen "Synovial Fluid" and "Caution: Don't Use Acid Diluents."

Normal findings
Routine examination includes gross analysis for color, clarity, quantity, viscosity, pH, and the presence of a mucin clot as well as microscopic analysis for WBC count and differential. Special examination includes microbiological analysis for formed elements (including crystals) and bacteria, serologic analysis, and chemical analysis for such components as glucose, protein, and enzymes.

Abnormal findings
Synovial fluid examination may reveal various joint diseases, including noninflammatory disease (traumatic arthritis and osteoarthritis), inflammatory disease (systemic lupus erythematosus, rheumatic fever, pseudogout, gout, and rheuma-

toid arthritis), and septic disease (tuberculous and septic arthritis).

Interfering factors
- Failure to adhere to dietary restrictions
- Specimen contamination
- Acid diluents added to the specimen for WBC count (alteration in cell count)
- Failure to adequately mix the specimen and the anticoagulant or to send the specimen to the laboratory immediately after collection

Selected readings

Barclay, L. "USPSTF Revises Recommendations for Osteoporosis Screening." *Medscape Medical News*, September 17, 2002. *www.medscape.com/viewarticle/441571.*

Cavanaugh, B.M. *Nurse's Manual of Laboratory and Diagnostic Tests*, 4th ed. Philadelphia: F.A. Davis Co., 2003.

Cummings, S.R., et al. "Clinical Use of Bone Densitometry: Scientific Review," *JAMA* 288(15):1889-97, October 2002.

Goldman, L., and Ausiello, D., eds. *Cecil Textbook of Medicine*, 22nd ed. Philadelphia: W.B. Saunders Co., 2004.

Guyton, A.C., and Hall, J.E. *Textbook of Medical Physiology*, 10th ed. Philadelphia: W.B. Saunders Co., 2001.

Henry, J.B., et al. *Clinical Diagnosis and Management by Laboratory Methods*, 20th ed. Philadelphia: W.B. Saunders Co., 2001.

Maher, A.B., et al. *Orthopaedic Nursing*, 3rd ed. Philadelphia: W.B. Saunders Co., 2002.

McClatchey, K.D. *Clinical Laboratory Medicine*, 2nd ed. Philadelphia: Lippincott Williams & Wilkins, 2002.

Pagana, K.D., and Pagana, T.J. *Mosby's Diagnostic and Laboratory Test Reference*, 6th ed. St. Louis: Mosby Year–Book, Inc., 2003.

Schnell, Z., et al. *Davis's Comprehensive Handbook of Laboratory and Diagnostic Tests with Nursing Implications*. Philadelphia: F.A. Davis Co., 2003.

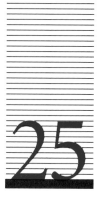

Reproductive system

Introduction

Diagnostic testing of the reproductive system may be performed to assess the organs and associated structures for abnormalities, to detect malignant tumors, or to determine the cause of infertility or sexual dysfunction. Some diagnostic tests are especially useful during pregnancy — first, to confirm pregnancy and, later, to detect genetic defects and monitor the fetus's well-being.

Reproductive organs

The reproductive system consists of essential and accessory organs for procreation. Essential organs are the gonads — the testes and the ovaries. In the male, the testes produce the germ cells known as spermatozoa and the hormone testosterone, which induces and maintains secondary sexual characteristics; in the female, the ovaries produce ova and the hormones estrogen and progesterone, which also promote and maintain secondary sexual characteristics.

Male accessory organs consist of the scrotum and a transport system of ducts

MALE REPRODUCTIVE SYSTEM

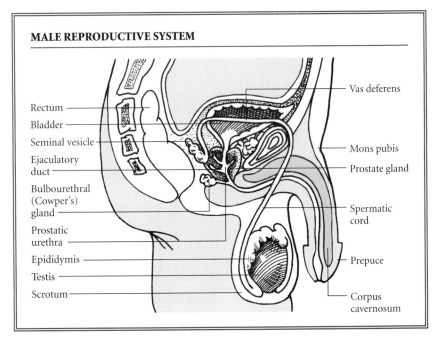

Rectum

Bladder

Seminal vesicle

Ejaculatory duct

Bulbourethral (Cowper's) gland

Prostatic urethra

Epididymis

Testis

Scrotum

Vas deferens

Mons pubis

Prostate gland

Spermatic cord

Prepuce

Corpus cavernosum

and glands, including the urethra, epididymis, vas deferens, ejaculatory duct, seminal vesicles, prostate, bulbourethral glands, and penis.

Female accessory organs include the fallopian tubes, uterus, and vagina. External structures of female genitalia, collectively called the vulva, include the mons pubis, labia majora, labia minora, clitoris, vestibule, urethral meatus, hymen, Bartholin's glands, Skene's glands, fourchette, and perineum. The mammary glands, whose primary function is lactation, are also generally considered part of the reproductive system. (See *Male reproductive system,* and *Female reproductive system.*)

Fetal development

Normally, the spermatozoon fertilizes the ovum in the upper to middle third of the fallopian tube. At fertilization, the sperm, which contains 22 autosomes and either an X or a Y chromosome, fuses with the ovum, which contains 22 autosomes and an X chromosome, to form a zygote made up of 44 autosomes and 2 sex chromosomes. The 44 autosomes determine genetic characteristics of the fetus; the sex chromosomes determine the sex of the fetus. Two X chromosomes produce a female zygote; an X and a Y produce a male zygote.

After fertilization, the fertilized ovum develops in two stages over a 40-week gestation period. During the *embryonic stage,* which begins at conception and lasts 8 weeks, the blastocyst develops and is implanted, and primitive chorionic villi start to form. The amnion begins to ensheathe the body stalk, which will become the umbilical cord. Embryonic heart chambers develop, and a primitive cardiovascular system begins to function. By the end of the embryonic stage, the eyes, ears, nose, and mouth are recognizable; the arms, legs, fingers, and toes are

FEMALE REPRODUCTIVE SYSTEM

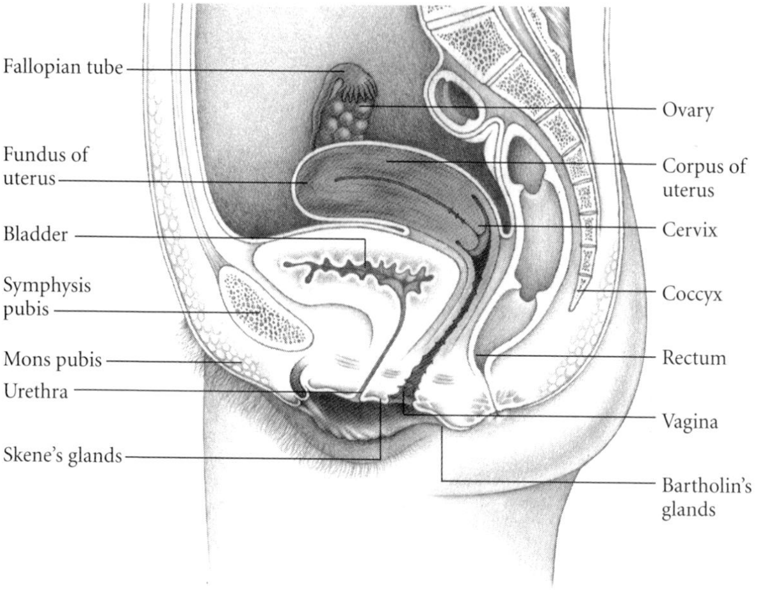

Fallopian tube

Fundus of
uterus

Bladder

Symphysis
pubis

Mons pubis

Urethra

Skene's glands

Ovary

Corpus of
uterus

Cervix

Coccyx

Rectum

Vagina

Bartholin's
glands

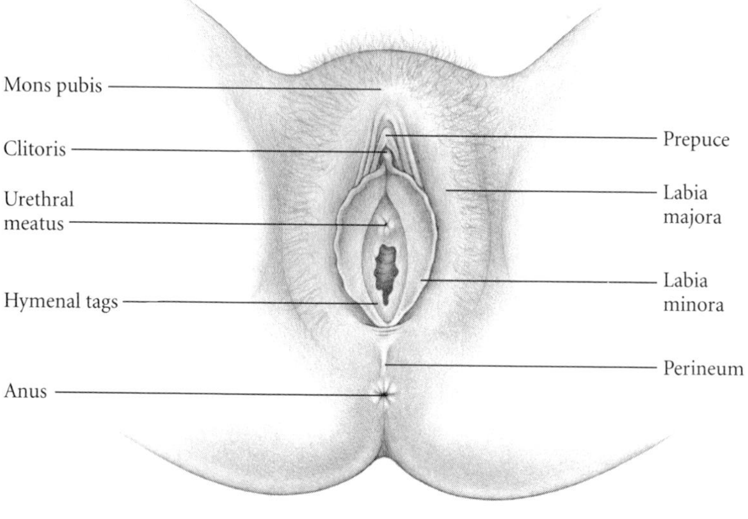

Mons pubis

Clitoris

Urethral
meatus

Hymenal tags

Anus

Prepuce

Labia
majora

Labia
minora

Perineum

REVIEWING FETAL GROWTH AND DEVELOPMENT

At the end of the first month, the embryo has a definite form, as seen in the illustration below. The head and trunk are apparent, and the tiny buds that will become the arms and legs are discernible. The cardiovascular system has begun to function, and the umbilical cord is visible in its most primitive form.

END OF FIRST MONTH
1 month
(10 times actual size)

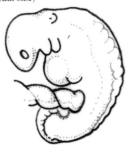

In the second month, the embryo — called a *fetus* from the 7th week on — grows to 1″ (2.5 cm) in length and weighs ⅓₀ oz. As seen in the illustration top right, the head and facial features develop as the eyes, ears, nose, lips, tongue, and tooth buds form. The arms and legs also take shape, with the elbows, forearms, hands, fingers, thighs, knees, ankles, and toes becoming visible. Although the gender of the fetus isn't yet discernible, all external genitalia are present. Cardiovascular function is complete, and the umbilical cord has a definite form. At the end of second month, the fetus resembles a full-term baby except for size.

END OF SECOND MONTH
2 months (actual size)

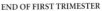

During the third month, as seen in the illustration below, the fetus grows to 3″ (8 cm) in length and weighs 1 oz (28 g). Teeth and bones begin to appear, and the kidneys start to function. Although the mother can't yet feel activity, the fetus is moving. It opens its mouth to swallow, grasps with its fully developed hands, and — even though its lungs aren't functioning — prepares for breathing by inhaling and exhaling. At the end of the first trimester, its gender is distinguishable.

END OF FIRST TRIMESTER
3 months
(actual size)

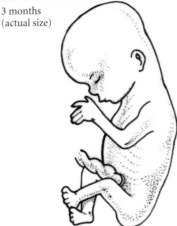

formed; and most organs have begun to develop.

During the *fetal stage*, a period lasting from 8 weeks after conception until delivery, the major structures and organs that are already developed grow and mature. (See *Reviewing fetal growth and development.*)

In the remaining 6 months, fetal growth continues as internal and external structures develop at a rapid rate. In the third trimester, the fetus stores the fats and minerals it needs to live outside the womb. At birth, as seen in the illustration below, the average full-term fetus measures 20″ (51 cm) and weighs 7 to 7½ lb (3 to 3.5 kg).

END OF THIRD TRIMESTER
9 months (one-third actual size)

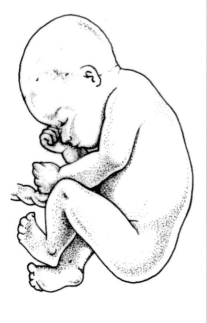

Stages of labor
- *Stage I* is the time between the beginning of regular contractions and full cervical dilation — usually about 12 hours

for a primigravida and about 6 hours for a multigravida.
- *Stage II*, the period lasting from full dilation until delivery, generally lasts about 2 to 3 hours for a primigravida and up to 1 hour for a multigravida.
- *Stage III* lasts from delivery to the expulsion of the placenta.

Special diagnostic tests
Evaluation of the reproductive system begins with a physical examination and a detailed history to detect abnormalities that may require further testing. Special tests using various techniques include:
- *Papanicolaou test* — the cytologic examination of cervical scrapings, allows for early detection of cervical cancer.
- *Colposcopy* — provides for direct visualization of cervical and vaginal abnormalities, such as benign lesions and invasive carcinoma.
- *Semen analysis* — evaluates male fertility (semen count and motility analysis), validates the effectiveness of a vasectomy, and detects the presence of semen for medicolegal investigations.
- *Sex chromatin test* — screens for abnormalities of the sex chromosomes.
- *Chromosomal analysis* — evaluates genetic defects in the fetus, thus aiding genetic counseling.
- *Amniotic fluid analysis, chorionic villi biopsy,* and *pelvic and vaginal ultrasonography* — facilitate early diagnosis of fetal abnormalities, some of which may be successfully treated in utero. (For instance, amniotic fluid analysis can identify Rh isoimmunization before birth, allowing treatment with intrauterine transfusions to prevent stillbirth.)
- *Laparoscopy* — determines if female infertility results from anatomic defects. It also can detect pathology of the ovaries, fallopian tubes, and uterus through direct

visualization, thus allowing early treatment of life-threatening conditions, such as cancers or severe hemorrhage.

- *Hysteroscopy*—investigates abnormal uterine bleeding and provides visualization of the interior of the uterus for other diagnoses, such as adhesions and fibroids.
- *Internal* and *external fetal monitoring* and *Doppler stethoscope testing*—rapidly assess fetal distress during pregnancy, labor, and delivery.
- *Mammography*—aids in the assessment of breast lumps.
- *Hysterosalpinography*—provides visualization of malformations, adhesions, and occlusions of the uterus and fallopian tubes through fluoroscopic examination.

Significance of emotional support

For the patient scheduled for diagnostic tests of the reproductive system, emotional support is especially important. Fertility or the ability to deliver a child can be closely related to self-image, which can conjure up emotions in the patient. Also, the tests themselves may cause anxiety. For example, a female patient scheduled for amniocentesis may fear having a deformed or retarded infant, or for mammography, she may likely fear cancer and mastectomy. Similarly, a male patient scheduled for a diagnostic test, such as a semen analysis, may pose a challenge to his quality of life, self-esteem, and sense of well-being. Therefore, it's important that you make sure you assess the patient's psychological state before the test so that you can deal with the patient appropriately. Remember that the patient has his own view of sexuality and reproduction. Take these views into account and remain nonjudgmental and supportive.

TISSUE ANALYSIS

Papanicolaou test

The Papanicolaou (Pap) test is a widely known cytologic test for early detection of cervical cancer. A physician or specially trained nurse scrapes secretions from the patient's cervix and spreads them on a slide, which is sent to the laboratory for cytologic analysis. The test relies on the ready exfoliation of malignant cells from the cervix and shows cell maturity, metabolic activity, and morphology variations.

Although cervical scrapings are the most common test specimen, the test may involve cytologic evaluation of the vaginal pool, prostatic secretions, urine, gastric secretions, cavity fluids, bronchial aspirations, sputum, or solid tumor cells obtained by fine needle aspiration. The American Cancer Society recommends a Pap test every 3 years for women between ages 20 and 40 who are not in a high-risk category and who have had negative results from three previous Pap tests. Yearly tests (or tests at physician-recommended intervals) are advised for women over age 40, for those in a high-risk category, and for those who have had a positive test previously. If a Pap test is positive or suggests malignancy, cervical biopsy can confirm the diagnosis.

Purpose
- To detect malignant cells
- To detect inflammatory tissue changes
- To assess the patient's response to chemotherapy and radiation therapy
- To detect viral, fungal and, occasionally, parasitic invasion

Patient preparation
- Explain to the patient that the Pap test allows for the study of cervical cells.

- Stress its importance as an aid for detection of cancer at a stage when the disease is commonly asymptomatic and still curable.
- The test shouldn't be scheduled during the menstrual period; the best time is midcycle.
- Instruct the patient to avoid having intercourse for 24 hours, not to douche for 48 hours, and not to insert vaginal medications for 1 week before the test because doing so can wash away cellular deposits and change the vaginal pH.
- Tell the patient that the test requires that the cervix be scraped, who will perform the procedure and when, and that she may experience slight discomfort but no pain from the speculum (but may feel some pain when the cervix is scraped).
- Inform her that the procedure takes 5 to 10 minutes or slightly longer if the vagina, pelvic cavity, and rectum are examined bimanually.
- Obtain an accurate patient history, and ask these questions: When did you last have a Pap test? Have you ever had an abnormal Pap test? When was your last menstrual period? Are your periods regular? How many days do they last? Is bleeding heavy or light? Have you taken or are you presently taking hormones or oral contraceptives? Do you use an intrauterine device? Do you have any vaginal discharge, pain, or itching? Which, if any, gynecologic disorders have occurred in your family? Have you ever had gynecologic surgery, chemotherapy, or radiation therapy? If so, describe it fully. Note the pertinent patient history data on the laboratory request.
- Provide emotional support if the patient is anxious; tell her that test results should be available in a few weeks.
- Ask the patient to empty her bladder before the test is performed.

Equipment
Gloves; drape; vaginal speculum; collection device, such as a Pap stick (wooden spatula), endocervical brush; saline solution; glass microscopic slides; fixative (commercial spray or 95% ethyl alcohol solution in a jar) for slides

Procedure and posttest care
- Instruct the patient to disrobe from the waist down and to drape herself.
- Ask the patient to lie on the examining table and to place her heels in the stirrups. (She may be more comfortable if she keeps her shoes or socks on.) Tell her to slide her buttocks to the edge of the table. Adjust the drape to minimize exposure.
- To avoid startling the patient, tell her when the examination will begin.
- The examiner puts on gloves and inserts an unlubricated speculum into the vagina. To make insertion easier, the speculum may be moistened with saline solution or warm water.
- After the examiner locates the cervix, he collects secretions from the cervix and material from the endocervical canal. He places the endocervical brush inside the endocervix and rolls it firmly inside the canal. If using a Pap stick (wooden spatula), it's placed against the cervix with the longest protrusion in the cervical canal, then rotates the stick clockwise 360 degrees firmly against the cervix.
- He then spreads the specimen on the slide according to laboratory recommendations and immediately immerses the slide in (or sprays it with) a fixative.
- Alternatively, posterior vaginal pool secretions and pancervical material may be collected and smeared on a single slide, which must be fixed immediately according to laboratory instructions.

TESTING FOR CERVICAL CANCER

To analyze cervical cells, the ThinPrep test may be collected in the same manner as a Papanicolaou (Pap) test using a cytobrush and plastic spatula. The specimens are deposited in a bottle provided with a fixative and sent to the laboratory. A filter is then inserted into the bottle and excess mucus, blood, and inflammatory cells are filtered out by centrifuge. Remaining cells are then placed on a slide in a uniform, thin layer and read as a Pap test. This causes fewer slides to be classified as unreadable, significantly reducing the incidence of false negatives and the need for repeat tests.

When using the ThinPrep test, screening can also be easily done for the human papillomavirus (HPV), of which certain strains have been identified as the primary cause of cervical cancer. The Digene hc2 HPV deoxyribonucleic acid (DNA) test has been approved by the Food and Drug Administration to determine if those identified at high risk for developing cervical cancer have been ex-posed to HPV. The specimen is collected as a Pap smear, but is dispersed with ThinPrep solution. Separate aliquots are used for each test, from brushings of the endocervix. The brush is then inserted into the specialized tube, snapped off at the shaft, and capped securely. The target solution in the tube disrupts the virus and releases target DNA, which combines with specific ribonucleic acid (RNA) probes creating RNA:DNA hybrids. The hybrids are captured, bound, and able to be magnified and measured using a luminometer.

If the patient is found to be positive for HPV, it means she has been infected with the virus. Depending on the type of HPV found through DNA testing, the patient harboring high-risk HPV strains has a higher risk of developing cervical cancer. It's recommended that the patient undergo colposcopy in which the cervix is viewed under microscope and a biopsy is taken from the tissue sample.

- Label the specimen appropriately, including the date, the patient's name, age, the date of her last menstrual period, and the collection site and method.
- A bimanual examination may follow after the removal of the speculum. Help the patient up and ask her to dress when the examination is completed.
- Supply the patient with a sanitary napkin if cervical bleeding occurs.
- Tell the patient when to return for her next Pap test.

- The specimen should be thick enough that it isn't transparent.
- Scrapings taken directly from the lesion are preferred if vaginal or vulval lesions are present.
- Use a small pipette, if necessary, in a patient whose uterus is involuting or atrophying from age, to aspirate cells from the squamocolumnar junction and the cervical canal.
- Preserve the slides immediately after the specimen is collected.

Precautions
- Make sure the cervical specimen is aspirated and scraped from the cervix. A vaginal pool sample isn't recommended for cervical or endometrial cancer screening.

Normal findings
Normally, no malignant cells or other abnormalities are present.

Abnormal findings

Malignant cells usually have relatively large nuclei and only small amounts of cytoplasm. They show abnormal nuclear chromatin patterns and marked variation in size, shape, and staining properties and may have prominent nucleoli.

A Pap smear may be graded in different ways, so check your laboratory's reporting format. In the Bethesda system, the current standardized method, potentially premalignant squamous lesions fall into three categories: atypical squamous cells of undetermined significance, low-grade squamous intraepithelial lesions, and high-grade squamous intraepithelial lesions. The low-grade category includes mild dysplasia and the changes of the human papillomavirus. The high-grade category includes moderate to severe dysplasia and carcinoma in situ.

To confirm a suggestive or positive cytology report, the test may be repeated or followed by a biopsy. (See *Testing for cervical cancer.*)

Interfering factors

- Douching within 48 hours or having intercourse within 24 hours before the test (can wash away cellular deposits)
- Excessive use of lubricating jelly on the speculum (false-negative)
- Collection of the specimen during menstruation
- Exclusive use of a specimen collected from the vaginal fornix (possible false-negative)
- Delay in fixing the specimen (difficult cytologic interpretation due to dehydration of cells)
- Too thin or thick a specimen

Colposcopy

In colposcopy, the cervix and vagina are visually examined by an instrument containing a magnifying lens and a light (colposcope). This test is primarily used to evaluate abnormal cytology or grossly suspicious lesions and to examine the cervix and vagina after a positive Papanicolaou (Pap) test.

During the examination, a biopsy may be performed and photographs taken of suspicious lesions with the colposcope and its attachments. Risks of biopsy include bleeding (especially during pregnancy) and infection.

Purpose

- To help confirm cervical intraepithelial neoplasia or invasive carcinoma after a positive Pap test
- To evaluate vaginal or cervical lesions
- To monitor conservatively treated cervical intraepithelial neoplasia
- To monitor the patient whose mother received diethylstilbestrol during pregnancy

Patient preparation

- Explain to the patient that the colposcopy magnifies the image of the vagina and cervix, providing more information than a routine vaginal examination.
- Inform the patient that she need not restrict food and fluids.
- Tell the patient who will perform the examination, where it will be done, and that it's safe and painless.
- Tell the patient that a biopsy may be performed during colposcopy and that this may cause minimal but easily controlled bleeding and mild cramping.
- Make sure that the patient or a responsible family member has signed an informed consent form.

Equipment
For colposcopy
Gloves, colposcope, vaginal speculum, 5% acetic acid solution, swabs

For biopsy
Gloves, biopsy forceps, endocervical curette, forceps for uterine dressing, tenaculum, ring forceps, Monsel's (ferric subsulfate) solution, biopsy bottle and preservative, sterile cotton balls, Pap test equipment (glass slide, wooden spatula, swabs, and fixative)

Procedure and posttest care
- The examiner puts on gloves. With the patient in the lithotomy position, the examiner inserts the speculum and, if indicated, performs a Pap test. Help the patient relax during insertion by telling her to breathe through her mouth and concentrate on relaxing her abdominal muscles.
- The cervix is gently swabbed with acetic acid solution to remove mucus.
- After the cervix and vagina are examined, biopsy is performed on areas that appear abnormal.
- Bleeding is stopped by applying pressure, hemostatic solutions, or by cautery.
- After a biopsy, instruct the patient to abstain from intercourse and to avoid inserting anything in her vagina (including a tampon) until healing of the biopsy site is confirmed (in approximately 10 days).

Normal findings
Surface contour of the cervical vessels should be smooth and pink; columnar epithelium appears grapelike. Different tissue types are sharply demarcated.

Abnormal findings
Abnormal colposcopy findings include white epithelium (leukoplakia) or punc-

tate and mosaic patterns, which may indicate underlying cervical intraepithelial neoplasia; keratinization in the transformation zone, which may indicate cervical intraepithelial neoplasia or invasive carcinoma; and atypical vessels, which may indicate invasive carcinoma.

Other abnormalities visible on colposcopic examination include inflammatory changes (usually from infection), atrophic changes (usually from aging or, less commonly, the use of oral contraceptives), erosion (probably from increased pathogenicity of vaginal flora due to changes in vaginal pH), and papilloma and condyloma (possibly from viruses).

Histologic study of the biopsy specimen confirms colposcopic findings. If the examination and biopsy results are inconsistent with the Pap test and biopsy of the squamocolumnar junction results, conization of the cervix for biopsy may be indicated.

Interfering factors
- Failure to clean the cervix of menstrual blood or foreign materials, such as creams and medications (possible obstruction to visualization)

Semen analysis

Semen analysis is a simple, inexpensive, and reasonably definitive test that's used in many applications, including evaluating a man's fertility. Fertility analysis usually includes measuring seminal fluid volume, performing sperm counts, and microscopic examination of spermatozoa. Sperm are counted in much the same way that white blood cells, red blood cells, and platelets are counted in a blood sample. Motility and morphology are studied microscopically after staining a drop of semen.

IDENTIFYING SEMEN FOR MEDICOLEGAL PURPOSES

Spermatozoa (or their fragments) persist in the vagina for more than 72 hours after sexual intercourse. This allows detection and positive identification of semen from vaginal aspirates or smears or from stains on clothing, other fabrics, skin, or hair, which is commonly necessary for medicolegal purposes, usually in connection with rape or homicide investigations. Spermatozoa taken from the vagina of an exhumed body that has been properly embalmed and remains reasonably intact can also be identified.

To determine which stains or fluids require further investigation, clothing or other fabrics can be scanned with ultraviolet light to detect the typical greenwhite fluorescence of semen. Soaking appropriate samples of clothing, fabric, or hair in physiologic saline solution elutes the semen and spermatozoa. Deposits of dried semen can be gently sponged from the victim's skin.

The two most common tests to identify semen are the determination of *acid phosphatase concentration* (the more sensitive test) and *microscopic examination* for the presence of spermatozoa. Acid phosphatase appears in semen in significantly greater concentrations than in other body fluids. In microscopic examination, spermatozoa or head fragments can be identified on stained smears prepared directly from vaginal scrapings or aspirates or from the concentrated sediment of eluates or lavages.

Like other body fluids, semen contains the soluble A, B, and H blood group substances in approximately 80% of males who are genetically determined secretors (males who have the dominant secretor gene in a homozygous or heterozygous state). Thus, the male who has group A blood and is a secretor has soluble blood group A substance in his seminal fluid and group A substance on the surface of his red blood cells. This fact can be of considerable medicolegal importance. Semen analysis can demonstrate that the semen of a suspect in a rape or homicide investigation is different from or consistent with semen found in or on the victim's body.

If analysis detects an abnormality, additional tests (for example, liver, thyroid, pituitary, or adrenal function tests) may be performed to identify the underlying cause and to screen for metabolic abnormalities (such as diabetes mellitus). Significant abnormalities—such as greatly decreased sperm count or motility or a marked increase in morphologically abnormal forms—may require testicular biopsy.

Semen analysis can also be used to detect semen on a rape victim , to identify the blood group of an alleged rapist, or to prove sterility in a paternity suit. (See *Identifying semen for medicolegal purposes.*) Some laboratories offer specialized semen tests such as screening for antibodies to spermatozoa.

Purpose

- To evaluate male fertility in an infertile couple
- To substantiate the effectiveness of a vasectomy
- To detect semen on the body or clothing of a suspected rape victim or elsewhere at the crime scene
- To identify blood group substances to exonerate or incriminate a criminal suspect
- To rule out paternity on grounds of complete sterility

Patient preparation
For fertility evaluation

■ Provide written instructions, and inform the patient that the most desirable specimen requires masturbation, ideally in a physician's office or laboratory.

■ Tell the patient to follow the instructions given to him regarding the period of sexual continence before the test because this may increase his sperm count. Some physicians specify a fixed number of days, usually between 2 and 5; others advise a period of continence equal to the usual interval between episodes of sexual intercourse.

■ If the patient prefers to collect the specimen at home, emphasize the importance of delivering the specimen to the laboratory within 1 hour after collection. Warn him not to expose the specimen to extreme temperatures or to direct sunlight (which can also increase its temperature). Ideally, the specimen should remain at body temperature until liquefaction is complete (about 20 minutes). To deliver a semen specimen during cold weather, suggest that the patient keep the specimen container in a coat pocket on the way to the laboratory to protect the specimen from exposure to cold.

■ Alternatives to collection by masturbation include coitus interruptus or the use of a condom. For collection by coitus interruptus, instruct the patient to withdraw immediately before ejaculation and to deposit the ejaculate in a suitable specimen container. For collection by condom, tell the patient to first wash the condom with soap and water, rinse it thoroughly, and allow it to dry completely. (Powders or lubricants applied to the condom may be spermicidal.) Special sheaths that don't contain spermicide are also available for semen collection. After collection, instruct him to tie the condom, place it in a glass jar, and promptly deliver it to the laboratory.

■ Fertility may also be determined by collecting semen from the woman after coitus to assess the ability of the spermatozoa to penetrate the cervical mucus and remain active. For the postcoital cervical mucus test, instruct the patient to report for examination 1 to 2 days before ovulation as determined by basal temperature records. A urine luteinizing hormone-releasing hormone test may help predict ovulation in the patient with an irregular cycle. Instruct the couple to abstain from intercourse for 2 days and then to have sexual intercourse 2 to 8 hours before the examination. Remind them to avoid using lubricants. Explain to the patient scheduled for this test that the procedure takes only a few minutes. Tell her that she'll be placed in the lithotomy position and that a speculum will be inserted into the vagina to collect the specimen. She may feel some pressure, but no pain.

For semen collection from a rape victim

■ Explain to the patient that the examiner will try to obtain a semen specimen from her vagina.

■ Prepare the victim for insertion of the speculum as you would the patient scheduled for postcoital examination.

■ Handle the victim's clothes as little as possible. If her clothes are moist, put them in a paper bag — not a plastic bag (which causes seminal stains and secretions to mold). Label the bag properly, and send it to the laboratory immediately.

■ Provide emotional support by speaking to the patient calmly and reassuringly. Encourage her to express her fears and anxieties. Listen sympathetically.

■ If the patient is scheduled for vaginal lavage, tell the rape victim to expect a

cold sensation when saline solution is instilled to wash out the specimen.
- Help the patient relax by instructing her to breathe deeply and slowly through her mouth.
- Instruct the victim to urinate just before the test, but warn her not to wipe the vulva afterward because this may remove semen.

Equipment
For semen collection by masturbation, coitus interruptus, or condom
Clean plastic specimen container (for example, disposable urine or sputum container with lid)

For a postcoital specimen collection
Clean plastic specimen container, vaginal speculum, rubber gloves, cotton applicator sticks, glass microscopic slides with frosted ends, 1-ml tuberculin syringe without a cannula or needle

For semen collection from a rape victim
Clean plastic specimen container, vaginal speculum, rubber gloves, cotton applicator sticks, glass microscopic slides with frosted ends, physiologic (0.85%) saline solution, Pap sticks, Coplin jars containing 95% ethanol, large syringe, rubber bulb or other device suitable for vaginal lavage

Procedure and posttest care
- Obtain a semen specimen for a fertility study by asking the patient to collect semen in a clean plastic specimen container.
- A specimen is obtained from the vagina of a rape victim by direct aspiration, saline lavage, or a direct smear of vaginal contents using a Pap stick or, less desir-

ably, a cotton applicator stick. Dried smears are usually collected from the suspected rape victim's skin by gently washing the skin with a small piece of gauze moistened with physiologic saline solution.
- Prepare direct smears on glass microscopic slides after labeling the frosted end. Immediately place smeared slides in Coplin jars containing 95% ethanol.
- Before postcoital examination, the examiner wipes excess mucus from the external cervix and collects the specimen by direct aspiration of the cervical canal using a 1-ml tuberculin syringe without a cannula or needle.
- Inform a patient who's undergoing infertility studies that test results should be available in 24 hours.
- Refer the suspected rape victim to an appropriate specialist for counseling—a gynecologist, psychiatrist, clinical psychologist, nursing specialist, member of the clergy, or representative of a community support group such as Women Organized Against Rape.

Precautions
- If the patient prefers to collect the specimen during coitus interruptus, tell him he must prevent any loss of semen during ejaculation.
- Deliver all specimens, regardless of the source or method of collection, to the laboratory within 1 hour.
- Protect semen specimens for fertility studies from extremes of temperature and direct sunlight during delivery to the laboratory.
- Never lubricate the vaginal speculum. Oil or grease hinders examination of spermatozoa by interfering with smear preparation and staining and by inhibiting sperm motility through toxic ingredi-

ents. Instead, moisten the speculum with water or physiologic saline solution.

■ Use extreme caution in securing, labeling, and delivering all specimens to be used for medicolegal purposes. You may be asked to testify as to when, where, and from whom the specimen was obtained; the specimen's general appearance and identifying features; steps taken to ensure the specimen's integrity; and when, where, and to whom the specimen was delivered for analysis. If your facility or clinic uses routing requests for such specimens, fill them out carefully and place them in the permanent medicolegal file.

Normal findings

Normal semen volume ranges from 0.7 to 6.5 ml. Paradoxically, the semen volume of many men in infertile couples is increased. Abstinence for 1 week or more results in progressively increased semen volume. (With abstinence of up to 10 days, sperm counts increase, sperm motility progressively decreases, and sperm morphology stays the same.) Liquefied semen is generally highly viscid, translucent, and gray-white, with a musty or acrid odor. After liquefaction, specimens of normal viscosity can be poured in drops. Normally, semen is slightly alkaline with a pH of 7.3 to 7.9.

Other normal characteristics of semen: It coagulates immediately and liquefies within 20 minutes; the normal sperm count is 20 to 150 million/ml and can be greater; 40% of spermatozoa have normal morphology; and 20% or more of spermatozoa show progressive motility within 4 hours of collection.

The normal postcoital cervical mucus test shows 10 to 20 motile spermatozoa per microscopic high-power field and spinnbarkeit (a measurement of the tenacity of the mucus) of at least 4″ (10 cm). These findings indicate adequate spermatozoa and receptivity of the cervical mucus. Shaking or dead sperm may indicate antisperm antibodies.

Abnormal findings

Abnormal semen is *not* synonymous with infertility. Only one viable spermatozoon is needed to fertilize an ovum. Although a normal sperm count is 20 million/ml or more, many men with sperm counts below 1 million/ml have fathered normal children. Only men who can't deliver *any* viable spermatozoa in their ejaculate during sexual intercourse are absolutely sterile. Nevertheless, subnormal sperm counts, decreased sperm motility, and abnormal morphology are usually associated with decreased fertility.

Other tests may be necessary to evaluate the patient's general health, metabolic status, or the function of specific endocrine glands (pituitary, thyroid, adrenal, or gonadal).

Interfering factors

■ Poor timing of test within the menstrual cycle (abnormal postcoital test results)
■ Previous cervical conization or cryotherapy and some medications such as clomiphene citrate (possible abnormal postcoital test results due to changes in cervical mucus)
■ Delayed transport of the specimen, exposure to extreme temperatures or direct sunlight, or the presence of toxic chemicals in the container or the condom (possible decrease in number of viable sperm)
■ An incomplete specimen — for example, from coitus interruptus or improper collection technique (decrease in specimen volume)

Sex chromosome tests

Although sex chromosome tests can screen for abnormalities in the number of sex chromosomes, the faster, simpler, and more accurate full karyotype (chromosome analysis) has all but replaced them. Sex chromosome tests are usually indicated for abnormal sexual development, ambiguous genitalia, amenorrhea, and suspected chromosomal abnormalities.

Purpose
■ To quickly screen for abnormal sexual development (X and Y chromatin tests)
■ To aid in the assessment of an infant with ambiguous genitalia (X chromatin test)
■ To determine the number of Y chromosomes in an individual (Y chromatin test)

Patient preparation
■ Explain to the patient or his parents, if appropriate, why the sex chromosome test is being performed.
■ Tell the patient that the test requires that the inside of his cheek be scraped to obtain a specimen and who will perform the test.
■ Assure the patient that the test takes only a few minutes, but may require a follow-up chromosome analysis.
■ Inform the patient that the laboratory generally requires as long as 4 weeks to complete the analysis.

Equipment
Wooden or metal spatula, clean glass slide, cell fixative

Procedure and posttest care
■ Scrape the buccal mucosa firmly with a wooden or metal spatula at least twice to obtain a specimen of healthy cells (vaginal mucosa is occasionally used in young women).
■ Rub the spatula over the glass slide, making sure the cells are evenly distributed.

■ Spray the slide with a cell fixative and send it to the laboratory with a brief patient history and indications for the test.

Precautions
■ Make sure the buccal mucosa is scraped firmly to ensure a sufficient number of cells.
■ Check that the specimen isn't saliva, which contains no cells.

Normal findings
A normal female (XX) has only one X chromatin mass (the number of X chromatin masses discernible is one less than the number of X chromosomes in the cells examined). For various reasons, an X chromatin mass is ordinarily discernible in only 20% to 50% of the buccal mucosal cells of a normal woman.

A normal male (XY) has only one Y chromatin mass (the number of Y chromatin masses equals the number of Y chromosomes in the cells examined).

Abnormal findings
In most laboratories, if less than 20% of the cells in a buccal smear contain an X chromatin mass, some cells are presumed to contain only one X chromosome, necessitating full karyotyping. A person with a female phenotype and a positive Y chromatin mass runs a high risk of developing a malignancy in the intra-abdominal gonads. In such cases, removal of these gonads is indicated and should generally be performed before age 5.

The patient or his parents require genetic counseling after the cause of chromosomal abnormal sexual development has been identified. A medical team comprised of physicians, psychologists, psychiatrists, and educators must decide the child's sex if a child is phenotypically of one sex and genotypically of the other. This careful evaluation should be made early to prevent developmental problems related to incorrect gender identification. (See *Sex chromosome anomalies.*)

Interfering factors
- Obtaining saliva instead of buccal cells (false specimen)
- Cell deterioration due to failure to apply cell fixative to the slide
- Presence of bacteria or wrinkles in the cell membrane, analysis of degenerative cells, or use of an outdated stain

Chromosome analysis

Chromosome analysis studies the relationship between the microscopic appearance of chromosomes and an individual's phenotype — the expression of the genes in physical, biochemical, or physiologic traits.

Ideally, chromosomes are studied during metaphase, the middle phase of mitosis, when new cell poles appear. During metaphase, colchicine (a cell poison) is added to arrest cell division. Cells are harvested, stained, and then examined under a microscope. These cells are then photographed to record the karyotype — the systematic arrangement of chromosomes in groupings according to size and shape.

Only rapidly dividing cells, such as bone marrow or neoplastic cells, permit direct, immediate study. In other cells, mitosis is stimulated by the addition of phytohemagglutinin. Indications for the test determine the specimen required (blood, bone marrow, amniotic fluid, skin, or placental tissue) and the specific analytic procedure. Umbilical cord sampling may also be used to perform chromosome analysis. (See *Percutaneous umbilical blood sampling,* page 666.)

SEX CHROMOSOMES ANOMALIES

Disorder and chromosomal aneuploidy

Klinefelter's syndrome
- 47,XXY
- 48,XXXY
- 49,XXXXY
- 48,XXYY
- 49,XXXYY

Polysomy Y
- 47,XYY

Turner's syndrome
- 45,XO
- Mosaics: XO/XX or XO/XXX
- Aberrations of X chromosomes, including deletion of short arm of one X chromosome, presence of a ring chromosome, or presence of an isochromosome on the long arm of an X chromosome

Other X polysomes

- 47,XXX

- 48,XXXX

- 49,XXXXX

Cause and incidence	Phenotypic features
• Nondisjunction or improper chromatid separation during anaphase I or II of oogenesis or spermatogenesis results in abnormal gamete • 1 per 1,000 male births	• Syndrome usually inapparent until puberty • Small penis and testes • Sparse facial and abdominal hair; feminine distribution of pubic hair • Somewhat enlarged breasts (gynecomastia) • Sexual dysfunction • Truncal obesity • Sterility • Possible mental retardation (greater incidence with increased X chromosomes)
• Nondisjunction during anaphase II of spermatogenesis causes both Y chromosomes to pass to the same pole and results in a YY sperm • 1 per 1,000 male births	• Above-average stature (commonly over 72″ [182.9 cm]) • Increased incidence of severe acne • May display aggressive, psychopathic, or criminal behavior • Normal fertility • Learning disabilities
• Nondisjunction during anaphase I or II of spermatogenesis results in sperm without any sex chromosomes • 1 per 3,500 female births (most common chromosome complement in first-trimester abortions)	• Short stature (usually under 57″ [144.8 cm]) • Webbed neck • Low posterior hairline • Broad chest with widely spaced nipples • Underdeveloped breasts • Juvenile external genitalia • Primary amenorrhea common • Congenital heart disease (30% with coarctation of the aorta) • Renal abnormalities • Sterility from underdeveloped internal reproductive organs (ovaries are only strands of connective tissue) • No mental retardation, but possible problems with space perception and orientation
• Nondisjunction at anaphase I or II of oogenesis	
• 1 per 1,400 female births	• Commonly, no obvious anatomic abnormalities • Normal fertility
• Rare	• Mental retardation • Ocular hypertelorism • Reduced fertility
• Rare	• Severe mental retardation • Ocular hypertelorism with uncoordinated eye movement • Abnormal sexual organ development • Various skeletal anomalies

PERCUTANEOUS UMBILICAL BLOOD SAMPLING

Useful in chromosome analysis, percutaneous umbilical blood sampling (PUBS) provides a fetal blood sample for karyotype, direct Coombs' test, or complete blood count. PUBS, sometimes called cordocentesis, can also be used to determine fetal blood type, check blood gas levels and acid-base status, and identify and treat isoimmunization.

To obtain a percutaneous umbilical blood sample, a needle is inserted transabdominally (using ultrasound guidance) into a fetal umbilical vessel. A blood sample is then tested to ensure that fetal and not maternal blood has been drawn. Possible complications include blood leakage at the puncture site, fetal bradycardia, or infection.

Purpose

■ To identify chromosomal abnormalities, such as hypoploidy or hyperploidy, as the underlying cause of malformation, maldevelopment, or disease

Patient preparation

■ Explain to the patient or his parents, if appropriate, the purpose of the chromosome analysis.
■ Tell the patient who will perform the test and what kind of specimen will be required.
■ Inform the patient when results will be available, according to the specimen required.

Procedure and posttest care

■ Collect a blood sample (in a 5- to 10-ml heparinized tube), a tissue specimen, 1 ml of bone marrow, or at least 20 ml of amniotic fluid.

■ Provide appropriate posttest care, depending on the procedure used to collect the specimen.
■ Explain the test results and their implications to the patient or his parents, if he's a child, with a chromosomal abnormality.
■ Recommend appropriate genetic or other counseling and follow-up care if necessary, such as an infant stimulation program for a patient with Down syndrome.

Precautions

■ Keep all specimens sterile, especially those requiring a tissue culture.
■ To facilitate interpretation of test results, send the specimen to the laboratory immediately after collection, with a brief patient history and the indication for the test.
■ Refrigerate the specimen if transport is delayed, but *never* freeze it.

▶ CLINICAL ALERT *Before a skin biopsy, make sure the povidone-iodine solution is thoroughly removed with alcohol. This solution could prevent cell growth.*

Normal findings

The normal cell contains 46 chromosomes: 22 pairs of nonsex chromosomes (autosomes) and 1 pair of sex chromosomes (Y for the male-determining chromosome, X for the female-determining chromosome). On a karyotype, chromosomes are arranged according to size and the location of their primary constrictions, or centromeres.

The centromere may be medial (metacentric), slightly to one end of the chromosome (submetacentric), or entirely to one end (acrocentric). The largest chromosomes are displayed first; the others are arranged in order of decreasing size, with the two sex chromosomes traditionally placed last. By convention, the centromere is always placed at the top in a karyotype. Thus, if the two pairs of chromosomal arms are of unequal length, the arm above the centromere will be shorter. The letter "p" designates the short arm; the letter "q," the long arm.

Special stains identify individual chromosomes and locate and enumerate particular portions of chromosomes. Trypsin, alkali, heat denaturation, and Giemsa stain are used for visible light microscopy; quinacrine stain, for ultraviolet microscopy. These techniques produce nonuniform staining of each chromosome in a repetitive, banded pattern. The mechanism of chromosome banding is unknown, but seems related to primary deoxyribonucleic acid sequence and protein composition of the chromosome.

Abnormal findings

Chromosomal abnormalities may be numerical or structural. Any numerical deviation from the norm of 46 chromosomes is called *aneuploidy.* Less than 46 chromosomes is called *hypoploidy; more* than 46, *hyperploidy.* Special designations exist for whole multiples of the haploid number 23: *diploidy* for the normal somatic number of 46, *triploidy* for 69, *tetraploidy* for 92, and so forth.

When the deviation occurs within a single pair of chromosomes, the suffix "–somy" is used, as in *trisomy* for the presence of three chromosomes instead of the usual pair or *monosomy* for the presence of only one chromosome.

Aneuploidy most commonly follows failure of the chromosomal pair to separate (nondisjunction) during anaphase, the mitotic stage that follows metaphase. It may also result from anaphase lag, in which one of the normally separated chromosomes fails to move to a pole and is left out of the daughter cells.

If nondisjunction or anaphase lag occurs during meiosis, the cells of the zygote will all be the same. Errors in mitotic division after zygote formation will produce more than one cell line (mosaicism).

Structural chromosomal abnormalities result from chromosome breakage. Intrachromosomal rearrangement occurs within a single chromosome in these forms:

- *deletion* — loss of an end (terminal) or middle (interstitial) portion of a chromosome
- *inversion* — end-to-end reversal of a chromosome segment, which may be pericentric inversion (including the centromere) or paracentric inversion (occurring in only one arm of the chromosome)
- *ring chromosome formation* — breakage of both ends of a chromosome and reunion of the ends
- *isochromosome formation* — abnormal splitting of the centromere in a transverse rather than a longitudinal plane.

Interchromosomal rearrangements (of more than one chromosome, usually two) also occur. The most common rearrangement is translocation, or exchange, of genetic material between two chromosomes. Translocations may be balanced, in which the cell neither loses nor gains genetic material; unbalanced, in which a piece of genetic material is gained or lost from each cell; reciprocal (in children), in which two chromosomes exchange material; or Robertsonian, in which two chromosomes join to form one combined chromosome with little or no loss of material.

Implications of chromosome analysis results depend on the specimen and indications for the test. (See *Chromosome analysis findings,* page 668.)

CHROMOSOME ANALYSIS FINDINGS

Specimen and indication	Result	Implication
Blood		
■ To evaluate abnormal appearance or development, suggesting chromosomal irregularity	■ Abnormal chromosome number (aneuploidy) or arrangement	■ Identifies specific chromosomal abnormality
■ To evaluate couples with a history of miscarriages or to identify balanced translocation carriers having unbalanced offspring	■ Normal chromosomes ■ Parental balanced translocation carrier	■ Miscarriage unrelated to parental chromosomal abnormality ■ Increased risk of repeated abortion or unbalanced offspring indicates need for amniocentesis in future pregnancies
■ To detect chromosomal rearrangements in rare genetic diseases predisposing the patient to malignant neoplasms	■ Chromosomal rearrangements, gaps, and breaks	■ Occurs in Bloom's syndrome, Fanconi's syndrome, telangiectasia; patient predisposed to malignant neoplasms
Blood or bone marrow		
■ To identify Philadelphia chromosome and confirm chronic myelogenous leukemia	■ Translocation of chromosome 22q (long arm) to another chromosome (often chromosome 9) ■ Aneuploidy (usually due to abnormalities in chromosomes 8 and 12) ■ Trisomy 21	■ Aids in the diagnosis of chronic myelogenous leukemia ■ Occurs in acute myelogenous leukemia ■ Occasionally occurs in chronic lymphocytic leukemia cells
Skin		
■ To evaluate abnormal appearance or development, suggesting chromosomal irregularity	■ All chromosomal abnormalities possible	■ Same as chromosomal abnormality in blood; rarely, mosaic individual has normal blood but abnormal skin chromosomes
Amniotic fluid		
■ To evaluate the developing fetus with possible chromosomal abnormality	■ All chromosomal abnormalities possible	■ Same as chromosomal abnormality in blood or fetus

CHROMOSOME ANALYSIS FINDINGS *(continued)*

Specimen and indication	Result	Implication
Placental tissue		
■ To evaluate products of conception after a miscarriage to determine if the abnormality is fetal or placental in origin	■ All chromosomal abnormalities possible	■ More than 50% of aborted tissue is chromosomally abnormal
Tumor tissue		
■ For research purposes only	■ Many chromosomal abnormalities possible	■ Although malignant tumors aren't associated with specific chromosomal aberrations, most are aneuploid, usually hyperploid

Interfering factors

■ Chemotherapy (possible abnormal results due to chromosome breaks)
■ Contamination of tissue with bacteria, fungus, or a virus (possible inhibition of culture growth)
■ Inclusion of maternal cells in a specimen obtained by amniocentesis, with subsequent culturing (possible false results)

Amniotic fluid analysis

Amniocentesis is the percutaneous transabdominal puncture of the uterus to obtain a 10- to 20-ml sample of amniotic fluid for laboratory analysis. It may be used to detect certain birth defects, such as Down syndrome or spina bifida; to determine fetal maturity; to detect hemolytic disease of the neonate; or, through karyotyping, to detect gender and chromosomal abnormalities. This test can be performed only when the amniotic fluid level reaches 150 ml, usually after 16 weeks' gestation.

Amniotic fluid reflects important metabolic changes in the fetus, the placenta, and the mother. It protects the fetus from external trauma, allows the fetus to move, and provides for the fetus an even body temperature and limited source of protein (10% to 15%). Although the origin of amniotic fluid is uncertain, its original composition is essentially the same as that of interstitial fluid. As the fetus matures, however, the amniotic fluid becomes progressively more diluted with hypotonic fetal urine.

One of the key differences between amniotic fluid and maternal plasma during intrauterine development is the amniotic fluid's relatively high levels of uric acid, urea, and creatinine. The volume of amniotic fluid steadily rises from 50 ml at the end of the first trimester to an average of 1,000 ml near term; at 40 weeks' gestation, the volume decreases to 700 to 800 ml.

CHORIONIC VILLI SAMPLING

Chorionic villi sampling (CVS) is a prenatal test for quick detection of fetal chromosomal and biochemical disorders that's performed during the first trimester of pregnancy. Preliminary results may be available within hours; complete results, within a few days. In contrast, amniocentesis can't be performed before 16 weeks' gestation, and the results aren't available for at least 2 weeks. Thus, CVS can detect fetal abnormalities as much as 10 weeks sooner than amniocentesis.

Chorionic villi are fingerlike projections that surround the embryonic membrane and eventually give rise to the placenta. Cells obtained from an appropriate sample are of fetal, rather than maternal, origin and thus can be analyzed for fetal abnormalities.

Collection time

Samples are best obtained between the 8th and 10th weeks of pregnancy. Before 7 weeks, the villi cover the embryo and make selective sampling difficult. After 10 weeks, maternal cells begin to grow over the villi, and the amniotic sac begins to fill the uterine cavity, making the procedure difficult and potentially dangerous.

Collection method

To collect a sample, the patient is placed in the lithotomy position. The physician checks the placement of the patient's uterus bimanually and then inserts a Graves speculum and swabs the cervix with an antiseptic solution. If necessary, he may use a tenaculum to straighten an acutely flexed uterus, permitting cannula insertion. Guided by ultrasound and possibly endoscopy, he directs the catheter through the cannula to the villi. Suction is applied to the catheter to remove about 30 mg of tissue from the villi. The sample is withdrawn, placed in a Petri dish, and examined with a dissecting microscope. Part of the specimen is then cultured for further testing.

Interpretation

CVS can be used to detect about 200 diseases prenatally. For example, direct analysis of rapidly dividing fetal cells can detect chromosome disorders, deoxyribonucleic acid analysis can detect hemoglobinopathies, and lysosomal enzyme assays can screen for lysosomal storage disorders such as Tay-Sachs disease.

The test appears to provide reliable results, except when the sample contains too

---

Amniocentesis is indicated if the patient is over age 35; has a family history of genetic, chromosomal, or neural tube defects; or has had a miscarriage. Although adverse effects are rare, potential complications include spontaneous abortion, trauma to the fetus or placenta, bleeding, premature labor, infection, and Rh sensitization from fetal bleeding into the maternal circulation. Because of the severity of possible complications, amniocentesis is contraindicated as a general screening test. Abnormal test results or failure of the

tissue cultures to grow may necessitate test repetition.

Another method of detecting fetal chromosomal and biochemical disorders in early pregnancy is chorionic villi sampling. (See *Chorionic villi sampling.*)

Purpose

■ To detect fetal abnormalities, particularly chromosomal and neural tube defects

■ To detect hemolytic disease of the neonate

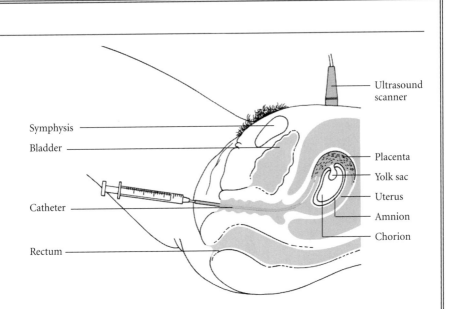

few cells or the cells fail to grow in culture. Patient risks for this procedure appear to be similar to those for amniocentesis: a small chance of spontaneous abortion, cramps, infection, and bleeding. However, recent research reports an incidence of limb malformations in neonates when CVS has been performed.

Unlike amniocentesis, CVS can't detect complications in cases of Rh sensitization, uncover neural tube defects, or determine pulmonary maturity. However, it may prove to be the best way to detect other serious fetal abnormalities early in pregnancy.

■ To diagnose metabolic disorders, amino acid disorders, and mucopolysaccharidosis
■ To determine fetal age and maturity, especially pulmonary maturity (See *Shake test*, page 672.)
■ To assess fetal health by detecting the presence of meconium or blood or measuring amniotic levels of estriol and fetal thyroid hormone
■ To identify fetal gender when one or both parents are carriers of a sex-linked disorder

Patient preparation

■ Describe the procedure to the patient and explain that amniocentesis detects fetal abnormalities.
■ Assess her understanding of the test and answer her questions.
■ Inform her that she need not restrict food and fluids.
■ Tell her that the test requires a specimen of amniotic fluid, who will perform the test, and when it will take place.

SHAKE TEST

Amniotic fluid from mature fetal lungs contains surfactants. In the shake test, also known as the *foam stability test*, bubbles should appear on the surface of a test tube of amniotic fluid that's shaken vigorously if adequate amounts of surfactants are present.

Using a chemically clean 13-mm × 100-mm glass tube with a Teflon-lined screw cap or a rubber stopper, combine 1 ml of amniotic fluid and 1 ml of 95% ethanol. In another tube, combine 0.5 ml of amniotic fluid, 0.5 ml of saline solution, and 1 ml of 95% ethanol. Shake both tubes vigorously for 15 seconds and place them upright in a rack for 15 minutes.

If a complete ring of bubbles is still evident in both tubes after 15 minutes, as shown, the test is positive and the risk of respiratory distress is low. A positive result in the second tube indicates pulmonary maturity. Negative results indicate a risk of respiratory distress. Blood or meconium in the fluid invalidates the test.

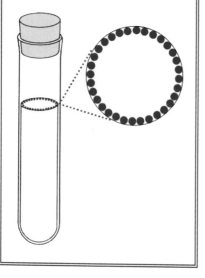

- Advise her that normal test results can't guarantee a normal fetus because some fetal disorders are undetectable.
- Make sure that the patient or a responsible family member has signed an informed consent form.
- Explain to the patient that she'll feel a stinging sensation when the local anesthetic is injected.
- Provide emotional support before and during the test.
- Ask the patient to void just before the test to minimize the risk of puncturing the bladder and aspirating urine instead of amniotic fluid.

Equipment
70% alcohol or povidone-iodine solution, sponge forceps, 2" × 2" gauze pads, local anesthetic (1% lidocaine), 25G sterile needle, 3-ml syringe, 20G sterile spinal needle with stylet, 10-ml syringe, amber or foil-covered sterile 10-ml test tube

Procedure and posttest care
- A pool of amniotic fluid is located after determining fetal and placental position, usually through palpation and ultrasonic visualization.
- The skin is prepared with antiseptic and alcohol, and then 1 ml of 1% lidocaine is injected with a 25G needle, first intradermally and then subcutaneously.
- Then a 20G spinal needle with a stylet is inserted into the amniotic cavity, and the stylet is withdrawn.
- A 10-ml syringe is attached to the needle, and then the fluid is aspirated and placed in an amber or foil-covered test tube.
- The needle is withdrawn and an adhesive bandage is placed over the needle insertion site.

■ Monitor fetal heart rate and maternal vital signs every 15 minutes for at least 30 minutes.

■ Position the patient on her left side if she sweats profusely or feels faint or nauseated to counteract uterine pressure on the vena cava.

■ Instruct the patient before she's discharged to immediately report abdominal pain or cramping, chills, fever, vaginal bleeding or leakage of serous vaginal fluid, or fetal hyperactivity or unusual fetal lethargy.

Precautions

■ Instruct the patient to fold her hands behind her head to prevent her from accidentally touching the sterile field and causing contamination.

■ Send the specimen to the laboratory immediately after collection.

Normal findings

Normal amniotic fluid is clear, but may contain white flecks of vernix caseosa when the fetus is near term. For an analysis of the appearance and components of amniotic fluid, see *Findings in amniotic fluid analysis,* page 674.

Abnormal findings

Blood, which is found in about 10% of amniocenteses, results from a faulty tap and doesn't indicate an abnormality. However, it does inhibit cell growth and changes the level of other amniotic fluid constituents. "Port wine" fluid, on the other hand, may be a sign of abruptio placentae, and blood of fetal origin may indicate damage to the fetal, placental, or umbilical cord vessels by the amniocentesis needle. (See *Apt test,* page 675.)

Large amounts of *bilirubin,* a breakdown product of red blood cells, may indicate hemolytic disease of the neonate.

Normally, the bilirubin level increases from 14 to 24 weeks' gestation, then declines as the fetus matures, essentially reaching zero at term. Testing for bilirubin usually isn't performed until the 26th week because that's the earliest time successful therapy for Rh sensitization can begin. Bilirubin level is determined by spectrophotometric measurement of the optic density of the amniotic fluid. The deviation of the scan at 450µ from a straight line drawn between 375µ and 525µ represents the bilirubin peak.

Meconium, a semisolid viscous material found in the fetal GI tract, consists of mucopolysaccharides, desquamated cells, vernix, hair, and cholesterol. Meconium passes into the amniotic fluid when hypoxia causes fetal distress and relaxation of the anal sphincter. Meconium is a normal finding in breech presentation. Meconium in the amniotic fluid produces a peak of 410 mµ on the spectrophotometric analysis. However, serial amniocentesis may show a clearing of meconium over a 2- to 3-week period. If meconium is present during labor, the neonate's nose and throat require thorough cleaning to prevent meconium aspiration.

Creatinine, a product of fetal urine, increases in the amniotic fluid as the fetal kidneys mature. Generally, the creatinine value exceeds 2 mg/dl in a mature fetus.

Alpha-fetoprotein (AFP) is a fetal alpha globulin produced first in the yolk sac and later in the parenchymal cells of the liver and GI tract. Fetal serum AFP levels are about 150 times higher than amniotic fluid levels; maternal serum AFP levels are far lower than amniotic fluid levels. High amniotic fluid levels indicate neural tube defects, but the AFP level may remain normal if the defect is small and closed. Elevated AFP levels may also occur in multiple pregnancy; in disorders

FINDINGS IN AMNIOTIC FLUID ANALYSIS

Test	Normal findings	Fetal implications of abnormal findings
Color	Clear, with white flecks of vernix caseosa in a mature fetus	Blood of maternal origin (usually harmless); "port wine" fluid indicating abruptio placentae; fetal blood indicating damage to the fetal, placental, or umbilical cord vessels
Bilirubin	Early: < 0.075 mg/dl (SI, < 1.3 µmol/L) Term: < 0.025 mg/dl (SI, < 0.41 µmol/L)	High levels indicating hemolytic disease of the neonate in isoimmunized pregnancy
Meconium	Absent (except in breech presentation)	Presence indicating fetal hypotension or distress
Creatinine	> 2 mg/dl (SI, 177 µmol/L)	Decreased levels indicating immature fetus (less than 37 weeks)
Lecithin-sphingomyelin ratio	> 2	< 2 indicating pulmonary immaturity
Phosphatidylglycerol	Present	Absence indicating pulmonary immaturity
Glucose	< 45 mg/dl (SI, 2.3 mmol/L)	Excessive increases at term or near term indicating hypertrophy of fetal pancreas
Alpha-fetoprotein	Variable, depending on gestation age and laboratory technique	Inappropriate increases indicating neural tube defects, such as spina bifida or anencephaly, impending fetal death, congenital nephrosis, or contamination by fetal blood
Bacteria	Absent	Presence indicating chorioamniotitis
Chromosome	Normal karyotype	Abnormal karyotype indicating fetal gender and chromosome disorders
Acetylcholinesterase	Absent	Presence indicating neural tube defects, exomphalos, or other serious malformations

such as omphalocele, congenital nephrosis, esophageal or duodenal atresia, cystic fibrosis, exomphalos, Turner's syndrome, and fetal bladder neck obstruction with hydronephrosis; and in impending fetal death.

The amount of *uric acid* in the amniotic fluid increases as the fetus matures, but these levels fluctuate widely and can't accurately predict maturity. Laboratory studies indicate that severe erythroblastosis fetalis, familial hyperuricemia, and Lesch-Nyhan syndrome tend to increase the uric acid level.

Estrone, estradiol, estriol, and *estriol conjugates* appear in amniotic fluid in varying amounts. Levels of estriol, the most prevalent estrogen, increase substantially at term. Severe erythroblastosis fetalis decreases the estriol level.

The type II cells lining the fetal lung alveoli produce *lecithin* slowly in early pregnancy and then markedly increase production around the 35th week.

The *sphingomyelin* level parallels that of lecithin until the 35th week, when it gradually decreases. Measuring the ratio of lecithin to sphingomyelin (L/S) confirms fetal pulmonary maturity (L/S ratio > 2) or suggests a risk of respiratory distress (L/S ratio < 2). However, fetal respiratory distress may develop in the fetus of a patient with diabetes, even though the L/S ratio is greater than 2, a level that usually indicates pulmonary maturity.

Phosphatidylglycerol levels are present with pulmonary maturity; *phosphatidylinositol* levels decrease.

Measuring *glucose* levels in the fluid can aid in assessing glucose control in the patient with diabetes, but this isn't done routinely. A level greater than 45 mg/dl (SI, > 2.6 mmol/L) indicates poor maternal and fetal control. *Insulin* levels normally increase slightly from the 27th to

---

APT TEST

Blood in the amniotic fluid can be of maternal or fetal origin. The Apt test, which is based on the premises that fetal hemoglobin is alkali-resistant and adult hemoglobin changes to alkaline hematin after the addition of alkali, can differentiate between the two. This test may be performed on all bloody amniotic fluid samples.

To perform this test, dilute 1 ml of amniotic fluid with water until it turns pink. Centrifuge for 10 minutes, then decant the supernatant. Add five parts supernatant to one part 0.25 N (1%) sodium hydroxide, and observe for 1 to 2 minutes. Fetal blood appears red; maternal blood, yellow-brown. To confirm the results, repeat the test with known maternal blood.

---

the 40th week, but increase sharply (up to 27 times normal) in a patient with poorly controlled diabetes.

Laboratory analysis can identify at least 25 different *enzymes* (usually in low concentrations) in amniotic fluid. The enzymes have few known clinical implications, although elevated acetylcholinesterase levels may occur with neural tube defects, exomphalos, and other serious malformations.

When the mother carries an *X-linked disorder,* determination of fetal sex is important. If chromosome karyotyping identifies a male fetus, there's a 50% chance he'll be affected; a female fetus won't be affected, but has a 50% chance of being a carrier.

Interfering factors

■ Use of plastic disposable syringes (possible toxicity to amniotic fluid cells)

- Failure to place the specimen in an appropriate amber or foil-covered tube (possible decrease in bilirubin)
- Blood or meconium in the fluid (effect on L/S ratio)
- Maternal blood in the fluid (possible decrease in creatinine)
- Any amount of fetal blood in the fluid specimen (possible doubling of AFP concentrations)
- Several disorders that aren't associated with pregnancy, including infectious mononucleosis, cirrhosis, hepatic cancer, teratoma, endodermal sinus tumor, gastric carcinoma, pancreatic carcinoma, and subacute hereditary tyrosinemia (possible increase in AFP levels)

ENDOSCOPY

Laparoscopy

Laparoscopy permits visualization of the peritoneal cavity by the insertion of a small fiber-optic telescope (laparoscope) through the anterior abdominal wall. This surgical technique may be used diagnostically to detect abnormalities, such as cysts, adhesions, fibroids, and infection. It can also be used therapeutically to perform procedures, such as adhesion lysis; ovarian biopsy; tubal sterilization; removal of ectopic pregnancies, fibroids, hydrosalpinx, and foreign bodies; and fulguration of endometriotic implants.

Although laparoscopy has largely replaced laparotomy, the latter is usually preferred when extensive surgery is indicated. Potential risks of laparoscopy include a punctured visceral organ, causing bleeding or spilling of intestinal contents into the peritoneum.

Purpose
- To identify the cause of pelvic pain
- To help detect endometriosis, ectopic pregnancy, and pelvic inflammatory disease (PID)
- To evaluate pelvic masses or the fallopian tubes of the infertile patient
- To stage carcinoma in selected cases

Patient preparation
- Explain the procedure to the patient and tell her that laparoscopy is used to detect abnormalities of the uterus, fallopian tubes, and ovaries.
- Instruct the patient to fast for at least 8 hours before surgery.
- Tell the patient who will perform the procedure and where it will take place.
- Tell the patient whether she'll receive a general anesthetic and whether the procedure will require an outpatient visit or overnight hospitalization.
- Warn the patient that she may experience pain at the puncture site and in the shoulder.
- Make sure that the patient or a responsible family member has signed an informed consent form.
- Check the patient's history for hypersensitivity to the anesthetic.
- Make sure laboratory work is completed and results are reported before the test.
- Instruct the patient to empty her bladder just before the test.

Equipment
Indwelling urinary or straight catheter; sterile tray with scalpel, hemostats, needle holder, suture, and suture scissors; Veress needle; gas insufflator; laparoscope; fiber-optic light source and cable; laparoscope sheath and trocar; electrosurgical generator; tenaculum and intrauterine manipulator; probes, scissors, or forceps; adhesive bandages

Procedure and posttest care

- The patient is anesthetized and placed in the lithotomy position.
- The examiner catheterizes the bladder and then performs a bimanual examination of the pelvic area to detect abnormalities that may contraindicate the test and to ensure that the bladder is empty.
- The tenaculum is placed on the cervix and a uterine manipulator is inserted; an incision is made at the inferior rim of the umbilicus.
- The Veress needle is inserted into the peritoneal cavity, and 2 to 3 L of carbon dioxide or nitrous oxide is insufflated to distend the abdominal wall and provide an organ-free space for trocar insertion; the needle is removed and a trocar and sheath are inserted into the peritoneal cavity; multiple trocars may be inserted at the pubic hairline to allow access for other instruments.
- After removal of the trocar, the laparoscope is inserted through the sheath to examine the pelvis and abdomen.
- To evaluate tubal patency, the examiner infuses a dye through the cervix and observes the tubes for spillage.
- After the examination, minor surgical procedures, such as ovarian biopsy, may be performed.
- Monitor the patient's vital signs and urine output. Report sudden changes immediately; they may indicate complications.
- Monitor the patient for adverse or allergic reactions. After administration of a general anesthetic, monitor her electrolyte balance, hemoglobin level, and hematocrit. Help her ambulate after recovery.
- Tell the patient that she may resume her usual diet.
- Instruct the patient to restrict activity for 2 to 7 days, as necessary.

- Reassure the patient that some abdominal and shoulder pain is normal and should disappear within 24 to 36 hours. If pain continues or worsens, notify the physician immediately as this may be a sign of bowel perforation. Provide analgesics, as ordered, and monitor her for adverse effects.

Precautions

- Laparoscopy is contraindicated in the patient with advanced abdominal wall cancer, advanced pulmonary or cardiovascular disease, intestinal obstruction, palpable abdominal mass, large abdominal hernia, chronic tuberculosis, or a history of peritonitis.
- During the procedure, check for proper catheter drainage.

Normal findings

The uterus and fallopian tubes are of normal size and shape, free from adhesions, and mobile. The ovaries are of normal size and shape; cysts and endometriosis are absent. Dye injected through the cervix flows freely from the fimbria.

Abnormal findings

An ovarian cyst appears as a bubble on the surface of the ovary. The cyst may be clear if filled with follicular fluid or serous or mucous material, or it may be red, blue, or brown if filled with blood. Adhesions may appear as thick and fibrous tissue or as almost transparent strands of tissue.

Endometriosis may resemble small, blue powder burns on the peritoneum or the serosa of any pelvic or abdominal structure; however, clear, red lesions are also possible. Fibroids appear as lumps on the uterus, hydrosalpinx as an enlarged fallopian tube, and ectopic pregnancy as an enlarged or ruptured fallopian tube. In PID, infection or abscess is evident.

Interfering factors
- Adhesions or marked obesity (possible obstruction to visualization)
- Tissue or fluid becoming attached to the lens (possible obstruction to visualization)

Hysteroscopy

In hysteroscopy, a small-diameter endoscope is used to visualize the interior of the uterus. Performed in the physician's office or a short procedure unit under local or general anesthesia, this procedure has become widely used to investigate abnormal uterine bleeding. It also aids in the removal of polyps and in the diagnosis and treatment of other uterine abnormalities. Other investigational uses for hysteroscopy are being studied, and it has recently been approved by the U.S. Food and Drug Administration for total sterilization.

Purpose
- To investigate abnormal uterine bleeding
- To remove polyps
- To evaluate an infertile patient
- To remove embedded intrauterine devices
- To aid in the diagnosis and treatment of intrauterine adhesions
- To diagnose uterine fibroids
- To resect fibroids and ablate the endometrium
- To provide total sterilization

Patient preparation
- Explain the procedure to the patient and tell her that hysteroscopy helps detect abnormalities in the uterus.

- Tell the patient that the physician will perform this procedure in his office, usually using a local anesthetic. (However, if the patient's problems appear extensive, an in-hospital operative hysteroscopy would be indicated.)
- Inform the patient that the test should take place within the first week after the end of her menstrual cycle. Ask her when her last Papanicolaou test was performed and obtain the results.
- Tell the patient that the physician will perform a complete pelvic examination before the hysteroscopy and that cultures of the vagina and cervix will be taken if necessary.
- Inform the patient that she'll be asked to empty her bladder before the test.
- Tell the patient that she may have some vaginal bleeding and mild abdominal cramping after the test.
- Explain to the patient that the physician may inflate her uterus with carbon dioxide gas so that he can see the interior of the uterus better. This gas will be absorbed and dispersed by her body and may cause upper abdominal or shoulder pain lasting 24 to 36 hours after the test.
- Recommend to the patient that she have a friend or relative drive her home.
- Make sure that the patient or a responsible family member has signed an informed consent form.
- Check the patient's history for hypersensitivity to the anesthetic.
- Make sure laboratory work is completed and results are reported before the test.

Equipment
Vaginal speculum, gas insufflator, hysteroscope, spinal needle, 1% lidocaine, sanitary pad (Equipment needs may vary, depending on the purpose of the procedure.)

Procedure and posttest care

- Place the patient in a modified dorsal lithotomy position with her legs held in the stirrups.
- The physician will expose the cervix using the smallest speculum possible, and then will suffuse the cervix with 1% lidocaine. Depending on the purpose of the procedure, a paracervical block, an anxiolytic, or an analgesic may also be used. In some cases, a regional or general anesthetic may be used.
- The physician will gently sound the endocervical canal and uterine cavity and will dilate the canal, as necessary, to insert the hysteroscope. (Modern hysteroscopes are 10″ [25 cm] long.) Visualization of the uterine cavity begins at the level of the internal os.
- The two primary types of hysteroscopy are contact and panoramic. In *contact hysteroscopy,* the uterus isn't distended and only the area in direct contact with the hysteroscope can be viewed. In *panoramic hysteroscopy,* the more common type, an external illumination source and media (such as carbon dioxide gas) for distention are needed. This method allows visualization of the tissue from a distance.
- Monitor the patient's vital signs.
- The patient may have slight vaginal bleeding and lower abdominal cramping. Provide a sanitary pad, if needed.
- Severe cramps, dyspnea, and upper abdominal and right shoulder pain can develop if carbon dioxide passes into the peritoneal cavity. Reassure the patient that some abdominal and shoulder pain is normal and should disappear within 24 to 36 hours. Recommend that she have a friend or relative drive her home.
- Provide analgesics, as needed.

Precautions

- Hysteroscopy requires experience in topographic interpretation of the uterus and skill in manipulating the required instruments.
- During the procedure, monitor the patient's vital signs and discomfort level.

Normal findings

The interior of the uterus is normal in size and shape and free from adhesions and lesions.

Abnormal findings

Hysteroscopy may detect polyps, uterine wall tumors, and other uterine abnormalities.

Interfering factors

- Heavy bleeding
- A distended bladder or improper patient positioning

DIRECT GRAPHIC RECORDING

External fetal monitoring

In external fetal monitoring, a noninvasive test, an electronic transducer and a cardiotachometer amplify and record fetal heart rate (FHR) while a pressure-sensitive transducer (tocodynamometer) records uterine contractions. Fetal monitoring records the baseline FHR (average FHR over two contraction cycles or 10 minutes), periodic fluctuations in the baseline FHR, and beat-to-beat heart rate variability. (See *Understanding fetal monitoring terminology,* page 680.) External fetal monitoring is also used during other tests of fetal health, notably the nonstress test and the contraction stress test (CST).

UNDERSTANDING FETAL MONITORING TERMINOLOGY

- Baseline fetal heart rate (FHR): Average FHR over two contraction cycles or 10 minutes
- Baseline changes: Fluctuations in FHR unrelated to uterine contractions
- Periodic changes: Fluctuations in FHR related to uterine contractions
- Amplitude: Difference in beats per minute between baseline readings and fluctuation in FHR
- Recovery time: Difference between the end of the contraction and the return to the baseline FHR
- Acceleration: Transient rise in FHR lasting longer than 15 seconds and associated with a uterine contraction
- Deceleration: Transient fall in FHR related to a uterine contraction
- Lag time: Difference between the peak of the contraction and the lowest point of deceleration

Purpose

- To measure FHR and the frequency of uterine contractions
- To evaluate antepartum and intrapartum fetal health during stress and nonstress situations
- To detect fetal distress
- To determine the necessity for internal fetal monitoring

Patient preparation

- Explain to the patient that external fetal monitoring assesses fetal health.
- Explain the procedure to the patient and answer all her questions. Assure her that external fetal monitoring is painless and won't hurt the fetus or interfere with normal labor.
- If monitoring is to be performed antepartum, instruct the patient to eat a meal just before the test to increase fetal activity, which decreases the test time.
- If the patient is still smoking, advise her to abstain for 2 hours before testing because smoking decreases fetal activity.
- Explain to the patient that she may have to restrict movement during baseline readings, but that she may change position between the readings.
- Make sure that the patient or a responsible family member has signed an informed consent form.

Equipment

Tocodynamometer (to measure uterine contractions); ultrasonic transducer (to amplify FHR); cardiotachymeter (to record FHR); mineral oil or ultrasound transmission jelly; elastic band, stockinette, or abdominal strap

Procedure and posttest care

- Place the patient in the semi-Fowler or left lateral position with her abdomen exposed. Cover the ultrasound transducer receiver crystal with ultrasound transmission jelly.
- Palpate the patient's abdomen to identify the fetal chest area, locate the most distinct fetal heart sounds, and then secure the ultrasound transducer over this area with the elastic band, stockinette, or abdominal strap.
- Check the recording equipment to ensure an adequate printout and verify the fetal monitor's alarm boundaries.
- During monitoring, check the elastic band, stockinette, or abdominal strap to ensure that the fit is comfortable yet tight enough to produce a good tracing.
- As labor progresses, reposition the pressure transducer as necessary so that it remains on the fundal portion of the

uterus. You may have to reposition the ultrasound transducer as fetal or maternal position changes.

For antepartum monitoring with nonstress tests

■ Tell the patient to hold the pressure transducer in her hand and to push it each time she feels the fetus move.

■ Within a 20-minute period, monitor baseline FHR until you record two fetal movements that last longer than 15 seconds each and cause heart rate accelerations of more than 15 beats/minute from the baseline. If you can't obtain two FHR accelerations within 30 minutes, shake the patient's abdomen to stimulate the fetus and repeat the test.

For antepartum monitoring with a CST

■ Induce contractions by oxytocin infusion or nipple stimulation (endogenous oxytocin).

■ When administering oxytocin, infuse a dilute solution at a rate of 1 mU/minute, increasing the oxytocin rate until the patient experiences three contractions within 10 minutes, each lasting longer than 45 seconds.

■ When using nipple stimulation, tell the patient to stimulate one nipple by hand until contractions begin. If a second contraction doesn't occur in 2 minutes, have her stimulate the nipple again. Stimulate both nipples if contractions don't occur in 15 minutes. Continue the test until contractions occur in 10 minutes.

■ If no decelerations occur during three contractions, the patient may be discharged. Late decelerations during any of the contractions require notification of the physician and further tests.

For intrapartum monitoring

■ Secure the pressure transducer with an elastic band, a stockinette, or an abdominal strap over the area of greatest uterine electrical activity during contractions (usually the fundus).

■ Adjust the machine to record 0 to 10 mm Hg of pressure between palpable contractions.

■ Reposition the ultrasound and pressure transducers as necessary to ensure continuous accurate readings. Review the tracings frequently for baseline abnormalities, periodic changes, variability of changes, and uterine contraction abnormalities.

■ Record maternal movement, administration of drugs, and procedures performed directly on the tracing to assist in the evaluation of changes in the tracing.

■ Report abnormalities immediately.

■ Repeat antepartum monitoring weekly as long as indications, such as pregnancy over 42 weeks' gestation or fetal growth retardation, persist.

Precautions

■ During a CST, watch for fetal distress with oxytocin infusion or nipple stimulation.

Normal findings

Normal baseline FHR ranges from 120 to 160 beats/minute, with a variability of 5 to 25 beats/minute. For the antepartum nonstress test, the fetus is considered healthy and should remain so for another week if two fetal movements causing a heart rate acceleration of more than 15 beats/minute from baseline FHR occur in a 20-minute period. Nonstress testing is also done for postdate fetal well-being. A normal, healthy fetus usually has three rises in FHR within 10 to 15 minutes, but fetuses may sleep up to 45 minutes at a time. If there's no change in FHR in a

COMPARING DECELERATED FETAL HEART RATES AND UTERINE CONTRACTIONS

Unlike variable decelerations, early and late decelerations in the fetal heart rate (FHR) correspond to uterine contractions.

Decelerations in FHR may be affected by uterine contractions. The three types of FHR decelerations — early, late, and variable — occur at different points in the contraction phase.

Early FHR decelerations occur at the onset of a uterine contraction and reach their lowest point at the peak of the contraction. In early deceleration, FHR returns to the average baseline by the end of the contraction. FHR produces a smooth wave pattern that mirrors the uterine contraction. There's a consistent relationship between the fall in FHR and the uterine contractions. Early deceleration is usually benign and is most commonly caused by compression of the fetal head. This pattern typically occurs with advanced dilation (more than 7 cm).

Late decelerations begin about 20 seconds after the onset of a contraction and reach their lowest point well after the contraction has peaked. In late decelera-

tion, FHR recovery occurs later than 15 seconds following the contraction. Although the FHR tracing in late deceleration resembles the smooth wave of early deceleration, its implications are far more serious. Late decelerations usually result from uteroplacental insufficiency and may lead to fetal death. When associated with increased variability or with tachycardia and no variability, late decelerations indicate fetal central nervous system depression and myocardial hypoxia.

Variable decelerations — sudden drops in the FHR — may occur at any time during a contraction. After the decline, baseline FHR recovery may be rapid or prolonged. Because the fall in FHR is unrelated to uterine contractions, wave patterns also vary. Variable decelerations occur in about 50% of all labors and are usually associated with transitory umbilical cord compression. But a severe drop (to less than 70 beats/minute for more than 60 seconds) may indicate fetal acidosis, hypoxia, and low Apgar scores.

10-minute period, consider shaking the patient's abdomen gently, clapping loudly, or having the patient drink ice water or apple juice. If the FHR remains unchanged, a contraction stress test or biophysical profile test should be ordered. The fetus is assessed by watching fetal movements, muscle tone, fetal breathing, and the amniotic fluid index.

For the CST, the fetus is assumed to be healthy and should remain so for another week if three contractions occur during a 10-minute period, with no late decelerations.

Abnormal findings

Bradycardia (FHR ≤ 120 beats/minute) may indicate fetal heart block, malposition, or hypoxia. Fetal bradycardia may also be drug-induced. Tachycardia (FHR >160 beats/minute) may result from maternal fever, tachycardia, hyperthyroidism, or use of vagolytic drugs or opioids; early fetal hypoxia; or fetal infection or arrhythmia.

Decreased variability (a fluctuation of < 5 beats/minute in the FHR) may be caused by fetal arrhythmia or heart block; fetal hypoxia, central nervous system malformation, or infections; or vagolytic

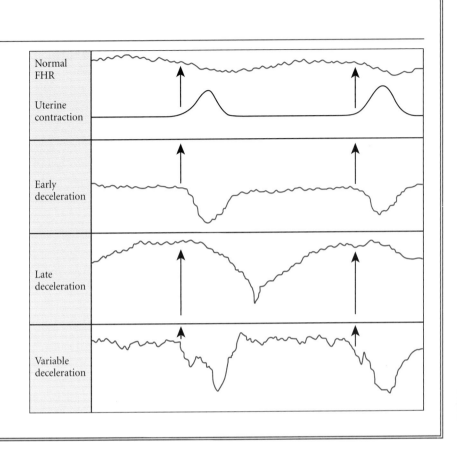

| Normal FHR |
| Uterine contraction |
| Early deceleration |
| Late deceleration |
| Variable deceleration |

drugs. FHR accelerations may result from early hypoxia. They may precede or follow variable decelerations and may indicate that the fetus is in a breech position. (See *Comparing decelerated fetal heart rates and uterine contractions.*)

For the antepartum nonstress test, a positive result (fewer than two accelerations of FHR that last longer than 15 seconds each, with a heart rate acceleration of over 15 beats/minute) indicates an increased risk of perinatal morbidity and mortality and usually requires a CST.

For the CST, persistent late decelerations during two or more contractions may indicate an increased risk of fetal morbidity or mortality. Hyperstimulation (long or frequent uterine contractions) or suspicious results require biophysical profile assessment. If findings are unsatisfactory, cesarean birth may be indicated.

Interfering factors

- Maternal position, particularly if supine (may cause artifactual fetal distress)
- Drugs that affect the sympathetic and parasympathetic nervous systems (possible low FHR)

- Excessive maternal or fetal activity (possible difficulty in recording uterine contractions or FHR)
- Maternal obesity (possible difficulty due to density of abdominal wall)
- Loose or dirty leads or transducer connections (possible production of artifacts)

Internal fetal monitoring

Internal fetal monitoring is an invasive procedure that involves attaching an electrode to the fetal scalp to directly monitor fetal heart rate (FHR). A catheter introduced into the uterine cavity measures the frequency and pressure of uterine contractions. Internal monitoring is performed only during labor, after the membranes have ruptured and the cervix has dilated 3 cm, with the fetal head lower than the −2 station and only if external monitoring provides inadequate data.

Internal monitoring provides more accurate information about fetal health than external monitoring and is especially useful in determining whether cesarean delivery is necessary. The procedure carries minimal risks to the patient (perforated uterus and intrauterine infection) and fetus (scalp abscess and hematoma).

Purpose

- To monitor FHR, especially beat-to-beat variability (short-term variability)
- To measure the frequency and pressure of uterine contractions to assess the progress of labor
- To evaluate intrapartum fetal health
- To supplement or replace external fetal monitoring

Patient preparation

- Explain to the patient that internal fetal monitoring accurately assesses fetal health and uterine activity and that it doesn't necessarily mean that there's a problem. Describe the procedure and answer all questions.
- Warn the patient that she may feel mild discomfort when the uterine catheter and scalp electrode are inserted.
- Make sure the patient or a responsible family member has signed an informed consent form.

Equipment

Sterile fetal scalp electrode and guide tube, intrauterine pressure catheter, catheter guide, pressure transducer, fetal heart monitor

Procedure and posttest care
For measuring FHR

- Place the patient in the dorsal lithotomy position and prepare her perineal area for a vaginal examination, explaining each step of the procedure as it's performed by a physician or certified nurse-midwife. As the procedure begins, ask the patient to breathe through her mouth and relax her abdominal muscles.
- After the vaginal examination, the fetal scalp is palpated and an appropriate site is identified. A plastic tube carrying the small electrode is introduced into the cervix, pressed firmly against the fetal scalp, and rotated clockwise to attach the electrode to the scalp. The electrode wire is tugged gently to ensure proper attachment and the tube is withdrawn, leaving the electrode in place.
- A conduction medium is applied to a leg plate, which is then strapped to the patient's thigh. Electrode wires are attached to the leg plate, and a cable from the leg plate is plugged into the fetal

UNDERSTANDING INTERNAL FETAL MONITORING

In internal fetal monitoring, an electrode is attached to the fetal scalp. The resultant fetal electrocardiograms (FECGs) are transmitted to an amplifier. Subsequently, a cardiotachometer measures the interval between FECGs and plots a continuous fetal heart rate (FHR) graph, which is displayed on a two-channel oscilloscope screen. Intrauterine catheters attached to a transducer in the leg plate measure the frequency and pressure of uterine contractions, which are plotted below the FHR graph.

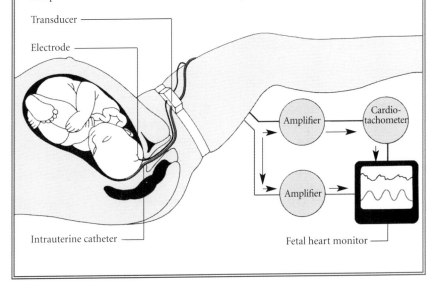

monitor. To check proper placement of the scalp electrode, the monitor is turned on and the electrocardiogram button is pressed; an FHR signal indicates proper electrode attachment. (See *Understanding internal fetal monitoring.*)

For measuring uterine contractions

■ Before inserting the uterine catheter, fill it with sterile normal saline solution to prevent air emboli. Explain each step of the procedure to the patient.

■ Ask the patient to breathe deeply through her mouth and to relax her abdominal muscles.

■ After the vagina has been examined and the presenting part of the fetus palpated, the catheter and guide are inserted ⅜″ to ¾″ (1 to 2 cm) into the cervix, usually between the fetal head and the posterior cervix.

■ The catheter is then gently advanced into the uterus until the black mark on the catheter is flush with the vulva. (The catheter guide should *never* be passed deeply into the uterus.)

■ The guide is removed and the catheter is connected to a transducer that converts the intrauterine pressure, as measured by the fluid in the catheter, to an electrical signal.

For both procedures

■ After removing the fetal scalp electrode, apply antiseptic or antibiotic solution to the attachment site.

NORMAL INTRAUTERINE PRESSURE READINGS DURING LABOR

Stage of labor	Frequency (number of contractions per 10 minutes)	Baseline pressure (mm Hg)	Pressure during contraction (mm Hg)
Prelabor	1 to 2	None	25 to 40
First stage	3 to 5	8 to 12	30 to 40 (or more)
Second stage	5	10 to 20	50 to 80

■ Watch for signs of fetal scalp abscess or maternal intrauterine infection.

Precautions

■ Internal fetal monitoring is contraindicated if there's uncertainty about the fetus's presenting part or a technical impediment to attaching the lead.
■ Prevent artifactual pressure readings by flushing the pressure transducer with normal saline solution; to relieve catheter obstruction (by vernix caseosa, for example), inject a small amount of sterile normal saline solution into the catheter while the transducer is isolated from the system.
■ Make sure a low heart rate is actually the FHR, not the maternal heart rate.
■ If FHR patterns indicate distress, fetal oxygenation commonly can be improved by loading maternal fluids to increase placental perfusion, turning the mother on her side (preferably left) to alleviate supine hypotension, and administering oxygen to the mother. If these measures return FHR patterns to normal, labor may continue. If abnormal patterns persist, cesarean birth may be necessary.
■ Make sure the fetal scalp electrode and the uterine catheter are removed before cesarean delivery.

Reference values

Normal FHR ranges from 120 to 160 beats/minute, with a variability of 5 to 25 beats/minute. (See *Normal intrauterine pressure readings during labor.*)

Abnormal findings

Bradycardia (FHR < 120 beats/minute) may indicate fetal heart block, malposition, or hypoxia. Fetal bradycardia may also result from maternal ingestion of certain drugs, such as propranolol and narcotic analgesics.

Tachycardia (FHR >160 beats/minute) may result from early fetal hypoxia, fetal infection or arrhythmia, prematurity, or maternal fever, tachycardia, hyperthyroidism, or use of vagolytic drugs.

Decreased variability (fluctuation of < 5 beats/minute from baseline) may result from fetal arrhythmia or heart block, hypoxia, central nervous system malformation, or infections or from maternal use of narcotics or vagolytic drugs.

Early decelerations (slowing of FHR at the onset of a contraction with recovery to baseline within no more than 15 seconds after the contraction ends) are related to fetal head compression and usually ensure fetal health.

Late decelerations (slowing of FHR after a contraction begins, a lag time of more than 20 seconds, and a recovery time of more than 15 seconds) may be related to uteroplacental insufficiency, fetal hypoxia, or acidosis. Recurrent and persistently late decelerations with decreased variability usually indicate serious fetal distress, possibly resulting from conduction (spinal, caudal, or epidural) anesthesia or fetal hypoxia.

Variable decelerations (sudden precipitous drops in FHR unrelated to uterine contractions) are commonly related to cord compression. A severe drop in FHR (to < 70 beats/minute for more than 60 seconds) with a decrease in variability indicates fetal distress and may result in a compromised neonate. Poor beat-to-beat variability without periodic patterns may indicate fetal distress, requiring further evaluation such as analysis of fetal blood gas levels.

Decreased intrauterine pressure during labor that isn't progressing normally may require oxytocin stimulation. Elevated intrauterine pressure readings may indicate abruptio placentae or overstimulation from oxytocin, possibly resulting in fetal distress due to decreased placental perfusion.

Interfering factors
■ Drugs that affect the parasympathetic and sympathetic nervous systems

RADIOGRAPHY

Mammography

Mammography is used as a screening test for breast cancer. It helps to detect breast cysts or tumors, especially those not palpable on physical examination. Biopsy of

USING ULTRASONOGRAPHY TO DETECT BREAST CANCER

Ultrasonography is especially useful for diagnosing tumors less than ¼" (0.6 cm) in diameter and in distinguishing cysts from solid tumors in dense breast tissue. As in other ultrasound techniques, a transducer sends a beam of high-frequency sound waves through the patient's skin and into the breast. The sound waves are then processed and displayed for interpretation.

A benefit to ultrasonography is that it can show all areas of the breast, including the area close to the chest wall, which is hard to study with X-rays. When used as an adjunct to mammography, ultrasound increases diagnostic accuracy; when used alone, it's more accurate than mammography in examining the denser breast tissue of a young patient.

suspicious areas may be required to confirm malignancy. Mammography may follow screening procedures, such as ultrasonography or thermography. (See *Using ultrasonography to detect breast cancer.*) Although mammography can detect 90% to 95% of breast cancers, this test produces many false-positive results.

The American College of Radiologists and the American Cancer Society have established separate guidelines for the use and potential risks of mammography. Both groups agree that despite low radiation levels, the test is contraindicated during pregnancy. Magnetic resonance imaging, which is highly sensitive, is becoming a more popular method of breast imaging; however, it isn't very specific and leads to biopsies of many benign lesions. A new digital image approved by the U.S.

DIGITAL MAMMOGRAPHY

Digital mammography produces pictures of the breast using X-rays. Instead of film, this process uses detectors that change the X-rays into electrical signals, which are then converted to an image. Digital mammography is used for screening and diagnosis. For the patient, the procedure is the same as with ordinary mammography.

Digital mammography may offer the following advantages over conventional mammography:

■ The images can be stored and retrieved electronically, which makes long-distance consultations with other mammography specialists easier.

■ Because the images can be adjusted by the radiologist, subtle differences between tissues may be noted.

■ The number of follow-up procedures that are necessary may be reduced.

■ The need for fewer exposures with digital mammography can reduce the already low levels of radiation.

The U.S. Food and Drug Administration has recently approved the Lorad Digital Breast Imager to be used in conjunction with the Lorad M-IV Mammography X-ray System for this digital procedure.

Digital mammography has been shown to be effective in the detection of breast cancer and other abnormalities.

large enough to form a tumor. (See *Ductal lavage.*)

Purpose

■ To screen for malignant breast tumors

■ To investigate palpable and unpalpable breast masses, breast pain, or nipple discharge

■ To help differentiate between benign breast disease and breast cancer

■ To monitor the patient with breast cancer who has been treated with breast-conserving surgery and radiation

Patient preparation

■ Assess the patient's understanding of the mammogram, answer her questions, and correct any misconceptions.

■ Tell the patient who will perform the test and where it will take place.

■ Tell the patient not to use underarm deodorant or powder on the day of the examination.

■ If the patient has breast implants, tell her to inform the staff when she schedules the mammogram so that a technologist familiar with imaging implants is on duty.

■ Inform the patient that although the test takes only about 15 minutes to perform, she may be asked to wait while the films are checked to make sure they're readable. Advise her that there's a high rate of false-positive results.

■ Just before the test, give the patient a gown to wear that opens in the front, and ask her to remove all jewelry and clothing above the waist.

Food and Drug Administration is similar in use as with mammography. (See *Digital mammography.*)

For the patient at high risk for breast cancer, a newer test, ductal lavage, may identify abnormal cells before they're

Procedure and posttest care

■ The patient stands and is asked to rest one of her breasts on a table above an X-ray cassette.

■ The compression plate is placed on the breast and the patient is told to hold her

DUCTAL LAVAGE

Ductal lavage is a minimally invasive procedure that's used to determine the existence of abnormal cells inside the milk ducts, where most breast cancer originates. Without the procedure, 8 to 10 years may pass before the abnormal cells, which indicate a significantly increased risk of breast cancer, grow into a tumor large enough to be detected by either mammogram or physical examination.

The procedure may be performed on an outpatient basis or in the physician's office. An anesthetic cream is applied to the patient's nipple area and gentle suction is used to draw tiny amounts of fluid from the milk ducts to the nipple surface, which helps the physician locate the milk duct's natural openings. A thin catheter is then inserted into a milk duct opening and a small amount of anesthetic is infused into it. Saline is introduced into the catheter to gently rinse the duct and collect cells. The ductal cell fluid is then withdrawn through the catheter, deposited into a collection vial, and sent to a cytology laboratory for analysis.

The high-risk patient can undergo repeated testing or may opt for early intervention, such as tamoxifen chemotherapy or surgical intervention.

breath. A radiograph is taken of the craniocaudal view. The machine is rotated, the breast is compressed again, and a radiograph of the lateral view is taken.
- The procedure is repeated on the other breast.
- After the films are developed, they're checked to make sure they're readable.

Normal findings

A normal mammogram reveals normal duct, glandular tissue, and fat architecture. No abnormal masses or calcifications should be seen.

Abnormal findings

Well-outlined, regular, and clear spots suggest benign cysts; irregular, poorly outlined, and opaque areas suggest a malignant tumor. Malignant tumors are generally solitary and unilateral; benign cysts tend to occur bilaterally. Findings that suggest cancer require further tests, such as biopsy, for confirmation.

Interfering factors

- Powders or salves on the breasts (possible false-positive results)
- Failure to remove jewelry and clothing (possible false-positive results or poor imaging)
- Glandular breasts (common under age 30), active lactation, and previous breast surgery (possible poor imaging)
- Breast implants (may hinder detection of masses)

Hysterosalpingography

Hysterosalpingography is a radiologic examination for visualizing the uterine cavity, the fallopian tubes, and the peritubal area. In this procedure, fluoroscopic X-ray films are taken as a contrast medium flows through the uterus and the fallopian tubes.

This test is generally performed as part of an infertility study. Although ultrasonography has virtually replaced hysterosalpingography in the detection of foreign bodies, such as a dislodged intrauterine device, it can't evaluate tubal patency, which is the main purpose of hysterosalpingography. Risks of this test include uterine perforation, intravascular injection of the contrast medium, and exposure to potentially harmful radiation.

Purpose

- To confirm tubal abnormalities, such as adhesions and occlusion
- To confirm uterine abnormalities, such as the presence of foreign bodies, congenital malformations, and traumatic injuries
- To confirm the presence of fistulas or peritubal adhesions

Patient preparation

- Explain to the patient that the hysterosalpingography confirms uterine and fallopian tube abnormalities.
- Tell the patient who will perform the test and where it will take place. The test should be performed 2 to 5 days after menstruation ends.
- Advise the patient that she may experience moderate cramping from the procedure; however, she may receive a mild sedative, such as diazepam, or a nonprescription prostaglandin inhibitor, if ordered, 30 minutes before the procedure.

Equipment

Antiseptic cleaning solution, sterile needle, contrast medium, vaginal speculum, tenaculum, cannula with acorn tip on one end and luer-lock on the other, radiograph machine with fluoroscopic capabilities

Procedure and posttest care

- With the patient in the lithotomy position, a scout film is taken.

- A speculum is inserted in the vagina, the tenaculum is placed on the cervix, and the cervix is cleaned.
- The cannula is inserted into the cervix and anchored to the tenaculum. After the contrast medium is injected through the cannula, the uterus and the fallopian tubes are viewed fluoroscopically and radiographs are taken. To take oblique views, the X-ray table may be tilted or the patient asked to change position. Films may also be taken later to evaluate spillage of contrast medium into the peritoneal cavity.
- Watch for signs of infection, such as fever, pain, increased pulse rate, malaise, and muscle ache.
- Assure the patient that cramps and vagal reaction (slow pulse rate, nausea, and dizziness) are transient.

Precautions

- Hysterosalpingography is contraindicated in the patient with menses, undiagnosed vaginal bleeding, or pelvic inflammatory disease.
- Watch for an allergic reaction to the contrast medium, such as urticaria, itching, or hypotension.

Normal findings

Normally, radiographs reveal a symmetrical uterine cavity; the contrast medium courses through fallopian tubes of normal caliber, spills freely into the peritoneal cavity, and doesn't leak from the uterus.

Abnormal findings

An asymmetrical uterus suggests intrauterine adhesions or masses, such as fibroids or foreign bodies; impaired contrast flow through the fallopian tubes suggests partial or complete blockage, resulting from intraluminal agglutination, extrinsic compression by adhesions, or perifimbrial adhesions; and leakage of the contrast medium through the uterine wall suggests fistulas. Laparoscopy with contrast medium confirms positive or equivocal findings.

Interfering factors
- Tubal spasm or excessive traction (may show as a stricture in normal fallopian tubes)
- Excessive traction (may displace adhesions, making the fallopian tubes appear normal)

ULTRASONOGRAPHY
Pelvic ultrasonography

In pelvic ultrasonography, high-frequency sound waves are reflected to a transducer to provide images of the interior pelvic area on a monitor. Techniques of sound imaging include A-mode (amplitude modulation, recorded as spikes), B-mode (brightness modulation), gray scale (a representation of organ texture in shades of gray), and real-time imaging (instantaneous images of the tissues in motion, similar to fluoroscopic examination). Selected views may be photographed for later examination and a permanent record of the test.

Purpose
- To detect foreign bodies and distinguish between cystic and solid masses (tumors)
- To measure organ size
- To evaluate fetal viability, position, gestational age, and growth rate
- To detect multiple pregnancy
- To confirm fetal and maternal abnormalities

- To guide amniocentesis by determining placental location and fetal position

Patient preparation
- Describe pelvic ultrasonography to the patient and tell her the reason it's being performed.
- Assure the patient that this procedure is safe, noninvasive, and painless.
- Because this test requires a full bladder as a landmark to define pelvic organs, instruct the patient to drink liquids and not to void before the test.
- Tell the patient who will perform the procedure and where it will take place.
- Explain that a water enema may be necessary to produce a better outline of the large intestine.
- Reassure the patient that the test won't harm the fetus and provide emotional support throughout.

Procedure and posttest care
- With the patient in a supine position, the pelvic area is coated with mineral oil or water-soluble conductive gel to increase sound wave conduction.
- The transducer is guided over the area, images are observed on the monitor, and good images are photographed.
- Remove the conductive gel from the patient's skin.
- Allow the patient to immediately empty her bladder after the test.

Normal findings
The uterus is normal in size and shape. The ovaries' size, shape, and sonographic density are normal. The body of the uterus lies on the superior surface of the bladder; the uterine tubes are attached laterally. The ovaries are located on the lateral pelvic walls, with the external iliac vessels above the ureter posteroinferiorly and covered by the fimbria of the uterine

tubes medially. No other masses are visible. If the patient is pregnant, the gestational sac and fetus are of normal size in relation to gestational age.

Abnormal findings

Cystic and solid masses have homogeneous densities, but solid masses (such as fibroids) appear denser. Inappropriate fetal size may indicate miscalculated conception or delivery date, fetal anomalies, or a dead fetus. Abnormal echo patterns may indicate foreign bodies (such as an intrauterine device), multiple pregnancy, maternal abnormalities (such as placenta previa or abruptio placentae), fetal abnormalities (such as molar pregnancy or abnormalities of the arms and legs, spine, heart, head, kidneys, and abdomen), fetal malpresentation (such as breech or shoulder presentation), and cephalopelvic disproportion.

Interfering factors

■ Failure to fill the bladder, obesity, or fetal head deep in the pelvis (possible poor imaging)

Vaginal ultrasonography

In vaginal ultrasonography, a probe inserted into the vagina reflects high-frequency sound waves to a transducer, forming an image of the pelvic structures. This study allows better evaluation of pelvic anatomy and earlier diagnosis of pregnancy. It also circumvents the poor visualization encountered with obese patients.

Purpose

■ To establish pregnancy with fetal heart motion as early as 5 to 6 weeks' gestation
■ To determine ectopic pregnancy
■ To evaluate abnormal pregnancy

■ To diagnose fetal abnormalities and placental location
■ To visualize retained products of conception
■ To evaluate adnexal pathology, such as tubo-ovarian abscess, hydrosalpinx, and ovarian masses
■ To evaluate the uterine lining (in cases of dysfunctional uterine bleeding and postmenopausal bleeding)
■ To monitor follicular growth during infertility treatment

Patient preparation

■ Describe the vaginal ultrasonography to the patient and explain the reason for the test.
■ Assure the patient that the procedure is safe.

Procedure and posttest care

■ The patient is placed in the lithotomy position. If the sonographer is a male, a female assistant should be present during the examination.
■ Water-soluble conductive gel is placed on the transducer tip to allow better sound transmission and a protective sheath is placed over the transducer.
■ Place more lubricant on the sheathed transducer tip to allow for its gentle insertion into the vagina by the patient or the sonographer. Allowing the patient to introduce the probe may decrease her anxiety.
■ To observe the pelvic structures, rotate the probe 90 degrees to one side and then the other.

Normal findings

If the patient isn't pregnant, the uterus and ovaries are normal in size and shape. The body of the uterus lies on the superior surface of the bladder; the uterine tubes are attached laterally. The ovaries are located on the lateral pelvic walls, with the external iliac vessels above the ureter posteroinferiorly and covered by the fimbria of the uterine tubes medially. If the patient is pregnant, the gestational sac and fetus are of normal size for the gestational date.

Abnormal findings

Vaginal ultrasonography may reveal an empty uterus if the patient was pregnant. Free peritoneal fluid may be visible in the pelvic cavity, indicating possible peritonitis. Ectopic pregnancies may also be visible in the pelvic cavity.

Interfering factors

- Mistaking the bowel for the ovaries
- Small tubal mass (possible difficulty in detecting ectopic pregnancies)

Selected readings

Fischbach, F. *A Manual of Laboratory and Diagnostic Tests,* 7th ed. Philadelphia: Lippincott Williams & Wilkins, 2004.

Guyton, A.C., and Hall, J.E. *Textbook of Medical Physiology,* 10th ed. Philadelphia: W.B. Saunders Co., 2001.

Hanratty, K., et al, eds. *Obstetrics Illustrated,* 6th ed. St. Louis: Mosby Year–Book, Inc., 2003.

Nursing Procedures, 4th ed. Springhouse, Pa.: Springhouse Corp., 2004.

Pagana, K.D., and Pagana, T.J. *Mosby's Diagnostic and Laboratory Test Reference,* 6th ed. St. Louis: Mosby Year–Book, Inc., 2003.

Phipps, W.J., et al, eds. *Medical Surgical Nursing: Health and Illness Perspectives,* 7th ed. St. Louis: Mosby Year–Book, Inc., 2003.

26

Nervous system

Introduction

The study of the human nervous system — neurology — comes closer than any other discipline to examining the fundamental mystery of life. It seeks to understand how we come to feel, think, and be aware of who and what we are. The field of neurodiagnostics faces an equally difficult challenge: to devise safe, effective methods of detecting the diseases and disorders that affect what is one of the most powerful body systems and yet contains some of its most fragile tissues. Sophisticated procedures, such as magnetic resonance imaging (MRI), help to meet this challenge.

The tests discussed in this chapter allow the diagnosis of the major disorders of the brain and its cavities, vasculature, and coverings; the brain stem and cranial nerves; the spinal cord and spinal roots; and the peripheral nerves and the major skeletal muscle groups they innervate. These disorders constitute the substance of clinical neurology, a clear understanding of which is essential to neurologic nursing practice.

The nervous system

The nervous system has three major divisions: the central nervous system (CNS), peripheral nervous system (PNS), and autonomic nervous system (ANS). The CNS consists of the brain, brain stem, and spinal cord; the PNS consists of cranial and spinal nerves; and the ANS has sympathetic and parasympathetic divisions that automatically modulate the function of the glands, blood vessels, smooth muscle, and internal organs.

Neurons, the basic structural unit of the nervous system, contain the necessary electrochemical potential for each body system. They are arranged in clusters that become centers (similar to the respiratory center) and have long strands of fibers called tracts (afferent and efferent). Neurons carry electrical impulses along their axons (or major processes) and transmit them electrochemically across junctions called synapses. These impulses are received by the branching dendrites of other neurons. Synaptic transmission is the basis for all cellular transactions within the CNS and in certain parts of the PNS and ANS.

Internal stimuli and external stimuli from the environment travel along the afferent fibers that bring electrical impulses into the CNS, where they are interpreted and generate a response. Electrical impulses (stimuli) travel away from the CNS along the efferent fibers to the appropriate site, where they generate a response. Movement is dependent upon efferent fibers that execute commands given by the CNS, which are transmitted to specific neuromuscular junctions. Disease in any one or combination of these elements can result in nervous system dysfunction.

Supporting cells

Within the brain, cells known as glia (from the Greek word for glue) support and help nourish nerve tissue. Glia may also be involved in myelin biosynthesis, the insulating material that surrounds certain portions of central and peripheral axons and that assist in nerve impulse conduction. Glia may undergo malignant metamorphosis, forming glia tumors.

Healthy brain function depends on the integrity of cerebral circulation and metabolism. Blood flows to the brain through two internal carotid arteries and two vertebral arteries. The carotid arteries supply 80% of blood to the brain, mainly to the cerebrum, and the vertebral arteries supply 20% of blood to the brain, mainly to the brain stem and cerebellum. The vertebral arteries unite posteriorly to form the basilar artery. The circle of Willis — consisting of six large vessels supplying the cortex — is situated at the base of the brain.

Venous drainage occurs by way of deep veins and large dural sinuses that empty into the internal jugular veins. Cerebral blood vessels are amply supplied by various nerve fibers. When a major cerebral artery is occluded, cerebral ischemia occurs distal to the occlusion. Collateral circulation may develop in the presence of gradual occlusion or reduced blood flow through certain areas of the brain, particularly during the aging process.

Blood-brain barrier

The brain has no lymph nodes. Instead, a complex combination of factors and structural elements exists to form a functional blood-brain barrier. This barrier consists mostly of tight endothelial junctions that prohibit passage of many substances through the capillary beds and cellular membranes that must also be traversed by substances leaving the circulation and entering the brain.

A healthy blood-brain barrier helps maintain a sterile, homeostatic environment for brain cells. Because a breakdown in the blood-brain barrier commonly occurs at the site of tumor growth, a tumor can be identified by substances that rapidly penetrate the tumor tissue (such as radioiodine-labeled albumin), allowing it to stand out radiographically. Acquired immunodeficiency syndrome (AIDS) has also been linked to a breakdown in the blood-brain barrier, and neuroscientists are attempting to clarify the role that the blood-brain barrier plays in the immune response.

Protective fluid

Cerebrospinal fluid (CSF) is formed mainly by the choroid plexuses within the brain's four ventricles. CSF composition, which depends on filtration and diffusion from the blood, is very similar to that of the brain's extracellular fluid.

Few conditions cause CSF volume and pressure to fall below normal (dehydration might be one), but many conditions can cause it to increase, sometimes under pressure. This may lead to hydrocephalus, in which the flow of CSF from one or more ventricles is blocked, causing CSF buildup and increased intracranial pressure. (See *Reviewing CSF circulation.*)

Along with the meninges, CSF protects and supports brain tissue, as evidenced by the pain generated by the withdrawal of spinal fluid. When this cushion of fluid is removed, the brain settles and its weight — combined with traction on pain-sensitive vessels — causes a severe headache.

Neurologic tests

Presented in this chapter are diagnostic tests that are performed to detect such brain diseases or disorders as congenital defects and anomalies, perinatal defects, ventricular abnormalities, epilepsies, degenerative diseases, and space-occupying lesions. This last category includes neoplasms, infections, and vascular lesions such as arteriovenous malformations.

These tests can diagnose infectious diseases, including those caused by bacteria (such as meningitis), viruses (such as encephalitis or polioencephalomyelitis), spirochetes (such as neutrosyphilis), parasitic infestations (such as toxoplasmosis, common in patients with AIDS), and fungal and related infections. Demyelinating diseases (such as multiple sclerosis), cerebrovascular disorders (including stroke, transient ischemic attacks, aneurysms of the blood vessels, and subdural and subarachnoid hemorrhages), and disorders of the skull, vertebral column, and other nonneural tissues may also be diagnosed using the tests presented in this chapter.

Disorders of the brain stem and cranial nerves that can be detected by these tests include vascular insufficiency due to obstruction to specific regions of the brain stem, cranial nerve syndromes (such as trigeminal neuralgia), headache disorders, and congenital disorders that occur as distortions of normal relationships between the skull and vertebral column or as abnormal formations of the skull base.

The spinal cord may be affected by metastasis from non-CNS primary tumors that spread to the vertebrae and meninges, producing extradural tumors that distort the spinal cord or interrupt CSF flow in the spinal subarachnoid spaces. This causes a block in CSF circulation accompanied by spinal cord dysfunc-

REVIEWING CSF CIRCULATION

Cerebrospinal fluid (CSF) is produced from blood in the capillary networks called the choroid plexus. Choroid plexuses are complex structures of vascular folds in the pia mater in the brain's lateral, third, and fourth ventricles. From these sites of origin, CSF passes into the lateral ventricles. It flows through the foramen of Monro into the third ventricle, through the aqueduct of Sylvius into the fourth ventricle, and through the foramina of Luschka and Magendie to the cisterna of the subarachnoid space. The cisterna is continuous with the subarachnoid space, surrounding the entire brain and spinal cord.

The fluid then passes under the base of the brain, upward over the brain's upper surface, and down around the spinal cord. When CSF reaches the arachnoid villi, it's absorbed into venous blood at the venous sinuses. Normally, the amount of CSF produced (500 to 800 ml/day) equals the amount absorbed. The average amount circulating at one time is 125 to 175 ml.

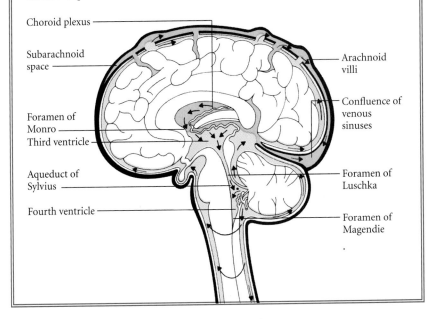

Choroid plexus

Subarachnoid space

Foramen of Monro

Third ventricle

Aqueduct of Sylvius

Fourth ventricle

Arachnoid villi

Confluence of venous sinuses

Foramen of Luschka

Foramen of Magendie

tion. The brain stem and the spinal cord may be affected by Guillain-Barré syndrome, which is typically a myeloradiculopathy.

Because disorders of the PNS are in many cases toxic or metabolic in origin, the tests covered in this chapter are generally not as useful for investigating exposure to toxins or as a systemic metabolic workup. In addition, the diagnosis of peripheral neuropathies commonly depends on nerve biopsy, which allows the identification of specific pathologic change in the nerve fibers. Similarly, when attempting to identify myopathies or muscle disorders, muscle biopsy is commonly the preferred diagnostic tool.

NEUROPSYCHOLOGICAL TESTING

Rather than documenting physiologic changes in the nervous system, neuropsychological testing evaluates the effects of neurologic disorders on a patient's ability to function.

Indications

Neuropsychological tests can evaluate cognitive functioning, including general intelligence, attention span, memory, and judgment as well as motor, sensory, and speech ability. Certain tests can assess emotional lability, quality of language production, abstraction, distractibility, persistence, or the ability to sequence learned activities. The neuropsychologist chooses the appropriate test based on the reason for the assessment and the skills being assessed.

Besides determining the type and extent of functional deficits in the patient with a known neurologic illness, neuropsychological tests can diagnose organic brain dysfunction and dementia. They're also used to determine whether an injured patient can return to a previous occupation or should be declared disabled. What's more, these tests can assess the extent of rehabilitation or vocational training required before the patient can fully function again. Neuropsychological tests may be performed before and after a major neurosurgical or radiologic procedure to obtain baseline information for comparison with postprocedural information. A neuropsychologist administers the series of paper-and-pencil tests, possibly in combination with other tests using puzzles, blocks, or word or recall games. The neuropsychologist explains each test to the patient before administration.

Precautions

Because these tests are mentally demanding and lengthy, they may tire the patient. If possible, withdraw medications that affect his ability to concentrate before the test. The patient should be well rested and free from sedatives, if possible, before testing. Any physiologic problem that may interfere with mental function or level of consciousness, such as fever or electrolyte imbalance, should be treated before testing to ensure that results are as accurate as possible.

The patient's ability to function with neurologic disorders can be evaluated by other tests. (See *Neuropsychological testing.*)

Noninvasive tests

Noninvasive tests that determine brain diseases or disorders, abnormalities, anomalies, infections, and many other conditions in the nervous system include:

■ *Skull radiography*—X-rays of the skull taken at various planes and from different angles—allows the examination of almost all intracranial structures.

■ *Computed tomography (CT) scanning* provides a computerized image of a section of the brain or spinal column as if sliced from front to back, in the horizontal plane or, alternatively, in the sagittal or coronal planes. Although generally considered a noninvasive test, CT scanning can become invasive if a radiopaque medium is injected into a peripheral vein, which allows for uptake by an intracranial or spinal lesion.

■ *Magnetic resonance imaging (MRI)* relies on the magnetic properties of the body's atoms. It uses radio-frequency energy and a powerful magnetic field to produce computerized multiplanar images of fine detail and resolution. New technology has adapted MRI for new types of diagnostic tests, such as magnetic resonance angiography, diffusion-perfusion imaging, and magnetic resonance spectroscopy.

■ *Electroencephalography* detects, records, and amplifies electrical potentials on the scalp that are generated by the brain's neurons using a noninvasive technique that requires small electrodes to be applied in carefully defined patterns on the scalp. The findings depict the electrical activity of the brain's surface, which reflects—and can be used to interpret—changes in electrical activity of deeper structures.

■ *Evoked potential studies* directly evaluate sensory and somatosensory neurologic pathways by recording the electrical response of the brain to external stimuli.

■ *Oculoplethysmography* indirectly measures ocular artery pressure and reflects the adequacy of cerebrovascular blood flow of the carotid arteries.

■ *Transcranial Doppler studies* measure blood flow velocity through the cerebral arteries and provide information about the quality and changing nature of circulation to an area of the brain.

Invasive tests

Invasive tests that determine brain diseases or disorders, abnormalities, anomalies, infections, and many other conditions in the nervous system include:

■ *Cerebral angiography* allows visualization of blood vessels through injection of a substance that's opaque to X-rays and therefore stands out as a white contrast. *Digital subtraction angiography* uses computers and video equipment to eliminate interfering images of bone and soft tissue and further reveal details of the opacified vessels. In addition to detecting disorders of cerebral blood vessels, angiography may also help detect displacement of

blood vessels by other lesions such as tumors.

■ *Electromyography* assesses the electrical potential across the muscle membrane through a needle electrode. This procedure yields information on nerve impulse conduction to the muscle as well as the muscle's response to the nerve impulse. The nerve conduction part of this test determines whether the velocity of propagation of the nerve impulse along a particular sensory, motor, or combined sensory-motor nerve is normal. This test also provides general information about the possibility of neuropathy.

■ *CSF analysis* provides a general profile of the cellular and chemical composition of CSF at a particular time. Because CSF is secreted and represents a highly refined distillate of the blood, concentrations of certain substances are different in CSF than in serum. The pressure under which CSF is circulating can be determined during lumbar puncture before the CSF specimen is obtained.

■ *Myelography* involves injection of a radiopaque contrast medium into the spinal subarachnoid space. CSF is removed for analysis at the time of myelography—thereby accomplishing two tests with one procedure—and is replaced by the heavier contrast medium, which gravitates toward the head or elsewhere within the spinal canal when the radiographic table is tilted.

■ In the *Tensilon test,* a short-acting potent anticholinesterase drug is administered I.V. to help diagnose myasthenia gravis.

Other tests

Additionally, there are other tests that have been used by laboratories for many years to conduct fundamental research on the nervous system. One such test is *positron emission tomography* (PET), which creates an image of a slice of the brain similar to a CT image, but is based on different biophysical and radiochemical techniques. (Because it's costly, PET is used mainly for research.) Another clinical application of electroencephalography is *somnography,* the scientific evaluation of sleep and its disorders. These techniques are essentially investigational and have limited clinical application.

NONINVASIVE TESTS

Skull radiography

Although skull radiography is of limited value in assessing patients with head injuries, skull X-rays are extremely valuable for studying abnormalities of the skull base and cranial vault, congenital and perinatal anomalies, and systemic diseases that produce bone defects of the skull. For more accurate assessment of head injuries as well as of skull and head abnormalities, nonenhanced computed tomography studies of the head are done.

Skull radiography evaluates the three groups of bones that comprise the skull: the calvaria (vault), the mandible (jaw bone), and the facial bones. The calvaria and the facial bones are closely connected by immovable joints with irregular serrated edges called sutures. The skull bones form an anatomic structure so complex that a complete skull examination requires several radiologic views of each area.

Purpose
■ To detect fractures in the patient with head trauma
■ To aid in the diagnosis of pituitary tumors

■ To detect congenital anomalies
■ To detect metabolic and endocrinologic disorders

Patient preparation
■ Explain to the patient that his head will be immobilized and that several X-rays of his skull will be taken from various angles.
■ Tell the patient that skull radiography helps to determine the presence of anomalies and helps establish a diagnosis.
■ Tell the patient who will perform the test and where it will take place.
■ Explain to the patient that he need not restrict food and fluids and that the test will cause no discomfort.
■ Tell the patient to remove glasses, dentures, jewelry, or any metallic objects that would be in the X-ray field.

Procedure and posttest care
■ Have the patient recline on the X-ray table or sit in a chair.
■ Tell the patient to remain still during the procedure.
■ Use foam pads, sandbags, or a headband to immobilize the patient's head and increase comfort.
■ Five views of the skull are routinely taken: left and right lateral, anteroposterior Towne's, posteroanterior Caldwell, and axial (or base). (See *Positioning the skull for radiography.*)
■ Films are developed and checked for quality before the patient leaves the area.

Normal findings
A radiologist interprets the X-rays, evaluating the size, shape, thickness, and position of the cranial bones as well as the vascular markings, sinuses, and sutures. All should be normal for the patient's age.

POSITIONING THE SKULL FOR RADIOGRAPHY

Right lateral and left lateral
The sagittal plane is parallel to the table-top and the film. A support, such as a folded towel or the patient's clenched fist, is placed under the chin. (Adequate film shows both halves of the mandible directly superimposed.)

Posteroanterior Caldwell
The patient lies in a prone position; his chin may be supported by a folded towel or his fist. The sagittal plane and the canthomeatal line are perpendicular to the tabletop and the film. The X-ray beam is angled 15 degrees toward the feet.

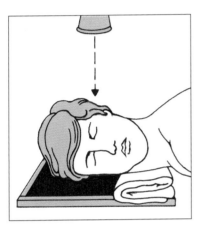

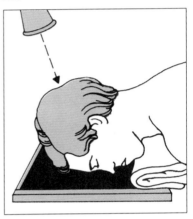

Anteroposterior Towne's
The patient lies in a supine position with his chin flexed toward the neck; the canthomeatal line is perpendicular to the tabletop and the film. The X-ray beam is angled 30 degrees toward the feet.

Axial (base)
The patient lies in a prone position with his chin fully extended; his head rests in such a way that the line of the face is perpendicular and the canthomeatal line is parallel to the tabletop and the film.

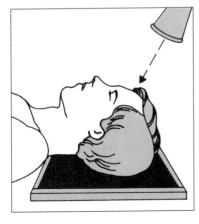

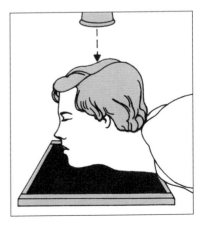

Abnormal findings

Skull radiography is commonly used to diagnose fractures of the vault or base, although basilar fractures may not show on the film if the bone is dense. This test may confirm congenital anomalies and may show erosion, enlargement, or decalcification of the sella turcica that result from increased intracranial pressure (ICP). A marked rise in ICP may cause the brain to expand and press against the inner bony table of the skull, yielding visible marks or impressions.

In conditions such as osteomyelitis (with possible skull calcification) and chronic subdural hematomas, X-rays may show abnormal areas of calcification. The X-rays can detect neoplasms within brain substances that contain calcium (such as oligodendrogliomas or meningiomas) or the midline shifting of a calcified pineal gland caused by a space-occupying lesion.

Radiography may also detect other changes in bone structure — for example, those that arise from metabolic disorders, such as acromegaly or Paget's disease.

Interfering factors

- Improper positioning of the patient and excessive head movement (possible poor imaging)
- Failure to remove radiopaque objects from the X-ray field (possible poor imaging)

Intracranial computed tomography

Intracranial computed tomography (CT) provides a series of tomograms, translated by a computer and displayed on a monitor, representing cross-sectional images of various layers of the brain. This technique can reconstruct cross-sectional, horizontal, sagittal, and coronal plane images. Hundreds of thousands of readings of radiation levels absorbed by brain tissues may be combined to depict anatomic slices of varying thickness. Specificity and accuracy are enhanced by the degree of resolution, which depends on the number of radiation density calculations made by the computer. Although magnetic resonance imaging (MRI) has surpassed CT scanning in diagnosing neurologic anatomy and pathology, the CT scan is more widely available and cost-effective and can be performed more easily in acute situations.

The increasing availability of CT scanners allows faster and safer diagnosis than in the past. In many cases, intracranial CT scanning eliminates the need for painful and hazardous invasive procedures, such as pneumoencephalography and cerebral angiography. CT scans, which usually use contrast enhancement, are especially valuable in assessing a patient with focal neurologic abnormalities and other clinical features that suggest an intracranial mass. In a patient with a suspected head injury, intracranial CT scans may allow the diagnosis of a subdural hematoma before characteristic symptoms appear.

Purpose

- To diagnose intracranial lesions and abnormalities
- To monitor the effects of surgery, radiation therapy, or chemotherapy on intracranial tumors
- To serve as a guide for cranial surgery

Patient preparation

- Explain to the patient that intracranial CT permits assessment of the brain.
- Unless contrast enhancement is scheduled, inform the patient that there are no food or fluid restrictions. If contrast en-

hancement is scheduled, instruct him to fast for 4 hours before the test.
- Tell the patient that a series of X-ray films will be taken of his brain. Describe who will perform the test and where it will take place. Explain that the test will cause minimal discomfort.
- Tell the patient that he'll be positioned on a moving CT bed with his head immobilized and his face uncovered. The head of the table will then be moved into the scanner, which rotates around his head and makes loud clacking sounds.
- If a contrast medium is used, tell the patient that he may feel flushed and warm and may experience a transient headache, a salty or metallic taste, or nausea and vomiting after the contrast medium is injected.
- Instruct the patient to wear a gown (outpatients may wear comfortable clothing) and to remove all metal objects from the CT scan field.
- If the patient is restless or apprehensive, a sedative may be prescribed.
- Check the patient's history for hypersensitivity to shellfish, iodine, or contrast media, and mark your findings in his chart. Inform the physician of any sensitivities because he may order prophylactic medications or may choose not to use contrast enhancement.

Equipment
CT scanner, oscilloscope, contrast medium (iothalamate meglumine or diatrizoate sodium), 60-ml syringe, 19G to 21G needle, I.V. tubing and I.V. insertion equipment, if needed

Procedure and posttest care
- Place the patient in a supine position on an X-ray table with his head immobilized by straps, if required, and ask him to lie still.

- The head of the table is moved into the scanner, which rotates around the patient's head, taking radiographs at 1-degree intervals in a 180-degree arc.
- When this series of radiographs is completed, contrast enhancement is performed. Usually 50 to 100 ml of contrast medium is administered by I.V. injection or I.V. drip over 1 to 2 minutes. Monitor the patient for hypersensitivity reactions, such as urticaria, respiratory difficulty, or rash. Reactions usually develop within 30 minutes.
- After injection of the contrast medium, another series of scans is taken. Information from the scans is stored on magnetic tapes, fed into a computer, and converted into images on an oscilloscope. Photographs of selected views are taken for further study.
- If a contrast medium was used, watch the patient for residual adverse reactions (headache, nausea, and vomiting) and inform him that he may resume his usual diet.

Precautions
- Intracranial CT scanning with contrast enhancement is contraindicated in the patient who's hypersensitive to iodine or contrast medium.
- Iodine or contrast medium may be harmful or fatal to a fetus, especially during the first trimester.

Normal findings
The tissue density determines the amount of radiation that passes through it. Tissue densities appear as white, black, or shades of gray on the computed image obtained by intracranial CT scanning. Bone, the densest tissue, appears white; ventricular and subarachnoid cerebrospinal fluid, the least dense, appears black. Brain matter appears in shades of gray. Structures are

UNDERSTANDING PET AND SPECT

Like computed tomography (CT) scanning and magnetic resonance imaging, positron emission tomography (PET) and single-photon emission computed tomography (SPECT) provide brain images through sophisticated computer reconstruction algorithms. However, PET and SPECT images detail brain function as well as structure and thus differ significantly from the images provided by these other advanced techniques. PET and SPECT combine elements of CT scanning and conventional radionuclide imaging. For example, they measure the emissions of injected radioisotopes and convert them to a tomographic image of the brain. SPECT scanning uses gamma radiation with radionucleotides within the brain, and PET uses radioisotopes of biologically important elements—oxygen, nitrogen, carbon, and fluorine—that emit particles called positrons.

How it works
During PET and SPECT, pairs of gamma rays are emitted; the scanner detects them and relays the information to a computer for reconstruction as an image. SPECT scanners use radionucleotides labeled with iodine or hexamethylpropyline amineoxime to detect blood flow. PET scanners omit positrons that can be chemically "tagged" to biological-

ly active molecules, such as carbon monoxide, neurotransmitters, hormones, and metabolites (especially glucose), enabling study of their uptake and distribution in brain tissue. For example, blood tagged with ^{11}C-carbon monoxide allows study of hemodynamic patterns in brain tissue; tagged neurotransmitters, hormones, and drugs allow mapping of receptor distribution.

Isotope-tagged glucose (which penetrates the blood-brain barrier rapidly) allows dynamic study of brain function because PET scans can pinpoint the sites of glucose metabolism in the brain under various conditions. Researchers expect SPECT and PET scanning to prove useful in the diagnosis of psychiatric disorders, transient ischemic attacks, amyotrophic lateral sclerosis, Parkinson's disease, Wilson's disease, multiple sclerosis, seizure disorders, cerebrovascular disease, and Alzheimer's disease. The reason is that all of these disorders may alter the location and patterns of cerebral glucose metabolism.

Cost factors
PET scanning is a costly test because the radioisotopes used have very short half-lives and must be produced at an on-site cyclotron and attached quickly to the desired tracer molecules.

evaluated according to their density, size, shape, and position.

Abnormal findings

Areas of altered density (they may be lighter or darker) or displaced vasculature or other structures may indicate an intracranial tumor, a hematoma, cerebral atrophy, an infarction, edema, or congenital anomalies such as hydrocephalus.

Intracranial tumors vary significantly in appearance and characteristics.

Metastatic tumors generally cause extensive edema in early stages and can usually be defined by contrast enhancement. Primary tumors vary in density and in their capacity to cause edema, displace ventricles, and absorb the contrast medium in contrast enhancement. Astrocytomas, for example, usually have low densities; meningiomas have higher densities and can generally be defined with contrast enhancement; glioblastomas, usually ill defined, are also enhanced after injection of a contrast medium.

Because the high density of blood contrasts markedly with low-density brain tissue, it's normally easy to detect subdural and epidural hematomas and other acute hemorrhages. Contrast enhancement helps locate subdural hematomas.

Cerebral atrophy customarily appears as enlarged ventricles with large sulci. Cerebral infarction may appear as low-density areas at the obstruction site or may not be apparent, especially within the first 24 hours or if the infarction is small or doesn't cause edema. With contrast enhancement, the infarcted area may not show in the acute phase, but will show clearly after resolution of the lesion. Cerebral edema usually appears as an area of marked generalized decreased density. In children, enlargement of the fourth ventricle generally indicates hydrocephalus.

Normally, the cerebral vessels don't appear on CT images. However, in the patient with arteriovenous malformation, cerebral vessels may appear with slightly increased density. Contrast enhancement allows a better view of the abnormal area, but MRI is now the preferred procedure for imaging cerebral vessels.

Another technology for obtaining brain images is positron emission tomography. (See *Understanding PET and SPECT*.)

Interfering factors

- Patient's head movement (possible poor imaging)
- Failure to remove metal objects from the scanning field (possible poor imaging)
- Hemorrhage (possible false-negative imaging due to change in hematoma)

Intracranial magnetic resonance imaging

Intracranial magnetic resonance imaging (MRI) produces highly detailed, cross-sectional images of the brain and spine in multiple planes. The primary advantage of MRI is its ability to "see through" bone and to delineate fluid-filled soft tissue. It has proved useful in the diagnosis of cerebral infarction, tumors, abscesses, edema, hemorrhage, nerve fiber demyelination (as in multiple sclerosis), and other disorders that increase the fluid content of affected tissues. It can also show irregularities of the spinal cord with a resolution and detail previously unobtainable. It can also produce images of organs and vessels in motion.

Exposed to an external magnetic field, positively charged atomic nuclei and their negatively charged electrons align uniformly in the field. Radiofrequency energy is then directed at the atoms, knocking them out of this magnetic alignment and causing them to precess, or spin. When the radiofrequency pulse is discontinued, the atoms realign themselves with the magnetic field, emitting radiofrequency energy as a tissue-specific signal based on the relative density of nuclei and the realignment time. These signals are monitored by the MRI computer, which processes them and displays the information on a video monitor as a high-resolution image.

MRI technology makes use of magnetic fields and radio-frequency waves, which are imperceptible by the patient; no harmful effects have been documented. Research continues on the optimal magnetic fields and radio-frequency waves for each type of tissue. (See *New methods of monitoring cerebral function*, page 706, and *MRI techniques*, page 707.)

NEW METHODS OF MONITORING CEREBRAL FUNCTION

Optical imaging

Optical imaging uses fiber-optic light and a camera to produce visual images of the brain as it responds to stimulation. This technique produces higher-resolution pictures of the brain than magnetic resonance imaging (MRI) or positron emission tomography scans. Researchers believe it may be valuable during neurosurgery to minimize damage to crucial areas of the brain that control speech, movement, and other activities. Because the procedure scans only the brain's surface, it's meant to be used in combination with other diagnostic techniques.

Fast MRI

Fast MRI produces pictures less than a second apart. These images display blood flow through the brain and the changes that occur in blood flow when the patient performs different tasks. Neuroscientists believe that active areas of the brain must consume more oxygen and that areas of the brain that are currently working become laden with oxygen. Fast MRI can distinguish between oxygen-laden and oxygen-depleted blood. Thus, this test may be used to help identify which areas of the normal brain are involved in certain activities and emotions. Possible applications for fast MRI include guiding neurosurgeons during surgery and helping researchers better understand epilepsy, brain tumors, and even psychiatric illnesses.

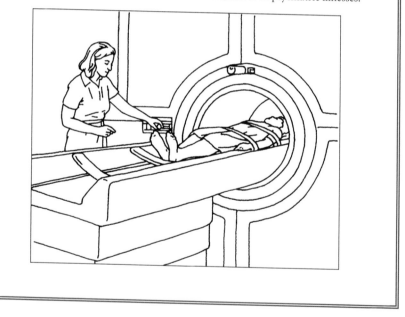

Purpose

■ To aid in the diagnosis of intracranial and spinal lesions and soft-tissue abnormalities

Patient preparation

■ Explain to the patient that intracranial MRI assesses bone and soft tissue. Tell

MRI TECHNIQUES

Magnetic resonance imaging (MRI) is used to provide clear images of parts of the brain, such as the brain stem and cerebellum, that are difficult to image by other methods. Four MRI techniques are available to examine other aspects of the brain.

Magnetic resonance angiography

Magnetic resonance angiography allows the visualization of blood flowing through the cerebral vessels. Images of blood vessels done with magnetic resonance angiography aren't as clear as those obtained by angiography, but this technique is less invasive.

Magnetic resonance spectroscopy

Magnetic resonance spectroscopy creates images over time that show the metabolism of certain chemical markers in a specific area of the brain. Some researchers have dubbed this test a "metabolic biopsy" because it reveals pathologic neurochemistry over time.

Diffusion-perfusion imaging

Diffusion-perfusion imaging uses a stronger-than-normal magnetic gradient to reveal areas of focal cerebral ischemia within minutes. Currently used in stroke research, this MRI technique may be used by diagnosticians to distinguish permanent from reversible ischemia.

Neurography

Neurograms provide a three-dimensional image of nerves. They may be used to find the exact location of nerves that are damaged, crimped, or in disarray.

him who will perform the test and where it will take place.

- Explain to the patient that MRI is painless and involves no exposure to radiation from the scanner. A radioactive contrast dye may be used, depending on the type of tissue being studied.
- Advise the patient that he'll have to remain still for the entire procedure.
- Inform the patient that the opening for the head and body is quite small and deep. Tell him that he'll hear the scanner clicking, whirring, and thumping as it moves inside its housing.
- Explain to the patient that sedation may be administered if he suffers from claustrophobia or if extensive time is required for scanning. As an alternative, an open MRI scanner may be used, which delivers accurate results, but may take longer to complete.

- Reassure the patient that he'll be able to communicate with the technician at all times.
- Instruct the patient to remove all metallic objects, including jewelry, hairpins, and a watch. Also ask him if he has any surgically implanted joints, pins, clips, valves, pumps, or pacemakers containing metal that could be attracted to the strong MRI magnet. If he does, he won't be able to undergo the test.
- Make sure that the patient or a responsible family member has signed an informed consent form, if required.

Procedure and posttest care

- The patient is placed in a supine position on a narrow bed, which then slides him to the desired position inside the scanner, where radio-frequency energy is directed at his head or spine.

- The resulting images are displayed on a monitor and recorded on film or magnetic tape for permanent storage.
- The radiologist may vary radio-frequency waves and use the computer to manipulate and enhance the images.
- During the procedure, the patient must remain still.
- Tell the patient that he may resume his usual activity after the test.
- If the patient was sedated, ensure that a responsible person drives him home.
- If the test took a long time and the patient was lying flat for an extended period, observe him for orthostatic hypotension.

Precautions
- Because MRI works through a powerful magnetic field, it can't be performed on the patient with a pacemaker, an intracranial aneurysm clip, or other ferrous metal implants or on a patient with gunshot wounds to the head.
- Because of the strong magnetic field, metallic or computer-based equipment (for example, ventilators and I.V. pumps) can't enter the MRI area.

Normal findings
MRI can show normal anatomic details of the central nervous system in any plane, without bone interference. Brain and spinal cord structures should appear distinct and sharply defined. Tissue color and shading will vary, depending on the radio-frequency energy, magnetic strength, and degree of computer enhancement.

Abnormal findings
Because MRI depicts the density (water content) of tissue, it clearly shows structural changes resulting from disorders that increase tissue water content, such as

cerebral edema, demyelinating disease, and pontine and cerebellar tumors. Edematous fluid, for example, generally appears cloudy or gray, whereas blood generally appears dark. Lesions of multiple sclerosis appear as areas of demyelination (curdlike, gray or gray-white areas) around the edges of ventricles. Tumors appear as changes in normal anatomy, which computer enhancement may further delineate.

Interfering factors
- Excessive patient movement (possible poor imaging)

Electroencephalography

In electroencephalography (EEG), electrodes attached to areas of the patient's scalp record the brain's electrical activity and transmit this information to an electroencephalograph, which records the resulting brain waves on recording paper. The procedure may be performed in a special laboratory or by a portable unit at the bedside. Ambulatory recording EEGs are available for the patient to wear at home or the workplace to record the patient as he performs his normal daily activities. Continuous-video EEG recording is available on an inpatient basis for identifying epileptic discharges during clinical events or for localization of a seizure focus during surgical evaluation of epilepsy. Intracranial electrodes are surgically implanted to record EEG changes for localization of the seizure focus.

Purpose
- To determine the presence and type of seizure disorder
- To aid in the diagnosis of intracranial lesions, such as abscesses and tumors

- To evaluate the brain's electrical activity in metabolic disease, cerebral ischemia, head injury, meningitis, encephalitis, mental retardation, psychological disorders, and drugs
- To evaluate altered states of consciousness or brain death

Patient preparation

- Explain to the patient that the EEG records the brain's electrical activity.
- Describe the procedure to the patient and family members and answer all her questions.
- Tell the patient that he must forgo caffeine before the test; other than this, there are no food or fluid restrictions. Tell him that skipping the meal before the test can cause relative hypoglycemia and alter the brain wave pattern.
- Inform the patient that smoking is prohibited for at least 8 hours before the test.
- Thoroughly wash and dry the patient's hair to remove hair sprays, creams, and oils.
- Explain to the patient that during the test, he'll relax in a reclining chair or lie on a bed and that electrodes will be attached to his scalp with a special paste. Assure him that the electrodes won't shock him.
- If needle electrodes are used, explain to the patient that he'll feel a pricking sensation as they're inserted; however, flat electrodes are more commonly used.
- Do your best to allay the patient's fears because nervousness can affect brain wave patterns.
- Check the patient's medication history for drugs that may interfere with test results. Anticonvulsants, tranquilizers, barbiturates, and other sedatives should be withheld for 24 to 48 hours before the test, as ordered by the physician. Infants and very young children occasionally require sedation to prevent crying and restlessness during the test, but sedation itself may alter test results.

- A patient with a seizure disorder may require a "sleep EEG." In this case, keep the patient awake the night before the test and administer a sedative (such as chloral hydrate) to help him sleep during the test.
- If the test is performed to confirm brain death, provide the patient's family members with emotional support.

Procedure and posttest care

- Position the patient on the bed or in a reclining chair. Reassure him as the electrodes are attached to his scalp.
- Before the recording procedure begins, instruct the patient to close his eyes, relax, and remain still.
- During the recording, observe the patient carefully; note blinking, swallowing, talking, or other movements and record these findings on the tracing. These activities may cause artifacts on the tracing and be misinterpreted as an abnormal tracing.
- The recording may be stopped at intervals to let the patient rest or reposition himself. This is important because restlessness and fatigue can alter brain wave patterns.
- After an initial baseline recording, the patient may be tested under various stress-producing conditions to elicit patterns not observable while he's at rest. For example, he may be asked to breathe deeply and rapidly for 3 minutes (hyperventilation), which may elicit brain wave patterns typical of seizure disorders or other abnormalities. This technique is commonly used to detect absence seizures. Also, photic stimulation tests central cerebral activity in response to bright light, accentuating abnormal activity in absence or myoclonic seizures. In this

procedure, a strobe light placed in front of the patient is flashed 1 to 20 times/second; recordings are made with the patient's eyes opened and closed.

■ Review carefully the reinstatement of anticonvulsant medication or other drugs withheld before the test.

■ Carefully observe the patient for seizure activity and provide a safe environment.

■ Help the patient remove electrode paste from his hair.

■ If the patient received a sedative before the test, take safety precautions such as raising the bed's side rails.

■ If brain death is confirmed, provide the patient's family members with emotional support.

■ If clinical events are found to be nonepileptic, a psychological evaluation may be needed.

Precautions

■ Observe the patient carefully for seizure activity.

■ If seizure activity occurs, record seizure patterns and be prepared to provide assistance. Have suction equipment readily available.

Normal findings

EEG records a portion of the brain's electrical activity as waves; some are irregular, whereas others demonstrate frequent patterns. Among the basic waveforms are the alpha, beta, theta, and delta rhythms.

Alpha waves occur at a frequency of 8 to 11 cycles/second in a regular rhythm. They're present only in the waking state when the patient's eyes are closed, but he's mentally alert; usually, they disappear with visual activity or mental concentration. *Beta waves* (13 to 30 cycles/second) — generally associated with anxiety, depression, and use of sedatives — are

seen most readily in the frontal and central regions of the brain. *Theta waves* (4 to 7 cycles/second) are most common in children and young adults and appear in the frontal and temporal regions. *Delta waves* (0.5 to 3.5 cycles/second) normally occur only in young children and during sleep. (See *Comparing EEG tracings.*)

Abnormal findings

Usually, about a 100′ to 200′ (30 to 60 m) strip of recordings is evaluated, with particular attention paid to basic waveforms, symmetry of cerebral activity, transient discharges, and responses to stimulation. A specific diagnosis depends on the patient's clinical status.

In the patient with epilepsy, EEG patterns may identify the specific disorder. In *absence seizures,* the EEG shows spikes and waves at a frequency of 3 cycles/second. In *generalized tonic-clonic seizures,* it generally shows multiple, high-voltage, spiked waves in both hemispheres. In *temporal lobe epilepsy,* the EEG usually shows spiked waves in the affected temporal region. In the patient with *focal seizures,* it usually shows localized, spiked discharges.

In the patient with an intracranial lesion, such as a tumor or abscess, the EEG may show slow waves (usually delta waves but possibly unilateral beta waves). Vascular lesions, such as cerebral infarcts and intracranial hemorrhages, generally produce focal abnormalities in the injured area.

Generally, any condition that causes a diminishing level of consciousness alters the EEG pattern in proportion to the degree of consciousness lost. For example, in a patient with a metabolic disorder, an inflammatory process (such as meningitis or encephalitis), or increased intracranial

COMPARING EEG TRACINGS

The following tracings are examples of regular and irregular brain electrical activity as recorded by an electroencephalogram.

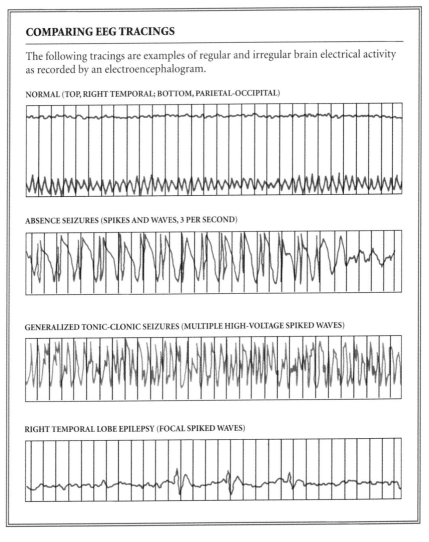

NORMAL (TOP, RIGHT TEMPORAL; BOTTOM, PARIETAL-OCCIPITAL)

ABSENCE SEIZURES (SPIKES AND WAVES, 3 PER SECOND)

GENERALIZED TONIC-CLONIC SEIZURES (MULTIPLE HIGH-VOLTAGE SPIKED WAVES)

RIGHT TEMPORAL LOBE EPILEPSY (FOCAL SPIKED WAVES)

pressure, the EEG shows generalized, diffuse, and slow brain waves.

The most pathologic finding of all is an absent EEG pattern — a "flat" tracing (except for artifacts), which may indicate brain death.

Interfering factors

■ Interference from extraneous electrical activity; head, body, eye, or tongue movement; or muscle contractions (possible production of excessive artifact)

■ Anticonvulsants, barbiturates, tranquilizers, and other sedatives (possible masking of seizure activity)

■ Acute drug intoxication or severe hypothermia, resulting in loss of consciousness (flat EEG)

Evoked potential studies

Evoked potential studies evaluate the integrity of visual, somatosensory, and auditory nerve pathways by measuring evoked potentials — the brain's electrical response to stimulation of the sensory organs or peripheral nerves. Evoked potentials are recorded as electronic impulses by surface electrodes attached to the scalp and skin over various peripheral sensory nerves. A computer extracts these low-amplitude impulses from background brain wave activity and averages the signals from repeated stimuli. (See *Visual and somatosensory evoked potentials.*)

Three types of responses are measured:
- *Visual evoked potentials,* produced by exposing the eye to a rapidly reversing checkerboard pattern, help evaluate demyelinating diseases, traumatic injury, and puzzling visual complaints.
- *Somatosensory evoked potentials,* produced by electrically stimulating a peripheral sensory nerve, help diagnose peripheral nerve disease and locate brain and spinal cord lesions.
- *Auditory brain stem evoked potentials,* produced by delivering clicks to the ear, help locate auditory lesions and evaluate brain stem integrity.

Evoked potential studies are also useful for monitoring comatose or anesthetized patients, monitoring spinal cord function during spinal cord surgery, and evaluating neurologic function in an infant whose sensory system normally can't be adequately assessed.

Purpose
- To aid in the diagnosis of nervous system lesions and abnormalities
- To assess the patient's neurologic function

Patient preparation
- Tell the patient that evoked potential studies measure the electrical activity of his nervous system. Explain who will perform the test and where it will take place.
- Tell the patient that he'll sit in a reclining chair or lie on a bed. If visual evoked potentials will be measured, electrodes will be attached to his scalp; if somatosensory evoked potentials will be measured, electrodes will be placed on his scalp, neck, lower back, wrist, knee, and ankle.
- Assure the patient that the electrodes won't hurt him. Encourage him to relax; tension can affect neurologic function and interfere with test results.
- Have the patient remove all jewelry and other metal objects.

Procedure and posttest care
- Position the patient in a reclining chair or on a bed and tell him to relax and remain still.

For visual evoked potentials
- Electrodes are attached to the patient's scalp at occipital, parietal, and vertex sites; a reference electrode is placed on the midfrontal area or ear.
- The patient is positioned 3′ (1 m) from the pattern-shift stimulator.
- One eye is occluded, and the patient is instructed to fix his gaze on a dot in the center of the screen.
- A checkerboard pattern is projected and then rapidly reversed or shifted 100 times, once or twice per second.
- A computer amplifies and averages the brain's response to each stimulus, and the results are plotted as a waveform.
- The procedure is repeated for the other eye.

VISUAL AND SOMATOSENSORY EVOKED POTENTIALS

Visual (pattern-shift) evoked potentials

In the visual (pattern-shift) evoked potentials test, visual neural impulses are recorded as they travel along the pathway from the eye to the occipital cortex. Wave P100 is the most significant component of the resultant waveform. Normal P100 latency is about 100 msec after the application of a visual stimulus, as shown in the top diagram. Increased P100 latency, shown in the bottom diagram, is an abnormal finding, indicating a lesion along the visual pathway.

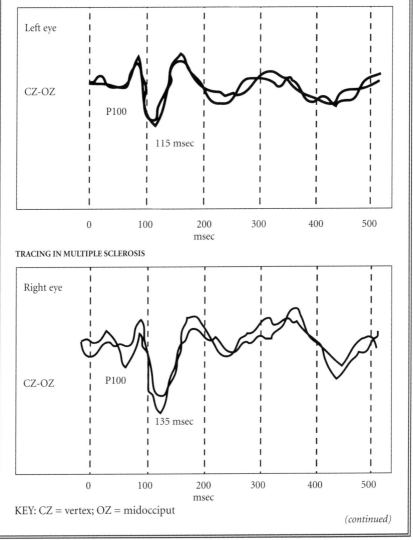

NORMAL TRACING

Left eye

CZ-OZ

P100

115 msec

0   100   200   300   400   500
              msec

TRACING IN MULTIPLE SCLEROSIS

Right eye

CZ-OZ

P100

135 msec

0   100   200   300   400   500
              msec

KEY: CZ = vertex; OZ = midocciput

(continued)

VISUAL AND SOMATOSENSORY EVOKED POTENTIALS *(continued)*

Somatosensory evoked potentials

The somatosensory evoked potentials tests measure the conduction time of an electrical impulse traveling along a somatosensory pathway to the cortex. Interwave latency is the most significant component of the resultant waveform. On the set of upper- and lower-limb tracings shown below, the top tracings represent normal interwave latencies; the bottom tracings, typical abnormal latencies found in a patient with multiple sclerosis. Because of the close correlation between waveforms and the anatomy of somatosensory pathways, such tracings allow precise location of lesions that produce conduction defects.

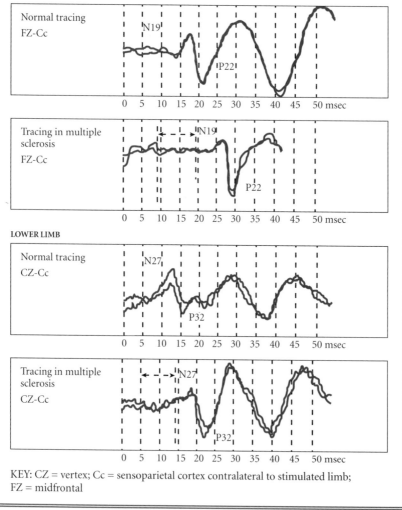

KEY: CZ = vertex; Cc = sensoparietal cortex contralateral to stimulated limb; FZ = midfrontal

For somatosensory evoked potentials

- Electrodes are attached to the patient's skin over somatosensory pathways—typically the wrist, knee, and ankle—to stimulate peripheral nerves. Recording electrodes are placed on the scalp over the sensory cortex of the hemisphere opposite the limb to be stimulated. Additional electrodes may be placed at Erb's point (above the clavicle overlying the brachial plexus), at the second cervical vertebra, and over the lower lumbar vertebrae. Midfrontal or noncephalic electrodes are placed for reference.
- Painless electrical stimulation is delivered to the peripheral nerve through the electrode. The intensity is adjusted to produce a minor muscle response such as a thumb twitch on median nerve stimulation at the wrist.
- Electrical stimuli are delivered 500 or more times at a rate of 5 per second.
- A computer measures and averages the time it takes for the electric current to reach the cortex; the results, expressed in milliseconds (msec), are recorded as waveforms.
- The test is repeated once to verify results, and then the electrodes are repositioned and the entire procedure is repeated for the other side.

Normal findings
Visual evoked potentials
On the waveform, the most significant wave is P100, a positive wave appearing about 100 msec after the pattern-shift stimulus is applied. The most clinically significant measurements are absolute P100 latency (the time between stimulus application and peaking of the P100 wave) and the difference between the P100 latencies of each eye. Because many physical and technical factors affect P100 latency, normal results vary greatly among laboratories and patients.

Somatosensory evoked potentials
Waveforms obtained vary, depending on locations of the stimulating and recording electrodes. The positive and negative peaks are labeled in sequence, based on normal time of appearance. For example, N19 is a negative peak normally recorded 19 msec after application of the stimulus. Each wave peak arises from a discrete location: N19 is generated mainly from the thalamus, P22 from the parietal sensory cortex, and so on. Interwave latencies (time between waves), rather than absolute latencies, are used as a basis for clinical interpretation. Latency differences between sides are significant.

Abnormal findings
Information from evoked potential studies is useful, but insufficient to confirm a specific diagnosis. Test data must be interpreted in light of clinical information.

Visual evoked potentials
Generally, abnormal (extended) P100 latencies confined to one eye indicate a visual pathway lesion anterior to the optic chiasm. A lesion posterior to the optic chiasm usually doesn't produce abnormal P100 latencies. Because each eye projects to both occipital lobes, the unaffected pathway transmits sufficient impulses to produce a normal latency response. Bilateral abnormal P100 latencies have been found in patients with multiple sclerosis, optic neuritis, retinopathies, amblyopia (although abnormal latencies don't correlate well with impaired visual acuity), spinocerebellar degeneration, adrenoleukodystrophy, sarcoidosis, Parkinson's disease, and Huntington's disease.

Somatosensory evoked potentials

Because somatosensory evoked potential components are assumed to be linked in series, an abnormal interwave latency indicates a conduction defect between the generators of the two peaks involved. This commonly identifies a precise location of a neurologic lesion. Abnormal upper-limb interwave latencies may indicate cervical spondylosis, intracerebral lesions, or sensorimotor neuropathies. Abnormalities in the lower limb demonstrate peripheral nerve and root lesions, such as those in Guillain-Barré syndrome, compressive myelopathies, multiple sclerosis, transverse myelitis, and traumatic spinal cord injury.

Interfering factors

- Incorrect electrode placement or equipment failure
- Patient tension, inability to relax, or failure to cooperate
- Poor patient vision

Spinal computed tomography

Much more versatile than conventional radiography, spinal computed tomography (CT) provides detailed high-resolution images in the cross-sectional, longitudinal, sagittal, and lateral planes. Multiple X-ray beams from a computerized body scanner are directed at the spine from different angles; these pass through the body and strike radiation detectors, producing electrical impulses. A computer then converts these impulses into digital information, which is displayed as a three-dimensional image on a monitor. Storage of the digital information allows electronic recreation and manipulation of the image, creating a permanent record of the images to enable

reexamination without repeating the procedure.

CT scans are helpful in defining the lesions causing spinal cord compression. Metastatic disease and discogenic disease with osteophyte formation and calcification are examples of pathologic processes diagnosed by CT scans. Since the advent of magnetic resonance imaging, CT scans are used less frequently to diagnose infection, abscesses, hematomas, and some disk herniations.

Purpose

- To diagnose spinal lesions and abnormalities
- To monitor the effects of spinal surgery or therapy

Patient preparation

- Explain to the patient that spinal CT allows visualization of his spine.
- If contrast medium isn't ordered, tell the patient that he need not restrict food and fluids. If contrast medium is ordered, instruct him to fast for 4 hours before the test.
- Tell the patient that a series of scans will be taken of his spine. Explain who will perform the procedure and where it will take place.
- Reassure the patient that the procedure is painless, but that he may find having to remain still for a prolonged period uncomfortable.
- Explain to the patient that he'll be positioned on an X-ray table inside a CT body scanning unit and he'll be told to lie still because movement during the procedure may cause distorted images. The computer-controlled scanner will revolve around him, taking multiple scans.
- If a contrast medium is used, tell the patient that he may feel flushed and warm and may experience a transient

headache, a salty taste, and nausea or vomiting after injection of the contrast medium. Reassure him that these reactions are normal.

■ Instruct the patient to wear a radiologic examining gown and to remove all metal objects and jewelry.

■ Check the patient's history for hypersensitivity reactions to iodine, shellfish, or contrast media. If such reactions have occurred, note them in the patient's chart and notify the physician, who may order prophylactic medications or choose not to use contrast enhancement.

■ If the patient appears restless or apprehensive about the procedure, a mild sedative may be prescribed.

■ Make sure that the patient or a responsible family member has signed an informed consent form, if required.

Equipment

CT body scanner, oscilloscope, recording equipment, contrast medium (iothalamate meglumine or diatrizoate sodium), 60-ml syringe, 19G or 20G needle

Procedure and posttest care

■ Place the patient in a supine position on an X-ray table and tell him to lie as still as possible.

■ The table slides into the circular opening of the CT scanner and the scanner revolves around the patient, taking radiographs at preselected intervals.

■ After the first set of scans is taken, the patient is removed from the scanner. Contrast medium may be administered. **CLINICAL ALERT** *Observe the patient for signs and symptoms of a hypersensitivity reaction, including pruritus, rash, and respiratory difficulty, for 30 minutes after the contrast medium has been injected.*

■ After contrast medium injection, the patient is moved back into the scanner, and another series of scans is taken. The images obtained from the scan are displayed on a monitor during the procedure and stored on magnetic tape.

■ After testing with contrast enhancement, observe the patient for residual effects, such as headache, nausea, and vomiting.

■ Inform the patient that he may resume his usual diet, as ordered.

Precautions

■ Body CT scanning with contrast enhancement is contraindicated in the patient who's hypersensitive to iodine, shellfish, or contrast media used in radiographic studies.

■ The patient may experience strong feelings of claustrophobia or anxiety when inside the CT body scanner. In such cases, a mild sedative to help reduce anxiety may be ordered.

■ For the patient with significant back pain, administer prescribed analgesics before the scan.

Normal findings

In the CT image, spinal tissue appears white, black, or gray, depending on its density. Vertebrae, the densest tissues, are white; cerebrospinal fluid is black; and soft tissues appear in shades of gray.

Abnormal findings

By highlighting areas of altered density and depicting structural malformation, CT scanning can reveal all types of spinal lesions and abnormalities. It's particularly useful in detecting and localizing tumors, which appear as masses varying in density. Measuring this density and noting the configuration and location relative to the spinal cord can usually identify the type of tumor. For example, a neurinoma (schwannoma) appears as a spherical mass dorsal to the cord. A darker, wider mass lying more laterally or ventrally to the cord may be a meningioma.

CT scans also reveal degenerative processes and structural changes in detail. Herniated nucleus pulposus shows as an obvious herniation of disk material with unilateral or bilateral nerve root compression; if the herniation is midline, spinal cord compression will be evident. Cervical spondylosis shows as cervical cord compression due to bony hypertrophy of the cervical spine; lumbar stenosis, as hypertrophy of the lumbar vertebrae, causing cord compression by decreasing space within the spinal column. Facet disorders show as soft-tissue changes, bony overgrowth, and spurring of the vertebrae, which result in nerve root compression. Fluid-filled arachnoidal and other paraspinal cysts show as dark masses displacing the spinal cord. Vascular malformations, evident after contrast enhancement, show as masses or clusters, usually on the dorsal aspect of the spinal cord.

Congenital spinal malformations, such as meningocele, myelocele, and spina bifida, show as abnormally large, dark gaps between the white vertebrae.

Interfering factors
- Excessive patient movement
- Failure to remove metallic objects from the scan area (possible poor imaging)

Oculoplethysmography

An important cerebrovascular test, oculoplethysmography (OPG) is a noninvasive procedure that indirectly measures blood flow in the ophthalmic artery. Because the ophthalmic artery is the first major branch of the internal carotid artery, its

blood flow accurately reflects carotid blood flow and ultimately that of cerebral circulation. Two techniques are used for this test. In OPG, pulse arrival times in the eyes and ears are measured and compared to detect carotid occlusive disease. In ocular pneumoplethysmography (OPG-Gee), ophthalmic artery pressures are measured indirectly and compared with the higher brachial pressure and with each other.

Indications for both of these tests include symptoms of transient ischemic attacks, asymptomatic carotid bruits, and nonhemispheric neurologic symptoms, such as dizziness, ataxia, or syncope. This test may also be performed as a follow-up procedure after carotid endarterectomy or with transcranial Doppler studies or carotid imaging. If indicated, it may be followed by cerebral angiography. Carotid phonoangiography is commonly a valuable complement to OPG. (See *Carotid phonoangiography.*)

Purpose
- To aid in the detection and evaluation of carotid occlusive disease

Patient preparation
- Explain to the patient that this test evaluates carotid artery function.
- Inform the patient that he need not restrict food and fluids.
- Tell the patient who will perform the test, where it will take place, and that the procedure takes only a few minutes.
- Warn the patient that his eyes may burn slightly after the eyedrops are instilled.
- If OPG-Gee is scheduled, warn the patient that he may experience transient loss of vision when suction is applied to the eyes.

CAROTID PHONOANGIOGRAPHY

Carotid phonoangiography graphically records the intensity of carotid bruits during systolic and diastolic phases. It thus helps identify the presence, site, and severity of carotid artery occlusive disease.

For this test, the patient assumes a supine position and holds his breath while a transducer is placed at several sites along the carotid artery. Soundings are made directly over the clavicle (common carotid artery), midway up the neck (carotid bifurcation), and directly below the mandible (internal carotid artery). Oscillographic recordings are obtained and stored on Polaroid film and magnetic tape for later study.

Absence of bruits generally indicates an absence of significant carotid artery disease. However, bruits may also be absent when stenosis nears total occlusion. Bruits heard at all three sites, but loudest over the clavicle, usually originate in the aortic arch or in the heart. Blood flow in the carotid artery itself is unobstructed. Bruits heard over the carotid bifurcation and internal carotid sites, but louder over the latter, indicate turbulent blood flow in the internal carotid artery and the probability of more than 40% occlusion.

Carotid phonoangiography is a quick test and relatively simple to perform, but it's less sensitive and less specific than other noninvasive techniques such as carotid imaging with Doppler ultrasound. Nevertheless, this test is approximately 85% accurate in detecting carotid artery stenosis of more than 40%.

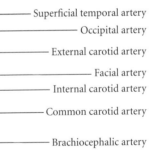

Superficial temporal artery

Occipital artery

External carotid artery

Facial artery

Internal carotid artery

Common carotid artery

Brachiocephalic artery

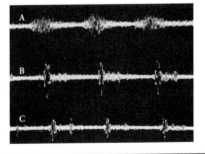

In this phonoangiogram of a patient with an internal carotid artery bruit, the bruit is loudest directly below the mandible (A), present midway up the neck (B), and absent directly over the clavicle (C).

OPG EXAMINATION AND TRACINGS

The patient shown here is undergoing oculoplethysmography (OPG). The eyecups on the patient's corneas detect ocular pulsations, which are compared with each other and with the blood flow in the ear. Blood flow in the ear is detected by a small photoelectric cell (not shown).

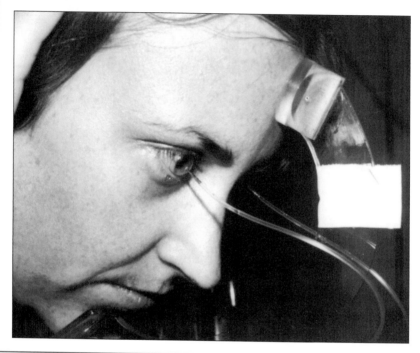

■ Instruct the patient not to blink or move during the procedure.

■ If the patient wears contact lenses, tell him to remove them before the test.

■ The patient with glaucoma may take his usual medications and eyedrops.

Equipment

Oculoplethysmograph or oculopneumo-plethysmograph, anesthetic eyedrops (such as proparacaine 0.5%), tissues

Procedure and posttest care
For OPG

■ Anesthetic eyedrops are instilled to minimize patient discomfort during the test.

■ Small photoelectric cells are attached to the earlobes; these cells can detect blood flow to the ear through the external carotid artery. Tracings for both ears are taken and compared, but only right ear tracings are compared with the eyes. (Tracings for the ears should be the same; if they aren't, this is considered during interpretation of test results.)

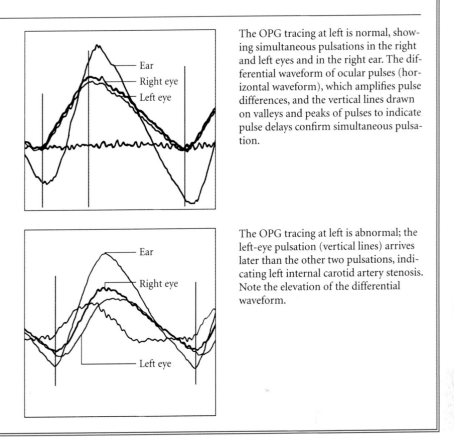

The OPG tracing at left is normal, showing simultaneous pulsations in the right and left eyes and in the right ear. The differential waveform of ocular pulses (horizontal waveform), which amplifies pulse differences, and the vertical lines drawn on valleys and peaks of pulses to indicate pulse delays confirm simultaneous pulsation.

The OPG tracing at left is abnormal; the left-eye pulsation (vertical lines) arrives later than the other two pulsations, indicating left internal carotid artery stenosis. Note the elevation of the differential waveform.

- Eyecups resembling contact lenses are applied to the corneas and held in place with light suction (40 to 50 mm Hg). Tracings of the pulsations within each eye are compared with each other and with tracings for the right ear.

For OPG-Gee
- Anesthetic eyedrops are instilled, and eyecups like those used in OPG are attached to the scleras of the eyes.
- A vacuum of 300 mm Hg is applied to each eye, corresponding to a mean pressure of 100 mm Hg in the ophthalmic artery, and then is gradually released.

- When suction is applied, the pulse in both eyes disappears; when suction is gradually released, pulses should return simultaneously. Pulse arrival times are converted to ophthalmic artery pressures and then compared.
- Both brachial pressures are taken. The higher systolic pressure is then compared with the ophthalmic artery pressures. (See *OPG examination and tracings.*)
- To prevent corneal abrasion, instruct the patient not to rub his eyes for 2 hours after the test. Observe for symptoms of corneal abrasion, such as pain or photophobia, and report them to the physician.

UNDERSTANDING CAROTID IMAGING

Carotid imaging is a diagnostic test that assesses the carotid arteries for occlusive disease. In this test, a pulsed Doppler ultrasonic flow transducer or a real-time imager produces images of the carotid artery and records them.

Real-time imaging (photo below) uses the echo technique to visualize the carotid artery. In this technique, a Doppler signal can be directed to specific points along the vessel. The audio signal is then evaluated.

Pulsed Doppler technique (photos at right) uses a transducer with a range-gating system that allows alternate transmission and reception of ultrasonic signals. The sound reflected from moving red blood cells within the lumen is then collected and stored in a computer for subsequent image reconstruction.

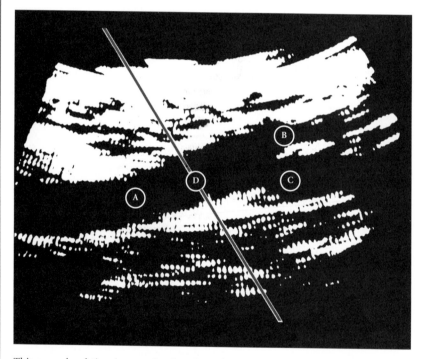

This normal real-time image, taken by echo technique, shows the common carotid artery (A), external carotid artery (B), internal carotid artery (C), and Doppler beam (D).

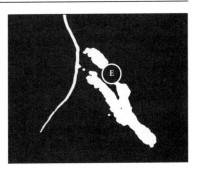

The abnormal pulsed Doppler image above shows total occlusion (E) of the internal carotid artery. Compare this to the normal pulsed Doppler image below.

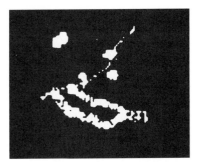

Procedure
The patient is placed in the supine position, and the probe is placed on his neck and moved slowly from the vicinity of the common carotid artery to that of the bifurcation and then to the site of the internal and external carotid arteries.

Advantages and disadvantages
Carotid imaging detects ulcerating plaques that can't be detected by other methods; it can also differentiate between total and near-total arterial occlusion.

Intramural calcification prevents sound penetration and may lead to false-positive results.

- Advise the patient that mild burning as the eyedrops wear off is normal. Tell him to report severe burning.
- If the patient wears contact lenses, instruct him not to reinsert them for about 2 hours after OPG; this will allow the effect of the anesthetic drops to wear off.

Precautions
- OPG is contraindicated in the patient who has had recent eye surgery (within 2 to 6 months), enucleation, or a history of retinal detachment or lens implantation and in the patient who's hypersensitive to the local anesthetic. Because of the risk of scleral hematoma or erythema, OPG-Gee is contraindicated in the patient receiving anticoagulants.
- To limit the risk of corneal abrasions, both techniques must be performed by specially trained personnel.

Normal findings
For OPG
All pulses should occur simultaneously.

For OPG-Gee
The difference between ophthalmic artery pressures should be less than 5 mm Hg. Ophthalmic artery pressure divided by the higher brachial systolic pressure should be greater than 0.67.

Abnormal findings
For OPG
Carotid occlusive disease reduces the rate of blood flow during systole and delays the arrival of a pulse in the ipsilateral eye or ear. When all pulses are compared, any delay can be measured and the degree of carotid artery stenosis estimated as mild, moderate, or severe. This test only estimates the extent of stenosis; it can't provide an exact percentage. (See *Understanding carotid imaging.*)

For OPG-Gee

A difference between ophthalmic artery pressures of more than 5 mm Hg suggests the presence of carotid occlusive disease on the side with the lower pressure. A ratio between the ophthalmic artery pressure and the higher brachial systolic pressure of less than 0.67 reinforces this finding. In other words, the ratio is related to the degree of stenosis: The lower the ratio, the more severe the stenosis. As with OPG, OPG-Gee only estimates the degree of stenosis present; angiography may be necessary to provide a precise evaluation.

Interfering factors

■ The patient with hypertension because of elevated ophthalmic artery pressures
■ Constant blinking or nystagmus causing an artifact
■ Severe cardiac arrhythmias

Transcranial Doppler studies

Transcranial Doppler studies provide information about the presence, quality, and changing nature of circulation to an area of the brain by measuring the velocity of blood flow through cerebral arteries. Narrowed blood vessels produce high velocities, indicating possible stenosis or vasospasm. High velocities may also indicate an arteriovenous malformation.

Purpose

■ To measure the velocity of blood flow through certain cerebral vessels
■ To detect and monitor the progression of cerebral vasospasm
■ To determine whether collateral blood flow exists before surgical ligation or radiologic occlusion of diseased vessels

Patient preparation

■ Explain the purpose of the transcranial Doppler study to the patient (or to his family).
■ Tell the patient that the test will be done while he lies on a bed or stretcher or sits in a reclining chair (or it can be performed at the bedside if he's too ill to be moved to the laboratory).
■ Describe the procedure. Explain that a small amount of gel will be applied to his skin and that a probe will be used to transmit a signal to the artery being studied. Tell the patient that it usually takes less than 1 hour, depending on the number of vessels to be examined and any interfering factors.
■ Tell the patient that he need not restrict food and fluids.

Equipment

Transcranial Doppler unit, probe, conductive gel

Procedure and posttest care

■ Have the patient recline in a chair or on a stretcher or bed.
■ A small amount of conductive gel is applied to the transcranial window (an area where bone is thin enough to allow the Doppler signal to enter and be detected); the most common approaches are temporal, transorbital, and through the foramen magnum.
■ The technician directs the signal toward the artery being studied and records the velocities detected. In a complete study, the middle cerebral arteries, anterior cerebral arteries, posterior cerebral arteries, ophthalmic arteries, carotid siphon, vertebral arteries, and basilar artery are studied.
■ The Doppler signal waveforms may be printed for later analysis and can be

COMPARING VELOCITY WAVEFORMS

A normal transcranial Doppler signal is usually characterized by mean velocities that fall within the normal reported values. Additional information can be gathered by evaluating the shape of the velocity waveform.

Effect of significant proximal vessel obstruction
A delayed systolic up-stroke can be seen in a waveform when significant proximal vessel obstruction is present.

NORMAL

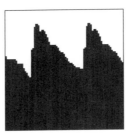

PROXIMAL VESSEL OBSTRUCTION

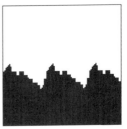

Effect of increased cerebrovascular resistance
Changes in cerebrovascular resistance, as occur with increased intracranial pressure, cause a decrease in diastolic flow.

NORMAL

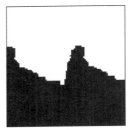

INCREASED RESISTANCE

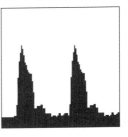

transmitted to varying depths (measured in millimeters).
■ When the study is completed, wipe away the conductive gel.

Precautions
■ Make sure to remove turban head dressings or thick dressings over the test site.

Normal findings
The type of waveforms and velocities obtained indicate whether pathology exists.

Abnormal findings
Although this test commonly isn't definitive, high velocities are typically abnormal and suggest that blood flow is too turbulent or the vessel is too narrow. (See *Comparing velocity waveforms*.)

After the transcranial Doppler study and before surgery, the patient may undergo cerebral angiography to further define cerebral blood flow patterns and locate the exact vascular abnormality.

Interfering factors
■ Failure to remove dressings over the test site (possible poor imaging)

INVASIVE TESTS

Cerebral angiography

Cerebral angiography involves injecting a contrast medium to allow radiographic examination of the cerebral vasculature. Possible injection sites include the femoral, carotid, and brachial arteries. Because it allows visualization of four vessels (the carotid and the vertebral arteries), the femoral artery is used most commonly.

Usually, this test is performed on patients with suspected abnormality of the cerebral vasculature; abnormalities may be suggested by intracranial computed tomography, lumbar puncture, magnetic resonance imaging, or magnetic resonance angiography.

Purpose

■ To detect cerebrovascular abnormalities, such as aneurysm or arteriovenous malformation (AVM), thrombosis, narrowing, or occlusion
■ To study vascular displacement caused by tumor, hematoma, edema, herniation, vasospasm, increased intracranial pressure (ICP), or hydrocephalus
■ To locate clips applied to blood vessels during surgery and to evaluate the postoperative status of affected vessels

Patient preparation

■ Explain to the patient that cerebral angiography shows blood circulation in the brain.
■ Describe the test, including who will administer it and where it will take place.
■ Tell the patient to fast for 8 to 10 hours before the test.
■ Make sure that any pretest blood work results are on the chart to determine bleeding tendency or kidney function.

■ Explain to the patient that he'll wear a gown and that he must remove all jewelry, dentures, hairpins, and other metallic objects in the radiographic field.
■ If ordered, administer a sedative and an anticholinergic drug 30 to 45 minutes before the test.
■ Make sure the patient voids before leaving his room.
■ Tell the patient that he'll be positioned on an X-ray table with his head immobilized and that he should remain still.
■ Explain that a local anesthetic will be administered (some patients — especially children — receive a general anesthetic).
■ Explain to the patient that he'll feel a transient burning sensation as the medium is injected; a warm, flushed feeling; a transient headache; a salty or metallic taste in his mouth; or nausea and vomiting after the dye is injected.
■ Make sure that the patient or a responsible family member has signed an informed consent form, if required.

▶ CLINICAL ALERT *Check the patient's history for hypersensitivity to iodine, iodine-containing substances (such as shellfish), or other contrast media. Note any hypersensitivities on his chart and report them as appropriate.*

Equipment

Contrast medium, automatic contrast injector, radiograph machine with rapid biplane cassette changes, arterial needles (18G or 19G, 2½″ needle for adults; 20G, 1½″ needle for children), femoral arterial catheters for femoral injection

Procedure and posttest care

■ Have the patient recline on an X-ray table and instruct him to lie still with his arms at his sides.

- Shave the injection site (femoral, carotid, or brachial artery) and clean it with alcohol and povidone-iodine.
- A local anesthetic is injected. Then the artery is punctured with the appropriate needle and catheterized.
- In the femoral artery approach, a catheter is threaded to the aortic arch.
- In the brachial artery approach (least common), a blood pressure cuff is placed distal to the puncture site and inflated before injection to prevent the contrast medium from flowing into the forearm and hand.
- After X-rays or fluoroscopy verifies placement of the needle or catheter, the contrast medium is injected. Observe the patient for an adverse reaction, such as hives, flushing, or laryngeal stridor.
- An initial series of lateral and anteroposterior X-rays is taken, developed, and reviewed. Depending on the results, more contrast medium may be injected and another series taken.
- During the test, maintain arterial catheter patency by continuous or periodic flushing. Monitor the patient's vital and neurologic signs.
- When a satisfactory series of X-rays is obtained, the needle (or catheter) is withdrawn. Apply firm pressure to the puncture site for 15 minutes.
- After the test, observe the patient for bleeding, check distal pulses, and apply a pressure bandage.
- Typically, the patient will be on bed rest for 6 to 8 hours. Administer prescribed pain medications and monitor his vital signs and neurologic status for 6 hours. The patient is usually discharged the same day.
- Observe the puncture site for signs of extravasation (redness, swelling) and apply an ice bag to ease the patient's discomfort and minimize swelling. If bleeding occurs, apply firm pressure to the puncture site and inform the physician.

⏵ **CLINICAL ALERT** *If the femoral approach was used, keep the patient's affected leg straight for 6 hours or longer and routinely check pulses distal to the site (dorsalis pedis, popliteal). Monitor the leg for temperature, color, and sensation. Thrombosis or hematoma can occlude blood flow; extravasation can also impede blood flow by exerting pressure on the artery.*

- Monitor the patient for disorientation and weakness or numbness in the extremities (signs of thrombosis or hematoma) and for arterial spasms, which may produce symptoms of transient ischemic attacks.
- If the brachial approach was used, immobilize the affected arm for 6 hours or longer and routinely check the radial pulse.
- Place a sign near the patient's bed warning personnel not to take blood pressure readings from the affected arm.
- Observe the patient's arm and hand for changes in color, temperature, or sensation. If they become pale, cool, or numb, report these changes at once.
- After the test, tell the patient he may resume his usual diet. Encourage him to drink fluids to help him pass the contrast medium.

Precautions

- Cerebral angiography is contraindicated in the patient with hepatic, renal, or thyroid disease.
- This test is also contraindicated in the patient with a hypersensitivity to iodine or contrast media.
- If the patient has been receiving aspirin or other anticoagulants daily, take extra care when compressing the puncture site.

Anticoagulants may need to be discontinued for 3 days before testing.

▶ **CLINICAL ALERT** *Monitor the catheter puncture site frequently and closely for hemorrhage or hematoma formation. If either occurs, notify the physician immediately.*

Normal findings

During the arterial phase of perfusion, the contrast medium fills and opacifies superficial and deep arteries and arterioles; it opacifies superficial and deep veins during the venous phase. The finding of apparently normal (symmetrical) cerebral vasculature must be correlated with the patient's history and clinical status.

Abnormal findings

Changes in the caliber of vessel lumina suggest vascular disease, possibly due to spasms, plaques, fistulas, AVM, or arteriosclerosis. Diminished blood flow to vessels may be related to increased ICP.

Vessel displacement may reflect the presence and size of a tumor, areas of edema, or obstruction of the cerebrospinal fluid pathway. Cerebral angiography may also show circulation within a tumor, usually giving precise information on its position and nature. Meningeal blood supply originating in the external carotid artery may indicate an extracerebral tumor, but usually designates a meningioma. Such a tumor may arise outside the brain substance, but it may still be within the cerebral hemisphere.

Interfering factors

■ Head movement during the test (possible poor imaging)
■ Failure to remove metallic objects from the X-ray field (possible poor imaging)

Digital subtraction angiography

Digital subtraction angiography (DSA) is a sophisticated radiographic technique that uses video equipment and computer-assisted image enhancement to examine the vascular systems. As in conventional angiography, X-ray images are obtained after injecting a contrast medium. However, unlike conventional angiography, in which images of bone and soft tissue commonly obscure vascular detail, DSA provides a high-contrast view of blood vessels without interfering images or shadows.

This unique view is made possible by digital subtraction, in which fluoroscopic images are taken before and after injection of a contrast medium. A computer converts these images into digital information and then "subtracts" the first image from the second, eliminating most information (mainly bone and soft tissue) common to both images. The result is a better image of the contrast-enhanced vasculature.

In addition to superior image quality, DSA has other advantages over conventional angiography. Because the digital subtraction process allows I.V., rather than intra-arterial, injection of the contrast medium, DSA avoids the risk of stroke associated with conventional angiography and reduces the pain and discomfort associated with arterial catheterization.

Although DSA has been used to study peripheral and renal vascular disease, it's probably most useful in diagnosing cerebrovascular disorders, such as carotid stenosis and occlusion, arteriovenous malformation, aneurysms, and vascular tumors. It's also useful in visualizing displacement of vasculature by other intracranial abnormalities or traumatic injuries and in detecting lesions typically missed by computed tomography scans such as thrombosis of the superior sagittal sinus.

Purpose

- To visualize extracranial and intracranial cerebral blood flow
- To detect and evaluate cerebrovascular abnormalities
- To aid postoperative evaluation of cerebrovascular surgery, such as arterial grafts and endarterectomies

Patient preparation

- Explain to the patient that DSA visualizes cerebral blood vessels.
- Tell the patient that he'll need to fast for 4 hours before the test, but he need not restrict fluids.
- Explain to the patient that he'll receive an injection of a contrast medium, either by needle or through a venous catheter inserted in his arm, and that a series of X-rays will be taken of his head. Tell him who will perform the test, where it will take place, and that it takes 30 to 90 minutes.
- Inform the patient that he'll be positioned on an X-ray table with his head immobilized and will be asked to lie still. (Some patients — especially children — may be given a sedative to prevent movement during the procedure.)
- Instruct the patient to remove all jewelry, dentures, and other radiopaque objects from the X-ray field.
- Tell the patient that he'll probably feel some transient pain from insertion of the needle or catheter and that he may experience a feeling of warmth, a headache, a metallic taste, and nausea or vomiting after the contrast agent is injected.

- Make sure that the patient or a responsible family member has signed an informed consent form, if required.
- Check the patient's history for hypersensitivity to iodine; iodine-containing substances, such as shellfish; and contrast media. If he's had such reactions, note them on the chart and inform the physician, who may order prophylactic medications or choose not to perform the test.

Equipment

X-ray machine with biplane cassette changer, computer and video monitor, video recorder, I.V. equipment and 250 ml normal saline solution, contrast medium, automatic contrast medium injector

Procedure and posttest care

- Place the patient in the supine position on an X-ray table and tell him to lie still with his arms at his sides.
- After an initial series of fluoroscopic pictures (mask images) of the patient's head is taken, the injection site — most commonly the antecubital basilic or cephalic vein — is shaved and cleaned with an antiseptic solution.
- If catheterization is ordered, a local anesthetic is administered, a venipuncture is performed, and a catheter is inserted and advanced to the superior vena cava.
- After placement is verified by X-ray, I.V. lines from a bag of normal saline solution and from an automatic contrast medium injector are connected. While the saline is administered, the injector delivers the contrast medium at a rate of about 14 ml/second. If a simple injection of the contrast medium is ordered, a bolus of 40 to 60 ml is administered I.V. by needle.
- Monitor the patient's vital signs and neurologic status and observe for signs of

a hypersensitivity reaction, such as urticaria, flushing, and respiratory distress.

■ After allowing time for the contrast medium to clear the pulmonary circulation and enter the cerebral vasculature, a second series of fluoroscopic images (contrast images) is taken. The computer digitizes the information received from both series and compares mask and contrast images, subtracting the information (images of bone and soft tissue) common to both. A detailed image of the contrast medium-filled vessels is displayed on a video monitor; the image may be stored on videotape or a videodisc for future reference.

■ Because the contrast medium acts as a diuretic, encourage the patient to increase his fluid intake for 24 hours after this test. Advise him that extra fluid intake will also speed excretion of the contrast medium. Monitor his intake and output, as ordered.

■ Check the venipuncture site for signs of extravasation, such as redness or swelling. If bleeding occurs, apply firm pressure to the puncture site. If a hematoma develops, elevate the arm and apply warm soaks.

■ Observe the patient for a delayed hypersensitivity reaction to the contrast medium. A delayed reaction can occur up to 18 hours after the procedure.

■ Tell the patient that he may resume his usual diet.

Precautions
■ DSA may be contraindicated in the patient with a hypersensitivity to iodine or contrast media; poor cardiac function; renal, hepatic, or thyroid disease; diabetes; or multiple myeloma.

Normal findings
The contrast medium should fill and opacify all superficial and deep arteries, arterioles, and veins, allowing visualization of normal cerebral vasculature. The digital subtraction process may intensify areas that should receive only contrast medium. However, conventional angiography provides a more detailed image of the carotid arteries than DSA.

Abnormal findings
Vascular filling defects, seen as areas of increased vascular opacity, may indicate arteriovenous occlusion or stenosis, possibly due to vasospasm, vascular malformation or angiomas, arteriosclerosis, or cerebral embolism or thrombosis. Outpouchings in vessel lumina may reflect cerebral aneurysms; such aneurysms frequently rupture, causing subarachnoid hemorrhage. Vessel displacement or vascular masses may indicate an intracranial tumor. DSA can clearly depict the vascular supply of some tumors, reflecting the tumor's position, size, and nature.

Interfering factors
■ Patient movement
■ Radiopaque objects in the fluoroscopic field

Electromyography

Electromyography (EMG) records the electrical activity of selected skeletal muscle groups at rest and during voluntary contraction. It involves percutaneous insertion of a needle electrode into a muscle. The electrical discharge of the muscle is then measured by an oscilloscope. Nerve conduction time is often measured simultaneously. (See *Nerve conduction studies.*)

Purpose

- To aid in differentiating between primary muscle disorders, such as the muscular dystrophies, and secondary disorders
- To help assess diseases characterized by central neuronal degeneration such as amyotrophic lateral sclerosis (ALS)
- To aid in the diagnosis of neuromuscular disorders such as myasthenia gravis
- To aid in the diagnosis of radiculopathies

Patient preparation

- Explain to the patient that EMG measures the electrical activity of his muscles.
- Tell the patient that there are usually no restrictions on food and fluids (in some cases, cigarettes, coffee, tea, and cola may be restricted for 2 to 3 hours before the test).
- Describe the test, including who will perform it and where it will take place.
- Tell the patient that he may wear a hospital gown or comfortable clothing that permits access to the muscles to be tested.
- Advise the patient that a needle will be inserted into selected muscles and that he may experience discomfort. Reassure him that adverse effects and complications are rare.
- Make sure that the patient or a responsible family member has signed an informed consent form, if required.
- Check the patient's history for medications that may interfere with the results of the test — for example, cholinergics, anticholinergics, and skeletal muscle relaxants. If the patient is receiving such medications, note this on the chart and withhold medications, as ordered.

Procedure and posttest care

- Position the patient on a stretcher or bed or in a chair, depending on the mus-

NERVE CONDUCTION STUDIES

Nerve conduction studies aid in the diagnosis of peripheral nerve injuries and diseases affecting the peripheral nervous system such as peripheral neuropathies. To measure nerve conduction time, a nerve is stimulated electrically through the skin and underlying tissues. The patient experiences a mild electric shock with each stimulation. At a known distance from the point of stimulation, a recording electrode detects the response from the stimulated nerve.

The time between stimulation of the nerve and the detected response is measured on an oscilloscope. The speed of conduction along the nerve is then calculated by dividing the distance between the point of stimulation and the recording electrode by the time between stimulus and response. In peripheral nerve injuries and diseases, such as peripheral neuropathies, nerve conduction time is abnormal.

cles to be tested. Position his arm or leg so that the muscle to be tested is at rest.

- The skin is cleaned with alcohol, the needle electrodes are quickly inserted, and a metal plate is placed under the patient to serve as a reference electrode. Then the muscle's electrical signal (motor unit potential), recorded during rest and contraction, is amplified 1 million times and displayed on an oscilloscope or computer screen.
- The recorder lead wires are attached to an audio amplifier so that the fluctuation of voltage within the muscle can be heard.

■ If the patient experiences residual pain, apply warm compresses and administer prescribed analgesics.

■ Tell the patient that he may resume his usual medications, as ordered.

Precautions
■ EMG is contraindicated in the patient with a bleeding disorder.

Normal findings
At rest, a normal muscle exhibits minimal electrical activity. During voluntary contraction, electrical activity increases markedly. A sustained contraction or one of increasing strength causes a rapid "train" of motor unit potentials that can be heard as a crescendo of sounds over the audio amplifier.

At the same time, the monitor displays a sequence of waveforms that vary in amplitude (height) and frequency. Waveforms that are close together indicate a high frequency, whereas waveforms that are far apart signify a low frequency.

Abnormal findings
In primary muscle diseases, such as muscular dystrophy, motor unit potentials are short (low amplitude), with frequent, irregular discharges. In disorders, such as ALS (as well as in peripheral nerve disorders), motor unit potentials are isolated and irregular, but show increased amplitude and duration. In myasthenia gravis, motor unit potentials initially may be normal, but progressively diminish in amplitude with continuing contractions. The interpreter distinguishes between waveforms that indicate a muscle disorder and those that indicate denervation. Findings must be correlated with the patient's history, clinical features, and the results of other neurodiagnostic tests.

Interfering factors
■ The patient's inability to comply with instructions
■ Drugs affecting myoneural junctions, such as cholinergics, anticholinergics, and skeletal muscle relaxants

Cerebrospinal fluid analysis

Cerebrospinal fluid (CSF), a clear substance that circulates in the subarachnoid space, has many vital functions. It protects the brain and spinal cord from injury and transports products of neurosecretion, cellular biosynthesis, and cellular metabolism through the central nervous system (CNS).

For qualitative analysis, CSF is most commonly obtained by lumbar puncture (usually between the third and fourth lumbar vertebrae) and, rarely, by cisternal or ventricular puncture. A CSF specimen may also be obtained during other neurologic tests such as myelography.

Purpose
■ To measure CSF pressure as an aid in detecting an obstruction of CSF circulation
■ To aid in the diagnosis of viral or bacterial meningitis, subarachnoid or intracranial hemorrhage, tumors, and brain abscesses
■ To aid in the diagnosis of neurosyphilis and chronic CNS infections
■ To check for Alzheimer's disease

Patient preparation
■ Describe the procedure to the patient and explain that CSF analysis analyzes the fluid around the spinal cord.
■ Inform the patient that he need not restrict food and fluids.

- Tell the patient who will perform the procedure and where it will take place.
- Advise the patient that a headache is the most common adverse effect of a lumbar puncture, but reassure him that his cooperation during the test helps minimize this effect.
- Make sure that the patient or a responsible family member has signed an informed consent form.
- If the patient is unusually anxious, assess and report his vital signs.

Equipment

Lumbar puncture tray, sterile gloves, face mask, local anesthetic (usually 1% lidocaine), povidone-iodine solution, small adhesive bandage

Procedure and posttest care

- Position the patient on his side at the edge of the bed with his knees drawn up to his abdomen and his chin on his chest. Provide pillows to support the spine on a horizontal plane. This position allows full flexion of the spine and easy access to the lumbar subarachnoid space. Help him maintain this position by placing one arm around his knees and the other arm around his neck.
- If the sitting position is preferred, have the patient sit up and bend his chest and head toward his knees. Help him maintain this position throughout the procedure.
- After the skin is prepared for injection, the area is draped. Warn the patient that he'll probably experience a transient burning sensation when the local anesthetic is injected.
- Tell the patient that when the spinal needle is inserted, he may feel slight local pain as the needle transverses the dura mater.

- Ask the patient to report pain or sensations that differ from or continue after this expected discomfort because such sensations may indicate irritation or puncture of a nerve root, requiring needle repositioning.
- Instruct the patient to remain still and breathe normally; movement and hyperventilation can alter pressure readings or cause injury.
- The anesthetic is injected, and the spinal needle is inserted in the midline, between the spinous processes of the vertebrae (usually between the third and fourth lumbar vertebra). At this point, initial (or opening) CSF pressure is measured and a specimen is obtained.
- After the specimen is collected, label the containers in the order in which they were filled and find out if specific instructions are required for the laboratory.
- Next, a final pressure reading is taken, and the needle is removed.
- Clean the puncture site with a local antiseptic, such as povidone-iodine solution, and apply a small adhesive bandage.
- Check whether the patient must lie flat or if the head of his bed may be slightly elevated. In most cases, you'll be instructed to keep the patient lying flat for 8 hours after lumbar puncture. Some physicians, however, allow a 30-degree elevation at the head of the bed. Remind the patient that although he must not raise his head, he can turn from side to side.
- Encourage the patient to drink fluids. Provide a flexible straw.
- Check the puncture site for redness, swelling, and drainage every hour for the first 4 hours, and then every 4 hours for the first 24 hours.
- If CSF pressure is elevated, assess the patient's neurologic status every 15 minutes for 4 hours. If he's stable, assess him every hour for 2 hours and then every

FINDINGS IN CEREBROSPINAL FLUID ANALYSIS

Test	Normal	Abnormality	Implications
Pressure	50 to 180 mm H_2O	Increase	Increased intracranial pressure
		Decrease	Spinal subarachnoid obstruction above puncture site
Appearance	Clear, colorless	Cloudy	Infection
		Xanthochromic or bloody	Subarachnoid, intracerebral, or intraventricular hemorrhage; spinal cord obstruction; traumatic tap (usually noted only in initial specimen)
		Brown, orange, or yellow	Elevated protein levels, red blood cell (RBC) breakdown (blood present for at least 3 days)
Protein	15 to 50 mg/dl (SI, 0.15 to 0.5 q/L)	Marked increase	Tumors, trauma, hemorrhage, diabetes mellitus, polyneuritis, blood in cerebrospinal fluid (CSF)
		Marked decrease	Rapid CSF production
Gamma globulin	3% to 12% of total protein	Increase	Demyelinating disease, neurosyphilis, Guillain-Barré syndrome
Glucose	50 to 80 mg/dl (SI, 2.8 to 4.4 mmol/L)	Increase	Systemic hyperglycemia
		Decrease	Systemic hypoglycemia, bacterial or fungal infection, meningitis, mumps, postsubarachnoid hemorrhage

FINDINGS IN CEREBROSPINAL FLUID ANALYSIS *(continued)*

Test	Normal	Abnormality	Implications
Cell count	0 to 5 white blood cells	Increase	Active disease: meningitis, acute infection, onset of chronic illness, tumor, abscess, infarction, demyelinating disease
	No RBCs	RBCs	Hemorrhage or traumatic lumbar puncture
Venereal Disease Research Laboratories, test for syphilis, and other serologic tests	Nonreactive	Positive	Neurosyphilis
Chloride	118 to 130 mEq/L (SI, 118 to 130 mmol/L)	Decrease	Infected meninges
Gram stain	No organisms	Gram-positive or gram-negative organisms	Bacterial meningitis

4 hours or according to the pretest schedule.

CLINICAL ALERT *Watch the patient for complications of lumbar puncture, such as reaction to the anesthetic, meningitis, bleeding into the spinal canal, and cerebellar tonsillar herniation and medullary compression. Signs of meningitis include fever, neck rigidity, and irritability; signs of herniation include decreased level of consciousness, changes in pupil size and equality, altered vital signs (including widened pulse pressure, decreased pulse rate, and irregular respirations), and respiratory failure.*

Precautions

■ Infection at the puncture site contraindicates removal of CSF; in a patient with increased intracranial pressure, CSF should be removed with extreme caution because the rapid reduction in pressure that follows withdrawal of fluid can cause cerebellar tonsillar herniation and medullary compression.

■ During the procedure, observe closely for adverse reactions, such as elevated pulse rate, pallor, or clammy skin. Report any significant changes immediately.

■ Record the collection time on the test request form. Send the form and labeled specimens to the laboratory immediately after collection.

Findings

For a summary of normal and abnormal findings in CSF analysis, see *Findings in cerebrospinal fluid analysis.*

Normally, the CSF pressure is recorded and the appearance of the specimen is checked. Three tubes are collected routinely and are sent to the laboratory for protein, sugar, and cell analysis as well as for serologic testing such as the Venereal Disease Research Laboratory test for neurosyphilis. A separate specimen is also sent to the laboratory for culture and sensitivity testing. Electrolyte analysis and Gram stain may be ordered as supplementary tests. CSF electrolyte levels are of special interest in the patient with abnormal serum electrolyte levels or CSF infection and in the patient receiving hyperosmolar agents.

Interfering factors
- Patient position and activity (possible increase or decrease in CSF pressure)
- Crying, coughing, or straining (possible increase in CSF pressure)
- Delay between collection time and laboratory testing (possible invalidation of test results, especially cell counts)

Myelography

Myelography uses fluoroscopy and radiography to evaluate the spinal subarachnoid space after injection of a contrast medium. Because the contrast medium is heavier than cerebrospinal fluid (CSF), it flows through the subarachnoid space to the dependent area when the patient, lying prone on a fluoroscopic table, is tilted up or down. The fluoroscope allows the physician to see the flow of the contrast medium and the outline of the subarachnoid space. X-rays are taken to provide a permanent record.

Myelography can help locate a spinal lesion, a ruptured disk, spinal stenosis, or an abscess. Sometimes it's performed to confirm the need for surgery; in such cases, a neurosurgeon may stand by. If this test confirms a spinal tumor, the patient may be taken directly to the operating room. Immediate surgery may also be necessary when the contrast medium causes a total block of the subarachnoid space.

Purpose
- To evaluate and determine the cause of neurologic symptoms (numbness, pain, weakness)
- To identify lesions, such as tumors and herniated intervertebral disks that partially or totally block the flow of CSF in the subarachnoid space
- To help detect arachnoiditis, spinal nerve root injury, or tumors in the posterior fossa of the skull

Patient preparation
- Explain to the patient that myelography reveals obstructions in the spinal cord.
- Tell the patient that his food and fluid intake will be restricted for 8 hours before the test. If the test is scheduled for the afternoon and facility policy permits, the patient may have clear liquids before the test.
- Describe the test, including who will administer it and where it will take place.
- Explain to the patient that he may feel a transient burning sensation as the contrast medium is injected; a warm, flushed feeling; transient headache; a salty taste; or nausea and vomiting after the dye is injected. Explain that he may feel some pain caused by his positioning, needle insertion and, in some cases, removal of the contrast medium.
- Make sure that the patient or a responsible family member has signed an informed consent form.

CLINICAL ALERT *Check the patient's history for hypersensitivity to iodine and iodine-containing substances (for example, shellfish), radiographic contrast media, and associated medications. Notify the radiologist if the patient has a history of epilepsy or phenothiazine use. If metrizamide is to be used as a contrast medium, discontinue phenothiazine 48 hours before the test.*

■ Tell the patient to remove all jewelry and other metallic objects in the X-ray field.

■ Tell the patient that the head of his bed must be elevated for 6 to 8 hours after the test and that he'll remain on bed rest for an additional 6 to 8 hours. If an oil-based contrast agent is used, inform the patient that it will be manually removed after the test and that he'll need to remain flat in bed for 6 to 24 hours.

■ Perform pretest procedures and administer prescribed medications. If the puncture is to be performed in the lumbar region, an enema may be prescribed. A sedative and anticholinergic (such as atropine sulfate) may be prescribed to reduce swallowing during the procedure. Make sure that pretest laboratory work (may include coagulation and kidney function studies) is present in the chart.

Equipment
Alcohol, 1% lidocaine solution, lumbar puncture tray, contrast medium (iophendylate or metrizamide), two 10-ml syringes, spinal needle (18G for iophendylate or 11G for metrizamide), X-ray machine capable of fluoroscopy, povidone-iodine solution, sterile gloves, small adhesive bandage

Procedure and posttest care
■ Position the patient on his side at the edge of the table with his chin on his chest and his knees drawn up to his abdomen. (If the patient has a lumbar deformity or an infection at the puncture site, a cisternal puncture may be done.)

■ After the lumbar puncture is performed, the fluoroscope is used to verify proper positioning of the needle in the subarachnoid space. Some CSF may be removed for routine laboratory analysis.

■ Turn the patient to the prone position and secure him with straps across his upper back, under his arms, and across his ankles. Hyperextend his chin to prevent the contrast medium from flowing into the cranium; place a towel under his chin for comfort.

■ If the patient complains of a headache or difficulty swallowing or reports that he isn't breathing deeply enough, provide reassurance and explain that he can rest periodically during the procedure.

■ The contrast medium is injected and the table tilted so that the dye flows through the subarachnoid space. (In rare circumstances, air is used as a negative contrast medium; however, this is typically reserved for a patient with suspected congenital abnormalities such as syringomyelia.)

■ The contrast medium flow is observed by fluoroscope, and X-rays are taken. If an obstruction in the subarachnoid space blocks the upward flow of the contrast medium, a cisternal puncture may be performed.

■ The contrast medium is withdrawn, if necessary, after satisfactory X-rays are obtained and the needle is removed. Clean the puncture site with povidone-iodine solution and apply a small adhesive bandage.

■ Based on the contrast medium used during the test, position the patient as follows: If metrizamide was used, tell him to stay in bed for the next 12 to 16 hours.

Keep the head of his bed elevated for at least 8 hours. If an oil-based contrast medium was used, tell him to remain flat in bed for 24 hours.

■ Monitor the patient's vital signs and neurologic status at least every 15 minutes for the first hour, every 30 minutes for the next 2 hours, and then every 4 hours for 24 hours. The patient may be discharged the same day.

■ Encourage the patient to drink extra fluids. He should void within 8 hours after returning to his room.

■ If there are no complications or adverse reactions, tell the patient that he may resume his usual diet and activities the day after the test.

■ Monitor the patient for radicular pain, fever, back pain, or signs of meningeal irritation, such as headache, irritability, or stiff neck. If these signs or symptoms occur, keep the room quiet and dark and administer an analgesic or antipyretic, as needed.

Precautions

■ Generally, myelography is contraindicated in the patient with increased intracranial pressure, hypersensitivity to iodine or contrast media, or an infection at the puncture site.

■ Improper positioning after the test may affect recovery.

Normal findings

Normally, the contrast medium flows freely through the subarachnoid space, showing no obstruction or structural abnormalities.

Abnormal findings

Myelography can identify and localize lesions within or surrounding the spinal cord or subarachnoid space. Examples of common extradural lesions include her-

niated intervertebral disks and metastatic tumors. Neurofibromas and meningiomas are common lesions within the subarachnoid space, and ependymomas and astrocytomas are common within the spinal cord.

If the test confirms a spinal tumor, the patient may be taken directly to the operating room. Immediate surgery may also be necessary if the contrast medium causes a total block of the subarachnoid space.

Myelography may help locate or confirm a ruptured or herniated disk, spinal stenosis, or abscess and, occasionally, confirm the need for surgery. This test may also detect syringomyelia (a congenital abnormality marked by fluid-filled cavities within the spinal cord and widening of the cord itself), arachnoiditis, spinal nerve root injury, and tumors in the posterior fossa of the skull. Other findings may include fractures, dislocations, thinning of bones (osteoporosis), deformities in the curvature of the spine, bone spurs, and vertebral degeneration. Test results must be correlated with the patient's history and clinical status.

Interfering factors

■ Incorrect needle placement
■ An uncooperative patient

Tensilon test

The Tensilon test involves careful observation of the patient after I.V. administration of Tensilon (edrophonium chloride), a rapid, short-acting anticholinesterase that improves muscle strength by increasing muscle response to nerve impulses.

It's especially useful in diagnosing myasthenia gravis, an abnormality of the myoneural junction in which nerve impulses fail to induce normal muscular responses. Patients with myasthenia gravis experience extreme fatigue at the end of the day and after repetitive activity or stress. Results of other procedures, including electromyography, may supplement Tensilon test findings in diagnosing this disease.

Purpose
- To aid in the diagnosis of myasthenia gravis
- To aid in differentiating between myasthenic and cholinergic crises
- To monitor oral anticholinesterase therapy

Patient preparation
- Explain to the patient that the Tensilon test helps determine the cause of muscle weakness.
- Describe the test, including who will perform it, where it will take place, and how long it will last.
- Don't describe the exact response that will be evaluated; foreknowledge can affect the test's objectivity.
- Explain to the patient that a small tube will be inserted into a vein in his arm and that a drug will be administered periodically. He'll be asked to make repetitive muscle movements and his reactions will be observed. To ensure accuracy, the test may be repeated several times.
- Advise the patient that the Tensilon may produce some unpleasant adverse effects, but reassure him that someone will be with him at all times and that any reactions will quickly disappear.
- Check the patient's history for medications that affect muscle function, anticholinesterase therapy, drug hypersensitivities, and respiratory disease. Withhold medications, as ordered. If the patient is receiving anticholinesterase therapy, note this on the requisition request; include the time of the most recent dose.

- Make sure that the patient or a responsible family member has signed an informed consent form.

Equipment
Standard
10 mg Tensilon, 0.4 mg atropine (may be prescribed for the patient with respiratory distress), one tuberculin and one 3-ml syringe, I.V. infusion set, 50-ml bag of I.V. solution (dextrose 5% in water [D_5W] or normal saline solution), tape, tourniquet, alcohol swabs

Emergency
0.5 to 1.0 mg atropine I.V. for cholinergic crisis, 0.5 to 2.0 mg neostigmine methylsulfate I.V. for myasthenic crisis (may be repeated up to a total of 5 mg), extra tuberculin and 3-ml syringes (for atropine or neostigmine injections), resuscitation equipment, including a tracheotomy tray

Procedure and posttest care
- Begin an I.V. infusion of D_5W or normal saline solution.
- When performing the test on an adult patient suspected of having myasthenia gravis, 2 mg of Tensilon are administered initially. Before the rest of the dose is administered, the physician may want to fatigue the muscles by asking the patient to perform various exercises, such as looking up until ptosis develops, counting to 100 until his voice diminishes, or holding his arms above his shoulders until they drop. When the muscles are fatigued, the remaining 8 mg of Tensilon are administered over 30 seconds.
- Some physicians may prefer to begin the test with a placebo injection to evaluate the patient's muscle response more accurately. The placebo isn't necessary if cranial muscles are being tested because

cranial strength can't be simulated voluntarily.

■ After Tensilon is administered, the patient is asked to perform repetitive muscle movements, such as opening and closing his eyes and crossing and uncrossing his legs. Closely observe the patient for improved muscle strength. If muscle strength doesn't improve within 3 to 5 minutes, the test may be repeated.

■ To differentiate between a myasthenic and cholinergic crisis, 1 to 2 mg of Tensilon is infused. After the infusion, continually monitor the patient's vital signs. Watch closely for respiratory distress and be prepared to provide respiratory assistance.

■ If muscle strength doesn't improve, more Tensilon is infused cautiously— 1 mg at a time up to a maximum of 5 mg w—and the patient is observed for distress.

■ Neostigmine is administered immediately if the test demonstrates myasthenic crisis; atropine is administered for cholinergic crisis.

■ To evaluate oral anticholinesterase therapy, 2 mg of Tensilon is infused 1 hour after the patient's last dose of the anticholinesterase. The patient is observed carefully for adverse effects and muscle response.

■ After Tensilon administration, the I.V. line is kept open at a rate of 20 ml/hour until all of the patient's responses have been evaluated.

■ When the test is complete, discontinue the I.V. and check the patient's vital signs.

■ Check the puncture site for hematoma, excessive bleeding, and swelling.

■ Tell the patient that he may resume his usual medications, as ordered.

Precautions

■ Because of the systemic adverse reactions Tensilon may produce, this test may be contraindicated in the patient with hypotension, bradycardia, apnea, or mechanical obstruction of the intestine or urinary tract.

■ The patient with a respiratory ailment, such as asthma, should receive atropine during the test to minimize adverse reactions to Tensilon.

■ Stay with the patient during the test and observe him closely for adverse reactions.

■ Keep resuscitation equipment handy in case of respiratory failure.

Normal findings

Someone who doesn't have myasthenia gravis usually develops fasciculation in response to Tensilon. The physician must interpret the responses carefully to distinguish a normal person from one with myasthenia gravis.

Abnormal findings

If the patient has myasthenia gravis, muscle strength should improve promptly after administration of Tensilon. The degree of improvement depends on the muscle group being tested; improvement is usually obvious within 30 seconds. Although the maximum benefit lasts only several minutes, lingering effects may persist—for example, up to 2 hours in a patient receiving prednisone. The patient with myasthenia gravis shows improved muscle strength in this test; in some cases, the patient responds slightly, and the test may need to be repeated to confirm the diagnosis.

The test may yield inconsistent results if myasthenia gravis affects only the ocular muscles, as in mild or early forms of the disorder. It may produce a positive response in motor neuron disease and in some neuropathies and myopathies. The response is usually less dramatic and less consistent than in myasthenia gravis. The patient in myasthenic crisis shows brief improvement in muscle strength after Tensilon administration. The patient in cholinergic crisis (anticholinesterase overdose) may experience exaggerated muscle weakness. If Tensilon increases the patient's muscle strength without increasing adverse effects, oral anticholinesterase therapy can be increased. If Tensilon decreases muscle strength in a person with severe adverse reactions, therapy should be reduced. If the test shows no change in muscle strength and only mild adverse effects occur, therapy should remain the same.

Interfering factors
- Prednisone (possible delay of Tensilon's effect on muscle strength)
- Quinidine and anticholinergics (inhibit the action of Tensilon)
- Procainamide and muscle relaxants (inhibit normal muscle response)

Selected readings

Braunwald, E., et al, eds. *Harrison's Principles of Internal Medicine*, 15th ed. New York: McGraw-Hill Book Co., 2001.

Fischbach, F. *A Manual of Laboratory and Diagnostic Tests*, 7th ed. Philadelphia: Lippincott Williams & Wilkins, 2004.

Guyton, A.C., and Hall, J.E. *Textbook of Medical Physiology*, 10th ed. Philadelphia: W.B. Saunders Co., 2001.

Nettina, S. *The Lippincott Manual of Nursing Practice*, 7th ed. Philadelphia: Lippincott Williams & Wilkins, 2000.

Nursing2004 Drug Handbook, 24th ed. Philadelphia: Lippincott Williams & Wilkins, 2004.

Nursing Procedures, 4th ed. Springhouse, Pa.: Springhouse Corp., 2004.

Pagana, K.D., and Pagana, T.J. *Mosby's Diagnostic and Laboratory Test Reference*, 6th ed. St. Louis: Mosby Year–Book, Inc., 2003.

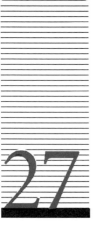

Gastrointestinal system

Introduction

The GI tract and the adjoining liver, gallbladder, and pancreas are responsible for the proper digestion and absorption of food and for the elimination of metabolic waste products. Numerous diagnostic tests evaluate this system to detect diseases, functional disorders, and abnormalities resulting from emotional stress. They range from laboratory analysis of stool and esophageal, gastric, and peritoneal contents to specialized invasive and noninvasive procedures, such as endoscopy, contrast radiography, nuclear imaging, ultrasonography, and computed tomography (CT). (See *Specialized tests in gastroenterology,* pages 744 and 745.) These specialized laboratory procedures are considered the most valuable because they produce results that are usually specific for a particular disease. However, the choice of an appropriate test or test battery always depends on the patient's signs and symptoms and on the results of a physical examination.

Anatomy and physiology

The GI tract includes the mouth, pharynx, esophagus, stomach (fundus, body, antrum), small intestine (duodenum, jejunum, ileum), and large intestine (cecum, colon, rectum, anal canal). Throughout the GI tract, peristalsis propels the ingested material along; sphincters prevent its reflux.

Digestion begins in the mouth through chewing and the action of the enzyme amylase, which is secreted in saliva and breaks down starches. Food is lubricated by the glycoprotein mucin, then swallowed as a bolus. While the food passes through the esophagus, it's also lubricated by mucous secretions. Digestion continues in the stomach through the action of glandular secretions, such as mucus, pepsinogen, hydrochloric acid, gastrin, and intrinsic factor, a glycoprotein essential in vitamin B_{12} absorption. The hormone gastrin, the most potent stimulus of gastric secretion, enhances the release of hydrochloric acid. In turn, hydrochloric acid lowers the pH of gastric contents, promoting the conversion of pepsinogen to pepsin, a proteolytic enzyme. Pepsin begins protein catabolism, breaking down dietary protein into products ranging from large polypeptides to amino acids.

Through a churning motion, the stomach breaks food into tiny particles, mixes them with gastric juices, and pushes the mass toward the pylorus. The liquid portion (chyme) enters the duodenum in small amounts; solid material remains in the stomach until it liquefies (usually in 1 to 6 hours). Although limited amounts of water, alcohol, and certain drugs are absorbed in the stomach, chyme passes unabsorbed into the duodenum.

Digestion and absorption occur primarily in the small intestine, where millions of villi increase the surface area. For digestion, the small intestine relies on the many enzymes produced by the pancreas and the intestinal lining. Pancreatic enzymes empty into the duodenum through the ampulla of Vater. These enzymes include trypsin, which digests protein to amino acids; lipase, which digests protein to amino acids and triglycerides (fat) to fatty acids and glycerol; and amylase, which digests starches to sugars. Intestinal enzymes include peptidases, which convert protein to amino acids; lactase, maltase, and sucrase, which digest complex sugars like glucose, fructose, and galactose; and enterokinase, which activates trypsin.

Bile also participates in digestion and absorption. After formation in the liver, bile is stored and concentrated in the gall-

SPECIALIZED TESTS IN GASTROENTEROLOGY

Test	Procedure	Clinical objectives
Endoscopy (direct visualization of the lining of a hollow viscus using an endoscope)	A cablelike cluster of glass fibers within the endoscope transmits light into the viscus, then returns an image to the scope's optical head.	■ To diagnose inflammatory, ulcerative, and infectious diseases; benign and malignant tumors; and other lesions of the esophageal, gastric, and intestinal mucosa
Radiography (passage of X-ray beams through the patient to create a radiograph)	X-ray films depict body structures and air in shades of gray, which reflect their density: Air appears black, fat appears dark gray, soft tissue appears light gray, and bone appears white. Use of contrast media accentuates density.	■ To detect obstructions, strictures, and deviations in the biliary tract ■ To detect inflammatory disease, tumors, ulcers, and other lesions ■ To diagnose hiatal hernia and other structural changes in the GI tract
Cineradiography (rapid-sequence X-ray examination that films motion)	Replay of cineradiography at slow speeds allows close observation of vascular perfusion and muscular contraction.	■ To detect vascular abnormalities by recording the stages of perfusion ■ To evaluate the condition of the pharynx by recording its muscular contraction
Fluoroscopy (projection of X-ray films into a fluoroscope, or specialized screen, to permit continuous observation of motion)	Spot films record significant findings.	■ To detect obstructions, strictures, and deviations in the biliary tract ■ To detect inflammatory disease, tumors, ulcers, and other lesions ■ To diagnose hiatal hernia and other structural changes in the GI tract ■ To check catheter placement in angiography by observing small injections of dye
Nuclear medicine imaging (use of a gamma camera or rectilinear scanner)	Distribution of a decaying radiopharmaceutical is recorded after I.V. injection.	■ To screen for hepatocellular disease and for focal disease in the liver and spleen ■ To detect hepatomegaly and splenomegaly ■ To diagnose liver or spleen hematoma after abdominal trauma ■ To detect the site of GI bleeding ■ To evaluate acute cholecystitis

SPECIALIZED TESTS IN GASTROENTEROLOGY *(continued)*

Test	Procedure	Clinical objectives
Ultrasonography (focused beam of high-frequency sound waves)	Sound waves pass through the patient, creating echoes that vary with tissue density. These echoes are converted into electrical energy and amplified by a transducer, and then they appear on an oscilloscope screen in shades of gray as spokes or dots.	■ To detect splenomegaly ■ To differentiate between tumors, cysts, and abscesses in the liver ■ To diagnose liver or spleen hematoma after abdominal trauma ■ To differentiate between obstructive and nonobstructive jaundice ■ To diagnose cholelithiasis
Computed tomography scan (multiple X-ray beams pass through the patient, detectors record tissue attenuation, and a computer then reconstructs this information as a three-dimensional image on an oscilloscope screen)	Attenuation varies with tissue density and appears in shades of gray on the oscilloscope screen. The use of contrast media accentuates density.	■ To differentiate between tumors, cysts, and abscesses in the liver, spleen, and pancreas ■ To detect liver metastasis ■ To diagnose liver or spleen hematoma after abdominal trauma ■ To evaluate, diagnose, or confirm pancreatitis ■ To distinguish obstructive from nonobstructive jaundice ■ To evaluate retroperitoneal disease

bladder. It's released in response to cholecystokinin, a hormone secreted by the duodenum, and is then emptied into the duodenum through the ampulla of Vater. Bile helps neutralize stomach acid and promotes the emulsification of fats and the absorption of the fat-soluble vitamins A, D, E, and K.

When food reaches the ileocecal valve and enters the large intestine (3 to 10 hours after ingestion), all its nutritional value has been absorbed. The first half of the large intestine absorbs water, sodium, and chloride, reducing bulk; the second half stores and further dehydrates the digestive material until defecation. The second half of the large intestine may also excrete water, potassium, and bicarbonate.

Bacterial action in the colon putrefies undigested foods; synthesizes vitamins K, B_{12}, B_2, (riboflavin), and B_1 (thiamine); and produces gas, which helps propel stool toward the anus. Intestinal gas may also result from swallowed air or diffusion of blood gases. Rectal distention by stool stimulates the defecation reflex, which is assisted by voluntary sphincter relaxation. The passage of stool through the large intestine normally takes 24 to 40 hours.

Analysis of esophageal, gastric, and peritoneal contents

Examination of esophageal and gastric contents reveals the secretory function of the mucosa in each organ; excessive or deficient mucosal secretions or the presence of blood commonly aids in diagnosis. Peritoneal fluid analysis provides a broader assessment of abdominal integrity because this fluid lubricates all organs within the peritoneum.

Esophageal contents consist entirely of mucus, whereas gastric contents (after a 12-hour fast) include water, hydrochloric acid, mucus, electrolytes, and pepsin. The fasting interval normally clears food particles from the stomach into the duodenum, but a small amount of food residue may be present.

Gastric contents may vary as well. For example, if excessive gagging accompanies nasogastric (NG) intubation, gastric juice may contain bile that gives it a lemon yellow to cloudy green color. It may contain mucus arising from stomach glandular secretions or from swallowed saliva and nasorespiratory secretions. Although gastric contents may normally contain flecks or streaks of bright red blood after minor trauma during intubation, a large amount of blood is abnormal. Partially digested blood appears as dark, coffee-colored particles and indicates chronic bleeding, as from ulceration or carcinoma.

Peritoneal fluid, normally clear and pale yellow, is removed from the abdominal cavity by paracentesis (needle aspiration). Less than 50 ml of this fluid normally lubricates the peritoneal surfaces; an excessive volume indicates disease.

Nasogastric intubation

Aspiration of gastric contents through an NG tube can help diagnose GI disorders by evaluating the secretory activity of the gastric mucosa and the efficiency of gastric emptying into the duodenum. Although intubation is somewhat unpleasant for the patient, it can be accomplished quickly, safely, and with minimal discomfort. Diagnostic intubation is contraindicated in the pregnant patient and in the patient with an aortic aneurysm, myocardial infarction, diverticula, esophageal varices, or head trauma; however, it may be performed cautiously in an emergency situation.

Fecal analysis

The GI tract processes about 10 qt (10 L) of chyme daily, of which 100 to 300 g are eventually expelled as stool. Normal defecation patterns—influenced by food and fluid intake, medications, exercise, and rate of digestion—vary from two or three times daily to two or three times weekly. Fecal analysis can evaluate digestive efficiency and stomach and intestinal integrity.

Stool normally consist of 75% water and 25% solids, such as cellulose and other indigestible fiber, bacteria, unabsorbed minerals, fat and fat derivatives, desquamated epithelial cells, mucus, and small amounts of digestive enzymes and secretions. Fecal analysis begins with gross examination of color, consistency, odor, and other characteristics and concludes with microscopic, chemical, or bacterial analysis.

Stool is usually light to dark brown, soft, and slightly acidic. Its normal brown color stems from the metabolism of bile pigments to stercobilin, but may also be affected by diet, drugs, absorption efficiency, and bilirubin concentration. Fecal pH depends on dietary influences: Acidic pH results from a high carbohydrate intake; alkaline pH results from a high protein intake. Fecal odor results from the presence of indole and skatole, end products of protein catabolism.

Stool is usually about 1" (2.5 cm) in diameter and has the tubular shape of the colon, but it may be larger or smaller, depending on the condition of the colon. If the colon is partially obstructed or loses its elasticity, the passage of stool commonly traumatizes the colon and may cause bleeding; blood in the stool may also result from hemorrhoids. A black, tarry stool can result from bleeding high in the intestinal tract. A large, bulky, foul-smelling stool that floats in water may indicate malabsorption of fat (steatorrhea) or a large quantity of air or other gases in the stool.

Diarrhea results from too-rapid passage of food through the GI tract, usually spurred by viral infection. Mucus-containing stool can indicate colitis or a mucus-producing tumor. Pus, detected in microscopic analysis, can result from rectal abscess or ulcerative colitis.

Stool specimen collection

Collection of a stool specimen is typically required for diagnosis of infectious diseases, GI bleeding, and other GI tract disorders. Because stool specimens can't be obtained on demand, close cooperation between the health care provider and patient is necessary to secure a suitable specimen. Stool specimens may be collected randomly or for a specified period; for example, a random specimen is required for urobilinogen, and a 72-hour specimen is required for lipids. Three specimens are usually required to test for occult blood.

Before collecting a stool specimen, have ready a clean (preferably sterile), dry bedpan; a specimen container; and tongue blades. Then teach the patient how to collect a random or timed stool specimen. Tell him to notify you when he feels the urge to defecate.

To collect a random stool specimen, provide the patient with a bedpan and instruct him to avoid contaminating the stool with urine or toilet tissue, which would interfere with test results. Observe standard precautions when obtaining the specimen. Using a tongue blade, carefully transfer the stool from the bedpan to the specimen container. Then tightly secure the container lid. If the patient passes blood or mucus with the stool, be sure to include these with the specimen. Carefully label the container and send it to the laboratory immediately because a fresh specimen produces the most accurate results. If the specimen can't be transported immediately, make sure to follow your facility's laboratory guidelines regarding storage; for example, some stool specimens require refrigeration while others should be kept at room temperature.

To collect a timed stool specimen, consider the first stool passed by the patient as the start of the collection period. Prepare this specimen and all other stools passed during the collection period in the same manner as for a random stool specimen. As ordered, send each specimen to the laboratory immediately, or follow your facility's laboratory guidelines regarding storage and send them when collection is completed.

Endoscopy, radiography, and ultrasonography

Accurate diagnosis of GI tract, hepatic, biliary, and pancreatic disorders commonly requires more than one test. Such tests usually follow a logical order:

■ *Fecal occult bleeding test* generally detects GI bleeding.

■ *Barium studies* (upper GI and small-bowel series and barium enema) visualize GI structures. They may reveal inflammation or ulcers, tumors, strictures, or other lesions.

■ *Endoscopies* (esophagogastroduodenoscopy, colonoscopy, and proctosigmoidoscopy) directly visualize an abnormality, locate sources of bleeding and, if necessary, provide a channel for biopsy.

The selection of a diagnostic test or test battery may depend on your facility's resources. If they're available, noninvasive procedures, such as ultrasonography and CT scans, are preferred over invasive procedures — such as endoscopic retrograde cholangiopancreatography — in evaluating pancreatic disorders. Similarly, oral cholecystography and ultrasonography commonly replace percutaneous transhepatic cholangiography in evaluating gallbladder and biliary tract disorders.

Other useful tests

Breath hydrogen analysis, a simple method of detecting lactose intolerance, measures the hydrogen content of breath samples in the fasting state before and after lactose ingestion. Lactose, a disaccharide composed of glucose and galactose, normally breaks down in the small intestine and is then absorbed. When lactase, the enzyme that breaks down lactose, is deficient, lactose passes unabsorbed into the large intestine. Bacteria then ferment and split lactose, producing hydrogen and other gases that the lungs exhale, causing the patient to experience abdominal pain, cramping, and diarrhea.

To produce a sample for this test, the patient exhales into an anesthesia balloon. The hydrogen content of the sample is then determined by gas chromatography and a thermistor detector. Increased hydrogen content after lactose ingestion

indicates lactose intolerance. Despite this test's widespread use, experts disagree about its specificity and sensitivity. False-negative test results have been reported in the patient who takes antibiotics or suffers from severe diarrhea.

Another test for detecting lactose intolerance measures the level of glucose in blood samples that are drawn over a 2-hour period after the patient ingests a liquid containing lactose. An elevated glucose level implies normal findings.

The *HIDA scan* (technetium-labeled iminodiacetic acid, or ^{99m}Tc HIDA) is a simple nuclear medicine procedure for evaluating hepatobiliary function. Because the scan requires only a 2-hour fast, it permits quicker diagnosis than oral cholecystography, particularly in the patient with severe abdominal pain, suggesting acute gallbladder disease.

The injected radioisotope, HIDA, is taken up by the liver and excreted into the biliary tree. Serial imaging with a gamma camera then depicts radioactivity in the liver, bile ducts, gallbladder, and duodenum. Adequate visualization of the gallbladder requires normal gallbladder and liver function as well as biliary tree patency. Failure to visualize the gallbladder can result from hepatocellular disease, which impairs the uptake of HIDA, or from biliary obstruction, which prevents the release of HIDA into the gallbladder. Abnormally diminished radioactivity in the liver characterizes hepatocellular disease; absence of radioactivity in the gallbladder and duodenum suggests biliary obstruction.

The *saline-load test,* a rarely used test that measures gastric retention during fasting, requires aspiration of stomach contents before and after instillation of 750 ml of normal saline solution through an NG tube. The amount of saline solution remaining in the stomach after 30 minutes provides an index of intrinsic gastric motility. Excessive saline solution retention (more than 300 ml) may indicate gastric outlet obstruction stemming from edema, tumor, or stenosis.

The *secretin test* assesses pancreatic exocrine function. It involves insertion of a double-lumen oral tube into the duodenum and aspiration of gastric and duodenal contents before and after I.V. injection of secretin, an intestinal hormone that stimulates liver and pancreatic secretions. After such injection, an abnormal volume of secretions or of bicarbonate or enzymes may indicate pancreatic carcinoma, ductal obstruction, chronic pancreatitis, or advanced pancreatic insufficiency. The secretin test may also be combined with pancreozymin (also called cholecystokinin), a polypeptide hormone secreted by the mucosa of the upper intestine that stimulates gallbladder contraction and pancreatic enzyme secretion, to detect cystic fibrosis. The *secretin pancreozymin test* is performed by first injecting pancreozymin intravenously, and then injecting secretin intravenously.

MONITORING PH WITH THE BRAVO SYSTEM

Traditional testing for esophageal acid levels typically uses an esophageal catheter that's inserted for a 24-hour period. Recently, a new technique called the Bravo pH Monitoring System was developed to measure acid levels in the esophagus via a capsule (about the size of a gel cap). The capsule is temporarily attached to the patient's esophageal wall using an endoscope and collects pH data, which are transmitted to a pager-sized receiver that the patient wears. Data are collected for 48 hours, downloaded from the receiver, and analyzed with special software.

The Bravo method is more accurate than catheter methods because the patient can eat normally and maintain regular activities during testing. The additional 24 hours also provides more information for diagnosing certain esophageal disorders.

In 7 to 10 days, the capsule spontaneously detaches from the esophageal wall and is passed through the patient's digestive system.

ESOPHAGEAL, GASTRIC, AND PERITONEAL CONTENT TESTS

Esophageal acidity

The esophageal acidity test evaluates the competence of the lower esophageal sphincter — the major barrier to reflux — by measuring intraesophageal pH with an electrode attached to a manometric catheter.

Recently, a newer method for measuring esophageal pH, called the Bravo pH monitoring system, was developed. This method uses a small capsule to monitor a patient's pH levels. (See *Monitoring pH with the Bravo system.*)

Purpose

■ To evaluate the competence of the lower esophageal sphincter

Patient preparation

■ Explain to the patient that the esophageal acidity test evaluates the function of the sphincter between the esophagus and

the stomach. Tell him to fast and avoid smoking after midnight before the test.
- Describe the test, including who will perform it and where it will take place.
- Tell the patient that a tube will be passed through his mouth into his stomach and that he may experience slight discomfort, a desire to cough, or a gagging sensation.
- Just before the test, check the patient's pulse rate and blood pressure and instruct him to void.
- Withhold antacids, anticholinergics, cholinergics, beta-adrenergic blockers, alcohol, corticosteroids, cimetidine, and reserpine for 24 hours before the test. If they must be continued, note this on the laboratory request.
- Make sure that the patient or a responsible family member has signed an informed consent form.

Procedure and posttest care
- After the patient is placed in high Fowler's position, the catheter with the electrode is introduced into his mouth.
- The patient is instructed to swallow when the electrode reaches the back of his throat.
- Using a manometer, the examiner locates the lower esophageal sphincter. The catheter is raised ¾″ (1.9 cm). The patient is told to perform Valsalva's maneuver or lift his legs to stimulate reflux. After he does so, intraesophageal pH is measured.
- If the pH is normal, the catheter is passed into the patient's stomach. A prescribed acid solution (300 ml of 0.1 NaHCl) is instilled over 3 minutes (100 ml/minute). Then the catheter is raised ¾″ above the sphincter. Again, the patient is asked to perform Valsalva's maneuver or lift his legs, and intraesophageal pH is measured.

- Tell the patient that he may resume his usual diet and medications, as ordered.
- Provide lozenges if the patient complains of a sore throat.

Precautions
- During insertion, the catheter may enter the trachea instead of the esophagus. If the patient develops cyanosis or paroxysmal coughing, move the catheter immediately.
- Observe the patient closely during insertion because arrhythmias may develop.
- Clamp the catheter before removing it to prevent fluid aspiration into the lungs.

Reference values
The pH of the esophagus normally exceeds 5.

Abnormal findings
An intraesophageal pH of 1.5 to 2.0 indicates gastric acid reflux resulting from incompetence of the lower esophageal sphincter. Persistent reflux leads to chronic reflux esophagitis. Additional studies, such as barium swallow and esophagogastroduodenoscopy, are necessary to diagnose and determine the extent of esophagitis.

Interfering factors
- Failure to observe pretest restrictions
- Antacids, anticholinergics, histamine-2 blockers, and proton pump inhibitors (possible lowering of intraesophageal pH because of decrease in gastric secretions or acidity)
- Alcohol, cholinergics, reserpine, adrenergic blockers, and corticosteroids (possible elevation of intraesophageal pH because of reflux from a relaxed lower esophageal sphincter or an increase in gastric secretions)

Acid perfusion

Also called the *Bernstein test,* the acid per-fusion test helps to distinguish pain caused by esophagitis (burning epigastric or retrosternal pain that radiates to the back or arms) from pain caused by angina pectoris or other disorders. It requires perfusion of saline and acidic solutions into the esophagus through a nasogastric (NG) tube.

Purpose
■ To distinguish chest pain caused by esophagitis from chest pain caused by cardiac disorders

Patient preparation
■ Tell the patient that the acid perfusion test helps determine the cause of heartburn.
■ Explain the following restrictions to the patient: no antacids for 24 hours before the test, no food for 12 hours before the test, and no fluids or smoking for 8 hours before the test.
■ Describe the test, including who will perform it, where it will take place, and how long it will last.
■ Explain to the patient that the test involves passing a tube through his nose into the esophagus and that he may experience some discomfort, a desire to cough, or a gagging sensation during tube passage.
■ Tell the patient that liquid is slowly perfused through the tube into the esophagus and that he should immediately report pain or burning during perfusion.
■ Just before the test, check the patient's pulse rate and blood pressure. Ask him whether he's experiencing any heartburn and, if so, to describe it.
■ Make sure that the patient or a responsible family member has signed an informed consent form.

Procedure and posttest care
■ After the patient is seated, insert an NG tube that has been marked 12″ (30.5 cm) from the tip into his stomach. Attach a 20-ml syringe to the tube and aspirate stomach contents. Withdraw the tube into the esophagus (to the 12″ mark).
■ Hang labeled containers of normal saline solution and a prescribed acidic solution (0.1 NaHCl) on an I.V. pole behind the patient, and then connect the NG tube to the I.V. tubing.
■ Open the line from the normal saline solution and infuse it at a rate of 60 to 120 drops/minute. Continue perfusion for 5 to 10 minutes.
■ Ask the patient whether he's experiencing any discomfort and record his response.
■ Without the patient's knowledge, close the line from the normal saline solution and open the line from the acidic solution. Infuse the acidic solution into the esophagus at the same rate used for the saline solution. Continue perfusion for 30 minutes.
■ Ask the patient again whether he's experiencing discomfort and record his response.
■ If the patient experiences discomfort, close the line from the acidic solution immediately and open the line from the normal saline solution. Continue to perfuse this solution until the discomfort subsides.
■ If ordered, repeat perfusion of the acidic solution to verify the patient's response. If this isn't required or if the patient experiences no discomfort after perfusion of the acidic solution for 30 minutes, stop the solution and withdraw the NG tube.
■ If the patient complains of pain or burning, administer an antacid, as ordered. If he complains of a sore throat,

provide soothing lozenges or obtain an order for an ice collar.

■ Instruct the patient that he may resume his usual diet and medications, as ordered.

Precautions

■ The acid perfusion test is contraindicated in the patient with esophageal varices, heart failure, acute myocardial infarction, or other cardiac disorders.

■ During intubation, make sure that the tube enters the esophagus and not the trachea. Withdraw the tube immediately if the patient develops cyanosis or paroxysmal coughing.

■ Assess the patient's pulse rate and rhythm to detect arrhythmias that may develop.

■ Clamp the tube before removing it to prevent fluid aspiration into the lungs.

Normal findings

Absence of pain or burning during perfusion of either solution indicates a healthy esophageal mucosa.

Abnormal findings

In the patient with esophagitis, the acidic solution causes pain or burning, and the normal saline solution should produce no adverse effects. Occasionally, both solutions cause pain in the patient with esophagitis, but they may not cause pain in the patient with asymptomatic esophagitis.

Interfering factors

■ Failure to observe pretest restrictions
■ Beta-adrenergic blockers, anticholinergics, reserpine, corticosteroids, histamine-2 blockers, and acid pump inhibitors

Basal gastric secretion

The basal gastric secretion test measures basal secretion during fasting by aspirating stomach contents through a nasogastric (NG) tube. It's indicated in the patient with obscure epigastric pain, anorexia, and weight loss. Because external factors — such as the sight or odor of food — and psychological stress stimulate gastric secretion, accurate testing requires that the patient be relaxed and isolated from all sources of sensory stimulation. Although abnormal basal secretion test results can suggest various gastric and duodenal disorders, a complete evaluation of secretions requires the gastric acid stimulation test.

Purpose

■ To determine gastric output while the patient is fasting

Patient preparation

■ Explain to the patient that the basal gastric secretion test measures the stomach's secretion of acid.

■ Instruct the patient to restrict food for 12 hours and fluids and smoking for 8 hours before the test.

■ Tell the patient who will perform the test and that the procedure takes approximately 1¼ hours (or 2¼ hours, if followed by the gastric acid stimulation test).

■ Inform the patient that the test requires insertion of a tube through the nose and into the stomach, that he may initially experience discomfort, and that he may cough or gag.

■ Notify the laboratory and physician of medications the patient is taking that may affect test results; they may need to be restricted. If these drugs must be continued, note this on the laboratory request.

- Check the patient's pulse rate and blood pressure just before the test. Then encourage him to relax.

Procedure and posttest care

- Insert the NG tube after seating the patient comfortably.
- Attach a 20-ml syringe to it and aspirate the stomach contents.
- To ensure complete emptying of the stomach, ask the patient to assume three positions in sequence—supine and right and left lateral decubitus—while stomach contents are aspirated.
- Label the specimen container RESIDUAL CONTENTS.
- Connect the NG tube to the suction machine. Aspirate gastric contents by continuous low suction for 1 hour. Aspiration can also be performed manually with a syringe.
- Collect a specimen every 15 minutes, but discard the first two; this eliminates the specimens that could be affected by the stress of the intubation.
- Record the color and odor of each specimen and note the presence of food, mucus, bile, or blood.
- Label these specimens BASAL CONTENTS, and number them 1 through 4.
- Next, measure secretion volume and acid concentration.
- If the NG tube is to be left in place, clamp it or attach it to low intermittent suction, as ordered.
- Watch for complications, such as nausea, vomiting, and abdominal distention or pain, following removal of the NG tube.
- If the patient complains of a sore throat, provide soothing lozenges.
- Instruct the patient that he may resume his usual diet and medications, as ordered, unless the gastric acid stimulation test will also be performed.

Precautions

- The basal gastric secretion test is contraindicated in the patient with a condition that prohibits NG intubation.
- During insertion, make sure that the NG tube enters the esophagus and not the trachea; remove it immediately if the patient develops cyanosis or paroxysmal coughing.
- Monitor the patient's vital signs during intubation and observe him carefully for arrhythmias.
- To prevent contamination of the specimens with saliva, instruct the patient to expectorate excess saliva.
- Send the specimens to the laboratory immediately after the collection is completed.

Reference values

Normally, basal secretion ranges from 1 to 5 mEq/hour in males and from 0.2 to 3.3 mEq/hour in females.

Abnormal findings

Abnormal basal secretion findings are nonspecific and must be considered with the results of the gastric acid stimulation test. Elevated secretion may suggest a duodenal or jejunal ulcer (after partial gastrectomy); markedly elevated secretion suggests Zollinger-Ellison syndrome. Depressed secretion may indicate gastric carcinoma or a benign gastric ulcer. Absence of secretion may indicate pernicious anemia.

Interfering factors

- Failure to observe pretest restrictions (increase)
- Psychological stress (possible increase)

- Cholinergics, reserpine, alcohol, adrenergic blockers, and adrenocorticosteroids (possible increase)
- Antacids, anticholinergics, histamine-2 blockers, and proton pump inhibitors (possible decrease)

Gastric acid stimulation

The gastric acid stimulation test measures the secretion of gastric acid for 1 hour after subcutaneous (S.C.) injection of pentagastrin or a similar drug that stimulates gastric acid output. This test is indicated when the basal secretion test suggests abnormal gastric secretion and is commonly performed immediately afterward. Although this test detects abnormal gastric secretion, radiographic studies and endoscopy are necessary to determine the cause.

Purpose

- To aid in the diagnosis of a duodenal ulcer, Zollinger-Ellison syndrome, pernicious anemia, and gastric carcinoma

Patient preparation

- Explain to the patient that the gastric acid stimulation test determines if the stomach is secreting acid properly.
- Instruct the patient to refrain from eating, drinking, and smoking after midnight before the test.
- Tell the patient who will perform the test, where it will take place, and that it takes 1 hour.
- Explain that the test requires passing a tube through the nose and into the stomach and an S.C. injection of pentagastrin.
- Describe the possible adverse effects of the test, such as abdominal pain, nausea, vomiting, flushing, and transitory dizziness, faintness, and numbness in the extremities. Instruct the patient to report such symptoms immediately.
- Check the patient's history for hypersensitivity to pentagastrin.
- Notify the laboratory and the physician of medications the patient is taking that may affect test results; they may need to be restricted. If these drugs must be continued, however, note this on the laboratory request.
- Record the patient's baseline vital signs before beginning the procedure.

Procedure and posttest care

- After basal gastric secretions have been collected, the nasogastric (NG) tube remains in place.
- Pentagastrin is injected S.C.; after 15 minutes, collect a specimen every 15 minutes for 1 hour.
- Record the color and odor of each specimen and note the presence of food, mucus, bile, or blood.
- Label the specimens STIMULATED CONTENTS, and number them 1 through 4.
- If the NG tube is kept in place, it should be clamped or attached to low intermittent suction, as ordered.
- Watch the patient for nausea, vomiting, and abdominal distention and pain after the NG tube is removed.
- If the patient complains of a sore throat, provide soothing lozenges.
- Instruct the patient that he may resume his usual diet and medications, as ordered.

Precautions

- The gastric acid stimulation test is contraindicated in the patient with hypersensitivity to pentagastrin or with conditions that prohibit NG intubation.
- Observe the patient for adverse effects of pentagastrin.

- To prevent contamination of the specimens with saliva, instruct the patient to expectorate excess saliva.
- Send the specimens to the laboratory immediately after the collection is completed.

Reference values

Following stimulation, gastric acid secretion ranges from 18 to 28 mEq/hour for males and from 11 to 21 mEq/hour for females.

Abnormal findings

Elevated gastric secretion may indicate a duodenal ulcer; markedly elevated secretion suggests Zollinger-Ellison syndrome. Depressed secretion may indicate gastric carcinoma; achlorhydria may indicate pernicious anemia.

Interfering factors

- Failure to observe pretest restrictions
- Cholinergics, adrenergic blockers, and reserpine (increase)
- Antacids, anticholinergics, histamine-2 blockers, and proton pump inhibitors (decrease)

Peritoneal fluid analysis

Peritoneal fluid analysis assesses a specimen of peritoneal fluid obtained by paracentesis. This procedure requires inserting a trocar and cannula through the abdominal wall while the patient receives a local anesthetic. If the fluid specimen is removed for therapeutic purposes, the trocar may be connected to a drainage system. However, if only a small amount of fluid is removed for diagnostic purposes, an 18G needle may be used in place of the trocar and cannula. In a four-quadrant tap, fluid is aspirated from each quadrant of the abdomen to verify abdo-

minal trauma and confirm the need for surgery.

Purpose

- To determine the cause of ascites
- To detect abdominal trauma

Patient preparation

- Explain to the patient that peritoneal fluid analysis helps determine the cause of ascites or detects abdominal trauma.
- Inform the patient that he need not restrict food and fluids.
- Tell the patient that the test requires a peritoneal fluid specimen, that he'll receive a local anesthetic to minimize discomfort, and that the procedure takes about 45 minutes to perform.
- Provide psychological support to decrease the patient's anxiety and assure him that complications are rare.
- If the patient has severe ascites, inform him that the procedure will relieve his discomfort and allow him to breathe more easily.
- Make sure that the patient or a responsible family member has signed an informed consent form.
- Record the patient's baseline vital signs, weight, and abdominal girth.
- Tell the patient that a blood sample may be taken for analysis.
- Tell the patient to void just before the test. This helps to prevent accidental bladder injury during needle insertion.
- X-rays may be performed before peritoneal analysis to ensure reliability.

Procedure and posttest care

- Have the patient sit on a bed or in a chair with his feet flat on the floor and his back well-supported. If he can't tolerate being out of bed, place him in high Fowler's position and make him as comfortable as possible.

- Except for the puncture site, keep the patient covered to prevent chilling.
- Provide a plastic sheet or absorbent pad to collect spillage and to protect the patient and bed linens.
- The puncture site is shaved, the skin prepared, and the area draped.
- The local anesthetic is injected.
- The examiner inserts the needle or trocar and cannula 1″ to 2″ (2.5 to 5 cm) below the umbilicus. (However, it may also be inserted through the flank, the iliac fossa, the border of the rectus, or at each quadrant of the abdomen.)
- If a trocar and cannula are used, a small incision is made to facilitate insertion. When the needle pierces the peritoneum, it "gives" with an audible sound. The trocar is removed and a sample of fluid is aspirated with a 50-ml luer-lock syringe.
- If additional fluid is to be drained, assist in attaching one end of an I.V. tube to the cannula and the other end to a collection bag. The fluid is then aspirated (no more than 1,500 ml). If aspirating is difficult, reposition the patient, as ordered.
- After aspiration, the trocar needle is removed and a pressure dressing is applied. Occasionally, the wound may be sutured first.
- Label the specimens in the order they were drawn. If the patient has received antibiotic therapy, note this on the laboratory request.
- Carefully and properly dispose of needles and contaminated articles according to the Centers for Disease Control and Prevention guidelines; incinerate disposable items and return reusable ones to the central supply area.
- Apply a gauze dressing to the puncture site. Make sure it's thick enough to absorb all drainage. Check the dressing frequently (for example, whenever you check vital signs) and reinforce or apply a pressure dressing, if needed.
- Monitor the patient's vital signs until they're stable. If his recovery is poor, check his vital signs every 15 minutes. Weigh him and measure his abdominal girth; compare these with his baseline values.
- Allow the patient to rest and, if possible, withhold treatment or procedures that may cause undue stress such as linen changes.
- Monitor the patient's urine output for at least 24 hours, and watch for hematuria, which may indicate bladder trauma.

► **CLINICAL ALERT** *Watch the patient for signs of hemorrhage or shock and for increasing pain or abdominal tenderness. These may indicate a perforated intestine or, depending on the site of the tap, puncture of the inferior epigastric artery, hematoma of the anterior cecal wall, or rupture of the iliac vein or bladder.*

- If a large amount of fluid was aspirated, watch the patient for signs of vascular collapse (color change, elevated pulse and respiratory rates, decreased blood pressure and central venous pressure, mental changes, and dizziness). Administer fluids orally if the patient is alert and can accept them.

► **CLINICAL ALERT** *Observe the patient with severe hepatic disease for signs of hepatic coma, which may result from sodium and potassium loss accompanying hypovolemia. Watch him for mental changes, drowsiness, and stupor. Such a patient is also prone to uremia, infection, hemorrhage, and protein depletion.*

- As ordered, administer I.V. infusions and albumin. Check the laboratory report for electrolyte (especially sodium) and serum protein levels.

NORMAL FINDINGS IN PERITONEAL FLUID ANALYSIS

Use the below chart to determine the normal findings in peritoneal fluid.

Element	Normal value or finding
Gross appearance	Sterile, odorless, clear to pale yellow color; scant amount (< 50 ml)
Red blood cells	None
White blood cells	< 300/µl (SI, < 300 x 10⁹/L)
Protein	0.3 to 4.1 g/dl (SI, 3 to 41 g/L)
Glucose	70 to 100 mg/dl (SI, 3.5 to 5 mmol/L)
Amylase	138 to 404 U/L (SI, 138 to 404 U/L)
Ammonia	< 50 µg/dl (SI, < 29 µmol/L)
Alkaline phosphatase	Males > age 18: 90 to 239 U/L (SI, 90 to 239 U/L) Females < age 45: 76 to 196 U/L (SI, 76 to 196 U/L) Females > age 45: 87 to 250 U/L (SI, 87 to 250 U/L)
Cytology	No malignant cells present
Bacteria	None
Fungi	None

Precautions

■ Peritoneal fluid analysis should be performed cautiously in a pregnant patient and in the patient with bleeding tendencies or unstable vital signs.

■ Check the patient's vital signs every 15 minutes during the procedure. Watch for deviations from baseline findings. Observe for dizziness, pallor, perspiration, and increased anxiety.

■ If rapid fluid aspiration induces hypovolemia and shock, reduce the vertical distance between the trocar and the collection bag to slow the drainage rate. If necessary, stop the drainage by turning off the stopcock or clamping the tubing.

■ Avoid contamination of the specimens, which alters their bacterial content. Send them to the laboratory immediately after collection.

Reference values

For normal peritoneal fluid values, see *Normal findings in peritoneal fluid analysis*.

Abnormal findings

Milk-colored peritoneal fluid may result from chyle or lymph fluid escaping from a thoracic duct that's damaged or blocked by a malignant tumor, lymphoma, tuberculosis, parasitic infestation, adhesion, or hepatic cirrhosis; a pseudochylous condition may result from the presence of leukocytes or tumor cells. Differential diagnosis of true chylous ascites depends on the presence of elevated triglyceride levels

($\geq$400 mg/dl [SI, $\geq$4.36 mmol/L]) and microscopic fat globules.

Cloudy or turbid fluid may indicate peritonitis due to primary bacterial infection, a ruptured bowel (after trauma), pancreatitis, a strangulated or an infarcted intestine, or an appendicitis. Bloody fluid may result from a benign or malignant tumor, hemorrhagic pancreatitis, or a traumatic tap; however, if the fluid fails to clear on continued aspiration, a traumatic tap isn't the cause. Bile-stained green fluid may indicate a ruptured gallbladder, acute pancreatitis, or a perforated intestine or duodenal ulcer.

A red blood cell count over 100/μl (SI, > 100/L) indicates neoplasm or tuberculosis; a count over 100,000/μl (SI, >100,000/L) indicates intra-abdominal trauma. An elevated white blood cell count with more than 25% neutrophils occurs in 90% of patients with spontaneous bacterial peritonitis and in 50% of those with cirrhosis. A high percentage of lymphocytes suggests tuberculous peritonitis or chylous ascites. Numerous mesothelial cells indicate tuberculous peritonitis.

Protein levels rise above 3 g/dl in malignancy (SI, > 3 g/L) and above 4 g/dl (SI, > 4 g/L) in tuberculosis. Peritoneal fluid glucose levels fall in the patient with tuberculous peritonitis or peritoneal carcinomatosis.

Amylase levels rise with pancreatic trauma, pancreatic pseudocyst, or acute pancreatitis and may also rise in intestinal necrosis or strangulation.

Peritoneal alkaline phosphatase levels rise to more than twice the normal serum levels in the patient with ruptured or strangulated small intestines. Peritoneal ammonia levels also exceed twice the normal serum levels in ruptured or strangu-lated large and small intestines and in a ruptured ulcer or an appendix.

A protein ascitic fluid to serum ratio of 0.5 or greater may suggest a malignancy or tuberculous or pancreatic ascites. The presence of this finding indicates a non-hepatic cause; its absence suggests uncomplicated hepatic disease. An albumin gradient between ascitic fluid and serum greater than 1 g/dl (SI, > 1 g/L) indicates chronic hepatic disease; a lesser value suggests malignancy.

Cytologic examination of peritoneal fluid accurately detects malignant cells. Microbiological examination can reveal coliforms, anaerobes, and enterococci, which can enter the peritoneum from a ruptured organ or from infections accompanying appendicitis, pancreatitis, tuberculosis, or ovarian disease. Gram-positive cocci commonly indicate primary peritonitis; gram-negative organisms, secondary peritonitis. The presence of fungi may indicate histoplasmosis, candidiasis, or coccidioidomycosis.

Interfering factors

■ Unsterile collection technique or failure to send the specimen to the laboratory immediately after collection
■ Contamination of the specimen with blood, bile, urine, or stool due to injury to underlying structures during paracentesis

FECAL CONTENT TESTS

Fecal occult blood

Fecal occult blood is detected by microscopic analysis or by chemical tests for hemoglobin, such as the guaiac test.

Normally, stool contains small amounts of blood (2 to 2.5 ml/day); therefore, tests for occult blood detect quantities larger than this. Testing is indicated when clinical symptoms and preliminary blood studies suggest GI bleeding. Additional tests are required to pinpoint the origin of the bleeding. (See *Common sites and causes of GI blood loss,* page 760.)

Purpose
- To detect GI bleeding
- To aid in the early diagnosis of colorectal cancer

Patient preparation
- Explain to the patient that the fecal occult blood test helps detect abnormal GI bleeding.

- Instruct the patient to maintain a high-fiber diet and to refrain from eating red meats, turnips, and horseradish for 48 to 72 hours before the test as well as throughout the collection period.

- Tell the patient that the test requires the collection of three stool specimens. Occasionally, only a random specimen is collected.

- Notify the laboratory and physician of medications the patient is taking that may affect test results; they may need to be restricted. If these drugs must be continued, note this on the laboratory request.

Procedure and posttest care
- Collect three stool specimens or a random stool specimen, as ordered. Obtain specimens from two different areas of each stool. Testing may take place in the laboratory or in a utility room on the nursing unit, depending on the facility's policy. Two of the most commonly used screening tests are Hematest and Hemoccult. Hematest uses orthotoluidine to de-

tect hemoglobin, and Hemoccult uses guaiac.

- After any of the tests described here are performed, tell the patient that he may resume his usual diet and medications.

Hematest reagent tablet test
- Use a wooden applicator to smear a bit of the stool specimen on the filter paper supplied with the kit. Alternatively, after performing a digital rectal examination, wipe the finger you used for the examination on a square of the filter paper. Place the filter paper with the stool smear on a glass plate.

- Remove a reagent tablet from the bottle, and immediately replace the cap tightly. Place the tablet in the center of the stool smear on the filter paper. Add one drop of water to the tablet, and allow it to soak in for 5 to 10 seconds. Add a second drop, letting it run from the tablet onto the specimen and filter paper. If necessary, tap the plate gently to dislodge any water from the top of the tablet.

- After 2 minutes, the filter paper will turn blue if the test is positive. Don't read the color that appears on the tablet itself or develops on the filter paper after the 2-minute period. Note the results and discard the filter paper. Remove and discard your gloves and wash your hands thoroughly.

Hemoccult slide test
- Open the flap on the slide pack and use a wooden applicator to apply a thin smear of the stool specimen to the guaiac-impregnated filter paper exposed in box A. Alternatively, after performing a digital rectal examination, wipe the finger you used for the examination on a square of filter paper. Apply a second smear from another part of the specimen to the filter paper exposed in box B because some

COMMON SITES AND CAUSES OF GI BLOOD LOSS

Illustrated here are potential areas that can cause blood loss, resulting in positive fecal occult blood testing. Further clinical assessment and testing is necessary to determine the area involved.

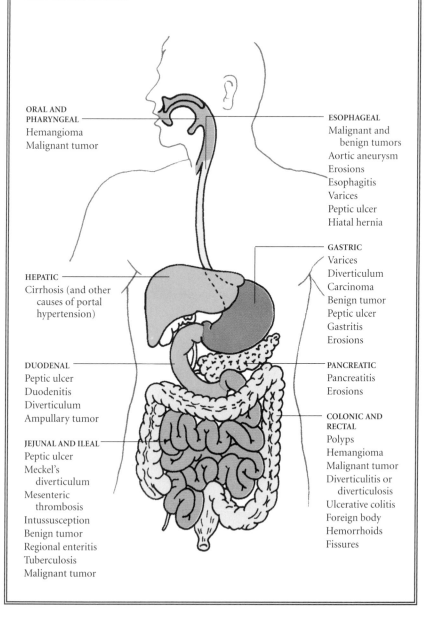

ORAL AND PHARYNGEAL
Hemangioma
Malignant tumor

ESOPHAGEAL
Malignant and
  benign tumors
Aortic aneurysm
Erosions
Esophagitis
Varices
Peptic ulcer
Hiatal hernia

HEPATIC
Cirrhosis (and other
  causes of portal
  hypertension)

GASTRIC
Varices
Diverticulum
Carcinoma
Benign tumor
Peptic ulcer
Gastritis
Erosions

DUODENAL
Peptic ulcer
Duodenitis
Diverticulum
Ampullary tumor

PANCREATIC
Pancreatitis
Erosions

JEJUNAL AND ILEAL
Peptic ulcer
Meckel's
  diverticulum
Mesenteric
  thrombosis
Intussusception
Benign tumor
Regional enteritis
Tuberculosis
Malignant tumor

COLONIC AND RECTAL
Polyps
Hemangioma
Malignant tumor
Diverticulitis or
  diverticulosis
Ulcerative colitis
Foreign body
Hemorrhoids
Fissures

parts of the specimen may not contain blood.

- Allow the specimen to dry for 3 to 5 minutes. Open the flap at the rear of the slide package and place 2 drops of Hemoccult developing solution on the paper over each smear. A blue reaction will appear in 30 to 60 seconds if the test is positive. Record the results and discard the slide package. Remove and discard your gloves and wash your hands thoroughly.

Instant-View fecal occult blood test
- Add a stool sample to the collection tube. Shake it to mix the sample with the extraction buffer, and then dispense 4 drops into the sample well of the cassette. Results will appear on the test region and the control region of the cassette in 5 to 10 minutes, indicating whether the level of hemoglobin is greater than 0.05 µg/ml of stool. Results will also indicate if the device is performing properly.

Precautions
- Instruct the patient to avoid contaminating the stool specimen with toilet tissue or urine.
- Send the specimen to the laboratory or perform the test immediately.

Normal findings
Less than 2.5 ml of blood should be present in stool, resulting in a green reaction.

Abnormal findings
A positive test indicates GI bleeding, which may result from many disorders, such as varices, a peptic ulcer, carcinoma, ulcerative colitis, dysentery, or hemorrhagic disease. This test is particularly important for the early diagnosis of colorectal cancer. Further tests, such as barium swallow, analyses of gastric contents, and

endoscopic procedures, are necessary to define the site and extent of bleeding.

Interfering factors
- Failure to observe pretest restrictions
- Failure to test the specimen immediately or to send it to the laboratory immediately after collection
- Iron preparations, bromides, rauwolfia derivatives, indomethacin, colchicine, phenylbutazone, and steroids (possible increase due to association with GI blood loss)
- Ascorbic acid (false-normal, even with significant bleeding)
- Ingestion of 2 to 5 ml of blood such as from bleeding gums
- Active bleeding from hemorrhoids (possible false-positive results)

Fecal lipids

Lipids excreted in stool include monoglycerides, diglycerides, triglycerides, phospholipids, glycolipids, soaps (fatty acids and fatty acid salts), sterols, and cholesterol esters. When biliary and pancreatic secretions are adequate, emulsified dietary lipids are almost completely absorbed in the small intestine.

Excessive excretion of fecal lipids (steatorrhea) occurs in several malabsorption syndromes. Qualitative and quantitative tests are used to detect excessive excretion of lipids in patients exhibiting signs of malabsorption, such as weight loss, abdominal distention, and scaly skin.

The qualitative test involves staining a specimen of stool with Sudan III dye and then examining it microscopically for evidence of malabsorption, such as undigested muscle fibers and various fats. The quantitative test involves drying and weighing a 72-hour specimen and then using a solvent to extract the lipids, which are subsequently evaporated and weighed. Only the quantitative test confirms steatorrhea.

Purpose
■ To confirm steatorrhea

Patient preparation
■ Explain to the patient that the fecal lipid test evaluates fat digestion.

■ Instruct the patient to abstain from alcohol and to maintain a high-fat diet (100 g/day) for 3 days before the test and during the collection period.

■ Tell the patient that the test requires a 72-hour stool collection.

■ Notify the laboratory and physician of medications the patient is taking that may affect test results; they may need to be restricted.

■ Teach the patient how to collect a timed stool specimen and provide him with the necessary equipment.

■ Inform the patient that the laboratory requires 1 or 2 days to complete the analysis.

Procedure and posttest care
■ Collect a 72-hour stool specimen.

■ Instruct the patient that he may resume his usual diet and medications.

Precautions
■ Don't use a waxed collection container because the wax may become incorporated in the stool and interfere with accurate testing.

■ Tell the patient to avoid contaminating the stool specimen with toilet tissue or urine.

■ Refrigerate the collection container and keep it tightly covered.

Normal findings
Fecal lipids normally comprise less than 20% of excreted solids, with excretion more than 7 g/24 hours.

Abnormal findings
Digestive and absorptive disorders cause steatorrhea. Digestive disorders may affect the production and release of pancreatic lipase or bile; absorptive disorders may affect the intestine's integrity.

In pancreatic insufficiency, impaired lipid digestion may result from insufficient lipase production. Pancreatic resection, cystic fibrosis, chronic pancreatitis, or ductal obstruction by stone or tumor may prevent the normal release or action of lipase.

In impaired hepatic function, faulty lipid digestion may result from inadequate bile salt production. Biliary obstruction, which may accompany gallbladder disease, may prevent the normal release of bile salts into the duodenum.

Extensive small-bowel resection or bypass may also interrupt normal enterohepatic bile salt circulation.

Diseases of the intestinal mucosa affect the normal absorption of lipids. Regional ileitis and atrophy due to malnutrition cause gross structural changes in the intestinal wall; celiac disease and tropical sprue produce mucosal abnormalities.

Scleroderma, radiation enteritis, fistulas, intestinal tuberculosis, small intestine diverticula, and altered intestinal flora may also cause steatorrhea.

Whipple's disease and lymphomas cause lymphatic obstruction that may inhibit fat absorption.

Interfering factors
■ Failure to observe pretest restrictions or the use of a waxed collection container

■ A contaminated or incomplete stool specimen (total weight < 300 g)

■ Azathioprine, bisacodyl, cholestyramine, kanamycin, neomycin, colchicine, aluminum hydroxide, calcium carbonate, alcohol, potassium chloride, and mineral oil (possible increase or decrease due to inhibited absorption or altered chemical digestion)

Fecal urobilinogen

Urobilinogen, the end product of bilirubin metabolism, is a brown pigment formed by bacterial enzymes in the small intestine. It's excreted in stool or reabsorbed into portal blood, where it's returned to the liver and excreted in bile. A small amount is excreted in urine. Proper bilirubin metabolism depends on normal hepatobiliary system functioning and a normal erythrocyte life span.

Although measuring fecal urobilinogen is a useful indicator of hepatobiliary and hemolytic disorders, the test is rarely performed because it's easier to measure serum bilirubin and urine urobilinogen.

Purpose

■ To aid in the diagnosis of hepatobiliary and hemolytic disorders

Patient preparation

■ Explain to the patient that the fecal urobilinogen test evaluates liver and bile duct function or detects red blood cell disorders.

■ Inform the patient that he need not restrict food and fluids.

■ Tell the patient that the test requires collection of a random stool specimen.

■ Notify the laboratory and physician of medications the patient is taking that may affect test results; they may need to be restricted.

Procedure and posttest care

■ Collect a random stool specimen.

■ Tell the patient that he may resume his usual medications.

Precautions

■ Tell the patient not to contaminate the stool specimen with toilet tissue or urine.

■ Use a light-resistant collection container because urobilinogen breaks down to urobilin when exposed to light.

■ Send the specimen to the laboratory immediately after collection.

■ Refrigerate the specimen if transport or testing is delayed more than 30 minutes; freeze the specimen if the test is to be performed by an outside laboratory.

Reference values

Normally, fecal urobilinogen values range from 50 to 300 mg/24 hours (SI, 100 to 400 EU/100 g).

Abnormal findings

Absent or low levels of urobilinogen in the stool indicate obstructed bile flow, the result of intrahepatic disorders (such as hepatocellular jaundice due to cirrhosis or hepatitis) or extrahepatic disorders (such as choledocholithiasis or tumor of the head of the pancreas, ampulla of Vater, or bile duct). Low fecal urobilinogen levels are also characteristic of depressed erythropoiesis such as in aplastic anemia.

Interfering factors

■ Contamination of the specimen or failure to use a light-resistant collection container

■ Broad-spectrum antibiotics (possible decrease due to inhibition of bacterial growth in the colon)

■ Sulfonamides, which react with the reagent used by the laboratory in this test, and large doses of salicylates (possible increase)

ENDOSCOPY

Esophagogastro-duodenoscopy

Esophagogastroduodenoscopy (EGD) permits visual examination of the lining of the esophagus, stomach, and upper duodenum using a flexible fiber-optic or video endoscope. It's indicated for patients with GI bleeding, hematemesis, melena, substernal or epigastric pain, gastroesophageal reflux disease, dysphagia, anemia, strictures, or peptic ulcer disease; those requiring foreign body retrieval; and postoperative patients with recurrent or new symptoms.

EGD eliminates the need for extensive exploratory surgery and can be used to detect small or surface lesions missed by radiography. Because the scope provides a channel for biopsy forceps or a cytology brush, it permits laboratory evaluation of abnormalities detected by radiography. Similarly, it allows for the removal of foreign bodies by suction (for small, soft objects) or by electrocautery snare or forceps (for large, hard objects).

Purpose
■ To diagnose inflammatory disease, malignant and benign tumors, ulcers, Mallory-Weiss syndrome, and structural abnormalities
■ To evaluate the stomach and duodenum postoperatively
■ To obtain emergency diagnosis of duodenal ulcer or esophageal injury such as that caused by chemical ingestion

Patient preparation
■ Explain to the patient that EGD permits visual examination of the lining of the esophagus, stomach, and upper duodenum.
■ Check the patient's medical history for allergies, medications, and information pertinent to the current complaint. Check for hypersensitivity to the medications and anesthetics ordered for the test.
■ Instruct the patient to fast for 6 to 12 hours before the test.
■ Tell the patient that a flexible instrument with a camera on the end will be passed through his mouth; explain who will perform this procedure, where it will take place, and that it takes about 30 minutes.
■ If emergency EGD is to be performed, tell the patient that stomach contents may be aspirated through a nasogastric tube.
■ Inform the patient that a bitter-tasting local anesthetic will be sprayed into his mouth and throat to calm the gag reflex and that his tongue and throat may feel swollen, making swallowing seem difficult. Advise him to let the saliva drain from the side of his mouth; a suction machine may be used to remove saliva if necessary.
■ Explain that a mouth guard will be inserted to protect his teeth and the endoscope; assure him that this won't obstruct his breathing.
■ Inform the patient that an I.V. line will be started and a sedative will be administered before the endoscope is inserted to help him relax. If the procedure is being done on an outpatient basis, advise the patient to arrange for someone to drive him home because he may feel drowsy from the sedative. Drugs that retard peristalsis of the upper GI tract may be administered in some circumstances.

- Tell the patient that he may experience pressure in the stomach as the endoscope is moved about and a feeling of fullness when air or carbon dioxide is insufflated. If he's apprehensive, administer meperidine or another analgesic I.M. about 30 minutes before the test as ordered; also administer atropine sulfate subcutaneously at this time, as ordered, to decrease gastric secretions, which would interfere with test results.
- Make sure that the patient or a responsible family member has signed an informed consent form.
- Just before the procedure, instruct the patient to remove dentures, eyeglasses, and constricting undergarments.

Procedure and posttest care
- Obtain the patient's baseline vital signs and leave the blood pressure cuff in place for monitoring throughout the procedure.
- If the patient has known cardiac disease, continuous electrocardiographic monitoring should be instituted. Continuous or periodic pulse oximetry is advisable, particularly in the patient with pulmonary compromise.
- Ask the patient to hold his breath while his mouth and throat are sprayed with a local anesthetic, if requested by the physician.
- Remind the patient to let saliva drain from the side of his mouth. Provide an emesis basin to spit out saliva and tissues to wipe saliva from his mouth or use oropharyngeal suction as needed.
- Place the patient in a left lateral position, bend his head forward, and ask him to open his mouth.
- The examiner guides the tip of the endoscope to the back of the patient's throat and downward. As the endoscope passes through the posterior pharynx and the

cricopharyngeal sphincter, the patient's neck is slowly extended. His chin must be kept at midline. The endoscope is then passed along the esophagus under direct vision.
- When the endoscope is well into the esophagus (about 12″ [30 cm]), the patient's head is positioned with his chin toward the table so that saliva can drain out of his mouth.
- After examination of the esophagus and the cardiac sphincter, the endoscope is rotated clockwise and advanced to allow examination of the stomach and duodenum. During the examination, air or water may be introduced through the endoscope to aid visualization, and suction may be applied to remove insufflated air and secretions.
- A camera may be attached to the endoscope to photograph areas for later study, or a measuring tube may be passed through the endoscope to determine the size of a lesion.
- Biopsy forceps or a cytology brush may be passed through the scope to obtain specimens for histologic or cytologic study.
- The endoscope is slowly withdrawn, and suspicious-looking areas of the gastric and esophageal lining are reexamined.
- Specimens should be collected in accordance with laboratory and pathology guidelines. Place tissue specimens immediately in a specimen bottle containing 10% formalin solution; cell specimens are smeared on glass slides and placed in a Coplin jar containing 95% ethyl alcohol.

CLINICAL ALERT *Observe the patient for possible perforation. Perforation in the cervical area of the esophagus produces pain on swallowing and with neck movement, thoracic perforation causes substernal or epigastric pain that increases* *with breathing or movement of the trunk, diaphragmatic perforation produces shoulder pain and dyspnea, and gastric perforation causes abdominal or back pain, cyanosis, fever, and pleural effusion.*

■ Observe the patient for evidence of aspiration of gastric contents, which could precipitate aspiration pneumonia.

■ Monitor the patient's vital signs and document them according to facility policy.

■ Test the patient's gag reflex by touching the back of the throat with a tongue blade. Withhold food and fluids until the gag reflex returns (usually in 1 hour), and then allow fluids and a light meal.

■ Tell the patient that he may burp some insufflated air and have a sore throat for 3 to 4 days. Throat lozenges and warm saline gargles may ease his discomfort.

■ If the patient experiences soreness at the I.V. site, apply warm soaks.

■ Because of sedation, an outpatient should avoid alcohol for 24 hours and shouldn't drive for 12 hours. Make sure the patient has transportation home.

■ Instruct the patient to notify the physician immediately if he experiences persistent difficulty with swallowing, pain, fever, black stools, or bloody vomitus.

Precautions

■ If tissue or cell specimens are obtained during the procedure, label and send them to the appropriate laboratory immediately.

■ This procedure is generally safe, but can cause perforation of the esophagus, stomach, or duodenum, especially if the patient is restless or uncooperative.

■ EGD is usually contraindicated in the patient with Zenker's diverticulum, a large aortic aneurysm, recent ulcer perforation (known as suspected viscus perfo-

ration), or an unstable cardiac or pulmonary condition.

■ EGD shouldn't be performed within 2 days after an upper GI series.

■ The patient requiring dental prophylaxis may also require antibiotics before this procedure.

▶ **CLINICAL ALERT** *Observe closely for adverse effects of the sedative: respiratory depression, apnea, hypotension, excessive diaphoresis, bradycardia, and laryngospasm. Have available emergency resuscitation equipment and an opioid antagonist such as naloxone. Be prepared to intervene as necessary.*

Normal findings

The smooth mucosa of the esophagus is normally yellow-pink and marked by a fine vascular network. A pulsation on the anterior wall of the esophagus between 8″ and 10″ (20 and 25.5 cm) from the incisor teeth represents the aortic arch. The orange-red mucosa of the stomach begins the "Z" line, an irregular transition line slightly above the esophagogastric junction.

Unlike the esophagus, the stomach has rugal folds, and its blood vessels aren't visible beneath the gastric mucosa. The reddish mucosa of the duodenal bulb is marked by a few shallow longitudinal folds. The mucosa of the distal duodenum has prominent circular folds, is lined with villi, and appears velvety.

Abnormal findings

EGD, coupled with the results of histologic and cytologic tests, may indicate acute or chronic ulcers, benign or malignant tumors, and inflammatory disease, including esophagitis, gastritis, and duodenitis. This test may demonstrate diverticula, varices, Mallory-Weiss syndrome, esophageal rings, esophageal and pyloric stenoses, and esophageal hiatal hernia. Although EGD can evaluate gross abnormalities of esophageal motility, as occur in achalasia, manometric studies are more accurate.

Interfering factors
- Anticoagulants (increased risk for bleeding)
- Failure to observe pretest restrictions
- Failure to send specimens to the laboratory immediately
- The patient's inability to cooperate, preventing optimal visualization

Colonoscopy

Colonoscopy uses a flexible fiber-optic video endoscope to permit visual examination of the lining of the large intestine. It's indicated for patients with a history of constipation or diarrhea, persistent rectal bleeding, and lower abdominal pain when the results of proctosigmoidoscopy and a barium enema test are negative or inconclusive.

Purpose
- To detect or evaluate inflammatory and ulcerative bowel disease
- To locate the origin of lower GI bleeding
- To aid in the diagnosis of colonic strictures and benign or malignant lesions
- To evaluate the colon postoperatively for recurrence of polyps and malignant lesions

Patient preparation
- Check the patient's medical history for allergies, medications, and information pertinent to the current complaint.
- Tell the patient that colonoscopy permits examination of the lining of the large intestine.
- Instruct the patient to maintain a clear liquid diet for 24 to 48 hours before the test and to take nothing by mouth after midnight the night before.
- Describe the procedure and tell the patient who will perform it and where it will take place.
- Explain that the large intestine must be thoroughly cleaned to be clearly visible. Instruct the patient to take a laxative, as ordered, or 1 gallon of GoLYTELY solution in the evening (drinking the chilled solutions at 8 oz [236.6 ml] every 10 minutes until the entire gallon is consumed).
- If fecal results aren't clear, the patient will receive a laxative, suppository, or tap water enema. Don't administer a soapsuds enema because this irritates the mucosa and stimulates mucus secretions that may hinder the examination.
- Inform the patient that an I.V. line will be started before the procedure and that a sedative will be administered just before the procedure. Advise him to arrange for someone to drive him home if he receives sedation.
- Assure the patient that the colonoscope is well lubricated to ease its insertion, that it initially feels cool, and that he may feel an urge to defecate when it's inserted and advanced.
- Explain to the patient that air may be introduced through the colonoscope to distend the intestinal wall and to facilitate viewing the lining and advancing the instrument. Tell him that flatus normally escapes around the instrument because of air insufflation and that he shouldn't attempt to control it.
- Tell the patient that suction may be used to remove blood or liquid stools that obscure vision, but that this won't cause discomfort.

■ Make sure that the patient or a responsible family member has signed an informed consent form.

Procedure and posttest care

■ Place the patient on his left side with his knees flexed and drape him.

■ Obtain the patient's baseline vital signs. Be prepared to monitor vital signs through the procedure. If the patient has known cardiac disease, continuous electrocardiographic monitoring should be instituted. Continuous or periodic pulse oximetry is advisable, particularly in the high-risk patient with possible respiratory depression secondary to sedation.

■ Instruct the patient to breathe deeply and slowly through his mouth as the physician palpates the mucosa of the anus and rectum and inserts the lubricated colonoscope through the patient's anus into the sigmoid colon under direct vision.

■ Insufflated a small amount of air to locate the bowel lumen and then advance the scope through the rectum.

■ When the instrument reaches the descending sigmoid junction, assist the patient to a supine position to aid the scope advance, if necessary. After passing the splenic flexure, the scope is advanced through the transverse colon, through the hepatic flexure, and into the ascending colon and cecum.

■ Abdominal palpation or fluoroscopy may be used to help guide the colonoscope through the large intestine.

■ Suction may be used to remove blood and secretions that obscure vision.

■ Biopsy forceps or a cytology brush may be passed through the colonoscope to obtain specimens for histologic or cytologic examination; an electrocautery snare may be used to remove polyps.

■ If the examiner removes a tissue specimen, immediately place it in a specimen bottle containing 10% formalin; immediately place cytology smears in a Coplin jar containing 95% ethyl alcohol. Send specimens to the laboratory immediately. Specimens should be collected in accordance with laboratory and pathology guidelines.

■ Observe the patient closely for signs of bowel perforation. Report such signs immediately.

■ Check the patient's vital signs and document them according to facility policy.

■ After the patient has recovered from sedation, he may resume his usual diet unless the physician orders otherwise.

■ Provide privacy while the patient rests after the test; tell him that he may pass large amounts of flatus after insufflation.

■ If a polyp has been removed, inform the patient that his stool may contain some blood, but excessive bleeding should be reported immediately.

Precautions

■ Although it's usually a safe procedure, colonoscopy can cause perforation of the large intestine, excessive bleeding, and retroperitoneal emphysema.

■ This procedure is contraindicated in the pregnant woman near term, the patient who has had a recent acute myocardial infarction or abdominal surgery, and one with ischemic bowel disease, acute diverticulitis, peritonitis, fulminant granulomatous colitis, perforated viscus, or fulminant ulcerative colitis. For these cases or for screening purposes, a virtual colonoscopy may be an option to help visualize polyps early before they became concerns. (See *Virtual colonoscopy*.)

▶ **CLINICAL ALERT** *Watch the patient closely for adverse effects of the sedative. Have available emergency resuscita-*

tion equipment and an opioid antagonist, such as naloxone, for I.V. use if necessary.
■ If a polyp is removed but not retrieved during the examination, give enemas and strain stools to retrieve it if the physician requests it.

Normal findings

Normally, the mucosa of the large intestine beyond the sigmoid colon appears light pink-orange and is marked by semilunar folds and deep tubular pits. Blood vessels are visible beneath the intestinal mucosa, which glistens from mucus secretions.

Abnormal findings

Visual examination of the large intestine, coupled with histologic and cytologic test results, may indicate proctitis, granulomatous or ulcerative colitis, Crohn's disease, and malignant or benign lesions. Diverticular disease or the site of lower GI bleeding can be detected through colonoscopy alone.

Interfering factors

■ Fixation of the sigmoid colon due to inflammatory bowel disease, surgery, or radiation therapy (may hinder passage of the colonoscope)
■ Blood from acute colonic hemorrhage (hinders visualization)
■ Insufficient bowel preparation or barium retained in the intestine from previous diagnostic studies (makes accurate visual examination impossible)
■ Failure to place histologic or cytologic specimens in the appropriate preservative or to send the specimens to the laboratory immediately

VIRTUAL COLONOSCOPY

Virtual colonoscopy combines computed tomography (CT) scanning and X-ray images with sophisticated image processing computers to generate three-dimensional (3-D) images of the patient's colon. These images are interpreted by a skilled radiologist to recreate and evaluate the colon's inner surface. Although this procedure isn't as accurate as a routine colonoscopy, it's less invasive and is useful in screening the patient with small polyps. The colon must be free from residue and fecal material. Bowel preparation consists of following a clear liquid diet for 24 hours before the procedure; also, the patient performs GoLYTELY bowel preparation the evening before and takes a rectal suppository on the morning of the test.

Before performing the CT scan, a thin red rectal tube is placed, and air is introduced into the colon to distend the bowel. This may produce mild cramping. The CT scan is done with the patient in the supine position and again while prone. The scans are then shipped over a network to a 3-D image processing computer, and a radiologist evaluates the images obtained. If polyps are identified, a colonoscopy may be scheduled to remove them.

Proctosigmoidoscopy

Proctosigmoidoscopy uses a proctoscope, sigmoidoscope, and digital examination to evaluate the lining of the distal sigmoid colon, rectum, and anal canal. It's indicated in patients with recent changes in bowel habits, lower abdominal and perineal pain, prolapse on defecation, pruritus, and passage of mucus, blood, or pus in the stool. Specimens may be obtained from suspicious areas of the mucosa by biopsy, lavage or cytology brush, or culture swab.

Possible complications of this procedure include rectal bleeding and, rarely, bowel perforation.

Purpose

■ To aid in the diagnosis of inflammatory, infectious, and ulcerative bowel disease

■ To detect hemorrhoids, hypertrophic anal papilla, polyps, fissures, fistulas, and abscesses in the rectum and anal canal

Patient preparation

■ Explain to the patient that proctosigmoidoscopy allows visual examination of the lining of the distal sigmoid colon, rectum, and anal canal.

■ Tell the patient that the test requires passage of two special instruments through the anus, who will perform the procedure, and where it will take place.

■ Check the patient's history for allergies, medications, and information pertinent to the current complaint. Find out if he has had a barium test within the past week because barium in the colon hinders accurate examination.

■ Because dietary and bowel preparations for this procedure vary according to the physician's preference, follow the orders carefully. If a special bowel preparation is ordered, explain to the patient that this clears the intestine to ensure a better view.

■ Instruct the patient to maintain a clear liquid diet for 24 to 48 hours before the test, to avoid eating fruits and vegetables before the procedure, and to fast the morning of the procedure, according to the physician's preference.

■ Describe the position the patient will be asked to assume and assure him that he'll be adequately draped.

■ As ordered, administer a warm tap water or sodium biphosphate enema 3 to 4 hours before the procedure. The procedure may be started without bowel preparation because enemas can alter intestinal markings and traumatize mucous membranes. For this reason, irritating soapsuds enemas are inappropriate before this test. If the examination is hindered by excessive fecal matter, an enema may be ordered before the examination proceeds.

■ Tell the patient that he may be secured to a tilting table that rotates into horizontal and vertical positions.

■ Tell the patient that the examiner's finger and the instrument are well lubricated to ease insertion, that the instrument initially feels cool, and that he may experience the urge to defecate when the instrument is inserted and advanced.

■ Inform the patient that the instrument may stretch the intestinal wall and cause transient muscle spasms or colicky lower abdominal pain.

■ Instruct the patient to breathe deeply and slowly through his mouth to relax the abdominal muscles; this reduces the urge to defecate and eases discomfort.

■ Explain to the patient that air may be introduced through the endoscope into the intestine to distend its walls. Tell him that this causes flatus to escape around the endoscope and that he shouldn't attempt to control it.

■ Inform the patient that a suction machine may remove blood, mucus, or liquid stool that obscures vision, but that it won't cause discomfort.

■ Inform the patient that an I.V. line may be started if an I.V. sedative is to be used. If the procedure is being done on an outpatient basis, advise him to arrange for someone to drive him home.

■ Make sure that the patient or a responsible family member has signed an informed consent form.

■ If the patient has rectal inflammation, provide a local anesthetic about 15 to 20 minutes before the procedure to minimize discomfort.

Procedure and posttest care

■ Obtain the patient's baseline vital signs and monitor him throughout the procedure.

■ Place the patient in a knee-chest or left lateral position with his knees flexed and drape him.

■ If a left lateral position is used, a sandbag may be placed under the patient's left hip so that the buttocks project over the edge of the table. The right buttock is gently raised, and the anus and perianal region are examined under good lighting.

■ Instruct the patient to breathe deeply and slowly through his mouth as the examiner palpates the anal canal, rectum, and rectal mucosa for induration and tenderness; the examiner then withdraws his finger and checks for the presence of blood, mucus, or stool.

■ The sigmoidoscope is lubricated, and the patient is told that the instrument is about to be inserted. The right buttock is raised, and the sigmoidoscope is inserted into the anus. As the scope is passed with steady pressure through the anal sphincters, instruct the patient to bear down as though defecating to aid its passage. The sigmoidoscope is advanced through the anal canal into the rectum.

■ At the rectosigmoid junction, a small amount of air may be insufflated to open the bowel lumen. The scope is then gently advanced to its full length into the distal sigmoid colon.

■ As the sigmoidoscope is slowly withdrawn, air is carefully insufflated, and the intestinal mucosa is thoroughly examined.

■ If stool obscures vision, the eyepiece on the scope is removed, a cotton swab is inserted through the scope, and the bowel lumen is swabbed. A suction machine may remove blood, excessive secretions, or liquid stool.

■ To obtain specimens from suspicious areas of the intestinal mucosa, a biopsy forceps, cytology brush, or culture swab is passed through the sigmoidoscope.

■ Polyps may be removed for histologic examination by inserting an electrocautery snare through the sigmoidoscope.

■ Specimens are collected in accordance with laboratory and pathology guidelines and immediately placed in a specimen bottle containing 10% formalin, cytology slides are placed in a Coplin jar containing 95% ethyl alcohol, and culture swabs are placed in a culture tube.

■ After the sigmoidoscope is withdrawn, the proctoscope is lubricated and the patient is told that it's about to be inserted. Assure him that he'll experience less discomfort during passage of the proctoscope.

■ The right buttock is raised, and the proctoscope is inserted through the anus and gently advanced to its full length.

■ The obturator is removed, and the light source is inserted through the proctoscope handle.

■ As the instrument is slowly withdrawn, the rectal and anal mucosa are carefully examined. Specimens may be obtained from suspicious areas of the intestinal mucosa.

■ If a biopsy of the anal canal is required, a local anesthetic may be administered first.

- Withdraw the proctoscope after the examination is completed.
- If the patient has been examined in a knee-chest position, instruct him to rest in a supine position for several minutes before standing to prevent orthostatic hypotension.
- Observe the patient closely for signs of bowel perforation and for vasovagal attack due to emotional stress. Report such signs immediately.
- Allow the patient nothing by mouth until he's alert.
- Monitor the patient's vital signs as per facility protocol until he's alert.
- If air was introduced into the intestine, tell the patient that he may pass large amounts of flatus. Provide privacy while he rests after the test.
- If a biopsy or polypectomy was performed, inform the patient that blood may appear in his stool.

Precautions

- If a tissue specimen or culture swab has been obtained, label it and send it to the appropriate laboratory immediately.
- In general, anticoagulant therapy isn't contraindicated; however, it may increase the risk of bleeding.
- If the patient received sedation, he should avoid alcohol for 24 hours and shouldn't drive for 12 hours, so make sure he has transportation home.

Normal findings

The mucosa of the sigmoid colon appears light pink-orange and is marked by semilunar folds and deep tubular pits. The rectal mucosa is redder due to its rich vascular network, deepens to a purple hue at the pectinate line (the anatomic division between the rectum and anus), and has three distinct valves. The lower two-thirds of the anus (anoderm) is lined with smooth gray-tan skin and joins with the hair-fringed perianal skin.

Abnormal findings

Visual examination and palpation demonstrate abnormalities of the anal canal and rectum, including internal and external hemorrhoids, hypertrophic anal papilla, anal fissures, anal fistulas, and anorectal abscesses. The examination may also reveal inflammatory bowel diseases, polyps, cancer, and other tumors. Biopsy, culture, and other laboratory tests are typically necessary to detect various disorders.

Interfering factors

- Barium in the intestine from previous diagnostic studies (hinders visualization)
- Large amounts of stool in the intestine (hinders visual examination and advancement of the endoscope)
- Failure to place histologic or cytologic specimens in the appropriate preservative or to send the specimens to the laboratory immediately

Endoscopic ultrasonography

Endoscopic ultrasonography (EUS) combines ultrasonography and endoscopy to visualize the GI wall and adjacent structures. The incorporation of the ultrasound probe at the distal end of the ultrasonic endoscope allows high-resolution ultrasound imaging.

Purpose

- To evaluate or stage lesions of the esophagus, stomach, duodenum, pancreas, ampulla, biliary ducts, and rectum
- To evaluate submucosal tumors and large folds
- To localize endocrine tumors

Patient preparation

- Explain to the patient that EUS permits visual examination of tumors and large folds in the GI tract.
- Check the patient's medical history for allergies, medications, and information pertinent to the current complaint.
- Instruct the patient to fast for 6 to 8 hours before the test.
- Describe the procedure to the patient. Tell him who will perform it and where it will take place.
- For esophagogastroduodenoscopy (EGD) EUS, explain that a flexible instrument will be passed through the mouth and into the esophagus, as in an EGD.
- If a sigmoid EUS is to be performed, tell the patient that the scope is well lubricated to ease its insertion through the anus, that it initially feels cool, and that he may feel an urge to defecate when it's inserted and advanced.
- For the sigmoid EUS, the patient may have to take a laxative the evening before if ordered.
- Inform the patient that he may receive an I.V. sedative to help him relax before the endoscope is inserted. If the procedure is being done on an outpatient basis, advise the patient to arrange for someone to drive him home because conscious sedation may affect his reaction time and reflexes, even though he may feel fine.
- Make sure that the patient or a responsible family member has signed an informed consent form.

Procedure and posttest care

- Obtain the patient's baseline vital signs and monitor him throughout the procedure according to facility policy.
- Follow the procedures for EGD or sigmoidoscopy, depending on which type of EUS will be performed.

Precautions

- This procedure is generally safe, but can cause perforation of the esophagus, stomach, or duodenum, as in EGD, or of the intestine, as in sigmoidoscopy or colonoscopy.

Normal findings

EUS usually reveals normal anatomy with no evidence of tumor.

Abnormal findings

Refer to the abnormal findings for EGD, colonoscopy, endoscopy, and sigmoidoscopy.

Interfering factors

- Esophageal stricture (hinders passage of the endoscope)
- All interfering factors listed under EGD, colonoscopy, and sigmoidoscopy

CONTRAST RADIOGRAPHY

Barium swallow

Barium swallow (esophagography) is the cineradiographic, radiographic, or fluoroscopic examination of the pharynx and the fluoroscopic examination of the esophagus after ingestion of thick and thin mixtures of barium sulfate. This test, most commonly performed as part of the upper GI series, is indicated in patients with histories of dysphagia and regurgitation. Further testing is usually required for definitive diagnosis. (See *Gastroesophageal reflux scanning*, page 774.)

Cholangiography and the barium enema test, if necessary, should precede the barium swallow because ingested barium

---

GASTROESOPHAGEAL REFLUX SCANNING

When the results of a barium swallow are inconclusive, gastroesophageal reflux scanning may be conducted to evaluate esophageal function and detect reflux. This test delivers less radiation than a barium swallow and is a much more sensitive indicator of reflux. It also allows reflux to be measured without insertion of an esophageal tube, an important consideration in testing infants, small children, and other patients for whom intubation is contraindicated.

Procedure

The patient is instructed to fast beginning at midnight the day of the test. As the test begins, he's placed in a supine or upright position and asked to swallow a solution containing a radiopharmaceutical such as technetium 99m (^{99m}Tc) sulfur colloid. A gamma counter placed over the patient's chest records its passage through the esophagus into the stomach to determine transit time and evaluate esophageal function.

If reflux is suspected, the patient is repositioned as his stomach distends, and continuous recordings visualize reflux and estimate its quantity. In reflux, radioactivity may be detected in the esophagus.

Findings and contraindications

Normally, ^{99m}Tc sulfur colloid descends through the esophagus in about 6 seconds; radioactivity is then detected only in the stomach and small bowel. However, diffuse spasm of the esophagus, achalasia, or other esophageal motility disorders may prolong transit time. In gastroesophageal reflux, radioactivity may be detected in the esophagus. As with other radionuclide studies, this scan is usually contraindicated during pregnancy and lactation. It can be modified for use in the infant or child.

---

may obscure anatomic detail on the X-rays.

Purpose

- To diagnose hiatal hernia, diverticula, and varices
- To detect strictures, ulcers, tumors, polyps, and motility disorders

Patient preparation

- Explain to the patient that the barium swallow test evaluates the function of the pharynx and esophagus.
- Instruct the patient to fast after midnight the night before the test. (If the patient is an infant, delay feeding to ensure complete digestion of barium.) He may also be given a restricted diet for 2 to 3 days before the test.

- Describe the test, including who will perform it and where it will take place.
- Describe the milk shake consistency and chalky taste of the barium preparation the patient is required to ingest. Although it's flavored, he may find it unpleasant to swallow. Tell the patient that he'll first receive a thick mixture, then a thin one, and that he must drink 12 to 14 oz (355 to 414 ml) during the examination.
- Inform the patient that he'll be placed in various positions on a tilting X-ray table and that X-rays will be taken. Reassure him that safety precautions will be maintained.
- Withhold antacids, histamine-2 blockers, and proton pump inhibitors, as ordered, if gastric reflux is suspected.

■ Just before the procedure, instruct the patient to put on a gown without snap closures and to remove jewelry, dentures, hair clips, or other radiopaque objects from the X-ray field.

Procedure and posttest care

■ The patient is placed in an upright position behind the fluoroscopic screen and his heart, lungs, and abdomen are examined.

■ The patient is then instructed to take one swallow of the thick barium mixture, and the pharyngeal action is recorded using cineradiography. (This action occurs too rapidly for adequate fluoroscopic evaluation.)

■ The patient is then told to take several swallows of the thin barium mixture. The passage of the barium is examined fluoroscopically, and spot films of the esophageal region are taken from lateral angles and from right and left posteroanterior angles. Esophageal strictures and obstruction of the esophageal lumen by the lower esophageal ring are best detected when the patient is upright. To accentuate small strictures or demonstrate dysphagia, the patient may be requested to swallow a special "barium marshmallow" (soft white bread that has been soaked in barium) or a barium pill.

■ The patient is then secured to the X-ray table and is rotated to the Trendelenburg position to evaluate esophageal peristalsis or demonstrate hiatal hernia and gastric reflux.

■ The patient is instructed to take several swallows of barium while the esophagus is examined fluoroscopically, and spot films of significant findings are taken when indicated. After the table is rotated to a horizontal position, the patient is told to take several swallows of barium so that the esophagogastric junction and peristalsis may be evaluated. The passage of the barium is fluoroscopically observed, and spot films of significant findings are taken with the patient in the supine and prone positions.

■ During fluoroscopic examination of the esophagus, the cardiac and fundus of the patient's stomach are also carefully studied because neoplasms in these areas may invade the esophagus and cause obstruction.

■ Check that additional spot films and repeat fluoroscopic evaluation haven't been ordered before allowing the patient to resume his usual diet.

■ Instruct the patient to drink plenty of fluids, unless contraindicated, to help eliminate the barium.

■ Administer a cathartic, if prescribed.

■ Inform the patient that stools will be chalky and light colored for 24 to 72 hours. Record a description of all stools passed by the patient in the hospital.

■ Barium retained in the intestine may harden, causing obstruction or fecal impaction. Notify the physician if the patient fails to expel barium in 2 or 3 days.

■ Check the patient for abdominal distention and absent bowel sounds, which are associated with constipation and may suggest barium impaction.

Precautions

■ Barium swallow is usually contraindicated in the patient with intestinal obstruction as well as in the pregnant patient because of radiation's possible teratogenic effects.

Normal findings

After the barium sulfate is swallowed, the bolus pours over the base of the tongue into the pharynx. A peristaltic wave propels the bolus through the entire length of the esophagus in about 2 seconds. When

GI MOTILITY STUDY

A GI motility study evaluates the intestinal motility and integrity of the mucosal lining by recording the passage of barium through the lower digestive tract. About 6 hours after the patient ingests the barium, the head of the barium column is usually in the hepatic flexure and the tail is in the terminal ileum; 24 hours after ingestion, the barium has completely opacified the large intestine. Spot films taken 24, 48, or 72 hours after ingestion are inferior to barium enema because the amount of barium passing through the large intestine isn't sufficient to fully extend the lumen. However, when spot films suggest intestinal abnormalities, barium enema and colonoscopy can provide more specific results and confirm diagnostic information.

the peristaltic wave reaches the base of the esophagus, the cardiac sphincter opens, allowing the bolus to enter the stomach. After passage of the bolus, the cardiac sphincter closes. Normally, the bolus evenly fills and distends the lumen of the pharynx and esophagus, and the mucosa appears smooth and regular.

Abnormal findings

Barium swallow may reveal hiatal hernia, diverticula, and varices. Aspiration into the lungs will also be revealed. Although strictures, tumors, polyps, ulcers, and motility disorders (pharyngeal muscular disorders, esophageal spasms, and achalasia) may be detected, definitive diagnosis commonly requires endoscopic biopsy or, for motility disorders, manometric studies. (See *GI motility study*.)

Interfering factors
- Aspiration of barium into lungs due to poor swallowing reflex

Upper GI and small-bowel series

The upper GI and small-bowel series is the fluoroscopic examination of the esophagus, stomach, and small intestine after ingestion of barium sulfate, a contrast agent. As the barium passes through the digestive tract, fluoroscopy outlines peristalsis and the mucosal contours of the respective organs, and spot films record significant findings. This test is indicated in patients who have upper GI symptoms (difficulty swallowing, regurgitation, burning or gnawing epigastric pain), signs of small-bowel disease (diarrhea, weight loss), and signs of GI bleeding (hematemesis, melena).

Although this test can detect various mucosal abnormalities, subsequent biopsy is typically necessary to rule out malignancy or distinguish specific inflammatory diseases. Oral cholecystography, barium enema, and routine X-rays should always precede this test because retained barium clouds anatomic detail on X-ray films.

Purpose
- To detect hiatal hernia, diverticula, and varices
- To aid in the diagnosis of strictures, blockages, ulcers, tumors, regional enteritis, and malabsorption syndrome
- To help detect motility disorders

Patient preparation
- Explain to the patient that the upper GI and small-bowel series uses ingested barium and X-ray films to examine the esophagus, stomach, and small intestine.

■ Tell the patient to consume a low-residue diet for 2 to 3 days before the test and then to fast and avoid smoking after midnight the night before the test.

■ Describe the test, including who will perform it and where it will take place.

■ Encourage the patient to bring reading material.

■ Inform the patient that he'll be placed on an X-ray table that rotates into vertical, semivertical, and horizontal positions.

■ Explain to the patient that he'll be adequately secured and assisted to the supine, prone, and side-lying positions.

■ Describe the milk shake consistency and chalky taste of the barium mixture. Although it's flavored, the patient may find its taste unpleasant, but tell him he must drink 16 to 20 oz (475 to 590 ml) for a complete examination.

■ Inform the patient that his abdomen may be compressed to ensure proper coating of the stomach or intestinal walls with barium or to separate overlapping bowel loops.

■ As ordered, withhold most oral medications after midnight and anticholinergics and opioids for 24 hours because these drugs affect small intestinal motility. Antacids, histamine-2 receptor antagonists, and proton pump inhibitors are also sometimes withheld for several hours if gastric reflux is suspected.

■ Just before the procedure, instruct the patient to put on a gown without snap closures and to remove jewelry, dentures, hair clips, or other objects that might obscure anatomic detail on the X-ray films.

Procedure and posttest care

■ After the patient is secured in a supine position on the X-ray table, the table is tilted until the patient is erect, and the

heart, lungs, and abdomen are examined fluoroscopically.

■ The patient is instructed to take several swallows of the barium suspension, and its passage through the esophagus is observed. (Occasionally, the patient is given a thick barium suspension, especially when esophageal pathology is strongly suspected.)

■ During fluoroscopic examination, spot films of the esophagus are taken from lateral angles and from right and left posteroanterior angles.

■ When barium enters the stomach, the patient's abdomen is palpated or compressed to ensure adequate coating of the gastric mucosa.

■ To perform a double-contrast examination, the patient is instructed to sip the barium through a perforated straw. As he does so, a small amount of air is also introduced into the stomach; this permits detailed examination of the gastric rugae, and spot films of significant findings are taken. The patient is then instructed to ingest the remaining barium suspension and the filling of the stomach and emptying into the duodenum are observed fluoroscopically.

■ Two series of spot films of the stomach and duodenum are taken from posteroanterior, anteroposterior, lateral, and oblique angles, with the patient erect and then in a supine position.

■ The passage of barium into the remainder of the small intestine is then observed fluoroscopically, and spot films are taken at 30- to 60-minute intervals until the barium reaches the region of the ileocecal valve. If abnormalities in the small intestine are detected, the area is palpated and compressed to help clarify the defect, and a spot film is taken. The examination ends when the barium enters the cecum.

- Make sure additional X-rays haven't been ordered before allowing the patient food, fluids, and oral medications (if applicable).
- Tell the patient to drink plenty of fluid (unless contraindicated) to help eliminate the barium.
- Administer a cathartic or enema to the patient. Tell the patient that his stool will be light colored for 24 to 72 hours. Record and describe any stool passed by the patient in the hospital. Barium retention in the intestine may cause obstruction or fecal impaction, so notify the physician if the patient doesn't pass the barium within 2 to 3 days. Also, barium retention may affect scheduling of other GI tests.
- Instruct the patient to tell the physician of abdominal fullness or pain or a delay in return to brown stools.

Precautions

- The upper GI and small-bowel series may be contraindicated in the patient with obstruction or perforation of the digestive tract. Barium may intensify the obstruction or seep into the abdominal cavity. Sometimes a small-bowel series is performed to find a "transition zone." If a perforation is suspected, Gastrografin (a water-soluble contrast medium) rather than barium may be used.
- The test is contraindicated in the pregnant patient because of radiation's possible teratogenic effects.

Normal findings

After the barium suspension is swallowed, it pours over the base of the tongue into the pharynx and is propelled by a peristaltic wave through the entire length of the esophagus in about 2 seconds. The bolus evenly fills and distends the lumen of the pharynx and esophagus, and the mucosa appears smooth and regular.

When the peristaltic wave reaches the base of the esophagus, the cardiac sphincter opens, allowing the bolus to enter the stomach. After passage of the bolus, the cardiac sphincter closes.

As barium enters the stomach, it outlines the characteristic longitudinal folds called *rugae*, which are best observed using the double-contrast technique. When the stomach is completely filled with barium, its outer contour appears smooth and regular without evidence of flattened, rigid areas suggestive of intrinsic or extrinsic lesions.

After barium enters the stomach, it quickly empties into the duodenal bulb through relaxation of the pyloric sphincter. Although the mucosa of the duodenal bulb is relatively smooth, circular folds become apparent as barium enters the duodenal loop. These folds deepen and become more numerous in the jejunum. The barium temporarily lodges between these folds, producing a speckled pattern on the X-ray film. As barium enters the ileum, the circular folds become less prominent and, except for their broadness, resemble those in the duodenum. The film also shows that the diameter of the small intestine tapers gradually from the duodenum to the ileum.

Abnormal findings

X-ray studies of the esophagus may reveal strictures, tumors, hiatal hernia, diverticula, varices, and ulcers (particularly in the distal esophagus). Benign strictures usually dilate the esophagus, whereas malignant ones cause erosive changes in the mucosa. Tumors produce filling defects in the column of barium, but only malignant ones change the mucosal contour. Nevertheless, biopsy is necessary for definitive diagnosis of esophageal strictures and tumors.

Motility disorders, such as esophageal spasm, are usually difficult to detect because spasms are erratic and transient; manometry, which measures the length and pressure of peristaltic contractions and evaluates cardiac sphincter function, is generally performed to detect such disorders. However, achalasia (cardiospasm) is strongly suggested when the distal esophagus has a beaklike appearance. Gastric reflux appears as a backflow of barium from the stomach into the esophagus.

X-ray studies of the stomach may reveal tumors and ulcers. Malignant tumors, usually adenocarcinomas, appear as filling defects on the X-ray film and usually disrupt peristalsis. Benign tumors, such as adenomatous polyps and leiomyomas, appear as outpouchings of the gastric mucosa and generally don't affect peristalsis. Ulcers occur most commonly in the stomach and duodenum (particularly in the duodenal bulb), and these two areas are thus examined together. Benign ulcers usually demonstrate evidence of partial or complete healing and are characterized by radiating folds extending to the edge of the ulcer crater. Malignant ulcers, usually associated with a suspicious mass, generally have radiating folds that extend beyond the ulcer crater to the edge of the mass. However, biopsy is necessary for definitive diagnosis of tumors and ulcers.

Occasionally, this test detects signs that suggest pancreatitis or pancreatic carcinoma. Such signs include edematous changes in the mucosa of the antrum or duodenal loop or dilation of the duodenal loop. These findings mandate further studies for pancreatic disease, such as endoscopic retrograde cholangiopancreatography, abdominal ultrasonography, or computed tomography scanning.

X-ray studies of the small intestine may reveal regional enteritis, malabsorption syndrome, and tumors. Although regional enteritis may not be detected in its early stages, small ulcerations and edematous changes develop in the mucosa as the disease progresses. Edematous changes, segmentation of the barium column, and flocculation characterize malabsorption syndrome. Filling defects occur with Hodgkin's disease and lymphosarcoma.

Interfering factors

- Failure to observe diet, smoking, and medication restrictions (may invalidate results)
- Excess air in the small bowel (possible poor imaging)
- Failure to remove metallic objects in the X-ray field (possible poor imaging)

Barium enema

Also called *lower GI examination,* barium enema is the radiographic examination of the large intestine after rectal instillation of barium sulfate (single-contrast technique) or barium sulfate and air (double-contrast technique). It's indicated in patients with histories of altered bowel habits, lower abdominal pain, or the passage of blood, mucus, or pus in the stool. It may also be indicated after colostomy or ileostomy; in these patients, barium (or barium and air) is instilled through the stoma. Complications include perforation of the colon, water intoxication, barium granulomas and, rarely, intraperitoneal and extraperitoneal extravasation of barium and barium embolism.

The single-contrast technique provides a profile view of the large intestine; the double-contrast technique provides profile and frontal views. The latter technique best detects small intraluminal tumors (especially polyps), the early mucosal changes of inflammatory disease, and subtle intestinal bleeding caused by ulcerated polyps or the shallow ulcerations of inflammatory disease.

Although barium enema clearly outlines most of the large intestine, proctosigmoidoscopy provides the best view of the rectosigmoid region. Barium enema should precede the barium swallow and upper GI and small-bowel series because barium ingested in the latter procedure may take several days to pass through the GI tract and thus may interfere with subsequent X-ray studies.

Purpose
- To aid in the diagnosis of colorectal cancer and inflammatory disease
- To detect polyps, diverticula, and structural changes in the large intestine

Patient preparation
- Explain to the patient that the barium enema test permits examination of the large intestine through X-ray films taken after a barium enema.
- Describe the test, including who will perform it and where it will take place.
- Because residual fecal material in the colon obscures normal anatomy on X-rays, instruct the patient to carefully follow the prescribed bowel preparation, which may include diet, laxatives, or an enema. However, in certain conditions, such as ulcerative colitis and active GI bleeding, their use may be prohibited.
- Stress that accurate test results depend on the patient's cooperation with prescribed dietary restrictions and bowel preparation. A common bowel preparation technique includes restricted intake of dairy products and maintenance of a liquid diet for 24 hours before the test. The patient is encouraged to drink five

8-oz glasses of water or clear liquids 12 to 24 hours before the test. Administer a bowel preparation supplied by the radiography department. (A GoLYTELY preparation isn't recommended because it leaves the bowel too wet for the barium to coat the walls of the bowel.)
- Advise the patient to administer prescribed enemas until return is clear.
- Tell the patient not to eat breakfast before the procedure; if the test is scheduled for late afternoon (or delayed), he may have clear liquids.
- Tell the patient that he'll be placed on a tilting X-ray table and adequately draped. Assure him that he'll be secured to the table and will be assisted to various positions.
- Tell the patient that he may experience cramping pains or the urge to defecate as the barium or air is introduced into the intestine. Instruct him to breathe deeply and slowly through his mouth to ease discomfort.
- Tell the patient to keep his anal sphincter tightly contracted against the rectal tube; this holds the tube in position and helps prevent leakage of barium. Stress the importance of retaining the barium enema; if the intestinal walls aren't adequately coated with barium, test results may be inaccurate.
- Assure the patient that the barium enema is fairly easy to retain because of its cool temperature.

Procedure and posttest care
- After the patient is in a supine position on a tilting X-ray table, spot films of the abdomen are taken.
- The patient is assisted to Sims' position, and a well-lubricated rectal tube is inserted through the anus. If the patient has anal sphincter atony or severe mental

or physical debilitation, a rectal tube with a retaining balloon may be inserted.

■ The barium is administered slowly and the filling process is monitored fluoroscopically. To aid filling, the table may be tilted or the patient assisted to supine, prone, and lateral decubitus positions.

■ As barium flow is observed, spot films are taken of significant findings. When the intestine is filled with barium, overhead films of the abdomen are taken. The rectal tube is withdrawn, and the patient is escorted to the toilet or provided with a bedpan and is instructed to expel as much barium as possible.

■ After evacuation, an additional overhead film is taken to record the mucosal pattern of the intestine and to evaluate the efficiency of colonic emptying.

■ A double-contrast barium enema may directly follow this examination or may be performed separately. If it's performed immediately, a thin film of barium remains in the patient's intestine, coating the mucosa, and air is carefully injected to distend the bowel lumen.

■ When the double-contrast technique is performed separately, a colloidal barium suspension is instilled, filling the patient's intestine to either the splenic flexure or the middle of the transverse colon. The suspension is then aspirated and air is forcefully injected into the intestine. If the intestine is filled to the lower descending colon, air is forcefully injected without previous aspiration of the suspension.

■ The patient is then assisted to erect, prone, supine, and lateral decubitus positions in sequence. Barium filling is monitored fluoroscopically, and spot films are taken of significant findings. After the required films are taken, the patient is escorted to the toilet or provided with a bedpan.

■ Make sure further studies haven't been ordered before allowing the patient food and fluids. Encourage extra fluid intake because bowel preparation and the test itself can cause dehydration.

■ Encourage rest because this test and the bowel preparation that precedes it is usually exhausting.

■ Because barium retention after this test can cause intestinal obstruction or fecal impaction, administer a mild cathartic or an enema. Tell the patient his stool will be light colored for 24 to 72 hours. Record and describe any stool passed by the patient in the hospital.

Precautions

■ Barium enema is contraindicated in the patient with tachycardia, fulminant ulcerative colitis associated with systemic toxicity and megacolon, toxic megacolon, or suspected perforation.

■ This test should be performed cautiously in the patient with obstruction, acute inflammatory conditions (such as ulcerative colitis and diverticulitis), acute vascular insufficiency of the bowel, acute fulminant bloody diarrhea, and suspected pneumatosis cystoides intestinalis.

■ Barium enema is contraindicated in the pregnant patient because of radiation's possible teratogenic effects.

Normal findings

In the single-contrast enema, the intestine is uniformly filled with barium, and colonic haustral markings are clearly apparent. The intestinal walls collapse as the barium is expelled, and the mucosa has a regular, feathery appearance on the postevacuation film. In the double-contrast enema, the intestines uniformly distend with air and have a thin layer of barium, providing excellent detail of the mucosal pattern. As the patient is assisted to various positions, the barium collects on the dependent walls of the intestine by the force of gravity.

Abnormal findings

Although most colonic cancers occur in the rectosigmoid region and are best detected by proctosigmoidoscopy, X-ray films may reveal adenocarcinoma and, rarely, sarcomas occurring higher in the intestine. Carcinoma usually appears as a localized filling defect, with a sharp transition between the normal and necrotic mucosa. If it's circumferential, it will have an "apple core" appearance. These characteristics help distinguish carcinoma from the more diffuse lesions of inflammatory disease, but endoscopic biopsy may be necessary to confirm the diagnosis.

X-ray studies demonstrate and define the extent of inflammatory disease, such as diverticulitis, ulcerative colitis, and granulomatous colitis. Ulcerative colitis usually originates in the anal region and ascends through the intestine; granulomatous colitis usually originates in the cecum and terminal ileum and then descends through the intestine. However, biopsy may be necessary to confirm diagnosis.

Barium X-ray films may also reveal saccular adenomatous polyps, broad-based villous polyps, structural changes in the intestine (such as intussusception, telescoping of the bowel, sigmoid volvulus [360-degree turn or greater], and sigmoid torsion [up to an 180-degree turn]), gastroenteritis, irritable colon, vascular injury due to arterial occlusion, and selected cases of acute appendicitis.

Interfering factors

■ Inadequate bowel preparation (possible poor imaging)

■ Barium retained from previous studies (possible poor imaging)
■ The patient's inability to retain barium

Hypotonic duodenography

Hypotonic duodenography is the fluoroscopic examination of the duodenum after instillation of barium sulfate and air through an intestinal catheter. This test is indicated in patients with symptoms of duodenal or pancreatic pathology such as persistent upper abdominal pain.

After the catheter is passed through the patient's nose into the duodenum, I.V. infusion of glucagon or I.M. injection of propantheline bromide (or another anticholinergic) induces duodenal atony. Instillation of barium and air distends the relaxed duodenum, flattening its deep circular folds; spot films then record the precise delineation of the duodenal anatomy. Although these films readily demonstrate small duodenal lesions and tumors of the head of the pancreas that impinge on the duodenal wall, differential diagnosis requires further studies.

Purpose

■ To detect small, postbulbar duodenal lesions, tumors of the head of the pancreas, and tumors of the ampulla of Vater
■ To aid in the diagnosis of chronic pancreatitis

Patient preparation

■ Explain to the patient that hypotonic duodenography permits examination of the duodenum and pancreas after the instillation of barium and air.
■ Instruct the patient to fast after midnight the night before the test.
■ Describe the test, including who will perform it and where it will take place.

- Inform the patient that a tube will be passed through his nose into the duodenum to serve as a channel for the barium and air.
- Tell the patient that he may experience a cramping pain as air is introduced into the duodenum. Instruct him to breathe deeply and slowly through his mouth if he experiences this pain to help relax the abdominal muscles.
- If glucagon or an anticholinergic is to be administered during the procedure, describe the possible adverse effects of glucagon (nausea, vomiting, hives, and flushing) or of anticholinergics (dry mouth, thirst, tachycardia, urine retention, and blurred vision). If an anticholinergic is administered to an outpatient, advise him to have someone accompany him home.
- Just before the test, tell the patient to remove dentures, glasses, necklaces, hairpins, combs, and constricting undergarments.
- Instruct the patient to void.

Procedure and posttest care

- While the patient is sitting, a catheter is passed through his nose into the stomach. He's then placed in a supine position on an X-ray table, and the catheter is advanced into the duodenum under fluoroscopic guidance.
- I.V. glucagon is administered, which quickly induces duodenal atony for approximately 20 minutes, or an anticholinergic is injected I.M.
- Barium is instilled through the catheter, and spot films are taken of the duodenum.
- Some of the barium is then withdrawn, air is instilled, and additional spot films are taken.
- When the required films have been obtained, the catheter is removed.

- After the procedure, encourage the patient to drink extra fluids (unless contraindicated) to help eliminate the barium.
- Throughout the procedure, observe the patient for adverse reactions. Be aware that such reactions may follow administration of glucagon or an anticholinergic. If an anticholinergic was given, make sure the patient voids within a few hours after the test. Advise the outpatient to rest in a waiting area until his vision clears (about 2 hours) unless someone can take him home.
- Administer a cathartic, as prescribed.
- Tell the patient that he may burp instilled air or pass flatus and that the barium colors the stool chalky white for 24 to 72 hours. Extra fluid may be ordered to aid barium elimination.
- Record a description of stool passed by the patient in the hospital and notify the physician if the patient hasn't expelled the barium after 2 to 3 days.

Precautions

- Anticholinergics are contraindicated in the patient with severe cardiac disorders or glaucoma.
- Glucagon is contraindicated in the patient with uncontrolled diabetes and should be used cautiously in the patient with type 1 diabetes mellitus.
- The patient with strictures in the upper GI tract, particularly those associated with ulcerations or large masses, should not undergo this procedure.
- Monitor the elderly or extremely ill patient for gastric reflux.
- This test is contraindicated in the pregnant patient because of radiation's possible teratogenic effects.

Normal findings

When barium and air distend the atonic duodenum, the mucosa normally appears smooth and even. The regular contour of the head of the pancreas also appears on the duodenal wall.

Abnormal findings

Irregular nodules or masses on the duodenal wall could mean duodenal lesions, tumors of the ampulla of Vater, tumors of the head of the pancreas, or chronic pancreatitis. Differential diagnosis requires further tests, such as endoscopic retrograde cholangiopancreatography, serum and urine amylase tests, ultrasonography of the pancreas, and computed tomography of the pancreas.

Interfering factors

■ Failure to fast

Oral cholecystography

Oral cholecystography is the radiographic examination of the gallbladder after administration of a contrast medium. This test is now commonly replaced by nuclear medicine ^{99}technetium-labeled scan, ultrasound, and computerized tomography. It's indicated in patients with symptoms of biliary tract disease, such as right upper quadrant epigastric pain, fat intolerance, and jaundice, and is most commonly performed to confirm gallbladder disease.

After the contrast medium is ingested, it's absorbed by the small intestine, filtered by the liver, excreted in the bile, and then concentrated and stored in the gallbladder. Full gallbladder opacification usually occurs 12 to 14 hours after ingestion, and a series of X-ray films then records gallbladder appearance. Additional information is obtained by giving the patient a fat stimulus, causing the gallbladder to contract and empty the

contrast-laden bile into the common bile duct and small intestine. Films are then taken to record this emptying and to evaluate common bile duct patency.

Oral cholecystography should precede barium studies because retained barium may cloud subsequent X-ray films.

Purpose

■ To detect gallstones
■ To aid in the diagnosis of inflammatory disease and gallbladder tumors

Patient preparation

■ Explain to the patient that oral cholecystography permits examination of the gallbladder through X-ray films taken after ingestion of a contrast medium.
■ Describe the test, including who will perform it and where it will take place.
■ Instruct the patient to eat a normal meal at noon the day before the test and a fat-free meal in the evening. The former stimulates release of bile from the gallbladder, preparing it to receive the contrast-laden bile; the latter inhibits gallbladder contraction, promoting bile accumulation.
■ Instruct the patient to restrict food and fluids (except water) after the evening meal.
■ Give the patient six tablets (3 g) of iopanoic acid 2 or 3 hours after the evening meal, as necessary. (Other commercial contrast agents are available, such as sodium ipodate, but iopanoic acid is most commonly used.) Have the patient swallow the tablets one at a time at 5-minute intervals, with one or two mouthfuls of water for a total of 8 oz (236.6 ml) of water. Thereafter, withhold water, cigarettes, and gum.

- Tell the patient that he'll be placed on an X-ray table and that films will be taken of his gallbladder.
- Check the patient's history for hypersensitivity to iodine, seafood, or contrast media used for other diagnostic tests.
- Inform the patient that the possible adverse effects of dye ingestion include diarrhea (common) and, rarely, nausea, vomiting, abdominal cramps, and dysuria. Tell him to report such symptoms immediately if they develop.
- Examine any vomitus or diarrhea for undigested tablets. If tablets were expelled, notify the X-ray department.
- Administer an enema the morning of the test, if prescribed. This clears the GI tract of interfering shadows that may obscure the gallbladder.

Procedure and posttest care
- After the patient is in a prone position on the radiographic table, the abdomen is examined fluoroscopically to evaluate gallbladder opacification, and films are taken of significant findings.
- The patient is then examined while in the left lateral decubitus and erect positions to detect possible layering or mobility of any filling defects, and additional films are taken.
- The patient may then be given a fat stimulus, such as a high-fat meal or a synthetic fat-containing agent (such as sincalide).
- Fluoroscopy is used to observe gallbladder emptying in response to the fat stimulus, and spot films are taken at 15- and 30-minute intervals to visualize the common bile duct. If the gallbladder empties slowly or not at all, these films are also taken at 60 minutes.
- If the test results are normal, tell the patient he may resume his usual diet.

- If gallstones are discovered during opacification, the patient will need an appropriate diet — usually one that restricts fat intake — to help prevent acute attacks.
- Nonopacification and repeat cholecystography require continuation of a low-fat diet until definitive diagnosis can be made.

Precautions
- Oral cholecystography is contraindicated in the patient with severe renal or hepatic damage and in the patient with hypersensitivity to iodine, seafood, or contrast media.
- This test is also contraindicated in the pregnant patient because of radiation's possible teratogenic effects.

Normal findings
The gallbladder is normally opacified and appears pear-shaped, with smooth, thin walls. Although its size is variable, its basic structure — neck, infundibulum, body, and fundus — is clearly outlined on film.

Abnormal findings
When the gallbladder is opacified, filling defects (typically appearing within the lumen as negative shadows that show mobility) indicate the presence of gallstones. Fixed defects, on the other hand, may indicate the presence of cholesterol polyps or a benign tumor such as an adenomyoma.

When the gallbladder fails to opacify or when only faint opacification occurs, inflammatory disease such as cholecystitis — with or without gallstone formation — may be present. Gallstones may obstruct the cystic duct and prevent the contrast medium from entering the gallbladder; inflammation may impair the concentrating ability of the gallbladder mucosa and prevent or diminish opacification.

When the gallbladder fails to contract following stimulation by a fatty meal, cholecystitis or common bile duct obstruction may be present. If the X-ray films are inconclusive, oral cholecystography is repeated the following day.

Interfering factors

- Inability to remain still
- Failure to follow dietary restrictions
- The patient's failure to ingest the full dose of contrast medium or partial loss of contrast medium through emesis or diarrhea (may invalidate test results)
- Inadequate absorption of the contrast medium in the small intestine or barium retained from previous studies (may invalidate test results)
- Decreased excretion of the contrast medium into the bile duct to impaired hepatic function and moderate jaundice (possible poor imaging)

Percutaneous transhepatic cholangiography

Percutaneous transhepatic cholangiography is the fluoroscopic examination of the biliary ducts after injection of an iodinated contrast medium directly into a biliary radicle. This test is especially useful for evaluating patients with persistent upper abdominal pain after cholecystectomy or severe jaundice.

Although a computed tomography scan or ultrasonography is usually performed first when obstructive jaundice is suspected, percutaneous transhepatic cholangiography may provide the most detailed view of the obstruction; however, this invasive procedure carries a potential risk of complications that include bleed-

ing, septicemia, bile peritonitis, extravasation of the contrast medium into the peritoneal cavity, and subcapsular injection.

Purpose

- To determine the cause of upper abdominal pain following cholecystectomy
- To distinguish between obstructive and nonobstructive jaundice
- To determine the location, the extent and, commonly, the cause of mechanical obstruction

Patient preparation

- Explain to the patient that percutaneous transhepatic cholangiography allows examination of the biliary ducts through X-ray films taken after a contrast medium is injected into the liver.
- Instruct the patient to fast for 8 hours before the test.
- Describe the test, including who will perform it and where it will take place.
- Inform the patient that he may receive a laxative the night before and an enema the morning of the test.
- Inform the patient that he'll be placed on a tilting X-ray table that rotates into vertical and horizontal positions during the procedure.
- Assure the patient that he'll be adequately secured to the table and assisted to supine and side-lying positions throughout the procedure.
- Warn the patient that injection of the local anesthetic may sting the skin and produce transient pain when it punctures the liver capsule.
- Advise the patient that injection of the contrast medium may produce a sensation of pressure and epigastric fullness and may cause transient upper back pain on his right side.

- Tell the patient that he must rest for at least 6 hours after the procedure.
- Make sure that the patient or a responsible family member has signed an informed consent form.
- Check the patient's history for hypersensitivity to iodine, seafood, contrast media used in other diagnostic tests, and the local anesthetic. Advise him of possible adverse effects of contrast medium administration, such as nausea, vomiting, excessive salivation, flushing, urticaria, sweating and, rarely, anaphylaxis; tachycardia and fever may accompany intraductal injection.
- Check the patient's history for normal bleeding, clotting, and prothrombin times and a normal platelet count. If prescribed, administer 1 g of I.V. ampicillin every 4 to 6 hours for 24 hours before the procedure.
- Just before the procedure, administer a sedative, if prescribed.

Procedure and posttest care

- After the patient is placed in a supine position on the X-ray table and is adequately secured, the right upper quadrant of the abdomen is cleaned and draped; the skin, subcutaneous tissue, and liver capsule are infiltrated with a local anesthetic.
- While the patient holds his breath at the end of expiration, the flexible needle is inserted under fluoroscopic guidance through the 10th or 11th intercostal space at the right midclavicular line.
- The needle is aimed toward the xiphoid process and is advanced through the liver parenchyma. It's then slowly withdrawn, injecting the contrast medium to locate a biliary radicle. When fluoroscopy reveals placement in a radicle, the needle is held in position and the remaining contrast medium is injected.

- Using a fluoroscope and television monitor, biliary duct opacification is observed, and spot films of significant findings are taken with the patient in supine and lateral recumbent positions. When the required films have been taken, the needle is removed.
- Apply a sterile dressing to the puncture site.
- Check the patient's vital signs until they're stable.
- Enforce bed rest for at least 6 hours after the test, preferably with the patient lying on his right side, to help prevent hemorrhage.
- Check the injection site for bleeding, swelling, and tenderness. Watch for signs of peritonitis: chills, temperature of 102° to 103° F (38.8° to 39.4° C), and abdominal pain, tenderness, and distention. Notify the physician immediately if such complications develop.
- Tell the patient that he may resume his usual diet.

Precautions

- Percutaneous transhepatic cholangiography is contraindicated in the patient with cholangitis, massive ascites, uncorrectable coagulopathy, or hypersensitivity to iodine as well as in the pregnant patient because of radiation's possible teratogenic effects.

Normal findings

The biliary ducts are of normal diameter and appear as regular channels homogeneously filled with contrast medium.

Abnormal findings

Distinguishing between obstructive and nonobstructive jaundice hinges on whether biliary ducts are dilated or of normal size. Obstructive jaundice is associated with dilated ducts; nonobstructive jaundice, with normal-sized ducts. When ducts are dilated, the obstruction site may be defined. Obstruction may result from cholelithiasis, biliary tract carcinoma, or carcinoma of the pancreas or papilla of Vater that impinges on the common bile duct, causing deviation or stricture.

When ducts are of normal size and intrahepatic cholestasis is indicated, liver biopsy may be performed to distinguish among hepatitis, cirrhosis, and granulomatous disease. If ducts are dilated as a result of obstruction, a drainage tube may be inserted to allow percutaneous drainage of bile into a collection bag.

Interfering factors
■ Marked obesity or gas overlying the biliary ducts (possible poor imaging)

Postoperative cholangiography

During cholecystectomy or common bile duct exploration, a T-shaped rubber tube may be inserted into the common bile duct to facilitate drainage. Postoperative cholangiography — radiographic and fluoroscopic examination of the biliary ducts — may be performed 7 to 10 days after surgery.

This procedure requires injection of contrast medium through the T-tube. The contrast medium flows through the biliary ducts and outlines the size and patency of the ducts, revealing any obstruction overlooked during surgery.

Purpose
■ To detect calculi, strictures, neoplasms, and fistulae in the biliary ducts

Patient preparation
■ Explain to the patient that postoperative cholangiography permits examination of the biliary ducts through X-ray films taken after the injection of a contrast medium.
■ Describe the test, including who will perform it and where it will take place.
■ Warn the patient that he may feel a bloating sensation (not pain) in the right upper quadrant as the contrast medium is injected.
■ Clamp the T-tube the day before the procedure, if necessary. Because bile fills the tube after clamping, this helps prevent air bubbles from entering the ducts.
■ Withhold the meal just before the test and administer an enema about 1 hour before the procedure.
■ Make sure that the patient or a responsible family member has signed an informed consent form.
■ Check the patient's history for hypersensitivity to iodine, seafood, or contrast media used in other diagnostic tests. Tell the patient that the adverse effects of intraductal administration may include nausea, vomiting, excessive salivation, flushing, urticaria, sweating and, rarely, anaphylaxis.

Procedure and posttest care
■ After the patient is in a supine position on the X-ray table, the injection area of the T-tube is cleaned with sponges soaked with povidone-iodine solution. The T-tube is held in a vertical position, which allows trapped air to surface, and a needle attached to a long transparent catheter is carefully inserted into the end of the T-tube. Care must be taken to avoid injecting air into the biliary tree because air bubbles may affect the clarity of the X-ray films.
■ Approximately 5 ml of contrast medium (usually sodium diatrizoate) is injected under fluoroscopic guidance, and a spot film is taken in the anteroposterior

position. Additional injections are then administered, and spot films and plain films are taken with the patient in supine and right lateral decubitus positions.

■ The T-tube is then clamped and the patient is assisted to an erect position for additional films; in this position, air bubbles may be distinguished from calculi or other pathology.

■ A final film is taken 15 minutes after contrast injection to record the emptying of contrast-laden bile into the duodenum. If emptying is delayed, additional films may be taken at 15- or 30-minute intervals until this action is demonstrated.

■ If a sterile dressing is applied after T-tube removal, observe and record any drainage. Change the dressing, as necessary.

■ If the T-tube is left in place, attach it to the drainage system.

■ Tell the patient that he may resume his usual diet and activity, as directed.

Precautions

■ Postoperative cholangiography is contraindicated in the patient who's hypersensitive to iodine, seafood, or contrast media used in other tests.

Normal findings

Biliary ducts demonstrate homogeneous filling with contrast medium and are normal in diameter. When Oddi's sphincter is functioning properly and the ducts are patent, the contrast flows unimpeded into the duodenum.

Abnormal findings

Negative shadows or filling defects within the biliary ducts associated with dilation may indicate calculi or neoplasms overlooked during surgery. Abnormal channels of contrast medium departing from the biliary ducts indicate fistulae.

Interfering factors

■ Marked obesity or gas overlying the biliary ducts (possible poor imaging)

Endoscopic retrograde cholangiopancreatography

Endoscopic retrograde cholangiopancreatography (ERCP) is the radiographic examination of the pancreatic ducts and hepatobiliary tree after injection of a contrast medium into the duodenal papilla. It's indicated in the patient with confirmed or suspected pancreatic disease or obstructive jaundice of unknown etiology. Complications may include cholangitis and pancreatitis.

Purpose

■ To evaluate obstructive jaundice
■ To diagnose cancer of the duodenal papilla, pancreas, and biliary ducts
■ To locate calculi and stenosis in the pancreatic ducts and hepatobiliary tree
■ To identify leaks from trauma or surgery

Patient preparation

■ Explain to the patient that ERCP permits examination of the liver, gallbladder, and pancreas through X-ray films taken after injection of a contrast medium.
■ Instruct the patient to fast after midnight before the test.
■ Describe the test, including who will perform it and where it will take place.
■ Inform the patient that a local anesthetic will be sprayed into his mouth to calm the gag reflex. Warn him that the spray has an unpleasant taste and makes

the tongue and throat feel swollen, causing difficulty swallowing.

■ Instruct the patient to let saliva drain from the side of his mouth and tell him that suction may be used to remove saliva. Tell him a mouth guard will be inserted to protect his teeth and the endoscope; assure him that it won't obstruct his breathing.

■ Tell the patient that he'll receive a sedative before insertion of the endoscope to help him relax, but that he'll remain conscious.

■ Tell the patient that he'll also receive an anticholinergic or I.V. glucagon after endoscope insertion. Describe the possible adverse effects of anticholinergics (dry mouth, thirst, tachycardia, urine retention, and blurred vision) or of glucagon (nausea, vomiting, urticaria, and flushing).

■ Warn the patient that he may experience transient flushing on injection of the contrast medium. Advise him that he may have a sore throat for 3 or 4 days after the examination.

■ Make sure that the patient or a responsible family member has signed an informed consent form.

■ Check the patient's history for hypersensitivity to iodine, seafood, or contrast media used for other diagnostic procedures and inform the physician of sensitivities.

■ Just before the procedure, obtain the patient's baseline vital signs. Instruct him to remove all metallic or other radiopaque objects and constricting undergarments. Then tell him to void to minimize the discomfort of urine retention that may follow the procedure.

Procedure and posttest care
■ An I.V. infusion is started with 150 ml of normal saline solution. The local anesthetic is then administered and usually takes effect in about 10 minutes.

■ If an anesthetic spray is used, ask the patient to hold his breath while his mouth and throat are sprayed.

■ Place the patient in a left lateral position and give him an emesis basin; provide tissues. Because the anesthetic causes the patient to lose some control of his secretions and thus increases the risk of aspiration, encourage him to allow saliva to drain from the side of his mouth.

■ Insert a mouth guard.

■ While the patient remains in the left lateral position, 5 to 20 mg of I.V. diazepam or midazolam is administered as well as an opioid analgesic, if needed.

■ When ptosis or dysarthria develops, the patient's head is bent forward and he's asked to open his mouth.

■ The examiner inserts his left index finger in the patient's mouth and guides the tip of the endoscope along his finger to the back of the patient's throat. The scope is then deflected downward with the left index finger and advanced. As the endoscope passes through the posterior pharynx and cricopharyngeal sphincter, the patient's head is slowly extended to assist the advance of the endoscope. The patient's chin must be kept midline. When the endoscope has passed the cricopharyngeal sphincter, the scope is advanced under direct vision. When it's well into the esophagus, the patient's chin is moved toward the table so saliva can drain from the mouth. The endoscope is advanced through the remainder of the esophagus and into the stomach under direct vision.

■ When the pylorus is located, a small amount of air is insufflated, and the tip of the endoscope is angled upward and passed into the duodenal bulb.

- After the endoscope is rotated clockwise to enter the descending duodenum, the patient is assisted to a prone position.
- An anticholinergic or I.V. glucagon is administered to induce duodenal atony and to relax the ampullary sphincter.
- A small amount of air is insufflated, and the endoscope is manipulated until the optic lies opposite the duodenal papilla. Then the cannula filled with contrast medium is passed through the biopsy channel of the endoscope, the duodenal papilla, and into the ampulla of Vater.
- The pancreatic duct is visualized first under fluoroscopic guidance with injection of contrast medium.
- The cannula is repositioned at a more cephalad angle, and the hepatobiliary tree is visualized with injection of contrast medium.
- After each injection, rapid-sequence X-ray films are taken.
- Instruct the patient to remain prone while the films are developed and reviewed. If necessary, additional films may be taken.
- When the required radiographs have been obtained, the cannula is removed. Before the endoscope is withdrawn, a tissue specimen may be obtained or fluid aspirated for histologic and cytologic examination, respectively.
- Observe the patient closely for signs of cholangitis and pancreatitis. Hyperbilirubinemia, fever, and chills are the immediate signs of cholangitis; hypotension associated with gram-negative septicemia may develop later. Left upper quadrant pain and tenderness, elevated serum amylase levels, and transient hyperbilirubinemia are the usual signs of pancreatitis. Draw blood samples for amylase and bilirubin determinations, if necessary, but remember that these levels usually rise after ERCP.
- Observe the patient for signs of perforation, such as abdominal pain, bleeding, and fever.
- Tell the patient that he may experience a feeling of fullness, some cramping, and passage of flatus several hours after the test.
- Continue to watch the patient for signs of respiratory depression, apnea, hypotension, excessive diaphoresis, bradycardia, and laryngospasm. Check his vital signs every 15 minutes for 1 hour, every 30 minutes for the next 2 hours, every hour for the next 4 hours, and then every 4 hours for 48 hours.
- Withhold food and fluids until the patient's gag reflex returns. Test the gag reflex by touching the back of his throat with a tongue blade. When the gag reflex returns, allow fluids and a light meal.
- Discontinue or maintain the I.V. infusion, as ordered.
- Check for signs of urine retention. Notify the physician if the patient hasn't voided within 8 hours.
- If the patient has a sore throat, provide soothing lozenges and warm saline gargles to ease discomfort.
- If a tissue biopsy or polypectomy occurred, a small amount of blood in the patient's first stool is normal. Report excessive bleeding immediately.
- If this test is performed on an outpatient basis, be sure that transportation is available. The patient who has undergone anesthesia or sedation shouldn't operate an automobile for at least 12 hours postprocedure. Alcohol should be avoided for 24 hours.

Precautions

- ERCP is contraindicated in the pregnant patient, due to risk of fetal harm secondary to radiation exposure.

- ERCP is contraindicated in the patient with infectious disease, pancreatic pseudocysts, stricture or obstruction of the esophagus or duodenum, or acute pancreatitis, cholangitis, or cardiorespiratory disease.
- The patient receiving anticoagulants has an increased risk of bleeding.
- Monitor the patient's vital signs and airway patency throughout the procedure. Watch him for signs of respiratory depression, apnea, hypotension, excessive diaphoresis, bradycardia, and laryngospasm. Be sure to have available emergency resuscitation equipment and an opioid antagonist such as naloxone.
- If the patient has known cardiac disease, continuous electrocardiographic monitoring should be instituted. Continuing periodic pulse oximetry is advisable, particularly in the patient with pulmonary compromise.

Normal findings

The duodenal papilla appears as a small red (or sometimes pale) erosion protruding into the lumen. Its orifice is commonly bordered by a fringe of white mucosa, and a longitudinal fold running perpendicular to the deep circular folds of the duodenum helps mark its location. Although the pancreatic and hepatobiliary ducts usually unite in the ampulla of Vater and empty through the duodenal papilla, separate orifices are sometimes present.

The contrast medium uniformly fills the pancreatic duct, hepatobiliary tree, and gallbladder.

Abnormal findings

Obstructive jaundice may result from various abnormalities of the hepatobiliary tree and pancreatic duct. Examination of the hepatobiliary tree may reveal stones, strictures, or irregular deviations that suggest biliary cirrhosis, primary sclerosing cholangitis, or carcinoma of the bile ducts.

Examination of the pancreatic ducts may also show stones, strictures, and irregular deviations that may indicate pancreatic cysts and pseudocysts, a pancreatic tumor, carcinoma of the head of the pancreas, chronic pancreatitis, pancreatic fibrosis, carcinoma of the duodenal papilla, and papillary stenosis.

Depending on test findings, a definitive diagnosis may require further studies. In addition, certain interventions, such as stent placement to allow drainage or a papillotomy to decrease scar tissue and allow light drainage, may be indicated.

Interfering factors

- Barium in the GI tract from previous studies (possible poor imaging)

Celiac and mesenteric arteriography

Celiac and mesenteric arteriography involves the radiographic examination of the abdominal vasculature after intra-arterial injection of a contrast medium through a catheter. Most commonly, the catheter is passed through the femoral artery into the aorta and then, using fluoroscopy, is positioned in the celiac, superior mesenteric, or inferior mesenteric artery. Injection of a contrast medium into one or more of these arteries provides a map of abdominal vasculature; injection into specific arterial branches, called superselective angiography, permits detailed visualization of a particular area. As the contrast medium flows through the abdominal vasculature, serial radiographs outline abdominal vessels in the arterial, capillary, and venous phases of perfusion.

Celiac and mesenteric arteriography is indicated when endoscopy can't locate the source of GI bleeding or when barium studies, ultrasonography, and nuclear medicine or computed tomography scanning prove inconclusive in evaluating neoplasms. It's also used to evaluate cirrhosis and portal hypertension (especially when a portacaval shunt is being considered); to evaluate vascular damage, particularly in the spleen and liver, after abdominal trauma; and to detect vascular abnormalities. Because arteriography can demonstrate the portal vein even when portal venous flow is reversed, it's used more often than splenoportography.

Complications associated with this test include hemorrhage, venous and intracardiac thrombosis, cardiac arrhythmia, and emboli caused by dislodging atherosclerotic plaques.

Purpose

■ To locate the source of GI bleeding
■ To help distinguish between benign and malignant neoplasms
■ To evaluate cirrhosis and portal hypertension
■ To evaluate vascular damage after abdominal trauma
■ To detect vascular abnormalities

Patient preparation

■ Explain to the patient that celiac and mesenteric arteriography permits examination of the abdominal blood vessels after injection of a contrast medium.
■ Instruct the patient to fast for 8 hours before the test.
■ Tell the patient that he'll receive I.V. conscious sedation and a local anesthetic and that he may feel a brief, stinging sensation as the anesthetic is injected. He

may also feel pressure when the femoral artery is palpated, but the local anesthetic will minimize the pain when the needle is introduced into the artery.
■ Tell the patient that he may feel a transient burning as the contrast medium is injected.
■ Tell the patient that the X-ray equipment makes a loud, clacking sound as the films are taken.
■ Instruct the patient to lie still during the test to avoid blurring the films and inform him that restraints may be used to help him remain still.
■ Warn the patient that he may feel some temporary stiffness after the test from lying still on the hard X-ray table.
■ Tell the patient who will perform the test, where it will take place, and that it takes 30 minutes to 3 hours, depending on the number of vessels studied.
■ Make sure that the patient or a responsible family member has signed an informed consent form.
■ Check the patient's history for hypersensitivity to iodine, shellfish, or the contrast medium.
■ Make sure blood studies (hemoglobin and hematocrit levels; clotting, prothrombin, and partial thromboplastin times; and platelet count) have been completed.
■ Just before the procedure, instruct the patient to put on a gown and to remove jewelry and other objects that might obscure anatomic detail on X-ray films.
■ Tell the patient to void, and then record his baseline vital signs.
■ Administer a sedative, if prescribed.

Procedure and posttest care

■ After the patient is placed in a supine position on the X-ray table, an I.V. infusion is started to maintain hydration and to permit emergency administration of medication. The patient is attached to a heart monitor and pulse oximeter and his blood pressure is monitored according to facility policy.

■ Spot films of the patient's abdomen are taken, and the peripheral pulses are palpated and marked.

■ The puncture site is cleaned with soap and water; the area is shaved, cleaned with povidone-iodine preparation, and surrounded by sterile drapes.

■ The local anesthetic is injected and the femoral artery is located by palpation. The needle is gently inserted until a pulsing blood flow is obtained.

■ A guide wire is passed through the needle into the aorta, and then the needle is removed, leaving the guide wire in place.

■ The catheter is inserted over the guide wire and then withdrawn to inject the contrast medium to check for catheter placement. The guide wire is again inserted into the selected artery for fluoroscopic guidance.

■ When the wire is in position, the catheter is advanced over it into the artery. The wire is then removed and placement verified by hand injection of contrast medium.

■ The automatic injector is then attached to the catheter. As the contrast medium is injected, a series of films is taken in rapid sequence.

■ After injecting into one or more major arteries, superselective catheterization may be performed. Using fluoroscopy, the catheter is repositioned in a specific branch of a major artery, contrast medium is injected, and rapid-sequence films are taken. If necessary, several specific branches may be catheterized.

■ If an occlusion is detected, balloon angioplasty is performed.

■ After filming, the catheter is withdrawn and firm pressure is applied to the puncture site for about 15 minutes.

■ Observe the puncture site for hematoma formation and check peripheral pulses.

■ Inform the patient that he'll be on bed rest for 4 to 6 hours and that he must keep the leg with the puncture site straight. Don't raise the bed further than 30 degrees. He'll be able to logroll and may use the unaffected leg to reposition himself to use the bedpan.

■ Monitor the patient's vital signs until stable and check peripheral pulses. Note the color and temperature of the leg that was used for the test.

■ Check the puncture site for bleeding and hematoma. If bleeding develops, apply pressure to the site. If a hematoma develops, apply warm soaks.

■ Confirm whether the patient can resume his usual diet. If the patient isn't receiving I.V. infusions, encourage intake of fluids to speed excretion of the contrast medium.

Precautions

■ Celiac and mesenteric arteriography should be performed cautiously in the patient with coagulopathy.

▶ **CLINICAL ALERT** *Most reactions to the contrast medium occur within ½ hour. Watch the patient carefully for cardiovascular shock or arrest, flushing, laryngeal stridor, or urticaria.*

■ This test is contraindicated in the pregnant patient because of radiation's possible teratogenic effects.

Normal findings

X-ray films show the three phases of perfusion — arterial, capillary, and venous. The arteries normally taper regularly, becoming gradually smaller with subsequent divisions. The contrast medium then spreads evenly within the sinusoids. The portal vein appears 10 to 20 seconds after the injection as the contrast medium empties from the spleen into the splenic vein or from the intestine into the superior mesenteric vein and further into the portal vein.

Abnormal findings

GI hemorrhage appears on the angiogram as the extravasation of contrast medium from the damaged vessels. Upper GI hemorrhage can result from such conditions as Mallory-Weiss syndrome, a gastric or peptic ulcer, hemorrhagic gastritis, and an eroded hiatal hernia. Esophageal hemorrhage rarely appears on the angiogram because the contrast medium usually fails to fill the esophageal vein. Lower GI hemorrhage can result from such conditions as bleeding diverticula, carcinoma, and angiodysplasia.

Abdominal neoplasms — carcinoid tumors, adenomas, leiomyomas, angiomas, and adenocarcinomas — can disrupt the normal vasculature in several ways. Neoplasms can invade or encase nearby arteries and veins, distorting their regular channel-like appearance and, in late stages, displacing them. Vessels within the neoplasm, known as neovasculature, appear as abnormal vascular areas. Areas of necrosis appear as puddles of contrast medium. Contrast medium may also remain in the neoplasm longer during capillary perfusion, producing a tumor blush or stain on the angiogram. Arteriovenous shunting may also be present, depending on the size and location of the tumor. Because these characteristics aren't uniformly present in all neoplasms, combinations of these characteristics can usually distinguish between benign and malignant neoplasms.

In early or mild cirrhosis, portal venous flow to the liver remains relatively unaffected, and the hepatic artery and its branches appear normal. As this disease progresses, portal venous flow diminishes, the hepatic artery and its branches become dilated and tortuous, and collateral veins develop. In advanced cirrhosis, portal venous flow reverses. However, the portal vein still appears on the X-ray film, which may also show thrombi.

Abdominal trauma commonly causes splenic injury; less commonly, hepatic injury. Splenic rupture usually displaces intrasplenic arterial branches, causing the contrast medium to leak from splenic arteries into the splenic pulp. When rupture occurs without subcapsular hematoma, the spleen usually maintains its normal size. However, in subcapsular hematoma, the spleen enlarges to displace the splenic artery and vein; the subcapsular hematoma itself appears as a large, avascular mass that stretches intrasplenic arteries and compresses the splenic pulp away from the capsule.

Hepatic injury causes similar vascular distortion such as displacement of the common hepatic artery and extrahepatic branches. Intrahepatic and subcapsular hematomas displace and stretch intrahepatic arteries. As the hepatic vascular supply is disrupted, an arteriovenous fistula may develop between the hepatic artery and portal vein.

Various abnormalities affecting the diameter and course of an artery may appear on the angiogram. Atherosclerotic plaques or atheromas — lipid deposits on the intima — narrow the arterial lumen and may even occlude it, resulting in collateral formation. Other identifiable vascular abnormalities include aneurysms, thrombi, and emboli.

Interfering factors
- The patient's inability to remain still during the procedure
- Barium, gas, or stool from a previous procedure (possible poor imaging)
- Presence of an atherosclerotic lesion in the vessel to be cannulated (prevents the entry and passage of catheter)

Small-bowel enema

Small-bowel enema, also called *enteroclysis*, is the fluoroscopic examination of the small bowel using a contrast medium. In this procedure, a small-lumen catheter is inserted through the nose or mouth and passed through the stomach into the distal duodenum or jejunum. A small balloon at the tip of the catheter may be inflated to prevent reflux of the contrast medium into the stomach. Barium is instilled by infusion, and then methylcellulose may be infused to obtain a double-contrast study of the small bowel.

The contrast media distend and opacify the bowel loops to allow evaluation and diagnosis. Metoclopramide may also be administered to facilitate peristalsis (which helps pass the catheter into the small bowel). Fluoroscopy and spot films are used to demonstrate and evaluate the small bowel.

Purpose
- To diagnose and evaluate Crohn's disease
- To diagnose Meckel's diverticulum
- To aid in the diagnosis of small-bowel obstruction
- To detect tumors

Patient preparation
- Explain to the patient that enteroclysis evaluates the small bowel.

- Tell the patient that contrast media will be instilled into his bowel and that X-ray films will then be taken to track the flow of the media and allow evaluation of small-bowel function.
- Inform the patient that he'll receive a laxative (such as bisacodyl) the afternoon before the examination, and then he'll receive nothing by mouth until the test. (If the test is being done on an emergency basis, no preparation is required.)
- Inform the patient that he shouldn't take peristalsis-inhibiting drugs (such as meperidine or oxycodone and aspirin) on the day of the test.
- Tell the patient that the examination will take about 45 minutes and that just before the test, he'll be asked to change into a gown, remove his undergarments and jewelry, and empty his bladder.
- Inform the patient that an I.V. line will be inserted for medication administration.
- Explain to the patient that he may receive an I.V. sedative, if needed, and that a local anesthetic will be injected inside his nose to make the catheter insertion more comfortable. A GI stimulant (such as metoclopramide) will be administered to aid passage of the tube and to speed the flow of barium by increasing peristalsis.
- Tell the patient that he'll be asked to turn from side to side and sometimes onto his abdomen during the procedure. Inform the patient that his cooperation will help the test proceed smoothly.
- After the test is completed, tell the patient that he'll go to a recovery area until he's ready for discharge.
- If the patient is having the procedure as an outpatient, make sure that he has someone to drive him home if he receives I.V. sedation.

■ Make sure that the patient or a responsible family member has signed an informed consent form.

Procedure and posttest care
■ Place the patient in the supine position on the X-ray table with his neck slightly extended.

■ Administer I.V. medication to help relax the patient and to aid in the tube passage, as ordered.

■ The local anesthetic is administered nasally; instruct the patient to swallow if he feels it at the back of his throat. The tube is passed through the nose into the nasopharynx, and the patient's chin is brought down to the chest; the tube is advanced into the stomach and duodenum and, if possible, into the jejunum.

■ A small balloon is inflated at the catheter tip to prevent reflux of the contrast agent into the patient's stomach.

■ The barium contrast is administered by infusion pump. Methylcellulose is then administered to help propel the barium into the distal bowel. This double-contrast administration distends the bowel walls and opacifies the bowel loops, allowing clearer evaluation.

■ Then spot films and overhead films are taken. Barium flow is followed on fluoroscopy.

■ The physician examines individual bowel loops as they are opacified and compresses the abdomen to better evaluate the loops.

■ The patient is asked to turn from side to side during the examination.

■ After the examination, the balloon is deflated and the catheter is removed.

■ Assist the patient to the bathroom to expel the barium through defecation.

■ Observe the patient in the recovery area until he's ready for discharge.

■ Monitor the patient's vital signs until he's alert.

Precautions
■ The patient may experience discomfort with the passage of the catheter. Provide reassurance as well as the prescribed anesthetic and sedative when needed.

Normal findings
The bowel loops and walls are visible and are free from tumors, ulcers, and constrictions.

Abnormal findings
Anatomy of the bowel loops can be evaluated by observing Kerckring's folds, lumen diameters, and wall thickness. Abnormalities may indicate Crohn's disease, tumors, partial or complete bowel obstruction, Meckel's diverticula, or congenital disorders.

Interfering factors
■ Complete gastric or duodenal obstruction

NUCLEAR MEDICINE

Liver-spleen scanning

In liver-spleen scanning, a gamma camera records the distribution of radioactivity within the liver and spleen after I.V. injection of a radioactive colloid. The colloid most commonly used, technetium 99m (^{99m}Tc) sulfide, concentrates in the reticuloendothelial cells through phagocytosis. About 80% to 90% of the injected colloid is taken up by Kupffer's cells in the liver, 5% to 10% by the spleen, and 3% to 5% by bone marrow. The gamma camera images either organ instantaneously without moving.

Although the indications for this test include the detection of focal disease, such as tumors, cysts, and abscesses, liver-spleen scanning demonstrates focal disease nonspecifically as a "cold spot" (a defect that fails to take up the colloid) and may fail to detect focal lesions smaller than $3/4''$ (2 cm) in diameter. Although clinical signs and symptoms may aid diagnosis, liver-spleen scanning frequently requires confirmation by ultrasonography, computed tomography (CT) scan, gallium scanning, or biopsy. CT scan is the fastest method of evaluating liver or splenic injury in abdominal trauma and is preferred to other scans.

Purpose
- To screen for hepatic metastases and hepatocellular disease, such as cirrhosis and hepatitis
- To detect focal disease, such as tumors, cysts, and abscesses, in the liver and spleen
- To demonstrate hepatomegaly or splenomegaly (in patients with palpable abdominal masses)
- To assess the condition of the liver and spleen after abdominal trauma

Patient preparation
- Explain to the patient that liver-spleen scanning permits examination of the liver and spleen through scintigrams or scans taken after I.V. injection of a radioactive substance.
- Inform the patient that he need not restrict food and fluids.
- Tell the patient who will perform the test and where it will take place.
- Explain to the patient that he may experience transient discomfort from the needle puncture.

- Make sure the patient isn't scheduled for more than one radionuclide scan on the same day.
- Assure the patient that the injection isn't dangerous because the test substance contains only trace amounts of radioactivity and allergic reactions to it are rare.
- Explain to the patient that the detector head of the gamma camera may touch his abdomen (if appropriate) and reassure him that this isn't dangerous.
- Advise the patient that he'll be asked to lie still and to breathe quietly during the procedure to ensure good quality images; he may also be asked to hold his breath briefly. Explain that this technique helps to evaluate liver mobility and pliability.
- Make sure that the patient or a responsible family member has signed an informed consent form.

Equipment
Scanner, ^{99m}Tc sulfide, I.V. insertion equipment if needed

Procedure and posttest care
- The ^{99m}Tc sulfide is injected by I.V.; after 10 to 15 minutes, the patient's abdomen is scanned with the patient placed in supine, left and right lateral, left and right anterior oblique, and prone positions to ensure optimal visualization of the liver and spleen.
- The left anterior oblique position provides the best view of the spleen separate from the left lobe of the liver. With the patient supine, liver mobility and pliability may be evaluated by marking the costal margin and scanning as the patient breathes deeply (fixation suggests disease).
- The scintigrams are reviewed for clarity before the patient is allowed to leave. If necessary, additional views are obtained.

- Watch for anaphylactoid reactions (shortness of breath, chest tightness, itching, headache) or pyrogenic (fever-producing) reactions, which may result from a stabilizer, such as dextran or gelatin, added to ^{99m}Tc sulfide.
- Inform the patient that the radioactive substance is eliminated from the body within 6 to 24 hours. Urge him to increase his fluid intake (unless contraindicated) to encourage this process.
- Instruct the patient to flush the toilet immediately after urinating to reduce exposure to radiation in the urine.

Precautions
- Liver-spleen scanning is usually contraindicated in a child and in the pregnant or lactating patient.

Normal findings
Because the liver and spleen contain equal numbers of reticuloendothelial cells, both organs normally appear equally bright on the image. However, distribution of radioactive colloid is generally more uniform and homogeneous in the spleen than in the liver. The liver has various normal indentations and impressions, such as the gallbladder fossa and falciform ligament, that may mimic focal disease. (See *Identifying liver indentations in nuclear imaging,* page 800.)

Abnormal findings
Although liver-spleen scanning may fail to detect early hepatocellular disease, it shows characteristic, distinct patterns such as disease progresses. The most prominent sign of hepatocellular disease is a shift of the radioactive colloid that's caused by reduced hepatic blood flow and impaired Kupffer's cell function. This inhibits distribution of the colloid in the liver, causing the liver colloid distribution to appear uniformly decreased or patchy. The spleen and bone marrow then take up the abnormally large amounts of the colloid unabsorbed by the liver, thus concentrating more radioactivity than in the liver, and appear brighter on the scan. This same distribution pattern (colloid shift) also accompanies portal hypertension due to extrahepatic causes.

Hepatitis and cirrhosis are associated with hepatomegaly and a colloid shift, but certain characteristics help distinguish them. In hepatitis, colloid distribution is usually uniformly decreased; in cirrhosis, it's patchy. Splenomegaly is typical in cirrhosis, but not in hepatitis.

Metastasis to the liver or spleen may appear on the scan as a focal defect and requires biopsy to confirm the diagnosis. Liver metastasis usually originates in the GI or genitourinary tract, the breasts, or the lungs and is more common than metastasis to the spleen. After metastasis is confirmed, serial liver-spleen studies are useful in evaluating the effectiveness of therapy.

Because cysts, abscesses, and tumors fail to take up the radioactive colloid, they appear on the scan as solitary or multiple focal defects. Hepatic cysts may appear as solitary defects; polycystic hepatic disease, as multiple defects. Splenic cysts are less common than hepatic cysts and may have a parasitic or nonparasitic origin. Ultrasonography can confirm hepatic or splenic cysts.

Intrahepatic abscesses are usually pyogenic or amebic. Subphrenic abscesses, located beneath the diaphragm, may distort the dome of the right lobe. Splenic abscesses are characteristic in bacterial endocarditis. All abscesses require gallium scanning or ultrasonography to confirm diagnosis.

IDENTIFYING LIVER INDENTATIONS IN NUCLEAR IMAGING

In nuclear imaging, normal indentations and impressions may be mistaken for focal lesions. These drawings of the liver — anterior and posterior view — identify the contours and impressions that may be misread.

ANTERIOR VIEW

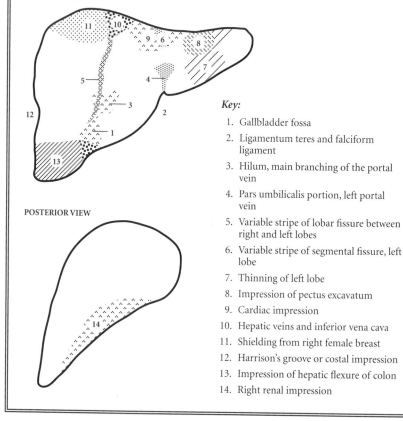

POSTERIOR VIEW

Key:
1. Gallbladder fossa
2. Ligamentum teres and falciform ligament
3. Hilum, main branching of the portal vein
4. Pars umbilicalis portion, left portal vein
5. Variable stripe of lobar fissure between right and left lobes
6. Variable stripe of segmental fissure, left lobe
7. Thinning of left lobe
8. Impression of pectus excavatum
9. Cardiac impression
10. Hepatic veins and inferior vena cava
11. Shielding from right female breast
12. Harrison's groove or costal impression
13. Impression of hepatic flexure of colon
14. Right renal impression

Benign hepatic tumors — such as hemangiomas, adenomas, and hamartomas — require confirming biopsy or flow studies. Primary malignant tumors, such as hepatomas, also require biopsy. Benign splenic tumors are rare and include hemangiomas, fibromas, myomas, and hamartomas. Primary malignant splenic tumors are also rare except in lymphoreticular malignancies such as Hodgkin's disease. Splenic tumors also require biopsy to confirm diagnosis. Although focal disease usually inhibits the uptake of the radioactive colloid, obstruction of the superior vena cava and Budd-Chiari syndrome cause markedly increased uptake.

Liver-spleen scanning can verify palpable abdominal masses and differentiate between splenomegaly and hepatomegaly.

A left upper quadrant mass may result from splenomegaly or, if the liver is grossly extended across the abdomen, from hepatomegaly. A right upper quadrant mass may result from hepatomegaly; a right lower quadrant mass may be a Riedel's lobe or a large dependent gallbladder. Splenic infarcts, commonly associated with bacterial endocarditis and massive splenomegaly, appear as peripheral defects, with decreased and irregular colloid distribution.

Scanning can assess hepatic injury after abdominal trauma. An intrahepatic hematoma appears as a focal defect; subcapsular hematoma, as a lentiform defect on the periphery of the liver; hepatic laceration, as a linear defect.

Scanning can also detect splenic injury after abdominal trauma. An intrahepatic hematoma appears as a focal defect; hepatic laceration appears as a linear defect. A splenic hematoma appears as a focal defect in or next to the spleen and may transect it. A subcapsular hematoma appears as a lentiform defect on the spleen's periphery.

Interfering factors
■ Radionuclides administered in other studies on the same day (possible poor imaging)
■ The patient's inability to remain still during the procedure

COMPUTED TOMOGRAPHY

Computed tomography of the liver and biliary tract

In computed tomography (CT) of the liver and biliary tract, multiple X-rays pass through the upper abdomen and are measured while detectors record differences in tissue attenuation. A computer reconstructs these data as a two-dimensional image on a monitor. CT scanning accurately distinguishes the biliary tract and the liver if the ducts are large. Use of I.V. contrast media during CT scanning can accentuate different densities.

Although CT scanning and ultrasonography detect biliary tract and liver disease equally well, the latter technique is performed more commonly. CT scanning is more expensive than ultrasonography and requires exposure to moderate amounts of radiation. However, it's the test of choice in patients who are obese and in those with livers positioned high under the rib cage because bone and excessive fat hinder ultrasound transmission.

Purpose
■ To distinguish between obstructive and nonobstructive jaundice
■ To detect intrahepatic tumors and abscesses, subphrenic and subhepatic abscesses, cysts, and hematomas

Patient preparation
■ Explain to the patient that CT scanning helps detect biliary tract and liver disease.
■ Tell the patient that he'll be given a contrast medium to drink and then he

should fast until after the examination. If contrast isn't ordered, fasting isn't necessary.

■ Explain to the patient who will perform the test and where it will take place.

■ Inform the patient that he'll be placed on an adjustable table, which is positioned inside a scanning gantry. Assure him that the test will be painless.

■ Tell the patient that he'll be asked to remain still during the test and to hold his breath when instructed. Stress the importance of remaining still during the test because movement can cause artifacts, thereby prolonging the test and limiting its accuracy.

■ If I.V. contrast medium is being used, inform the patient that he may experience transient discomfort from the needle puncture and a localized feeling of warmth on injection as well as a salty or metallic taste. Tell him to immediately report nausea, vomiting, dizziness, headache, and hives.

■ Check the patient's history for hypersensitivity to iodine, seafood, or the contrast media used in other diagnostic tests.

■ If a contrast medium has been ordered, give the patient the oral contrast medium supplied by the radiology department.

■ Make sure that the patient or a responsible family member has signed an informed consent form.

Procedure and posttest care

■ The patient is placed in a supine position on an X-ray table, and the table is positioned within the opening in the scanning gantry.

■ A series of transverse X-ray films is taken and recorded on magnetic tape. This information is reconstructed by a computer and appears as images on a television screen.

■ These images are studied, and selected ones are photographed. When the first series of films is completed, the images are reviewed.

■ Contrast enhancement may be performed. After the contrast medium is injected, a second series of films is taken, and the patient is carefully observed for an allergic reaction.

Precautions

■ CT scanning of the biliary tract and liver is usually contraindicated during pregnancy.

■ Use of an I.V. contrast medium is contraindicated in the patient with hypersensitivity to iodine or with severe renal or hepatic disease.

Normal findings

Normally, the liver has a uniform density that's slightly greater than that of the pancreas, kidneys, and spleen. Linear and circular areas of slightly lower density, representing hepatic vascular structures, may interrupt this uniform appearance. The portal vein is usually visible; the hepatic artery usually isn't. I.V. contrast medium enhances the isodensity of vascular structures and liver parenchyma.

Typically, intrahepatic biliary radicles aren't visible, but the common hepatic and bile ducts may be visible as low-density structures. Because bile has the same density as water, use of an I.V. contrast medium improves demarcation of the biliary tract by enhancing the surrounding parenchyma and vascular structures.

Like the biliary ducts, the gallbladder is visible as a round or elliptic low-density structure. A contracted gallbladder may be impossible to visualize.

Abnormal findings

Most focal hepatic defects appear less dense than the normal parenchyma, and CT scans can detect small lesions. Use of rapid-sequence scanning with an I.V. contrast medium helps distinguish between the two because the normal parenchyma shows greater enhancement than focal defects.

Primary and metastatic neoplasms may appear as well-circumscribed or poorly defined areas of slightly lower density than the normal parenchyma. However, some lesions have the same density as the liver parenchyma and may be undetectable. Neoplasms that are especially large may distort the liver's contour. Hepatic abscesses appear as relatively low-density, homogeneous areas, usually with well-defined borders. Hepatic cysts appear as sharply defined round or oval structures and have a density lower than abscesses and neoplasms.

The density of a hepatic hematoma varies with its age. A recent clot is as dense as or slightly more dense than the normal parenchyma; a resolving clot is somewhat less dense than the normal parenchyma. Intrahepatic hematomas vary in shape; subcapsular hematomas are usually crescent-shaped and compress the liver away from the capsule.

When distinguishing between obstructive and nonobstructive jaundice, biliary duct dilation indicates the former and an absence of dilation indicates the latter. Dilated intrahepatic bile ducts appear as low-density linear and circular branching structures. Dilation of the common hepatic duct, common bile duct, and gallbladder may also be apparent, depending on the site and severity of obstruction. Use of an I.V. contrast medium helps detect biliary dilation, especially when the ducts are only slightly dilated.

Usually, CT scanning can identify the cause of obstruction — for example, calculi or pancreatic carcinoma. However, if the site of obstruction must be located before surgery, percutaneous transhepatic cholangiography or endoscopic retrograde cholangiopancreatography (less common) may be performed as well.

Interfering factors

■ Presence of oral or I.V. contrast media, including barium, in the bile duct from earlier tests (possible poor imaging)

Computed tomography of the pancreas

In computed tomography (CT) of the pancreas, multiple X-rays penetrate the upper abdomen while a detector records the differences in tissue attenuation, which is then displayed as an image on a television screen. A series of cross-sectional views can provide a detailed look at the pancreas. CT scanning accurately distinguishes the pancreas and surrounding organs and vessels if enough fat is present between the structures. Use of an I.V. or oral contrast medium can further accentuate differences in tissue density.

CT scanning is replacing ultrasonography as the test of choice for examining the pancreas. Although ultrasonography costs less and involves less risk for the patient, it's also less accurate. In retroperitoneal disorders, specifically when pancreatitis is suspected, CT scanning goes beyond ultrasonography by showing the general swelling that accompanies acute inflammation of the gland. In chronic cases, CT scanning easily detects calcium deposits commonly missed by simple radiography, particularly in obese patients.

Purpose
- To detect pancreatic carcinoma or pseudocysts
- To detect or evaluate pancreatitis
- To distinguish between pancreatic disorders and disorders of the retroperitoneum

Patient preparation
- Explain to the patient that CT scanning helps detect disorders of the pancreas.
- Instruct the patient to fast after administration of the oral contrast medium.
- Describe the test, including who will perform it and where it will take place.
- Tell the patient that he'll be placed on an adjustable table that's positioned inside a scanning gantry. Assure him that the procedure is painless.
- Explain to the patient that he'll need to remain still during the test and periodically hold his breath.
- Inform the patient that he may be given an I.V. contrast medium, an oral contrast medium, or both to enhance visualization of the pancreas. Describe possible adverse reactions to the medium, such as nausea, flushing, dizziness, and sweating, and tell him to report these symptoms.
- Check the patient's history for recent barium studies and for hypersensitivity to iodine, seafood, or contrast media used in previous tests.
- Make sure that the patient or a responsible family member has signed an informed consent form.
- Administer the oral contrast medium.

Procedure and posttest care
- Help the patient into the supine position on the X-ray table and position the table within the opening in the scanning gantry.
- A series of transverse X-rays is taken and recorded on magnetic tape. The vary-

ing tissue absorption is calculated by a computer, and the information is reconstructed as images on a television screen. These images are studied, and selected ones are photographed.
- After the first series of films is completed, the images are reviewed. Then contrast enhancement may be ordered. After the contrast medium is administered, another series of films is taken, and the patient is observed for an allergic reaction, such as itching, hypotension, hypertension, diaphoresis, or dyspnea.
- After the procedure, tell the patient he may resume his usual diet.
- Observe for a delayed allergic reaction to the contrast dye, such as urticaria, headache, and vomiting.

Precautions
- CT scanning of the pancreas is contraindicated in the pregnant patient.
- If a contrast medium is used, the test is contraindicated in the patient with a history of hypersensitivity to iodine or severe renal or hepatic disease.

Normal findings
Usually, the pancreatic parenchyma displays a uniform density, especially when an I.V. contrast medium is used. The gland normally thickens from tail to head and has a smooth surface. A contrast medium administered orally opacifies the adjacent stomach and duodenum and helps outline the pancreas, particularly in the patient with little peripancreatic fat, such as a child or a thin adult. (See *Normal CT scan of the pancreas.*)

Abnormal findings
Because the tissue density of pancreatic carcinoma resembles that of the normal parenchyma, changes in pancreatic size and shape help demonstrate carcinoma

NORMAL CT SCAN OF THE PANCREAS

This normal pancreatic computed tomography (CT) scan shows the pancreas opacified by contrast medium.

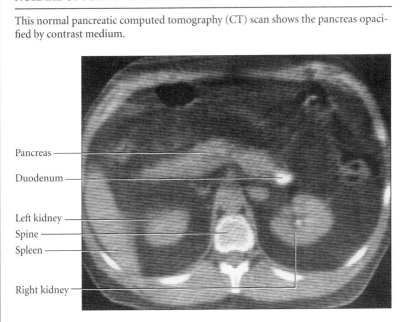

Pancreas

Duodenum

Left kidney

Spine

Spleen

Right kidney

and pseudocysts. Usually, carcinoma first appears as a localized swelling of the head, body, or tail of the pancreas and may spread to obliterate the fat plane, dilate the main pancreatic duct and common bile duct by obstructing them, and produce low-density focal lesions in the liver from metastasis. Use of an I.V. contrast medium helps detect metastases by opacifying the pancreatic and hepatic parenchyma.

Adenocarcinoma and islet cell tumors are the most common carcinomas of the pancreas. Cystadenomas and cystadenocarcinomas, usually multilocular, occur most frequently in the body and tail of the pancreas and appear as low-density focal lesions marked by internal septa. Contrast medium administered by mouth helps distinguish between bowel loops and tumors in the tail of the pancreas.

Acute pancreatitis, either edematous (interstitial) or necrotizing (hemorrhagic), produces diffuse enlargement of the pancreas. In acute edematous pancreatitis, parenchyma density is uniformly decreased. In acute necrotizing pancreatitis, the density is nonuniform because of the presence of necrosis and hemorrhage. The areas of tissue necrosis have diminished density. In acute pancreatitis, inflammation typically spreads into the peripancreatic fat, causes stranding in the mesenteric fat, and blurs the gland margin.

Abscesses, phlegmons, and pseudocysts may occur as complications of acute pancreatitis. Abscesses, either within or outside the pancreas, appear as low-density areas and are most readily detected when they contain gas. Pseudocysts, which may be unilocal or multilocal, appear as sharply circumscribed, low-density areas that may contain debris. Ascites and pleural effusion may also be apparent in acute pancreatitis.

In chronic pancreatitis, the pancreas may appear normal, enlarged (localized or generalized), or atrophic, depending on disease severity. Duct calcification and dilation of the main pancreatic duct are characteristic. Pseudocysts, obliteration of the fat plane, and secondary complications, such as biliary obstruction, may occur.

Interfering factors
- Barium or other contrast media in the GI tract from earlier tests (possible poor imaging)
- Excessive peristalsis or excessive patient movement

Given diagnostic imaging system

The given diagnostic imaging system (also called the *camera pill*) is a tiny video camera with a light source and transmitter inside a capsule, allowing recording of images along its path. The "capsule endoscope" measures 11 × 30 mm and is propelled along the digestive tract by peristalsis. The clear end records images of the stomach walls and, particularly, the small intestine, where many other diagnostic techniques may not reach or otherwise visualize. (See *Detecting disorders in the stomach and small intestine.*) The images are transmitted to a data recorder on a belt placed around the patient's waist. After swallowing the pill, the patient doesn't need to stay at the hospital and can return to work or other activities of daily living.

Purpose
- To detect polyps or cancer
- To detect causes of bleeding and anemia

Patient preparation
- Explain to the patient that this test helps visualize the stomach and small intestine, helping to detect disorders.
- Tell the patient who will perform the test and where it will take place.
- Inform the patient that he may need to fast for 12 hours before the test, but may have fluids for up to 2 hours before the test, unless ordered otherwise. (Usually no preparation is involved, but some patients may benefit from it.)
- Explain to the patient that he'll need to swallow the camera pill and that it will send information to a receiver he'll wear on his belt.
- Tell the patient that the procedure is painless and after swallowing the pill he can go home or go to work.
- Explain to the patient that walking helps facilitate movement of the pill.
- Tell the patient that he'll need to return to the facility in 24 hours (or as directed) so the recorder can be removed from his belt.
- Tell the patient that the pill will be excreted normally in his stool in 8 to 72 hours.

Procedure and posttest care
- The patient ingests the camera pill, as ordered, and a receiver is attached to his belt.
- The pill records images for up to 6 hours along its path of the stomach, small intestine, and mouth of the large intestine, transmitting the information to the receiver.
- The patient returns to the facility, as ordered, so the images can be transmitted

DETECTING DISORDERS IN THE STOMACH AND SMALL INTESTINE

In the given system, after the patient swallows the capsule, it travels through the body by the natural movement of the digestive tract. A receiver worn outside the body records the images. The strength of the signal indicates the capsule's location.

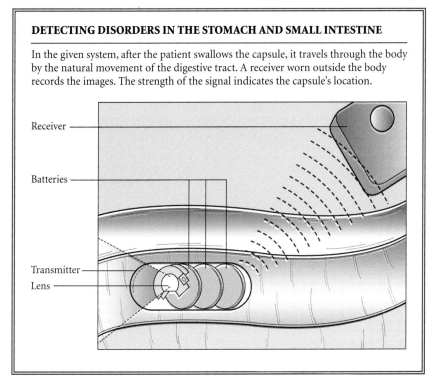

into the computer, where they're displayed on the screen.

- Tell the patient that he may resume his usual diet after the images are obtained.
- The pill is excreted normally in the stool.

Precautions

- The procedure is contraindicated in the patient with a suspected obstruction, fistula, or stricture and in the patient who can't swallow (an infant, a young child, or someone with a swallowing impairment).
- The battery is short-lived, so images of the large intestine are unobtainable.
- The pill can't be used to stop bleeding, take tissue samples, remove growths, or repair any problems detected. Other invasive studies may be needed.

Normal findings

The camera illustrates normal anatomy of the stomach and small intestine.

Abnormal findings

The camera may detect bleeding sites or abnormalities of the stomach and small bowel, such as erosions, Crohn's disease, celiac disease, benign and malignant tumors of the small intestine, vascular disorders, medication-related small-bowel injuries, and pediatric small-bowel disorders.

Interfering factors

- Narrowing or obstruction of the intestine, causing the pill to become lodged

ULTRASONOGRAPHY

Ultrasonography of the gallbladder and biliary system

In ultrasonography of the gallbladder and biliary system, a focused beam of high-frequency sound waves passes into the right upper quadrant of the abdomen, creating echoes that vary with changes in tissue density. These echoes are converted to images on a screen, indicating the size, shape, and position of the gallbladder and biliary system.

Purpose

- To confirm a diagnosis of cholelithiasis
- To diagnose acute cholecystitis
- To distinguish between obstructive and nonobstructive jaundice

Patient preparation

- Explain to the patient that ultrasonography allows examination of the gallbladder and the biliary system.
- Instruct the patient to eat a fat-free meal in the evening and then to fast for 8 to 12 hours before the procedure, if possible; this promotes accumulation of bile in the gallbladder and enhances ultrasonic visualization.
- Tell the patient who will perform the procedure and where it will take place.
- Tell the patient that the room may be darkened slightly to aid visualization on the screen.
- Describe the procedure. Tell the patient that a transducer will pass smoothly over his abdomen in direct contact with his skin, but assure him that he'll feel only mild pressure.
- Instruct the patient to remain as still as possible during the procedure and to hold his breath when requested to ensure that the gallbladder is in the same position for each scan.

Procedure and posttest care

- The patient is placed in a supine position.
- A water-soluble conductive gel is applied to the face of the transducer.
- Transverse and longitudinal oblique scans of the gallbladder are taken at ⅜″ (1-cm) intervals, starting at the level of the xiphoid and moving laterally to the right subcostal area. Longitudinal oblique scans are taken at 5-mm intervals parallel to the long axis of the gallbladder marked on the patient's skin, beginning medial to the gallbladder and continuing through to its lateral border.
- During each scan, the patient is asked to inhale deeply and to hold his breath. (If the gallbladder is positioned deeply under the right costal margin, a scan may be taken through the intercostal spaces while the patient holds his breath.)
- The patient is then placed in a left lateral decubitus position and is scanned beneath the right costal margin. (This position and scanning angle may displace and allow detection of stones lodged in the gallbladder neck and cystic duct region.)
- Scanning with the patient erect helps demonstrate mobility or fixity of suspicious echogenic areas. Views may be photographed for later study.
- Remove the conductive gel from the patient's skin.
- Inform the patient that he may resume his usual diet.

Precautions

- Keep the patient in a fasting state to prevent the excretion of bile in the gallbladder. Even smelling greasy foods, such as popcorn, can cause the gallbladder to empty.

Normal findings

The normal gallbladder is sonolucent; it appears circular on transverse scans and pear-shaped on longitudinal scans. Although the size of the gallbladder varies, its outer walls normally appear sharp and smooth. Intrahepatic radicles seldom appear because the flow of sonolucent bile is very fine. The cystic duct may also be indistinct — the result of folds known as Heister's valves that line the cystic duct lumen. When visualized, the cystic duct has a serpentine appearance. The common bile duct, in contrast, has a linear appearance, but is sometimes obscured by overlying bowel gas.

Abnormal findings

Gallstones within the gallbladder lumen or the biliary system typically appear as mobile, echogenic areas, usually associated with an acoustic shadow. The size of gallstones generally parallels the size of their shadows; gallstones 5 mm or larger usually produce shadows. However, if the gallbladder is distended with bile, gallstones as small as 1 mm can be detected because of the acoustic contrast between liquid bile and solid gallstones. Detecting stones in the biliary ducts, which contain little bile, may be difficult. When the gallbladder is shrunken or fully impacted with gallstones, inadequate bile may likewise make gallstone detection difficult, and the gallbladder itself might not be detectable. In this case, an acoustic shadow in the gallbladder fossa indicates cholelithiasis; the presence of such a shadow in the cystic and common bile ducts can also indicate cholelithiasis.

Polyps and carcinoma within the gallbladder lumen are distinguished from gallstones by their fixity. Polyps usually appear as sharply defined, echogenic areas; carcinoma appears as a poorly defined mass, commonly associated with a thickened gallbladder wall.

Biliary sludge within the gallbladder lumen appears as a fine layer of echoes that slowly gravitates to the dependent portion of the gallbladder as the patient changes position. Although biliary sludge may arise without accompanying pathology, it may also result from obstruction and can predispose the patient to gallstone formation.

Acute cholecystitis is indicated by an enlarged gallbladder with thickened, double-rimmed walls, usually with gallstones within the lumen. There may also be precholecystic fluid. In chronic cholecystitis, the walls of the gallbladder appear thickened; the organ itself, however, is generally contracted. In obstructive jaundice, ultrasonography readily demonstrates a dilated biliary system and, usually, a dilated gallbladder. Dilated intrahepatic radicles appear tortuous and irregular; a dilated gallbladder usually loses its characteristic pear shape, becoming spherical.

Biliary obstruction may result from intrinsic factors, such as a gallstone or small carcinoma within the biliary system. (Ultrasonography can't distinguish between these two echogenic masses.) Alternatively, it may result from extrinsic factors, such as a mass in the hepatic portal vein that compresses the cystic duct and interferes with bile drainage from the intrahepatic radicles, or from pathology in the head of the pancreas that obstructs the common bile duct. Such pathology includes carcinoma and pancreatitis, although ultrasonography can't distinguish between the two. When ultrasonography fails to clearly define the site of biliary obstruction, percutaneous transhepatic cholangiography or endoscopic retrograde cholangiopancreatography should be performed.

Interfering factors
- Failure to observe pretest dietary restrictions
- Overlying bowel gas or retained barium from a previous test (possible poor imaging)
- Deficiency of body fluids in a dehydrated patient, obscuring boundaries between organs and tissue structures (possible poor imaging)

Ultrasonography of the liver

Ultrasonography of the liver produces images by channeling high-frequency sound waves into the right upper quadrant of the abdomen. Resultant echoes are converted to cross-sectional images on a monitor; different shades of gray depict various tissue densities. Ultrasonography can show intrahepatic structures and organ size, shape, and position.

This procedure is indicated in patients with jaundice of unknown etiology, unexplained hepatomegaly and abnormal biochemical test results, suspected metastatic tumors and elevated serum alkaline phosphatase levels, and recent abdominal trauma.

When used with liver-spleen scanning, ultrasonography can define cold spots (focal defects that fail to pick up the radionuclide) as tumors, abscesses, or cysts; it also provides better views of the periportal and perihepatic spaces than liver-spleen scanning. If ultrasonography fails to provide definitive diagnosis, computed tomography (CT), gallium scanning, or liver biopsy may yield more information.

Purpose
- To distinguish between obstructive and nonobstructive jaundice
- To screen for hepatocellular disease
- To detect hepatic metastases and hematomas
- To define cold spots as tumors, abscesses, or cysts

Patient preparation
- Explain to the patient that ultrasonography allows examination of the liver. Tell him who will perform the test and where it will take place.
- Instruct the patient to fast for 8 to 12 hours before the test to reduce bowel gas, which hinders ultrasound transmission.
- Describe the procedure. Tell the patient a transducer will pass smoothly over his abdomen, channeling sound waves into the liver, but assure him that he'll feel only mild pressure.
- Instruct the patient to remain as still as possible during the procedure and to hold his breath when requested.

Procedure and posttest care
- The patient is placed in a supine position.
- A water-soluble conductive gel is applied to the face of the transducer.
- Transverse scans are taken at $\frac{3}{8}''$ (1-cm) intervals, using a single-sweep technique between the costal margins. Although this technique demonstrates the left lobe of the liver and part of the right lobe, sector scans through the intercostal spaces are used to view the remainder of the right lobe.
- Scans are taken longitudinally from the right border of the liver to the left.
- For better demonstration of the right lateral dome, oblique cephalad-angled scans may be taken beneath the right costal margin.

- Scans are then taken parallel to the hepatic portal, at a 45-degree angle toward the superior right lateral dome, to examine the peripheral anatomy, portal venous system, common bile duct, and biliary tree. Clear images are photographed for later study.
- During each scan, ask the patient to hold his breath briefly in deep inspiration to displace the liver caudally from the costal margin and the ribs to aid visualization.
- Remove the conductive gel from the patient's skin.
- Inform the patient that he may resume his usual diet.

Normal findings

The liver normally demonstrates a homogeneous, low-level echo pattern, interrupted only by the different echo patterns of its portal and hepatic veins, the aorta, and the inferior vena cava. Hepatic veins appear completely sonolucent; portal veins have margins that are highly echogenic.

Abnormal findings

In obstructive jaundice, ultrasonography shows dilated intrahepatic biliary radicles and extrahepatic ducts. Conversely, in nonobstructive jaundice, ultrasonography shows a biliary tree of normal diameter.

Ultrasonographic characteristics of hepatocellular disease are generally nonspecific, and disorders in early stages can escape detection; liver-spleen scanning is a more sensitive diagnostic tool. In cirrhosis, ultrasonography may demonstrate variable liver size; dilated, tortuous portal branches associated with portal hypertension; and an irregular echo pattern with increased echo amplitude, causing overall increased attenuation. Demonstration of splenomegaly by spleen ultrasonography

or liver-spleen scanning aids diagnosis. In fatty infiltration of the liver, ultrasonography may show hepatomegaly and a regular echo pattern that, although greater in echo amplitude than that of a normal parenchyma, doesn't alter attenuation.

Ultrasonographic characteristics of metastases in the liver vary widely; metastases may appear either hypoechoic or echogenic, poorly defined or well defined. For example, metastatic lymphomas and sarcomas are generally hypoechoic; mucin-secreting adenocarcinoma of the colon is highly echogenic. Liver biopsy is necessary to confirm the tumor type. Serial ultrasonography may be used to monitor the effectiveness of therapy.

Primary hepatic tumors also present a varied appearance and may mimic metastases, requiring angiography and liver biopsy for definitive diagnosis. Hepatomas are the most common malignant tumors in adults; hepatoblastomas are most common in children. Benign tumors are far less common than malignant ones.

Abscesses usually appear as sonolucent masses with ill-defined, slightly thickened borders and accentuated posterior wall transmission; scattered internal echoes, caused by necrotic debris, may also be present. Because they produce similar echo patterns, intrahepatic abscesses are occasionally mistaken for hematomas, necrotic metastases, or hemorrhagic cysts. Gas-containing intrahepatic abscesses, which may be echogenic, are sometimes confused with solid intrahepatic lesions. Subphrenic abscesses occur between the diaphragm and the liver; subhepatic abscesses appear inferior to the liver and anterior to the upper pole of the right kidney. Ascitic fluid resembles a subhepatic abscess, but lacks internal echoes and has a more regular border.

Cysts usually appear as spherical, sonolucent areas with well-defined borders and accentuated posterior wall transmission. When a cyst can't be distinguished from an abscess or necrotic metastases, gallium scanning, CT, and angiography should be performed.

Hematomas—either intrahepatic or subcapsular—usually result from trauma. Intrahepatic hematomas appear as poorly defined, relatively sonolucent masses and may have scattered internal echoes due to clotting; serial ultrasonography can differentiate between a hematoma and a cyst or tumor as the hematoma becomes smaller. Subcapsular hematoma may appear as a focal, sonolucent mass on the periphery of the liver or as a diffuse, sonolucent area surrounding part of the liver.

Interfering factors

- Overlying ribs and gas or residual barium in the stomach or colon (possible misleading results)
- Deficiency of body fluids in a dehydrated patient, obscuring boundaries between organs and tissue structures (possible misleading results)

Ultrasonography of the spleen

In ultrasonography of the spleen, a focused beam of high-frequency sound waves passes into the left upper quadrant of the abdomen, creating echoes that vary with changes in tissue density. These are displayed on a monitor as real-time images that indicate the size, shape, and position of the spleen and surrounding viscera.

Ultrasonography is indicated in patients with an upper left quadrant mass of unknown origin; with known spleno-megaly, to evaluate changes in splenic size; with left upper quadrant pain and local tenderness; and with recent abdominal trauma.

Purpose

- To demonstrate splenomegaly
- To monitor the progression of primary and secondary splenic disease and to evaluate the effectiveness of therapy
- To evaluate the spleen after abdominal trauma
- To help detect splenic cysts and subphrenic abscesses

Patient preparation

- Explain to the patient that ultrasonography allows examination of the spleen.
- Tell the patient who will perform the test, where it will take place, and that the room may be darkened slightly to aid visualization on the monitor.
- Instruct the patient to fast for 8 to 12 hours before the procedure, if possible; this reduces the amount of gas in the bowel, improving sound wave transmission.
- Describe the procedure. Tell the patient that a transducer will pass smoothly over his abdomen in direct contact with his skin, but assure him that he'll feel only mild pressure.
- Instruct the patient to remain as still as possible during the procedure and to hold his breath when requested to aid visualization.

Procedure and posttest care

- Because the procedure for ultrasonography varies depending on the size of the spleen and the patient's physique, the patient is usually repositioned several times; the transducer scanning angle or path is also changed.

■ Generally, the patient is first placed in a supine position, with his chest uncovered.

■ A water-soluble conductive gel is applied to the face of the transducer, and transverse scans of the spleen are taken at ⅜″ to ¾″ (1- to 2-cm) intervals, beginning at the level of the diaphragm and moving posteriorly, while the transducer is angled anteromedially.

■ The patient is then placed in a right lateral decubitus position, and transverse scans are taken through the intercostal spaces using a sectoring motion.

■ A pillow may be placed under the patient's right side to help separate the intercostal spaces, making it easier to position the transducer face between them.

■ Longitudinal scans are taken from the axilla toward the iliac crest.

■ To prevent rib artifacts and to obtain the best view of the splenic parenchyma, oblique scans are taken by passing the transducer face along the intercostal spaces.

■ During each scan, the patient may be asked to hold his breath briefly at various stages of inspiration.

■ Good views are photographed for later study.

■ Remove the conductive gel from the patient's skin.

■ Inform the patient that he may resume his usual diet.

Normal findings

The splenic parenchyma normally demonstrates a homogeneous, low-level echo pattern; its individual vascular channels aren't usually apparent. The superior and lateral splenic borders are clearly defined, each having a convex margin. The undersurface and medial borders, in contrast, show indentations from surrounding organs (stomach, left kidney, and pancreas). The hilar region, where the vascular pedicle enters the spleen, commonly produces an area of highly reflective echoes. The medial surface is generally concave, which helps differentiate between left upper quadrant masses and an enlarged spleen. Even when splenomegaly is present, the spleen generally remains concave medially unless a space-occupying lesion distorts this contour.

Abnormal findings

Ultrasonography can show splenomegaly, but it usually doesn't indicate the cause; a computed tomography (CT) scan can provide more specific information. Splenomegaly is generally accompanied by increased echogenicity. Enlarged vascular channels are commonly visible, especially in the hilar region. If spaceoccupying lesions distort the splenic contour, liver-spleen scanning should be performed to confirm splenomegaly.

Abdominal trauma may result in splenic rupture or subcapsular hematoma. In splenic rupture, ultrasonography demonstrates splenomegaly and an irregular, sonolucent area (the presence of free intraperitoneal fluid); however, these findings must be confirmed by arteriography. In subcapsular hematoma, ultrasonography shows splenomegaly as well as a double contour, altered splenic position, and a relatively sonolucent area on the spleen's periphery. The double contour results from blood accumulation between the splenic parenchyma and the intact splenic capsule. As the spleen enlarges, a transverse section shows its anterior margin extending more anteriorly than the aorta. Ultrasonography may be difficult and painful after abdominal trauma because the transducer may have to pass across fractured ribs and contusions; CT scanning, which differentiates blood and fluid in the peritoneal space, should be used instead.

In subphrenic abscess, ultrasonography shows a sonolucent area beneath the diaphragm. Clinical findings may differentiate between abscess and blood or fluid accumulation.

Used with liver-spleen scanning, ultrasonography differentiates cold spots as cystic or solid lesions. It shows cysts as spherical, sonolucent areas with well-defined, regular margins with acoustic enhancement behind them. When ultrasonography fails to identify a cyst as splenic or extrasplenic — especially if the cyst is located in the upper pole of the left kidney and the adrenal gland or in the tail of the pancreas — a CT scan and arteriography are used. Ultrasonography can readily clarify cystic cold spots, but using a CT scan with a contrast medium is superior for evaluating primary and metastatic tumors. Ultrasonography usually fails to identify tumors associated with lymphoma and chronic leukemias because these resemble tumors of the splenic parenchyma.

Interfering factors

- Overlying ribs, an aerated left lung, or gas or residual barium in the colon or stomach (possible poor imaging)
- Deficiency of body fluids in a dehydrated patient, obscuring boundaries between organs and tissue structures (possible poor imaging)
- Body physique affecting the spleen's shape or adjacent masses displacing the spleen (possible poor imaging, may be mistaken for splenomegaly)
- Splenic trauma (possible difficulty in tolerating the procedure)

Ultrasonography of the pancreas

In ultrasonography of the pancreas, cross-sectional images are produced by channeling high-frequency sound waves into the epigastric region and converting the resultant echoes to real-time images, which are displayed on a monitor. The pattern varies with tissue density and indicates the size, shape, and position of the pancreas and surrounding viscera.

Purpose

- To aid in the diagnosis of pancreatitis, pseudocysts, and pancreatic carcinoma

Patient preparation

- Explain to the patient that ultrasonography permits examination of the pancreas.
- Instruct the patient to fast for 8 to 12 hours before the procedure to reduce bowel gas.
- Tell the patient who will perform the procedure, where it will take place, and that the room may be darkened slightly to aid visualization on the monitor.
- If the patient is a smoker, ask him to abstain before the test; this eliminates the risk of swallowing air while inhaling, which interferes with test results.
- Describe the procedure. Tell the patient a transducer will pass smoothly over his epigastric region, channeling sound waves into the pancreas, but assure him that he'll only feel mild pressure.
- Tell the patient he'll be asked to inhale deeply during scanning, and instruct him to remain still during the procedure.

Procedure and posttest care

- The patient is placed in a supine position.
- A water-soluble conductive gel or mineral oil is applied to the abdomen and, with the patient at full inspiration, transverse scans are taken at 1-cm intervals, starting from the xiphoid and moving caudally; longitudinal scans are taken to view the head, body, and tail of the pancreas in sequence; scanning the right anterior oblique view allows imaging of the head and body of the pancreas; oblique sagittal scans are used to view the portal vein; and scanning from the sagittal view images the vena cava.
- When good ultrasonography views are obtained, they're photographed for later study.
- Remove the conductive gel from the patient's skin.
- Inform the patient that he may resume his usual diet.

Normal findings

The pancreas normally demonstrates a coarse, uniform echo pattern and usually appears more echogenic than the adjacent liver.

Abnormal findings

Alterations in the size, contour, and parenchymal texture of the pancreas characterize pancreatic disease. An enlarged pancreas with decreased echogenicity and distinct borders suggests pancreatitis. A well-defined mass with an essentially echo-free interior indicates pseudocyst; an ill-defined mass with scattered internal echoes or a mass in the head of the pancreas (obstructing the common bile duct) and a large noncon-tracting gallbladder suggest pancreatic carcinoma.

Subsequent computed tomography scan and biopsy of the pancreas may be necessary to confirm a diagnosis.

Interfering factors

- Gas or residual barium in the stomach and intestine (possible poor imaging)
- Deficiency of body fluids in a dehydrated patient, obscuring boundaries between organs and tissue structures (possible poor imaging)
- Obesity (possible poor imaging)
- Fatty infiltration of the pancreas (possible poor imaging)

Selected readings

Cavanaugh, B.M. *Nurse's Manual of Laboratory and Diagnostic Tests,* 4th ed. Philadelphia: F.A. Davis Co., 2003.

Goldman, L., and Ausiello, D., eds. *Cecil Textbook of Medicine,* 22nd ed. Philadelphia: W.B. Saunders Co., 2004.

Guyton, A.C., and Hall, J.E. *Textbook of Medical Physiology,* 10th ed. Philadelphia: W.B. Saunders Co., 2001.

Henry, J.B., et al. *Clinical Diagnosis and Management by Laboratory Methods,* 20th ed. Philadelphia: W.B. Saunders Co., 2001.

McClatchey, K.D. *Clinical Laboratory Medicine,* 2nd ed. Philadelphia: Lippincott Williams & Wilkins, 2002.

Pagana, K.D., and Pagana, T.J. *Mosby's Diagnostic and Laboratory Test Reference,* 6th ed. St. Louis: Mosby Year–Book, Inc., 2003.

Schnell, Z., et al. *Davis's Comprehensive Handbook of Laboratory and Diagnostic Tests with Nursing Implications.* Philadelphia: F.A. Davis Co., 2003.

28

Cardiovascular system

Introduction

According to the American Heart Association, cardiovascular system disorders afflict nearly 70 million people in North America. Because many diagnostic tests can detect these disorders, it's important to understand the indications for each test and its clinical implications to prepare the patient physically and psychologically before the test, assist the physician during the test, and implement proper care after the test.

Cardiovascular dysfunction tests fall into six major groups: cardiac enzyme analysis, radiography, graphic recording, ultrasonography, nuclear medicine, and catheterization. *Cardiac enzyme analysis* proves most useful in detecting acute myocardial infarction (MI). *Radiography,* including X-rays of the heart, is one of the first diagnostic tests used to assess myocardial or vascular dysfunction. *Graphic recording,* such as electrocardiography (ECG), is a noninvasive technique for evaluating cardiac electrical activity performed by specially trained personnel. *Ultrasonography,* another noninvasive technique, now holds an important place in cardiovascular testing—for example, echocardiography has superseded cardiac series fluoroscopy for most diagnostic applications. *Nuclear medicine imaging* is one of the most rapidly changing areas of diagnostic testing, partly because of the development of new radiopharmaceuticals. *Catheterization* is an effective invasive method for evaluating cardiac and vascular dysfunction.

Choosing a specific diagnostic test depends on the physician's clinical suspicions, the kind of information needed, and the risk to the patient. As a rule, noninvasive tests precede invasive tests because the latter are usually more hazardous and more costly. However, invasive tests are commonly necessary to obtain the most diagnostic information.

The pump

The heart is the mechanism and the arteries, veins, and capillaries are the pathway by which blood circulates throughout the body. Together they act to deliver oxygen and vital nutrients to the body cells and to remove carbon dioxide and other waste products.

The heart is a hollow, muscular organ located in the mediastinum between the lungs. It's enclosed by a membranous sac called the *pericardium,* which consists of two layers, one inside the other: an external fibrous (parietal) layer attached to the great vessels leaving the heart and an internal serous (visceral) sac that envelops the heart and lines the fibrous portion. Space between these layers is filled with 10 to 50 ml of pericardial fluid, which lubricates the layers as they glide over each other during heart movement.

The heart pump consists of four chambers. The *atria*—the two smaller upper chambers—receive blood from the systemic and pulmonary circulation. The two larger, thicker lower chambers—the *ventricles*—receive blood from the atria. The interventricular septum divides the heart into right and left halves. Two valves separate the atria from the ventricles: the tricuspid valve in the right side and the mitral valve in the left side of the heart. The mitral valve has two movable leaflets; the tricuspid has three. Two semilunar valves, each with three fibrous cusps, guard the entrances to the aortic and pulmonary arteries. (See *The conduction system,* page 818.)

The vascular system

The vascular system consists of the arteries, arterioles, capillaries, venules, and

THE CONDUCTION SYSTEM

The heart's conduction system contains specialized muscle fibers that generate and conduct their own electrical impulses.

SA node

The sinoatrial (SA) node—located in the right atrium beneath the orifice of the superior vena cava—normally controls heart rate and is called the *pacemaker*. The SA node sends an impulse through the internodal pathways and atrial muscle to the atrioventricular (AV) node in the lower posterior part of the right atrium near the lumen of the coronary sinus. As an impulse passes through the atrial muscles, the atria contract.

After a short delay in the AV node, the impulse continues down the bundle His—which divides into right and left bundle branches—and finally, into the subendothelial Purkinje fibers, which transmit the impulse into the ventricular myocardium, causing it to contract.

Repolarization

After this contraction, the myocardium repolarizes while the ventricles relax and begin to fill with blood in preparation for the next impulse from the SA node. Evidence of this conduction of electric currents through the heart may be picked up on the skin surface and graphically recorded by an electrocardiogram.

Automaticity

The SA node discharges 60 to 100 impulses per minute. If it fails to generate the expected impulses, the AV node can also discharge, but at a slower rate of 40 to 60 impulses per minute. If both nodes fail to discharge, the Purkinje fibers can discharge at a rate of 15 to 40 impulses per minute. The heart's ability to spontaneously generate and maintain its own impulse rate is known as *automaticity*.

When any part of the heart other than the SA node takes over to pace the heart, this part is known as an *ectopic pacemaker*. If the electrical impulse is too weak, it won't excite the muscle fiber at all; if it's strong enough to cause the fiber to reach its electrical threshold potential, excitation occurs. The current then spreads to neighboring fibers by virtue of the low resistance of their cell walls, and the entire muscle mass reacts as a unit. This response is known as the "all-or-nothing" principle.

veins. Arteries and veins have three layers: the tunica intima (inner coat), consisting of endothelial, connective, and elastic tissues; the tunica media (middle coat), consisting of smooth-muscle fibers and elastic and collagenous tissue; and the tunica adventitia (external coat), consisting of connective, smooth muscle, and elastic tissue. *Capillaries* consist of endothelial tissues one cell thick, whereas venules and arterioles have a variable composition depending on their size.

Arteries, which contain 15% of circulating blood volume, carry blood away from the heart. Normally, the aorta (the largest artery) and its branches can withstand significant changes in cardiac pressure that distend them during ventricular contraction; these pressure changes are detectable as a palpable wave (pulse) in certain arteries near the skin. The aorta and other large arteries add little to total peripheral vascular resistance because they don't ordinarily impede blood flow. By their ability to dilate and contract, the

THE HEART'S BLOOD SUPPLY

The heart's blood supply system is shown in these schematic anterior and posterior views. Coronary angiography—a cardiac catheterization procedure—evaluates coronary artery function. Coronary artery disease results mainly from atherosclerosis, which impedes blood flow and thus interferes with the oxygen and nutrient supply to the myocardium.

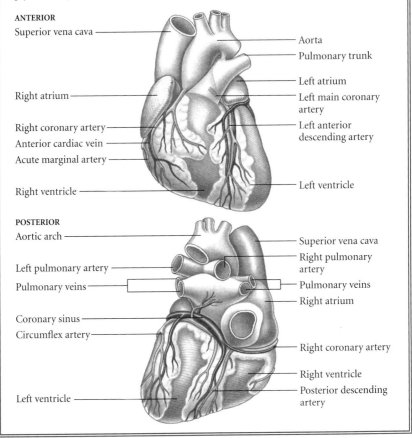

ANTERIOR

Superior vena cava

Right atrium

Right coronary artery

Anterior cardiac vein

Acute marginal artery

Right ventricle

Aorta

Pulmonary trunk

Left atrium

Left main coronary artery

Left anterior descending artery

Left ventricle

POSTERIOR

Aortic arch

Left pulmonary artery

Pulmonary veins

Coronary sinus

Circumflex artery

Left ventricle

Superior vena cava

Right pulmonary artery

Pulmonary veins

Right atrium

Right coronary artery

Right ventricle

Posterior descending artery

arterioles largely control the degree of total peripheral resistance and, consequently, the amount of blood flow to and in the tissues.

The *veins* carry blood toward the heart and contain 50% of total circulating blood volume. The superior and inferior venae cavae, which empty into the right atrium, are the body's largest veins. In the venous system, pressure changes only slightly with vessel dilation or constriction. However, total circulating blood volume, heart and lung function, venomotor tone, and the condition of the one-way venous valves in the limbs may affect the capacitance and pressure of the venous system. (See *The heart's blood supply.* See also *The cardiac cycle,* page 820.)

THE CARDIAC CYCLE

The schematic drawings here show events during a single cardiac cycle.

■ **Period of rapid ventricular filling (1):** Unoxygenated blood returning from the tissues enters the right atrium at the same time that oxygenated blood from the lungs enters the left atrium. The atria and ventricles are passively filled.

■ **Atrial kick (2):** About 70% of incoming blood flows through the atria directly into the ventricles before the atria contract; when they do, they force an

additional 30% of blood into the ventricles — the atrial kick.

■ **Period of isovolumic contraction (3):** The ventricles begin contracting before emptying.

■ **Period of ejection (4):** The ventricles contract, pushing the unoxygenated blood into pulmonary arteries and the oxygenated blood into the aorta.

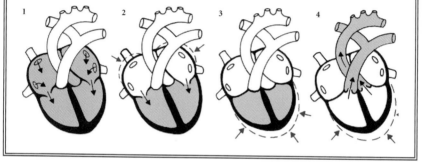

In the coronary circulation, blood flow occurs mainly during diastole and depends directly on the perfusion pressure (the pressure gradient between the coronary arteries and the right atrium). (See *Stroke volume and Starling's law.*) Coronary blood flow may diminish if aortic pressure decreases or right-sided heart pressure increases. It may also be influenced by tachycardias, which reduce diastolic flow time, and by conditions that reduce diastolic perfusion pressure such as hypotension.

Coronary circulation, which constitutes 50% of total cardiac output in the resting heart, uses 70% of the arterial oxygen. Increases oxygen demand requires increased coronary blood flow because the heart extracts virtually all oxygen from the blood, even at rest.

Radiography

Cardiac radiography permits visualization of the position, size, and contour of the heart and great vessels of the circulatory system. Chest X-rays can show heart enlargement, interstitial and alveolar edema, aortic dilation, left-sided heart failure, and intracardiac calcification.

Cardiac series (chest fluoroscopy) shows the heart's motion and the pulsations of the heart and great vessels during systole and diastole; it also helps detect and confirm malfunctioning prosthetic heart valves. Although largely replaced by echocardiography, the cardiac series is used in some cases for placing temporary

STROKE VOLUME AND STARLING'S LAW

Total ventricular volume in each cardiac cycle reaches 120 to 130 ml during diastolic filling (end-diastolic volume) and falls to 50 to 60 mg as the ventricles empty during contraction; this 70-ml difference represents the *stroke volume.* The stroke volume multiplied by heart rate per minute equals *cardiac output,* or the volume of blood pumped in 1 minute. Normally, the cardiac output for a resting person is about 5 L, but this amount varies with body size, heart rate, and stroke volume.

The heart's remarkable ability to deliver equal volumes of blood each minute, even when the right and left ventricles deliver very different volumes of blood per stroke, is explained by *Starling's law:* The force of contraction of each heartbeat depends on the length of the muscle fibers of the walls of the heart. Thus, if right ventricular output exceeds left ventricular output, the fibers of the left ventricle lengthen at end-diastole to increase the contraction force.

In the diagrams on the left (A), normal filling during diastole causes normal fiber stretch, normal contractile force, and normal stroke volume. In the diagrams on the right (B), increased filling during diastole increases fiber stretch, force of contraction, and stroke volume.

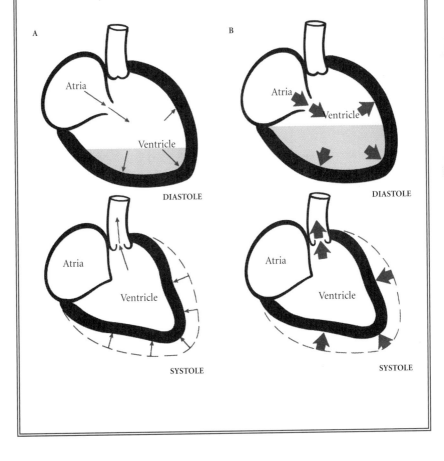

A

Atria

Ventricle

Ventricle

DIASTOLE

Atria

Ventricle

SYSTOLE

B

Atria

Ventricle

Ventricle

DIASTOLE

Atria

Ventricle

SYSTOLE

pacemakers or pulmonary artery catheters.

By injecting a contrast medium into the veins for filming, *lower limb venography* may confirm deep vein thrombosis (DVT), identify the causes of edema, and assess preoperative vascular status. The benefits of the test must outweigh the risks of radiation exposure.

Graphic monitoring

ECG records the conduction, magnitude, and duration of the heart's electrical activity to identify rhythm disturbances, conduction abnormalities, and electrolyte imbalances. It reveals the size of the heart's chambers and the heart's relative position in the chest. ECG is used to diagnose and document the progression of MI, ischemia, and pericarditis and to evaluate artificial pacemakers and cardiotonic drug therapy.

Exercise ECG measures the cardiovascular effects of controlled physical stress (bike riding or treadmill walking). An ergometer (a push wheel with handlebars) is used for exercise stress testing for the patient who can't physically walk or ride a bike. The exercise ECG may reveal ischemia, arrhythmias, or conduction abnormalities. It can also find the cause of chest pain and thus help the staff plan appropriate therapy. A thorough clinical workup must precede exercise ECG.

Holter monitoring (ambulatory ECG) records the heart's electrical activity for 24 hours or longer as the patient performs his usual activities and encounters normal physical and emotional stress. This portable ECG can detect intermittent arrhythmias, evaluate antiarrhythmic drugs, and assess recovery after an MI. It can also detect the cause of vertigo, palpitations, and chest pain. A thorough clinical workup must precede Holter monitoring.

Impedance plethysmography evaluates changes in blood volume in the limbs. Less reliable than venography in detecting small thrombi, it can confirm a diagnosis of DVT.

Ultrasonography

Echocardiography directs ultra-high-frequency sound waves into the heart, which reflects these waves at various frequencies, depending on the density of cardiac tissue. By assessing cardiac structure and function, this test can reveal valve deformities, tumors, septal defects, and pericardial effusion. It can also assess left ventricular function after an MI, prosthetic valve functioning, and hypertrophic obstructive cardiomyopathy (also known as idiopathic hypertrophic subaortic stenosis).

Transesophageal echocardiography uses ultrasonography and endoscopy to view the heart posteriorly. This test helps diagnose thoracic aortic disease, valvular disease, congenital heart disease, cardiac tumors, and intracardiac thrombi.

Doppler ultrasonography — in which sound waves are reflected from moving blood cells in underlying blood vessels — evaluates the major vascular network of the arms and legs and the extracranial cerebrovascular system. This test helps detect DVT, peripheral arterial aneurysms, congenital defects, and carotid arterial occlusive disease and can be used to assess valve function.

Ultrasonography of the abdominal aorta is used to detect and monitor the progression of abdominal aortic aneurysms, to evaluate the inferior vena cava, and to locate visceral arteries.

Nuclear medicine

Positron emission tomography images the extent of myocardial contractility to help distinguish viable tissue from infarcted tissue. After the appropriate positron emitter is injected, a scan is obtained.

Magnetic resonance imaging uses a strong magnetic field to image cardiac anatomic structures and their functions noninvasively. This test is rarely used to diagnose cardiac disease because of its high cost.

Technetium 99m pyrophosphate scanning reveals damaged myocardial tissue as hot spots—areas where the radioisotope accumulates. This test helps to detect an acute MI and define its location and size.

Thallium imaging evaluates myocardial blood flow and the status of myocardial cells after I.V. injection of the radioisotope thallium-201; healthy myocardial tissue absorbs this radioisotope, but ischemic or necrotic tissue does not. This test can detect abnormalities from perfusion defects in the coronary arteries and myocardium. *Stress testing* after thallium injection can reveal areas of ischemia.

Radiopharmaceutical myocardial perfusion imaging (also called chemical stress imaging and persantine-thallium scanning) is an alternative to exercise ECG. A persantine injection may stimulate an ischemic event, and then a thallium injection helps record cardiac vessels' response to this event.

Cardiac blood pool imaging, in which a radioisotope is tagged to red blood cells or albumin and injected intravenously, outlines the heart cavities to detect left ventricular regional wall motion abnormalities (commonly seen after an MI). In this test, a scintillation camera records the first pass of the radioisotope through the heart and then, in subsequent gated or timed imaging, the camera records two or more points in the cardiac cycle, allowing study of left ventricular function. Blood pool imaging also aids in the diagnosis of left ventricular aneurysm, cardiomyopathies, and intracardiac shunts.

Catheterization

Cardiac catheterization permits visualization of cardiac contraction and coronary artery anatomy through the insertion of a catheter into the right or left side of the heart and the injection of a contrast medium. *Left-sided heart catheterization* helps evaluate aortic and mitral valve function, cardiac output, and coronary artery patency. It also helps assess candidates for coronary artery bypass surgery or interventional procedures, such as percutaneous transluminal coronary angioplasty, stent placement, and directional coronary atherectomy.

Right-sided heart catheterization permits evaluation of pulmonic and tricuspid valve function, cardiac output, right-sided heart pressures, and pulmonary artery wedge pressure (PAWP). It can demonstrate valvular efficiency or defects, assess the causes of chest pain, and detect congenital heart defects.

In *electrophysiology studies,* an electrode-tipped catheter is passed into the right atrium and ventricle to record and study the activity of the heart's electrical conduction system. These studies allow precise location of bundle-branch blocks, detection of arrhythmias, and evaluation of the effects of antiarrhythmic drugs. Electrophysiology studies are contraindicated in the patient with severe coagulopathy or acute pulmonary embolism.

Pulmonary artery catheterization permits measurement of PAWP after passage of a balloon-tipped, flow-directed catheter into a small branch of the pulmonary artery; PAWP reflects left atrial and left ventricular end-diastolic pressure. This test, performed primarily in the patient who has suffered an acute MI, helps assess left-sided heart failure and monitors the effects of therapy after complications develop. It should be performed cautiously in the patient with left bundle-branch block because the catheter could cause right bundle-branch block, resulting in complete heart block.

Miscellaneous tests
The *cold stimulation test for Raynaud's syndrome,* performed by immersing a patient's hand in ice water and checking digital temperatures after removing the hand from the water, can verify Raynaud's syndrome in the patient who doesn't exhibit arterial-tree occlusion.

Pericardial fluid analysis, performed after needle aspiration of fluid from the pericardial sac, helps detect the cause of pericardial effusion. After aspiration, the fluid specimen is sent to the laboratory for biochemical analysis and bacterial culture.

RADIOGRAPHY

Cardiac radiography

Among the most frequently used tests for evaluating cardiac disease and its effects on the pulmonary vasculature, cardiac radiography provides images of the thorax, mediastinum, heart, and lungs. In a routine evaluation, posteroanterior and left lateral views are taken. The posteroanterior view is preferable to the anteroposterior view because it places the heart slightly closer to the plane of the film, providing a sharper, less distorted image. Cardiac radiography may be performed on a bedridden patient using portable equipment, but such equipment can provide only anteroposterior views.

Purpose
- To help detect cardiac disease and abnormalities that change the size, shape, or appearance of the heart and lungs
- To ensure correct positioning of pulmonary artery and cardiac catheters and of pacemaker wires

Patient preparation
- Explain to the patient that cardiac radiography reveals the size and shape of the heart. Tell him who will perform the test and where it will take place. Reassure him that the test uses little radiation and is harmless.
- Instruct the patient to remove jewelry, other metallic objects, and clothing above his waist and to put on a gown that has ties instead of metal snaps.

Procedure and posttest care
Posteroanterior view
- The patient stands erect about 6′ (2 m) from the X-ray machine with his back to the machine and his chin resting on top of the film cassette holder.
- The holder is adjusted to slightly hyperextend the patient's neck. The patient places his hands on his hips, with his shoulders touching the holder, and centers his chest against it.
- The patient is asked to take a deep breath and hold it during the X-ray film exposure.

Left lateral view
- The patient is positioned with his arms extended over his head and his left torso flush against the cassette and centered.
- The patient is asked to take a deep breath and hold it during the X-ray film exposure.

*Anteroposterior view of a
bedridden patient*
- The head of the bed is elevated as
much as possible.
- The patient is assisted to an upright
position to reduce visceral pressure on
the diaphragm and other thoracic structures.
- The film cassette is centered under the
patient's back. Although the distance between the patient and the X-ray machine
may vary a little, the path between the
two should be clear.
- The patient is instructed to take a deep
breath and hold it during the X-ray film
exposure.

Precautions
- Cardiac radiography is usually contraindicated during the first trimester of
pregnancy. If it's performed during pregnancy, a lead shield or apron should cover
the patient's abdomen and pelvic area
during the X-ray exposure.
- When testing an ambulatory patient,
make sure the radiographic order stipulates a posteroanterior view and not an
anteroposterior view. Include on the order any pertinent findings from previous
cardiac radiographs as well as the indication for this test.
- When testing a bedridden patient,
make sure anyone else in the room is protected from X-rays by a lead shield, a
room divider, or sufficient distance.

Normal findings
Normally, in the posteroanterior view, the
thoracic cage appears at least twice as
wide as the heart. However, in the anteroposterior view, relative heart size and position may look different, and the cardiac
silhouette and vascular markings may increase.

If cardiac radiography is performed to
evaluate the position of cardiac catheters
and pacemakers, the films should confirm
accurate placement.

Abnormal findings
Cardiac X-ray films must be evaluated
based on the patient's history, physical examination, electrocardiography results,
and results of previous radiographic tests
for cardiac abnormalities.

An abnormal cardiac silhouette usually
reflects left or right ventricular or left
atrial enlargement, or even a multichamber enlargement. In left ventricular enlargement, the posteroanterior view
shows the border of the left side of the
heart to be rounded and convex, with lateral extension of the lower left border; the
lateral view shows posterior bulging of
the left ventricle. In right ventricular enlargement, the posteroanterior view
shows secondary prominence of the pulmonary artery segment at the border of
the left side of the heart; the lateral view
shows anterior bulging in the region of
the right ventricular outflow tract.

In left atrial enlargement, the posteroanterior view shows double density of
the enlarged left atrium, straightening of
the border of the left side of the heart, elevation of the left mainstem bronchus
and, rarely, lateral extension of the border
of the right side of the heart superior to
the right ventricle; the lateral view shows
a posterior bulge at the level of the left
atrium.

In the posteroanterior view, dilation of
pulmonary venous shadows in the superior lateral aspect of the hilus and vascular
shadows horizontally and inferiorly along
the margin of the right side of the heart
may be the first signs of pulmonary vascular congestion. Chronic pulmonary venous hypertension produces an antler

pattern, caused by dilated superior pulmonary veins and normal or constricted inferior pulmonary veins. Acute alveolar edema may produce a butterfly appearance, with increased densities in central lung fields; interstitial pulmonary edema, a cloudy or cotton-puff appearance.

Interfering factors

- The patient's failure to maintain inspiration or to remain motionless
- The patient's chest off-center on the film cassette (may hinder viewing of costophrenic angle on X-ray)
- Thoracic deformity such as scoliosis (possible misleading results)
- Underexposure or overexposure of films

Lower limb venography

Lower limb venography, or ascending contrast phlebography, is the radiographic examination of a vein. Commonly used to assess the condition of the deep leg veins after injection of a contrast medium, it's the definitive test for deep vein thrombosis (DVT), an acute condition marked by inflammation and thrombus formation in the deep veins of the legs. Such thrombi usually develop in valve pockets — venous junctions or sinuses of the calf muscle — then travel to the deep calf veins; if untreated, they may occlude the popliteal, femoral, and iliac vein systems, which may lead to pulmonary embolism, a potentially lethal complication. Predisposing factors to DVT include vein wall injury, prolonged bed rest, coagulation abnormalities, surgery, childbirth, and use of hormonal contraceptives. Venography shouldn't be used for routine screening because it exposes the patient to relatively high doses of radiation and can cause complications, such as phle-

bitis, local tissue damage and, occasionally, DVT itself.

Venography is also expensive and not easily repeated. A combination of three noninvasive tests — Doppler ultrasonography, impedance plethysmography, and ^{125}I fibrinogen scan — is an acceptable though less accurate alternative to venography. Radionuclide tests, such as the ^{125}I fibrinogen scan, are used to screen for DVT or to attempt to detect the disorder in a patient who is too ill for venography or is hypersensitive to the contrast medium.

Purpose

- To confirm a diagnosis of DVT
- To distinguish clot formation from venous obstruction (for example, a large tumor of the pelvis impinging on the venous system)
- To evaluate congenital venous abnormalities
- To assess deep vein valvular competence (especially helpful in identifying underlying causes of leg edema)
- To locate a suitable vein for arterial bypass grafting

Patient preparation

- Explain to the patient that lower limb venography helps detect abnormal conditions in the veins of the legs.
- Instruct the patient to restrict food and to drink only clear liquids for 4 hours before the test.
- Describe the test, including who will perform it and where it will take place. Tell the patient pretest blood work for coagulation and kidney function may be needed.
- Warn the patient that he may feel a burning sensation in his leg on injection of the contrast medium and some discomfort during the procedure.

PATIENT POSITIONING FOR LOWER LIMB VENOGRAPHY

In lower limb venography, the patient lies on an X-ray table that's inclined 40 to 60 degrees, while keeping his weight off the leg being tested. Fluoroscopy monitors the progress of the contrast medium, and spot films are taken as the contrast circulates through the venous system of the leg.

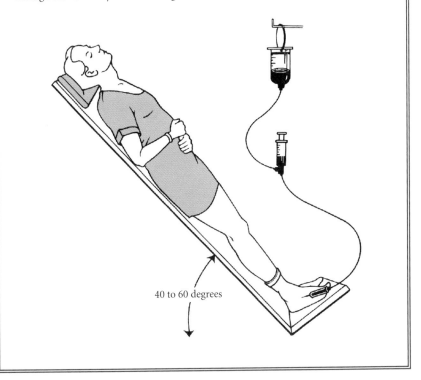

40 to 60 degrees

- Make sure that the patient or a responsible family member has signed an informed consent form.
- Check the patient's history for hypersensitivity to iodine or iodine-containing foods or to contrast media. Mark any sensitivities on the chart and notify the physician.
- Reassure the patient that contrast media complications are rare, but tell him to report nausea, severe burning or itching, constriction in the throat or chest, or dyspnea immediately. Restrict anticoagulant therapy, if ordered.

- Just before the test, instruct the patient to void, to remove all clothing below the waist, and to put on a gown.
- If ordered, administer a prescribed sedative to an anxious or uncooperative patient.

Procedure and posttest care
- The patient is positioned on a tilting radiographic table so that the leg being tested doesn't bear any weight. (See *Patient positioning for lower limb venography.*) He's instructed to relax this leg and keep it still; a tourniquet may be tied

around the ankle to expedite venous filling.

■ A superficial vein in the dorsum of the patient's foot is injected with normal saline solution.

■ When needle placement is correct, 100 to 150 ml of the contrast medium is slowly injected over 90 seconds to 3 minutes and the presence of extravasation is checked.

■ If a suitable superficial vein can't be found (due to edema), a surgical cutdown of the vein may be performed.

■ Using a fluoroscope, the distribution of the contrast medium is monitored, and spot films are taken from the anteroposterior and oblique projections and over the thigh and femoroiliac regions. Then, overhead films are taken of the calf, knee, thigh, and femoral area.

■ After filming, the patient is repositioned horizontally, the leg is quickly elevated, and normal saline solution is infused to flush the contrast medium from the veins.

■ The fluoroscope is checked to confirm complete emptying. Then the needle is removed.

■ Apply an adhesive bandage to the injection site.

■ Monitor the patient's vital signs until he's stable; check his pulse rate and quality on the dorsalis pedis, popliteal, and femoral arteries.

■ Administer prescribed analgesics, as ordered, to counteract the irritating effects of the contrast medium.

■ Watch for an allergic reaction to the contrast medium, hematoma, redness, bleeding, or infection (especially if a vein cutdown was performed) at the puncture site, and replace the dressing when necessary. Notify the physician if complications develop.

■ If the venogram indicates DVT, initiate the prescribed therapy (heparin infusion, bed rest, leg elevation or support, or blood chemistry tests).

■ Tell the patient that he may resume his usual diet and medications, as ordered.

■ Observe the patient for signs and symptoms of a latent reaction to the dye. Encourage fluids to flush the dye from the kidneys.

Precautions

▶ **CLINICAL ALERT** *Most allergic reactions to the contrast medium occur within 30 minutes of injection. Carefully observe the patient for signs of anaphylaxis (flushing, urticaria, laryngeal stridor).*

Normal findings

A normal venogram shows steady opacification of the superficial and deep vasculature with no filling defects.

Abnormal findings

A venogram that shows consistent filling defects on repeat views, abrupt termination of a column of contrast material, unfilled major deep veins, or diversion of flow (for example, through collateral veins) is diagnostic of DVT.

Interfering factors

■ The patient placing weight on the leg being tested (possible filling of leg veins with contract medium)

■ Movement of the leg being tested

■ Excessive tourniquet constriction

■ Insufficient injection or dilution of contrast medium

■ Delay between injection and radiography

■ Previous thrombosis, severe edema or obesity, or cellulitis (may limit visualization of the deep venous system)

GRAPHIC MONITORING

Electrocardiography

A common test for evaluating cardiac status, electrocardiography (ECG) graphically records the electric current (electrical potential) generated by the heart. This current radiates from the heart in all directions and, on reaching the skin, is measured by electrodes connected to an amplifier and strip chart recorder. The standard resting (scalar) ECG uses 5 electrodes to measure the electrical potential from 12 leads: the standard limb leads (I, II, III), the augmented limb leads (aV_R, aV_L, and aV_F), and the precordial, or chest, leads (V_1 through V_6).

New computerized ECG machines don't routinely use gel and suction bulbs. The electrodes are small tabs that peel off a sheet and adhere to the patient's skin. The leads coming from the ECG machine are clearly marked and applied to the electrodes with alligator clamps. The entire tracing is displayed on a screen so that abnormalities (loose leads or artifacts) can be corrected before the tracing is printed or transmitted to a central computer. The electrode tabs can remain on the patient's chest, arms, and legs to provide continuous lead placement for serial ECG studies.

Purpose
- To help identify primary conduction abnormalities, cardiac arrhythmias, cardiac hypertrophy, pericarditis, electrolyte imbalances, myocardial ischemia, and the site and extent of myocardial infarction (MI)
- To monitor recovery from an MI
- To evaluate the effectiveness of cardiac medication (cardiac glycosides, antiarrhythmics, antihypertensives, and vasodilators)
- To assess pacemaker performance
- To determine the effectiveness of thrombolytic therapy and the resolution of ST-segment depression or elevation and T-wave changes

Patient preparation
- Explain to the patient that an ECG evaluates the heart's electrical activity.
- Tell the patient that he need not restrict food and fluids.
- Describe the test, including who will perform it, where it will take place, and how long it will last.
- Tell the patient that electrodes will be attached to his arms, legs, and chest and that the procedure is painless. Explain that during the test, he'll be asked to relax, lie still, and breathe normally.
- Advise the patient not to talk during the test because the sound of his voice may distort the ECG tracing.
- Check the patient's medication history for use of cardiac drugs and note the use of such drugs on the test request form.

Equipment
ECG machine, recording paper, pregelled disposable electrodes, shaving supplies (if necessary), marking pen, moist cloth towel, sterile drape

Procedure and posttest care
- Place the patient in the supine position. If he can't tolerate lying flat, help him to assume semi-Fowler's position.
- Have the patient expose his chest, both ankles, and both wrists for electrode placement. If the patient is a woman, provide a chest drape until the chest leads are applied.
- Turn on the machine and check the paper supply.

NORMAL ECG WAVEFORMS

Because each lead takes a different view of heart activity, it generates its own characteristic tracing. The traces shown here are representative of each of the 12 leads. Leads aV_R, V_1, V_2, V_3, and V_4 normally show strong negative deflections. Negative deflections indicate that the current is moving away from the positive electrode; positive deflections, that the current is moving toward the positive electrode.

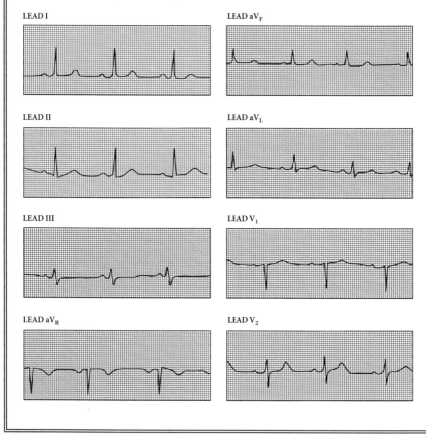

LEAD I   LEAD aV_F

LEAD II   LEAD aV_L

LEAD III   LEAD V_1

LEAD aV_R LEAD V_2

Multichannel ECG

■ Place electrodes on the inner aspect of the wrists, the medial aspect of the lower legs, and the chest. If using disposable electrodes, remove the paper backing before positioning.

■ Connect the leadwires after all electrodes are in place.

■ If frequent ECGs will be necessary, use a marking pen to indicate lead positions on the patient's chest to ensure consistent placement.

■ Press the START button and record any required information (for example, the patient's name and room number).

■ The machine produces a printout showing all 12 leads simultaneously.

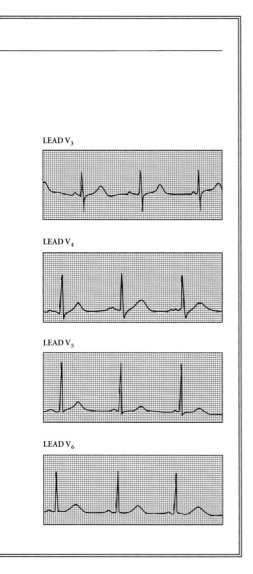

LEAD V₃

LEAD V₄

LEAD V₅

LEAD V₆

Check to make sure all leads are represented in the tracing. If not, determine which one has come loose, reattach it, and restart the tracing.

■ Make sure the wave doesn't peak beyond the top edge of the recording grid. If it does, adjust the machine to bring the wave inside the boundaries.

■ When the machine finishes the tracing, remove the electrodes and reposition the patient's gown and bed covers.

Single-channel ECG

■ Apply either disposable or standard electrodes to the inner aspect of the wrists and the medial aspect of the lower legs. Connect each leadwire to the corresponding electrode by inserting the wire prong into the terminal post and tightening the screw, if required.

■ Set the paper speed, if required (usually 25 mm/second), and calibrate the machine by adjusting the sensitivity to normal. Recalibrate the machine after running each lead to provide a consistent test standard.

■ Turn the lead selector to I. Then mark the lead by writing "I" on the paper strip or by depressing the marking button on the machine (some machines do this automatically). Record for 3 to 6 seconds, and then return the machine to the standby mode. Repeat this procedure for leads II, III, aV_R, aV_L, and aV_F.

■ Determine proper placement for the chest electrodes. (If frequent ECGs are necessary, mark these spots on the patient's chest to ensure consistent placement.)

■ Connect the chest leadwire to the suction bulb, apply gel to each of the six chest positions, and then firmly press the suction bulb to attach the chest lead to the V_1 position. Mark the strips as before.

■ Turn the lead selector to V_1, and record V_1 for 3 to 6 seconds. Return the lead selector to standby. Reposition the electrode, and repeat the procedure for V_2 through V_6.

■ After completing V_6, run a rhythm strip on lead II for at least 6 seconds. Assess the quality of the tracings and repeat any that are unclear.

■ Disconnect the equipment, remove the electrodes, and wipe the gel from the patient with a moist cloth towel. Wash the gel from the electrodes and dry them thoroughly.

Both types
■ Label each ECG strip with the patient's name and room number (if applicable), date and time of the procedure, and physician's name. Note whether the ECG was performed during or on resolution of a chest pain episode.
■ Disconnect the equipment. The electrode patches are usually left in place if the patient is having recurrent chest pain or if serial ECGs are ordered, as with the use of thrombolytics.
■ Report any abnormal ECG findings to the physician.

Precautions
■ The recording equipment and other nearby electrical equipment should be properly grounded to prevent electrical interference.
■ Double-check color codes and lead markings to be sure connectors match.
■ Make sure that the electrodes are firmly attached, and reattach them if loose skin contact is suspected. Don't use cables that are broken, frayed, or bare.
■ Make sure that the patient is quiet and motionless during the test because talking and movement distort the recordings.
■ If the patient has a pacemaker in place, an ECG may be performed with or without a magnet. Indicate the presence of a pacemaker and whether a magnet is used. (Many pacemakers function only when the heartbeat falls below a preset rate; a magnet makes the pacemaker fire regularly, which permits evaluation of pacemaker performance.)

Normal findings
The lead II waveform, known as the rhythm strip, depicts the heart's rhythm more clearly than any other waveform. In lead II, the normal P wave doesn't exceed 2.5 mm (0.25 mV) in height or last longer than 0.12 second. The PR interval, which includes the P wave plus the PR segment, persists for 0.12 to 0.2 second for heart rates above 60 beats/minute. The QT interval varies with the heart rate and lasts 0.4 to 0.52 second for heart rates above 60 beats/minute; the voltage of the R wave in the V_1 through V_6 leads doesn't exceed 27 mm. The total QRS complex lasts 0.06 to 0.1 second. The ST segment is also useful for assessing myocardial ischemia. (See *Normal ECG waveforms,* pages 830 and 831.)

Abnormal findings
An abnormal ECG may show an MI, right or left ventricular hypertrophy, arrhythmias, right or left bundle-branch block, ischemia, conduction defects or pericarditis, electrolyte abnormalities (such as hypokalemia), and the effects of cardioactive drugs. Sometimes an ECG may reveal abnormal waveforms only during angina episodes or during exercise. (See *Abnormal ECG waveforms.*)

Interfering factors
■ Inaccurate test results because of improper placement of electrodes, patient movement or muscle tremors, strenuous exercise before the test, or medication reactions
■ Mechanical difficulties, such as ECG machine malfunction, faulty adherence of electrode patches (for example, due to diaphoresis), and electromagnetic interference (production of artifact)

(Text continues on page 836.)

ABNORMAL ECG WAVEFORMS

Premature ventricular contractions (PVCs) originate in an ectopic focus of the ventricular wall. They can be unifocal (having the same single focus), as shown in this tracing from lead V_1, or multifocal (arising from more than one ectopic focus). In PVCs, the P wave is absent and the QRS complex shows considerable distortion, usually deflecting in the opposite direction from the patient's normal QRS complex. The T wave also deflects in the opposite direction from the QRS complex, and the PVC usually precedes a compensatory pause. Some examples of abnormalities causing PVCs include electrolyte imbalances (especially hypokalemia), myocardial infarction (MI), reperfusion of a new MI or injury, hypoxia, and drug toxicity (cardiac glycosides, beta-adrenergics).

PVC — LEAD V_1

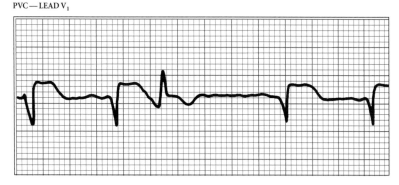

First-degree heart block, the most common conduction disturbance, occurs in healthy hearts as well as diseased hearts and usually is clinically insignificant. It's typically characteristic in elderly patients with chronic degeneration of the cardiac conduction system, and it occasionally occurs in patients receiving cardiac glycosides or antiarrhythmic drugs, such as procainamide and quinidine. In children, first-degree heart block may be the earliest sign of acute rheumatic fever. In this lead V_1 tracing, the interval between the P wave and the QRS complex (the PR interval) exceeds 0.20 second.

FIRST-DEGREE HEART BLOCK — LEAD V_1

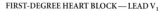

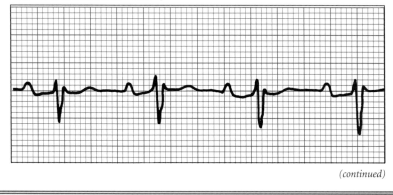

(continued)

ABNORMAL ECG WAVEFORMS *(continued)*

Hypokalemia is a common electrolyte imbalance that's caused by low serum potassium levels and affects the electrical activity of the myocardium. Mild hypokalemia may cause only muscle weakness, fatigue and, possibly, atrial or ventricular irritability; a severe imbalance causes pronounced muscle weakness, paralysis, atrial tachycardia with varying degrees of block, and PVCs that may progress to ventricular tachycardia and fibrillation.

Early signs of hypokalemia, as shown on this lead V_1 tracing, include prominent U waves, a prolonged QU interval, and flat or inverted T waves. Usually, T waves don't flatten or invert until potassium depletion becomes severe.

HYPOKALEMIA — LEAD V_1

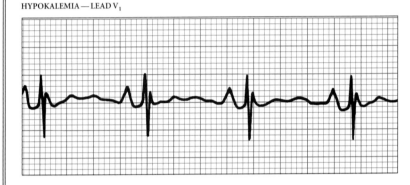

MI produces typical ECG changes in several leads at once, enabling the physician to accurately determine the location and extent of tissue damage. MI causes three changes: an inner zone of tissue necrosis (infarction), a surrounding zone of inflamed tissue, and an outer zone of ischemia. As the infarction progresses, the first ECG change is an elevated ST segment, which indicates formation of an ischemic zone. Then the T wave begins to flatten and finally inverts, and enlarged Q waves appear, indicating developing necrosis — a true infarction. (Abnormal Q waves should be larger than one small square on the chart — 0.04 second by 0.1 mV.) The T wave may stay inverted for the rest of the patient's life or it can revert to normal, whereas the deep Q wave remains as a permanent indicator of necrosis. The infarction can be located by studying the characteristic ST-segment, T-wave, and Q-wave changes in various lead combinations. In the three tracings shown here, the ST-segment elevations in leads II, III, and aV_F indicate an infarction in the inferior (diaphragmatic) area of the heart.

ABNORMAL ECG WAVEFORMS *(continued)*

Stages of MI

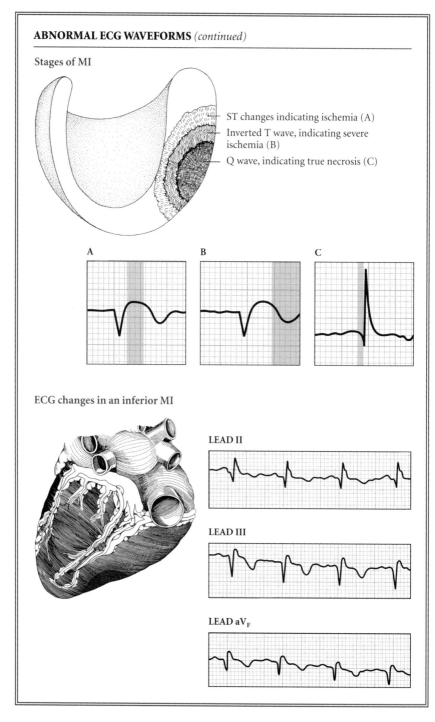

ST changes indicating ischemia (A)

Inverted T wave, indicating severe ischemia (B)

Q wave, indicating true necrosis (C)

A   B   C

ECG changes in an inferior MI

LEAD II

LEAD III

LEAD aV_F

Exercise electrocardiography

Also referred to as *a stress test,* an exercise electrocardiogram (ECG) evaluates the heart's response to physical stress, providing important diagnostic information that can't be obtained from a resting ECG alone.

An ECG and blood pressure readings are taken while the patient walks on a treadmill or pedals a stationary bicycle, and his response to a constant or an increasing workload is observed. Unless complications develop, the test continues until the patient reaches the target heart rate (determined by an established protocol) or experiences chest pain or fatigue. The patient who has recently had a myocardial infarction (MI) or coronary artery surgery may walk the treadmill at a slow pace to determine his activity tolerance before discharge.

Purpose
- To help diagnose the cause of chest pain or other possible cardiac pain
- To determine the functional capacity of the heart after surgery or an MI
- To screen for asymptomatic coronary artery disease (CAD), particularly in men over age 35
- To help set limitations for an exercise program
- To identify arrhythmias that develop during physical exercise
- To evaluate the effectiveness of antiarrhythmic or antianginal therapy
- To evaluate myocardial perfusion

Patient preparation
- Explain to the patient that the exercise ECG records the heart's electrical activity and performance under stress.

- Instruct the patient not to eat, smoke, or drink alcoholic or caffeinated beverages for 3 hours before the test, but to continue his prescribed drug regimen unless directed otherwise.
- Describe to the patient who will perform the test, where it will take place, and how long it will last.
- Tell the patient that the test will cause fatigue and that he'll be slightly breathless and sweaty, but assure him that the test poses few risks. He may, in fact, stop the test if he experiences fatigue or chest pain.
- Advise the patient to wear comfortable socks and shoes and loose, lightweight shorts or slacks. Men usually don't wear a shirt during the test, and women generally wear a bra and a lightweight short-sleeved blouse or a patient gown with a front closure.
- Explain to the patient that electrodes will be attached to several areas on his chest and, possibly, his back after the skin areas are cleaned and abraded. Reassure him that he won't feel current from the electrodes; however, they may itch slightly.
- Tell the patient that his blood pressure will be checked periodically throughout the procedure and assure him that his heart rate will be monitored continuously.
- If the patient is scheduled for a multi-stage *treadmill test,* explain that the speed and incline of the treadmill will increase at predetermined intervals and that he'll be informed of each adjustment.
- If the patient is scheduled for a *bicycle ergometer test,* explain that the resistance he experiences in pedaling increases gradually as he tries to maintain a specific speed.
- Encourage the patient to report his feelings during the test. Tell him that his

blood pressure and ECG will be monitored for 10 to 15 minutes after the test.

■ Check the patient's history for a recent physical examination (within 1 week) and for baseline 12-lead ECG results.

■ Make sure that the patient or a responsible family member has signed an informed consent form.

Procedure and posttest care

■ The electrode sites are cleaned with an alcohol swab, and superficial epidermal cell layers and excess skin oils are removed with a gauze pad, fine sandpaper, or a dental burr. After thorough cleaning and abrading, adequately prepared sites will appear slightly red.

■ Chest electrodes are placed according to the lead system selected and are secured with adhesive tape, if necessary. The leadwire cable is placed over the patient's shoulder, and the leadwire box is placed on his chest. The cable is secured by pinning it to the patient's clothing or taping it to his shoulder or back. Then the leadwires are connected to the chest electrodes.

■ The monitor is started, and a stable baseline tracing is obtained and checked for arrhythmias. A blood pressure reading is taken, and the patient is auscultated for the presence of S_3 or S_4 gallops or crackles.

■ In a treadmill test, the treadmill is turned on to a slow speed, and the patient is shown how to step onto it and how to use the support railings to maintain balance, but not support weight. Then the treadmill is turned off. The patient is instructed to step onto the treadmill, and it's turned on to slow speed until he gets used to walking on it. Exercise intensity is then increased every 3 minutes by slightly increasing the speed of the machine and

at the same time increasing the incline by 3%.

■ For a bicycle ergometer test, the patient is instructed to sit on the bicycle while the seat and handlebars are adjusted to comfortable positions. He's instructed not to grip the handlebars tightly, but to use them only for maintaining balance and to pedal until he reaches the desired speed, as shown on the speedometer.

■ In both tests, a monitor is observed continuously for changes in the heart's electrical activity. The rhythm strip is checked at preset intervals for arrhythmias, premature ventricular contractions (PVCs), and ST-segment and T-wave changes. The test level and the time elapsed in the test level are marked on each strip. Blood pressure is monitored at predetermined intervals, usually at the end of each test level, and changes in systolic readings are noted. Some common responses to maximal exercise are dizziness, light-headedness, leg fatigue, dyspnea, diaphoresis, and a slightly ataxic gait. If symptoms become severe, the test is stopped.

■ Usually, testing stops when the patient reaches the target heart rate. As the treadmill speed slows, he may be instructed to continue walking for several minutes to cool down. Then the treadmill is turned off, the patient is helped to a chair, and his blood pressure and ECG are monitored for 10 to 15 minutes or until the ECG returns to baseline.

■ Auscultate for the presence of an S_3 or S_4 gallop. An S_4 gallop commonly develops after exercise because of increased blood flow volume and turbulence. An S_3 gallop is more significant than an S_4 gallop, indicating transient left ventricular dysfunction.

- Tell the patient that he may resume any activities and medications discontinued before the test, as ordered.
- Remove the electrodes and clean the electrode sites before the patient leaves.

Precautions

- Because an exercise ECG places considerable stress on the heart, it may be contraindicated in the patient with ventricular aneurysm, dissecting aortic aneurysm, uncontrolled arrhythmias, pericarditis, myocarditis, severe anemia, uncontrolled hypertension, unstable angina, or heart failure.
- Stop the test immediately if the ECG shows three consecutive PVCs or a significant increase in ectopy, if the systolic blood pressure falls below resting level, if the heart rate falls to 10 beats/minute below resting level, or if the patient becomes exhausted. Depending on the patient's condition, the test may be stopped if the ECG shows bundle-branch block, ST-segment depression that exceeds 1.5 mm, persistent ST-segment elevation, or frequent or complicated PVCs; if blood pressure fails to rise above the resting level; if systolic pressure exceeds 220 mm Hg; or if the patient experiences angina.

Normal findings

In a normal exercise ECG, the P and T waves, the QRS complex, and the ST segment change minimally; a slight ST-segment depression occurs in some cases, especially a woman. The heart rate rises in direct proportion to the workload and metabolic oxygen demand; blood pressure also rises as workload increases. The patient attains the endurance levels predicted by his age and the appropriate exercise protocol. (See *Exercise ECG tracings.*)

Abnormal findings

Although criteria for judging test results vary, two findings strongly suggest an abnormality: a flat or downsloping ST-segment depression of 1 mm or more for at least 0.08 second after the junction of the QRS and ST segments (J point) and a markedly depressed J point, with an upsloping but depressed ST segment of 1.5 mm below the baseline 0.08 second after the J point. T-wave inversion also signifies ischemia. Initial ST-segment depression on the resting ECG must be further depressed by 1 mm during exercise to be considered abnormal.

Hypotension resulting from exercise, ST-segment depression of 3 mm or more, downsloping ST segments, and ischemic ST segments appearing within the first 3 minutes of exercise and lasting 8 minutes into the posttest recovery period may indicate multivessel or left CAD. ST-segment elevation may indicate dyskinetic left ventricular wall motion or severe transmural ischemia.

The predictive value of this test for CAD varies with the patient's history and sex; false-negative and false-positive test results are common. This is usually related to the effects of drugs, such as digoxin, or caffeine ingestion before testing. To detect CAD accurately, thallium imaging and stress testing, exercise multiple-gated acquisition scanning, or coronary angiography may be necessary.

Interfering factors

- Failure to observe pretest restrictions
- The patient's inability to exercise to the target heart rate due to fatigue or failure to cooperate
- Wolff-Parkinson-White syndrome (anomalous atrioventricular excitation), electrolyte imbalance, or use of a cardiac glycoside (possible false-positive)

EXERCISE ECG TRACINGS

These tracings are from an abnormal exercise electrocardiogram (ECG) obtained during a treadmill test performed on a patient who had just undergone a triple coronary artery bypass graft. The first tracing shows the heart at rest, with a blood pressure reading of 124/80 mm Hg. In the second tracing, the patient worked up to a 10% grade at 1.7 miles per hour before experiencing angina at 2 minutes, 25 seconds. The tracing shows a depressed ST segment; heart rate was 85 beats/minute, and blood pressure was 140/70 mm Hg. The third tracing shows the heart at rest 6 minutes after the test; blood pressure was 140/90 mm Hg.

RESTING

ANGINA

RECOVERY

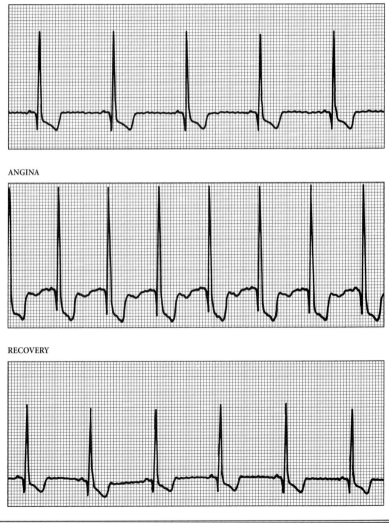

- Conditions that affect left ventricular hypertrophy, such as congenital abnormalities and hypertension (possible interference with testing for ischemia)
- Beta-adrenergic blockers (may make test results difficult to interpret)

Holter monitoring

Holter monitoring, also called *dynamic monitoring* and *ambulatory electrocardiography* (ECG), involves the continuous recording of heart activity over a 24-hour period as the patient follows his normal routine. During this period, the patient wears a small reel-to-reel or cassette tape recorder connected to electrodes placed on his chest and keeps a diary of his activities and any associated symptoms. After the recording period, the tape is analyzed by a computer and a physician to correlate cardiac irregularities, such as arrhythmias and ST-segment changes, with the activities noted in the patient's diary.

Purpose
- To detect cardiac arrhythmias
- To evaluate chest pain
- To evaluate cardiac status after an acute myocardial infarction (MI) or a pacemaker implantation
- To evaluate the effectiveness of antiarrhythmic drug therapy
- To assess and correlate dyspnea, central nervous system (CNS) symptoms (such as syncope and light-headedness), and palpitations with actual cardiac events and the patient's activities

Patient preparation
- Explain to the patient that Holter monitoring helps determine how the heart responds to normal activity or, if appropriate, to cardioactive medication. Tell him that electrodes will be attached to his chest, that his chest may be shaved, and that he may experience some discomfort during preparation of the electrode sites.
- Explain to the patient that he'll wear a small tape recorder for 24 hours (for 5 to 7 days, if a patient-activated monitor is being used).
- Mention that a shoulder strap or a special belt will be provided to carry the recorder, which weighs about 2 lb (1 kg). Show him how to position the recorder when he lies down.
- Encourage the patient to continue his routine activities during the monitoring period. Stress the importance of logging his usual activities (such as walking, climbing stairs, urinating, sleeping, and having sex), emotional upsets, physical symptoms (dizziness, palpitations, fatigue, chest pain, and syncope), and ingestion of medication; show the patient a sample diary.
- Tell the patient to wear loose-fitting clothing with front-buttoning tops during monitoring.
- Demonstrate the proper use of specific equipment, including how to mark the tape (if applicable) at the onset of symptoms.
- If a patient-activated monitor is being used, show the patient how to press the event button to activate the monitor if he experiences an unusual sensation. Instruct him not to tamper with the monitor or disconnect the leadwires or electrodes.
- Bathing instructions depend on the type of recorder being worn (certain equipment must not get wet).
- Advise the patient to avoid magnets, metal detectors, high-voltage areas, and electric blankets. Show him how to check the recorder to make sure it's working properly. Instruct him how to trouble-

shoot problems if the monitor alarm sounds. Explain that if the monitor light flashes, one of the electrodes may be loose and he should depress the center of each one. Tell him to notify you if one comes off.

■ If the patient won't be returning to the health care facility immediately after the monitoring period, show him how to remove and store the equipment. Remind him to bring the diary when he returns.

Procedure and posttest care
■ Clean and gently abrade the electrode sites. Peel the backings from the electrodes and apply them to the correct sites, making sure to press the sides and center of each electrode firmly to ensure proper adhesion.
■ Attach the electrode cable securely to the monitor.
■ Position the monitor and case as the patient will wear it, and then attach the leadwires to the electrodes. There shouldn't be too much slack or pull on the wires.
■ Make sure the recorder has a new or fully charged battery, insert the tape, and turn on the recorder.
■ Test the electrode attachment circuit by connecting the recorder to a standard ECG machine. Watch for artifacts while the patient moves normally (stands, sits).
■ Remove all chest electrodes and clean the electrode sites after the test.

Precautions
■ To eliminate muscle artifact, make sure the lead cable is plugged in firmly. Check to ensure that electrodes aren't placed over large muscle masses such as the pectorals.

Normal findings
When correlated with the patient's diary, the ECG pattern shows normal sinus

rhythm with no significant arrhythmias or ST-segment changes. Changes in heart rate normally occur during various activities.

Abnormal findings
Cardiac abnormalities detected by ambulatory ECG include premature ventricular contractions (PVCs), conduction defects, tachyarrhythmias, bradyarrhythmias, and brady-tachy syndrome. Arrhythmias may be associated with dyspnea and CNS symptoms, such as dizziness and syncope.

During recovery from an MI, this test can monitor for PVCs to determine the prognosis and effectiveness of drug therapy.

ST-T wave changes associated with ischemia may coincide with chest pain or increased patient activity. ST-segment changes associated with an acute MI require careful study because smoking, eating, postural changes, certain drugs, Wolff-Parkinson-White syndrome, bundle-branch block, myocarditis, myocardial hypertrophy, anemia, hypoxemia, and abnormal hemoglobin binding can produce a similar tracing on the ECG. Monitoring the patient with an MI for 1 to 3 days before discharge and again 4 to 6 weeks after discharge may detect ST-T wave changes associated with ischemia or arrhythmias; such information aids patient therapy and rehabilitation and refines the prognosis. Monitoring a patient with an artificial pacemaker may detect an arrhythmia, such as bradycardia, that the pacemaker fails to override.

Although ambulatory ECG correlates patient symptoms and ECG changes, it doesn't always identify the symptoms' causes. If initial monitoring proves inconclusive, the test may be repeated.

Interfering factors

- Electrode placement over a large muscle mass, poor electrode contact with skin, or other failure to correctly apply the electrodes (possible muscle or movement artifact)
- The patient's failure to carefully record daily activities and symptoms, to maintain his normal routine, or to turn on the monitor during symptoms (if using a patient-activated monitor)
- Physiologic variation in arrhythmia frequency and severity (possible failure to detect arrhythmias during 24-hour Holter monitoring)

Signal-averaged electrocardiography

Signal averaging is the amplification, averaging, and filtering of an electrocardiogram (ECG) signal that's recorded on the body surface by orthogonal leads. The recording detects high-frequency, low-amplitude cardiac electrical signals in the last part of the QRS complex and in the ST segment. In patients who have survived an acute myocardial infarction (MI), these distinctive signals, called late potentials, may represent delayed disorganized activity in abnormal areas of the myocardium at the interface of fibrous scar tissue and normal tissue. This activity can lead to life-threatening ventricular arrhythmias.

In this computerized procedure, each electrode lead input is amplified, its voltage is measured or sampled at intervals of 1 msec or less, and each sample is converted into a digital number. The ECG is thereby converted from an analogue voltage waveform into a series of digital numbers that are, in essence, a computer-readable ECG of 100 or more QRS complexes.

Purpose

- To detect late potentials and evaluate the risk of life-threatening arrhythmias

Patient preparation

- Explain to the patient that signal-averaged ECG is used to evaluate his heart's electrical activity and the potential for developing a life-threatening arrhythmia.
- Inform the patient that the test will be performed by a technician who has been specially trained to monitor recording and computerized equipment used to analyze the signal-averaged ECG.
- Describe the test, including who will perform it, where it will take place, and how long it will last.
- Tell the patient that electrodes will be attached to his arms, legs, and chest and that the procedure is painless.
- Explain to the patient that during the test, he'll be asked to lie still and breathe normally. This is important because limb movement or the sound of his voice will distort the recording.
- Inform the patient that he need not restrict food and fluids.
- Record on the patient's chart any use of antiarrhythmics.

Equipment

Recording paper, disposable electrodes or reusable electrodes with suction bulbs, conductive gel, rubber straps, 4″ × 4″ gauze pads, moist cloth towel, sterile drape, computer equipment for analyzing the recorded ECG

Procedure and posttest care

- Place the patient in the supine position. If he can't tolerate lying flat, help him into semi-Fowler's position.
- Have the patient expose his chest, both ankles, and both wrists for electrode

placement. If the patient is a woman, provide a chest drape until the chest leads are applied.

■ The test is performed by a technician who's specially trained to operate the recording and computer equipment used in analyzing the signal-averaged ECG.

■ The technician gathers the multiple inputs necessary for signal averaging from standard orthogonal bipolar X, Y, and Z leads over a series of ECG cycles. The average is taken over a large number of beats, typically 100 or more.

■ After the test is completed, disconnect the equipment. If suction cups were used, be sure to wash the conductive gel from the patient's skin.

Precautions

■ The recording equipment and other nearby electrical equipment should be properly grounded to prevent electrical interference.

■ Tissue-electrode artifacts can be minimized by lightly sanding the skin with fine sandpaper (no. 220), wiping with alcohol, and using silver-silver chloride electrodes.

■ Urge the patient to lie as quiet and motionless as possible to avoid signal distortion.

Normal findings

A QRS complex without low potentials is considered normal.

The areas of interest in the signal-averaged ECG are:

■ the duration of the filtered QRS complex (QRST), which indicates how long the completion of the QRS complex is delayed by late potentials

■ the amount of energy in the late potentials, as indicated by the root mean square (RMS) voltage in the terminal 40 msec of the QRS complex (RMS40)

■ the duration of the late potentials, as indicated by the duration of the low-amplitude signals of less than 40 μV in the terminal QRS region.

The preceding values can be read either from the signal-averaged ECG itself or from the computer system.

Defining a late potential and scoring a signal-averaged ECG as normal or abnormal are highly dependent on technique. Representative criteria include when late potentials exist when the filtered QRS complex is longer than 114 msec, when there's less than 20 μV RMS of signal in the terminal 40 msec of the filtered QRS, or when the terminal portion of the filtered QRS remains below 40 μV for longer than 38 msec.

Abnormal findings

Identifying late potentials after the QRS complex indicates a risk of ventricular arrhythmias. Late potentials are most common and of greater prognostic value in the patient who has sustained an MI. The patient who doesn't have late potentials is at low risk for serious ventricular arrhythmias and sudden death. Although the predictive accuracy of a positive signal-averaged ECG is relatively low, it has been advocated as a screening test for the patient who should undergo electrophysiologic testing.

Interfering factors

■ Artifact from skeletal muscle movement (possible need to administer a muscle relaxant)

■ Electromagnetic interference (possible need to shield and twist input cables to reduce noise)

■ Poor tissue-electrode contact (production of artifact)

■ Antiarrhythmic drugs

Impedance plethysmography

Also called *occlusive impedance phlebography,* impedance plethysmography is a reliable, widely used, noninvasive test that measures venous flow in the limbs. Electrodes from a plethysmograph are applied to the patient's leg to record changes in electrical resistance (impedance) caused by blood volume variations that may result from respiration or venous occlusion.

Purpose

- To detect deep vein thrombosis (DVT) in the proximal deep veins of the leg
- To screen the patient at high risk for thrombophlebitis
- To evaluate the patient with suspected pulmonary embolism (because most pulmonary emboli are complications of DVT in the leg)

Patient preparation

- Explain to the patient that impedance plethysmography helps detect DVT.
- Inform the patient that he need not restrict food, fluids, and medications.
- Explain that the test requires that both legs be tested and that three to five tracings may be made for each leg.
- Tell the patient who will perform the test and where it will take place.
- Assure the patient that the test is painless and safe.
- Emphasize that accurate testing requires that leg muscles be relaxed and breathing be normal. Reassure the patient that if he experiences pain that interferes with leg relaxation, a mild analgesic will be administered, if ordered.
- Just before the test, instruct the patient to void and to put on a hospital gown.

Procedure and posttest care

- Place the patient in the supine position, elevating the leg to be tested 30 to 35 degrees. To promote venous drainage, place the calf above the patient's heart level.
- Ask the patient to flex his knee slightly and to rotate his hips by shifting weight to the same side as the leg being tested.
- After the electrodes (connected to the plethysmograph) have been loosely attached to the calf about 3″ to 4″ (7.5 to 10 cm) apart, the pressure cuff (connected to the air pressure system) is wrapped snugly around the thigh about 2″ (5 cm) above the knee.
- The pressure cuff is inflated to 45 to 60 cm H_2O, allowing full venous distention without interfering with arterial blood flow. Pressure is maintained for 45 seconds or until the tracing stabilizes. (In a patient with reduced arterial blood flow, pressure is maintained for 2 minutes or longer, after which the pressure cuff is rapidly deflated.)
- The strip chart tracing, which records the increase in venous volume after cuff inflation and the decrease in venous volume 3 seconds after deflation, is checked. Then the test is repeated for the other leg. If necessary, three to five tracings for each leg are obtained to confirm full venous filling and outflow; the tracing showing the greatest rise and fall in venous volume is used as the test result.
- If the result is ambiguous, the position of the patient's leg as well as cuff and electrode placement are checked.
- Make sure that the conductive gel is removed from the patient's skin after the test.

Precautions

- Urge the patient to lie quietly and relax and much as possible.

■ Keep the room temperature as warm as possible to help prevent the patient's extremities from becoming cold.

Normal findings

Temporary venous occlusion normally produces a sharp rise in venous volume; release of the occlusion produces rapid venous outflow.

Abnormal findings

When clots in a major deep vein obstruct venous outflow, the pressure in the distal leg (calf) veins rises, and these veins become distended. Such veins are unable to expand further when additional pressure is applied with an occlusive thigh cuff. Blockage of major deep veins also decreases the rate at which blood flows from the leg. If significant thrombi are present in a major deep vein of the lower leg (popliteal, femoral, or iliac), calf vein filling and venous outflow rates are reduced. In such cases, the physician will evaluate the need for further treatment, such as anticoagulant therapy, taking the patient's overall condition into consideration.

Interfering factors

■ Decreased peripheral arterial blood flow due to shock, increased vasoconstriction, low cardiac output, or arterial occlusive disease

■ Extrinsic venous compression, as from pelvic tumors, large hematomas, constricting clothing, or bandages

■ The patient's failure to breathe normally or to completely relax his leg muscles due to pain

■ Cold extremities due to cold room temperature

ULTRASONOGRAPHY

Echocardiography

Echocardiography is a noninvasive test that shows the size, shape, and motion of cardiac structures. It's useful for evaluating patients with chest pain, enlarged cardiac silhouettes on X-ray films, electrocardiographic (ECG) changes unrelated to coronary artery disease (CAD), and abnormal heart sounds on auscultation.

In this test, a transducer directs ultra-high-frequency sound waves toward cardiac structures, which reflect these waves. The echoes are converted to images that are displayed on a monitor and recorded on a strip chart or videotape. Results are correlated with clinical history, physical examination, and findings from additional tests.

The techniques most commonly used in echocardiography are M-mode (motion-mode), for recording the motion and dimensions of intracardiac structures, and two-dimensional (cross-sectional), for recording lateral motion and providing the correct spatial relationship between cardiac structures. (See *M-mode echocardiograms*, page 846.)

Purpose

■ To diagnose and evaluate valvular abnormalities

■ To measure the size of the heart's chambers

■ To evaluate chambers and valves in congenital heart disorders

■ To aid in the diagnosis of hypertrophic and related cardiomyopathies

■ To detect atrial tumors

■ To evaluate cardiac function or wall motion after myocardial infarction

■ To detect pericardial effusion

■ To detect mucal thrombi

M-MODE ECHOCARDIOGRAMS

In the normal motion-mode (M-mode) echocardiogram of the mitral valve shown below (top), valve movement appears as a characteristic lopsided M-shaped tracing. The anterior and posterior mitral valve leaflets separate (D) in early diastole, quickly reach maximum separation (E), and then close during rapid ventricular filling (E-F).

Leaflet separation varies during mid-diastole, and the valve opens widely again (A) following atrial contraction. The valve starts to close with atrial relaxation (A-B) and is completely closed during the start of ventricular systole (C). The steepness of the E-F slope indirectly shows the speed of ventricular filling, which is normally rapid.

NORMAL ECHOCARDIOGRAM

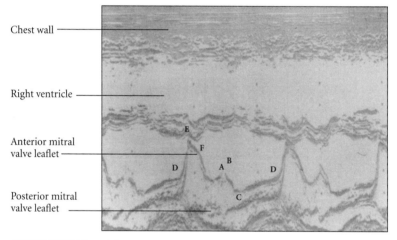

Chest wall

Right ventricle

Anterior mitral valve leaflet

Posterior mitral valve leaflet

ABNORMAL ECHOCARDIOGRAM

Mitral stenosis is evident in the abnormal echocardiogram shown at right. The E-F slope (line) is very shallow, indicating slowed left ventricular filling.

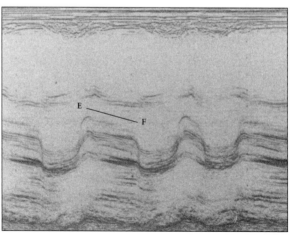

Patient preparation

- Explain to the patient that echocardiography is used to evaluate the size, shape, and motion of various cardiac structures.
- Inform the patient that he need not restrict food and fluids.
- Tell the patient who will perform the test, where it will take place, and that it's safe, painless, and noninvasive.
- Explain that the room may be darkened slightly to aid visualization on the monitor screen and that other procedures (ECG and phonocardiography) may be performed simultaneously to time events in the cardiac cycle.
- Describe the procedure to the patient and instruct him to remain still during the test because movement may distort results.
- Tell the patient that conductive gel will be applied to his chest and a quarter-sized transducer will be placed directly over it. Warn him that he may feel minor discomfort because pressure is exerted to keep the transducer in contact with the skin.
- Explain to the patient that the transducer is angled to observe different parts of the heart and that he may be repositioned on his left side during the procedure.
- Inform the patient that he may be asked to inhale a gas with a slightly sweet odor (amyl nitrite) while changes in heart function are recorded; describe the possible adverse effects (dizziness, flushing, and tachycardia), but assure him that such symptoms quickly subside.

Procedure and posttest care

- The patient is placed in a supine position.
- Conductive gel is applied to the third or fourth intercostal space to the left of the sternum, and the transducer is placed directly over it.
- The transducer is systematically angled to direct ultrasonic waves at specific parts of the patient's heart.
- During the test, the oscilloscope screen, which displays the returning echoes, is observed.
- Significant findings are recorded on a strip chart recorder (M-mode echocardiography) or on a videotape recorder (two-dimensional echocardiography).
- For a different view of the heart, the transducer is placed beneath the xiphoid process or directly above the sternum.
- For a left lateral view, the patient may be positioned on his left side.
- To record heart function under various conditions, the patient is asked to inhale and exhale slowly, to hold his breath, or to inhale amyl nitrite.
- Doppler echocardiography may be used in this examination to assess speed and direction of blood flow. The sound of blood flow may be heard as the continuous-wave and pulsed-wave Doppler sampling of cardiac valves is performed. This technique is used primarily to assess heart sounds and murmurs as they relate to cardiac hemodynamics.
- When the test is completed, remove the conductive gel from the patient's skin.

Normal findings

An echocardiogram can reveal the motion pattern and structure of the four cardiac valves. Anterior and posterior mitral valve leaflets normally separate in early diastole, with the anterior leaflet moving toward the chest wall and the posterior leaflet moving away from it. The leaflets attain maximum excursion rapidly, and then move toward each other during ventricular diastole; after atrial contraction, they come together and remain so during ventricular systole. On an M-mode echocardiogram, the leaflets appear as two fine lines within the echo-free, blood-filled left ventricular cavity.

The aortic valve cusps lie between the parallel walls of the aortic root, which move anteriorly during systole and posteriorly during diastole. During ventricular systole, these cusps separate and appear as a boxlike configuration on an M-mode echocardiogram. They remain open throughout systole and normally demonstrate a characteristic fine fluttering motion. During diastole, the cusps come together and appear as a single or double line within the aortic root on an M-mode echocardiogram.

The motion of the tricuspid valve resembles that of the mitral valve. The motion of the pulmonic valve—particularly the posterior cusp—is different: During diastole, this cusp gradually moves posteriorly; during atrial systole, it's displaced posteriorly; during ventricular systole, it quickly moves posteriorly; and during right ventricular ejection, the cusp moves anteriorly, attaining its most anterior position during diastole.

The left ventricular cavity normally appears as an echo-free space between the interventricular septum and the posterior left ventricular wall. Echoes produced by the chordae tendineae and the mitral leaflet appear within this cavity. The right ventricular cavity normally appears as an echo-free space between the anterior chest wall and the interventricular septum.

Abnormal findings

Valvular abnormalities readily appear on the echocardiogram. In mitral stenosis, the valve narrows abnormally due to the leaflets' thickening and disordered motion. Instead of moving in opposite directions during diastole, both mitral valve leaflets move anteriorly. In mitral valve prolapse, one or both leaflets balloon into the left atrium during systole.

Aortic valve abnormalities—especially aortic insufficiency—can also affect the mitral valve because the anterior mitral leaflet is just below the aortic cusps. When blood regurgitates through the aortic valve during diastole, it strikes this leaflet, causing the flutter seen in M-mode echocardiography. Although the aortic valve may appear normal, this characteristic fluttering confirms aortic insufficiency. In stenosis, due to conditions such as rheumatic fever or bacterial endocarditis, the aortic valve thickens and thus generates more echoes. However, in rheumatic fever, the valve may thicken slightly and allow normal motion during systole, or it may thicken severely and curtail motion. In bacterial endocarditis, valve motion is disrupted, and shaggy or fuzzy echoes usually appear on or near the valve.

Other chamber or valve abnormalities may indicate a congenital heart disorder, such as aortic stenosis, which may require further tests. A large chamber size may indicate cardiomyopathy, valvular disorders, or heart failure; a small chamber, restrictive pericarditis.

Hypertrophic obstructive cardiomyopathy can also be identified by the echocardiogram, with systolic anterior motion of the mitral valve and asymmetric septal hypertrophy.

Left atrial tumors are usually on a pedicle and can thus shift in and out of the mitral opening. During diastole, the tumor appears as a mass of echoes against the anterior mitral valve leaflet. During ventricular systole, these echoes shift back into the body of the atrium.

In CAD, ischemia or infarction may cause absent or paradoxical motion in ventricular walls that normally move together and thicken during systole. These affected areas may also fail to thicken or may become thinner, particularly if scar tissue is present.

The echocardiogram is especially sensitive in detecting pericardial effusion. Normally, the epicardium and pericardium are continuous membranes and thus produce a single or near-single echo. When fluid accumulates between these membranes, it causes an abnormal echo-free space to appear. In large effusions, pressure exerted by excess fluid can restrict pericardial motion.

An echocardiogram should be correlated with the patients' history, physical examination findings, and results of additional tests. For a patient with a suboptimal echocardiogram, an agent composed of human albumin microspheres filled with perfluorocarbon gas (Optison) can be used. This agent can enhance the contrast of the ultrasound scans to opacify the left ventricle and improve the delineation of the left ventricular endocardial borders.

Interfering factors

- Incorrect transducer placement and excessive movement
- Thick chest or chest wall abnormalities or chronic obstructive pulmonary disease (possible poor imaging)

Transesophageal echocardiography

Transesophageal echocardiography combines ultrasound with endoscopy to give a better view of the heart's structures. In this procedure, a small transducer is attached to the end of a gastroscope and inserted into the esophagus, allowing images to be taken from the posterior aspect of the heart. This causes less tissue penetration and interference from chest wall structures and produces high-quality images of the thoracic aorta, except for the superior ascending aorta, which is shadowed by the trachea.

This test is appropriate for inpatients and outpatients, for patients under general anesthesia, and for critically ill, intubated patients.

Purpose

To visualize and evaluate:

- thoracic and aortic disorders, such as dissection and aneurysm
- valvular disease, especially in the mitral valve and in prosthetic devices
- endocarditis
- congenital heart disease
- intracardiac thrombi
- cardiac tumors
- valvular repairs

Patient preparation

- Explain to the patient that transesophageal echocardiography allows visual examination of heart function and structures.
- Tell the patient who will perform the test, when it's scheduled, and that he'll need to fast for 6 hours before the test.
- Review the patient's medical history for possible contraindications to the test, such as esophageal obstruction or varices, GI bleeding, previous mediastinal radiation therapy, or severe cervical arthritis.
- Ask the patient about any allergies and note them on the chart.
- Before the test, have the patient remove any dentures or oral prostheses and note any loose teeth.
- Explain to the patient that his throat will be sprayed with a topical anesthetic

and that he may gag when the tube is inserted.

- Tell the patient that an I.V. line will be inserted to administer sedation before the procedure and that he may feel slight discomfort from the needle puncture and the tourniquet. Reassure him that he'll be made as comfortable as possible and that his blood pressure and heart rate will be monitored continuously.
- Make sure that the patient or a responsible family member has signed an informed consent form.

Equipment
Cardiac monitor, sedative, topical anesthetic, bite block, gastroscope, ultrasonography equipment, suction equipment, resuscitation equipment

Procedure and posttest care
- Connect the patient to a cardiac monitor, the automated blood pressure cuff, and pulse oximetry probe so that all parameters can be assessed during the procedure.
- Help the patient lie down on his left side and administer the prescribed sedative.
- The back of the patient's throat is sprayed with a topical anesthetic.
- A bite block is placed in his mouth and he's instructed to close his lips around it.
- A gastroscope is introduced and advanced 12″ to 14″ (30 to 35 cm) to the level of the right atrium. To visualize the left ventricle, the scope is advanced 16″ to 18″ (40 to 45 cm).
- Ultrasound images are recorded and then reviewed after the procedure.
- Monitor the patient's vital signs and oxygen levels for any changes.
- Keep the patient in a supine position until the sedative wears off.

- Encourage the patient to cough after the procedure while lying on his side or sitting upright.
- Don't give food or water until the gag response returns.
- If the procedure is done on an outpatient basis, make sure someone is available to drive the patient home.
- Treat sore throat symptomatically.

Precautions
- Keep resuscitation equipment readily available.
- Have suction equipment nearby to avoid aspiration if vomiting occurs.
- Vasovagal responses may occur with gagging, so observe the cardiac monitor closely.
- Use pulse oximetry to detect hypoxia.
- If bleeding occurs, stop the procedure immediately.
- Laryngospasm, arrhythmias, or bleeding increase the risk of complications. If any of these occurs, postpone the test.

Normal findings
Transesophageal echocardiography should reveal no cardiac problems.

Abnormal findings
Transesophageal echocardiography can reveal thoracic and aortic disorders, endocarditis, congenital heart disease, intracardiac thrombi, or tumors and it can evaluate valvular disease or repairs. Findings may include aortic dissection or aneurysm, mitral valve disease, or congenital defects such as patent ductus arteriosus.

Interfering factors
- An uncooperative patient
- Using a transesophageal approach (restricted visualization of the left atrial ap-

pendage and ascending or descending aorta)

■ Hyperinflation of lungs due to such causes as chronic obstructive pulmonary disease or mechanical ventilation (possible poor imaging)

Doppler ultrasonography

Doppler ultrasonography is a noninvasive test used to evaluate blood flow in the major veins and arteries of the arms and legs and in the extracranial cerebrovascular system. An alternative to arteriography and venography, it's safer, less costly, and faster than invasive tests.

In Doppler ultrasonography, a handheld transducer directs high-frequency sound waves to the artery or vein being tested. The sound waves strike moving red blood cells and are reflected back to the transducer, allowing direct listening and graphic recording of blood flow.

Measurement of systolic pressure during this test is used to detect the presence, location, and extent of peripheral arterial occlusive disease. Changes in sound wave frequency during respiration are observed to detect venous occlusive disease. Compression maneuvers detect occlusion of the veins and occlusion or stenosis of carotid arteries.

Pulse volume recorder testing may be performed with Doppler ultrasonography to record changes in blood volume or flow in an extremity or organ.

Purpose

■ To aid in the diagnosis of venous insufficiency and superficial and deep vein thrombosis (popliteal, femoral, iliac)

■ To aid in the diagnosis of peripheral artery disease and arterial occlusion

■ To monitor the patient who has had arterial reconstruction and bypass grafts

■ To detect abnormalities of carotid artery blood flow associated with conditions such as aortic stenosis

■ To evaluate possible arterial trauma

Patient preparation

■ Explain to the patient that Doppler ultrasonography is used to evaluate blood flow in the arms and legs or neck.

■ Tell the patient who will perform the test.

■ Reassure the patient that the test doesn't involve risk or discomfort.

■ Tell the patient that he'll be asked to move his arms to different positions and to perform breathing exercises as measurements are taken. A small ultrasonic probe resembling a microphone is placed at various sites along veins or arteries, and blood pressure is checked at several sites.

■ Check with the vascular laboratory about special equipment or instructions.

Procedure and posttest care

■ Water-soluble conductive gel is applied to the tip of the transducer.

Peripheral arterial evaluation

■ Peripheral arterial evaluation is always performed bilaterally. The usual test sites in each leg are the common femoral, superficial femoral, popliteal, posterior tibial, and dorsalis pedis arteries; in each arm, the test sites are usually the subclavian, brachial, radial, ulnar and, occasionally, the palmar arch and digital arteries.

■ The patient is instructed to remove all clothing above or below the waist, depending on the test site, and he's placed in a supine position on the examining table or bed, with his arms at his sides.

■ Brachial blood pressure is measured, and the transducer is placed at various points along the test arteries.

- The signals are monitored and the waveforms recorded for later analysis.
- Segmental limb blood pressure is obtained to localize arterial occlusive disease.
- During lower extremity tests, a blood pressure cuff is wrapped around the calf, pressure readings are obtained, and waveforms are recorded from the dorsalis pedis and posterior tibial arteries. Then the cuff is wrapped around the thigh, and waveforms are recorded at the popliteal artery.
- In upper extremity tests, examination is performed on one arm, with the patient first placed in a supine position and then sitting; it's then repeated on the other arm. A blood pressure cuff is wrapped around the forearm, pressure readings are taken, and waveforms are recorded over the radial and ulnar arteries. Then, the cuff is wrapped around the upper arm, pressure readings are taken, and waveforms are recorded with the transducer over the brachial artery.
- Blood pressure readings and waveform recordings are repeated with the arm in extreme hyperextension and hyperabduction to check for possible compression factors that may interfere with arterial blood flow. The upper extremity examination is performed on one arm, with the patient first placed in a supine position and then sitting; it's then repeated on the other arm.

Peripheral venous evaluation
- Usual test sites for peripheral venous evaluation include the popliteal, superficial femoral, and common femoral veins in the leg and the posterior tibial vein at the ankle; the brachial, axillary, and subclavian veins in the arm; jugular veins; and, occasionally, the inferior and superior vena cava.

- The patient is instructed to remove all clothing above or below the waist, depending on the test site.
- He's placed in a supine position and instructed to breathe normally.
- The transducer is placed over the appropriate vein, waveforms and compressibility are recorded, and respiratory modulations are noted.
- Proximal limb compression maneuvers are performed and augmentation is noted after release of compression, to evaluate venous valve competency.
- Changes in respiration are monitored.
- During lower extremity tests, the patient is asked to perform Valsalva's maneuver, and venous blood flow is recorded.
- The procedure is repeated for the other arm or leg.

Extracranial cerebrovascular evaluation
- Usual test sites for extracranial cerebrovascular evaluation include the supraorbital, common carotid, external carotid, internal carotid, and vertebral arteries.
- The patient is placed in a supine position on the examining table or bed, with a pillow beneath his head for support.
- Brachial blood pressure is then recorded using the Doppler probe.
- The transducer is positioned over the test artery, and blood flow velocity is monitored and recorded.
- The influence of compression maneuvers on blood flow velocity is measured, and the procedure is repeated on the opposite side. (See *How to detect thrombi with a Doppler probe.*)

All procedures
- Remove the conductive gel from the patient's skin.

HOW TO DETECT THROMBI WITH A DOPPLER PROBE

The Doppler probe is typically used to detect venous thrombi by first positioning the transducer and then occluding the blood vessel by compression (as shown in the illustration of the normal leg below). Water-soluble conductive gel is applied to the tip of the transducer to provide coupling between the skin and transducer.

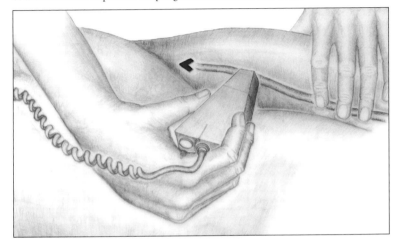

When pressure is released, allowing blood flow to resume, the transducer picks up the sudden augmentation of the flow sound and permits graphic recording of blood flow. If a thrombus is present, a compression maneuver fails to produce the augmented flow sound because the blood flow (as shown below in the femoral vein) is significantly impaired.

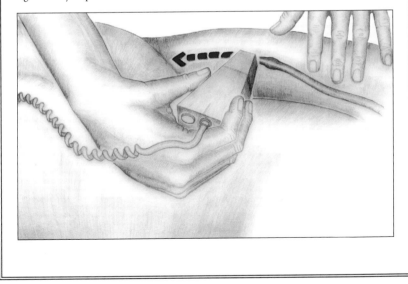

Precautions

- Don't place the Doppler probe over an open or draining lesion.

Normal findings

Arterial waveforms of the arms and legs are triphasic, with a prominent systolic component and one or more diastolic sounds. The ankle-arm pressure index — the ratio between ankle systolic pressure and brachial systolic pressure — is normally equal to or greater than 1. (The ankle-arm pressure index is also known as the arterial ischemia index, the ankle-brachial index, or the pedal-brachial index.) Proximal thigh pressure is normally 20 to 30 mm Hg higher than arm pressure, but pressure measurements at adjacent sites are similar. In the arms, pressure readings should remain unchanged despite postural changes.

Venous blood flow velocity is normally phasic with respiration and is of a lower pitch than arterial flow. Distal compression or release of proximal limb compression increases blood flow velocity. In the legs, abdominal compression eliminates respiratory variations, but release increases blood flow; Valsalva's maneuver also interrupts venous flow velocity.

In cerebrovascular testing, a strong velocity signal is present. In the common carotid artery, blood flow velocity increases during diastole due to low peripheral vascular resistance of the brain. The direction of periorbital arterial flow is normally anterograde out of the orbit.

Abnormal findings

Arterial stenosis or occlusion diminishes the blood flow velocity signal, with no diastolic sound and a less prominent systolic component distal to the lesion. At the lesion, the signal is high-pitched and, occasionally, turbulent. If complete occlusion is present and collateral circulation hasn't taken over, the velocity signal may be absent.

A pressure gradient exceeding 20 mm Hg at adjacent sites of measurement in the leg may indicate occlusive disease. Specifically, low proximal thigh pressure signifies common femoral or aortoiliac occlusive disease. An abnormal gradient between the proximal thigh and the above- or below-knee cuffs indicates superficial femoral or popliteal artery occlusive disease; an abnormal gradient between the below-knee and ankle cuffs indicates tibiofibular disease. Abnormal gradients of arm and forearm pressure readings may indicate brachial artery occlusion.

An abnormal ankle-arm pressure index is directly proportional to the degree of circulatory impairment: mild ischemia, 1.0 to 0.75; claudication, 0.75 to 0.50; pain at rest, 0.50 to 0.25; and pregangrene, 0.25 to 0.

If venous blood flow velocity is unchanged by respirations, doesn't increase in response to compression or Valsalva's maneuver, or is absent, venous thrombosis is indicated. In chronic venous insufficiency and varicose veins, the flow velocity signal may be reversed. Confirmation of results may require venography.

Inability to identify Doppler signals during cerebrovascular examination implies total arterial occlusion. Reversed periorbital arterial flow indicates significant arterial occlusive disease of the extracranial internal carotid artery. In addition, the audible signal may take on the acoustic characteristics of a normal peripheral artery. Internal carotid artery stenosis causes turbulent signals. Collateral circulation can be assessed by compression maneuvers.

Oculoplethysmography, carotid phonoangiography, or carotid imaging can further evaluate cerebrovascular disease. Retrograde blood velocity in the vertebral artery can indicate subclavian steal syndrome. A weak velocity signal on comparison of contralateral vertebral arteries can indicate diffuse vertebral artery disease.

Interfering factors
■ An uncooperative patient

Ultrasonography of the abdominal aorta

In ultrasonography of the abdominal aorta, a transducer directs high-frequency sound waves into the abdomen over a wide area from the xiphoid process to the umbilical region. The echoing sound waves are displayed on a monitor to indicate internal organs, the vertebral column, and the size and course of the abdominal aorta and other major vessels.

Purpose
■ To detect and measure a suspected abdominal aortic aneurysm (findings may be supported and refined by angiography or computed tomography angiography)
■ To detect and measure the expansion of a known abdominal aortic aneurysm

Patient preparation
■ Explain to the patient that ultrasonography allows examination of the abdominal aorta.
■ Instruct the patient to fast for 12 hours before the test to minimize bowel gas and motility.
■ Tell the patient who will perform the test, where it will take place, that the lights may be lowered, and that he'll feel only slight pressure.

■ Describe the procedure. Tell the patient that mineral oil or a gel, which may feel cool, will be applied to his abdomen.
■ Explain that a transducer will pass over his skin, from the costal margins to the umbilicus or slightly below, directing safe, painless, and inaudible sound waves into the abdominal vessels and organs.
■ Reassure the patient with a known aneurysm that the sound waves won't cause rupture.
■ Instruct the patient to remain still during scanning and to hold his breath when requested.
■ If ordered, give simethicone to reduce bowel gas.

Procedure and posttest care
■ The patient is placed in a supine position, and conductive gel or mineral oil is applied to his abdomen.
■ Longitudinal scans are made at ⅛″ to ¾″ (0.5- to 2-cm) intervals left and right of the midline until the entire abdominal aorta is outlined; transverse scans are made at ⅜″ to ¾″ (1- to 2-cm) intervals from the xiphoid to the bifurcation at the common iliac arteries.
■ The patient may be placed in the right and left lateral positions.
■ Appropriate views are photographed or videotaped.
■ Remove the conductive gel from the patient's skin.
■ Instruct the patient that he may resume his usual diet and medications, as ordered.

◀ **CLINICAL ALERT** *Aneurysms may expand and dissect rapidly, so check the patient's vital signs frequently. Remember that the sudden onset of constant abdominal or back pain accompanies rapid expansion of the aneurysm; sudden, excruciating pain with weakness, sweating,* *tachycardia, and hypotension signals rupture.*

Normal findings

In adults, the normal abdominal aorta tapers from about 1″ to ⅝″ (2.5 to 1.5 cm) in diameter along its length from the diaphragm to the bifurcation. It descends through the retroperitoneal space, anterior to the vertebral column and slightly left of the midline. Four of its major branches are usually well visualized: the celiac trunk, the renal arteries, the superior mesenteric artery, and the common iliac arteries.

Abnormal findings

The luminal diameter of the abdominal aorta greater than 1½″ (3.8 cm) suggests aneurysm; greater than 2¾″ (7 cm), aneurysm with high risk of rupture.

Interfering factors

- Bowel gas and motility, excessive body movement, surgical wounds, and severe dyspnea
- Residual barium from GI contrast studies within the past 24 hours
- Air introduced during endoscopy within the past 12 to 24 hours
- Mesenteric fat in the obese patient

NUCLEAR MEDICINE

Cardiac positron emission tomography

Cardiac positron emission tomography (PET) scanning combines elements of computed tomography scanning and conventional radionuclide imaging. Like radionuclide imaging, cardiac PET scans measure emissions of injected radioisotopes and convert these values to tomographic images. PET uses radioisotopes of biologically important elements — oxygen, nitrogen, carbon, and fluorine — which emit particles called positrons. During positron emissions, gamma rays are detected by the PET scanner and reconstructed to form an image. One distinct advantage of PET scans is that positron emitters can be chemically "tagged" to biologically active molecules, such as carbon monoxide, neurotransmitters, hormones, and metabolites (particularly glucose), enabling study of their uptake and distribution in tissue.

Purpose

- To detect coronary artery disease
- To evaluate myocardial metabolism and contractility
- To distinguish viable from infarcted cardiac tissue, especially during the early stages of myocardial infarction

Patient preparation

- If cardiac PET is ordered to assess myocardial contractility, explain to the patient that the test distinguishes viable tissue from tissue injured by infarction and also may help the physician assess mitochondrial impairment associated with ischemia or evaluate coronary artery obstruction.
- Describe the test to the patient, including who will perform it and where it will take place. Take the time to describe the equipment.
- Tell the patient that the test is painless, unless an I.V. infusion is planned, in which case he may experience slight discomfort from the needle puncture and the tourniquet. If the radioisotope will be inhaled, explain to the patient that this procedure is painless.

- If fasting is ordered, describe food and fluid restrictions to the patient.
- Explain to the patient that he'll be given a radioactive substance, either by injection, inhalation, or I.V. infusion, and that a highly specialized camera will detect the radioactive decay of this substance and send these data to a computer, which converts the data to an image.
- Tell the patient that he'll undergo an attenuation scan for about 30 minutes. Then he'll receive the appropriate positron emitter and undergo PET scanning.

🏵 **AGE ISSUE** *Because the radioisotope may be harmful to a fetus, the female patient of child-bearing age should be screened carefully before undergoing cardiac PET.*

Procedure and posttest care
- The patient is placed in a supine position with his arms above his head.
- An attenuation scan, lasting about 30 minutes, is performed.
- The appropriate positron emitter is administered and scanning is completed.
- An additional positron emitter may be given if comparative studies are needed.
- Instruct the patient to move slowly after the procedure to avoid postural hypotension.
- Encourage increased oral fluid intake to flush the radioisotope from the bladder.

Precautions
- Stress to the patient the importance of remaining still during the study.

Normal findings
Normally, no areas of ischemic tissue are present. If the patient receives two tracers, the flow and distribution should match, indicating normal tissue.

Abnormal findings
Reduced blood flow, with increased glucose use, indicates ischemia. Reduced blood flow, with decreased glucose use, indicates necrotic, scarred tissue.

Interfering factors
- The patient's failure to maintain proper positioning

Cardiac magnetic resonance imaging

A great asset in the diagnosis of cardiac disorders, cardiac magnetic resonance imaging (MRI) has the ability to "see through" bone and to delineate fluid-filled soft tissue in great detail as well as produce images of organs and vessels in motion.

In this noninvasive procedure, the patient is placed in a magnetic field, into which a radiofrequency beam is introduced. Resulting energy changes are measured and used by the MRI computer to generate images on a monitor. Cross-sectional images of the anatomy are viewed in multiple planes and recorded for the permanent record.

Purpose
- To identify anatomic sequelae related to myocardial infarction, such as formation of ventricular aneurysm, ventricular wall thinning, and mural thrombus
- To detect and evaluate cardiomyopathy
- To detect and evaluate pericardial disease
- To identify paracardiac or intracardiac masses
- To detect congenital heart disease, such as atrial or ventricular septal defects, and the degree of malposition of the great vessel

■ To identify vascular disease, such as thoracic aneurysm and thoracic dissection

■ To assess the structure of the pulmonary vasculature

Patient preparation

■ Explain to the patient that cardiac MRI assesses the heart's function and structure.

■ Tell the patient who will perform the test and where it will take place.

■ Inform the patient that he'll be positioned on a narrow bed, which slides into a large cylinder that houses the MRI magnets. Tell him that the scanner will make clicking, whirring, and thumping noises as it moves inside its housing and that he may receive earplugs.

■ Explain to the patient who's claustrophobic or anxious about the test's duration that he'll receive a mild sedative to reduce his anxiety or he may need to be scanned in an open MRI scanner, which may take longer, but is less confining.

■ Explain to the patient the need to lie flat.

■ Reassure the patient that he'll be able to communicate with the technician at all times and that the procedure will be stopped if he feels claustrophobic.

■ Immediately before the test, have the patient remove all metal objects. Double-check to make sure that he doesn't have a pacemaker or any surgically implanted joints, pins, clips, valves, or pumps containing metal that could be attracted to the strong MRI magnet. If he does, he won't be able to undergo the test.

■ Make sure that the patient or a responsible family member has signed an informed consent form.

■ Administer the prescribed sedative.

Procedure and posttest care

■ At the scanner room door, check the patient one last time for metal objects.

■ The patient is placed supine on a narrow, padded, nonmetallic bed that slides to the desired position inside the scanner. Radiofrequency waves are directed at his chest. The resulting images are displayed on a monitor and recorded on film or magnetic tape for permanent storage.

■ The radiologist may vary the waves and use the computer to manipulate and enhance the images.

■ Remind the patient to remain still throughout the procedure.

■ Assess how the patient responds to the enclosed environment. Provide reassurance, if necessary.

▶ **CLINICAL ALERT** *If the patient is sedated, monitor his hemodynamic, cardiac, respiratory, and mental status until the effects of the sedative have worn off.*

Precautions

■ The claustrophobic patient may experience anxiety. Monitor the cardiac patient for signs of ischemia (chest pressure, shortness of breath, or changes in hemodynamic status).

■ MRI can't be performed on the patient with a pacemaker or an intracranial aneurysm clip.

■ If the patient is unstable, make sure an I.V. line with no metal components is in place and that all equipment is compatible with MRI imaging. If necessary, monitor the patient's oxygen saturation, cardiac rhythm, and respiratory status during the test.

■ An anesthesiologist may be needed to monitor a heavily sedated patient.

■ A nurse or radiology technician should maintain verbal contact with the conscious patient.

Normal findings

MRI should reveal no anatomic or structural dysfunctions in cardiovascular tissue.

Abnormal findings

MRI can detect cardiomyopathy and pericardial disease. It can also detect atrial or ventricular septal defects or other congenital defects. MRI is useful for identifying paracardiac or intracardiac masses. In addition, it can evaluate the extent of pericardial or vascular disease.

Interfering factors

■ The patient's inability to remain still during the procedure

Technetium pyrophosphate scanning

Technetium pyrophosphate scanning (also called *hot spot myocardial imaging* or *infarct avid imaging*) is used to detect a recent myocardial infarction (MI) and to determine its extent. This test uses an I.V. tracer isotope (technetium 99m [^{99m}Tc] pyrophosphate). This isotope accumulates in damaged myocardial tissue (possibly by combining with calcium in the damaged myocardial cells), where it forms a "hot spot" on a scan made with a scintillation camera. Such hot spots first appear within 12 hours of infarction, are most apparent after 48 to 72 hours, and usually disappear after 1 week. Hot spots that persist longer than 1 week usually suggest ongoing myocardial damage.

Purpose

■ To confirm a recent MI
■ To help define the size and location of an MI
■ To assess the prognosis after an acute MI

Patient preparation

■ Explain to the patient that technetium pyrophosphate scanning helps assess if the heart muscle is injured.
■ Inform the patient that he need not restrict food and fluids. Tell him who will perform the test and where it will take place.
■ Inform the patient that he'll receive an I.V. tracer isotope 2 or 3 hours before the procedure and that multiple images of his heart will be made.
■ Reassure the patient that the injection causes only slight discomfort, that the scan itself is painless, and that the test involves less exposure to radiation than a chest X-ray.
■ Instruct the patient to remain quiet and motionless while he's being scanned.
■ Make sure that the patient or a responsible family member has signed an informed consent form.

Equipment

Scanner, ^{99m}Tc pyrophosphate; I.V. equipment, if needed

Procedure and posttest care

■ Usually, 20 millicuries of ^{99m}Tc pyrophosphate are injected intravenously into the antecubital vein.
■ After 2 or 3 hours, the patient is placed in a supine position and electrocardiography electrodes are attached for continuous monitoring during the test.
■ Generally, scans are taken with the patient in several positions, including anterior, left anterior oblique, right anterior oblique, and left lateral. Each scan takes 10 minutes.

Precautions

■ Monitor the patient for adverse reactions to the injected contrast medium.

Normal findings

A normal technetium pyrophosphate scan shows no isotope in the myocardium.

Abnormal findings

The isotope is taken up by the sternum and ribs, and their activity is compared with the heart's; 2+, 3+, and 4+ activity (equal to or greater than bone) indicates a positive myocardial scan. The technetium pyrophosphate scan can reveal areas of isotope accumulation, or hot spots, in damaged myocardium, particularly 48 to 72 hours after onset of an acute MI; however, hot spots are apparent as early as 12 hours after an acute MI. In most cases, hot spots disappear after 1 week; in some, they persist for several months if necrosis continues in the area of infarction.

Knowing where the infarct is makes it possible to anticipate complications and to plan care. About one-fourth of patients with unstable angina pectoris show hot spots due to subclinical myocardial necrosis and may require coronary arteriography and bypass grafting.

Interfering factors

■ Isotope accumulation (in about 10% of patients, may result from ventricular aneurysm associated with dystrophic calcification, pulmonary neoplasm, recent cardioversion, or valvular heart disease due to severe calcification)

Thallium imaging

Also called *cold spot myocardial imaging* or *thallium scintigraphy,* thallium imaging evaluates myocardial blood flow after I.V. injection of the radioisotope thallium-201 or Cardiolite. The main difference between these tracers is that Cardiolite has a better energy spectrum for imaging.

Cardiolite requires living myocardial cells for uptake and allows for imaging the myocardial blood flow before and after reperfusion. This allows for better estimation of myocardial salvage. Because thallium, the physiologic analogue of potassium, concentrates in healthy myocardial tissue but not in necrotic or ischemic tissue, areas of the heart with a normal blood supply and intact cells rapidly take it up. Areas with poor blood flow and ischemic cells fail to take up the isotope and appear as "cold spots" on a scan.

This test is performed in a resting state or after stress. Resting imaging can detect acute myocardial infarction (MI) within the first few hours of symptoms, but doesn't distinguish an old from a new infarct. Stress imaging, performed after the patient exercises on a treadmill until he experiences angina or rate-limiting fatigue, can assess known or suspected coronary artery disease (CAD) and can evaluate the effectiveness of antianginal therapy or balloon angioplasty and the patency of grafts after coronary artery bypass surgery. Possible complications of stress testing include arrhythmias, angina pectoris, and MI.

Purpose

■ To assess myocardial scarring and perfusion
■ To demonstrate the location and extent of acute or chronic MI, including transmural and postoperative infarction (resting imaging)
■ To diagnose CAD (stress imaging)
■ To evaluate the patency of grafts after coronary artery bypass surgery
■ To evaluate the effectiveness of antianginal therapy or balloon angioplasty (stress imaging)

Patient preparation

■ Explain to the patient that thallium imaging helps determine if any areas of the heart muscle aren't receiving an adequate blood supply.

■ If the patient is undergoing stress imaging, instruct him to restrict alcohol, tobacco, and nonprescribed medications for 24 hours before the test and to have nothing by mouth for 3 hours before the test.

■ Describe the test, including who will perform it and where it will take place. Explain that additional scans may be required.

■ Tell the patient that he'll receive an I.V. radioactive tracer and that multiple images of his heart will be scanned.

■ Explain to the patient that it's important to lie still when images are taken.

■ Warn the patient that he may experience discomfort from skin abrasion during preparation for electrode placement. Assure him that the test involves minimal radiation exposure.

■ Make sure that the patient or a responsible family member has signed an informed consent form.

■ Tell the patient undergoing stress imaging to wear walking shoes during the treadmill exercise and to report fatigue, pain, or shortness of breath immediately.

Equipment

Scanner; I.V. insertion equipment, if needed; radioactive tracer

Procedure and posttest care
Resting imaging

■ Optimally, within the first few hours of symptoms of a MI, the patient receives an injection of I.V. thallium or Cardiolite and scanning begins after 10 minutes.

■ If further scanning is required, have the patient rest and restrict food and beverages other than water.

Stress imaging

■ The patient, wired with electrodes, walks on a treadmill at a regulated pace that's gradually increased, while the electrocardiogram (ECG), blood pressure, and heart rate are monitored.

■ When the patient reaches peak stress, the examiner injects 1.5 to 3 millicuries of thallium into the antecubital vein and then flushes it with 10 to 15 ml of normal saline solution or an infusion of Cardiolite.

■ The patient exercises an additional 45 to 60 seconds to permit circulation and uptake of the isotope, and then lies on his back under the scintillation camera.

■ If the patient is asymptomatic, the precordial leads are removed. Scanning begins after 10 minutes with the patient in the anterior, left anterior oblique, and left lateral positions.

■ Additional scans may be taken after the patient rests and occasionally after 24 hours. Taking a scan after the patient rests is helpful in differentiating between an ischemic area and an infarcted or scarred area of the myocardium.

Precautions

■ Contraindications include impaired neuromuscular function, pregnancy, locomotor disturbances, acute MI or myocarditis, aortic stenosis, acute infection, unstable metabolic conditions (such as diabetes), digoxin toxicity, and recent pulmonary infarction.

■ Emergency medical equipment should be readily available, if needed.

⏵ **CLINICAL ALERT** *Stop stress imaging at once if the patient develops chest pain, dyspnea, fatigue, syncope, hy-*

potension, ischemic ECG changes, significant arrhythmias, or critical signs (pale, clammy skin, confusion, or staggering).

Normal findings

Imaging should show normal distribution of the isotope throughout the left ventricle and no defects (cold spots). The results may be normal if the patient has narrowed coronary arteries but adequate collateral circulation.

Abnormal findings

Persistent defects indicate an MI; transient defects (those that disappear after 3 to 6 hours of rest) indicate ischemia from CAD. After coronary artery bypass surgery, improved regional perfusion suggests patency of the graft. Increased perfusion after taking antianginal drugs can show that they relieve ischemia. Improved perfusion after balloon angioplasty suggests increased coronary flow.

Interfering factors

■ Cold spots (possible result of sarcoidosis, myocardial fibrosis, cardiac contusion, attenuation due to soft tissue, apical cleft, coronary spasm, and artifacts, such as implants and electrodes)
■ Absence of cold spots in the presence of CAD (possibly due to insignificant obstruction, inadequate stress, delayed imaging, collateral circulation, or single-vessel disease, particularly of the right or left circumflex coronary arteries)

Radiopharmaceutical myocardial perfusion imaging

Also known as *chemical stress imaging*, radiopharmaceutical myocardial perfusion imaging is an alternative method of assessing coronary vessel function in the patient who can't tolerate exercise electrocardiography (ECG).

In this test, I.V. infusion of a selected drug—for example, adenosine, dobutamine, or dipyridamole—is used to simulate the effects of exercise by increasing blood flow in the coronary arteries. Next, a radiopharmaceutical is injected intravenously to allow imaging that assists in evaluating the cardiac vessel's response to the drug-induced stress. Resting and stress images are obtained to evaluate coronary perfusion.

Purpose

■ To assess the presence and degree of coronary artery disease (CAD)
■ To evaluate therapeutic procedures, such as bypass surgery or coronary angioplasty
■ To evaluate myocardial perfusion

Patient preparation

■ Describe to the patient what the radiopharmaceutical myocardial perfusion imaging test is, including who will perform it and where it will take place.
■ Tell the patient that he'll need to arrive 1 hour before the test and that an I.V. line will be initiated before the test.
■ If the patient will receive adenosine or dipyridamole, instruct him to avoid taking all theophylline medications for 24 to 36 hours and all caffeinated drinks for 12 hours before the test.
■ If the patient will receive dobutamine, instruct him to withhold beta-adrenergic blockers for 48 hours before the test. Also tell him not to eat for 3 to 4 hours before the test, although he may have water. Instruct him to take his other medications, as prescribed, with sips of water.
■ Tell the patient to continue taking antihypertensive medications. If his systolic blood pressure is higher than 200 mm

Hg, the dobutamine stress test can't be done until his blood pressure is under control.

🌀 **AGE ISSUE** *Confirm that the female patient of childbearing age isn't pregnant before performing radiopharmaceutical myocardial perfusion imaging.*

■ Tell the patient that a cardiologist, a nurse, an ECG technician, and a nuclear medicine technologist will be present for the medication infusion. Advise him that he'll be weighed first to determine the proper drug dose.

■ Inform the patient that he may experience flushing, shortness of breath, dizziness, headache, chest pain, and increased heart rate during the infusion, but that these will end as soon as the infusion ends and that emergency equipment will be available, if needed.

■ Screen the patient for bronchospastic lung disease or asthma. Adenosine and dipyridamole are contraindicated in these cases; use dobutamine instead. Weigh the patient to determine the appropriate dosage.

■ Make sure that the patient or a responsible family member has signed an informed consent form.

Procedure and posttest care

■ Place the patient on a bed or an examination table in the ECG or medical imaging department and start an I.V. line.

■ Apply 12 ECG leadwires to appropriate sites and obtain baseline ECG and blood pressure readings.

■ The selected chemical stress medication is infused, and blood pressure, pulse, and cardiac rhythm are monitored continuously.

■ Tell the patient to report the symptoms he's feeling.

■ At the appropriate time, the selected radiopharmaceutical is injected.

■ Depending on which radiopharmaceutical is used, the patient either undergoes imaging immediately or is instructed to return for imaging 45 minutes to 2 hours later. Resting imaging may be done before stress imaging or 3 to 4 hours afterward, depending on the radiopharmaceutical used.

■ Tell the patient when he needs to return and whether he should continue to fast.

■ Remove the I.V. line after the images are completed.

■ When all scans are completed, tell the patient that he may resume his usual diet.

■ If the patient must return for further scanning, tell him to rest; he may also need to restrict foods and fluids in the interim.

Precautions

■ This test is usually contraindicated in a pregnant patient.

■ The use of adenosine or dipyridamole is contraindicated in the patient with bronchospastic lung disease or asthma.

◀ **CLINICAL ALERT** *Keep resuscitation equipment available in case the patient experiences arrhythmias, angina, ST-segment depression, or bronchospasm.*

■ Aminophylline, the reversal agent for adenosine and dipyridamole, can be administered to reverse severe adverse reactions.

■ Contraindications include a myocardial infarction within 10 days of testing, acute myocarditis and pericarditis, unstable angina, arrhythmias, hypertension or hypotension, aortic or mitral stenosis, hyperthyroidism, and severe infection.

■ Beta-adrenergic blockers, calcium channel blockers, and angiotensin-converting enzyme inhibitors should be withheld up to 36 hours before testing, as ordered. Nitrates should be withheld 6 hours before testing.

Normal findings
Imaging should reveal characteristic distribution of the radiopharmaceutical throughout the left ventricle and show no visible defects.

Abnormal findings
Cold spots are usually due to CAD, but may result from myocardial fibrosis, attenuation due to soft tissue (for example, breasts and diaphragm), or coronary spasm. The absence of cold spots in the presence of CAD may result from insignificant artifact obstruction, single-vessel disease, or collateral circulation.

Interfering factors
■ Certain drugs such as digoxin (may produce a false-positive reading)
■ Cold spots due to artifacts, such as implants and electrodes
■ Delayed imaging (may cause absence of cold spots in the presence of CAD)

Persantine-thallium imaging

Persantine-thallium imaging is an alternative method of assessing coronary vessel function for the patient who can't tolerate exercise or stress electrocardiography (ECG). Dipyridamole (Persantine) infusion simulates the effects of exercise by increasing blood flow to the collateral circulation and away from the coronary arteries, thereby inducing ischemia. Thallium infusion allows the examiner to evaluate the cardiac vessels' response. The heart is scanned immediately after the thallium infusion and again 2 to 4 hours later. Diseased vessels can't deliver thalli-

um to the heart, and thallium lingers in diseased areas of the myocardium.

Purpose
■ To identify exercise- or stress-induced arrhythmias
■ To assess the presence and degree of cardiac ischemia

Patient preparation
■ Tell the patient that a painless, 5- to 10-minute baseline ECG will precede Persantine-thallium imaging.
■ Explain to the patient that he'll need to restrict food and fluids before the test. Tell him to avoid caffeine and other stimulants (which may cause arrhythmias).
■ Instruct the patient to continue to take all his regular medications, with the possible exception of beta-adrenergic blockers, as prescribed.
■ Explain to the patient that an I.V. line infuses the medications for the study. Tell him who will start the I.V. and when and that he may experience slight discomfort from the needle insertion and the tourniquet.
■ Inform the patient that he may experience mild nausea, headache, dizziness, or flushing after Persantine administration. Reassure him that these adverse reactions are usually temporary and rarely need treatment.
■ Make sure that the patient or a responsible family member has signed an informed consent form.

Procedure and posttest care
■ The patient reclines or sits while a resting ECG is performed. Then Persantine is given either orally or intravenously over 4 minutes. Blood pressure, pulse rate, and cardiac rhythm are monitored continuously.

■ After Persantine administration, the patient is asked to get up and walk. After it takes effect, thallium is injected.

■ The patient is placed in a supine position for about 40 minutes while the scan is performed. Then the scan is reviewed. If necessary, a second scan is performed.

■ If the patient must return for further scanning, tell him to rest and to restrict food and fluids in the interim.

Precautions

■ The patient may experience arrhythmias, angina, ST-segment depression, or bronchospasm. Make sure resuscitation equipment is readily available.

■ More common adverse reactions are nausea, headache, flushing, dizziness, and epigastric pain.

Normal findings

Imaging should reveal characteristic distribution of the isotope throughout the left ventricle and no visible defects.

Abnormal findings

The presence of ST-segment depression, angina, and arrhythmias strongly suggests coronary artery disease (CAD). Persistent ST-segment depression generally indicates a myocardial infarction. In contrast, transient ST-segment depression indicates ischemia from CAD.

Cold spots usually indicate CAD, but may result from sarcoidosis, myocardial fibrosis, cardiac contusion, attenuation due to soft tissue (for example, breast and diaphragm), apical cleft, and coronary spasm. The absence of cold spots in the presence of CAD may result from insignificant obstruction, single-vessel disease, or collateral circulation.

Interfering factors

■ Failure to observe pretest restrictions

■ Artifacts, such as implants and electrodes (possible false-positive)

■ Absence of cold spots with CAD (possible delay in imaging)

Cardiac blood pool imaging

Cardiac blood pool imaging evaluates regional and global ventricular performance after I.V. injection of human serum albumin or red blood cells (RBCs) tagged with the isotope technetium 99m (^{99m}Tc) pertechnetate. In first-pass imaging, a scintillation camera records the radioactivity emitted by the isotope in its initial pass through the left ventricle. Higher counts of radioactivity occur during diastole because there's more blood in the ventricle; lower counts occur during systole as the blood is ejected. The portion of isotope ejected during each heartbeat can then be calculated to determine the ejection fraction; the presence and size of intracardiac shunts can also be determined.

Gated cardiac blood pool imaging, performed after first-pass imaging or as a separate test, has several forms; however, most forms use signals from an electrocardiogram (ECG) to trigger the scintillation camera. In two-frame gated imaging, the camera records left ventricular endsystole and end-diastole for 500 to 1,000 cardiac cycles; superimposition of these gated images allows assessment of left ventricular contraction to find areas of hypokinesia or akinesia.

In multiple-gated acquisition (MUGA) scanning, the camera records 14 to 64 points of a single cardiac cycle, yielding sequential images that can be studied like motion picture films to evaluate regional wall motion and determine the ejection fraction and other indices of cardiac function. In the stress MUGA test, the same test is performed at rest and after exercise to detect changes in ejection fraction and cardiac output. In the nitroglycerin MUGA test, the scintillation camera records points in the cardiac cycle after sublingual nitroglycerin administration to assess its effect on ventricular function.

Blood pool imaging is more accurate and involves less risk to the patient than left ventriculography in assessing cardiac function.

Purpose
- To evaluate left ventricular function
- To detect aneurysms of the left ventricle and other motion abnormalities of the myocardial wall (areas of akinesia or dyskinesia)
- To detect intracardiac shunting

Patient preparation
- Explain to the patient that cardiac blood pooling imaging permits assessment of the heart's left ventricle.
- Describe the test, including who will perform it, where it will take place, and its expected duration.
- Tell the patient that he need not restrict food and fluids.
- Explain to the patient that he'll receive an I.V. injection of a radioactive tracer and that a detector positioned above his chest will record the circulation of this tracer through the heart.
- Reassure the patient that the tracer poses no radiation hazard and rarely produces adverse effects.
- Inform the patient that he may experience slight discomfort from the needle puncture, but that the imaging itself is painless.
- Instruct the patient to remain silent and motionless during imaging, unless otherwise instructed.

- Make sure that the patient or a responsible family member has signed an informed consent form.

Equipment
Scanner, ECG recorder, nitroglycerin, I.V. insertion equipment, if necessary

Procedure and posttest care
- The patient is placed in a supine position beneath the detector of a scintillation camera, and 15 to 20 millicuries of albumin or RBCs tagged with ^{99m}Tc pertechnetate are injected intravenously.
- For the next minute, the scintillation camera records the first pass of the isotope through the heart so that the aortic and mitral valves can be located.
- Then, using an ECG, the camera is gated for selected 60-msec intervals, representing end-systole and end-diastole, and 500 to 1,000 cardiac cycles are recorded on X-ray or Polaroid film.
- To observe septal and posterior wall motion, the patient may be assisted to modified left anterior oblique position or he may be assisted to a right anterior oblique position and given 0.4 mg of nitroglycerin sublingually. The scintillation camera then records additional gated images to evaluate abnormal contraction in the left ventricle.
- The patient may be asked to exercise as the scintillation camera records gated images.

AGE ISSUE *If the patient is elderly or physically compromised, assist him to a sitting position and make sure he isn't dizzy. Then provide assistance in getting off the examination table.*

Precautions
- Cardiac blood pool imaging is contraindicated during pregnancy.

Normal findings

Normally, the left ventricle contracts symmetrically, and the isotope appears evenly distributed in the scans. Normal ejection fraction is 55% to 65%.

Abnormal findings

The patient with coronary artery disease usually has asymmetrical blood distribution to the myocardium, which produces segmental abnormalities of ventricular wall motion; such abnormalities may also result from preexisting conditions such as myocarditis. In contrast, the patient with a cardiomyopathy shows globally reduced ejection fractions. In the patient with a left-to-right shunt, the recirculating radioisotope prolongs the downslope of the curve of scintigraphic data; early arrival of activity in the left ventricle or aorta signifies a right-to-left shunt.

Interfering factors

■ None significant

CATHETERIZATION

Cardiac catheterization

Cardiac catheterization involves passing a catheter into the right or left side of the heart. Catheterization can determine blood pressure and blood flow in the chambers of the heart, permit blood sample collection, and record films of the heart's ventricles (contrast ventriculography) or arteries (coronary arteriography or angiography).

In catheterization of the left side of the heart, a catheter is inserted into an artery in the antecubital fossa or into the femoral artery through a puncture or cutdown procedure. Guided by fluoroscopy, the catheter is advanced retrograde through the aorta into the coronary artery orifices and left ventricle. Then a contrast medium is injected into the ventricle, permitting radiographic visualization of the ventricle and coronary arteries and filming (cineangiography) of heart activity.

Catheterization of the left side of the heart assesses the patency of the coronary arteries, mitral and aortic valve function, and left ventricular function. It aids in the diagnosis of left ventricular enlargement, aortic stenosis and insufficiency, aortic root enlargement, mitral insufficiency, aneurysm, and intracardiac shunt.

In catheterization of the right side of the heart, the catheter is inserted into an antecubital vein or the femoral vein and is advanced through the inferior vena cava or right atrium into the right side of the heart and the pulmonary artery. Catheterization of the right side of the heart assesses tricuspid and pulmonic valve function and pulmonary artery pressures.

Purpose

■ To evaluate valvular insufficiency or stenosis, septal defects, congenital anomalies, myocardial function and blood supply, and cardiac wall motion

Patient preparation

■ Explain to the patient that cardiac catheterization evaluates the function of the heart and its vessels.

■ Instruct the patient to restrict food and fluids for at least 6 hours before the test, but to continue his prescribed drug regimen unless directed otherwise.

■ Describe the test, including who will perform it and where it will take place.

■ Make sure that the patient or a responsible family member has signed an informed consent form.

868 CARDIOVASCULAR SYSTEM

- Inform the patient that he may receive a mild sedative, but will remain conscious during the procedure. He'll lie on a padded table as the camera rotates so that his heart can be examined from different angles.
- Tell the patient that the catheterization team will wear gloves, masks, and gowns to protect him from infection.
- Inform the patient that he'll have an I.V. needle inserted in his arm to administer medication. Assure him that the electrocardiography (ECG) electrodes attached to his chest during the procedure will cause no discomfort.
- Tell the patient that the catheter will be inserted into an artery or a vein in his arm or leg; if the skin above the vessel is hairy, it will be shaved and cleaned with an antiseptic.
- Explain to the patient that he'll experience a slight stinging sensation when a local anesthetic is injected to numb the incision site for catheter insertion and that he may experience pressure as the catheter moves along the blood vessel. Assure him that these sensations are normal.
- Inform the patient that injection of a contrast medium through the catheter may produce a hot, flushing sensation or nausea that quickly passes; instruct him to follow directions to cough or breathe deeply.
- Explain to the patient that he'll be given medication if he experiences chest pain during the procedure and that he may also receive nitroglycerin periodically to dilate coronary vessels and aid visualization. Reassure him that complications, such as a myocardial infarction or thromboembolism, are rare.
- Check the patient's history for hypersensitivity to shellfish, iodine, or the contrast media used in other diagnostic tests;

notify the physician of any hypersensitivities.
- Discontinue any anticoagulant therapy, as ordered, to reduce the risk of complications from venous bleeding.
- Just before the procedure, tell the patient to void and put on a hospital gown.

Procedure and posttest care
- The patient is placed in the supine position on a tilt-top table and secured by restraints. ECG leads are applied for continuous monitoring, and an I.V. line, if not already in place, is started with dextrose 5% in water or normal saline solution at a keep-vein-open rate.
- After a local anesthetic is injected at the catheterization site, a small incision or percutaneous puncture is made into the artery or vein, and the catheter is passed through the needle into the vessel; the catheter is guided to the cardiac chambers or coronary arteries using fluoroscopy.
- When the catheter is in place, the contrast medium is injected through it to visualize the cardiac vessels and structures.
- The patient may be asked to cough or breathe deeply. Coughing helps counteract nausea or light-headedness caused by the contrast medium and can correct arrhythmias produced by its depressant effect on the myocardium; deep breathing can ease catheter placement into the pulmonary artery or the wedge position and moves the diaphragm downward, making the heart easier to visualize.
- During the procedure, the patient may be given nitroglycerin to eliminate catheter-induced spasm or to measure its effect on the coronary arteries.
- Monitor the patient's heart rate and rhythm, respiratory and pulse rates, and blood pressure frequently during the procedure.

- After completion of the procedure, the catheter is removed and pressure should be applied to the incision site for about 30 minutes either manually or with a mechanical compression device. An adhesive bandage or clear occlusive dressing should be applied to protect the site and permit visualization for detection of bleeding or hematoma formation.

- Monitor the patient's vital signs every 15 minutes for 2 hours after the procedure, every 30 minutes for the next 2 hours, and then every hour for 2 hours. If no hematoma or other problems arise, begin checking every 4 hours. If vital signs are unstable, check every 5 minutes and notify the physician.

- Observe the insertion site for a hematoma or blood loss. Additional compression may be necessary to control bleeding.

- Check the patient's color, skin temperature, and peripheral pulse below the puncture site. The brachial approach is associated with a higher incidence of vasospasm (characterized by cool fingers and hands and weak pulses on the affected side); this usually resolves within 24 hours.

- Enforce bed rest for 8 hours. If the femoral route was used for catheter insertion, keep the patient's leg extended for 6 to 8 hours; if the antecubital fossa was used, keep the patient's arm extended for at least 3 hours.

- If medications were withheld before the test, check with the physician about resuming administration.

- Administer prescribed analgesics.

- Unless the patient is scheduled for surgery, encourage intake of fluids high in potassium, such as orange juice, to counteract the diuretic effect of the contrast medium.

- Make sure a posttest ECG is scheduled to check for possible myocardial damage.

Precautions

- Coagulopathy, impaired renal function, and debilitation usually contraindicate catheterization of both sides of the heart. Unless a temporary pacemaker is inserted to counteract induced ventricular asystole, left bundle-branch block contraindicates catheterization of the right side of the heart.

- If the patient has valvular heart disease, prophylactic antimicrobial therapy may be indicated to guard against subacute bacterial endocarditis.

Normal findings

Cardiac catheterization should reveal no abnormalities of heart chamber size or configuration, wall motion or thickness, direction of blood flow, or valve motion; the coronary arteries should have a smooth and regular outline and vessels should be patent.

Cardiac catheterization provides information on pressures in the heart's chambers and vessels. Higher pressures than normal are clinically significant; lower pressures, except in shock, usually aren't significant. (See *Normal pressure curves,* page 870, and *Upper limits of normal pressures in cardiac chambers and great vessels in recumbent adults,* page 871.)

Abnormal findings

Common abnormalities confirmable by cardiac catheterization include coronary artery disease (CAD), myocardial incompetence, valvular heart disease, and septal defects.

In CAD, catheterization shows constriction of the lumen of the coronary arteries. Constriction greater than 70% is especially significant, particularly in prox-

NORMAL PRESSURE CURVES

Chambers of the right side of the heart
Two pressure complexes are represented
for each chamber. Complexes at the far
right in this diagram represent simultaneous recordings of pressures from the
right atrium, right ventricle, and pulmonary artery.

Chambers of the left side of the heart
Overall pressure configurations are similar to those of the right side of the
heart, but pressures in the left side of the
heart are significantly higher because
systemic flow resistance is much greater
than pulmonary resistance.

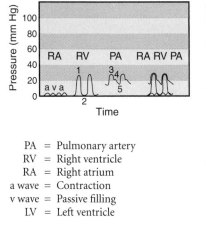

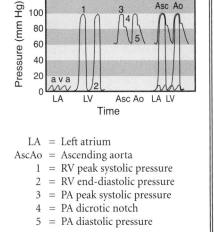

PA   = Pulmonary artery
RV   = Right ventricle
RA   = Right atrium
a wave = Contraction
v wave = Passive filling
LV   = Left ventricle

LA   = Left atrium
AscAo = Ascending aorta
1   = RV peak systolic pressure
2   = RV end-diastolic pressure
3   = PA peak systolic pressure
4   = PA dicrotic notch
5   = PA diastolic pressure

imal lesions. Narrowing of the left main
coronary artery and occlusion or narrowing high in the left anterior descending
artery are commonly indications for
revascularization surgery. (This lesion
responds best to coronary artery bypass
grafting.)

Impaired wall motion can indicate
myocardial incompetence from CAD,
aneurysm, cardiomyopathy, or congenital
anomalies. Comparing the size of the left
ventricle in systole and diastole helps assess the efficiency of cardiac muscle contraction, segmental wall motion, chamber
size, and ejection fraction. An ejection
fraction under 35% generally increases
the risk of complications and decreases
the probability of successful surgery.

Valvular heart disease is indicated by a
gradient, or difference in pressures, above
and below a heart valve. For example, systolic pressure measurements on both
sides of a stenotic aortic valve show a gradient across the valve. The higher the gradient, the greater the degree of stenosis. If
left ventricular systolic pressure measures
200 mm Hg and aortic systolic pressure
measures 120 mm Hg, the gradient across
the valve is 80 mm Hg. Because these
pressures should normally be equal during systole, when the aortic valve is open,
a gradient of this magnitude indicates the
need for corrective surgery. Incompetent
valves can be visualized during ventriculography by watching retrograde flow of
the contrast medium across the valve
during systole.

UPPER LIMITS OF NORMAL PRESSURES IN CARDIAC CHAMBERS AND GREAT VESSELS IN RECUMBENT ADULTS

This chart details the upper limits of normal pressures within the cardiac chambers and great vessels in recumbent adults. Higher-than-normal pressures usually are clinically significant.

Chamber or vessel	Pressure (mm Hg)
Right atrium	6 (mean)
Right ventricle	30/6*
Pulmonary artery	30/12* (mean, 18)
Left atrium	12 (mean)
Left ventricle	140/12*
Ascending aorta	140/90* (mean, 105)
Pulmonary artery wedge	Almost identical (±1 to 2 mm Hg) to left atrial mean pressure

* Peak systolic and end-diastolic

Septal defects (atrial and ventricular) can be confirmed by measuring blood oxygen content in both sides of the heart. Elevated blood oxygen levels on the right side indicate a left-to-right atrial or ventricular shunt; decreased oxygen levels on the left side indicate a right-to-left shunt.

Cardiac output can be measured by analyzing blood oxygen levels in the cardiac chambers. This may be accomplished by drawing blood from cardiac chambers or by injecting contrast medium into the venous circulation and measuring its concentration as it moves past a thermodilution catheter.

Interfering factors
- Improperly functioning equipment and poor technique
- Patient anxiety (increase in heart rate and cardiac chamber pressures)

Electrophysiology studies

Electrophysiology studies (also known as *bundle of His electrography*) permit measurement of discrete conduction intervals by recording electrical conduction during the slow withdrawal of a bipolar or tripolar electrode catheter from the right ventricle through the bundle of His to the sinoatrial node. The catheter is introduced into the femoral vein, passing through the right atrium and across the septal leaflet of the tricuspid valve.

Purpose
- To diagnose arrhythmias and conduction anomalies
- To determine the need for an implanted pacemaker, an internal cardioverter-defibrillator, and cardioactive drugs and to evaluate their effects on the conduction system and ectopic rhythms

- To locate the site of a bundle-branch block, especially in an asymptomatic patient with conduction disturbances
- To determine the presence and location of accessory conducting structures

Patient preparation
- Explain to the patient that electrophysiology studies help to evaluate his heart's conduction system.
- Tell the patient not to eat or drink anything for at least 6 hours before the test.
- Describe the test, including who will perform it and where it will take place.
- Inform the patient that after the groin area is shaved, a catheter will be inserted into the femoral vein and an I.V. line may be started. Assure him that the electrocardiography (ECG) electrodes attached to his chest during the test will cause no discomfort.
- Explain to the patient that he'll experience a stinging sensation when a local anesthetic is injected to numb the incision site for catheter insertion and that he may experience pressure on catheter insertion.
- Inform the patient that he'll be conscious during the test, and urge him to report any discomfort or pain.
- Make sure that the patient or a responsible family member has signed an informed consent form.
- Check the patient's history, and inform the physician of any ongoing drug therapy.
- Just before the procedure, ask the patient to void and to put on a hospital gown.

Procedure and posttest care
- Help the patient into the supine position on a padded table.
- Limb electrodes and precordial leads are applied for continuous monitoring. If not already in place, an I.V. line is started and dextrose 5% in water or normal saline solution is administered at a keep-vein-open rate.
- After a local anesthetic is injected at the catheterization site, a small incision or percutaneous puncture is made, and a J-tip electrode is introduced intravenously into the femoral vein (or into the antecubital fossa). The catheter is guided to the cardiac chambers using fluoroscopy. It's advanced until it crosses the tricuspid valve and enters the right ventricle. Then the catheter is slowly withdrawn from the tricuspid area, and recordings of conduction intervals are made from each pole of the catheter, either simultaneously or sequentially.
- Monitor the patient's vital signs frequently during the test, noting especially a drop in blood pressure during an arrhythmia.
- The catheter is removed, and a pressure dressing is applied after completion of the procedure.
- Monitor the patient's vital signs every 15 minutes for 1 hour after the procedure and then every hour for 4 hours until he's stable. If he's unstable, check every 15 minutes and notify the physician.
- Observe the patient for shortness of breath, chest pain, pallor, or changes in pulse or blood pressure.
- Enforce bed rest for 4 to 6 hours.
- Check the catheter insertion site for bleeding, as ordered, usually every 30 minutes for 8 hours. If bleeding occurs, notify the physician and apply a pressure bandage until the bleeding stops.
- Advise the patient that he may resume his usual diet.
- Make sure a 12-lead resting ECG is scheduled to assess for changes.

Precautions

- Electrophysiology studies are contraindicated in the patient with severe coagulopathy, recent thrombophlebitis, or acute pulmonary embolism.

▶ **CLINICAL ALERT** *Have emergency medication and resuscitation equipment available in case the patient develops arrhythmias during the electrophysiology study.*

Normal findings

Normal conduction intervals in an adult are as follows: HV interval, 35 to 55 msec; AH interval, 45 to 150 msec; and PA interval, 20 to 40 msec.

Abnormal findings

Abnormalities in electrophysiology studies may reveal a prolonged HV interval (the conduction time from the bundle of His to the Purkinje fibers) that can result from acute or chronic disease. Atrioventricular nodal (AH interval) delays can also occur that stem from atrial pacing, chronic conduction system disease, carotid sinus pressure, recent myocardial infarction, and taking certain drugs. In addition, intra-atrial (PA interval) delays can result from acquired, surgically induced, or congenital atrial disease and atrial pacing.

Interfering factors

- Malfunctioning recording equipment and improper catheter positioning

Pulmonary artery catheterization

In pulmonary artery (PA) catheterization, also known as *Swan-Ganz catheterization,* a balloon-tipped, flow-directed catheter is threaded through the right atrium to provide intermittent occlusion of the pulmonary artery. PA catheterization permits measurement of pulmonary artery pressure (PAP) and pulmonary artery wedge pressure (PAWP).

The PAWP reading accurately reflects left atrial pressure (LAP) and left ventricular end-diastolic pressure, although the catheter itself never enters the left side of the heart. Obtaining this information is possible because the heart momentarily relaxes during diastole as it fills with blood from the pulmonary veins; at this instant, the pulmonary vasculature, left atrium, and left ventricle act as a single chamber, and all have identical pressures. Thus, changes in PAP and PAWP reflect changes in left ventricular filling pressure, permitting detection of left ventricular impairment.

The procedure is usually performed at bedside in an intensive or coronary care unit. The catheter is inserted through the cephalic vein in the antecubital fossa or the subclavian (sometimes femoral) vein. In addition to measuring atrial and PA pressures, this procedure evaluates pulmonary vascular resistance and tissue oxygenation, as indicated by mixed venous oxygen content. It should be performed cautiously in the patient with left bundle-branch block or an implanted pacemaker.

Purpose

- To help assess right and left ventricular function
- To monitor therapy for myocardial infarction, cardiogenic shock, septic shock, pulmonary edema, fluid-related hypovolemia and hypotension, systolic murmur, unexplained sinus tachycardia, and various cardiac arrhythmias
- To monitor fluid status in the patient with serious burns, renal disease, noncar-

diogenic pulmonary edema, or acute respiratory distress syndrome
- To monitor the effects of cardiovascular drugs, such as nitroglycerin and nitroprusside
- To establish baseline pressures preoperatively in the patient with existing cardiac disease and then adjust I.V. medications for optimal surgical success
- To differentiate between pulmonary and cardiac pulmonary edema

Patient preparation
- Explain to the patient that PA catheterization evaluates heart function and provides data necessary to determine appropriate therapy or manage fluid status.
- Tell the patient that he need not restrict food and fluids.
- Describe the test, including who will perform it and where it will take place.
- Tell the patient that he'll be conscious during catheterization and that he may experience discomfort from administration of the local anesthetic.
- Explain that catheter insertion takes about 30 minutes, but that the catheter will remain in place, causing little or no discomfort.
- Instruct the patient to report any discomfort immediately.
- Explain that after insertion, he'll need to have a portable chest X-ray to confirm proper placement of the PA catheter.
- Make sure that the patient or a responsible family member has signed an informed consent form.

Equipment
Pressure cuff; balloon-tipped, flow-directed PA catheter; bag of heparinized normal saline solution (usually 500 ml of normal saline solution with 500 to 1,000 units of heparin, if ordered); alcohol pads; medication-added label; pressure bag; pressure tubing with flush device and disposable transducer; monitor and monitor cable; I.V. pole with transducer mount; electrocardiography (ECG) monitor and electrodes; emergency resuscitation equipment; armboard (for antecubital insertion); lead aprons (if fluoroscope is used during insertion); sutures; 4″ × 4″ gauze pads or other dry occlusive dressing material; prepackaged introducer kit; optional: dextrose 5% in water, shaving materials

If a prepackaged introducer kit is unavailable, obtain the following: introducer (one size larger than the catheter), sterile tray containing instruments for procedure, masks, sterile gowns and gloves, povidone-iodine ointment, sutures, two 10-ml syringes, local anesthetic (1% to 2% lidocaine), one 5-ml syringe, 25G needle, ½″ needle, 1″ and 3″ tape.

Procedure and posttest care
- Choose an appropriate flexible PA catheter. Catheters used in this test come in 2- to 5-lumen modes and in various lengths. In the 2-lumen catheter, one lumen contains the balloon, 1 mm behind the catheter tip; the other lumen, which opens at the tip, measures pressure in front of the balloon. The 2-lumen catheter measures PAP and PAWP and can be used to sample mixed venous blood and infuse I.V. solutions. The 3-lumen catheter has another proximal lumen that opens 12″ (30.5 cm) behind the tip; when the tip is in the main pulmonary artery, the proximal lumen lies in the right atrium, permitting fluid administration or right atrial pressure (RAP; central venous pressure) monitoring. The 4-lumen type includes a transistorized thermistor for monitoring blood temperature and allows for cardiac output measurement. A 4-lumen catheter with thermodilution and

pacer port mode is used in critical care settings to allow for pacing, if necessary. The introducer part of the system may also be used to infuse large amounts of fluids.

■ Before catheterization, set up the equipment according to the manufacturer's directions and the facility's protocol.

■ If the insertion site is being prepared for a cutdown procedure, prepare the patient's skin and cover it with a sterile drape.

■ Assist the patient to the supine position. For antecubital insertion, his arm is abducted with the palm upward on an overbed table for support; for subclavian insertion, the patient is placed in the supine position with his head and shoulders slightly lower than his trunk to make the vein more accessible. If the patient can't tolerate the supine position, assist him to semi-Fowler's position. During the test, monitor all pressures with the patient in the same position.

■ Check the catheter balloon for defects, using sterile technique, and flush all ports to ensure patency.

■ The catheter introducer is inserted into the vein percutaneously or by cutdown. Then the catheter is inserted through the introducer and directed to the right atrium, and the catheter balloon is partially inflated so that venous flow carries the catheter tip through the right atrium and tricuspid valve into the right ventricle and the pulmonary artery.

■ Observe the monitor for characteristic waveform changes. Obtain a printout of each stage of catheter insertion. (See *PA catheterization: Insertion sites and associated waveforms,* pages 876 and 877.)

■ Instruct the patient to extend the appropriate arm (or leg, if the catheter is inserted into the femoral vein).

CLINICAL ALERT *During PA catheterization—as the catheter is passed into the chambers of the right side of the heart—observe the monitor for frequent premature ventricular contractions or tachycardia (including ventricular tachycardia), which may result from right ventricular catheter irritation. If irritation occurs, the catheter may be partially withdrawn or medication administered to suppress the arrhythmia or right bundle-branch block.*

■ To record the PAWP, carefully inflate the catheter balloon with the specified amount of air; the catheter tip will float into the wedge position, as indicated by an altered waveform on the monitor. If a PAWP waveform occurs with less than the recommended inflation volume, don't inflate the balloon further.

■ After the balloon is inflated, record the PAWP. Then allow the balloon to deflate passively. This allows the catheter to float back into the pulmonary artery. Observe the monitor for a PA waveform.

■ The 1.5-ml syringe that comes in the introducer kit has an indentation along the barrel that won't allow you to inject more than 1.5 cc of air, to prevent overinflation. The stopcock should be turned so that it's perpendicular to the insertion port to prevent air from the syringe from accidentally inflating the balloon.

CLINICAL ALERT *Don't overinflate the balloon catheter. Overinflation could distend the pulmonary artery, causing vessel rupture.*

■ If the balloon can't be fully deflated after recording the PAWP, don't reinflate it unless the physician is present; balloon rupture may cause a life-threatening air embolism. Check all connections for air leaks that may have prevented balloon inflation, particularly if the patient is confused or uncooperative.

PA CATHETERIZATION: INSERTION SITES AND ASSOCIATED WAVEFORMS

As the pulmonary artery (PA) catheter is directed through the chambers on the right side of the heart to its wedge position, it produces distinctive waveforms on the oscilloscope screen that are important indicators of the catheter's position in the heart.

Right atrial pressure	**Right ventricular pressure**
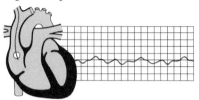	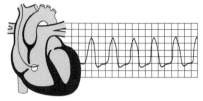

When the catheter tip reaches the right atrium from the superior vena cava, the waveform on the oscilloscope screen or readout strip resembles the one shown above. When this waveform appears, the physician inflates the catheter balloon, which floats the tip through the tricuspid valve into the right ventricle.

When the catheter tip reaches the right ventricle, the waveform looks like the one shown above.

■ When the catheter's correct positioning and function are established, it's sutured to the skin. Antimicrobial ointment and an airtight dressing are applied to the insertion site according to facility policy.

■ A chest X-ray is obtained, as ordered, to verify catheter placement.

■ Set alarms on the ECG and pressure monitors.

■ Monitor the patient's vital signs, as ordered or per facility protocol.

■ Document PAP waveforms at the beginning of each shift and monitor them frequently throughout each shift and with changes in treatment. Check PAWP and cardiac output, as ordered (usually every 6 to 8 hours).

■ Take routine aseptic precautions to prevent infection.

■ When the catheter is no longer needed, the dressing is removed and the catheter is slowly withdrawn after ensuring that the balloon is deflated. The ECG is monitored for arrhythmias. In some facilities, the physician is required to remove the catheter.

■ After the catheter is withdrawn, the catheter tip is usually sent to the laboratory for analysis.

■ Apply a sterile dressing over the catheter introducer.

■ Observe the site for signs of infection, such as redness, swelling, and discharge.

■ Watch for complications, such as pulmonary emboli, PA perforation, heart murmurs, thrombi, and arrhythmias.

Precautions

■ Before obtaining a PAWP reading, flush the monitoring system and recalibrate the system per facility protocol.

Pulmonary artery pressure

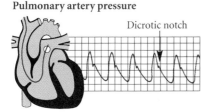

Dicrotic notch

A waveform that resembles the one shown above indicates that the balloon has floated the catheter tip through the pulmonic valve into the pulmonary artery. A dicrotic notch should be visible in the waveform, indicating the closing of the pulmonic valve.

Pulmonary artery wedge pressure

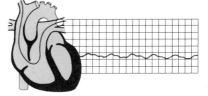

Blood flow in the pulmonary artery then carries the catheter balloon into one of the pulmonary artery's many smaller branches. When the vessel becomes too narrow for the balloon to pass through, the balloon wedges in the vessel, occluding it. The monitor then displays a pulmonary artery wedge pressure waveform such as the one shown above.

■ After obtaining a PAWP reading, make sure the balloon is completely deflated.
■ Maintain 300 mm Hg of pressure in the pressure bag to permit a fluid flow of 3 to 6 ml/hour. Instruct the patient to extend the appropriate arm (or leg, if the catheter is inserted in the femoral vein).
■ If a damped waveform occurs, the catheter may need to be adjusted. Pulmonary infarct may occur if the catheter is allowed to remain in a wedged position.
■ Make sure that the stopcocks are properly positioned and the connections are secure. Loose connections may introduce air into the system or cause blood backup, leakage of deoxygenated blood, or inaccurate pressure readings.
■ Make sure that the lumen hubs are properly identified to serve the appropriate catheter ports.

CLINICAL ALERT *Don't add or remove fluids from the distal PA port; this could cause pulmonary extravasation or damage the artery.*
■ If the catheter hasn't been sutured to the skin, tape it securely to prevent dislodgment.
■ If the patient shows signs of sepsis, treat the catheter as the source of infection and send it to the laboratory for culture when removed.

Reference values
Normal pressures are as follows:
■ *RAP:* 1 to 6 mm Hg
■ *systolic right ventricular pressure:* 20 to 30 mm Hg
■ *end-diastolic right ventricular pressure:* < 5 mm Hg
■ *systolic PAP:* 20 to 30 mm Hg
■ *diastolic PAP:* 10 to 15 mm Hg

- *mean PAP:* < 20 mm Hg
- *PAWP:* 6 to 12 mm Hg
- *LAP:* about 10 mm Hg.

Abnormal findings

An abnormally high RAP can indicate pulmonary disease, right-sided heart failure, fluid overload, cardiac tamponade, tricuspid stenosis and insufficiency, or pulmonary hypertension.

Elevated right ventricular pressure can result from pulmonary hypertension, pulmonary valvular stenosis, right-sided heart failure, pericardial effusion, constrictive pericarditis, chronic heart failure, or ventricular septal defects.

An abnormally high PAP is characteristic in increased pulmonary blood flow, as occurs in a left-to-right shunt secondary to atrial or ventricular septal defect; increased PA resistance, as occurs in pulmonary hypertension or mitral stenosis; chronic obstructive pulmonary disease; pulmonary edema or embolus; and left-sided heart failure from any cause. PA systolic pressure is the same as right ventricular systolic pressure. PA diastolic pressure is the same as LAP, except in the patient with severe pulmonary disease causing pulmonary hypertension; in such cases, catheterization is still important diagnostically.

An elevated PAWP can result from left-sided heart failure, mitral stenosis and insufficiency, cardiac tamponade, or cardiac insufficiency; a depressed PAWP can result from hypovolemia.

Interfering factors

- Malfunctioning monitoring and recording devices, loose connections, clot formation at the catheter tip, air in the fluid column, or a ruptured balloon

- Mechanical ventilation with positive pressure, causing increased intrathoracic pressure (increase in catheter pressure)
- Incorrect catheter placement, causing excessive movement called *catheter fling* (damped pressure tracing)
- Migration of the catheter against a vessel wall (possible constant occlusion, or wedging, of the pulmonary artery)
- Extreme patient agitation

MISCELLANEOUS TESTS

Cold stimulation test for Raynaud's syndrome

The cold stimulation test for Raynaud's syndrome demonstrates Raynaud's syndrome by recording temperature changes in the patient's fingers before and after submersion in ice water. Note that digital blood pressure recording or examination of the arteries in the arm and palmar arch should precede this test to rule out arterial occlusive disease.

Purpose

- To detect Raynaud's syndrome, an arteriospastic disorder characterized by intense vasospasm of the small cutaneous arteries and arterioles of the hands after exposure to cold or stress

Patient preparation

- Explain to the patient that the cold stimulation test for Raynaud's syndrome detects vascular disorders.
- Tell the patient that he need not restrict food and fluids.

- Describe the test, including who will perform it, where it will take place, and how long it will last.
- Explain to the patient that he may experience discomfort when his hands are briefly immersed in ice water.
- Have the patient remove his watch and other jewelry and encourage him to relax.

Procedure and posttest care

- To minimize extraneous environmental stimuli, make sure the test room is neither too warm nor too cold.
- Tape a thermistor to each of the patient's fingers and record the temperature.
- Have the patient submerge his hands in an ice-water bath for 20 seconds.
- When the patient removes his hands from the water, record the temperature of his fingers immediately and every 5 minutes thereafter until it returns to the baseline temperature.

Precautions

- The cold stimulation test is contraindicated in the patient with gangrenous fingers or open, infected wounds.

Normal findings

Normally, digital temperature returns to baseline levels within 15 minutes.

Abnormal findings

If digital temperature takes longer than 20 minutes to return to the baseline level, Raynaud's syndrome is indicated. Its benign form, Raynaud's disease, requires no specific treatment and has no serious sequelae. Its more serious form, Raynaud's phenomenon, is associated with connective tissue disorders that may not be clinically apparent for several years, such as scleroderma, systemic lupus erythematosus, and rheumatoid arthritis. Distin-guishing between Raynaud's phenomenon and Raynaud's disease is difficult.

Interfering factors

- Excessively warm or cold test environment

Pericardial fluid analysis

Analysis of the fluid inside the pericardial sac of the heart is usually done for the patient with pericardial effusion (an accumulation of excess pericardial fluid), which may result from inflammation (as in pericarditis), rupture, or penetrating trauma.

Obtaining a specimen for analysis requires needle aspiration of pericardial fluid, a procedure called *pericardiocentesis*. This procedure must be performed cautiously because of the risk of potentially fatal complications, such as myocardial or coronary artery laceration, ventricular fibrillation or vasovagal arrest, pleural infection, or accidental puncture of the lung, liver, or stomach. If possible, echocardiography should determine the effusion site before pericardiocentesis is performed to minimize the risk of complications. (See *Aspirating pericardial fluid,* page 880.)

Purpose

- To assist in identifying the cause of pericardial effusion and to help determine appropriate therapy

Patient preparation

- Explain to the patient that pericardial fluid analysis detects excessive fluid around the heart, determines its cause, and helps determine appropriate therapy.
- Inform him that he need not restrict food and fluids.

ASPIRATING PERICARDIAL FLUID

In pericardiocentesis, a needle and syringe assembly is inserted through the chest wall into the pericardial sac, as illustrated here. Electrocardiographic (ECG) monitoring with a leadwire attached to the needle and electrodes placed on the limbs (right arm [RA], right leg [RL], left arm [LA], and left leg [LL]) helps to ensure proper needle placement and to avoid damage to the heart.

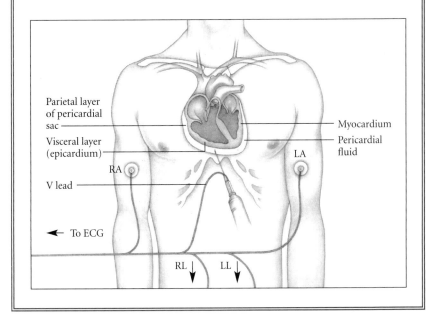

■ Tell him who will perform the test and where it will take place.

■ Inform the patient that a local anesthetic will be injected before the aspiration needle is inserted.

■ Warn him that although fluid aspiration isn't painful, he may experience pressure upon needle insertion into the pericardial sac.

■ Advise him that he may be asked to briefly hold his breath to aid needle insertion and placement.

■ Tell the patient that an I.V. line will be started at a slow rate in case medications need to be administered.

■ Assure him that someone will remain with him during the test and that his pulse and blood pressure will be monitored after the procedure.

■ Check the patient's history for current antimicrobial usage and record such usage on the test request form.

■ Make sure that the patient or a responsible family member has signed an informed consent form.

■ Explain the test to the family if pericardiocentesis is performed to relieve cardiac tamponade and the patient is in shock.

Equipment

70% alcohol or povidone-iodine solution; local anesthetic (1% procaine or 1% lidocaine); sterile 25G needle for the anesthetic; sterile 14G, 16G, and 18G 4″ or 5″

cardiac needles; 50-ml syringe with luer-lock tip; 7-ml sterile test tubes (one clot-activator, one heparin, and one with EDTA); sterile specimen container for culture; vial of heparin 1:1,000; 4″ × 4″ gauze pads; bandage; three-way stopcock (All of these items may be included in a prepackaged pericardiocentesis tray.)

Also needed: electrocardiograph (ECG) or bedside monitor, Kelly clamp, alligator clips, defibrillator, emergency drugs

Procedure and posttest care

- Place the patient in the supine position with the thorax elevated 60 degrees.
- When the patient is comfortable and well supported, instruct him to remain still during the procedure.
- A local anesthetic is administered at the insertion site after the skin is prepared with alcohol or povidone-iodine solution from the left costal margin to the xiphoid process.
- With the three-way stopcock open, a 50-ml syringe is aseptically attached to one end and the cardiac needle to the other end.
- The ECG leadwire is attached to the needle hub with an alligator clip. The ECG is set to lead V and turned on (or the patient is connected to a bedside monitor).
- The needle is inserted through the chest wall into the pericardial sac, main-taining gentle aspiration until fluid appears in the syringe.
- The needle is angled 35 to 45 degrees toward the tip of the right scapula between the left costal margin and the xiphoid process. A Kelly clamp is attached at the skin surface after the needle is properly positioned so it won't advance further.
- While the fluid is being aspirated, label and number the specimen tubes.

- When the needle is withdrawn, apply pressure to the site *immediately* with sterile gauze pads for 3 to 5 minutes. Then apply a bandage.
- Check blood pressure readings, pulse, respiration, and heart sounds every 15 minutes until stable, every 1½ hours for 2 hours, every hour for 4 hours, and then every 4 hours thereafter. Reassure the patient that such monitoring is routine.

◆ **CLINICAL ALERT** *Be alert for respiratory or cardiac distress. Watch especially for signs of cardiac tamponade: muffled and distant heart sounds, distended neck veins, paradoxical pulse, and shock. Cardiac tamponade may result from rapid reaccumulation of pericardial fluid or puncture of a coronary vessel, causing bleeding into the pericardial sac.*

Precautions

- Carefully observe the ECG tracing during insertion of the cardiac needle; an ST-segment elevation indicates that the needle has reached the epicardial surface and should be retracted slightly; an abnormally shaped QRS complex may indicate perforation of the myocardium. Premature ventricular contractions usually indicate that the needle has touched the ventricular wall.
- Watch for grossly bloody aspirate — a sign of inadvertent puncture of a cardiac chamber.
- Be sure to use specimen tubes with the proper additives. Although fibrin isn't a normal component of pericardial fluid, it does appear in fluid in some pericardial diseases and in carcinoma, and clotting is possible.
- Clean the top of the culture and sensitivity tube with povidone-iodine solution to reduce the risk of extrinsic contamination.

- If bacterial culture and sensitivity tests are scheduled, record any antimicrobial therapy the patient is receiving on the laboratory request.
- If anaerobic organisms are suspected, consult the laboratory concerning the proper collection technique to avoid exposing the aspirate to air. The aspirate may be placed in an anaerobic collection tube, or the syringe may be filled completely, displacing all air, and the collection tube capped tightly with a sterile rubber tip.
- Send all specimens to the laboratory immediately after collection.
- Have resuscitation equipment on hand.

Normal findings

Normally, 10 to 50 ml of sterile fluid is present in the pericardium. Pericardial fluid is clear and straw-colored, without evidence of pathogens, blood, or malignant cells. It normally contains fewer than 1,000/μl (SI, < 1.0 × 10⁹/L) white blood cells (WBCs). Its glucose concentration approximately equals the levels in whole blood.

Abnormal findings

Generally, pericardial effusions are classified as transudates or exudates. Transudates are protein-poor effusions that usually arise from mechanical factors altering fluid formation or resorption, such as increased hydrostatic pressure, decreased plasma oncotic pressure, or obstruction of the pericardial lymphatic drainage system by a tumor.

Most exudates result from inflammation and contain large amounts of protein. In these effusions, inflammation damages the capillary membrane, allowing protein molecules to leak into the pericardial fluid. Exudate effusions may occur in pericarditis, neoplasms, acute

myocardial infarction, tuberculosis (TB), rheumatoid disease, and systemic lupus erythematosus.

An elevated WBC count or neutrophil fraction may also accompany inflammatory conditions, such as bacterial pericarditis; a high lymphocyte fraction may indicate fungal or tuberculous pericarditis. Turbid or milky effusions may result from lymph or pus accumulation in the pericardial sac or from TB or rheumatoid disease.

Bloody pericardial fluid may indicate hemopericardium, hemorrhagic pericarditis, or a traumatic tap. Hemopericardium, the accumulation of blood in the pericardium, may result from myocardial rupture after infarction or aortic rupture secondary to a dissecting aortic aneurysm or thoracic trauma. In hemopericardium, the fluid has a hematocrit level similar to that of whole blood; in hemorrhagic pericarditis, it has a relatively low hematocrit and doesn't clot on standing.

Hemorrhagic effusions may indicate a malignant tumor, closed chest trauma, Dressler's syndrome, or postcardiotomy syndrome. A traumatic tap is easily distinguished from hemopericardium or hemorrhagic pericarditis because the fluid becomes progressively clearer.

Glucose concentrations below whole blood levels may reflect increased local metabolism due to malignancy, inflammation, or infection. Possible causes of bacterial pericarditis include *Staphylococcus aureus*, *Haemophilus influenzae*, and various gram-negative organisms; possible causes of granulomatous pericarditis include *Mycobacterium tuberculosis* or various fungal agents; and possible causes of viral pericarditis include coxsackieviruses, echoviruses, and others.

Interfering factors
- Failure to use aseptic collection technique, allowing skin contaminants to be mistaken for the causative organism
- Failure to use proper additives in test tubes
- Antimicrobial therapy (can prevent isolation of the causative organisms)

Selected readings

Braunwald, E., et al., eds. *Harrison's Principles of Internal Medicine,* 15th ed. New York: McGraw-Hill Book Co., 2001.

Fischbach, F. *A Manual of Laboratory and Diagnostic Tests,* 7th ed. Philadelphia: Lippincott Williams & Wilkins, 2004.

Guyton, A.C., and Hall, J.E. *Textbook of Medical Physiology,* 10th ed. Philadelphia: W.B. Saunders Co., 2001.

Nursing Procedures, 4th ed. Philadelphia: Lippincott Williams & Wilkins, 2004.

Ott, K., et al. "New Technologies in the Assessment of Hemodynamic Parameters," *Journal of Cardiovascular Nursing* 15(2):41-55, January 2001.

Pagana, K.D., and Pagana, T.J. *Mosby's Diagnostic and Laboratory Test Reference,* 6th ed. St. Louis: Mosby Year–Book, Inc., 2003.

Phipps, W.J., et al, eds. *Medical-Surgical Nursing, Health and Illness Perspectives,* 7th ed. St. Louis: Mosby Year–Book, Inc., 2003.

Quaal, S.J. "Improving the Accuracy of Pulmonary Artery Catheter Measurements," *Journal of Cardiovascular Nursing* 15(2):71-82, January 2001.

Urden, L.D., et al., eds. *Thelan's Critical Care Nursing: Diagnosis and Management,* 4th ed. St. Louis: Mosby Year–Book, Inc., 2002.

29
Urinary system

Introduction

Two groups of diagnostic tests exist for the detection and evaluation of urologic abnormalities in the urinary system. One group of tests analyzes the properties of urine, the end product of the urinary system; these tests, which include the invaluable routine urinalysis, are discussed in Section II, Chapters 12 to 17. The other group of tests — which is detailed in this chapter — is used to study the structures and functions of the components of the urinary system.

Structure of the kidneys
The urinary system consists of the kidneys, ureters, bladder, and urethra. The kidneys are reddish brown, bean-shaped organs situated in the back of the abdomen, flanking the vertebral column. Each kidney is about 4″ to 5″ (10 to 12.5 cm) long, 3″ (7.5 cm) wide, a little more than 1″ (2.5 cm) thick and weighs 4 to 6 oz (113 to 170 g). It has an upper and a lower pole, anterior and posterior surfaces, convex lateral margins, and concave medial margins (or *hila*) that open into a

fat-filled pocket called the *renal sinus,* through which pass the renal blood vessels, nerves, and pelvis. A fibrous capsule encloses the kidney and is continuous with internal connective tissues, which also line the sinus and calyces of the renal pelvis.

The kidneys consist of the *cortex* and the *medulla.* The outer cortical substance is light and granular, while the inner medullary substance is dark and striated. The cortex and the medulla contain uriniferous tubules — *nephrons* — and collecting tubules. Each nephron is made up of a renal corpuscle and a renal tubule. Each kidney contains about 1 million of these functional units.

The cortex, containing vascular glomeruli and convoluted tubules, forms a series of arches, supported on renal columns extending toward the central sinus. The arches and columns enclose the medulla, forming *renal pyramids* (8 to 12 per kidney). The bases of these pyramids project toward the cortex, ending in *papillae* toward the sinus. The minor *calyces* cap these papillae, collecting the urine that oozes through them. Urine drains from the minor calyces into three major calyces, which empty into the renal pelvis, ureteropelvic junction, and from there into the ureter. (See *The urinary system,* pages 886 and 887.)

Renal blood supply

Blood flows from the aorta into the two renal arteries, each of which divides into two main branches. Just outside the sinus, these main branches subdivide into more branches to supply blood to the entire kidney. These branches are end arteries without anastomoses, so if one of them is obstructed, the result is infarction of the segment it supplies. Straight *interlobular arteries,* too small to be seen with the un-

aided eye, supply blood to the renal columns and cortical arches. Each of these tiny arteries, in turn, supplies a group of lobules with a series of fine, twiglike *afferent arterioles.*

These minute arterioles enter the renal corpuscle, break into capillary tufts or glomeruli, and emerge as *efferent arterioles,* each of which ends in a *capillary intertubular plexus* along the convoluted tubules of its own nephron. The arterial and venous sets of capillaries are called *vasa recta* because they run parallel to the straight tubules. Venous blood from the cortex and medulla returns to the interlobular veins and retraces the course of the arterial branches back to the sinus, ending in the *renal vein.*

Ureters and bladder

The *ureters* are narrow, muscular tubes that transport urine from the kidneys to the bladder. They are 10″ to 11″ (25 to 28 cm) long and nearly ¼″ (6 mm) in diameter. The *renal pelvis* narrows to form the top of the ureters; the tubes terminate at the posterior aspect of the bladder. The ureters enter the bladder wall obliquely, so that the ureteral openings in the bladder are normally only about 1″ (2.5 cm) apart.

An expansile, muscular sac, the *bladder* lies in the space between the pubic bones and the rectum and serves as a reservoir for urine. When empty, the bladder has an apex (behind the symphysis pubis), a base, a superior aspect, and two inferolateral aspects. The base of the bladder faces downward and backward in both sexes. In males, the ampullae of the vas deferens, the seminal vesicles, and the rectovesical fascia separate the base from the rectum. In females, the uterus and vagina intervene. Superiorly, the peritoneum loosely covers the bladder, with loops of intestine

(Text continues on page 888.)

THE URINARY SYSTEM

The urinary system consists of the kidneys, ureters, bladder, and urethra. The kidneys house over 2 million uriniferous tubules (nephrons and collecting tubules), which perform these vital renal functions: cleaning the blood of metabolic wastes and regulating the retention of substances required to preserve the body's fluid, electrolyte, and acid-base balances.

The glomeruli, tufts of capillaries within each nephron's renal corpuscle, accomplish the actual filtration of fluids and solutes from the blood, and the renal tubules reabsorb needed fluids and secrete excess electrolytes. The end product that reaches the collecting tubule is urine.

OVERVIEW

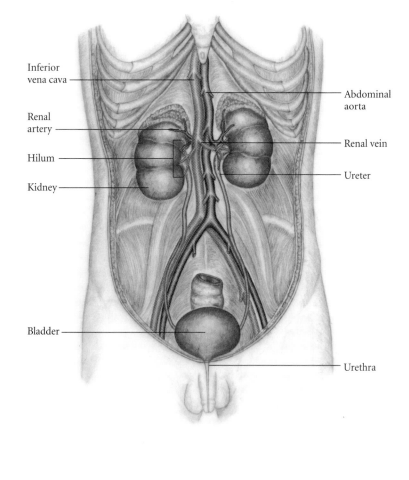

Inferior vena cava

Renal artery

Hilum

Kidney

Bladder

Abdominal aorta

Renal vein

Ureter

Urethra

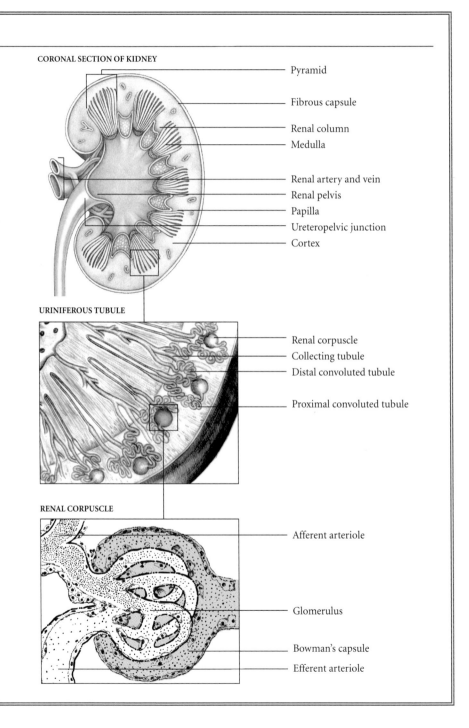

CORONAL SECTION OF KIDNEY

Pyramid

Fibrous capsule

Renal column
Medulla

Renal artery and vein
Renal pelvis
Papilla
Ureteropelvic junction
Cortex

URINIFEROUS TUBULE

Renal corpuscle
Collecting tubule
Distal convoluted tubule

Proximal convoluted tubule

RENAL CORPUSCLE

Afferent arteriole

Glomerulus

Bowman's capsule
Efferent arteriole

above it in males and the uterus over it in females. Inferolaterally, in males and females, the bladder abuts the pubic bones and the internal obturator and levator ani muscles.

The bladder consists of two basic parts: the *trigone* and the *detrusor muscle*. The trigone occupies the space between the internal urethral orifice and the two ureteral openings. The detrusor muscle — a meshwork of muscular fibers — forms most of the bladder wall, encircling the neck of the bladder and running inferiorly adjacent to the proximal urethra.

Urethra

In an adult male, the *urethra* is an S-shaped tube about 9″ (23 cm) long, extending from the internal urethral orifice through the prostate gland, the deep perineal pouch, and the corpus spongiosum of the penis. The urethra is anatomically divided into three sections: the prostatic urethra (about 2½″ [6.5 cm] long), the membranous urethra (½″ to ¾″ [1.3 to 2 cm] long), and the spongy (or cavernous) urethra (about 6″ [15 cm] long). The first two sections, which easily become infected because of their vascularity and lymph drainage, are clinically considered to be one part — the *prostatic urethra*. The membranous segment — the thin-walled, least mobile part of the urethra — is susceptible to injury on catheterization or pelvic fracture. The male urethra serves as a conduit for urine and for the products of the genital system.

In an adult female, the urethra serves one function: to conduit urine out of the body. The female urethra is only 1½″ (4 cm) long and can dilate to a diameter of ¼″ (6 mm). It runs downward and forward, from the neck of the bladder to the pudendal cleft, with a slight anterior concavity behind the symphysis pubis. The lower fibers of the urethral sphincter muscle bind the urethra tightly to the anterior vaginal wall, in which it's embedded. The epithelial lining of the urethra, subject to diverse hormonal activity, undergoes postmenopausal attrition along with adjacent structures. Adventitious organisms commonly colonize the external meatus because it's so close to the vagina and the rectum, which largely accounts for the higher incidence of urinary tract infections in females.

Diagnostic applications

The diagnostic tests discussed in this chapter are recommended after a complete history and physical examination have established the presence of clinical abnormalities associated with urologic disease. For example, the patient may complain of hematuria or flank pain, and the history may reveal urinary urgency or frequency, dysuria, nocturia, enuresis, or incontinence. The physical examination may detect fever, hypertension, and weight gain related to fluid retention.

Associated changes in skin color and texture may include pallor, jaundice, excoriation, redness, pitting edema, easy bruising, and urate crystals. Ocular changes may reflect hemorrhage, exudates, and papilledema. Abnormal oral findings include stomatitis and a fetid breath odor. Fluid retention may also cause edema in the eyelids, face, abdomen, arms, and legs. Palpation of the abdomen may reveal tender or enlarged kidney masses or a distended bladder. Examination of the genitalia may reveal phimosis, paraphimosis, or testicular masses; a rectal examination may reveal prostatic hypertrophy.

Urologic tests

Diagnostic testing of urinary structures includes:

- kidney-ureter-bladder radiography
- nephrotomography
- renal computed tomography
- renal ultrasonography
- cystourethroscopy
- retrograde urethrography
- retrograde cystography
- retrograde ureteropyelography
- antegrade pyelography
- magnetic resonance imaging of the urinary tract
- excretory urography (I.V. pyelography)
- radionuclide renal imaging
- renal angiography
- renal venography.

Urodynamic tests include:

- uroflometry
- cystometry
- voiding cystourethrography
- Whitaker test
- external sphincter electromyography.

Special considerations

When caring for a patient who's scheduled for or has undergone urologic testing, remember these points:

- Make sure the fluid intake of a patient with a suspected urinary tract lesion is adequate (except when underlying medical conditions dictate fluid restriction). Adequate hydration is also necessary to help flush out contrast media.
- Administer a laxative, as ordered, to a patient scheduled for a radiographic test because overlying gas or stool in the lumen of the GI tract may interfere with the quality of X-ray films.
- After an invasive procedure, such as retrograde cystography, monitor the patient's fluid intake and output. Inability to void may necessitate catheterization. No-

tify the physician if hematuria persists after the third voiding.

- Watch for signs of urinary sepsis (such as fever, chills, or hypotension) after any test that involves urinary system instrumentation (such as cystourethroscopy).
- Because many urologic tests are embarrassing to the patient, minimize his anxiety by clearly describing the procedures he'll undergo.

STRUCTURAL TESTS

Kidney-ureter-bladder radiography

Usually the first step in diagnostic testing of the urinary system, kidney-ureter-bladder (KUB) radiography surveys the abdomen to determine the position of the kidneys, ureters, and bladder and to detect gross abnormalities.

This test doesn't require intact renal function and may aid differential diagnosis of urologic and GI diseases, which commonly produce similar signs and symptoms. However, KUB radiography has many limitations and usually must be followed by more elaborate tests, such as excretory urography or renal computed tomography. KUB radiography shouldn't follow recent instillation of barium.

Purpose

- To evaluate the size, structure, and position of the kidneys
- To screen for abnormalities, such as calcifications, in the region of the kidneys, ureters, and bladder

Patient preparation

■ Explain to the patient that KUB radiography helps detect urinary system abnormalities.

■ Inform the patient that he need not restrict food and fluids. Tell him who will perform the test, where it will take place, and that it takes only a few minutes.

Procedure and posttest care

■ The patient is placed in a supine position in correct body alignment on an X-ray table. His arms are extended overhead, and the iliac crests are checked for symmetrical positioning.

■ If the patient can't extend his arms or stand, he may lie on his left side with his right arm up.

■ A single X-ray is taken.

Precautions

■ A male patient should have gonadal shielding to prevent irradiation of the testes. A female patient's ovaries can't be shielded because they're too close to the kidneys, ureters, and bladder.

Normal findings

The shadows of the kidneys appear bilaterally, the right slightly lower than the left. They should be approximately the same size, with the superior poles tilted slightly toward the vertebral column, paralleling the shadows (or stripes) produced by the psoas muscles. The ureters are only visible when an abnormality, such as calcification, is present. Visualization of the bladder depends on the density of its muscular wall and on the amount of urine in it. Generally, the bladder's shadow can be seen, but not as clearly as the kidneys' shadows.

Abnormal findings

Bilateral renal enlargement may result from polycystic disease, multiple myeloma, lymphoma, amyloidosis, diabetes, hydronephrosis, or compensatory hypertrophy. A tumor, a cyst, or hydronephrosis may cause unilateral enlargement. Abnormally small kidneys may suggest end-stage glomerulonephritis or bilateral atrophic pyelonephritis. An apparent decrease in the size of one kidney suggests possible congenital hypoplasia, atrophic pyelonephritis, or ischemia. Renal displacement may be due to a retroperitoneal tumor such as an adrenal tumor. Obliteration or bulging of a portion of the psoas muscle stripe may result from a tumor, an abscess, or a hematoma.

Congenital anomalies, such as abnormal location or absence of a kidney, may be detected. Horseshoe kidney may be suggested by renal axes that parallel the vertebral column, especially if the inferior poles of the kidneys can't be clearly distinguished. A lobulated edge or border may suggest polycystic kidney disease or patchy atrophic pyelonephritis.

Opaque bodies may reflect calculi or vascular calcification due to aneurysm or atheroma; opacification may also suggest cystic tumors, fecaliths, foreign bodies, or abnormal fluid collection. Calcifications may appear anywhere in the urinary system, but positive identification requires further testing. The lone exception is staghorn calculus, which forms a perfect cast of the renal pelvis and calyces.

Interfering factors

■ Gas, stool, contrast medium, or foreign bodies in the intestine (possible poor imaging)

■ Calcified uterine fibromas or ovarian lesions

- Obesity or ascites (possible poor imaging)

Nephrotomography

In nephrotomography, special films are exposed before and after opacification of the renal arterial network and parenchyma with contrast medium. The resulting tomographic slices clearly delineate various linear layers of the kidneys, while blurring structures in front of and behind these selected planes.

Nephrotomography can be performed as a separate procedure or as an adjunct to excretory urography. Nephrotomography is particularly helpful in visualizing space-occupying lesions suggested by excretory urography or retrograde ureteropyelography. Additional films are exposed to define the wall thickness of the mass and its interior. Other tests that may resolve nephrotomographic findings include renal angiography and radionuclide renal imaging.

Purpose

- To differentiate between a simple renal cyst and a solid neoplasm
- To assess renal lacerations as well as posttraumatic nonperfused areas of the kidneys
- To localize adrenal tumors when laboratory tests indicate their presence

Patient preparation

- Explain to the patient that nephrotomography provides images of sections or layers of the kidney tissues and blood vessels.
- Instruct the patient to fast for 8 hours before the test. Tell him who will perform the test and where it will take place.
- Tell the patient that he'll be positioned on an X-ray table and that he may hear loud, clacking sounds as the films are exposed. Tell him that he may experience transient adverse effects from the contrast medium injection — usually a burning or stinging sensation at the injection site, flushing, and a metallic taste.
- Make sure that the patient or a responsible family member has signed an informed consent form.

CLINICAL ALERT *Check the patient's history for hypersensitivity to iodine or iodine-containing foods or to contrast media used in other diagnostic tests. If he has a history of sensitivity, provide antiallergenic prophylaxis (such as diphenhydramine) or use a non–iodine-containing contrast medium, as necessary.*

AGE ISSUE *An elderly or a dehydrated patient is at increased risk for contrast-induced renal failure. Check serum creatinine levels and inform the physician if they're elevated. I.V. fluids may be ordered before the test to ensure hydration and decrease nephrotoxic potential.*

Procedure and posttest care

- The test may be performed using either the infusion method or bolus method. Complications resulting from either technique are minor and infrequent.
- A plain film of the kidneys is exposed to provide general information about their position, size, and shape, and preliminary anteroposterior tomograms are made to determine tomographic levels. Posterior oblique tomograms are made to rule out the presence of radiopaque renal calculi, which would be masked by the contrast medium.

Infusion method

- After test tomograms are reviewed, five vertical slices of renal parenchyma ⅜″ (1 cm) apart are selected for filming.

SIMPLE CYST OR SOLID TUMOR: DIFFERENTIAL DIAGNOSIS IN NEPHROTOMOGRAPHY

Feature	Cyst	Tumor
Consistency	Homogeneous	Irregular
Contact with healthy renal tissue	Sharply distinct	Poorly resolved
Density	Radiolucent	Variable radiolucent patches (or same as normal renal parenchyma)
Shape	Spheric	Variable
Wall of lesion	Thin and well defined	Thick and irregular

■ Contrast medium is then administered through the antecubital vein—the first half in 4 to 5 minutes (rapid phase) and the second half in the following 8 to 10 minutes (slow phase). Serial tomograms are made as soon as the slow phase begins.

Bolus method

■ After test tomograms are reviewed, circulation time from arm to tongue is determined by injecting a bolus of a bitter-tasting agent (dehydrocholic acid or sodium dehydrocholate) into the antecubital vein. Arm-to-tongue circulation time is close to arm-to-kidney circulation time.

■ With the needle still in place, a loading dose of a conventional urographic contrast medium is injected to perform excretory urography.

■ Five minutes after this injection, a loading dose of a contrast medium is quickly injected to ensure a high concentration of the contrast medium in the kidneys. A multifilm tomographic cassette, exposed at the predetermined arm-to-kidney circulation time, visualizes the main renal vessels and possible vessels within tumors.

■ A series of individual tomograms measuring 1 cm are then made in rapid succession through the opacified kidneys.

■ If the exposures are poor, this method requires a second infusion of contrast medium because normal kidneys quickly clear the substance.

Both methods

■ If a hematoma develops at the injection site, apply warm soaks.

■ Monitor the patient's vital signs and urine output for 24 hours after the test.

■ Ensure adequate hydration (unless contraindicated) and monitor serum creatinine levels because of the risk of contrast-induced renal failure.

▶ **CLINICAL ALERT** *Observe for signs of a posttest allergic reaction (flushing, nausea, urticaria, and sneezing). Have epinephrine (1:1,000) and an antihistamine readily available to counter allergic reactions.*

Precautions

■ Nephrotomography should be performed with extreme caution in the patient with hypersensitivity to iodine-based compounds, cardiovascular disease, or multiple myeloma and in an elderly or a dehydrated patient with impaired renal function, as evidenced by elevated serum creatinine.

Normal findings

The size, shape, and position of the kidneys appear within normal range, with no space-occupying lesions or other abnormalities.

Abnormal findings

Among the abnormalities detectable through nephrotomography are simple cysts and solid tumors, renal sinus–related lesions, ectopic renal lobes, adrenal tumors, areas of nonperfusion, and renal lacerations following trauma. (See *Simple cyst or solid tumor: Differential diagnosis in nephrotomography.*)

Interfering factors

■ Residual barium from a recent enema or other GI studies (possible poor imaging)

Renal computed tomography

Renal computed tomography (CT) provides a useful image of the kidneys made from a series of tomograms or cross-sectional slices, which are then translated by a computer and displayed on a monitor. The image density reflects the amount of radiation absorbed by renal tissue and permits identification of masses and other lesions. An I.V. contrast medium may be injected to accentuate the renal parenchyma's density and help differentiate renal masses. This highly accurate test is usually performed to investigate diseases found by other diagnostic procedures such as excretory urography.

Purpose

■ To detect and evaluate renal abnormalities, such as a tumor, an obstruction, calculi, polycystic kidney disease, congenital anomalies, and abnormal fluid accumulation around the kidneys
■ To evaluate the retroperitoneum

Patient preparation

■ Explain to the patient that renal CT permits examination of the kidneys.
■ If contrast enhancement isn't scheduled, inform the patient that he need not restrict food and fluids. If contrast enhancement is scheduled, instruct him to fast for 4 hours before the test.
■ Tell the patient who will perform the test and where it will take place.
■ Inform the patient that he'll be positioned on an X-ray table and that a scanner will take films of his kidneys.
■ Warn the patient that the scanner may make loud, clacking sounds as it rotates around his body.
■ Tell the patient that he may experience transient adverse effects, such as flushing, a metallic taste, and headache, after contrast medium injection.
■ Make sure that the patient or a responsible family member has signed an informed consent form.

▶ **CLINICAL ALERT** *Check the patient's history for hypersensitivity to shellfish, iodine, or contrast media. Mark any sensitivities in his chart.*
■ Just before the procedure, instruct the patient to put on a gown and to remove any metallic objects that could interfere with the scan.
■ Administer prescribed sedatives.

Equipment

CT scanner; contrast medium, if ordered; I.V. insertion equipment, if necessary

Procedure and posttest care

- The patient is placed in a supine position on the X-ray table and secured with straps.
- The table is moved into the scanner.
- Instruct the patient to lie still.
- The scanner then rotates around the patient, taking multiple images at different angles within each cross-sectional slice.
- When one series of tomograms is complete, I.V. contrast enhancement may be performed. Another series of tomograms is then taken.
- After the I.V. contrast medium is administered, monitor the patient for allergic reactions, such as respiratory difficulty, urticaria, or skin eruptions.
- Information from the scan is stored on a disk or magnetic tape, fed into a computer, and converted into an image for display on a monitor. Radiographs and photographs are taken of selected views.
- If the procedure was performed with contrast enhancement, observe the patient for hypersensitivity to the contrast medium.
- After the test, tell the patient that he may resume his usual diet.
- If calculi are present, strain urine, hydrate the patient, and discuss nutritional adaptations as indicated.
- Support the patient and his family if surgery is indicated for a neoplasm.
- Monitor the patient's vital signs if a sedative was administered.

Precautions

- Watch for signs of hypersensitivity to the contrast medium if contrast enhancement is required.

Normal findings

Normally, the density of the renal parenchyma is slightly higher than that of the liver, but is much less dense than bone, which appears white on a CT scan. The density of the collecting system is generally low (black), unless a contrast medium is used to enhance it to a higher (whiter) density. The position of the kidneys is evaluated according to the surrounding structures; their size and shape are determined by counting cuts between the superior and inferior poles and following the contour of the kidneys' outline.

Abnormal findings

Renal masses appear as areas of different density than normal parenchyma, possibly altering the kidneys' shape or projecting beyond their margins. Renal cysts, for example, appear as smooth, sharply defined masses with thin walls and a lower density than normal parenchyma. Tumors, such as renal cell carcinoma, however, are usually not as well delineated; they tend to have thick walls and nonuniform density. With contrast enhancement, solid tumors show a higher density than renal cysts, but lower density than normal parenchyma. Tumors with hemorrhage, calcification, or necrosis show higher densities. Vascular tumors are more clearly defined with contrast enhancement. Adrenal tumors are confined masses, usually detached from the kidneys and from other retroperitoneal organs.

Renal CT scanning may also identify other abnormalities, including obstructions, calculi, polycystic kidney disease, congenital anomalies, and abnormal accumulations of fluid around the kidneys, such as hematomas, lymphoceles, and abscesses. After nephrectomy, CT scanning can detect abnormal masses, such as recurrent tumors, in a renal fossa that should be empty.

Interfering factors
- Inability to remain still
- Presence of contrast media from other recent tests or of foreign bodies such as catheters or surgical clips (possible poor imaging)

Renal ultrasonography

In renal ultrasonography, high-frequency sound waves are transmitted from a transducer to the kidneys and perirenal structures. The resulting echoes are displayed on a monitor as anatomic images.

Renal ultrasonography can be used to detect abnormalities or clarify those detected by other tests. It's especially useful in cases in which excretory urography is ruled out. Unlike excretory urography, this test isn't dependent on renal function and therefore may be useful in the patient with renal failure. Ultrasonography of the ureter, bladder, and gonads also may be used to evaluate urologic disorders.

Purpose
- To determine the size, shape, and position of the kidneys, their internal structures, and perirenal tissues
- To evaluate and localize urinary obstruction and abnormal fluid accumulation
- To assess and diagnose complications after kidney transplantation
- To detect renal or perirenal masses
- To differentiate between renal cysts and solid masses
- To verify placement of a nephrostomy tube

Patient preparation
- Explain to the patient that renal ultrasonography is used to detect kidney abnormalities.
- Inform the patient that he need not restrict food and fluids.
- Tell the patient who will perform the test, where it will take place, and that it's safe and painless.

Procedure and posttest care
- The patient is placed in the prone position, the area to be scanned is exposed, and conductive gel is applied.
- The longitudinal axis of the kidneys is located by using measurements from excretory urography or by performing transverse scans through the upper and lower renal poles.
- These points are marked on the skin and connected with straight lines. Sectional images $\frac{3}{8}''$ to $\frac{3}{4}''$ (1 to 2 cm) apart can then be obtained by moving the transducer longitudinally, transversely, or at any other angle required.
- During the test, the patient may be asked to breathe deeply to visualize upper portions of the kidney.
- After the test, remove the conductive gel from the patient's skin.
- If bladder abnormalities are found, prepare the patient for further testing.
- If rejection of a transplanted kidney is suspected or diagnosed, monitor the patient's intake and output, blood pressure, blood urea nitrogen and creatinine levels, and vital signs. In addition, monitor for adrenal dysfunction (hypotension, decreased urine output, and electrolyte imbalances) if a tumor is detected on the gland.
- If ultrasonography is used as a guide for nephrostomy tube placement or abscess drainage, monitor the amount and

Normal findings

The kidneys are located between the superior iliac crests and the diaphragm. The renal capsule should be outlined sharply; the cortex should produce more echoes than the medulla. In the center of each kidney, the renal collecting systems appear as irregular areas of higher density than surrounding tissue. The renal veins and, depending on the scanner, some internal structures can be visualized. If the bladder is also being evaluated, its size, shape, position, and urine content can be determined.

Abnormal findings

Cysts are usually fluid-filled, circular structures that don't reflect sound waves. Tumors produce multiple echoes and appear as irregular shapes. Abscesses found within or around the kidneys usually echo sound waves poorly; their boundaries are slightly more irregular than those of cysts. A perirenal abscess may displace the kidney anteriorly.

Generally, acute pyelonephritis and glomerulonephritis aren't detectable unless the renal parenchyma is significantly scarred and atrophied. In such cases, the renal capsule appears irregular and the kidney may appear smaller than normal; also, an increased number of echoes may arise from the parenchyma due to fibrosis.

In the patient with hydronephrosis, renal ultrasonography may show a large, echo-free, central mass that compresses the renal cortex. Calyceal echoes are usually circularly diffused and the pelvis significantly enlarged. This test can also be used to detect congenital anomalies, such as horseshoe, ectopic, or duplicated kidneys. Ultrasonography clearly detects renal hypertrophy.

Following kidney transplantation, compensatory hypertrophy of the transplanted kidney is normal, but an acute increase in size indicates rejection.

This test allows identification of abnormal accumulations of fluid within or around the kidneys that sometimes arise from an obstruction. It also allows evaluation of perirenal structures and can identify abnormalities of the adrenal glands, such as tumors, cysts, and adrenal dysfunction. However, a normal adrenal gland is difficult to define ultrasonically because of its small size.

Renal ultrasonography can be used to detect changes in the shape of the bladder that result from masses and can assess urine volume. Increased urine volume or residual urine after voiding may indicate bladder outlet obstruction.

Interfering factors

■ Retained barium from a previous test (possible poor imaging)
■ An obese patient (possible poor imaging)

Cystourethroscopy

Cystourethroscopy, a test that combines two endoscopic techniques, allows visual examination of the bladder and urethra. One of the instruments used in this test is the cystoscope, which has a fiber-optic light source, a magnification system, a right-angled telescopic lens, and an angled beak for smooth passage into the bladder. The other instrument, the urethroscope (or panendoscope), is similar, but has a straight-ahead lens and is used for examination of the bladder neck and urethra. The lenses of the cystoscope and urethroscope use a common sheath inserted into the urethra to obtain the desired view.

Other invasive procedures, such as biopsies, lesion resection, calculi removal, dilatation of a constricted urethra, and catheterization of the ureteral orifices for retrograde pyelography, may also be performed through this sheath.

Kidney-ureter-bladder radiography and excretory urography usually precede this test.

Purpose

■ To diagnose and evaluate urinary tract disorders by direct visualization of urinary structures

Patient preparation

■ Explain to the patient that cystourethroscopy permits examination of the bladder and urethra.

■ Unless a general anesthetic has been ordered, inform the patient that he need not restrict food and fluids. If a general anesthetic will be administered, instruct the patient to fast for 8 hours before the test.

■ Tell the patient who will perform the test, where it will take place, and that it takes about 20 to 30 minutes.

■ Inform the patient that he may experience some discomfort after the procedure, including a slight burning when he urinates.

■ Make sure that the patient or a responsible family member has signed an informed consent form.

■ Before the procedure, administer a sedative, if ordered, and instruct the patient to urinate.

Equipment

Cystourethroscopy (components include sheath, cystoscope, and urethroscope); light source; bougie à boule (for urethral calibration); urethral sounds (for urethral dilatation); filiforms and followers (for severe stricture); preparatory tray; local anesthetic set; irrigating solution and administration set; sterile gloves, gown, and drape; sterile specimen containers

Procedure and posttest care

■ After a general or regional anesthetic (as required) has been administered, the patient is placed in the lithotomy position on a cystoscopic table. The genitalia are cleaned with an antiseptic solution, and the patient is draped. (Local anesthetic is instilled at this point.)

■ The instrument is moved toward the bladder to visually examine the urethra. A urethroscope is inserted into the well-lubricated sheath (instead of an obturator), and both are passed gently through the urethra into the bladder. The urethroscope is then removed, and a cystoscope is inserted through the sheath into the bladder.

■ After the bladder is filled with irrigating solution, the scope is rotated to inspect the entire surface of the bladder wall and ureteral orifices with the right-angled telescopic lens.

■ The cystoscope is then removed, the urethroscope reinserted, and the urethroscope and sheath are slowly withdrawn, permitting examination of the bladder neck and the various portions of the urethra, including the internal and external sphincters. (See *Using a cystourethroscope,* page 898.)

■ During cystourethroscopy, a urine specimen is routinely taken from the bladder for culture and sensitivity testing, and residual urine is measured.

■ If a tumor is suspected, a urine specimen is sent to the laboratory for cytologic examination; if a tumor is found, biopsy may be performed. If a urethral stricture

USING A CYSTOURETHROSCOPE

This cross-sectional illustration shows how a urologic examination is performed with a cystourethroscope, a device that allows direct visualization of the tissues of the lower urinary tract. The sheath of the cystourethroscope permits passage of a cystoscope and urethroscope for illuminating the urethra, bladder, and ureters. This instrument also provides a channel for minor surgical procedures, such as biopsies, excision of small lesions, and calculi removal.

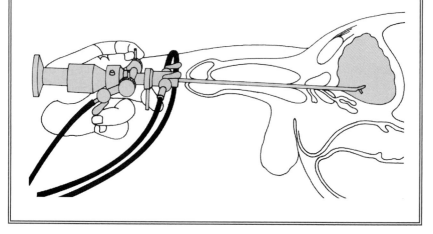

is present, urethral dilatation may be necessary before cystourethroscopy.

■ If the patient has received only a local anesthetic, he may complain of a burning sensation when the instrument is passed through the urethra. He may also feel an urgent need to urinate as the bladder fills with irrigating solution. Reassure the patient that these sensations are common and generally transient.

■ Monitor the patient's vital signs for 15 minutes for the first hour after the test, and then every hour until they stabilize.

■ If local anesthesia was used, keep the patient supine for several minutes, and then help him to sit or stand. Watch for orthostatic hypotension.

■ Instruct the patient to drink lots of fluids (or increase I.V. fluids, if ordered) and to take the prescribed analgesic. Reassure

him that burning and frequency will soon subside.

■ Administer antibiotics, as ordered, to prevent bacterial sepsis due to urethral tissue trauma.

■ Report flank or abdominal pain, chills, fever, an elevated white blood cell count, or low urine output to the physician immediately.

■ Record the patient's intake and output for 24 hours, and observe him for distention. If he doesn't void within 8 hours after the test or if bright red blood continues to appear after three voidings, notify the physician.

■ Instruct the patient to abstain from alcohol for 48 hours.

■ Apply heat to the lower abdomen to relieve pain and muscle spasm (if ordered). A warm sitz bath may be ordered.

Precautions

- Cystourethroscopy is contraindicated in the patient with acute forms of urethritis, prostatitis, or cystitis because instrumentation can lead to sepsis.
- The test is also contraindicated in the patient with bleeding disorders because instrumentation can lead to increased bleeding.

Normal findings

The urethra, bladder, and ureteral orifices appear normal in size, shape, and position. The mucosa lining the lower urinary tract should appear smooth and shiny, with no evidence of erythema, cysts, or other abnormalities. The bladder should be free from obstructions, tumors, and calculi.

Abnormal findings

One of the most common abnormal findings detected in cystourethroscopy is an enlarged prostate gland in older men. In males and females, urethral stricture, calculi, tumors, diverticula, ulcers, and polyps are also common findings. This test also may detect bladder wall trabeculation and various congenital anomalies, such as ureteroceles, duplicate ureteral orifices, or urethral valves in children.

Interfering factors

- None significant

Retrograde urethrography

Used almost exclusively in men, retrograde urethrography requires instillation or injection of a contrast medium into the urethra and permits visualization of its membranous, bulbar, and penile portions.

Although visualization of the anterior portion of the urethra is excellent with this test alone, the posterior portion is more effectively outlined by retrograde urethrography in tandem with voiding cystourethrography.

Purpose

- To diagnose urethral strictures, diverticula, and congenital anomalies
- To assess urethral lacerations or other trauma
- To assist with follow-up examination after surgical repair of the urethra

Patient preparation

- Explain to the patient that retrograde urethrography diagnoses urethral structural problems. Inform him that he need not restrict food and fluids.
- Describe the test, including who will perform it and where it will take place.
- Inform the patient that he may experience some discomfort when the catheter is inserted and when the contrast medium is instilled through the catheter.
- Tell the patient that he may hear loud, clacking sounds as the X-ray films are made.
- Make sure that the patient or a responsible family member has signed an informed consent form.
- Check the patient's history for hypersensitivity to iodine-containing foods, such as shellfish, or contrast media.
- Administer any prescribed sedatives just before the procedure and instruct the patient to void before leaving the unit.

Equipment

Radiograph machine and table, penile clamp, 50-ml syringe with tapered universal adapter, indwelling urinary catheter, 1″ roller gauze, contrast medium (half-strength preparation)

Procedure and posttest care
For men

■ The patient is placed in a recumbent position on the examining table. Anteroposterior exposures of the bladder and urethra are made, and the resulting films studied for radiopaque densities, foreign bodies, or calculi.

■ The glans and meatus are cleaned with an antiseptic solution. The catheter is filled with the contrast medium before insertion to eliminate air bubbles.

■ Although no lubricant should be used, the tip of the catheter may be dipped in sterile water to facilitate insertion.

■ The catheter is inserted until the balloon portion is inside the meatus; the balloon is then inflated with 1 to 2 ml of water, which prevents the catheter from slipping during the procedure.

■ The patient then assumes the right posterior oblique position, with his right thigh drawn up to a 90-degree angle and the penis placed along its axis. The left thigh is extended.

■ The contrast medium is injected through the catheter. After three-fourths of the contrast medium has been injected, the first X-ray film is exposed while the remainder of the contrast medium is being injected. Left lateral oblique views may also be taken.

■ Fluoroscopic control may be helpful, especially for evaluating urethral injury.

For women and children

■ In women, this test may be used when urethral diverticula are suspected. A double-balloon catheter is used, which occludes the bladder neck from above and the external meatus from below.

■ In children, the procedure is the same as for adults except that a smaller catheter is used.

For all patients

◀ **CLINICAL ALERT** *Watch for chills and fever related to extravasation of contrast medium into the general circulation for 12 to 24 hours after retrograde urethrography. Also observe for signs of sepsis and allergic manifestations.*

Precautions

■ Retrograde urethrography should be performed cautiously in the patient with a urinary tract infection (UTI).

■ Monitor the patient for a UTI. If urethral trauma is present, monitor for stricture, infection, and urinary extravasation. Prepare him for surgery, if indicated.

Normal findings

The membranous, bulbar, and penile portions of the urethra — and occasionally the prostatic portion — appear normal in size, shape, and course.

Abnormal findings

Radiographs obtained during retrograde urethrography may show the following abnormalities: urethral diverticula, fistulas, strictures, false passages, calculi, and lacerations; congenital anomalies, such as urethral valves and perineal hypospadias; and, rarely, tumors (in less than 1% of cases).

Interfering factors

■ None significant

Retrograde cystography

Retrograde cystography involves the instillation of contrast medium into the bladder, followed by radiographic examination. This procedure is used to diagnose bladder rupture without urethral involvement because it can determine the location and extent of the rupture. Other indications for retrograde cystography include neurogenic bladder; recurrent urinary tract infections (UTIs), especially in children; suspected vesicoureteral reflux; and vesical fistulas, diverticula, and tumors. This test is also performed when cystoscopic examination is impractical, as in male infants, or when excretory urography hasn't adequately visualized the bladder. Voiding cystourethrography is commonly performed concomitantly.

Purpose

■ To evaluate the structure and integrity of the bladder

Patient preparation

■ Explain to the patient that retrograde cystography permits radiographic examination of the bladder.

■ Inform the patient that he need not restrict food and fluids.

■ Tell the patient who will perform the test and where it will take place.

■ Inform the patient that he may experience some discomfort when the catheter is inserted and when the contrast medium is instilled through the catheter.

■ Tell the patient that he may hear loud, clacking sounds as the X-ray films are made.

■ Make sure that the patient or a responsible family member has signed an informed consent form.

■ Check the patient's history for hypersensitivity to contrast media, iodine, or shellfish; mark it on the chart and inform the physician.

Equipment

Radiographic equipment, drip infusion set or syringes, standard contrast medium, urethral indwelling urinary catheters

Procedure and posttest care

■ The patient is placed in a supine position on the X-ray table and a preliminary kidney-ureter-bladder radiograph is taken.

■ The radiograph is developed immediately and scrutinized for renal shadows, calcifications, contours of the bone and psoas muscles, and gas patterns in the lumen of the GI tract.

■ The bladder is catheterized and 200 to 300 ml of sterile contrast medium (50 to 100 ml for an infant) is instilled by gravity or gentle syringe injection. The catheter is then clamped.

■ With the patient in a supine position, an anteroposterior film is taken. The patient is then tilted to one side, then the other, and two posterior oblique (and sometimes lateral) views are taken.

■ If the patient's condition permits, he's placed in the jackknife position and a posteroanterior film is taken. A space-occupying vesical lesion may require additional exposures. Rarely, to enhance visualization, 100 to 300 ml of air may be insufflated into the bladder by syringe after removal of the contrast medium (double-contrast technique).

■ The catheter is then unclamped, the bladder fluid is allowed to drain, and a radiograph is obtained to detect urethral diverticula, reflux into the ureters, fistulous tracts into the vagina, or intraperitoneal or extraperitoneal extravasation of the contrast medium.

■ Monitor the patient's vital signs every 15 minutes for the first hour, every 30 minutes during the second hour, and then every 2 hours for up to 24 hours.

■ Record the time of the patient's voidings and the color and volume of the urine. Observe for hematuria that persists after the third voiding and notify the physician.

- Watch for signs of urinary sepsis from UTIs (chills, fever, elevated pulse and respiration rates, and hypotension) or similar signs related to extravasation of contrast medium into the general circulation.
- Prepare the patient for surgery and urinary diversion, if indicated. Strain urine if calculi are detected.
- Monitor for retention or distention if neurogenic bladder is diagnosed and administer medication, as ordered (baclofen for spasms; bethanechol chloride for hypotonic bladder).
- Discuss the use of a percutaneous stimulator if one is being contemplated. Teach self-catheterization, if indicated for neurogenic bladder.

Precautions

- Retrograde cystography is contraindicated during exacerbation of an acute UTI or in the patient with an obstruction that prevents passage of a urinary catheter.
- This test shouldn't be performed in the patient with urethral evulsion or transection, unless catheter passage and flow of contrast medium are monitored fluoroscopically.

Normal findings

Retrograde cystography shows a bladder with normal contours, capacity, integrity, and urethrovesical angle and with no evidence of a tumor, diverticula, or a rupture. Vesicoureteral reflux should be absent. The bladder shouldn't be displaced or externally compressed; the bladder wall should be smooth, not thick.

Abnormal findings

Retrograde cystography can identify vesical trabeculae or diverticula, space-occupying lesions (tumors), calculi or gravel, blood clots, high- or low-pressure vesicoureteral reflux, and a hypotonic or hypertonic bladder.

Interfering factors

- Gas, stool, or residual barium from recent diagnostic tests in the bowel (possible poor imaging)

Retrograde ureteropyelography

Retrograde ureteropyelography allows radiographic examination of the renal collecting system after injection of a contrast medium through a ureteral catheter during cystoscopy. The contrast medium is usually iodine-based and although some of it may be absorbed through the mucous membranes, this test is preferred for the patient with hypersensitivity to iodine (in whom I.V. administration of an iodine-based contrast medium, as in excretory urography, is contraindicated). This test is also indicated when visualization of the renal collecting system by excretory urography is inadequate due to inferior films or marked renal insufficiency because retrograde ureteropyelography isn't influenced by impaired renal function.

Purpose

- To assess the structure and integrity of the renal collecting system (calyces, renal pelvis, and ureter) (See *Sites and types of obstruction indicated by ureteropyelography.*)

Patient preparation

- Explain to the patient that retrograde ureteropyelography permits visualization of the urinary collecting system.
- If a general anesthetic is to be used, instruct the patient to fast for 8 hours be-

SITES AND TYPES OF OBSTRUCTION INDICATED BY URETEROPYELOGRAPHY

Ureteropyelography may detect a stricture, neoplasm, blood clot, or calculus that obstructs urine flow in the calyces, pelvis, or ureter. Small calculi may remain in the calyces and pelvis or pass down the ureter. A staghorn calculus (a cast of the calyceal and pelvic collecting system) may form from a calculus that stays in the kidney.

Staghorn calculus

Blood clot (due to hemangioma)

Neoplasm

Calculus

Stricture

fore the test. Generally, he should be well hydrated to ensure adequate urine flow.
■ Tell the patient who will perform the test and where it will take place.
■ Inform the patient that he'll be positioned on an examination table, with his legs in stirrups, and that the position may be tiring.
■ If the patient will be awake throughout the procedure, tell him that he may feel pressure as the instrument is passed and a pressure sensation in the kidney area when the contrast medium is introduced. Also, he may feel an urgency to void.
■ Make sure that the patient or a responsible family member has signed an informed consent form.
■ Administer prescribed premedication just before the procedure.

Equipment

Cystoscopy setup, ureteral catheters, 10-ml syringes with ureteral adapters, contrast medium, radiographic equipment, tilt table with stirrups

Procedure and posttest care

■ Place the patient in the lithotomy position. Care must be taken to avoid pressure points or impairment to circulation while his legs are in the stirrups.

■ After the patient is anesthetized, the urologist first performs a cystoscopic examination.

■ After visual inspection of the bladder, one or both ureters are catheterized with opaque catheters, depending on the condition or abnormality suspected. Radiographic monitoring allows correct positioning of the catheter tip in the renal pelvis.

■ The renal pelvis is emptied by gravity drainage or aspiration. About 5 ml of contrast medium is then slowly injected through the catheter using the syringe with the special adapter.

■ When adequate filling and opacification have occurred, anteroposterior radiographic films are taken and immediately developed. Lateral and oblique films can be taken, as needed, after the injection of more contrast medium.

■ After the radiographs of the renal pelvis are examined, a few more milliliters of contrast medium are injected to outline the ureters as the catheter is slowly withdrawn.

■ Delayed films (10 to 15 minutes after complete catheter removal) are then taken to check for contrast medium retention, indicating urinary stasis.

■ If ureteral obstruction is present, the ureteral catheter may be kept in place and, together with an indwelling urinary catheter, connected to a gravity drainage system until posttest urinary flow is corrected or returns to normal.

■ Check the patient's vital signs every 15 minutes for the first hour, every 30 minutes for 1 hour, every hour for the next 2 hours, and then every 4 hours for 24 hours.

■ Monitor the patient's fluid intake and urine output for 24 hours. Observe each specimen for hematuria. Gross hematuria or hematuria after the third voiding is abnormal and should be reported. If the patient doesn't void for 8 hours after the procedure or if the patient immediately feels distress and his bladder is distended, urethral catheterization may be necessary.

■ Be especially attentive to catheter output if ureteral catheters have been left in place because inadequate output may reflect catheter obstruction, requiring irrigation. Protect ureteral catheters from dislodgment. Note output amounts for each catheter (indwelling, urinary, urethral) separately; this helps determine the location of an obstruction that's causing reduced output.

■ Administer prescribed analgesics, tub baths, and increased fluid intake for dysuria, which commonly occurs after retrograde ureteropyelography.

▶ **CLINICAL ALERT** *Watch for and report severe pain in the area of the kidneys as well as any signs of sepsis (such as chills, fever, and hypotension). If irrigation is ordered, never use more than 10 ml of sterile saline solution.*

Precautions

■ Retrograde ureteropyelography must be done carefully in the patient with urinary stasis caused by ureteral obstruction to prevent further injury to the ureter.

■ This test is contraindicated in the pregnant patient unless the benefits of the procedure outweigh the risks to the fetus.

Normal findings

Following a normal cystoscopic examination, ureteral catheterization, and injection of contrast medium through the catheters, opacification of the pelves and calyces should occur immediately. Normal structures should be outlined clearly and should appear symmetrical in bilateral testing. Ureters should fill uniformly and appear normal in size and course. Inspiratory and expiratory exposures, when superimposed, normally create two outlines of the renal pelvis ¾″ (2 cm) apart.

Abnormal findings

Incomplete or delayed drainage reflects an obstruction, most commonly at the ureteropelvic junction. Enlargement of the components of the collecting system or delayed emptying of contrast medium may indicate obstruction due to a tumor, a blood clot, a stricture, or calculi.

Perinephric inflammation or suppuration commonly causes fixation of the kidney on the same side, resulting in a single sharp radiographic outline of the collecting system when inspiratory and expiratory exposures are superimposed. Upward, downward, or lateral renal displacement can result from a renal abscess or tumor or from a perinephric abscess. Neoplasms can cause displacement of either pole or of the entire kidney.

Interfering factors

■ Previous contrast studies or presence of stool or gas in the bowel (possible poor imaging)

Antegrade pyelography

Antegrade pyelography allows examination of the upper collecting system when ureteral obstruction rules out retrograde ureteropyelography or when cystoscopy is contraindicated. It depends on percutaneous needle puncture for injection of contrast medium into the renal pelvis or calyces.

Renal pressure can be measured during this procedure. Also, urine can be collected for cultures and cytologic studies and for evaluation of renal functional reserve before surgery.

After completing radiographic studies, a nephrostomy tube can be inserted to provide temporary drainage or access for other therapeutic or diagnostic procedures.

Purpose

■ To evaluate obstruction of the upper collecting system by stricture, calculus, clot, or tumor
■ To evaluate hydronephrosis revealed during excretory urography or ultrasonography and to enable placement of a percutaneous nephrostomy tube
■ To evaluate the function of the upper collecting system after ureteral surgery or urinary diversion
■ To assess renal functional reserve before surgery

Patient preparation

■ Explain to the patient that antegrade pyelography allows radiographic examination of the kidney.
■ Tell the patient that he may be required to fast for 6 to 8 hours before the test.
■ Tell the patient that he may receive antimicrobial drugs before and after the procedure.
■ Tell the patient who will perform the test and where it will take place.
■ Explain to the patient that a needle will be inserted into the kidney after he's given a sedative and local anesthetic. Explain that urine may be collected from the kidney for testing and that, if necessary, a

tube will be left in the kidney for drainage.

■ Tell the patient that he may feel mild discomfort during injection of the local anesthetic and contrast medium and that he may also feel transient burning and flushing from the contrast medium.

■ Warn the patient that the X-ray machine makes loud, clacking sounds as films are taken.

■ Check the patient's history for hypersensitivity reactions to contrast media, iodine, or shellfish. Mark any sensitivities clearly on the chart. Also check his history and recent coagulation studies for indications of bleeding disorders.

■ Make sure that the patient or a responsible family member has signed an informed consent form.

■ Administer a sedative just before the procedure, if needed, and check that pretest blood work, such as kidney function, has been performed, if ordered.

Equipment

Radiographic equipment, including a fluoroscope and, possibly, ultrasound equipment; percutaneous nephrostomy tray; manometer; preparatory tray; gloves and sterile containers for specimens; syringes and needles; contrast medium; local anesthetic; emergency resuscitation equipment

Procedure and posttest care

■ The patient is placed in a prone position on the X-ray table. The skin over the kidney is cleaned with antiseptic solution, and a local anesthetic is injected.

■ Previous urographic films or ultrasound recordings are studied for anatomic landmarks. (It's important to determine if the kidney to be studied is in the normal position. If not, the angle of the needle entry must be adjusted during percutaneous puncture.)

■ Under guidance of fluoroscopy or ultrasonography, the percutaneous needle is inserted below the 12th rib at the level of the transverse process of the 2nd lumbar vertebra. Aspiration of urine confirms that the needle has reached the dilated collecting system, which is usually $2\frac{3}{4}''$ to $3\frac{1}{8}''$ (7 to 8 cm) below the skin surface in adults.

■ Flexible tubing is connected to the needle to prevent displacement during the procedure. If intrarenal pressure is to be measured, the manometer is connected to the tubing as soon as it's in place. Urine specimens are then taken, if needed.

■ An amount of urine equal to the amount of contrast medium to be injected is withdrawn to prevent overdistention of the collecting system.

■ The contrast medium is injected under fluoroscopic guidance. Posteroanterior, oblique, and anteroposterior radiographs are taken. Ureteral peristalsis is observed on the fluoroscope screen to evaluate obstruction.

■ A percutaneous nephrostomy tube is inserted if drainage is needed because of increased renal pressure, dilation, or intrarenal reflux. If drainage isn't needed, the catheter is withdrawn and a sterile dressing is applied.

■ Check the patient's vital signs every 15 minutes for the first hour, every 30 minutes for the second hour, and then every 2 hours for the next 24 hours.

■ Check dressings for bleeding, hematoma, or urine leakage at the puncture site at each vital signs check. For bleeding, apply pressure. For a hematoma, apply warm soaks. Report urine leakage or the patient's failure to void within 8 hours.

■ Monitor the patient's fluid intake and urine output for 24 hours. Observe each specimen for hematuria. Report hematuria if it persists after the third voiding.

■ Watch for and report signs of sepsis or extravasation of contrast medium (chills, fever, rapid pulse or respirations, and hypotension).

🔴 **CLINICAL ALERT** *Also watch for and report signs that adjacent organs have been punctured, such as pain in the abdomen or flank, or pneumothorax (sudden onset of pleuritic chest pain, dyspnea, tachypnea, decreased breath sounds on the affected side, and tachycardia).*

■ If a nephrostomy tube is inserted, check to make sure it's patent and draining well. Irrigate with 5 to 7 ml of sterile saline solution, as ordered, to maintain patency.

■ Administer prescribed antibiotics for several days after the procedure and prescribed analgesics.

■ If hydronephrosis is present, monitor intake and output, edema, hypertension, flank pain, acid-base status, and glucose level.

Precautions

■ Antegrade pyelography is contraindicated in the patient with bleeding disorders.

■ Watch for signs of hypersensitivity to the contrast medium.

■ This procedure is contraindicated in the pregnant patient unless the benefits outweigh the risks to the fetus.

Normal findings

After injection of contrast medium, the upper collecting system should fill uniformly and appear normal in size and course. Normal structures should be outlined clearly.

Abnormal findings

Enlargements of the upper collecting system and parts of the ureteropelvic junction indicate obstruction. Antegrade pyelography shows the degree of dilation, clearly defines obstructions, and demonstrates intrarenal reflux. In hydronephrosis, the ureteropelvic junction shows marked distention. Results of recent surgery or urinary diversion will be obvious; for example, a ureteral stent or a dilated stenotic area will be clearly visualized.

Intrarenal pressure greater than 20 cm H_2O indicates obstruction. Cultures or cytologic studies of urine specimens taken during antegrade pyelography can confirm antegrade pyelonephrosis or malignancy.

Interfering factors

■ Recent barium procedures or stool or gas in the bowel (possible poor imaging)

■ An obese patient (possible difficulty in needle placement)

Magnetic resonance imaging of the urinary tract

Magnetic resonance imaging (MRI) is becoming more commonly used for diagnosing urinary tract disorders. It's unclear at present whether MRI is better than computed tomography or ultrasound for imaging the urinary system. In most cases, MRI is used when these alternative tests fail to produce a clear image. MRI uses radio-frequency waves and magnetic fields to visualize specific structures (kidney or prostate), which are then converted to computer-generated images.

Purpose

- To evaluate genitourinary tumors and abdominal or pelvic masses
- To detect prostate stones and cysts
- To detect cancer invasion into seminal vesicles and pelvic lymph nodes

Patient preparation

- Explain to the patient that MRI of the urinary tract helps evaluate abnormalities in the urinary system.
- Advise the patient to avoid alcohol, caffeine-containing beverages, and smoking for at least 2 hours and food for at least 1 hour before the test.
- Tell the patient who will perform the test, where it will take place, and that it takes about 30 to 90 minutes.
- Explain to the patient that he can continue taking medications, except for iron, which interferes with the imaging.
- Before the test, tell the patient that he'll need to remove all clothing, jewelry, and metallic objects and wear a special hospital gown without snaps or closures.
- Inform the patient that he won't feel pain, but may feel claustrophobic while lying supine in the tubular MRI chamber. If so, the physician may order an antianxiety medication.
- Tell the patient that he'll hear loud, crushing noises throughout the test. However, he'll probably receive a headset with a choice of music to decrease the loud noise.
- If contrast media will be used, obtain a history of allergies or hypersensitivity to these agents. Mark any sensitivities on the chart and notify the physician.
- Ask the patient if he has any implanted metal devices or prostheses, such as vascular clips, shrapnel, pacemakers, joint implants, filters, and intrauterine devices. If so, he may not be able to have the test.

- Make sure that the patient or a responsible family member has signed an informed consent form.
- Just before the procedure, have the patient urinate.

Equipment

MRI machine (which contains a circular magnet and a radio-frequency coil), headset with music

Procedure and posttest care

- If a contrast medium is used, start an I.V. line so that the medium is administered before the procedure.
- The patient is placed in the supine position on a narrow, flat table, and the table is then moved into the enclosed cylindrical scanner.
- Varying radio-frequency waves are directed at the area being scanned.
- The patient is told to lie very still in the scanner while the images are being produced.
- Although his face remains uncovered to allow him to see out, the patient is advised to keep his eyes closed to promote relaxation and prevent a closed-in feeling.
- If nausea occurs because of claustrophobia, the patient is encouraged to take deep breaths.
- If sedatives were given, monitor the patient's vital signs until he's awake and responsive.
- Advise the patient that he may resume his usual diet, fluids, and medications, as ordered.
- Monitor the patient for adverse reactions to the contrast medium (flushing, nausea, urticaria, and sneezing).
- Watch the I.V. site for a hematoma, if applicable. If a hematoma occurs, apply warm soaks.

Precautions

- This test is contraindicated in the patient with metal implants, rods, or screws or prosthetic devices.
- This test is contraindicated in the pregnant patient unless its benefits greatly outweigh the possible risks to the fetus.
- The scanner can't be used with an extremely obese patient.
- All metal objects, such as jewelry, hairpins, and dentures, are removed before the test.

Normal findings

In visualizing the soft-tissue structures of the kidneys, MRI can determine blood vessel size and anatomy. However, this test hasn't proved useful for detecting calculi or calcified tumors.

Abnormal findings

MRI can reveal tumors, strictures, stenosis, thrombosis, malformations, abscess, inflammation, edema, fluid collection, bleeding, hemorrhage, and organ atrophy.

Interfering factors

- Uncooperative behavior, unstable medical conditions (confusion, combativeness), or inability to remain still during the procedure
- Use of I.V. pumps or assistive life-support equipment

STRUCTURAL AND FUNCTIONAL TESTS

Excretory urography

The cornerstone of a urologic workup, excretory urography (also called I.V. pyelography) requires I.V. administration of a contrast medium and allows visualization of the renal parenchyma, calyces, and pelvis as well as the ureters, bladder and, in some cases, the urethra.

In some facilities, a nonenhanced computed tomography scan of the urinary tract is commonly performed instead of this test if urinary tract stones are suspected.

Purpose

- To evaluate the structure and excretory function of the kidneys, ureters, and bladder
- To support a suspected differential diagnosis of renovascular hypertension

Patient preparation

- Explain to the patient that excretory urography helps to evaluate the structure and function of the urinary tract.
- Make sure that the patient is well hydrated; then instruct him to fast for 8 hours before the test. Tell him who will perform the test and where it will take place. Obtain blood urea nitrogen (BUN) and creatinine levels, as ordered.
- Inform the patient that he may experience a transient burning sensation and metallic taste when the contrast medium is injected. Tell him to report other sensations he may experience.
- Warn the patient that the X-ray machine may make loud, clacking sounds during the test.
- Make sure that the patient or a responsible family member has signed an informed consent form.
- Check the patient's history for hypersensitivity to iodine, iodine-containing foods, or contrast media containing iodine. Mark sensitivities on the chart and notify the physician.
- Administer a laxative, if necessary, the night before the test, to minimize poor

resolution of X-ray films due to stool and gas in the GI tract.

Equipment

Contrast medium (sodium diatrizoate or iothalamate, or meglumine diatrizoate or iothalamate); 50-ml syringe (or I.V. container and tubing); 19G to 21G needle, catheter, or butterfly needle; venipuncture equipment (tourniquet, antiseptic, adhesive bandage); X-ray table; X-ray and tomographic equipment; emergency resuscitation equipment

Procedure and posttest care

- The patient is placed in a supine position on the X-ray table.
- A kidney-ureter-bladder radiograph is exposed, developed, and studied for gross abnormalities of the urinary system. Contrast medium is injected (dosage varies according to age), and the patient is observed for signs of hypersensitivity (flushing, nausea, vomiting, hives, or dyspnea).
- The first radiograph, visualizing the renal parenchyma, is obtained about 1 minute after the injection, possibly supplemented by tomography if small space-occupying masses, such as cysts or tumors, are suspected.
- Films are then exposed at regular intervals — usually 5, 10, and 15 or 20 minutes after the injection.
- Ureteral compression is performed after the 5-minute film is exposed. This can be accomplished through inflation of two small rubber bladders placed on the abdomen on both sides of the midline, secured by a fastener wrapped around the patient's torso. The inflated bladders occlude the ureters without causing the patient discomfort and facilitate retention of the contrast medium by the upper urinary tract. (Ureteral compression is contraindicated by ureteral calculi, aortic aneurysm, pregnancy, or recent abdominal trauma or surgical procedure.)
- After the 10-minute film is exposed, ureteral compression is released. As the contrast flows into the lower urinary tract, another film is taken of the lower halves of both ureters and then, finally, one is taken of the bladder.
- At the end of the procedure, the patient voids, and another film is made immediately to visualize residual bladder content or mucosal abnormalities of the bladder or urethra.
- If a hematoma develops at the injection site, apply warm soaks.
- Observe the patient for delayed reactions to the contrast medium.
- Continue I.V. fluids or provide oral fluid to increase hydration. Administer medications, as ordered.

Precautions

- Premedication with corticosteroids may be indicated for the patient with severe asthma or a history of sensitivity to the contrast medium.
- This test may be contraindicated in the patient with abnormal renal function (as evidenced by increased creatinine and BUN levels) and in a child or an elderly patient with actual or potential dehydration.

Normal findings

The kidneys, ureters, and bladder show no gross evidence of soft- or hard-tissue lesions. Prompt visualization of the contrast medium in the kidneys demonstrates bilateral renal parenchyma and pelvicalyceal systems of normal conformity. The ureters and bladder should be outlined, and the postvoiding radiograph should show no mucosal abnormalities and minimal residual urine.

Abnormal findings

Excretory urography can demonstrate many abnormalities of the urinary system, including renal or ureteral calculi; abnormal size, shape, or structure of kidneys, ureters, or bladder; a supernumerary or an absent kidney; polycystic kidney disease associated with renal hypertrophy; a redundant pelvis or ureter; a space-occupying lesion; pyelonephrosis; renal tuberculosis; hydronephrosis; and renovascular hypertension.

Interfering factors

■ End-stage renal disease or stool or gas in the colon (possible poor imaging)
■ Insufficient injection of contrast medium, a recent barium enema, or GI or gallbladder series (possible poor imaging)

Radionuclide renal imaging

Radionuclide renal imaging, which involves I.V. injection of a radionuclide followed by scintigraphy, provides a wealth of information for evaluating the kidneys. Observing the uptake concentration and transit of the radionuclide during this test allows assessment of renal blood flow, renal structure, and nephron and collecting system function. Depending on the patient's clinical presentation, this procedure may include dynamic scans to assess renal perfusion and function or static scans to assess structure.

The radioisotope injected depends on the specific information required and the examiner's preference. However, this procedure commonly includes double isotope technique to obtain a sequence of perfusion and function studies, followed by static images. This test may also be substituted for excretory urography in the patient with hypersensitivity to contrast agents.

Purpose

■ To detect and assess functional and structural renal abnormalities (such as lesions and renovascular hypertension) and acute or chronic disease (such as pyelonephritis or glomerulonephritis)
■ To assess renal transplantation or renal injury due to trauma to the urinary tract or obstruction

Patient preparation

■ Explain to the patient that radionuclide renal imaging permits the evaluation of the structure, blood flow, and function of the kidneys.
■ Tell the patient who will perform the test and where. (If static scans are ordered, there will be a delay of several hours before the images are taken.)
■ Inform the patient that he'll receive an injection of a radionuclide and that he may experience transient flushing and nausea.
■ Emphasize to the patient that only a small amount of radionuclide is administered and that it's usually excreted within 24 hours.
■ Tell the patient several series of films will be taken of his bladder.
■ Make sure that the patient or a responsible family member has signed an informed consent form.
■ Make sure that the patient isn't scheduled for other radionuclide scans on the same day as this test.
■ If the patient receives antihypertensive medication, ask the physician if it should be withheld before the test.
■ A pregnant patient or a young child may receive supersaturated solution of potassium iodide 1 to 3 hours before the test to block thyroid uptake of iodine.

Equipment

Computerized gamma scintillation camera, technetium 99m (^{99m}Tc) for perfusion study, iodohippurate sodium I 131 (Hippuran) for function study, oscilloscope, magnetic tape, I.V. equipment

Procedure and posttest care

■ The patient is commonly placed in a prone position so that posterior views may be obtained. If the test is being performed to evaluate transplantation, the patient is positioned supine for anterior views.

■ Instruct the patient not to change his position.

■ A perfusion study (radionuclide angiography) is performed first to evaluate renal blood flow. The ^{99m}Tc is administered intravenously, and rapid-sequence photographs (one per second) are taken for 1 minute.

■ Next, a function study is performed to measure the transit time of the radionuclide through the kidneys' functional units. After Hippuran is administered intravenously, images are obtained at a rate of one per minute for 20 minutes. Alternatively, this entire procedure can be recorded on computer-compatible magnetic tape, and concurrent renogram curves can be plotted.

■ Finally, static images are obtained 4 or more hours later, after the radionuclide has drained through the pelvicaliceal system.

■ Instruct the patient to flush the toilet immediately after each voiding for 24 hours as a radiation precaution.

■ If the patient is incontinent, change bed linens promptly and wear gloves to maintain standard precautions and prevent unnecessary skin contact.

■ Monitor the infection site for signs of hematoma, infection, and discomfort. Apply warm compresses for comfort.

■ Monitor the patient's intake and output and electrolyte, acid-base, blood urea nitrogen, and creatinine levels, as indicated.

Precautions

■ This test is contraindicated in a pregnant woman unless the benefits to the mother outweigh the risk to the fetus.

Normal findings

Because 25% of cardiac output goes directly to the kidneys, renal perfusion should be evident immediately following uptake of the ^{99m}Tc in the abdominal aorta. Within 1 to 2 minutes, a normal pattern of renal circulation should appear. The radionuclide should delineate the kidneys simultaneously, symmetrically, and with equal intensity.

Hippuran administered for the function study rapidly outlines the kidneys — which should be normal in size, shape, and position — and also defines the collecting system and bladder. Maximum counts of the radionuclide in the kidneys occur within 5 minutes after injection (and within 1 minute of each other) and should fall to approximately one-third or less of the maximum counts in the same kidney within 25 minutes. Within this time, kidney function can be compared as the concentration of radionuclide shifts from the cortex to the pelvis and, finally, to the bladder.

Renal function is best evaluated by comparing these images with the renogram curves. Total function is considered normal when the effective renal plasma flow is 420 ml/minute or greater and the percentage of the dose excreted in the urine at 30 to 35 minutes is greater than 66%.

Abnormal findings

Images from the perfusion study can identify impeded renal circulation, such as that caused by trauma and renal artery stenosis or renal infarction. These conditions may occur in the patient with renovascular hypertension or abdominal aortic disease. Because malignant renal tumors are usually vascular, these images can help differentiate tumors from cysts.

In evaluating a kidney transplant, abnormal perfusion may indicate obstruction of the vascular grafts. The function study can detect abnormalities of the collecting system and urine extravasation. Markedly decreased tubular function causes reduced radionuclide activity in the collecting system; outflow obstruction causes decreased radionuclide activity in the tubules, with increased activity in the collecting system. This test can also define the level of ureteral obstruction.

Static images can demonstrate lesions, congenital abnormalities, and traumatic injury. These images also detect space-occupying lesions within or surrounding the kidney, such as tumors, infarcts, and inflammatory masses (abscesses, for example); they can also identify congenital disorders, such as horseshoe kidney and polycystic kidney disease. They can define regions of infarction, rupture, or hemorrhage after trauma.

A lower-than-normal total concentration of the radionuclide, as opposed to focal defects, suggests a diffuse renal disorder, such as acute tubular necrosis, severe infection, or ischemia. In a patient who has had a kidney transplant, decreased radionuclide uptake generally indicates organ rejection. Failure of visual-ization may indicate congenital ectopia or aplasia.

Definitive diagnosis usually requires the combined analysis of static images, perfusion studies, and function studies.

Interfering factors

- Antihypertensives (possible masking of abnormalities)
- Scans of different organs performed on the same day (possible poor imaging)

Renal angiography

Renal angiography requires arterial injection of a contrast medium and permits radiographic examination of the renal vasculature and parenchyma. As the contrast pervades the renal vasculature, rapid-sequence radiographs show the vessels during three phases of filling: arterial, nephrographic, and venous.

This procedure usually follows standard bolus aortography, which shows individual variations in number, size, and condition of the main renal arteries, aberrant vessels, and the relationship of the renal arteries to the aorta.

Purpose

- To demonstrate the configuration of total renal vasculature before surgical procedures
- To determine the cause of renovascular hypertension, such as from stenosis, thrombotic occlusions, emboli, and aneurysms
- To evaluate chronic renal disease or renal failure
- To investigate renal masses and renal trauma
- To detect complications following kidney transplantation, such as a nonfunctioning shunt or rejection of the donor organ

■ To differentiate highly vascular tumors from avascular cysts

Patient preparation

■ Explain to the patient that renal angiography permits visualization of the kidneys, blood vessels, and functional units and aids in diagnosing renal disease or masses.

■ Instruct the patient to fast for 8 hours before the test and to drink extra fluids the day before the test and the day after the test to maintain adequate hydration (or to start an I.V. line, if needed). Oral medication may be continued; a special order is needed for the patient with diabetes.

■ Tell the patient he may receive a laxative or an enema the evening before the test.

■ Tell the patient who will perform the test and where it will take place.

■ Describe the procedure to the patient and inform him that he may experience transient discomfort (flushing, burning sensation, and nausea) during injection of the contrast medium.

■ Make sure that the patient or a responsible family member has signed an informed consent form.

▶ **CLINICAL ALERT** *Check the patient's history for hypersensitivity to iodine-based contrast media or iodine-containing foods such as shellfish. Mark sensitivities on the chart and inform the physician because the patient may require prophylactic antiallergenics (diphenhydramine or corticosteroids).*

■ Administer prescribed medications (usually a sedative and a narcotic analgesic) before the test.

■ Instruct the patient to put on a gown and to remove all metallic objects that may interfere with test results.

■ Ask the patient to void before leaving the unit.

■ Record the patient's baseline vital signs. Ensure that recent laboratory test results (blood urea nitrogen and serum creatinine levels and bleeding studies) are documented on the patient's chart. Verification of adequate renal function and adequate clotting ability is vital.

■ Evaluate peripheral pulse sites and mark them for easy access in postprocedure assessment.

Equipment

Image-intensified fluoroscope with television monitor, high-powered radiographic equipment, pressure-injection device, rapid cassette changer, polyethylene radiopaque vascular catheters, guide wire, contrast material (such as diatrizoate), preparation tray with 70% alcohol or povidone-iodine solution, emergency resuscitation equipment

Procedure and posttest care

■ The patient is placed in a supine position, and a peripheral I.V. infusion is started. The skin over the arterial puncture site is cleaned with antiseptic solution, and a local anesthetic is injected.

■ The femoral artery is punctured and, under fluoroscopic visualization, cannulated. (If a femoral pulse is absent or the artery is convoluted or plaque-ridden, percutaneous transaxillary, transbrachial, or translumbar catheterization may be performed instead.)

■ After passing the flexible guide wire through the artery, the cannula is withdrawn, leaving several inches of wire in the lumen.

■ A polyethylene catheter is passed over the wire and advanced, under fluoroscopic guidance, up the femoroiliac vessels to the aorta. The guide wire is removed, and the catheter is flushed with heparin flush solution.

■ The contrast medium is injected, and screening aortograms are taken before proceeding.

■ On completion of the aortographic study, a renal catheter is exchanged for the vascular catheter.

■ To determine the position of the renal arteries and ensure that the tip of the catheter is in the lumen, a test bolus (3 to 5 ml) of contrast medium is injected immediately.

■ If the patient has no adverse reaction to the contrast medium, 20 to 25 ml of the substance is injected just below the origin of the renal arteries.

■ A series of rapid-sequence X-ray films of the filling of the renal vascular tree is exposed.

■ If additional selective studies are required, the catheter remains in place while the films are examined. If the films are satisfactory, the catheter is removed.

■ Apply a sterile pad firmly to the puncture site for 15 minutes.

■ Before the patient is returned to his room, observe the puncture site for a hematoma.

■ Keep the patient flat in bed and instruct him to keep the punctured leg straight for at least 6 hours or as otherwise ordered.

■ Check the patient's vital signs every 15 minutes for 1 hour, every 30 minutes for 2 hours, and then every hour until they stabilize.

■ Monitor popliteal and dorsalis pedis pulses for adequate perfusion at least every hour for 4 hours. Note the color and temperature of the involved extremity and compare with the uninvolved extremity. Watch for signs of pain or paresthesia in the involved limb.

■ Watch for bleeding or hematomas at the injection site. Keep the pressure dressing in place and check for bleeding when you check the patient's vital signs. If bleeding occurs, promptly notify the physician and apply direct pressure or a sandbag to the site.

■ Apply cold compresses to the puncture site to reduce edema and lessen pain.

▶ **CLINICAL ALERT** *Provide extra fluids (2,000 to 3,000 ml) in the 24-hour period after the test to prevent nephrotoxicity from the contrast medium. Also monitor the patient for anaphylaxis from the contrast medium. (Signs include cardiorespiratory distress, renal failure, and shock.)*

■ Monitor the patient for atrial arrhythmias and evaluate aspartate aminotransferase and lactate dehydrogenase activity if renal stenosis is observed.

Precautions

■ Renal angiography is contraindicated during pregnancy and in the patient with bleeding tendencies, allergy to contrast media, or renal failure caused by end-stage renal disease.

Normal findings

Renal arteriographs show normal arborization of the vascular tree and normal architecture of the renal parenchyma.

Abnormal findings

Renal tumors usually show hypervascularity; renal cysts typically appear as clearly delineated, radiolucent masses. Renal artery stenosis caused by arteriosclerosis produces a noticeable constriction in the blood vessels, usually within the proximal portion of its length; this is a crucial finding in confirming renovascular hypertension. Renal artery dysplasia, unlike renal artery stenosis, usually affects the middle and distal portions of the vessel. Alternating aneurysms and stenotic regions give this rare disorder a characteristic beads-on-a-string appearance.

In renal infarction, blood vessels may appear to be absent or cut off, with the normal tissue replaced by scar tissue. Another typical finding is the appearance of triangular areas of infarcted tissue near the periphery of the affected kidney. The kidney itself may appear shrunken due to tissue scarring.

Renal angiography may also detect renal artery aneurysms (saccular or fusiform) and renal arteriovenous fistula with abnormal widening of and direct passage between the renal artery and renal vein. Destruction, distortion, and fibrosis of renal tissue with areas of reduced and tortuous vascularity may be noted in severe or chronic pyelonephritis, and an increase in capsular vessels with abnormal intrarenal circulation may indicate renal abscesses or inflammatory masses.

When angiography is used to evaluate renal trauma, it may detect an intrarenal hematoma, a parenchymal laceration, shattered kidneys, and areas of infarction. Renal angiography may also be useful in distinguishing pseudotumors from tumors or cysts, in evaluating the volume of residual functioning renal tissue in hydronephrosis, and in evaluating donors and recipients before and after renal transplantation.

Interfering factors
■ Patient movement
■ Recent contrast studies, such as barium enema or an upper GI series (possible poor imaging)
■ Presence of stool or gas in the GI tract (possible poor imaging)

Renal venography

Renal venography is a relatively simple procedure allowing radiographic examination of the main renal veins and their tributaries. In this test, contrast medium is injected by percutaneous catheter passed through the femoral vein and inferior vena cava into the renal vein. Indications for renal venography include renal vein thrombosis, a tumor, and venous anomalies.

Purpose
■ To detect renal vein thrombosis
■ To evaluate renal vein compression due to extrinsic tumors or retroperitoneal fibrosis
■ To assess renal tumors and detect invasion of the renal vein or inferior vena cava
■ To detect venous anomalies and defects
■ To differentiate renal agenesis from a small kidney
■ To collect renal venous blood samples for evaluation of renovascular hypertension

Patient preparation
■ Explain to the patient that renal venography permits radiographic study of the renal veins.
■ If prescribed, instruct the patient to fast for 4 hours before the test.
■ Tell the patient who will perform the test and where it will take place.
■ Inform the patient that a catheter will be inserted into a vein in the groin area after he's given a sedative and a local anesthetic.
■ Tell the patient that he may feel mild discomfort during injection of the local anesthetic and contrast medium and that he may also feel transient burning and flushing from the contrast medium.

- Warn the patient that the X-ray equipment may make loud, clacking noises as the films are taken.

⏵ **CLINICAL ALERT** *Check the patient's history for hypersensitivity to contrast media, iodine, or iodine-containing foods such as shellfish. Mark sensitivities on the chart and report them to the physician.*

- Check the patient's history and any coagulation studies for indications of bleeding disorders.

- If renin assays will be done, check the patient's diet and medications and consult with the health care team. As ordered, restrict the patient's salt intake and discontinue antihypertensive drugs, diuretics, estrogen, and hormonal contraceptives.

- Make sure that the patient or a responsible family member has signed an informed consent form.

- Administer a sedative, if necessary, just before the procedure.

- Record the patient's baseline vital signs. Make sure pretest blood urea nitrogen and urine creatinine levels are adequate because the kidneys clear contrast media.

Equipment

Radiographic equipment, renal venography tray with flexible guide wires, polyethylene radiopaque vascular catheters, needle and cannula or 18G needle, three-way stopcock, and flexible tubing; preparatory tray; syringes and needles; contrast medium; local anesthetic; emergency resuscitation equipment

Procedure and posttest care

- The patient is placed in a supine position on the X-ray table, with his abdomen centered over the film. The skin over the right femoral vein near the groin is cleaned with antiseptic solution and

draped. (The left femoral vein or jugular veins may be used.)

- A local anesthetic is injected and the femoral vein is cannulated.

- Under fluoroscopic guidance, a guide wire is threaded a short distance through the cannula, which is then removed. A catheter is passed over the wire into the inferior vena cava.

- When catheterization of the femoral vein is contraindicated, the right antecubital vein is punctured, and the catheter is inserted and advanced through the right atrium of the heart into the inferior vena cava.

- A test bolus of contrast medium is injected to determine that the vena cava is patent. If so, the catheter is advanced into the right renal vein and contrast medium (usually 20 to 40 ml) is injected.

- When studies of the right renal vasculature are completed, the catheter is withdrawn into the vena cava, rotated, and guided into the left renal vein.

- If visualization of the renal venous tributaries is indicated, epinephrine can be injected into the ipsilateral renal artery by catheter before contrast medium is injected into the renal vein. Epinephrine temporarily blocks arterial flow and allows filling of distal intrarenal veins. Obstructing the artery briefly with a balloon catheter produces the same effect.

- After anteroposterior films are made, the patient lies prone for posteroanterior films.

- For renin assays, blood samples are withdrawn under fluoroscopy within 15 minutes after venography. After catheter removal, apply pressure to the site for 15 minutes and put on a dressing.

- Check the patient's vital signs and distal pulses every 15 minutes for the first hour, every 30 minutes for the second hour, and then every 2 hours for 24 hours. Keep the patient on bed rest for 2 hours.

■ Observe the puncture site for bleeding or a hematoma when checking the patient's vital signs; if bleeding occurs, apply pressure. Report bleeding as soon as possible.

⬤ **CLINICAL ALERT** *Report signs of vein perforation, embolism, and extravasation of contrast medium. These include chills, fever, rapid pulse and respiration, hypotension, dyspnea, and chest, abdominal, or flank pain. Also report complaints of paresthesia or pain in the catheterized limb—symptoms of nerve irritation or vascular compromise.*

■ Administer prescribed sedatives and antimicrobials.

■ Prepare for further arteriography or surgery, as ordered.

■ As ordered, instruct the patient that he may resume his usual diet and medications.

■ Instruct the patient to increase fluid intake (unless contraindicated) to help clear contrast media.

Precautions

■ Renal venography is contraindicated in severe thrombosis of the inferior vena cava.

■ The guide wire and catheter should be advanced carefully if severe renal vein thrombosis is suspected.

■ Watch the patient for signs of hypersensitivity to the contrast medium.

Normal findings

After injection of the contrast medium, opacification of the renal vein and tributaries should occur immediately. Normal renin content of venous blood in an adult in a supine position is 1.5 to 1.6 ng/ml/hour.

Abnormal findings

Renal vein occlusion near the inferior vena cava or the kidney indicates renal vein thrombosis. If the clot is outlined by contrast medium, it may look like a filling defect. However, a clot can usually be identified because it's within the lumen and less sharply outlined than a filling defect. Collateral venous channels, which opacify with retrograde filling during contrast injection, commonly surround the occlusion. Complete occlusion prolongs transit of the contrast medium through the renal veins.

A filling defect of the renal vein may indicate obstruction or compression by an extrinsic tumor or retroperitoneal fibrosis. A renal tumor that invades the renal vein or inferior vena cava usually produces a filling defect with a sharply defined border.

Venous anomalies are indicated by opacification of abnormally positioned or clustered vessels. Absence of a renal vein differentiates renal agenesis from a small kidney.

Elevated renin content in renal venous blood usually indicates essential renovascular hypertension when assay results correspond for both kidneys. Elevated renin levels in one kidney indicate a unilateral lesion and usually require further evaluation by arteriography.

Interfering factors

■ Recent contrast studies or stool or gas in the bowel

■ Failure to restrict salt, antihypertensive drugs, diuretics, estrogen, and hormonal contraceptives

URODYNAMIC TESTS

Uroflometry

Uroflometry, a simple, noninvasive test, uses a uroflometer to detect and evaluate dysfunctional voiding patterns. The uroflometer, contained in a funnel into which the patient voids, measures flow rate (volume of urine voided per second), continuous flow (time of measurable flow), and intermittent flow (total voiding time, including any interruptions).

Types of uroflometers include rotary disc, electromagnetic, spectrophotometric, and gravimetric systems. The gravimetric system, which weighs urine as it's voided and plots the weight against time, is the simplest to use.

Purpose

■ To evaluate lower urinary tract function

■ To demonstrate bladder outlet obstruction

Patient preparation

■ Explain to the patient that uroflometry evaluates his pattern of urination. Advise him not to urinate for several hours before the test and to increase fluid intake so that he'll have a full bladder and a strong urge to void.

■ Describe the test, including who will perform it and where it will take place.

■ Instruct the patient to remain still while voiding during the test to help ensure accurate results. Assure him that he'll have complete privacy during the test.

■ As ordered, discontinue drugs that may affect bladder and sphincter tone, such as urinary spasmolytics and anticholinergics.

Equipment

Commode chair with funnel containing a uroflometer, beaker to hold urine, transducer, start and flow cables, data recording module

Procedure and posttest care

■ Check cable connections before the test.

■ Remind the patient not to strain while voiding.

■ Ask the male patient to void while standing and the female patient to void while sitting.

■ The patient pushes the START button on the commode chair, counts for 5 seconds (1 one-thousand, 2 one-thousand, and so on), and voids. When finished, he counts for 5 seconds and pushes the button again. The volume of urine voided is then recorded and plotted as a curve over the time of voiding. The patient's position and the route of fluid intake (oral or I.V.) are noted.

■ Instruct the patient that he may resume any medications discontinued for the test.

■ Monitor the patient for urine retention or bladder distention. Also monitor his intake and output. If neurogenic bladder is diagnosed, teach self-catheterization, if indicated; provide bladder training as needed.

Precautions

■ The transducer must be level, and the beaker must be centered beneath the funnel.

■ The beaker must be large enough to hold all urine; overflow can invalidate results and damage the transducer.

MINIMUM VOLUME FLOW RATES

This chart lists the minimum volume flow rates needed to obtain adequate recordings.

Age	Min. vol. (ml/sec)	Male (ml/sec)	Female (ml/sec)
4 to 7	100	10	10
8 to 13	100	12	15
14 to 45	200	21	18
46 to 65	200	12	15
66 to 80	200	9	10

CHARACTERISTIC UROFLOW CURVES

The graphs below illustrate common uroflow curves that may be seen with conditions such as hesitancy, incontinence, abdominal straining, and detrusor muscle weakness and obstruction.

Normal curve

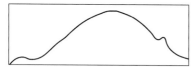

Normal peak with hesitancy may result from the patient's embarrassment or advanced age.

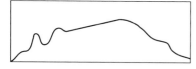

High peak flow over short voiding time may indicate incontinence.

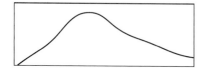

Many peaks over normal voiding time indicate abdominal straining and detrusor muscle weakness.

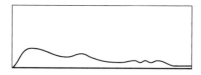

Low peak with long voiding time and urethral dribbling indicates obstruction.

Normal findings

Flow rate varies according to the patient's age and sex and the volume of urine voided. (See *Minimum volume flow rates.*)

Abnormal findings

Increased flow rate indicates reduced urethral resistance, possibly associated with external sphincter dysfunction. (See *Characteristic uroflow curves*) A high peak on the curve plotted over the voiding time indicates decreased outflow resistance, possibly due to stress incontinence. Decreased flow rate indicates outflow obstruction or hypotonia of the detrusor muscle. More than one distinct peak in a normal curve indicates abdominal straining, possibly due to pushing against an obstruction to empty the bladder.

Interfering factors

■ Drugs that affect bladder and sphincter tone, such as urinary spasmolytics and anticholinergics
■ Strong drafts (possible effect on transducer function)
■ Patient movement while seated on the commode chair (possible inaccuracy of flow recording)
■ Presence of toilet tissue in the beaker (invalidation)
■ Straining to void

Cystometry

Cystometry assesses the bladder's neuromuscular function by measuring the efficiency of the detrusor muscle reflex, intravesical pressure and capacity, and the bladder's reaction to thermal stimulation. Because results from cystometry can be ambiguous, they're typically supported by results of other tests, such as cystourethrography, excretory urography, and voiding cystourethrography.

Purpose

■ To evaluate detrusor muscle function and tonicity
■ To help determine the cause of bladder dysfunction

Patient preparation

■ Explain to the patient that cystometry evaluates bladder function.
■ Tell the patient that he need not restrict food and fluids.
■ Describe the procedure, including who will perform it, where it will take place, and how long it will last.
■ Tell the patient that he'll feel a strong urge to void during the test and that he may feel embarrassed or uncomfortable. Provide reassurance.
■ Make sure that the patient or a responsible family member has signed an informed consent form.
■ Check the patient's medication history for drugs that may affect test results such as antihistamines.
■ Tell the patient to urinate just before the procedure.

Equipment

Four-channel gas cystometer, set of catheters

Procedure and posttest care

■ Place the patient in a supine position on the examination table.
■ A catheter is passed into the bladder to measure the residual urine level. Any difficulty with insertion of the catheter may reflect meatal or urethral obstruction.
■ To test the patient's response to thermal sensation, 30 ml of room-temperature physiologic saline solution or sterile water is instilled into the bladder. Then an equal volume of warm (110° to 115° F [43.3° to 46.1° C]) fluid is instilled into the bladder. The patient is asked to report

his sensations, such as the need to void, nausea, flushing, discomfort, and a feeling of warmth.

■ After the fluid is drained from the patient's bladder, the catheter is connected to the cystometer, and normal saline solution, sterile water, or gas (usually carbon dioxide) is slowly introduced into the bladder. The flow of gas is adjusted automatically to the desired reading (100 ml/minute) by a four-channel cystometer.

■ The patient is asked to indicate when he *first* feels an urge to void and then when he feels he *must* urinate. The related pressure and volume are automatically plotted on the graph.

■ When the bladder reaches its full capacity, the patient is asked to urinate so that the maximal intravesical voiding pressure can be recorded. The patient's bladder is then drained and, if no additional tests are required, the catheter is removed; otherwise, the catheter is left in place to measure urethral pressure profile or to provide supplemental findings.

■ If abnormal bladder function is caused by muscle incompetence or disrupted innervation, an anticholinergic (atropine) or cholinergic (bethanechol) medication may be injected and the study repeated in 20 to 30 minutes.

■ Encourage the patient to drink lots of fluids, unless contraindicated, to relieve burning on urination, a common adverse effect of the procedure.

■ Short-term antibiotics are commonly given to prevent infection.

■ Administer a sitz bath or warm tub bath if the patient experiences discomfort after the test.

■ Measure fluid intake and urine output for 24 hours. Watch for hematuria that persists after the third voiding and for signs of sepsis (such as fever or chills).

Precautions

■ Cystometry is contraindicated in the patient with an acute urinary tract infection because uninhibited contractions may cause erroneous readings and the test may lead to pyelonephritis and septic shock.

■ Tell the patient not to strain at voiding; it can cause ambiguous cystometric readings.

■ If the patient has a spinal cord injury that has caused motor impairment, transport him on a stretcher so that the test can be performed without transferring him to the examination table.

Normal findings

For characteristic findings, see *Normal and abnormal cystometry findings.*

Interfering factors

■ Failure to follow instructions because of misunderstanding or embarrassment

■ Inability to urinate in the supine position

■ Concurrent use of drugs such as antihistamines (possible interference with bladder function)

■ Cystometry performed within 6 to 8 weeks after surgery for spinal cord injury (inconclusive results)

Voiding cystourethrography

In voiding cystourethrography, a contrast medium is instilled by gentle syringe pressure or gravity into the bladder through a urethral catheter. Fluoroscopic films or overhead radiographs demonstrate bladder filling and then show excretion of the contrast medium as the patient voids.

NORMAL AND ABNORMAL CYSTOMETRY FINDINGS

Because cystometry assesses micturition and vesical function, it can aid diagnosis of neurogenic bladder dysfunction. The five main types of neurogenic bladder, as presented in the following chart, result from lesions of the central or peripheral nervous system. Uninhibited neurogenic bladder results from a lesion to the upper motor neuron and causes frequent, usually uncontrollable micturition in the presence of even a small amount of urine. A complete upper motor neuron lesion characterizes reflex neurogenic bladder and causes total loss of conscious sensation and vesical control.

Feature or response	Normal bladder function	Uninhibited neurogenic bladder (mildly spastic, incomplete upper motor neuron lesion)	Reflex neurogenic bladder (completely spastic, complete upper motor neuron lesion)
Micturition			
Start	+	+/0	0
Stop	+	0	0
Residual urine	0	0	+
Vesical sensation	+	+	0
First urge to void	150 to 200 ml	E (< 150 ml)	0
Bladder capacity	400 to 500 ml	↓	↓
Bladder contractions	0	+	+
Intravesical pressure	L	↑	↑
Bulbocavernosus reflex	+	+	↑
Saddle sensation	+	+	0
Bethanechol test (exaggerated response)	0	+	0
Ice water test	+	+	+
Anal reflex	+	+	+
Heat sensation and pain	+	+	0

KEY:

+ = Present/Positive	↓ = Decreased	D = Delayed
0 = Absent/Negative	V = Variable	L = Low
↑ = Increased	E = Early	

(continued)

NORMAL AND ABNORMAL CYSTOMETRY FINDINGS *(continued)*

In autonomous neurogenic bladder, a lower motor neuron lesion produces a flaccid bladder that fills without contracting. The patient can't perceive bladder fullness or initiate and maintain urination without applying external pressure. Lower motor neuron lesions can cause sensory or motor paralysis of the bladder. In sensory paralysis, the patient experiences chronic urine retention because he can't perceive bladder fullness. In motor paralysis, the patient has full sensation, but can't initiate or control urination.

Feature or response	Autonomous neurogenic bladder (flaccid, incomplete lower motor neuron lesion)	Sensory paralytic bladder (lower motor neuron lesion)	Motor paralytic bladder (lower motor neuron lesion)
Micturition			
Start	0	+	0
Stop	0	+	0
Residual urine	+	+	++
Vesical sensation	0	0	+
First urge to void	0	D	+
Bladder capacity	↑	↑ (< 1 L)	V
Bladder contractions	0	0	0
Intravesical pressure	↓	↓	L
Bulbocavernosus reflex	0	+/↓/0	+
Saddle sensation	0	V	+
Bethanechol test (exaggerated response)	+	+	0
Ice water test	0	0	0
Anal reflex	0	V	V
Heat sensation and pain	0	0	+

KEY:

+ = Present/Positive   ↓ = Decreased   D = Delayed
0 = Absent/Negative   V = Variable   L = Low
↑ = Increased   E = Early

Purpose

- To detect abnormalities of the bladder and urethra, such as vesicoureteral reflux, neurogenic bladder, prostatic hyperplasia, urethral strictures, or diverticula

Patient preparation

- Explain to the patient that voiding cystourethrography permits assessment of the bladder and the urethra.
- Inform the patient that he need not restrict food and fluids.
- Tell the patient who will perform the test and where it will take place.
- Inform the patient that a catheter will be inserted into his bladder and that a contrast medium will be instilled through the catheter.
- Tell the patient that he may experience a feeling of fullness and an urge to void when the contrast medium is instilled. Explain that X-rays will be taken of his bladder and urethra and that he'll be asked to assume various positions.
- Make sure that the patient or a responsible family member has signed an informed consent form.
- ◤ **CLINICAL ALERT** *Check the patient's history for hypersensitivity to contrast media or iodine-containing foods such as shellfish; note sensitivities on the chart and notify the physician.*
- Administer a sedative, if prescribed, just before the procedure.

Equipment

Radiographic equipment (fluoroscope and screen and accessories for spot-film radiography), indwelling urinary catheter, standard urographic contrast medium (up to 1,000 ml of 15% solution), 50-ml syringe (for infants) or gravity-feed apparatus

Procedure and posttest care

- The patient is placed in a supine position, and an indwelling urinary catheter is inserted into the bladder.
- The contrast medium is instilled through the catheter until the bladder is full.
- The catheter is clamped, and X-ray films are exposed with the patient in supine, oblique, and lateral positions.
- The catheter is removed, and the patient assumes the right oblique position (right leg flexed to 90 degrees, left leg extended, penis parallel to right leg) and begins to void.
- Four high-speed exposures of the bladder and urethra, coned down to reduce radiation exposure, are usually made on one film during voiding.
- If the right oblique view doesn't delineate both ureters, the patient is asked to stop urinating and to begin again in the left oblique position.
- The most reliable voiding cystourethrograms are obtained with the patient recumbent. The patient who can't void recumbent may do so standing (not sitting).
- Expression cystourethrography may have to be performed, under a general anesthetic, for a young child who can't void on command.
- ◤ **CLINICAL ALERT** *Observe and record the time, color, and volume of the patient's voidings. Report hematuria if present after the third voiding.*
- Encourage the patient to drink large quantities of fluids to reduce burning on urination and to flush out residual contrast medium.
- ◤ **CLINICAL ALERT** *Monitor the patient for chills and fever related to extravasation of contrast material or urinary sepsis.*

- If stricture is present, prepare for surgery, as indicated.
- Monitor the patient for symptoms of urinary tract infection.

Precautions

- Voiding cystourethrography is contraindicated in the patient with an acute or exacerbated urethral or bladder infection or an acute urethral injury.
- Hypersensitivity to the contrast medium may also contraindicate this test.

Normal findings

Delineation of the bladder and urethra shows normal structure and function, with no regurgitation of contrast medium into the ureters.

Abnormal findings

Voiding cystourethrography may show urethral stricture, vesical or urethral diverticula, ureterocele, cystocele, prostate enlargement, vesicoureteral reflux, or neurogenic bladder. The severity and location of such abnormalities are then evaluated to determine whether surgical intervention is necessary.

Interfering factors

- Embarrassment (inhibits the patient from voiding on command)
- Interrupted or less vigorous voiding, muscle spasm, or incomplete sphincter relaxation (due to urethral trauma during catheterization)
- Presence of contrast media from recent tests, stool, or gas in the bowel (possible poor imaging)

Whitaker test

Also called a *pressure* or *flow study,* the Whitaker test correlates radiographic findings with measurements of pressure and flow in the kidneys and ureters and facilitates assessment of the upper urinary tract's efficiency in emptying.

In this procedure, radiographs are taken after urethral catheterization, I.V. administration of a contrast medium, percutaneous cannulation of the kidney, and renal perfusion of the contrast medium. Intrarenal and bladder pressures are then measured.

Purpose

- To identify and evaluate renal obstruction

Patient preparation

- Explain to the patient that the Whitaker test helps to evaluate kidney function.
- Instruct the patient to avoid food and fluids for at least 4 hours before the test.
- Tell the patient who will perform the test, where it will take place, and that it will take about 1 hour.
- Describe the procedure to the patient. Inform him that he'll be given a mild sedative before the test, that he may feel some discomfort during insertion of the urethral catheter and injection of the local anesthetic, and that he may also feel transient burning and flushing after injection of the contrast medium.
- Warn the patient that the X-ray machine makes loud clacking sounds as films are exposed.
- Make sure that the patient or a responsible family member has signed an informed consent form.
- Check the patient's history and recent coagulation studies for bleeding disorders. Also check for hypersensitivity reactions to iodine; iodine-containing foods such as shellfish; and contrast media. Mark sensitivities on the chart and inform the physician.

- Instruct the patient to void and administer prescribed sedatives just before the procedure. Check that pretest blood work (such as kidney function) was done, if ordered.
- Administer prophylactic antimicrobials, as prescribed, to prevent infection from instrumentation.

Equipment

Radiographic equipment, perfusion pump with 50-ml luer-lock syringe, transducer and recorder, manometer, three-way and four-way stopcocks, I.V. extension set, manometer lines, one double-male connector to connect urethral catheter and stopcock, sterile water and normal saline solution, contrast medium, local anesthetic, percutaneous puncture tray with 4″ to 6″ 18G Longdwel cannula, gloves, preparatory tray, emergency resuscitation equipment

Procedure and posttest care

- Place the patient in a supine position on the X-ray table. The table must be horizontal and must remain at the same height throughout the test.
- To prepare for measurement of bladder pressure, a urethral catheter is placed in the bladder. The patient's bladder may be emptied, depending on his suspected condition. (If an obstruction is suspected, the patient will be asked to void before the test. If a condition, such as a bladder hypertonia, is the suspected cause of insufficient emptying, he shouldn't void.)
- A plain film of the urinary tract is taken to obtain anatomic landmarks.
- The catheter is then connected to a three-way stopcock on a manometer line linked to the transducer and recorder. The line is then filled with sterile water.
- Contrast medium is injected intravenously.

- The patient is placed prone and made comfortable with pillows. When urography demonstrates contrast medium in the kidney, the skin is cleaned with antiseptic solution and draped.
- Pressure recording equipment is calibrated. The renal perfusion tubing is filled with sterile water or normal saline solution and held at the level of the kidney.
- Local anesthetic is injected, and an incision is made through the flank for cannulation of the kidney.
- The patient is asked to hold his breath while the needle is inserted into the renal pelvis. Aspiration of urine confirms that the needle is in position.
- The cannula is then connected by a four-way stopcock to the perfusion tubing and the manometer line.
- Perfusion of the contrast medium is begun, serial X-rays are taken, and intrarenal pressure is measured. Bladder pressure is then measured.
- Perfusion continues at a steady rate of 10 ml/minute until bladder pressure is constant. When pressure holds steady for a few minutes and adequate films have been taken, perfusion is discontinued. Residual fluid is aspirated from the kidney, the cannula is removed, and the wound is dressed.
- Keep the patient in a supine position for 12 hours after the test.
- Check the patient's vital signs every 15 minutes for the first hour, every 30 minutes for the next hour, and then every 2 hours for 24 hours.
- Check the puncture site for bleeding, hematoma, or urine leakage each time vital signs are checked. If bleeding occurs, apply pressure. If a hematoma develops, apply warm soaks. Report urine leakage.

■ Monitor fluid intake and urine output for 24 hours. Report hematuria that persists after the third voiding.

▶ **CLINICAL ALERT** *Watch the patient for signs of sepsis (chills, fever, tachycardia, tachypnea, or hypotension) or similar signs of contrast medium extravasation.*

■ Inform the patient that colicky pains are transient.

■ Administer prescribed analgesics.

■ Administer antimicrobials for several days after the test, as ordered, to prevent infection.

■ If an obstruction is present, prepare the patient for surgery.

Precautions

■ Contraindications include bleeding disorders and severe infection.

Normal findings

Visualization of the kidney after gradual perfusion of the contrast medium shows normal outlines of the renal pelvis and calyces. The ureter should fill uniformly and appear normal in size and course.

The normal value for intrarenal pressure is 15 cm H_2O. The normal value for bladder pressure may range from 5 to 10 cm H_2O.

Abnormal findings

Enlargement of the renal pelvis, calyces, or ureteropelvic junction may indicate obstruction. Subtraction of bladder pressure from intrarenal pressure results in a differential that aids diagnosis. A differential of 12 to 15 cm H_2O indicates obstruction. A differential of less than 10 cm H_2O indicates a bladder abnormality, such as hypertonia or neurogenic bladder.

Interfering factors

■ Recent barium studies or stool or gas in the bowel (hinders accurate needle placement and visualization of the upper urinary tract)

■ Patient movement

External sphincter electromyography

External sphincter electromyography (EMG) measures electrical activity of the external urinary sphincter using needle electrodes inserted in perineal or periurethral tissues, electrodes in an anal plug, or skin electrodes. Skin electrodes are the most common method used.

Incontinence is the primary indication for external sphincter EMG. Usually, the test is done with cystometry and voiding urethrography as part of a full urodynamic study.

Purpose

■ To assess neuromuscular function of the external urinary sphincter

■ To assess the functional balance between bladder and sphincter muscle activity

Patient preparation

■ Explain to the patient that external sphincter EMG will determine how well his bladder and sphincter muscles work together.

■ Describe the test, including who will perform it, where it will take place, and how long it will last.

■ If skin electrodes are used, describe their placement and explain the preparatory procedure, which may include shaving a small area.

■ If needle electrodes are used, describe their placement to the patient and explain that the discomfort is equivalent to an I.M. injection. Assure him that he'll feel discomfort only during insertion. Explain that wires connect the needles to the recorder, but pose no danger of electric shock. If the patient is a woman, tell her that she may notice slight bleeding at the first voiding.

■ If an anal plug is used, tell the patient that only the tip of the plug will be inserted into the rectum and that he may feel fullness, but no discomfort.

■ Check the patient's history for use of cholinergic or anticholinergic drugs and note such use.

■ Make sure that the patient or a responsible family member has signed an informed consent form.

Equipment

Electromyograph and recorder; skin, needle, or anal plug electrodes; ground plate; electrode paste; tape; antiseptic solution such as povidone-iodine; preparatory tray if shaving is necessary.

Procedure and posttest care

■ Place the patient in the lithotomy position for electrode placement. After placement, he may lie in the supine position. Record the patient's position, the type of electrode and measuring equipment used, and other tests done at the same time.

■ Electrode paste is applied to the ground plate, which is taped to the thigh and grounded. The electrodes are positioned and connected to electrode adapters.

■ When using skin electrodes, clean the skin with antiseptic solution and then dry the area. If necessary, shave a small area to optimize electrode contact. Apply electrode paste and tape the electrodes in place. For a woman, electrodes are placed in the periurethral area; for a man, in the perineal area beneath the scrotum.

■ To position needle electrodes on a male patient, a gloved finger is inserted in the rectum. The needles and wires are inserted through the perineal skin toward the apex of the prostate. Needle positions are 3 o'clock and 9 o'clock. The needles are withdrawn, and the wires are held in place and then taped to the thigh.

■ To position needle electrodes on a female patient, the labia are spread and the needles and wires are inserted periurethrally at the 2 o'clock and 10 o'clock positions. The needles are withdrawn, and the wires are taped to the thigh.

■ When using anal plug electrodes, the plug is lubricated, and the patient is asked to breathe slowly and deeply and to relax the anal sphincter to accommodate the plug by bearing down.

■ After electrode placement, the adapters are inserted in the preamplifier, and recording starts. The patient is asked to alternately relax and tighten the sphincter.

■ When sufficient data have been recorded, the patient is asked to bear down and exhale while the anal plug and needle electrodes are removed. Remove skin electrodes gently to avoid pulling hair and tender skin.

■ Clean and dry the area before the patient dresses.

■ In some urodynamic laboratories, cystometrography is done with EMG for a thorough evaluation of detrusor and sphincter coordination.

■ For women, watch for and report hematuria after the first voiding if needle electrodes were used.

■ Watch for and report symptoms of mild urethral irritation, such as dysuria, hematuria, and urinary frequency.

■ Advise the patient to take a warm sitz bath and encourage him to drink 2 to 3 L (2 to 3 qt) of fluids daily, unless contraindicated.

Precautions

- Insert the needles quickly to minimize discomfort.
- The ground plate should be properly applied and anchored; wires should be taped securely to prevent artifacts.

Normal findings

The EMG shows increased muscle activity when the patient tightens the external urinary sphincter and decreased muscle activity when he relaxes it. If EMG and cystometrography are performed simultaneously, a comparison of results shows that muscle activity of the normal sphincter increases as the bladder fills. During voiding and bladder contraction, muscle activity decreases as the sphincter relaxes. This comparison is important in assessing external sphincter efficiency and functional balance between bladder and sphincter muscle activity.

Abnormal findings

Failure of the sphincter to relax or increased muscle activity during voiding demonstrates detrusor–external sphincter dyssynergia. Confirmation of such muscle activity by EMG may indicate neurogenic bladder, spinal cord injury, multiple sclerosis, Parkinson's disease, or stress incontinence.

Interfering factors

- Patient movement (possible distortion)
- Effect of anticholinergic or cholinergic drugs on detrusor and sphincter activity
- Improperly placed and anchored electrodes

Selected readings

Cavanaugh, B.M. *Nurse's Manual of Laboratory and Diagnostic Tests,* 4th ed. Philadelphia: F.A. Davis Co., 2003.

Chapple, C.R., and MacDiarmid, S.A. *Urodynamics Made Easy,* 2nd ed. London: Churchill-Livingstone, 2000.

Goldman, L., and Ausiello, D., eds. *Cecil Textbook of Medicine,* 22nd ed. Philadelphia: W.B. Saunders Co., 2004.

Guyton, A.C., and Hall, J.E. *Textbook of Medical Physiology,* 10th ed. Philadelphia: W.B. Saunders Co., 2001.

McClatchey, K.D. *Clinical Laboratory Medicine,* 2nd ed. Philadelphia: Lippincott Williams & Wilkins, 2002.

Pagana, K.D., and Pagana, T.J. *Mosby's Diagnostic and Laboratory Test Reference,* 6th ed. St. Louis: Mosby Year-Book, Inc., 2003.

Retik, A.B., et al. *Campbell's Urology,* 8th ed. Philadelphia: W.B. Saunders Co., 2002.

Schnell, Z., et al. *Davis's Comprehensive Handbook of Laboratory and Diagnostic Tests with Nursing Implications.* Philadelphia: F.A. Davis Co., 2003.

SECTION VI.
MISCELLANEOUS
TESTS

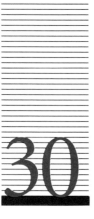

30
Miscellaneous tests

Introduction

Some important diagnostic tests resist easy classification. For example, skin tests evaluate the immune response using different procedures from other immunologic tests. The contrast radiography and nuclear medicine tests found elsewhere in this book apply specifically to certain organs or body systems, but others, such as lymphangiography and gallium scanning, apply more widely. D-xylose absorption is the only diagnostic test that uses serum and urine samples to detect the cause of malabsorption syndrome. And the dexamethasone suppression test is the standard screening test for Cushing's syndrome.

Skin tests

Skin tests evaluate cellular immunity by determining patient response to the intradermal injection or topical application of one or more antigens. Anergy — the inability to react to a battery of common antigens — suggests immunodeficiency. The anergic patient may require additional hypersensitivity skin tests using greater concentrations of the same antigens.

Radiology and nuclear medicine

Lymphangiography is rarely used today for detecting obstruction, disease, and neoplasm in the lymphatic system. This system transports lymph — derived from tissue fluids — throughout the body and eventually empties it into the veins. The lymphatic system can spread inflammation and disease throughout the body.

In gallium scanning, a gamma camera or rectilinear scanner records distribution of radioactivity after I.V. injection of radioactive gallium citrate. Because gallium concentrates at sites of inflammation, such as abscesses and carcinomas, it can help detect them or determine the extent of metastases and help evaluate the effectiveness of treatment.

The red blood cell (RBC) survival time test measures the life span of RBCs tagged with radioactive chromium 51 to help evaluate unexplained anemia. Serial blood tests and gamma camera scans help identify the type and site of RBC destruction.

Malabsorption test

The D-xylose absorption test distinguishes intestinal disease from other disorders that cause malabsorption. Blood and urine samples are analyzed after ingestion of a standard dose of D-xylose. In malabsorption due to intestinal disease, D-xylose absorption decreases; in malabsorption due to pancreatic insufficiency, cystic fibrosis, or liver disease, absorption remains normal.

Dexamethasone suppression test

The dexamethasone suppression test helps to diagnose Cushing's syndrome. It also helps detect and monitor major depression by measuring the body's level of adrenal steroid hormones.

SKIN TESTS

Delayed hypersensitivity skin tests

Skin testing for delayed-type hypersensitivity (DTH) is an important method for evaluating T-cell mediated immune response in a patient. (However, positive reactions don't indicate protection against the antigen.) This response requires previous exposure to the antigen and an intact immune system. After initial exposure to the antigen, the body produces antibodies and sensitized T cells. When re-exposed to the antigen (recall antigen), the antibodies react immediately, causing a hypersensitivity reaction; however, the T cells respond over the next few days, causing a delayed hypersensitivity reaction. The immediate response is typically erythema, while the delayed response is induration (hardening). The lack of response to a recall antigen is termed anergy and, in the absence of underlying disease or immunosuppressive therapy, may indicate T-cell immunodeficiency disease.

The most commonly used recall antigen is *Mycobacterium tuberculosis* (purified protein derivative [PPD] Mantoux test). Other antigens used in the clinical setting include *Candida*, *Trichophyton*, and mumps. Some antigens previously used for DTH testing, such as fungi and streptococci, are no longer available or recommended for clinical use.

DTH-like reactions may occur with topical contact to *Rhus* species plants (poison ivy, oak, and sumac), nickel, dinitrochlorobenzene (DNCB), dinitrofluo-

---

PERFORMING A PATCH TEST

A patch test confirms allergic contact sensitivity and can help identify its cause. In this test, a sample series of common allergens (antigens) is applied to the skin in the hope that one or more will produce a positive reaction. A positive patch test proves that the patient has a contact sensitivity, but doesn't necessarily confirm that the test substance caused the clinical eruption.

If the patient has an acute inflammation, the patch test should be postponed until the inflammation subsides to avoid exacerbating the inflammation.

Keep the following points in mind when performing a patch test:

■ Use only *potentially* irritating substances for a patch test. Testing with primary irritants isn't possible.

■ To avoid skin irritation, dilute substances that may be irritating to 1% to 2% in petroleum jelly, mineral oil or, as a last choice, water. When there are no clues to a likely allergen in a person with possible contact dermatitis, use a series of common allergens available in standard patch tests.

■ Apply the allergens to normal, hairless skin on the back or on the ventral surface of the forearm. First, apply them to a small disk of filter paper attached to aluminum and coated with plastic. Tape the paper to the skin, or use a small square of soft cotton and cover it with occlusive tape. Apply liquids and ointments to the disk or cotton. Apply volatile liquids to the skin and allow the areas to dry before covering. Before application, powder solids and moisten powders and fabrics.

■ Make sure that patches remain in place for 48 hours. However, remove the patch immediately if pain, pruritus, or irritation develops. Positive reactions may take time to develop, so check findings 20 to 30 minutes after removing the patch and again 96 hours (4 days) after the application.

■ To relieve the effects of a positive reaction, tell the patient to apply topical corticosteroids, as ordered.

---

robenzene (DNFB), and picryl chloride. Contact sensitivity to *Rhus* and nickel is determined clinically, and skin testing isn't considered necessary. There's a risk of local tissue necrosis when using chemical antigens, specifically DNCB and DNFB, so their use is discouraged; in vitro assessment of cell-mediated immunity is preferred in those circumstances.

DTH testing can be used to assess the status of an individual's immune system in severe infection, cancer, pretransplantation, and malnutrition. Antigens used for this testing must be antigens the patient has been previously exposed to. For example, *C. albicans*, tetanus, or mumps can be used.

DTH testing is performed by injecting a small amount of antigenic material intradermally or applying it topically and measuring the reaction after 48 to 72 hours. Skin testing has limited value in infants due to their immature immune system and lack of previous sensitization. In addition, patch testing may be used. This involves applying antigenic material topically to the skin, helping to confirm allergic contact sensitization and isolate the causative agent. (See *Performing a patch test.*)

Purpose

■ To assess for exposure to or activation of certain diseases, most commonly tuberculosis (TB)

- To assess the status of a patient's immune system during illness (cancer, transplantation)
- To evaluate sensitivity to environmental antigens in the patient with persistent symptoms (for example, asthma, seasonal rhinitis, recurrent or persistent urticaria)

Patient preparation

- Explain to the patient that a small amount of antigenic material will be injected superficially or applied to the skin.
- Inform the patient that testing takes only a few minutes for each antigen. Reactions will be evaluated 48 to 72 hours later. Occasionally, the test must be repeated in 2 to 3 weeks when a negative result is displayed initially. The first test "reminds" the body that it was previously exposed to the antigen and a response is noted on retesting. This is commonly done for TB testing and is called the *two-step test*.
- Be sure to ask the patient about sensitivity to the test antigens, whether he has had previous skin testing, and what the outcomes of that testing were. When performing TB testing, ask about previous TB disease or exposure and bacille Calmette-Guérin vaccination.
- Be aware that the U.S. Food and Drug Administration hasn't approved all vaccines for use in skin testing, though nonapproved substances are commonly used. Currently approved antigens include PPD to *M. tuberculosis* and mumps.

Procedure and posttest care

- Inject each antigen being tested intradermally, using a separate tuberculin syringe, on the patient's forearm. (See *Administering test antigens.*)
- Circle each injection site with a pen, and label each according to the antigen given.

ADMINISTERING TEST ANTIGENS

The illustration here shows the arm of a patient undergoing a recall antigen test, which determines whether he has previously been exposed to certain antigens. A sample panel of four (4) test antigens has been injected into his forearm, and the test site has been marked and labeled for each antigen.

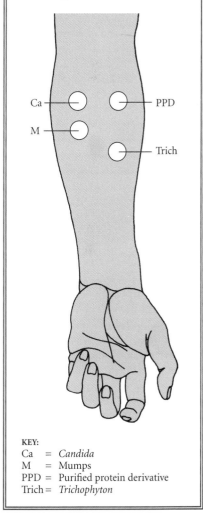

KEY:
Ca = *Candida*
M = Mumps
PPD = Purified protein derivative
Trich = *Trichophyton*

■ Instruct the patient to avoid washing off the circles until the test is completed.

■ Inject the control allergy diluent on the other forearm.

■ Inspect the injection sites for reactivity after 48 to 72 hours. Record induration and erythema in millimeters. A negative test at the first concentration of antigen should be confirmed using a higher concentration.

■ Watch the patient closely for severe local reactions that may occur at the test site, such as pain, blistering, swelling, induration, itching, and ulceration. Scarring or hyperpigmentation also may result. Also observe for swelling and tenderness in the lymph nodes at the elbow or axillary region. Check for tachycardia and fever, although these rarely occur. Symptoms typically appear in 15 to 30 minutes.

■ Tell the patient experiencing hypersensitivity that steroids will control the reaction, but that skin lesions may persist for 10 to 14 days. Instruct him to avoid scratching or otherwise disturbing the affected area.

Precautions

■ If appropriate, store antigens in lyophilized (freeze-dried) form at 39.2° F (4° C) and protected from light. Reconstitute them shortly before use and check their expiration dates. If the patient is suspected of being hypersensitive to the antigens, apply them first in low concentrations.

■ If the forearms are not free from disease (for example, if the patient has atopic dermatitis), use other sites such as the back.

▶ **CLINICAL ALERT** *Observe the patient carefully for signs of anaphylactic shock — urticaria, respiratory distress,*

and hypotension. If such signs develop, administer epinephrine, as ordered, and notify the physician immediately.

Normal findings

In the recall antigen test, a positive response (5 mm or more of induration at the test site) appears 48 hours after injection.

Abnormal findings

In the recall antigen test, a positive response to less than two of the test antigens, a persistent unresponsiveness to intradermal injection of higher-strength antigens, or a generalized diminished reaction (causing less than 10 mm combined induration) indicates diminished delayed hypersensitivity.

Diminished delayed hypersensitivity can result from Hodgkin's disease (common); sarcoidosis; liver disease; congenital immunodeficiency disease, such as ataxia-telangiectasia, DiGeorge syndrome, and Wiskott-Aldrich syndrome; uremia; acute leukemia; viral diseases, such as influenza, infectious mononucleosis, measles, mumps, and rubella; fungal diseases, such as coccidioidomycosis and cryptococcosis; bacterial diseases, such as leprosy and TB; and terminal cancer. Diminished delayed hypersensitivity can also result from immunosuppressive or steroid therapy or viral vaccination.

Interfering factors

■ Use of antigens that have expired or that have been exposed to heat and light or to bacterial contamination

■ Poor injection technique (subcutaneous instead of intradermal injection)

■ Inaccurate dilution of antigens or an error in reading or timing test results

- A strong immediate reaction to the antigen at the injection site
- Oral contraceptives (may cause false-negative results by inhibiting lymphocyte mitosis)

RADIOLOGY AND NUCLEAR MEDICINE TESTS

Lymphangiography

Lymphangiography (or lymphography) is the radiographic examination of the lymphatic system after the injection of an oil-based contrast medium into a lymphatic vessel in each foot or, less commonly, in each hand. This test is no longer used widely.

Injection into the foot allows visualization of the lymphatics of the leg, inguinal and iliac regions, and the retroperitoneum up to the thoracic duct.

Injection into the hand allows visualization of the axillary and supraclavicular nodes. This procedure may also be used to study the cervical region (retroauricular area), but this is less useful and less common.

X-ray films are taken immediately after injection to demonstrate the filling of the lymphatic system and then again 24 hours later to visualize the lymph nodes. Because the contrast medium remains in the nodes for up to 2 years, subsequent X-ray films can assess progression of disease and monitor effectiveness of treatment.

Purpose
- To detect and stage lymphomas and to identify metastatic involvement of the lymph nodes (Computed tomography [CT] is used more commonly for staging.)
- To distinguish primary from secondary lymphedema
- To suggest surgical treatment or evaluate the effectiveness of chemotherapy and radiation therapy in controlling malignancy
- To investigate enlarged lymph nodes detected by CT or ultrasonography

Patient preparation
- Explain to the patient that lymphangiography permits examination of the lymphatic system through X-ray films taken after the injection of a contrast medium.
- Inform the patient that he need not restrict food and fluids.
- Tell the patient who will perform the procedure and where it will take place.
- Mention to the patient that additional X-ray films are also taken the following day, but that these take less than 30 minutes.
- Inform the patient that blue contrast medium will be injected into each foot to outline the lymphatic vessels, that the injection causes transient discomfort, and that the contrast medium discolors urine and stool for 48 hours and may give his skin and vision a bluish tinge for 48 hours.
- Tell the patient that a local anesthetic will be injected before a small incision is made in each foot.
- Inform the patient that the contrast medium is then injected for the next 1¼ hours using a catheter inserted into a lymphatic vessel.
- Advise the patient that he must remain as still as possible during injection of the contrast medium and that he may experience some discomfort in the popliteal or

inguinal areas at the beginning of the injection.

■ If this test is performed on an outpatient basis, advise the patient to have a friend or relative accompany him.

■ Warn the patient that the incision site may be sore for several days after lymphangiography.

■ Make sure that the patient or a responsible family member has signed an informed consent form.

■ Check the patient's history to determine if he's hypersensitive to iodine, seafood, or the contrast media used in other diagnostic tests such as excretory urography. Alert the physician to any sensitivities.

■ Just before the procedure, instruct the patient to void and check his vital signs for a baseline. If prescribed, administer a sedative and an oral antihistamine (if hypersensitivity to the contrast medium is suspected).

Procedure and posttest care

■ A preliminary X-ray of the chest is taken with the patient in an erect or a supine position.

■ The skin over the dorsum of each foot is cleaned with antiseptics.

■ Blue contrast dye is injected intradermally into the area between the toes, usually the first and fourth toe webs.

■ The contrast medium infiltrates the lymphatic system, and within 15 to 30 minutes, the lymphatic vessels appear as small blue lines on the upper surface of the instep of each foot.

■ A local anesthetic is then injected into the dorsum of each foot and a transverse incision is made to expose the lymphatic vessel.

■ Each vessel is cannulated with a 30G needle attached to polyethylene tubing and a syringe filled with ethiodized oil.

■ After the needles are positioned, the patient is instructed to remain still throughout the injection period to avoid dislodging the needles.

■ The syringe is then placed within an infusion pump that injects the contrast medium at a constant rate of 0.1 to 0.2 ml/minute for about 1½ hours to avoid injury to delicate lymphatic vessels.

■ Fluoroscopy may be used to monitor filling of the lymphatic system.

■ The needles are removed, the incisions are sutured, and sterile dressings are applied.

■ X-ray films of the legs, pelvis, abdomen, and chest are taken.

■ The patient is then taken to his room, but must return 24 hours later for additional films.

■ Check the patient's vital signs every 4 hours for 48 hours.

CLINICAL ALERT *Watch for pulmonary complications, such as shortness of breath, pleuritic pain, hypotension, low-grade fever, and cyanosis caused by embolization of the contrast medium.*

■ Enforce bed rest for 24 hours, with the patient's feet elevated to help reduce swelling.

■ Apply ice packs to the incision sites to help reduce swelling and administer prescribed analgesics.

■ Check the incision sites for infection and leave the dressings in place for 2 days, making sure the wounds remain dry. Tell the patient that the sutures will be removed in 7 to 10 days.

■ Prepare the patient for follow-up X-rays, as needed.

Precautions

■ Lymphangiography is contraindicated in the patient with hypersensitivity to iodine, pulmonary insufficiencies, cardiac diseases, or severe renal or hepatic disease.

Normal findings

The lymphatic system normally demonstrates homogeneous and complete filling with contrast medium on the initial films. On the 24-hour films, the lymph nodes are fully opacified and well circumscribed; the lymphatic channels are emptied a few hours after injection of the contrast medium.

Abnormal findings

Enlarged, foamy-looking nodes indicate Hodgkin's disease or malignant lymphoma. Filling defects or lack of opacification indicates metastatic involvement of the lymph nodes. The number of nodes affected, unilateral or bilateral involvement, and the extent of extranodal involvement help determine staging of lymphoma. However, definitive staging may require additional diagnostic tests, such as CT, ultrasonography, selective biopsy, and laparotomy.

In differential diagnosis of primary and secondary lymphedema, shortened lymphatic vessels and a deficient number of vessels indicate primary lymphedema. Abruptly terminating lymphatic vessels, caused by retroperitoneal tumors impinging on the vessels, inflammation, filariasis, and trauma resulting from surgery or radiation, indicate secondary lymphedema.

Interfering factors

■ Inability to cannulate the lymphatic vessels (precludes use of this test)

Gallium scanning

A gallium scan is a total body scan used to assess certain neoplasms and inflam-matory lesions that attract gallium. It's usually performed 24 to 48 hours after the I.V. injection of radioactive gallium (^{67}Ga) citrate; occasionally, it's performed 72 hours after the injection or, in acute inflammatory disease, 4 to 6 hours after the injection.

Because gallium has an affinity for benign and malignant neoplasms and inflammatory lesions, exact diagnosis requires additional confirming tests, such as ultrasonography and computed tomography scanning. Also, be aware that many neoplasms and a few inflammatory lesions may fail to demonstrate abnormal gallium activity.

Purpose

■ To detect primary or metastatic neoplasms and inflammatory lesions when the site of the disease hasn't been clearly defined
■ To evaluate malignant lymphoma and identify recurrent tumors following chemotherapy or radiation therapy
■ To clarify focal defects in the liver when liver-spleen scanning and ultrasonography prove inconclusive
■ To evaluate bronchogenic carcinoma

Patient preparation

■ Explain to the patient that gallium scanning helps detect abnormal or inflammatory tissue.
■ Tell the patient that he need not restrict food and fluids.
■ Explain to the patient that the test requires a total body scan (usually performed 24 to 48 hours after the I.V. injection of ^{67}Ga citrate).
■ Tell the patient who will perform the test and where it will take place.
■ Warn the patient that he may experience transient discomfort from the needle puncture during injection of the ^{67}Ga cit-

rate. Reassure him, however, that the dosage is only slightly radioactive and isn't harmful.

■ If a gamma scintillation camera is to be used, assure the patient that although the uptake probe and detector head may touch his skin, he'll experience no discomfort.

■ If a rectilinear scanner is to be used, mention to the patient that it makes a soft, irregular clicking noise as it registers the radiation emissions.

■ Make sure that the patient or a responsible family member has signed an informed consent form.

■ Administer a laxative, an enema, or both, as ordered.

Procedure and posttest care

■ The patient may be positioned erect or recumbent or in an appropriate combination of these positions, depending on his physical condition.

■ Scans or scintigrams of the patient are taken 24 to 48 hours after ^{67}Ga citrate injection, from anterior and posterior views and, occasionally, lateral views.

■ If the initial gallium scan suggests bowel disease and additional scans are necessary, give the patient a cleaning enema before continuing the test.

Precautions

■ This test should precede barium studies because barium retention may hinder visualization of gallium activity in the bowel.

■ Gallium scanning is usually contraindicated in a child and during pregnancy or lactation; however, it may be performed if the potential diagnostic benefit outweighs the risks of exposure to radiation.

Normal findings

Gallium activity is normally demonstrated in the liver, spleen, bones, and large bowel. Activity in the bowel results from mucosal uptake of gallium and fecal excretion of gallium.

Abnormal findings

Gallium scanning may reveal inflammatory lesions — discrete abscesses or diffuse infiltration. In pancreatic or perinephric abscess, gallium activity is relatively localized; in bacterial peritonitis, gallium activity is spread diffusely within the abdomen.

Abnormally high gallium accumulation is characteristic in inflammatory bowel diseases, such as ulcerative colitis and regional ileitis (Crohn's disease), and in carcinoma of the colon. However, because gallium normally accumulates in the colon, the detection of inflammatory and neoplastic diseases is sometimes difficult.

Abnormal gallium activity may be present in various sarcomas, Wilms' tumor, and neuroblastomas; carcinoma of the kidney, uterus, vagina, and stomach; and testicular tumors, such as seminoma, embryonal carcinoma, choriocarcinoma, and teratocarcinoma, which commonly metastasize via the lymphatic system. In Hodgkin's disease and malignant lymphoma, gallium scanning can demonstrate abnormal activity in one or more lymph nodes or in extranodal locations. However, gallium scanning supported by results of lymphangiography can gauge the extent of metastases more accurately than either test alone because neither test consistently identifies all neoplastic nodes.

After chemotherapy or radiation therapy, gallium scanning may be used to detect new or recurrent tumors. However, these forms of therapy tend to diminish tumor affinity for gallium without necessarily eliminating the tumor.

In the differential diagnosis of focal hepatic defects, abnormal gallium activity may help narrow the diagnostic possibilities. Gallium localizes in hepatomas, but not in pseudotumors; in abscesses, but not in pleural effusions; and in tumors, but not in cysts or hematomas.

In examining patients with suspected bronchogenic carcinoma, abnormal activity confirms the presence of a tumor. However, because gallium also localizes in inflammatory pulmonary diseases, such as pneumonia and sarcoidosis, a chest X-ray should be performed to distinguish a tumor from an inflammatory lesion.

Interfering factors
■ Hepatic and splenic intake (possible false-negative scans due to possible obscuring of abnormal para-aortic nodes in Hodgkin's disease)
■ Fecal accumulation in the bowel (poor imaging of retroperitoneal space)
■ Residual barium from other tests done 1 week before the scan (possible poor imaging)

Red blood cell survival time

Normally, red blood cells (RBCs) are destroyed only when they reach senility. However, in hemolytic diseases, RBCs of all ages are randomly destroyed, resulting in anemia. The RBC survival time test measures the survival time of circulating RBCs and detects sites of abnormal RBC sequestration and destruction.

Survival time is measured by labeling a random sample of RBCs with radioactive chromium-51 sodium chromate (^{51}Cr). This labeled group of RBCs is then injected back into the patient. Serial blood samples measure the percentage of labeled cells per unit volume over 3 to 4 weeks until 50% of the cells disappear. (The disappearance rate corresponds to destruction of a random cell population.)

A normal RBC survives about 120 days (half-life of 60 days); the ^{51}Cr-labeled RBCs have a shorter half-life (25 to 30 days) because about 1% of senescent RBCs are removed from the circulation each day and about 1% of ^{51}Cr is spontaneously eluted from the labeled RBCs each day.

During the test period, a gamma camera scans the body for sites of abnormally high radioactivity, which indicates sites of excessive RBC sequestration and destruction. Other tests performed with the RBC survival time test may include spot-checks of the stool to detect GI blood loss, hematocrit, blood volume studies, and radionuclide iron uptake and clearance tests to aid in the differential diagnosis of anemia.

Purpose
■ To help evaluate unexplained anemia, particularly hemolytic anemia
■ To identify sites of abnormal RBC sequestration and destruction

Patient preparation
■ Explain to the patient that the RBC survival time test helps identify the cause of his anemia.
■ Advise the patient that he need not restrict food and fluids.
■ Explain to the patient that the test involves labeling a blood sample with a radioactive substance and requires regular blood samples at 3-day intervals for 3 to 4 weeks. Tell him who will perform the test and where it will take place.
■ Tell the patient that he may experience discomfort from the needle punctures

and the tourniquet. Reassure him that collecting each sample takes less than 3 minutes and that the small amount of radioactive substance used is harmless.

■ If stool collection is required to test for GI bleeding, teach the patient the proper collection technique.

■ Make sure that the patient or a responsible family member has signed an informed consent form.

Procedure and posttest care

■ A 30-ml blood sample is drawn and mixed with 100 microcuries of ^{51}Cr for an adult (less for a child).

■ After an incubation period, the mixture is injected intravenously into the patient. A blood sample is drawn 30 minutes after injection to determine blood and RBC volumes.

■ A 6-ml sample is collected in a heparinized tube after 24 hours; follow-up samples are collected at 3-day intervals for 3 to 4 weeks. (Intervals between samples may vary, depending on the laboratory.)

■ To avoid error from physical decay of the ^{51}Cr, each sample is measured with a scintillation well counter on the day it's drawn.

■ Radioactivity per milliliter of RBCs is calculated, and the values are plotted to determine mean RBC survival time. Simultaneous gamma camera scans of the precordium, sacrum, liver, and spleen detect radioactivity at sites of excess RBC sequestration. A hematocrit test is done on a small portion of each blood sample to check for blood loss.

■ At the end of the study, a sample is drawn to compare ending blood and RBC volumes with beginning volumes.

■ If a hematoma develops at the venipuncture site, apply warm soaks.

Precautions

■ This test is contraindicated during pregnancy because it exposes the fetus to radiation.

■ Because excess blood loss can invalidate test results, this test is usually contraindicated for a patient with active bleeding or poor clotting function. However, if the test is necessary for a patient with poor clotting function, observe the venipuncture sites carefully for signs of hemorrhage.

■ The patient shouldn't receive blood transfusions during the test period and shouldn't have blood samples drawn for other tests.

Normal findings

The normal half-life for RBCs labeled with ^{51}Cr is 25 to 30 days. Normal gamma camera scans reveal slight radioactivity in the spleen, liver, and sometimes the bone marrow.

Abnormal findings

Decreased RBC survival time indicates a hemolytic disease, such as chronic lymphocytic leukemia, congenital nonspherocytic hemolytic anemia, hemoglobin C disease, hereditary spherocytosis, idiopathic acquired hemolytic anemia, paroxysmal nocturnal hemoglobinuria, elliptocytosis, pernicious anemia, sickle cell anemia, sickle cell hemoglobin C disease, or hemolytic-uremic syndrome. If hemolytic anemia is diagnosed, additional tests using cross-transfusion of labeled RBCs can determine whether anemia results from an intrinsic RBC defect or an extrinsic factor.

A gamma camera scan that detects a site of excess RBC sequestration provides direction for treatment. For example, abnormally high RBC sequestration in the spleen may require a splenectomy.

Interfering factors
- Dehydration, overhydration, or blood loss (possible invalidation of results due to changed circulating RBC volume)
- Blood transfusions during the test period (alters proportion of labeled RBCs to total RBCs)

OTHER TESTS

D-xylose absorption

The D-xylose absorption test evaluates the patient with symptoms of malabsorption, such as weight loss and generalized malnutrition, weakness, and diarrhea. D-xylose is a pentose sugar that's absorbed in the small intestine without the aid of pancreatic enzymes, passes through the liver without being metabolized, and is excreted in the urine. Because of its absorption in the small intestine without digestion, measurement of D-xylose in the urine and blood indicates the absorptive capacity of the small intestine.

Purpose
- To aid in the differential diagnosis of malabsorption
- To determine the cause of malabsorption syndrome

Patient preparation
- Tell the patient that the D-xylose absorption test helps evaluate digestive function by analyzing blood samples and urine specimens after ingestion of a sugar solution.
- Explain to the patient that he must fast overnight before the test and that he'll have to fast and remain in bed during the test.
- Tell the patient that the test requires several blood samples. Explain who will perform the venipunctures and when.
- Explain to the patient that he may experience discomfort from the needle punctures and the tourniquet.
- Inform the patient that all his urine will be collected for 5 or 24 hours, as ordered.
- Withhold medications that alter test results, such as aspirin and indomethacin, as ordered. Record any medications the patient is taking on the laboratory request.

Procedure and posttest care
- Perform a venipuncture to obtain a fasting blood sample and collect the sample in a 10-ml tube without additives. Collect a first-voided morning urine specimen. Label these specimens and send them to the laboratory immediately to serve as a baseline.
- Give the patient 25 g of D-xylose dissolved in 8 oz (240 ml) of water, followed by an additional 8 oz of water. If the patient is a child, administer 0.5 g of D-xylose per pound of body weight, up to 25 g. Record the time of D-xylose ingestion.
- For an adult, draw a blood sample 2 hours after D-xylose ingestion; for a child, 1 hour after ingestion. Collect the sample in a 10-ml tube without additives. Occasionally, a 5-hour sample may be drawn to support the findings of the 1- or 2-hour sample.
- Collect and pool all urine during the 5 or 24 hours after D-xylose ingestion.
- If a hematoma develops at the venipuncture site, apply warm soaks.
- Observe the patient for abdominal discomfort or mild diarrhea caused by D-xylose ingestion.

■ Instruct the patient that he may resume his usual diet and medications, as ordered.

Precautions
■ Handle the sample gently to prevent hemolysis.
■ Tell the patient not to contaminate the urine specimens with toilet tissue or stool.
■ Be sure to collect all urine and refrigerate the specimen during the collection period.
■ Because patients age 65 and older and those with borderline or elevated creatinine levels tend to have low 5-hour urine levels but normal 24-hour levels, the physician will have to establish the length of the collection period. At the end of the collection period, send the urine specimen to the laboratory immediately.
■ Maintain bed rest and withhold food and fluids (other than D-xylose) throughout the test period.

Reference values
AGE ISSUE *Normal values are as follows:*
■ *children:* blood concentration > 30 mg/dl in 1 hour; urine, 16% to 33% of ingested D-xylose excreted in 5 hours
■ *adults:* blood concentration 25 to 40 mg/dl in 2 hours; urine, 3.5 g excreted in 5 hours (age 65 or older, > 5 g in 24 hours).

Abnormal findings
Depressed blood and urine D-xylose levels most commonly result from malabsorption disorders that affect the proximal small intestine, such as sprue and celiac disease. Depressed levels may also result from regional enteritis involving the jejunum, Whipple's disease, multiple jejunal diverticula, myxedema, diabetic neuropathic diarrhea, rheumatoid arthritis, alcoholism, severe heart failure, and ascites.

Interfering factors
■ Failure to observe pretest restrictions
■ Aspirin (decreased D-xylose excretion by the kidneys)
■ Indomethacin (decreased intestinal D-xylose absorption)
■ Failure to obtain a complete urine specimen or to collect blood samples at designated times
■ Intestinal overgrowth of bacteria, renal insufficiency, or renal retention of urine (possible drop in urine levels)

Dexamethasone suppression

The dexamethasone suppression test requires administration of dexamethasone, an oral steroid. Dexamethasone suppresses levels of circulating adrenal steroid hormones in normal people, but fails to suppress them in patients with Cushing's syndrome and some forms of clinical depression.

Purpose
■ To diagnose Cushing's syndrome
■ To aid in the diagnosis of clinical depression

Patient preparation
■ Explain to the patient the purpose of the dexamethasone suppression test.
■ Inform the patient that the test requires two blood samples drawn after administration of dexamethasone. Explain who will perform the venipunctures and when.
■ Explain to the patient that he may experience discomfort from the needle punctures and the tourniquet.

- Restrict food and fluids for 10 to 12 hours before the test.

Procedure and posttest care
- On the first day, give the patient 1 mg of dexamethasone at 11 p.m. On the next day, collect blood samples at 4 p.m. and 11 p.m. More frequent sampling may increase the likelihood of measuring a nonsuppressed cortisol peak.
- If a hematoma develops at the venipuncture site, apply warm soaks.

Precautions
- Many medications, including corticosteroids, oral contraceptives, lithium, methadone, aspirin, diuretics, morphine, and monoamine oxidase (MAO) inhibitors, can affect the accuracy of test results. If possible, don't administer any of these medications for 24 to 48 hours before the test, as ordered.

Normal findings
A cortisol level of 5 g/dl (140 nmol/L) or greater indicates failure of dexamethasone suppression.

Abnormal findings
A normal test result doesn't rule out major depression, but an abnormal result strengthens a clinically based diagnosis. Failure of suppression occurs in the patient with Cushing's syndrome, severe stress, and depression that's likely to respond to treatment with antidepressants.

Interfering factors
- Diabetes mellitus, pregnancy, and severe stress, such as trauma, severe weight loss, dehydration, and acute alcohol withdrawal (possible false-positive)
- Certain drugs, particularly barbiturates or phenytoin, within 3 weeks of the test (possible false-positive)

- Caffeine consumed after midnight the night before the test (possible false-positive)
- Failure to withhold corticosteroids, oral contraceptives, lithium, methadone, aspirin, diuretics, morphine, or MAO inhibitors for 24 to 48 hours before the test

Selected readings

Cavanaugh, B.M. *Nurse's Manual of Laboratory and Diagnostic Tests,* 4th ed. Philadelphia: F.A. Davis Co., 2003.

Goldman, L., and Ausiello, D., eds. *Cecil Textbook of Medicine,* 22nd ed. Philadelphia: W.B. Saunders Co., 2004.

Guyton, A.C., and Hall, J.E. *Textbook of Medical Physiology,* 10th ed. Philadelphia: W.B. Saunders Co., 2001.

McClatchey, K.D. *Clinical Laboratory Medicine,* 2nd ed. Philadelphia: Lippincott Williams & Wilkins, 2002.

Pagana, K.D., and Pagana, T.J. *Mosby's Diagnostic and Laboratory Test Reference,* 6th ed. St. Louis: Mosby Year-Book, Inc., 2003.

Schnell, Z., et al. *Davis's Comprehensive Handbook of Laboratory and Diagnostic Tests with Nursing Implications.* Philadelphia: F.A. Davis Co., 2003.

Williams, P.B., et al. "Are Our Impressions of Allergy Test Performances Correct?" *Annals of Allergy, Asthma, and Immunology* 91(1):26-33, July 2003.

Appendices
Index

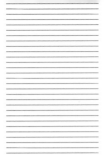

Collection techniques:
Blood and urine samples

Blood

The type of blood sample that's required for a test — whole blood, plasma, or serum — depends on the nature of the test. *Whole blood* — containing all blood elements — is the sample of choice for blood gas analysis, determination of hemoglobin derivatives, and measurement of red blood cell (RBC) constituents. In addition, most routine hematologic studies, such as complete blood count, erythrocyte sedimentation rate, reticulocyte and platelet counts, and the osmotic fragility test, require whole blood samples.

Plasma is the liquid part of whole blood, which contains all the blood proteins; *serum* is the liquid that remains after whole blood clots. Plasma and serum samples, which contain most of the physiologically and clinically significant substances found in blood, are used for most biochemical, immunologic, and coagulation studies. They also provide electrolyte evaluation, enzyme analysis, glucose concentration, protein determination, and bilirubin level.

Venous, arterial, and capillary blood

Venous blood returns to the heart through the veins. It carries a high concentration of carbon dioxide from the cells back to the lungs for exhalation. Because venous blood represents physiologic conditions throughout the body and is relatively easy to obtain, it's used for most laboratory procedures.

Arterial blood, replenished with oxygen from the lungs, leaves the heart through the arteries to distribute nutrients throughout the capillary network. Although an arterial puncture increases the risks of hematoma and arterial spasm, arterial blood samples are necessary for determining pH, partial pressure of arterial oxygen, partial pressure of carbon dioxide, and oxygen saturation.

Capillary, or peripheral, blood does the real work of the circulatory system — exchanging fluids, nutrients, and wastes between blood and tissues. Capillary blood samples are most useful for such studies as hemoglobin and hematocrit determinations; blood smears; microtechniques for clinical chemistry; and platelet, RBC, and white blood cell counts requiring only small amounts of blood. (See *Common arterial and venous puncture sites*, page 950.)

Quantities and containers

The most recent guidelines from the Centers for Disease Control and Prevention mandate that gloves always be worn when obtaining and handling blood and urine specimens as well as any other body fluid. (See *Standard precautions*, pages 951 and 952.)

Sample quantities needed for diagnostic studies depend on the laboratory, available equipment, and the type of test. Some laboratories, for example, use automated analyzer systems that require a serum sample of 100 µl or less; others use manual systems that require a larger amount. The desired sample quantity de-

termines the collection procedure and the type and size of the container. A single venipuncture with a conventional glass or disposable plastic syringe can provide 10 ml of blood — sufficient for many hematologic, immunologic, chemical, and coagulation tests, but hardly enough for a series of tests.

To avoid multiple venipunctures when tests require a large blood sample, use an evacuated tube system (Vacutainer, Corvac) with interchangeable glass tubes, optional draw capacities, and a selection of additives. Evacuated tubes are commercially prepared with or without additives (indicated by their color-coded stopper) and with enough vacuum to draw a predetermined blood volume (2 to 20 ml per tube). (See "Guide to color-top collection tubes," page 967.)

Microanalysis of minute amounts of capillary blood collected with micropipettes or glass capillary tubes allows numerous hemtologic and routine laboratory studies to be performed on infants, children, and patients with severe burns or poor veins. Micropipettes are color-coded by sample capacity and hold 30 to 50 µl of whole blood; glass capillary tubes hold 80 to 130 µl of serum or plasma.

Equipment

For venipuncture: gloves; tourniquet; 70% alcohol or povidone-iodine solution; sterile syringes or evacuated tubes; sterile needle (20G or 21G for forearm; 25G for wrist, hand, or ankle and for children); color-coded tubes with appropriate additives; identification labels; small adhesive bandage; sterile 2″ × 2″ gauze pads.

For arterial blood: gloves; 1.0 ml vented, heparinized syringe; 20G 1½″ short-bevel needle; 23G 1″ short-bevel needle; rubber stopper or cork; antiseptic swabs; 70% alcohol or povidone-iodine solution; sterile 2″ × 2″ gauze pads; tape or adhesive bandage; iced specimen container; labels (for syringe and specimen

(Text continues on page 953.)

COMMON ARTERIAL AND VENOUS PUNCTURE SITES

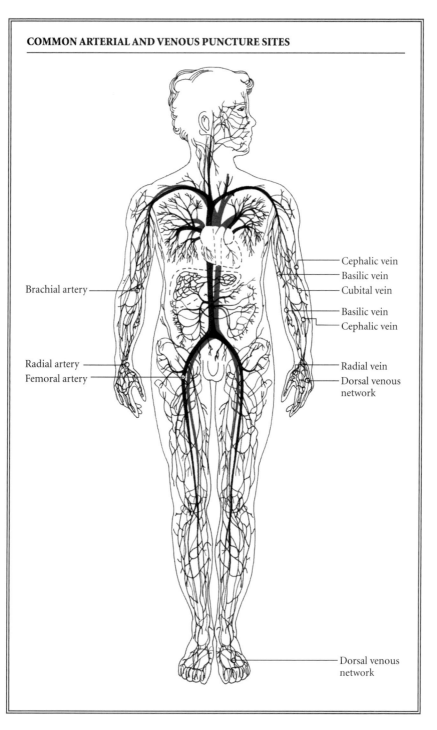

Brachial artery

Radial artery
Femoral artery

Cephalic vein
Basilic vein
Cubital vein

Basilic vein
Cephalic vein

Radial vein
Dorsal venous
network

Dorsal venous
network

STANDARD PRECAUTIONS

The Centers for Disease Control and Prevention (CDC) and the Hospital Infection Control Practices Advisory Committee have developed two categories of guidelines for preventing the transmission of nosocomial infections. These latest guidelines — *standard precautions* and *transmission-based precautions* — have replaced the previous *universal precautions* and *category-specific guidelines.* The transmission-based precautions are further divided into three types, based on the mode of transmission: *airborne precautions, droplet precautions,* and *contact precautions.*

Standard precautions are designed to decrease the risk of transmitting organisms from both recognized and unrecognized sources of infection in hospitals. They should be followed at all times, with every patient.

Standard precautions combine the major features of the former universal precautions, which were developed in response to the increasing incidence of human immunodeficiency virus (HIV), hepatitis B virus (HBV), and other blood-borne diseases, and the former *body-substance isolation precautions,* which were developed to reduce the risk of pathogen transmission from moist body surfaces. Because standard precautions reduce the risk of transmitting blood-borne and other pathogens, many patients with diseases that previously required category-specific or disease-specific isolation precautions now require only standard precautions.

The specific substances covered by standard precautions include blood and all other body excretions, except sweat, even if blood isn't visible. Standard precautions should also be followed in the presence of nonintact skin or exposed mucous membranes.

Transmission-based precautions should be followed — in addition to standard precautions — whenever a pa-

tient is known or suspected to be infected with a highly contagious and epidemiologically important pathogen that's transmitted by air, by droplets, or by contact with dry skin or other contaminated surfaces. Examples include the pathogens that cause measles (transmitted by air), influenza (transmitted by droplets), and GI, respiratory, skin, and wound infections (transmitted by contact).

Transmission-based precautions replace all previous categories of isolation precautions, including strict isolation, contact isolation, respiratory isolation, enteric precautions, and drainage and secretion precautions, as well as other disease-specific precautions. One or more transmission-based precautions may be combined when a patient has a disease with multiple modes of transmission.

Equipment
Gloves, masks, goggles, or face shields; gowns or aprons; resuscitation masks; bags for specimens; 1:10 dilution of bleach to water (mixed daily) or hospital-strength disinfectant certified effective against HIV and HBV.

Implementation
■ Wash your hands immediately if they become contaminated with blood or body fluids; also wash them before and after patient care and after removing gloves (as shown below). Hand washing

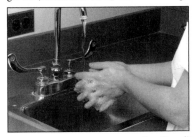

(continued)

STANDARD PRECAUTIONS *(continued)*

retards the growth of organisms on your skin.

■ Wear a gown and face shield (or goggles and a mask) during procedures that are likely to generate droplets of blood or bodily fluids, such as surgery, endoscopic procedures, and dialysis (as shown below).

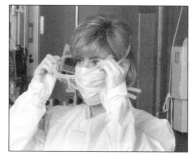

■ Wear gloves if you will, or could, come in contact with blood, specimens, tissue, body fluids, or excretions as well as contaminated surfaces or objects (as shown below). Change your gloves between patient contacts to prevent cross-contamination.

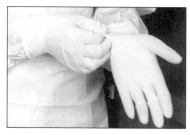

■ Handle used needles and other sharp implements carefully. Don't bend or break them, reinsert them into their original sheaths, or handle them unnecessarily. Discard them intact immediately after use in a sharps biohazard container. These measures reduce the risk of accidental injury or infection.

■ Notify your employee health provider immediately about all needle-stick injuries, mucosal splashes, and contamination of open wounds with blood or body fluids to allow investigation of the accident and appropriate care and documentation.

■ Properly label all specimens collected from patients, and place them in plastic biohazard bags at the collection site.

■ Promptly clean all blood and body fluids with a 1:10 dilution of bleach to water (mixed daily) or with an approved hospital-strength disinfectant that's effective against HIV and HBV.

■ Disposable food trays and dishes aren't necessary.

■ If you have an exudative lesion, avoid all direct patient contact until the condition has resolved and you've been cleared by your employee health provider. Intact skin is your best defense against infection.

Special considerations
Standard precautions are intended to supplement — not replace — recommendations for routine infection control, such as hand washing and wearing gloves.

Keep mouthpieces, resuscitation bags, and other ventilation devices nearby to minimize the need for emergency mouth-to-mouth resuscitation, thus reducing the risk of exposure to body fluids.

Because precautions can't be specified for every clinical situation, you must use your judgment in individual cases. If your job requires you to be exposed to blood, make sure you receive an HBV vaccine.

Complications
Failure to follow standard precautions may lead to exposure to blood-borne diseases and all the complications they may incur.

bag) for patient's name and identification number, physician's name, date, collection time, and details of oxygen therapy.

For capillary blood: gloves; sterile, disposable blood lancet; sterile 2″ × 2″ gauze pads; 70% alcohol or povidone-iodine solution; glass slides, heparinized capillary tubes or pipettes; appropriate solutions.

Venous sample

The nature of the test and the patient's age and condition determine the appropriate blood sample, collection site, and technique. Most tests require a venous sample. Although a relatively simple procedure, venipuncture must be performed carefully to avoid hemolysis or hemoconcentration of the sample, to prevent hematoma formation, and to prevent damage to the patient's veins. (See *How to collect a venous sample,* pages 954 and 955.) Label all test tubes clearly with the patient's name, date, and collection time.

Select a venipuncture site. The most common site is the antecubital fossa area; other sites are the wrist and the dorsum of the hand or foot. When drawing the sample at bedside, instruct the patient to lie on his back, with his head slightly elevated and his arms resting at his sides. When drawing blood from an ambulatory patient, have him sit in a chair, with his arm supported on an armrest or a table. Restrain small children if necessary.

Always wash your hands and put on gloves before drawing a blood sample. When using an evacuated tube, attach the needle to the holder before applying the tourniquet. Unless cautioned otherwise, apply a soft rubber tourniquet above the puncture site to increase venous pressure, which makes the veins more prominent. Make sure the tourniquet is snug but not constrictive. If the patient's veins appear distinct, you may not need to apply a tourniquet. Using a tourniquet for a patient with large, distended, and highly visible veins increases the risk of hema-toma. Do the venipuncture below all I.V. sites or in the opposite arm. Instruct the patient to make a fist several times to enlarge the veins. Select a vein by palpation and inspection. If you can't feel a vein distinctly, *don't* attempt the venipuncture. (See *Safeguards for venipuncture,* pages 954 and 955.)

Working in a circular motion from the center outward, clean the puncture site with alcohol or povidone-iodine solution, and dry it with a gauze pad. If you must touch the cleaned puncture site again to relocate the vein, palpate with an antiseptically clean finger, and wipe the area again with an alcohol pad. Draw the skin tautly over the vein by pressing just below the pressure site with your thumb to keep the vein from moving.

Hold the syringe tube with the needle bevel up and the shaft parallel to the path of the vein at a 15-degree angle to the arm. Enter the vein with a single direct puncture of the skin and vein wall. If you use a syringe, venous blood will appear in the hub. Withdraw the blood slowly, gently pulling on the syringe to create steady suction until you obtain the desired amount. If you're using an evacuated tube, when a drop of blood appears just inside the needle holder, grasp the needle holder securely and push down on the collection tube until the needle punctures the rubber stopper; blood will then flow into the tube automatically. When the tube is filled, remove it; if you're drawing multiple samples, repeat the procedure with additional tubes.

To prevent stasis, release the tourniquet as soon as you establish adequate blood flow. If the flow is sluggish, you may want to leave the tourniquet in place longer. However, always remove the tourniquet before withdrawing the needle.

After drawing the sample, ask the patient to open his fist as soon as you collect the desired amount. Release the tourniquet. Place a gauze pad over the

HOW TO COLLECT A VENOUS SAMPLE

Gather the necessary equipment. Wash your hands thoroughly and put on gloves. Screw the Vacutainer needle into the sleeve (as shown).

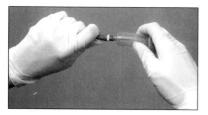

Select a venipuncture site, usually the antecubital fossa. Apply a soft rubber tourniquet above the venipuncture site. Then, using a circular motion, clean the area first with povidone-iodone solution (as shown) and then with alcohol.

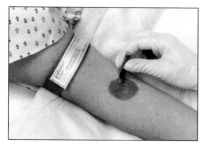

Remove the needle cover from the Vacutainer needle. With the bevel facing up, insert the needle into the patient's vein at a 15-degree angle (as shown).

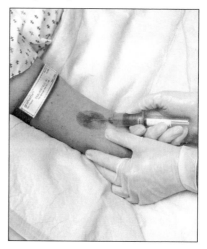

When a drop of blood appears just inside the needle holder, gently push the Vacutainer tube into the needle sleeve, so the blood enters the tube. Try to keep the needle still to prevent it from penetrating the patient's vein. When the tube is filled, remove the tourniquet.

SAFEGUARDS FOR VENIPUNCTURE

■ Make sure the patient is adequately supported in case of syncope.
■ To avoid injecting air into a vein when using a syringe to withdraw a sample, first make sure that the plunger is fully depressed.
■ Avoid drawing blood from an arm or leg used for I.V. infusion of blood, dextrose, or electrolyte solutions because this dilutes the blood sample. If you must collect blood near an I.V. site, choose a location below it.

■ For easier identification of veins in patients with tortuous or sclerosed veins or veins damaged by repeated venipuncture, antimicrobial therapy, or chemotherapy, apply warm, wet compresses 15 minutes before attempting venipuncture.
■ If you aren't successful after two attempts, ask another nurse to do the venipuncture.
■ When you can't find a vein quickly, release the tourniquet temporarily to avoid tissue necrosis and circulation problems.

If another specimen is needed, gently remove the filled Vacutainer tube and place another tube into the needle. When collection is complete, remove the tourniquet and place a 1″ × 1″ gauze pad over the venipuncture site (as shown), apply direct pressure, and remove the needle.

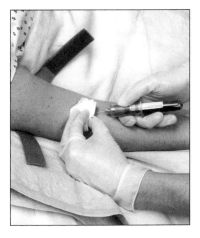

After 2 to 3 minutes, cover the site with an adhesive bandage.

■ Be sure to insert the needle at the correct angle to reduce the risk of puncturing the opposite wall of the vein and causing a hematoma.
■ Always release the tourniquet before withdrawing the needle to prevent a hematoma. When drawing multiple samples, release the tourniquet within 1 minute after beginning to draw blood to prevent a hemoconcentration sample.

puncture site; then withdraw the needle slowly and gently. Apply gentle pressure to the puncture site. If the patient is alert and cooperative, tell him to hold the gauze pad in place for several minutes until the bleeding stops to prevent hematoma. If the patient isn't alert or cooperative, hold the pad in place or apply a small adhesive bandage.

After collection with a syringe, remove the needle and carefully empty the sample into the appropriate test tube without delay. To prevent foaming and hemolysis, *don't* eject the blood through the needle or force it out of the syringe. Place the appropriate color-coded stoppers on the tubes. Gently invert a tube containing an anticoagulant several times to mix the sample thoroughly. Examine the sample for clots or clumps; if none appear, send the sample to the laboratory. *Don't* shake the tube.

Before leaving the patient, check his condition. If a hematoma develops at the puncture site, apply warm soaks. If the patient has lingering discomfort or excessive bleeding, instruct him to lie down. Watch for anxiety or signs of shock, such as hypotension and tachycardia. Send the sample to the laboratory immediately.

Many laboratories use automated electronic systems that can perform multiple tests on a blood sample. (See *Automatic test series: SMA 12/60 and SMAC,* page 956.)

Arterial sample

Arterial blood is rarely required for routine studies. Because arterial puncture carries risks, samples are usually collected by a physician or a specially trained nurse. Before drawing an arterial blood sample, administer a local anesthetic at the puncture site, if necessary. If available, you may use an arterial blood gas (ABG) kit, which contains all the necessary equipment, including a heparinized syringe. Perform Allen's test to assess radial artery circulation. (See *Performing Allen's test,* page 957.) Try to obtain the

AUTOMATIC TEST SERIES: SMA 12/60 AND SMAC

Many laboratories use automated electronic systems, such as the sequential multiple analyzer (SMA) 12/60 and the sequential multiple analyzer with computer (SMAC), to perform chemistry, blood banking, serologic, and bacteriologic tests. (Many laboratories have SMA 6, 12, and 20.)

The SMA 12/60 can make 12 determinations on 60 serum specimens in 1 hour: glucose, cholesterol, albumin, total protein levels (nutritional status); bilirubin levels (liver function); blood urea nitrogen (BUN) and uric acid levels (kidney function); aspartate aminotransferase (AST) and lactate dehydrogenase (LD) enzyme levels (tissue injury); alkaline phosphatase levels (bone tissue injury); and calcium and phosphate levels (parathyroid function).

The SMAC can perform 20 to 40 biochemical determinations on 120 serum specimens in 1 hour. It can analyze selected blood components, singly or in combination, and provide an entire test profile on each specimen. This system also automatically reports special cardiac, renal, hepatic, lipid, bone, enzyme, and electrolyte profiles.

Tests performed on a 450-μl sample include cholesterol, triglycerides, glucose, BUN, calcium, phosphorus, sodium, potassium, chloride, carbon dioxide, total protein, total bilirubin, albumin, creatinine, gammaglutamyltransferase, AST, alanine aminotransferase, LD, uric acid, acid and alkaline phosphatase, and iron.

specimen from the radial artery; use the brachial artery only when necessary. Don't use the arm if the patient has had a vascular graft or has an arterioventricular fistula in situ.

Next, using a circular motion, clean the puncture site with povidone-iodine solution. Then wipe the site with alcohol to remove any povidone-iodine solution, which is sticky and may hinder palpation. Palpate the artery with the forefinger and middle finger of one hand while holding the syringe over the puncture site with the other hand. With the needle bevel up, puncture the skin at a 45-degree angle for the radial artery and a 60-degree angle for the brachial artery. For a femoral arterial puncture, the needle is inserted at a 90-degreee angle.

Advance the needle, but don't pull the plunger back. When you've punctured the artery, blood will pulsate into the syringe. Allow 5 to 10 ml to fill the syringe. If the syringe doesn't fill immediately, you may have pushed the needle through the artery. If so, pull the needle back slightly, but don't pull the plunger back. If the syringe still doesn't fill, withdraw the needle and start over with a fresh heparinized needle. Never make more than two attempts to draw blood from one site.

After drawing the sample, remove the needle and apply firm pressure to the puncture site with a gauze pad for at least 5 minutes to prevent hematoma (a significant risk after arterial puncture). If the patient is receiving an anticoagulant or has a bleeding disorder, apply pressure for at least 15 minutes. *Don't* ask the patient to apply pressure to the site; he may not apply the continuous, firm pressure that's needed.

Rotate the syringe to mix the heparin with the sample. Try to remove air bubbles by holding the syringe upright and tapping it lightly with your finger. If the

PERFORMING ALLEN'S TEST

Before obtaining a specimen from an arterial site, assess the blood supply to your patient's hand. If the radial artery is blocked by a blood clot — a common complication — the ulnar artery alone must supply blood to the hand. The Allen's test is a simple, reliable procedure that quickly assesses arterial function.

Just follow these steps:

1. Have the patient rest his arm on the bedside table. Support his wrist with a rolled towel. Ask him to clench his fist. Use your index and middle fingers to exert pressure over both the radial and the ulnar arteries (as shown).

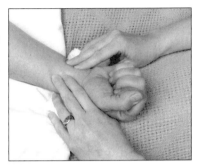

2. Without removing your fingers, ask the patient to unclench his fist (as shown). You'll notice his palm is blanched because you've impaired the normal blood flow with your fingers.

Nursing tip: If your patient is unconscious or unable to clench his fist for some other reason, you can encourage his palm to blanch by occluding both arteries, elevating his hand, and massaging his palm.

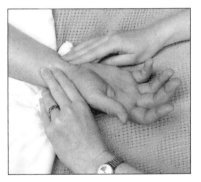

3. Release the pressure on the ulnar artery and ask the patient to open his fist (as shown).

If the ulnar artery is functioning well, his palm will turn pink in about 5 seconds, even though the radial artery is still occluded. But if blood return is slow and his fingers begin to contract, blood supply from the ulnar artery may not be adequate. In that case, try Allen's test on his other wrist; you may get better results. *Note:* Slow blood return may indicate poor cardiac output or poor capillary refill due to shock.

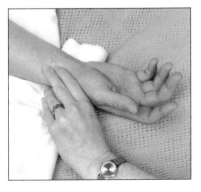

bubbles don't disappear, hold the syringe upright and pierce a 2″ × 2″ gauze pad or alcohol pad with the needle. (Slowly forcing some of the blood out of the syringe eliminates the bubbles, and the gauze pad catches the ejected blood.) After removing air bubbles, plunge the needle into a rubber stopper to seal it, or remove the needle and apply the syringe stopper from the ABG kit, if available. Transfer the sample to the iced specimen container.

Note on the laboratory request the type and amount of oxygen the patient is receiving. In certain instances (such as hypothermia), you may also be asked to provide the patient's temperature and hemoglobin count. Send the sample to the laboratory immediately.

After releasing pressure on the puncture site, tape a bandage firmly over it. (Don't tape the entire wrist.)

▶ **CLINICAL ALERT** After arterial puncture, observe the patient closely for signs of circulatory impairment distal to the puncture site, such as swelling or discoloration. Ask if he feels pain, numbness, or tingling in the extremity.

Before drawing an arterial blood sample for ABG analysis, check the patient's oxygen therapy. If ABG levels are being measured to monitor his response to withdrawal of oxygen but the patient continues to receive it, results will be misleading. For the same reason, wait 15 to 30 minutes before drawing an arterial sample after suctioning the patient or placing him on a ventilator to allow circulating blood levels to reflect mechanical ventilation. Blood gases shouldn't be drawn during dialysis.

Capillary sample
Collection of a capillary blood sample requires puncturing the fingertip or earlobe of adults or the great toe or heel of neonates. To facilitate collection of a capillary sample, first dilate the vessels by applying warm, moist compresses to the area for about 10 minutes. Select the puncture site, wipe it with gauze and alcohol pads, and dry it thoroughly with another gauze pad so the blood will well up. Avoid cold, cyanotic, or swollen sites to ensure an adequate blood sample. To draw a sample from the fingertip, use an automatic lancing device and make the puncture perpendicular to the lines of the patient's fingerprints.

After drawing the sample, wipe away the first drop of blood and avoid squeezing the puncture to reduce the risk of diluting the sample with tissue fluid. After collecting the sample, apply pressure to the puncture site briefly to prevent painful extravasation of blood into the subcutaneous tissues. Ask the adult patient to hold a sterile gauze pad over the puncture site until bleeding has stopped. Then apply a small adhesive bandage.

Interfering factors
Because food and medications can interfere with test methods, be sure to check the patient's diet and medication history before testing, and schedule tests after an overnight fast of 12 to 14 hours. Although the concentration of most blood constituents doesn't change significantly after a meal, fasting is customary because blood collected shortly after eating often appears cloudy (turbid) from a temporary increase in triglyceride levels, which can interfere with many chemical reactions. Transient, food-related lipemia usually disappears in 4 to 6 hours after a meal, making such short fasts acceptable before blood collection. Baseline studies often depend on the patient's diet. For example, valid glucose tolerance test results require an adequate daily carbohydrate intake (250 mg) for 3 days before testing. Similarly, recent protein and fat consumption influences uric acid, urea, and lipid levels.

Numerous drugs and their metabolites can affect test results by pharmacologic or chemical interference. Pharmacologic interference results from temporary or permanent drug-induced physiologic changes in a blood component. For example, long-term administration of aminoglycosides can damage the kidneys and alter the results of renal function studies. Chemical interference results from a drug's physical characteristic that alters the test reaction. For example, high doses of ascorbic acid may raise blood glucose levels. To identify such interference with test results, all unexpected changes in blood values require a meticulous review of the patient's drug and dietary history and of his clinical status.

Urine

The type of urine specimen required—random, second-voided, clean-catch midstream, first morning, fasting, or timed—depends on the patient's condition and the purpose of the test. Random, second-voided, and clean-catch midstream specimens can be collected at any time; first morning, fasting, and timed specimens require collection at specific times.

To collect a *random specimen* (for such routine tests as urinalysis), the patient simply collects urine from one voiding in a specimen container. Although this method provides quick laboratory results, the information it supplies is less reliable than that from a controlled specimen.

To collect a *second-voided specimen,* the patient voids, discards the urine, and then voids again 30 minutes later into a specimen container.

To collect a *clean-catch specimen,* the patient voids first into either a bedpan or toilet and then collects a sample in midstream. Originally used mainly to test for bacteriuria and pyuria, this type of specimen is now replacing the random specimen because it's aseptic.

First morning and *fasting specimens* must be collected when the patient awakens. Because the first morning specimen is the most concentrated of the day, it's the specimen of choice for nitrate, protein, and urinary sediment analyses. To obtain this specimen, the patient voids and discards the urine before going to bed, then collects the urine from the first voiding of the morning. For the fasting specimen, which is used for glucose testing, the patient maintains an overnight fast and collects a first morning specimen.

A *timed specimen* determines the urinary concentration of such substances as hormones, proteins, creatinine, and electrolytes over a specified period—usually 2, 12, or 24 hours. The 24-hour collection, the most common duration, provides a measure of average excretion for substances eliminated in variable amounts during the day, such as hormones. A timed specimen may also be collected after administration of a challenge dose of a chemical, to measure physiologic efficiency—for example, ingestion of glucose to test for incipient diabetes mellitus or hypoglycemia. This type of specimen is also preferred for quantitative analysis of urobilogen, amylase, or dye excretion.

Equipment

For random, second-voided, first morning, or fasting collections: clean, dry bedpan or urinal (for nonambulatory patients); gloves; specimen container; specimen labels; laboratory request.

For clean-catch midstream collection: commercially prepared kit containing necessary equipment and directions for the patient in several languages (English, Spanish, French); or antiseptic solution (green soap or povidone-iodine solution); water; cotton balls; sterile gloves; specimen labels; laboratory request.

For timed collection (24-hour specimen): clean, dry gallon containers or commercial urine collection containers; preservative, as ordered; labels for collection container; display signs.

For pediatric urine collection: gloves; plastic disposable collection bags; specimen containers; laboratory request; cotton swabs; soap and water; diapers.

Random and second-voided collections

For random collection, tell the ambulatory patient to urinate directly into a clean, dry specimen container. Tell the nonambulatory patient to void into a clean bedpan or urinal to minimize bacterial or chemical contamination; then put on gloves, transfer about 30 ml of urine to the specimen container, and secure the cap.

For second-voided collection, instruct the patient to void and discard the urine. Then offer him at least one glass of water to stimulate urine production. Collect urine 30 minutes later, using the random collection technique.

Label the specimen container with the patient's name and room number (if applicable), physician's name, date, and collection time. Send the labeled container to the laboratory immediately. On the chart, record the procedure and the time the specimen was sent.

First morning and fasting collections

Unless the patient is an infant or is catheterized or unable to urinate, use these collection techniques.

For fasting specimen collection, instruct the patient to restrict food and fluids after midnight before the test. For both collection procedures, instruct the patient to void and discard the urine before retiring for the night and then collect the first voiding of the next day in a clean, dry specimen container. (If the patient must void during the night, note it on the specimen label—for example, "Urine specimen, 2:15 a.m. to 8:00 a.m.")

Label the container with the patient's name and room number (if applicable), physician's name, date, and collection time. Send the specimen and a completed request to the laboratory immediately. On the chart, record the procedure and the time the specimen was sent.

Clean-catch midstream collection

This aseptic technique for obtaining a clean-catch midstream urine specimen has become the acceptable procedure for collecting a random urine specimen. It's especially valuable for collecting urine specimens from women because it provides a specimen that's virtually free of bacterial contamination.

Teach the patient how to obtain a clean-catch midstream specimen. Send the specimen to the laboratory immediately or refrigerate it to prevent proliferation of bacteria. On the chart, record the procedure and the time the specimen was sent.

Timed collection

All timed specimens—2-, 12-, and 24-hour—are collected in virtually the same way. The procedure is used for uncatheterized adults and continent children.

Explain the procedure to the patient, and instruct him to collect all urine during the test period, to notify you after each voiding, and to avoid contaminating the specimen with toilet tissue or stool. Also, provide him with written instructions for home collection. Explain any necessary dietary, drug, or activity restrictions.

Obtain the proper preservative from the laboratory. Write down the test requirements on the nursing care Kardex. Label a gallon jug or a commercial urine collection container with the patient's name and room number (if applicable); the physician's name, the date and time the collection begins and ends; a "Do Not Discard" warning; and instructions to keep the container refrigerated. Prominently display signs indicating that a 24-hour urine collection is in progress: one at the head of the patient's bed, a second over the toilet bowl in his bathroom, and a third over the utility room bedpan hopper.

Tell the patient to void and discard the urine; then begin a 24-hour collection with the next voiding. After placing the urine from the first voiding in the container, add the preservative. Add each subsequent urine specimen to the container immediately. If any urine is lost, restart the test, but remember that the test should end at a time when the laboratory is open. Just before the end of the collection period, instruct the patient to void, and add the urine to the gallon jug.

Send the labeled container to the laboratory as soon as the collection period has ended. On the chart, record the time that urine collection ended and when the specimen was sent to the laboratory.

Special timed collection

Some tests require specimen collection at specified times — for example, the glucose tolerance test requires collection of urine at 30 minutes, 1 hour, 2 hours, 3 hours and, occasionally, 4 and 5 hours after a test meal. To ensure that the patient can void at the specified times, have him drink water at least every hour. Other tests, including urea clearance, require only 2-hour collection periods. For these tests, give the patient at least 20 oz (600 ml) of water 30 minutes before the test, and instruct him to drink at least one full glass each hour during the test.

Pediatric urine collection

Pediatric urine collection is used to obtain a random, second-voided, first morning, fasting, or timed specimen from infants.

Position the infant on his back, with his hips externally rotated and abducted, and knees flexed. Put on gloves. Clean the perineal area with cotton swabs, soap, and water. Rinse the area with warm water and dry it thoroughly.

For *boys,* apply the collection device over the penis and scrotum with gloved hands, and closely press the flaps of the bag against the perineum to secure it. For *girls,* put on gloves, and tape the pediatric collection device to the perineum, starting between the anus and the vagina and working anteriorly. (See *Applying a pediatric urine collector,* page 962.) Place a diaper over the collection bag to discourage the child from tampering with it. Elevate the head of the bed to facilitate drainage.

Remove the bag immediately after collection is complete to prevent skin excoriation. Transfer the urine to a clean, dry specimen container. Label the container with the patient's name and room number (if applicable), physician's name, date, and collection time. Send the specimen and the completed request to the laboratory immediately, and note the collection time on the chart.

Catheter collection

Although catheter collection increases the risk of bacterial infection in the lower genitourinary tract, it may be necessary to obtain a random, second-voided, first morning, fasting, or timed specimen in a patient who can't void voluntarily.

Have the necessary equipment available: sterile catheterization set (sterile gloves, sterile catheter [#16F for adults or appropriate size catheter according to the size of the child]); sterile forceps; soap, water, towelette; sterile water-soluble lubricant; sterile cotton balls; antiseptic solution; sterile drapes; sterile specimen container; labels for specimen container.

Tell the patient you'll collect a urine specimen by inserting a small tube into the bladder through the urethra and that, although the procedure may cause some discomfort, it takes only a few minutes. (See *Inserting a straight urinary catheter,* page 963.)

APPLYING A PEDIATRIC URINE COLLECTOR

To attach a plastic urine collector to an infant girl (left), stretch the perineum to smooth the skin around the vagina. Working upward from the perineum, press the bag's adhesive ring inside the labia. To attach the collector to an infant boy (right), make sure the adhesive seal attaches firmly to the skin and doesn't pucker.

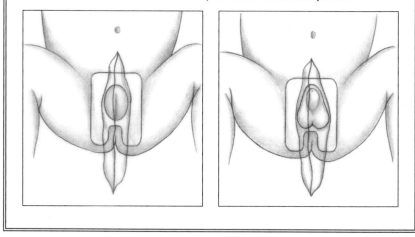

Male catheterization: Put on gloves and wash the perineal area with soap and water. Place a sterile drape under the patient's buttocks and around the penis, making sure that you don't contaminate the drape. Remove the contaminated gloves, and put on sterile gloves. Place the antiseptic solution on the cotton balls. Arrange all sterile articles within easy reach on a sterile wrapper. Open the sterile specimen container, and lubricate the sterile catheter. Grasp the shaft of the penis in one hand and elevate it about 90 degrees to the upright position: hold it in this position until the procedure is completed.

Retract the foreskin and, with the forceps, grasp an antiseptic-moistened cotton ball. Clean the urethral meatus, wiping with a circular motion away from the urethral opening toward the glans. Repeat twice, each time with a clean cotton ball. Hold the penis straight and *gently* insert the lubricated catheter into the urinary meatus until urine flows. Allow a few milliliters to drain into the basin; then collect 10 to 60 ml in a sterile plastic container, depending on test requirements. After gently removing the catheter, clean and dry the periurethral area.

Send the specimen and the laboratory request to the laboratory within 10 minutes, or refrigerate the specimen. On the chart, record the procedure and the time the specimen was sent.

Female catheterization: Put on gloves. After washing the perineal area with soap and water, place the patient in the supine position, with knees flexed and feet on the bed. Place a sterile drape under her buttocks and around the perineal area, making sure that you don't contaminate the drape. Remove the contaminated gloves, and put on sterile gloves. Place the antiseptic solution on the cotton balls, and lubricate the sterile catheter. Arrange all sterile articles within easy reach on a

INSERTING A STRAIGHT URINARY CATHETER

1. Obtain a prepackaged sterile insertion kit, which contains sterile gloves, drapes (regular and fenestrated), cotton balls, forceps, water-soluble lubricant, a urine collection basin, a sterile urine specimen container with label, and povidone-iodine or another antiseptic solution. If the prepackaged kit doesn't contain a urinary catheter, obtain one in the proper size. You should also gather a washcloth and towel, gloves, soap and water, a biohazard bag, and a reliable light source.

Explain the procedure to the patient and reassure him.

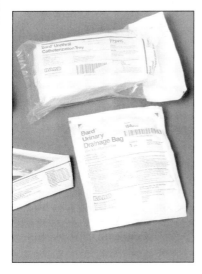

2. Position a female patient flat on her back, with her knees bent and her legs abducted. Place a linen-saver pad under her buttocks, and position her feet about 2′ (160 cm) apart (as shown). Direct the light source toward the perineum.

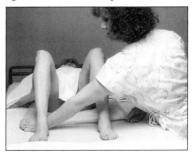

3. Put on gloves and wash the patient's perineum with soap and water, pat it dry with a towel. Then remove your gloves.

Place the sterile catheter insertion kit between the patient's legs (as shown). Open the kit, using aseptic technique. If

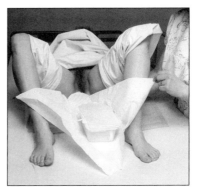

the catheter is packaged separately, open the package and drop the catheter into the open kit.
4. Still using aseptic technique, put on sterile gloves and pick up the sterile, fenestrated drape. Ask the patient to raise her pelvis by pushing down on her feet. Slide the drape under her buttocks with your gloved hand. Now tell her to lower her pelvis onto the drape. Position the

(continued)

INSERTING A STRAIGHT URINARY CATHETER *(continued)*

drape so that the opening is over the perineum (as shown).

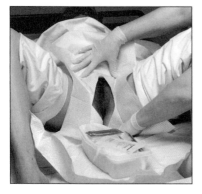

5. To clean the perineal area, use your nondominant hand to spread apart the patient's labia. With the thumb and index finger of the same hand, separate the labia to expose the urethral meatus (as shown).

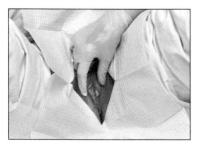

Be careful not to confuse the urethral opening with the vaginal opening. Look for the meatus between the clitoris and the vagina. If you can't see it, it may be hidden in the anterior part of the vagina. If you can't find it there, exert gentle downward pressure when you clean between the labia (see step 5); this should open the meatus briefly.

Caution: The hand used to clean the labia is now considered contaminated. *Don't* use it to insert the catheter.

6. With your uncontaminated hand, use the forceps to pick up a cotton ball saturated with the antiseptic solution. Clean the labia minora with a downward stroke (as shown). Discard the cotton ball in the biohazard bag. Then clean the other side with another saturated cotton ball, and discard the cotton ball. Pick up another cotton ball and wipe directly over the meatus. Discard the cotton ball and the forceps.

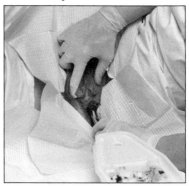

6a. If the patient is male, hold the penis in your nondominant hand. With your uncontaminated hand, use the forceps to pick up a saturated cotton ball (as shown). Clean around the meatus using a circular motion. Then, with another cotton ball, clean in a spiral motion to the corona of the glans penis.

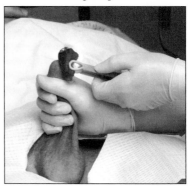

INSERTING A STRAIGHT URINARY CATHETER *(continued)*

7. Now, with your uncontaminated hand, grasp the catheter (as shown). Making sure that the catheter doesn't touch the unprepped areas of the perineum, gently insert it 2″ to 3″ (5 to 8 cm) into the meatus. Angle the catheter slightly upward as you advance it.

Caution: Never force the catheter.

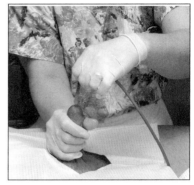

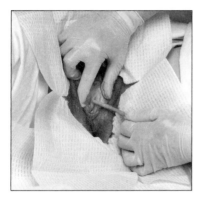

7a. For a male patient, hold the penis at a 90-degree angle to his thighs. Grasp the catheter with your uncontaminated hand, and gently insert it into the meatus (as shown). Advance it 7″ to 10″ (18 to 25 cm) along the anterior wall of the urethra. A few inches into the urethra (at the internal sphincter, just below the prostate), you'll encounter resistance from most patients. If your patient indicates discomfort, reassure him.

Caution: Never forcibly insert a catheter. If you encounter an obstruction, call the physician. He'll introduce the catheter using a guide.

8. As the catheter enters the patient's bladder, urine begins to flow. Release the labia. Using your sterile hand, place the free end of the catheter in the specimen container (as shown). Make sure you grasp the catheter high enough to avoid contaminating the specimen. Let the container fill to the three-quarters mark. When the container has filled, allow the remaining urine to drain.

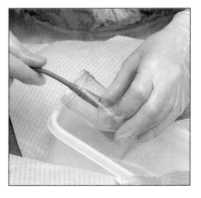

sterile wrapper, and open the sterile specimen container.

Separate the labia majora and keep them open with one hand. With the forceps, grasp an antiseptic-moistened cotton ball. Make two vertical swipes on the labia minora. (Use a new cotton ball for

each swipe, cleaning from the urethral meatus toward the anus.) Position the sterile tray with the lubricated catheter on the sterile field between the patient's legs. *Gently* insert the catheter into the urethra until urine flows. Allow a few milliliters of urine to flow into a basin;

then collect 10 to 60 ml in a sterile plastic container, depending on the test requirements. After gently removing the catheter, clean and dry the urethral area.

Send the specimen and a laboratory request to the laboratory within 10 minutes after collection, or refrigerate the specimen. On the chart, record the procedure and the time that the specimen was sent.

Collection from an indwelling urinary catheter

You can minimize the risk of bacterial contamination by aspirating a urine specimen from an indwelling urinary catheter made of self-sealing rubber or from a collection tube with a special sampling port. (However, *don't* aspirate a Silastic, silicone, or plastic catheter.) This technique can provide a random, second-voided, first morning, fasting, or timed specimen.

Have the necessary equipment available: gloves; sterile syringe (10 to 20 ml); sterile needle (21G to 25G); alcohol pad; sterile specimen container; specimen labels; laboratory request.

About 30 minutes before collecting the specimen, clamp the collection tube. (This procedure is contraindicated for patients who have just undergone genitourinary surgery). Put on gloves. After wiping the sampling port with an alcohol pad, insert the needle at a 90-degree angle and aspirate the urine into the syringe. If the collection tube has a rubber catheter but not a port, obtain the specimen from the catheter. Insert the needle at a 45-degree angle into the catheter, and withdraw the urine specimen. Never insert the needle into the shaft of the catheter because this may puncture the lumen leading to the balloon.

Failure to unclamp the tube after collecting the specimen can cause bladder distention and may predispose the patient to a bladder infection. If you can't draw any urine, lift the tube a little, but make sure urine doesn't return to the bladder. Aspirate urine, transfer the specimen to a sterile container, and cap the container securely. Send it to the laboratory in a plastic bag.

Interfering factors

A common interfering factor in urine collection, especially in timed collections, is the patient's failure to follow the correct collection procedure. Inaccurate test results may be due to *overcollection,* by failing to discard the last voiding before the test period; *undercollection,* by failing to include all urine voided during the test; *contamination,* by including toilet tissue or stool in the specimen; or, for procedures requiring collection at specified times or for the second-voided collection, the patient's inability to urinate on demand. In urine specimens collected from females, vaginal drainage (such as menses, which elevates the RBC count) can alter the results of a urinalysis.

Improper collection or handling of the specimen can also produce unreliable results. For instance, failure to thoroughly clean the urethral meatus and glans before collection can contaminate a clean-catch midstream specimen. Similarly, failure to send a urine specimen to the laboratory immediately allows bacterial proliferation and thus invalidates the colony count on bacterial culture.

Foods and drugs can affect test results by changing the composition of the urine. For example, ingestion of sugar increases urine glucose levels. Drugs can cause chemical or pharmacologic interference with the laboratory analysis. For example, corticosteroids tend to elevate glucose levels.

Guide to color-top collection tubes

The colors of collection tubes can vary from laboratory to laboratory. This guide lists the most commonly used collection tubes. Consult your laboratory for its specific collection tube requirements.

Marble
(gold or light green)

Marble-top tubes contain a silicone gel to separate serum from cells.

Acid phosphatase
Alanine aminotransferase
Alkaline phosphatase
Amylase
Aspartate aminotransferase
Bilirubin
Blood urea nitrogen
Calcium
Carcinoembryonic antigen
Cardiac glycosides
Chloride
Cholesterol, total
Cholinesterase
Creatine
Creatine kinase
Creatinine
Cryoglobulins
Folic acid
Follicle-stimulating hormone
Free thyroxine and free triiodothyronine
Gamma-glutamyltransferase
Gastrin
Growth hormone/somatropic hormone
Growth hormone suppression test (glucose loading)
Hepatitis B surface antigen
Hydroxybutyric dehydrogenase
Lactate dehydrogenase
Lipase
Lipoprotein-cholesterol fractionation
Magnesium
Phosphates
Phospholipids
Potassium
Prolactin
Protein electrophoresis
Sodium
Triiodothyronine resin uptake
Testosterone
Thyroid-stimulating hormone
Triglycerides
Tubular reabsorption of phosphate
Urea clearance
Uric acid
Vitamin B_{12}

Red

Red-top tubes contain no additives. Draw volume may be 2 to 20 ml. These tubes are used for tests performed on serum samples.

ABO blood typing
Acetaminophen
Acetylcholine receptor antibodies
Alpha-fetoprotein
Androstenedione
Angiotensin-converting enzyme
Antibody screening test
Anticonvulsants
Antidepressants, plasma
Antidiuretic hormone
Antideoxyribonucleic acid antibodies
Antiglobulin, direct
Antimicrobials
Antimitochondrial antibodies
Anti–smooth-muscle antibodies
Antistreptolysin-O test
Antithyroid antibodies
Arginine test
Barbiturates
Bronchodilators
Ceruloplasmin
Cold agglutinins
Complement assays
C-reactive protein
Crossmatching
D-xylose absorption
Estrogens
Ethanol, blood
Extractable nuclear antigen antibodies
Febrile agglutination tests
Ferritin
Fluorescent treponemal antibody absorption test
Fungal serology
Haptoglobin
Heterophil agglutination tests
Hexosaminidase A and B
Human chorionic gonadotropin
Human placental lactogen
Hypnotics
Immunoglobulins A, G, and M
Immune complex assays
Insulin

Iron and total iron-binding
capacity
Isocitrate dehydrogenase
Isopropanol
Leucine aminopeptidase
Leukoagglutinins
Long-acting thyroid stimulator
Lupus erythematosus cell
preparation
Luteinizing hormone, plasma
Lyme test
Methanol
Myoglobin
5'-Nucleotidase
Ornithine carbamoyltrans-
ferase
Parathyroid hormone
(parathormone)
Phenothiazines
Prothrombin consumption
Radioallergosorbent test
Rh typing
Rheumatoid factor
Rubella antibodies
Salicylates
Thyroid-stimulating hormone,
neonatal
Thyroxine
Thyroxine-binding globulin
Tranquilizers
Transferrin
Triiodothyronine
Venereal Disease Research
Laboratory test
Vitamin A and carotene
Vitamin B$_2$
Vitamin D$_3$

Lavender

Lavender-top *tubes contain
EDTA. Draw volume may be 2
to 10 ml. These tubes are used
for tests performed on whole
blood samples.*

ABO blood typing
Adrenocorticotropic hormone
Antidiuretic hormone
Coombs' direct
Erythrocyte sedimentation
rate
Glucagon
Glucose-6-phosphate dehydro-
genase
Heinz bodies
Hematocrit
Hemoglobin, glycosylated
Hemoglobin, total

Hemoglobins, unstable
Hemoglobin electrophoresis
Lead
Lipoprotein phenotyping
Plasma renin activity
Platelet count
Platelet survival
Pyruvate kinase
Red blood cell count
Red cell indices
Reticulocyte count
Rh typing
Sickle cell test (hemoglobin S)
White blood cell count
White blood cell differential

Dark green

Dark green-top *tubes contain
heparin (sodium, lithium, or
ammonium). Draw volume
may be 2 to 15 ml. These tubes
are used for tests performed on
plasma samples.*

Amino acid scan
Ammonia
Androstenedione
Angiotensin-converting
enzyme
Calcitonin (thyrocalcitonin)
Catecholamines
Chromosomal analysis
Erythropoietic porphyrins
Galactose 1-phosphate uridyl-
transferase
Insulin tolerance test
Inulin clearance
Lymphocyte transformation
tests
Osmotic fragility
Para-aminohippuric acid
excretion
Rapid adrenocorticotropic
hormone
Red blood cell survival time
Terminal deoxynucleotidyl
transferase
Uroporphyrinogen I synthase

Blue

Blue-top *tubes contain sodium
citrate and citric acid. Draw
volume may be 2.7 or 4.5 ml.
These tubes are used for coagulation studies requiring plasma
samples.*

Euglobulin lysis time
Fibrinogen
Hemoglobin derivatives
One-stage assay: Extrinsic
coagulation system
One-stage assay: Intrinsic
coagulation system
Partial thromboplastin time
Plasminogen
Platelet aggregation
Protein C
Protein S
Prothrombin time
Thrombin time
Tissue thromboplastin
inhibitor study (lupus anti-
coagulation)

Black

Black-top *tubes contain sodium oxalate. Draw volume may
be 2.7 or 4.5 ml. These tubes are
used for coagulation studies
performed on plasma samples.*

Plasma vitamin C
Fibrin split products

Gray

Gray-top *tubes contain a gly-
colytic inhibitor (such as sodium fluoride, powdered oxalate,
or glycolytic/microbial inhibitor). Draw volume may be 3 to
10 ml. These tubes are used
most often for glucose determinations in serum or plasma
samples.*

Serum glucose levels (all
types)
Insulin tolerance test
Lactic acid and pyruvic acid
Tolbutamide tolerance test

Guide to selected reagent strip tests

Substance detected

Reagent strips	Bilirubin	Blood	Glucose	Ketones	Nitrite	pH	Protein	Urobilinogen
Albustix							●	
Bili-Labstix	●	●	●	●		●	●	
Chemstrip GK			●	●				
Chemstrip GP			●				●	
Chemstrip 5		●	●	●		●	●	
Chemstrip 6	●	●	●	●		●	●	
Chemstrip 7	●	●	●	●		●	●	●
Chemstrip 8	●	●	●	●	●	●	●	●
Clinistix			●					
Combistix			●			●	●	
Dextrostix (use fingerstick or venous blood)			●					
Diastix			●					
Hema-Combistix		●	●			●	●	
Hemastix (may also test fecal matter)		●						
Hemoccult		●						
Keto-Diastix			●	●				
Ketostix				●				
Labstix		●	●	●		●	●	
Microstix-Nitrite					●			
Multistix	●	●	●	●		●	●	●
Nitrazine paper						●		
N-Multistix	●	●	●	●	●	●	●	●
N-Uristix			●		●		●	
Tes-Tape			●					
Uristix			●				●	
Urobilistix								●

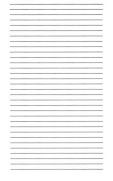

Laboratory value changes
in elderly patients

Standard normal laboratory values reflect the physiology of adults ages 20 to 40. However, normal values for older patients usually differ because of age-related physiologic changes.

Certain test results, however, remain unaffected by age. These include partial thromboplastin time, prothrombin time, serum acid phosphatase, serum carbon dioxide, serum chloride, aspartate aminotransferase, and total serum protein. You can use this chart to interpret other changeable test values in your elderly patients.

Test values ages 20 to 40	Age-related changes	Considerations
Serum		
Albumin 3.5 to 5 g/dl (SI, 35 to 50 g/L)	Younger than age 65: Higher in males Older than age 65: Equal levels that then decrease at same rate	Increased dietary protein intake needed in older patients if liver function is normal; edema — a sign of low albumin level
Alkaline phosphatase 30 to 85 IU/L (SI, 42 to 128 U/L)	Increases 8 to 10 IU/L	May reflect liver function decline or vitamin D malabsorption and bone demineralization
Beta globulin 0.7 to 1.1 g/dl (SI, 7 to 11 g/L)	Increases slightly	Increases in response to decrease in albumin if liver function is normal; increased dietary protein intake needed
Blood urea nitrogen Men: 10 to 25 mg/dl (SI, 3.6 to 9.3 mmol/L) Women: 8 to 20 mg/dl (SI, 2.9 to 7.5 mmol/L)	Increases, possibly to 69 mg/dl (SI, 25.8 mmol/L)	Slight increase acceptable in absence of stressors, such as infection or surgery
Cholesterol Men: < 205 mg/dl (SI,< 5.30 mmol/L) Women: < 190 mg/dl (SI, < 4.90 mmol/L)	Men: Increases to age 50, then decreases Women: Lower than men until age 50, increases to age 70, then decreases	Rise in cholesterol level (and increased cardiovascular risk) in women as a result of postmenopausal estrogen decline; dietary changes, weight loss, and exercise needed

Test values ages 20 to 40	Age-related changes	Considerations
Serum (continued)		
Creatine kinase 55 to 170 U/L (SI, 0.94 to 2.89 µkat/L)	Increases slightly	May reflect decreasing muscle mass and liver function
Creatinine 0.6 to 1.3 mg/dl (SI, 53 to 115 µmol/L)	Increases, possibly to 1.9 mg/dl (SI, 168 µmol/L) in men	Important factor to prevent toxicity when giving drugs excreted in urine
Creatinine clearance Men: 94 to 140 ml/min/1.73 m² (SI, 0.91 to 1.35 ml/s/m²) Women: 72 to 110 ml/min/1.73 m² (SI, 0.69 to 1.06 ml/s/m²)	Men: Decreases; formula: ([140 – age]) × kg body weight)/(72 × serum creatinine) Women: 85% of men's rate	Reflects reduced glomerular filtration rate; important factor to prevent toxicity when giving drugs excreted in urine
Hematocrit Men: 45% to 52% (SI, 0.45 to 0.52) Women: 37% to 48% (SI, 0.37 to 0.48)	May decrease slightly (unproven)	Reflects decreased bone marrow and hematopoiesis, increased risk of infection (because of fewer and weaker lymphocytes and immune system changes that diminish antigen-antibody response)
Hemoglobin Men: 14 to 18 g/dl (SI, 140 to 180 g/L) Women: 12 to 16 g/dl (SI, 120 to 160 g/L)	Men: Decreases by 1 to 2 g/dl Women: Unknown	Reflects decreased bone marrow, hematopoiesis, and (for men) androgen levels
High-density lipoprotein Men: 37 to 70 mg/dl (SI, 0.96 to 1.8 mmol/L) Women: 40 to 85 mg/dl (SI, 1.03 to 2.2 mmol/L)	Levels higher in women than in men but equalize with age	Compliance with dietary restrictions required for accurate interpretation of test results
Lactate dehydrogenase 71 to 207 U/L (SI, 1.2 to 3.52 µkat/L)	Increases slightly	May reflect declining muscle mass and liver function
Leukocyte count 4,000 to 10,0000/µl (SI, 4 to 10 < 10⁹/L)	Decreases to 3,100 to 9,000/µl (SI, 3.1 to 9 × 10⁹/L)	Decrease proportionate to lymphocyte count
Lymphocyte count 25% to 40% (SI, 0.25 to 0.4)	Decreases	Decrease proportionate to leukocyte count
Platelet count 140,000 to 400,000/µl (SI, 140 to 400 × 10⁹/L)	Change in characteristics; decreased granular constituents, increased platelet-release factors	May reflect diminished bone marrow and increased fibrinogen levels

Test values ages 20 to 40	Age-related changes	Considerations
Serum (continued)		
Potassium 3.5 to 5.5 mEq/L (SI, 3.5 to 5.5 mmol/L)	Increases slightly	Requires avoidance of salt substitutes composed of potassium, vigilance in reading food labels, and knowledge of hyperkalemia's signs and symptoms
Thyroid-stimulating hormone 0 to 15 µlU/ml (SI, 15 mU/L)	Increases slightly	Suggests primary hypothyroidism or endemic goiter at much higher levels
Thyroxine 5 to 13.5 µg/dl (SI, 60 to 165 mmol/L)	Decreases 25%	Reflects declining thyroid function
Triglycerides Men: 44 to 180 mg/dl (SI, 0.44 to 2.01 mmol/L) Women: 10 to 190 mg/dl (SI, 0.11 to 2.21 mmol/L)	Increases slightly	Suggests abnormalities at any other levels, requiring additional tests such as serum cholesterol
Triiodothyronine 80 to 220 ng/dl (SI, 1.2 to 3 nmol/L)	Decreases 25%	Reflects declining thyroid function
Urine		
Glucose 0 to 15 mg/dl (SI, 0 to 8 mmol/L)	Decreases slightly	May reflect renal disease or urinary tract infection (UTI); unreliable check for older diabetics because glucosuria may not occur until plasma glucose level exceeds 300 mg/dl
Protein 50 to 80 mg/24 hours (SI, 50 to 80 mg/d)	Increases slightly	May reflect renal disease or UTI
Specific gravity 1.032 (SI, 1.032)	Decreases to 1.024 (SI, 1.024) by age 80	Reflects 30% to 50% decrease in number of nephrons available to concentrate urine

Drug interference with test results

Drugs can interfere with the results of laboratory tests in two ways. A drug in a blood or urine specimen may interact with the chemicals used in the laboratory test, causing a false result. Or a drug may cause a physiologic change in the patient, resulting in an actual increased or decreased blood or urine level of the substance being tested. This chart identifies drugs that can cause these two types of interference in some common blood and urine tests.

Test	Chemical reaction	Physiologic change	
		Increased test values	*Decreased test values*
alkaline phosphatase	▪ albumin ▪ fluorides	▪ anticonvulsants ▪ hepatotoxic drugs ▪ ticlopidine	▪ clofibrate ▪ estrogen ▪ vitamin D ▪ zinc supplements
ammonia, blood		▪ acetazolamide ▪ alcohol ▪ ammonium chloride ▪ asparaginase ▪ barbiturates ▪ diuretics, loop and thiazide	▪ kanamycin, oral ▪ lactulose ▪ neomycin, oral ▪ potassium salts ▪ tetracycline
amylase, serum	▪ chloride salts ▪ fluorides	▪ asparaginase ▪ cholinergic agents ▪ contraceptives, hormonal ▪ contrast media with iodine ▪ drugs inducing acute pancreatitis: azathioprine, corticosteroids, loop and thiazide diuretics ▪ methyldopa ▪ opioids	▪ somatostatin

Test	Chemical reaction	Physiologic change	
		Increased test values	*Decreased test values*
aspartate aminotransferase	■ erythromycin ■ methyldopa	■ cholinergic agents ■ hepatotoxic drugs ■ opium alkaloids	■ interferon ■ naltrexone
bilirubin, serum	■ ascorbic acid ■ barbiturates ■ dextran ■ epinephrine ■ levodopa ■ pindolol ■ theophylline	■ hemolytic agents ■ hepatotoxic drugs ■ methyldopa ■ rifampin	■ barbiturates ■ sulfonamides
blood urea nitrogen	■ chloral hydrate ■ chloramphenicol ■ streptomycin	■ anabolic steroids ■ nephrotoxic drugs	■ tetracyclines
calcium, serum	■ aspirin ■ heparin ■ hydralazine ■ sulfisoxazole	■ asparaginase ■ calcium salts ■ diuretics, loop and thiazide ■ lithium ■ thyroid hormones ■ vitamin D	■ acetazolamide ■ anticonvulsants ■ calcitonin ■ cisplatin ■ contraceptives, hormonal ■ corticosteroids ■ laxatives ■ magnesium salts ■ plicamycin
chloride, serum		■ acetazolamide ■ androgens ■ estrogens ■ nonsteroidal anti-inflammatory drugs	■ corticosteroids ■ diuretics, loop and thiazide ■ laxatives
cholesterol, serum	■ androgens ■ aspirin ■ corticosteroids ■ nitrates ■ phenothiazines ■ vitamin D	■ alcohol ■ beta-adrenergic blocking agents ■ contraceptives, hormonal ■ corticosteroids ■ cyclosporine ■ diuretics, thiazide ■ phenothiazines ■ sulfonamides ■ ticlopidine	■ androgens ■ captopril ■ chlorpropamide ■ cholestyramine ■ clofibrate ■ colestipol ■ haloperidol ■ neomycin, oral
creatine kinase (CK)		■ aminocaproic acid ■ amphotericin B ■ chlorthalidone ■ clofibrate ■ ethanol, chronic use ■ gemfibrozil	

Test	Chemical reaction	Physiologic change	
		Increased test values	*Decreased test values*
creatinine, serum	■ cefoxitin (Jaffe method) ■ cephalothin ■ flucytosine	■ cimetidine ■ flucytosine ■ nephrotoxic drugs	
glucose, serum	■ acetaminophen ■ ascorbic acid (urine) ■ cephalosporins (urine)	■ antidepressants, tricyclic ■ beta-adrenergic blocking agents ■ corticosteroids ■ cyclosporine ■ dextrothyroxine ■ diazoxide ■ diuretics, loop and thiazide ■ epinephrine ■ estrogens ■ isoniazid ■ lithium ■ phenothiazines ■ phenytoin ■ salicylates, toxic levels ■ somatostatin ■ thiabendazole	■ acetaminophen ■ alcohol ■ anabolic steroids ■ clofibrate ■ disopyramide ■ gemfibrozil ■ monoamine oxidase inhibitors ■ pentamidine
magnesium, serum		■ lithium ■ magnesium salts	■ alcohol ■ aminoglycosides ■ amphotericin B ■ calcium salts ■ cardiac glycosides, toxic levels ■ cisplatin ■ diuretics, loop and thiazide
phosphates, serum		■ vitamin D, excessive amounts	■ antacids, phosphate-binding (such as aluminum phosphate gel) ■ lithium ■ mannitol
potassium, serum		■ aminocaproic acid ■ angiotensin-converting enzyme (ACE) inhibitors ■ antineoplastic agents ■ cyclosporine ■ diuretics, potassium-sparing ■ isoniazid ■ lithium ■ mannitol ■ nephrotoxic drugs ■ succinylcholine	■ aminoglycosides ■ ammonium chloride ■ amphotericin B ■ corticosteroids ■ diuretics, potassium-wasting ■ glucose ■ insulin ■ laxatives ■ penicillins, extended-spectrum ■ salicylates

Test	Chemical reaction	Physiologic change	
		Increased test values	*Decreased test values*
protein, serum		■ anabolic steroids ■ corticosteroids ■ phenazopyridine	■ contraceptives, hormonal ■ estrogens ■ hepatotoxic drugs
protein, urine	■ aminoglycosides ■ cephalosporins ■ contrast media with iodine ■ magnesium sulfate, large doses ■ miconazole ■ nafcillin ■ phenazopyridine ■ sulfonamides ■ tolbutamide ■ tolmetin	■ ACE inhibitors ■ cephalosporins ■ contrast media with iodine ■ corticosteroids ■ nafcillin ■ nephrotoxic drugs ■ sulfonamides	
prothrombin time		■ abciximab ■ anticoagulants ■ asparaginase ■ aspirin ■ azathioprine ■ cefamandole ■ cefoperazone ■ cephalosporins ■ cephalothin ■ chloramphenicol ■ cholestyramine ■ cilostazol ■ clopidogrel ■ colestipol ■ cyclophosphamide ■ dipyridamole ■ eptifibatide ■ hepatotoxic drugs ■ moxalactam ■ propylthiouracil ■ quinidine ■ quinine ■ sulfonamides ■ tetracyclines ■ ticlopidine	■ anabolic steroids ■ contraceptives, hormonal ■ estrogens ■ vitamin K

Test	Chemical reaction	Physiologic change	
		Increased test values	*Decreased test values*
sodium, serum		▪ anabolic steroids ▪ carbamazepine ▪ clonidine ▪ contraceptives, hormonal ▪ corticosteroids ▪ diazoxide ▪ estrogens ▪ guanabenz ▪ guanadrel ▪ guanethidine ▪ methyldopa ▪ nonsteroidal antiinflammatory drugs ▪ sulfonylureas	▪ ammonium chloride ▪ carbamazepine ▪ desmopressin ▪ diuretics ▪ lithium ▪ lypressin ▪ vasopressin ▪ vincristine
uric acid, serum	▪ ascorbic acid ▪ caffeine ▪ levodopa ▪ theophylline	▪ acetazolamide ▪ alcohol ▪ cisplatin ▪ cyclosporine ▪ diazoxide ▪ diuretics ▪ epinephrine ▪ ethambutol ▪ levodopa ▪ niacin ▪ phenytoin ▪ propranolol ▪ spironolactone	▪ acetohexamide ▪ allopurinol ▪ clofibrate ▪ contrast media with iodine ▪ diflunisal ▪ glucose infusions ▪ guaifenesin ▪ phenothiazines ▪ phenylbutazone ▪ salicylates, small doses ▪ uricosuric agents

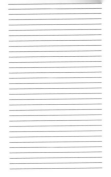

Quick-reference guide to laboratory test results

A

Acetylcholine receptor antibodies, serum
Negative

Acid mucopolysaccharides, urine
Adults: < 13.3 μg glucuronic acid/mg/creatinine/24 hours

Acid phosphatase, serum
0 to 3.7 U/L (SI, 0 to 3.7 U/L)

Adrenocorticotropic hormone, plasma
< 120 pg/ml (SI, < 26.4 pmol/L)

Alanine aminotransferase
8 to 50 IU/L (SI, 0.14 to 0.85 μkat/L)

Aldosterone, serum
Supine individuals: 3 to 16 ng/dl (SI, 80 to 440 pmol/L)
Upright individuals: 7 to 30 ng/dl (SI, 190 to 832 pmol/L)

Aldosterone, urine
3 to 19 μg/24 hours (SI, 8 to 51 nmol/d)

Alkaline phosphatase, peritoneal fluid
Males > 18 years: 90 to 239 U/L (SI, 90 to 239 U/L)
Females < 45 years: 76 to 196 U/L (SI, 76 to 196 U/L); *> 45 years:* 87 to 250 U/L (87 to 250 U/L)

Alkaline phosphatase, serum
30 to 85 IU/ml (SI, 42 to 128 U/L)

Alpha-fetoprotein, serum
Males and nonpregnant females: < 15 ng/ml (SI, < 15 mg/L)

Ammonia, peritoneal fluid
< 50 μg/dl (SI, < 29 μmol/L)

Amniotic fluid analysis
Lecithin-sphingomyelin ratio: > 2
Meconium: absent (except in breech presentation)
Phosphatidylglycerol: present

Amylase, peritoneal fluid
138 to 404 U/L (SI, 138 to 404 U/L)

Amylase, serum
Adults ≥ 18 years: 25 to 85 U/L (SI, 0.39 to 1.45 μkat/L)

Amylase, urine
1 to 17 U/hour (SI, 0.017 to 0.29 μkat/h)

Androstenedione (radioimmunoassay)
Males: 75 to 205 ng/dl (SI, 2.6 to 7.2 nmol/L)
Females: 85 to 275 ng/dl (SI, 3.0 to 9.6 nmol/L)

Angiotensin-converting enzyme
Adults ≥ 20 years: 8 to 52 U/L (SI, 0.14 to 0.88 μkat/L)

Anion gap
8 to 14 mEq/L (SI, 8 to 14 mmol/L)

Antibody screening, serum
Negative

Antidiuretic hormone, serum
1 to 5 pg/ml (SI, 1 to 5 mg/L)

Antiglobulin test, direct
Negative

Antimitochondrial antibodies, serum
Negative

Anti–smooth-muscle antibodies, serum
Negative

Antistreptolysin-O, serum
Preschoolers and adults: 85 Todd units/ml
School-age children: 170 Todd units/ml

Antithrombin III
80% to 120% of normal control values

Antithyroid antibodies, serum
Normal titer < 1:100

Arginine test
Human growth hormone levels
– *Males:* increase to >10 ng/ml (SI, >10 μg/L)
– *Females:* increase to >15 ng/ml (SI, >15 μg/L)
– *Children:* increase to > 48 ng/ml (SI, > 48 μg/L)

Arterial blood gases
pH: 7.35 to 7.45 (SI, 7.35 to 7.45)
PaO_2: 80 to 100 mm Hg (SI, 10.6 to 13.3 kPa)
$PaCO_2$: 35 to 45 mm Hg (SI, 4.7 to 5.3 kPa)
O_2CT: 15% to 23% (SI, 0.15 to 0.23)
SaO_2: 94% to 100% (SI, 0.94 to 1)
HCO_3^-: 22 to 25 mEq/L (SI, 22 to 25 mmol/L)

Arylsulfatase A, urine
Random: 16 to 42 U/g creatinine
24-hour: 0.37 to 3.60 U/day creatinine
1-hour test: 2 to 19 U/1 hour (SI, 2 to 19 U/h)
2-hour test: 4 to 37 U/2 hours(SI, 4 to 37 U/h)
24-hour test: 170 to 2,000 U/24 hours (SI, 2.89 to 34.0 μkat/L)

Aspartate aminotransferase
Males: 8 to 46 U/L (SI, 0.14 to 0.78 μkat/L)
Females: 7 to 34 U/L (SI, 0.12 to 0.58 μkat/L)

Aspergillosis antibody, serum
Normal titer < 1:8

Atrial natriuretic factor, plasma
20 to 77 pg/ml

B

Bacterial meningitis antigen
Negative

Bence Jones protein, urine
Negative

Beta-hydroxybutyrate
< 0.4 mmol/L (SI, 0.4 mmol/L)

Bilirubin, amniotic fluid
Early: < 0.075 mg/dl (SI, < 1.3 Umol/L)
Term: < 0.025 mg/dl (SI, < 0.41 Umol/L)

Bilirubin, serum
Adults
– *Direct:* < 0.5 mg/dl (SI, < 6.8 μmol/L)
– *Indirect:* 1.1 mg/dl (SI, 19 μmol/L)
Neonates
– *Total:* 1 to 12 mg/dl (SI, 34 to 205 μmol/L)

Bilirubin, urine
Negative

Blastomycosis antibody, serum
Normal titer < 1:8

Bleeding time
Template: 3 to 6 minutes (SI, 3 to 6 m)
Ivy: 3 to 6 minutes (SI, 3 to 6 m)
Duke: 1 to 3 minutes (SI, 1 to 3 m)

Blood urea nitrogen
8 to 20 mg/dl (SI, 2.9 to 7.5 mmol/L)

B-lymphocyte count
270 to 640/μl

C

Calcitonin, plasma
Baseline
– *Males:* 40 pg/ml (SI, 40 ng/L)
– *Females:* 20 pg/ml (SI, 20 ng/L)
Calcium infusion
– *Males:* 190 pg/ml (SI, 190 ng/L)
– *Females:* 130 pg/ml (SI, 130 ng/L)
Pentagastrin infusion
– *Males:* 110 pg/ml (SI, 110 ng/L)
– *Females:* 30 pg/ml (SI, 30 ng/L)

Calcium, serum
Adults: 8.2 to 10.2 mg/dl (SI, 2.05 to 2.54 mmol/L)
Children: 8.6 to 11.2 mg/dl (SI, 2.15 to 2.79 mmol/L)
Ionized: 4.65 to 5.28 mg/dl (SI, 1.1 to 1.25 mmol/L)

Calcium, urine
100 to 300 mg/24 hours (SI, 2.50 to 7.50 mmol/d)

Candida antibodies, serum
Negative

Capillary fragility
Petechiae per 5 cm:	Score:
11 to 20	2+
21 to 50	3+
over 50	4+

Carbon dioxide, total, blood
22 to 26 mEq/L (SI, 22 to 26 mmol/L)

Carcinoembryonic antigen, serum
< 5 ng/ml (SI, < 5 mg/L)

Catecholamines, plasma
Supine
– *Epinephrine:* undetectable to 110 pg/ml (SI, undetectable to 600 pmol/L)
– *Norepinephrine:* 70 to 750 pg/ml (SI, 413 to 4,432 pmol/L)
Standing
– *Epinephrine:* undetectable to 140 pg/ml (SI, undetectable to 764 pmol/L)
– *Norepinephrine:* 200 to 1,700 pg/ml (SI, 1,182 to 10,047 pmol/L)

Catecholamines, urine
Epinephrine: 0 to 20 μg/24 hours (SI, 0 to 109 nmol/24 h)
Norepinephrine: 15 to 80 μg/24 hours (SI, 89 to 473 nmol/24 h)
Dopamine: 65 to 400 μg/24 hours (SI, 425 to 2,610 nmol/24 h)

Cerebrospinal fluid
Pressure: 50 to 180 mm H_2O
Appearance: clear, colorless
Gram stain: no organisms

Ceruloplasmin, serum
22.9 to 43.1 g/dl (SI, 0.22 to 0.43 g/L)

Chloride, cerebrospinal fluid
118 to 130 mEq/L (SI, 118 to 130 mmol/L)

Chloride, serum
100 to 108 mEq/L (SI, 100 to 108 mmol/L)

Chloride, urine
Adults: 110 to 250 nmol/24 hours (SI, 110 to 250 mmol/d)
Children: 15 to 40 nmol/24 hours (SI, 15 to 40 mmol/d)
Infants: 2 to 10 mmol/24 hours (SI, 2 to 10 mmol/d)

Cholinesterase (pseudocholinesterase)
204 to 532 IU/dl (SI, 2.04 to 5.32 kU/L)

Coccidioidomycosis antibody, serum
Normal titer < 1:2

Cold agglutinins, serum
Normal titer < 1:64

Complement, serum
Total
– 40 to 90 U/ml (SI, 0.4 to 0.9 g/L)
C3
– *Males:* 80 to 180 mg/dl (SI, 0.8 to 1.8 g/L)
– *Females:* 76 to 120 mg/dl (SI, 0.76 to 1.2 g/L)
C4
– *Males:* 15 to 60 mg/dl (SI, 0.15 to 0.6 g/L)
– *Females:* 15 to 52 mg/dl (SI, 0.15 to 0.52 g/L)

Copper, urine
3 to 35 μg/24 hours (SI, 0.05 to 0.55 μmol/d)

Cortisol, free, urine
< 50 μg/24 hours (SI, < 138 mmol/d)

Cortisol, plasma
Morning: 9 to 35 μg/dl (SI, 250 to 690 nmol/L)
Afternoon: 3 to 12 μg/dl (SI, 80 to 330 nmol/L)

C-reactive protein, serum
< 0.8 mg/dl (SI, < 8 mg/L)

Creatine kinase
– *Males:* 55 to 170 U/L (SI, 0.94 to 2.89 μkat/L)
– *Females:* 30 to 135 U/L (SI, 0.51 to 2.3 μkat/L)

Creatinine clearance
Males: 94 to 140 ml/min/1.73 m² (SI, 0.91 to 1.35 ml/s/m²)
Females: 72 to 110 ml/min/1.73 m² (SI, 0.69 to 1.06 ml/s/m²)

Creatinine, serum
Males: 0.8 to 1.2 mg/dl (SI, 62 to 115 μmol/L)
Females: 0.6 to 0.9 mg/dl (SI, 53 to 97 μmol/L)

Creatinine, urine
Males: 14 to 26 mg/kg body weight/24 hours (SI, 124 to 230 μmol/kg body weight/d)
Females: 11 to 20 mg/kg body weight/24 hours (SI, 97 to 177 μmol/kg body weight/d)

Cryoglobulins, serum
Negative

Cyclic adenosine monophosphate, urine
0.3 to 3.6 mg/day (SI, 100 to 723 μmol/d)
or
0.29 to 2.1 mg/g creatinine (SI, 100 to 723 μmol/mol creatinine)

Cytomegalovirus antibodies, serum
Negative

D

D-xylose absorption
Blood
– *Adults:* 25 to 40 mg/dl in 2 hours
– *Children:* > 30 mg/dl in 1 hour
Urine:
– *Adults:* > 3.5 g excreted in 5 hours (age 65 or older, > 5 g in 24 hours)
– *Children:* 16% to 33% excreted in 5 hours

E

Epstein-Barr virus antibodies
Negative

Erythrocyte sedimentation rate
Males: 0 to 10 mm/hour (SI, 0 to 10 mm/h)
Females: 0 to 20 mm/hour (SI, 0 to 20 mm/h)

Esophageal acidity
pH > 5.0

Estrogens, serum
Females
– *Menstruating:* 26 to 149 pg/ml (SI, 90 to 550 pmol/L)
– *Postmenopausal:* 0 to 34 pg/ml (SI, 0 to 125 pmol/L)
Males
– 12 to 34 pg/ml (SI, 40 to 125 pmol/L)
Children
– *< 6 years:* 3 to 10 pg/ml (SI, 10 to 36 pmol/L)

Euglobulin lysis time
2 to 4 hours (SI, 2 to 4 h)

F

Factor assay, one-stage
50% to 150% of normal activity (SI, 0.5 to 1.5)

Febrile agglutination, serum
Salmonella *antibody:* < 1:80
Brucellosis antibody: < 1:80
Tularemia antibody: < 1:40
Rickettsial antibody: < 1:40

Ferritin, serum
Males
–20 to 300 ng/ml (SI, 20 to 300 µg/L)
Females
–20 to 120 ng/ml (SI, 20 to 120 µg/L)
Infants
– *1 month:* 200 to 600 ng/ml (SI, 200 to 600 µg/L)
– *2 to 5 months:* 50 to 200 ng/ml (SI, 50 to 200 µg/L)
– *6 months to 15 years:* 7 to 140 ng/ml (SI, 7 to 140 µg/L)
Neonates
–25 to 200 ng/ml (SI, 25 to 200 µg/L)

Fibrinogen, plasma
200 to 400 mg/dl (SI, 2 to 4 g/L)

Fibrin split products
Screening assay: < 10 µg/ml (SI, < 10 mg/L)
Quantitative assay: < 3 µg/ml (SI, < 3 mg/L)

Fluorescent treponemal antibody absorption, serum
Negative

Folic acid, serum
1.8 to 9 ng/ml (SI, 4 to 20 nmol/L)

Follicle-stimulating hormone, serum
Menstruating females
– *Follicular phase:* 5 to 20 mIU/ml (SI, 5 to 20 IU/L)
– *Ovulatory phase:* 15 to 30 mIU/ml (SI, 15 to 30 IU/L)
– *Luteal phase:* 5 to 15 mIU/ml (SI, 5 to 15 IU/L)
Menopausal females
– 5 to 100 mIU/ml (SI, 50 to 100 IU/L)
Males
– 5 to 20 mIU/ml (5 to 20 IU/L)

Free thyroxine, serum
0.9 to 2.3 ng/dl (SI, 10 to 30 nmol/L)

Free triiodothyronine
0.2 to 0.6 ng/dl (SI, 0.003 to 0.009 nmol/L)

G

Galactose 1-phosphate uridyl transferase
Qualitative: negative
Quantitative: 18.5 to 28.5 U/g of hemoglobin (SI, 1.19 to 1.84 mU/mol Hb)

Gamma-glutamyltransferase
Males
– ≥ *16 years:* 6 to 38 U/L (SI, 0.10 to 0.63 µkat/L)
Females
– *16 to 45 years:* 4 to 27 U/L (SI, 0.08 to 0.46 µkat/L)
– *> 45 years:* 6 to 38 U/L (SI, 0.10 to 0.63 µkat/L)
Children
– 3 to 30 U/L (SI, 0.05 to 0.51 µkat/L)

Gastric acid stimulation
Males: 18 to 28 mEq/hour
Females: 11 to 21 mEq/hour

Gastric secretion, basal
Males: 1 to 5 mEq/hour
Females: 0.2 to 3.3 mEq/hour

Gastrin, serum
50 to 150 pg/ml (SI, 50 to 150 ng/L)

Globulin, peritoneal fluid
30% to 45% of total protein

Glucose, amniotic fluid
< 45 mg/dl (SI, < 2.3 mmol/L)

Glucose, cerebrospinal fluid
50 to 80 mg/dl (SI, 2.8 to 4.4 mmol/L)

Glucose, peritoneal fluid
70 to 100 mg/dl (SI, 3.5 to 5 mmol/L)

Glucose, plasma, fasting
70 to 100 mg/dl (SI, 3.9 to 6.1 mmol/L)

Glucose-6-phosphate dehydrogenase
4.3 to 11.8 U/g (SI, 0.28 to 0.76 mU/mol) of hemoglobin

Glucose tolerance, oral
Peak at 160 to 180 mg/dl (SI, 8.8 to 9.9 mmol/L) 30 to 60 minutes after challenge dose

Growth hormone suppression
Undetectable to 3 ng/ml (SI, undetectable to 3 µg/L) after 30 minutes to 2 hours

H

Ham test
Negative

Haptoglobin, serum
40 to 180 mg/dl (SI, 0.4 to 1.8 g/L)

Heinz bodies
Negative

Hematocrit
Males
– 42% to 52% (SI, 0.42 to 0.52)
Females
– 36% to 48% (SI, 0.36 to 0.48)
Children
– *10 years:* 36% to 40% (SI, 0.36 to 0.4)
Infants
– *3 months:* 30% to 36% (SI, 0.3 to 0.36)
– *1 year:* 29% to 41% (SI, 0.29 to 0.41)
Neonates
– *At birth:* 55% to 68% (SI, 0.55 to 0.68)
– *1 week:* 47% to 65% (SI, 0.47 to 0.65)
– *1 month:* 37% to 49% (SI, 0.37 to 0.49)

Hemoglobin (Hb) electrophoresis
Hb A: 95% (SI, 0.95)
Hb A$_2$: 1.5% to 3% (SI, 0.015 to 0.03)
Hb F: < 2% (SI, < 0.02)

Hemoglobin, unstable
Heat stability: negative
Isopropanol: stable

Hemoglobin, urine
Negative

Hemosiderin, urine
Negative

Hepatitis B surface antigen, serum
Negative

Herpes simplex antibodies, serum
Negative

Heterophil agglutination, serum
Normal titer < 1:56

Hexosaminidase A and B, serum
Total: 5 to 12.9 U/L (hexosaminidase A constitutes 55% to 76% of total)

Histoplasmosis antibody, serum
Normal titer < 1:8

Homovanillic acid, urine
< 10 mg/24 hours (SI, < 55 µmol/d)

Human chorionic gonadotropin, serum
< 4 IU/L

Human chorionic gonadotropin, urine
Pregnant women
– *First trimester:* 500,000 IU/24 hours
– *Second trimester:* 10,000 to 25,000 IU/24 hours
– *Third trimester:* 5,000 to 15,000 IU/24 hours

Human growth hormone, serum
Males: undetectable to 5 ng/ml (SI, undetectable
to 5 µg/L)
Females: undetectable to 10 ng/ml (SI, undetectable to 10 µg/L)
Children: undetectable to 16 ng/ml (SI, undetectable to 16 µg/L)

**Human immunodeficiency virus antibody,
serum**
Negative

Human placental lactogen, serum
Males and nonpregnant females: < 0.5 µg/ml
Pregnant females at term: 9 to 11 µg/ml

17-hydroxycorticosteroids, urine
Males
– 4.5 to 12 mg/24 hours (SI, 12.4 to 33.1
µmol/d)
Females
– 2.5 to 10 mg/24 hours (SI, 6.9 to 27.6 µmol/d)
Children
– *8 to 12 years:* < 4.5 mg/24 hours
(SI, < 12.4 µmol/d)
– *< 8 years:* < 1.5 mg/24 hours
(SI, < 4.14 µmol/d)

5-hydroxyindoleacetic acid, urine
2 to 7 mg/24 hours (SI, 10.4 to 36.6 µmol/d)

Hydroxyproline, total, urine
1 to 9 mg/24 hours (SI, 1.0 to 3.4 IU/d)

IJ

Immune complex, serum
Negative

Immunoglobulins (Ig), serum
IgG: 800 to 1,800 mg/dl (SI, 8 to 18 g/L)
IgA: 100 to 400 mg/dl (SI, 1 to 4 g/L)
IgM: 55 to 150 mg/dl (SI, 0.55 to 1.5 g/L)

Insulin, serum
0 to 35 µU/ml (SI, 144 to 243 pmol/L)

Insulin tolerance test
10- to 20-ng/dl (SI, 10- to 20-µg/L) increase
over baseline levels of human growth hormone and adrenocorticotropic hormone

Iron, serum
Males: 60 to 170 µg/dl (SI, 10.7 to 30.4 µmol/L)
Females: 50 to 130 µg/dl (SI, 9 to 23.3 µmol/L)

Iron, total binding capacity, serum
300 to 360 µg/dl (SI, 54 to 64 µmol/L)

K

17-ketogenic steroids, urine
Males: 4 to 14 mg/24 hours (SI, 13 to 49
µmol/d)
Females: 2 to 12 mg/24 hours (SI, 7 to 42
µmol/d)
Infants to 11 years: 0.1 to 4 mg/24 hours (SI, 0.3
to 14 µmol/d)
11 to 14 years: 2 to 9 mg/24 hours (SI, 7 to
31 µmol/d)

Ketones, urine
Negative

17-ketosteroids, urine
Males: 10 to 25 mg/24 hours (SI, 35 to 87 μmol/d)
Females: 4 to 6 mg/24 hours (SI, 4 to 21 μmol/d)
Infants to 10 years: < 3 mg/24 hours (SI, < 10 μmol/d)
10 to 14 years: 1 to 6 mg/24 hours (SI, 2 to 21 μmol/d)

L

Lactate dehydrogenase
Total: 71 to 207 IU/L (SI, 1.2 to 3.52 μkat/L)
LD_1: 14% to 26% (SI, 0.14 to 0.26)
LD_2: 29% to 39% (SI, 0.29 to 0.39)
LD_3: 20% to 26% (SI, 0.2 to 0.26)
LD_4: 8% to 16% (SI, 0.08 to 0.16)
LD_5: 6% to 16% (SI, 0.06 to 0.16)

Lactic acid, blood
0.93 to 1.65 mEq/L (SI, 0.93 to 1.65 mmol/L)

Leucine aminopeptidase
Males: 80 to 200 U/ml (SI, 80 to 200 kU/L)
Females: 75 to 185 U/ml (SI, 75 to 185 kU/L)

Leukoagglutinins
Negative

Lipase, serum
< 160 U/L (SI, < 2.72 μkat)

Lipids, fecal
Constitute < 20% of excreted solids; < 7 g excreted in 24 hours

Lipoproteins, serum
High-density lipoprotein cholesterol
– *Males:* 37 to 70 mg/dl (SI, 0.96 to 1.8 mmol/L)
– *Females:* 40 to 85 mg/dl (SI, 1.03 to 2.2 mmol/L)
Low-density lipoprotein cholesterol:
– *In individuals who don't have coronary artery disease:* < 130 mg/dl (SI, < 3.36 mmol/L)

Long-acting thyroid stimulator, serum
Negative

Lupus erythematosus cell preparation
Negative

Luteinizing hormone, serum
Menstruating women
– *Follicular phase:* 5 to 15 mIU/ml (SI, 5 to 15 IU/L)
– *Ovulatory phase:* 30 to 60 mIU/ml (SI, 30 to 60 IU/L)
– *Luteal phase:* 5 to 15 mIU/ml (SI, 5 to 15 IU/L)
Postmenopausal women
– 50 to 100 mIU/ml (SI, 50 to 100 IU/L)
Males
– 5 to 20 mIU/ml (SI, 5 to 20 IU/L)
Children
– 4 to 20 mIU/ml (SI, 4 to 20 IU/L)

Lyme disease serology
Nonreactive

Lysozyme, urine
0 to 3 mg/24 hours

M

Magnesium, serum
1.3 to 2.1 mg/dl (SI, 0.65 to 1.05 mmol/L)

Magnesium, urine
6 to 10 mEq/24 hours (SI, 3.0 to 5.0 mmol/d)

Manganese, serum
0.4 to 1.4 μg/ml

Melanin, urine
Negative

Myoglobin, urine
Negative

N

5′-nucleotidase
2 to 17 U/L (SI, 0.034 to 0.29 μkat/L)

O

Occult blood, fecal
< 2.5 ml

Oxalate, urine
≤ 40 mg/24 hours (SI, ≤ 456 μmol/d)

PQ

Parathyroid hormone, serum
Intact: 10 to 50 pg/ml (SI, 1.1 to 5.3 pmol/L)
N-terminal fraction: 8 to 24 pg/ml (SI, 0.8 to 2.5 pmol/L)
C-terminal fraction: 0 to 340 pg/ml (SI, 0 to 35.8 pmol/L)

Partial thromboplastin time
21 to 35 seconds (SI, 21 to 35 s)

Pericardial fluid
Amount: 10 to 50 ml
Appearance: clear, straw-colored
White blood cell count: < 1,000/μl (SI, < 1.0 × 10^9/L)
Glucose: approximately whole blood level

Peritoneal fluid
Amount: < 50 ml
Appearance: clear, straw-colored

Phenylalanine, serum
< 2 mg/dl (SI, < 121 μmol/L)

Phosphates, serum
Adults: 2.7 to 4.5 mEq/L (SI, 0.87 to 1.45 mmol/L)
Children: 4.5 to 6.7 mEq/L (SI, 1.45 to 1.78 mmol/L)

Phosphates, urine
< 1,000 mg/24 hours

Phospholipids, plasma
180 to 320 mg/dl (SI, 1.80 to 3.20 g/L)

Plasma renin activity
Normal sodium diet: 1.1 to 4.1 ng/ml/hour (SI, 0.30 to 1.14 ng LS)
Restricted sodium diet: 6.2 to 12.4 ng/ml/hour (SI, 1.72 to 3.44 ng LS)

Phosphate, tubular reabsorption, urine and plasma
80% reabsorption

Plasminogen, plasma
Immunologic method: 10 to 20 mg/dl (SI, 0.10 to 0.20 g/L)

Platelet aggregation
3 to 5 minutes (SI, 3 to 5 m)

Platelet count
Adults: 140,000 to 400,000/µl (SI, 140 to 400 × 10^9/L)
Children: 150,000 to 450,000/µl (SI, 150 to 450 × 10^{9}L)

Potassium, serum
3.5 to 5 mEq/L (SI, 3.5 to 5mmol/L)

Potassium, urine
Adults: 25 to 125 mmol/24 hours (SI, 25 to 125 mmol/d)
Children: 22 to 57 mmol/24 hours (SI, 22 to 57 mmol/d)

Pregnanediol, urine
Nonpregnant females
– 0.5 to 1.5 mg/24 hours (during the follicular phase of the menstrual cycle)
Pregnant females
– *First trimester:* 10 to 30 mg/24 hours
– *Second trimester:* 35 to 70 mg/24 hours
– *Third trimester:* 70 to 100 mg/24 hours
Postmenopausal females
– 0.2 to 1 mg/24 hours
Males
– 0 to 1 mg/24 hours

Pregnanetriol, urine
Males ≥ 16 years: 0.4 to 2.5 mg/24 hours (SI, 1.2 to 7.5 µmol/d)
Females ≥ 16 years: 0 to 1.8 mg/hours (SI, 0.3 to 5.3 µmol/d)

Progesterone, plasma
Menstruating females
– *Follicular phase:* < 150 ng/dl (SI, < 5 nmol/L)
– *Luteal phase:* 300 to 1,200 ng/dl (SI, 10 to 40 nmol/L)
Pregnant women
– *First trimester:* 1,500 to 5,000 ng/dl (SI, 50 to 160 nmol/L)
– *Second and third trimesters:* 8,000 to 20,000 ng/dl (SI, 250 to 650 nmol/L)

Prolactin, serum
Undetectable to 23 ng/ml (SI, undetectable to 23 µg/L)

Prostate-specific antigen
40 to 50 years: 2 to 2.8 mg/ml (SI, 2 to 2.8 µg/L)
51 to 60 years: 2.9 to 3.8 mg/ml (SI, 2.9 to 3.8 µg/L)
61 to 70 years: 4 to 5.3 mg/ml (SI, 4 to 5.3 µg/L)
≥ 71 years: 5.6 to 7.2 mg/ml (SI, 5.6 to 7.2 µg/L)

Protein, cerebrospinal fluid
15 to 50 mg/dl (SI, 0.15 to 0.5 g/L)

Protein C, plasma
70% to 140% (SI, 0.7 to 1.4)

Protein, total peritoneal fluid
0.3 to 4.1 g/dl (SI, 3 to 41 g/L)

Protein, urine
50 to 80 mg/24 hours (SI, 50 to 80 mg/d)

Prothrombin time
10 to 14 seconds (10 to 14 s)

Pulmonary artery pressures
Right atrial: 1 to 6 mm Hg
Left atrial: approximately 10 mm Hg
Systolic: 20 to 30 mm Hg
Systolic right ventricular: 20 to 30 mm Hg
Diastolic: 10 to 15 mm Hg
End-diastolic right ventricular: < 5 mm Hg
Mean: < 20 mm Hg
Pulmonary artery wedge pressure: 6 to 12 mm Hg

Pyruvate kinase
Ultraviolet: 9 to 22 U/g of hemoglobin
Low substrate assay: 1.7 to 6.8 U/g of hemoglobin

Pyruvic acid, blood
0.08 to 0.16 mEq/L (SI, 0.08 to 0.16 mmol/L)

R

Red blood cell count
Males: 4.5 to 5.5 million/µl (SI, 4.5 to 5.5 × 10^{12}/L)
Females: 4 to 5 million/µl (SI, 4 to 5 × 10^{12}/L)
Neonates: 4.4 to 5.8 million/µl (SI, 4.4 to 5.8 × 10^{12}/L)
2 months: 3 to 3.8 million/µl (SI, 3 to 3.8 × 10^{12}/L) (increasing slowly)
Children: 4.6 to 4.8 million/µl (SI, 4.6 to 4.8 × 10^{12}/L)

Red blood cell survival time
25 to 35 days

Red blood cells, urine
0 to 3 per high-power field

Red cell indices
Mean corpuscular volume: 84 to 99 μm^3
Mean corpuscular hemoglobin: 26 to 32 pg/cell
Mean corpuscular hemoglobin concentration: 30 to 36 g/dl

Respiratory syncytial virus antibodies, serum
Negative

Reticulocyte count
Adults: 0.5% to 2.5% (SI, 0.005 to 0.025)
Infants (at birth): 2% to 6% (SI, 0.02 to 0.06), decreasing to adult levels in 1 to 2 weeks

Rheumatoid factor, serum
Negative or titer < 1:20

Ribonucleoprotein antibodies
Negative

Rubella antibodies, serum
Titer of 1:8 or less indicates little or no immunity; titer more than 1:10 indicates adequate protection against rubella

S

Semen analysis
Volume: 0.7 to 6.5 ml
pH: 7.3 to 7.9
Liquefaction: within 20 minutes
Sperm count: 20 to 150 million/ml

Sickle cell test
Negative

Sjögren's antibodies
Negative

Sodium chloride, urine
110 to 250 mEq/L (SI, 100 to 250 mmol/d)

Sodium, serum
135 to 145 mEq/L (SI, 135 to 145 mmol/L)

Sodium, urine
Adults: 40 to 220 mEq/L/224 hours (SI, 40 to 220 mmol/d)
Children: 41 to 115 mEq/L/24 hours (SI, 41 to 115 mmol/d)

Sporotrichosis antibody, serum
Normal titers < 1:40

T

Terminal deoxynucleotidyl transferase, serum
Bone marrow: < 2%
Blood: undetectable

Testosterone, plasma or serum
Males: 300 to 1,200 ng/dl (SI, 10.4 to 41.6 nmol/L)
Females: 20 to 80 ng/dl (SI, 0.7 to 2.8 nmol/L)

Thrombin time, plasma
10 to 15 seconds (10 to 15 s)

Thyroid-stimulating hormone, neonatal
≤2 *days:* 25 to 30 μIU/ml (SI, 25 to 20 mU/L)
>2 *days:* < 25 μIU/ml (SI, < 25 mU/L)

Thyroid-stimulating hormone, serum
Undetectable to 15 μIU/ml (SI, undetectable to 15 mU/L)

Thyroid-stimulating immunoglobulin, serum
Negative

Thyroxine-binding globulin, serum
Immunoassay: 16 to 32 μg/dl (SI, 120 to 180 mg/ml)

Thyroxine, total, serum
5 to 13.5 μg/dl (SI, 60 to 165 nmol/L)

T-lymphocyte count
1,500 to 3,000/μl

Transferrin, serum
200 to 400 mg/dl (SI, 2 to 4 g/L)

Triglycerides, serum
Males: 44 to 180 mg/dl (SI, 0.44 to 2.01 nmol/L)
Females: 11 to 190 mg/dl (SI, 0.11 to 2.21 mmol/L)

Triiodothyronine, serum
80 to 200 ng/dl (SI, 1.2 to 3 nmol/L)

U

Uric acid, serum
Males: 3.4 to 7 mg/dl (SI, 202 to 42 μmol/L)
Females: 2.3 to 6 mg/dl (SI, 143 to 357 μmol/L)

Uric acid, urine
250 to 750 mg/24 hours (SI, 1.48 to 4.43 mmol/d)

Urinalysis, routine
Color: straw to dark yellow
Appearance: clear
Specific gravity: 1.005 to 1.035
pH: 4.5 to 8.0
Epithelial cells: 0 to 5 per high-power field
Casts: none, except 1 to 2 hyaline casts per low-power field
Crystals: present

Urine osmolality
24-hour urine: 300 to 900 mOsm/kg
Random urine: 50 to 1,400 mOsm/kg

Urobilinogen, fecal
50 to 300 mg/24 hours (SI, 100 to 400 EU/100 g)

Urobilinogen, urine
0.1 to 0.8 EU/2 hours (SI 0.1 to 0.8 EU/2h)
or
0.5 to 4.0 EU/24 hours (SI, 0.5 to 4.0 EU/d)

Uroporphyrinogen I synthase
≥ 7 nmol/second/L

V

Vanillylmandelic acid, urine
1.4 to 6.5 mg/24 hours (SI, 7 to 33 µmol/day)

Venereal Disease Research Laboratory test, cerebrospinal fluid
Negative

Venereal Disease Research Laboratory test, serum
Negative

Vitamin A, serum
30 to 80 µg/dl (SI, 1.05 to 2.8 µmol/L)

Vitamin B_2, serum
3 to 15 µg/dl

Vitamin B_{12}, serum
200 to 900 pg/ml (SI, 148 to 664 pmol/L)

Vitamin C, plasma
0.2 to 2 mg/dl (SI, 11 to 114 µmol/L)

Vitamin C, urine
30 mg/24 hours

Vitamin D_3, serum
10 to 60 ng/ml (SI, 25 to 150 nmol/L)

WXY

White blood cell count, blood
4,000 to 10,000/µl (SI, 4 to 10 $\times$ 10^9/L)

White blood cell count, peritoneal fluid
< 300/µl (SI, < 300 $\times$ 10^9/L)

White blood cell count, urine
0 to 4 per high-power field

White blood cell differential, blood
Adults
– *Neutrophils:* 54% to 75% (SI, 0.54 to 0.75)
– *Lymphocytes:* 25% to 40% (SI, 0.25 to 0.40)
– *Monocytes:* 2% to 8% (SI, 0.02 to 0.08)
– *Eosinophils:* 1% to 4% (SI, 0.01 to 0.04)
– *Basophils:* 0 to 1% (SI, 0 to .01)

Z

Zinc, serum
70 to 120 µg/dl (SI, 10.7 to 18.4 µmol/L)

Patient guide to test preparation

The experience of having a diagnostic test may be new to your patient. Even if he has had tests before, your teaching can help reassure him. If he knows what to expect, he'll be more cooperative and relaxed, which may help the procedure go more smoothly.

Here are teaching aids for some of the most common tests. They explain what the patient needs to know before, during, and after his test.

You'll find a diet to prepare the patient for an oral glucose tolerance test as well as preparation guides for imaging tests, such as cardiac catheterization, computed tomography (CT) scans, breast ultrasonography, barium enema, and endoscopic retrograde cholangiopancreatography. Also included are pointers for undergoing a stress test, cystoscopy, needle aspiration of the breast, liver biopsy, and pulmonary function tests.

When you review the test with your patient, remember to:
- name the test and describe what the patient may see, hear, smell, feel, or taste (be honest about discomfort he may experience)
- define unfamiliar terms
- outline home preparation that's required, such as fasting, bowel preparation, or fluid restriction
- tell the patient where the test will be performed (physician's office, hospital, or other medical facility) and who will perform it
- inform him if he'll have an I.V. line or receive an anesthetic or a sedative
- suggest that he practice what he'll be asked to do during the test — for example, lying perfectly still for a CT scan
- tell him how long the procedure will take and whether he'll need help getting home
- review possible adverse effects, if any, including which ones require him to call the physician
- discuss recommendations for follow-up visits, if applicable
- tell him when to expect test results.

If your patient feels anxious and overwhelmed with information, he may have difficulty remembering everything he's been taught. By giving him an easy-to-read teaching aid, you reinforce your teaching and provide your patient with a handy reference.

GETTING READY FOR AN ORAL GLUCOSE TOLERANCE TEST

Dear Patient:
To prepare for an oral glucose tolerance test and to ensure accurate results, you need to follow a high-carbohydrate diet for 3 days before the test. Here's a sample diet you can use. If you find it too restrictive, follow your regular diet, but eat 12 additional slices of bread each day.

Breakfast
1 serving fruit
Eggs, as desired
5 bread exchanges
1 cup milk
Butter or margarine
Coffee or tea, if desired

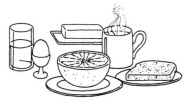

Lunch and dinner
Meat, as desired
5 bread exchanges
2 vegetables
1 serving fruit
1 cup milk
Butter or margarine
Coffee or tea, if desired

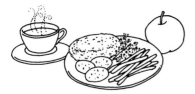

What are bread exchanges?
One of these items equals one bread exchange:
1 slice bread, white or whole wheat
1½-inch cube of corn bread
½ hamburger or hotdog roll
½ cup cooked cereal
¾ cup dry cereal (avoid sugar-coated varieties)
½ cup noodles, spaghetti, or macaroni
½ cup cooked dried beans or peas
⅓ cup corn or ½ small ear of corn
1 biscuit
½ corn muffin
1 roll
5 saltine crackers
2 graham crackers
½ cup grits or rice
1 small white potato
½ cup mashed potato
¼ cup sweet potato
¼ cup baked beans
¼ cup pork and beans

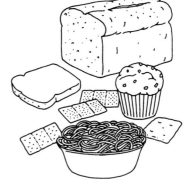

FOLLOWING A CLEAR LIQUID DIET

Dear Patient:
Your doctor has ordered a clear liquid diet to prepare you for certain intestinal tests that you'll be having. A clear liquid diet consists of foods that are transparent and liquid or that liquefy at room temperature. This type of diet reduces the amount of stools in your bowels, which helps the doctor to better see the inside of your bowels.

The foods listed here are the *only* foods you should eat or drink on a clear liquid diet:

- water
- ice chips
- clear tea (no milk or lemon)
- strained and clear fruit juices, such as apple, grape, and cranberry (no pulp)
- decaffeinated coffee (may vary with institution)
- clear carbonated beverages
- plain fruit gelatin (no fruit added)
- chicken or beef broth (fat-free only)
- chicken or beef bouillon
- frozen ice pops (no fruit or pulp)
- clear, fruit-flavored drink mixes.

FOLLOWING A LOW-SODIUM DIET FOR RENIN TESTING

Dear Patient:
Before undergoing renin testing, you must drastically restrict your intake of sodium for 3 days to ensure accurate test results. If you're following this diet at home, observe these precautions:

■ Eat only the foods included in the meal plan provided by the doctor. You may delete foods from the diet, but you may not add foods.

■ Measure all portions using standard measuring cups and spoons.

■ Use 4 oz (112 g) *unsalted* beefsteak or ground beef for lunch and 4 oz *unsalted* chicken for dinner. (Amount refers to weight before cooking.)

■ You may eat these *unsalted* (fresh or frozen) vegetables: asparagus, green or wax beans, cabbage, cauliflower, lettuce, and tomatoes.

■ Use only the specified amount of coffee.

■ If you're thirsty between meals, drink distilled water (but no other food or beverages).

■ Prepare all foods without salt; don't use salt at the table.

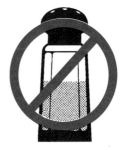

Breakfast
1 egg, poached or boiled, or fried in *unsalted* fat
2 slices *unsalted* toast
1 shredded wheat biscuit or ⅔ cup *unsalted* cooked cereal
4 oz (120 ml) milk
8 oz (240 ml) coffee
1 cup orange juice
Sugar, jam or jelly, and *unsalted* butter, as desired

Lunch
4 oz (120 ml) *unsalted* tomato juice
4 oz (112 g) *unsalted* beefsteak or ground beef; may be broiled or fried in *unsalted* fat
½ cup *unsalted* potato
½ cup *unsalted* green beans or other allowed vegetable
1 serving fruit
8 oz (240 ml) coffee
1 slice *unsalted* bread
Sugar, jam or jelly, and *unsalted* butter, as desired

Dinner
4 oz (112 g) *unsalted* chicken; may be baked or broiled, or fried in *unsalted* fat
½ cup *unsalted* potato
Lettuce salad (vinegar and oil dressing)
½ cup *unsalted* green beans or other allowed vegetable
1 serving fruit
8 oz (240 ml) coffee
1 slice *unsalted* bread
Sugar, jam or jelly, and *unsalted* butter, as desired

LEARNING ABOUT A STRESS TEST

Dear Patient:
Don't be intimidated by the name *stress test.* The only stress involved is some carefully controlled physical exercise.

What the test does
A stress test tells your doctor how your heart functions while you're exercising. It may be combined with another test, called a *thallium scan,* to evaluate blood flow through your coronary arteries to the heart muscle itself.

What happens during the test
After not eating or drinking (except for normal medications) for at least 2 hours before the test, you'll go to the cardiology lab. There, a nurse will attach electrocardiogram (ECG) monitors to your chest and arms, along with a blood pressure cuff. Then, you'll either ride a stationary bike or walk on a treadmill at gradually increasing speeds and slopes. While you're exercising, your blood pressure will be checked frequently and an ECG will be run continuously. Be sure to inform the doctor as soon as you feel tired, short of breath, or dizzy, or experience chest pain.

Thallium scan
If the test includes a thallium scan, the doctor will inject thallium into a vein in your arm while you're exercising (see illustration). Then, he'll ask you to continue exercising for several minutes.

Next, you'll be taken to the scanner room, where the doctor will take pic-

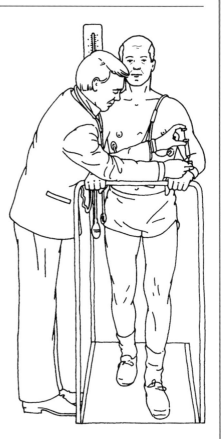

tures of your heart with a special scanner. These pictures will show how well your coronary arteries supply blood to your heart during exercise.

About 4 hours after you finish exercising, the doctor may take more pictures of your heart. They'll show how well your coronary arteries supply blood to your heart after a rest period.

PREPARING FOR CARDIAC CATHETERIZATION

Dear Patient:
Your doctor has scheduled you for cardiac catheterization, a procedure that allows him to look inside of your heart. He does this by first making a small incision in a blood vessel near your elbow or groin and then inserting a long, thin, flexible tube called a *catheter* into the vessel.

After inserting the catheter, the doctor will slowly thread it through your bloodstream into your heart. When the catheter is in place, the doctor will perform certain tests that may include injection of a special dye. What the doctor sees will help him to decide what additional treatment might improve your heart's functioning.

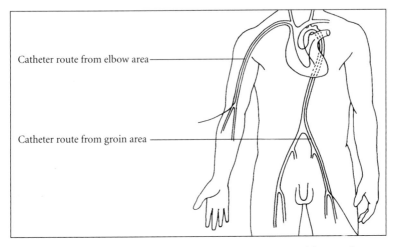

Catheter route from elbow area

Catheter route from groin area

Before the procedure
If your catheterization is scheduled for early morning, you probably won't be allowed to eat or drink anything after midnight the day before the test.

To protect against infection, the nurse will shave the area where the incision will be made. Before you go to the catheterization lab, she'll ask you to urinate, then help you into a hospital gown. Depending on the doctor's orders, she also may start an I.V. line in your arm.

When you reach the catheterization lab, you'll be placed on a padded table and probably be strapped to it. During the test, the doctor will tilt the table to view your heart from different angles. The straps will keep you from slipping out of position. Special foam pads, called *leads*, may be put on your chest so that your heartbeat can be monitored.

Cardiac catheterization usually takes 1 to 2 hours. You'll be awake throughout the procedure, although the doctor may order medication to help you relax. (Some patients even doze off.) You may feel pain in your chest, flushing, or nausea during catheterization, but these sensations should pass quickly.

During the procedure
First, the doctor will inject a local anesthetic at the catheter insertion site to numb the area before he puts in the catheter. When the catheter is going in, you should feel a little pressure but no pain. You may receive nitroglycerin dur-

PREPARING FOR CARDIAC CATHETERIZATION *(continued)*

ing the test to enlarge your heart's blood vessels and help the doctor get a better view.

If the catheter's passage is blocked — because of a narrowed blood vessel, for example — the doctor will pull back the catheter and start from another insertion area.

When the catheter enters your heart, you may feel a fluttering sensation. Tell the doctor if you do, but don't worry; this is a normal reaction. You're also likely to feel a warm sensation, some nausea, or the urge to urinate if dye is injected, but these feelings will quickly pass. Throughout the catheterization, remember to let the doctor or the nurse know if you have chest pain.

During the test, your doctor may give you oxygen and ask you to cough or to breathe deeply.

When the test is finished, the doctor will slowly remove the catheter and put a special bandage on your arm or groin. You may need a few stitches at the insertion site. Because the anesthetic will still be working, you shouldn't feel anything.

After the procedure

When you're back in your room, the nurse will probably do an electrocardiogram if you aren't already on a cardiac monitor. She'll check your bandage and your temperature, pulse, breathing, and blood pressure frequently.

Your bandaged arm or leg must stay completely still for up to 8 hours. To help keep you from moving, the nurse may splint your arm or leg or weigh it down with a sandbag. She'll check the site frequently for swelling as well as check the blood flow in your arm or leg. She'll probably ask you to wiggle your toes or fingers once an hour or more.

As your anesthetic wears off, you'll probably feel some pain at the insertion site. Let the nurse know so she can give you pain medication.

As soon as the test results are available, the doctor will talk to you and your family about them. Don't hesitate to ask him or the nurse any questions you may have.

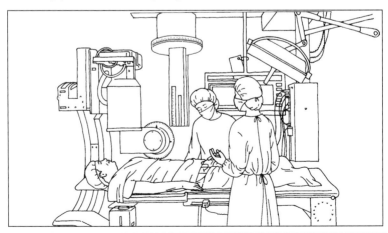

PREPARING FOR PULMONARY FUNCTION TESTS

Dear Patient:
Your doctor has ordered pulmonary (or lung) function tests for you. These tests measure how well your lungs work. Here's what to expect.

How the tests work
You'll be asked to breathe as deeply as possible into a mouthpiece that's connected to a machine called a *spirometer*. This device measures and records the rate and amount of air that you inhale and exhale. Or, you may sit in a small, boothlike enclosure for a test called *body plethysmography*. Again, you'll be asked to breathe in and out, and the measurements will be recorded.

Before the tests
Avoid smoking for at least 4 hours before the tests. Eat lightly and drink only a small amount of fluid. Wear loose, comfortable clothing, and urinate before the tests.

To make the tests go quickly, you'll need to cooperate fully. Tell the technician if you don't understand the instructions. If you wear dentures, keep them in — they'll help you to keep a tight seal around the spirometer's mouthpiece.

During the tests
During spirometry, you'll sit upright and you'll wear a noseclip to make sure you breathe only through your mouth. During body plethysmography, you won't need a noseclip.

If you feel too confined in the small chamber, keep in mind that you can't suffocate. And you can talk to the nurse or technician through a window.

The tests have several parts. For each test, you'll be asked to breathe a certain way — for example, to inhale deeply and exhale completely or to inhale quickly. You may need to repeat some tests after inhaling a medication to expand the airways in your lungs. Also, the nurse may take a sample of blood from an artery in your arm. This sample will be used to measure how well your body uses the air you breathe.

How will you feel?
During the tests, you may feel tired or short of breath. However, you'll be able to rest between measurements. Tell the technician right away if you feel dizzy, begin wheezing, or have chest pain, a racing or pounding heart, an upset stomach, or severe shortness of breath. Also tell him if your arm swells, if you're bleeding from the spot where the blood sample was taken, or if you experience weakness or pain in that arm.

After the tests
When the tests are over, rest if you feel like it. You may resume your usual activities when you regain your energy.

PREPARING FOR MAGNETIC RESONANCE IMAGING

Dear Patient:
Your doctor wants you to have a painless test called *magnetic resonance imaging*—*MRI* for short. Unlike an X-ray, this test produces images of your body's organs and tissues without exposing you to radiation. Instead, MRI uses a powerful magnetic field and radio-frequency energy to produce computerized pictures. Here's how to prepare for it.

Before the test
You may eat, drink, and take your usual medicines. Try to use the bathroom just before the test because MRI may take up to 90 minutes.

Take off any metal objects you may be carrying or wearing, such as a watch, rings, eyeglasses, and a hearing aid. Metal can be damaged by the strong magnetic field. Also empty your pockets of any coins and plastic card keys or charge cards with metallic strips. The scanner will erase the strips.

Let the doctor know if you have any metal objects inside your body, such as a pacemaker, an aneurysm clip, a joint prosthesis, a metal pin, or bullet fragments, so the scanner can be adjusted.

During the test
You'll lie on a narrow, padded table throughout the test. The technician will tell you to stay still to prevent blurred images. To help you stay still, your head, chest,

and arms may be secured with straps. Remember that MRI is painless and involves no exposure to radiation.

The table on which you're lying will slowly glide into the scanner's narrow tunnel. You'll notice the walls are just a few inches from your body. Inside, you'll hear fans and feel air circulating around you, and you may hear thumping noises made by the machine. The technician will probably offer you earphones, or you may request earplugs before the test.

The technician, located in an adjacent room, can see and hear you. Mirrors above your head will enable you to see the technician.

After the test
You may resume your usual activities. If you've been lying down for a long time, however, don't get up too quickly or you may feel slightly dizzy. Rise slowly to give your body a chance to adjust.

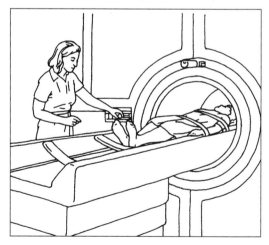

PREPARING FOR A CT SCAN

Dear Patient:
The doctor has scheduled you for a computed tomography (CT) scan. This test uses X-rays and a computer to create detailed images of the body part being scanned. It involves the use of a large machine called a *CT scanner*. The test is painless and takes between 30 and 60 minutes.

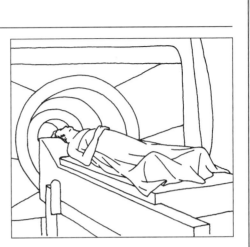

Before the test
You may receive an injection of a contrast dye in your arm. This substance highlights certain areas of your body. If the test requires this dye, don't eat or drink anything for 4 hours before the test.

Tell your doctor if you've ever had an allergic reaction to X-ray contrast material or if you're allergic or sensitive to shellfish or iodine-containing solutions. Let him know if you have other allergies, too.

Remove all metal objects and jewelry, such as a watch, hairpins, and earrings. Also remember to remove objects that might obstruct the X-ray beam, such as glasses, dentures, and a hearing aid. Wear loose, comfortable clothing or a hospital gown. You may be given a mild sedative to help you relax.

During the test
A technician will position you on an X-ray table. Then the table will slide into the tubelike scanner, which looks like a giant thermos bottle lying on its side. Every few seconds, the table will move a small distance and an X-ray image will be taken. You'll hear clicking or buzzing noises from the scanner as it revolves, obtaining images from many angles.

Remember to lie still. To prevent blurring of the X-ray images, your body will be steadied with straps or a support. You'll be alone in the scanner room during the test, but you can talk to the technician through a two-way intercom.

If you received contrast material, you may develop a headache, have a salty taste in your mouth, or feel warm or flushed and nauseous. These reactions usually subside rapidly, but be sure to mention them to the technician.

After the test
You may resume your usual activities and diet. If you received a contrast dye, drink plenty of fluids for the rest of the day to help flush it from your system. Tell your doctor or nurse if you feel sick, vomit, or have a headache after the test.

Within 1 to 2 days, your doctor will have the full test results. He'll review the scan and discuss the results with you.

PREPARING FOR BREAST ULTRASONOGRAPHY

Dear Patient:
Your doctor wants you to undergo breast ultrasonography—commonly called *ultrasound*. This test provides an image of the inside of your breasts and is helpful for detecting and evaluating breast lumps. It can usually determine whether a lump is fluid-filled or solid, but it can't distinguish whether a lump is cancerous.

How the test works

This test uses a small instrument called a *transducer* that sends a beam of high-frequency sound waves toward your breast. When the sound waves bounce back from breast tissue, they're picked up again by the transducer. This information is then processed by a computer and displayed as an image of the inner breast on a TV screen.

Ultrasound is painless and poses no known health risk. It's also safe it you're pregnant because it uses no radiation.

Before the test

You'll be asked to remove your clothes from the waist up and to put on a hospital gown. In most cases, you won't need to restrict your diet, medications, or activities. If you have questions, ask them now. During the test, you'll need to rest quietly so the operator can concentrate on the images.

During the test

The procedure varies at different hospitals and clinics, so check with your doctor about how the test will be performed at the facility where you'll be examined.

Either a doctor or an ultrasonographer will perform the test.

In most places, you'll be asked to lie on your back, with a pillow placed under the shoulder on the same side as the breast to be examined. Then a water-soluble gel will be applied to your breast. The test operator will glide the handheld transducer back and forth over your breast. Unless your breasts are very tender, the test should be painless and feel like a light massage.

In some hospitals and clinics, you'll be asked to lie on your back while a water-filled chamber is lowered over your breasts. Or you may be asked to lie on your stomach with your breasts submerged in a warm-water bath. In these methods, the sound waves are sent through water. You should feel no discomfort, although if you're asked to immerse your breasts in a water bath, the water may feel a bit cool.

During the test, don't expect to hear the high-frequency sound waves, which are inaudible to the human ear.

You'll probably be able to see images of your breast on the TV screen, but they'll look obscure, something like a satellite weather map.

After the test

You may resume your normal activities immediately. To find out your test results, you'll typically wait a day or two until a report is sent to the doctor who referred you for the test.

PREPARING FOR A BARIUM ENEMA TEST

Patient:

Your doctor has ordered a barium enema test to help find the cause of your gastrointestinal (GI) symptoms. This test, which is also called a *lower GI exam*, involves taking an X-ray of your large intestine (colon).

To make the intestine visible on an X-ray, liquid barium will be inserted through your anus to fill your colon. The barium makes your colon appear as a white shadow on the X-ray.

Getting ready

For the test to be accurate, your large intestine must be empty, so you'll need to follow a special diet for 1 to 3 days before the test. You'll also need to drink plenty of water or clear liquids for 12 to 24 hours beforehand.

The afternoon before the test, you'll receive a laxative and possibly a suppository. Then the night before or the morning of the test, you'll receive a cleansing enema.

Don't take oral medications after midnight on the day of the test unless your doctor tells you otherwise.

During the test

The test will be done in the X-ray department and will take about 1 hour. You'll be asked to lie on an X-ray table that tilts while holding you secured. First, the radiologist will take an X-ray to make sure your intestine is completely empty.

Then, as you lie on your side, he'll insert a well-lubricated tube gently into your rectum. The barium, stored in a bag, will flow slowly through the tube into your intestine, along with some air. The air and the barium make your intestine more visible on the X-ray.

As the barium and air enter your intestine, you may experience slight cramps or feel as though you need to move your bowels. To ease this discomfort, try to breathe deeply and slowly through your mouth. Tell the radiologist if the cramping increases.

Tighten your anal spincter muscle against the tube. This will help to hold the tube in place and prevent the barium from leaking out. If too much liquid barium leaks out of the tube, your intestine won't be well coated, and the test will be inaccurate.

After the test

Once the enema tube is removed, you'll be allowed to empty your bowels in the toilet or a bedpan. You should drink lots of fluids, and you may be given a mild laxative or an enema to help you rid your intestine of the extra barium. You may resume your normal diet and medications.

Plan to rest because the test may be tiring. Expect your stools to look chalky for the next 24 to 72 hours. If you have trouble having a bowel movement after the test, call your doctor.

PREPARING FOR ERCP

Dear Patient:

You're about to undergo endoscopic retrograde cholangiopancreatography — called *ERCP* for short. This procedure uses a dyelike substance, a flexible tube called an *endoscope,* and X-rays to outline your gallbladder and pancreatic structures.

Performed in the radiology department, ERCP may take up to 1 hour to complete. Read the information here to help you prepare.

Before the test

The day before ERCP, you can eat and drink as usual. Then after midnight before the procedure, don't eat or drink anything unless your doctor directs otherwise. (He may tell you to continue taking certain medications.) Before you enter the test room, be sure to urinate because ERCP can cause you to retain urine.

During the test

You'll lie on an X-ray table for this test. The nurse will take your temperature, blood pressure, and pulse rate. Then she'll insert an I.V. line into your hand or arm to administer medication. You'll receive a sedative to relax you and to ease the procedure. You may be aware of noises around you but you won't be fully awake.

The doctor will spray your throat with a bitter-tasting anesthetic, which will make your mouth and throat feel swollen and numb. Because you'll have difficulty swallowing, the doctor may give you a device to suction your saliva, or may tell you to let it drain from your mouth.

Next, the nurse will give you a mouthguard to keep your mouth open and to protect your teeth during ERCP. Though you'll be unable to talk, you'll have no trouble breathing.

When the doctor passes the endoscope down your throat, you may gag a little, but this reflex is normal.

As the tube reaches the duodenum (small intestine), the doctor may inject some air through it. You'll also receive medication through your I.V. line to relax the duodenum. Next, the doctor will insert a thinner tube through the endoscope to the billiary structures and the duodenum.

When the second tube is in place, the doctor will inject dye and quickly take X-ray images from several angles. After the doctor views the images, he may obtain a tissue sample. Then he'll gently remove the endoscope, tube, and mouthpiece.

After the test

The nurse will check your blood pressure, pulse rate, and temperature frequently for several hours.

When you regain feeling in your throat and your gag reflex returns, you'll be allowed to have a light meal and liquids. You can resume your regular diet the next day.

Expect to have a sore throat for a few days. Call the doctor if you can't urinate or if you experience chills, abdominal pain, nausea, or vomiting.

LEARNING ABOUT CYSTOSCOPY

Dear Patient:
Your doctor has scheduled you for cystoscopy. During this procedure, he can look inside your bladder through an instrument called a *cystoscope*. He'll insert the cystoscope through your urethra (the opening through which you urinate).

Cystoscopy allows the doctor to diagnose and, sometimes, treat your urinary disorder. The test may be done in a hospital or the doctor's office and takes 15 to 45 minutes.

What to expect before the test
You may receive a local anesthetic before the procedure. This means that the doctor will numb the area around the urethra before inserting the cystoscope. Or you may have general anesthesia. In this case, don't eat or drink anything after midnight on the night before the procedure. If the doctor plans to take X-rays of your bladder during the cystoscopy, he may prescribe medication that will clean your bowels to ensure sharper, clearer images.

Just before the procedure begins, an intravenous line will be inserted in your arm to deliver fluids and medications if you need them. You'll also receive a sedative to help you relax.

What to expect during the test
After the anesthetic takes effect, you'll be positioned on your back. Then the doctor will insert the cystoscope. Remember to take deep breaths and try to relax. This will allow the test to proceed smoothly.

If you received a local anesthetic, you may feel a strong urge to urinate as the instrument is inserted and removed. If the doctor instills an irrigant into your bladder, you may feel some pressure. Again, try to relax. If you experience any pain or feel your heart beating irregularly, let your doctor know.

What to expect after the test
Your condition will be monitored until you're fully alert. If you received a local anesthetic, you'll be awake but you may feel weak; so don't chance walking by yourself. Wait for someone to assist you.

For several days after the procedure, your urine may be tinged with blood. You may also have bladder spasms, a feeling that your bladder is full, or a burning sensation when you urinate. Take acetaminophen (Tylenol) or a medication your doctor prescribes, drink plenty of fluids, and lie in a tub of warm water to help relieve these adverse effects.

When to call the doctor
Call your doctor if you have heavy bleeding or blood clots in your urine, bladder pain or spasms that aren't relieved by medication, or burning and a frequent urge to urinate that persists for more than 24 hours. Also notify your doctor at once if you can't urinate within 8 hours after the test.

PREPARING FOR A LIVER BIOPSY

Dear Patient:
Your doctor wants you to have a liver biopsy, which helps diagnose cirrhosis and other liver disorders. The test involves removing a small sample of liver tissue and studying it under a microscope. Usually, it takes about 15 minutes and the results are available within a day.

Before the test
Don't eat or drink anything for 4 to 8 hours before the test, as your doctor orders. You'll probably have a blood test to measure your blood's clotting ability and other factors. Just before the test, be sure to empty your bladder.

During the test
You'll lie on your back with your right hand under your head. You'll need to remain in this position and keep as still as you can. The doctor will drape and clean an area on your abdomen. Then he'll inject a local anesthetic, which may sting and cause brief discomfort.

You'll be told to hold your breath and lie still as the doctor inserts the biopsy needle into the liver (as shown below). The needle will remain in your liver for only about 1 second, but it may cause a sensation of pressure and some discomfort in your right upper back.

After the needle is withdrawn, resume normal breathing. The doctor will apply pressure to the biopsy site to stop bleeding. Then he'll apply a pressure bandage.

After the test
You'll be told to lie on your right side for 2 hours, with a small pillow tucked under your side. For the next 24 hours, you should rest in bed. Your vital signs will be checked periodically.

Tell your doctor or nurse right away if you experience problems, such as chest pain, persistent shoulder pain, or difficulty breathing. You can resume your normal diet.

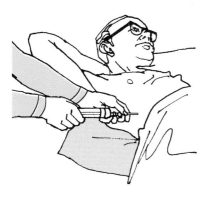

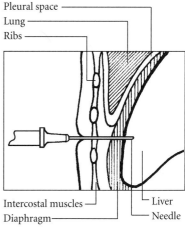

Pleural space
Lung
Ribs
Intercostal muscles
Diaphragm
Liver
Needle

Illustrated guide to home testing

In recent years, the number of diagnostic tests that people can perform themselves at home has greatly increased. The teaching aids on these pages describe how to accurately perform several of the most common home tests, including tests for blood cholesterol levels, pacemaker function, and the presence of human immunodeficiency virus.

When you review these tests with your patient, remember to:
- stress the importance of following the manufacturer's instructions exactly
- explain unfamiliar terms
- review special forms that the patient must complete such as the diary needed when using a Holter monitor
- discuss how to follow up on test results.

TESTING YOUR BLOOD GLUCOSE LEVEL

Dear Patient:
Testing your blood glucose levels daily will tell you whether your diabetes is under control. Follow these steps to learn how to obtain blood for testing and how to perform the test.

Getting ready
1. Begin by assembling the necessary equipment: your glucose meter, a lancet, an alcohol pad, gauze pads, and a vial with reagent strips.
2. Remove a reagent strip from the vial. Then replace the cap, making sure that it's tight.
3. Turn on the glucose meter and, if necessary, calibrate the machine according to the manufacturer's instructions. Then wait for the display window to show that the meter is ready for the blood sample.

Obtaining blood
1. Wash your hands thoroughly and dry them. Choose a site on the end or side of a fingertip. To enhance blood flow, hold your finger under warm water for a minute or two.
2. Hold your hand below your heart, and press the blood toward the fingertip you plan to pierce by squeezing that fingertip with the thumb of the same hand. Wipe the designated fingertip with an alcohol pad, and dry it with a gauze pad. Then place your fingertip (with your

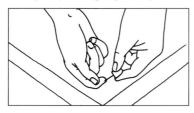

thumb still pressed against it) on a firm surface such as a table.
3. Twist off the lancet's protective cap. Then grasp the lancet and quickly pierce your fingertip just to the side of the finger pad, where you have more blood vessels and fewer nerve endings.
4. Next, push the sharp end of the lancet into the protective cap to avoid accidental sticks. Place the device in a sharps container (a coffee can or a 2-L plastic soda bottle).
5. Remove your thumb from your fingertip to permit blood flow. Then gently press your finger until you get a large, hanging drop of blood.

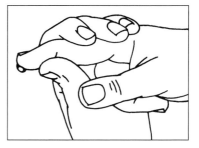

Testing blood
1. When the display window indicates that the meter is ready, touch the drop of blood to the reagent strip at the indicated spot, and insert the strip into the glucose meter. In most cases, the drop of blood will automatically start the meter's timer. Apply pressure to the puncture site with a dry gauze pad to stop the bleeding.
2. After the meter has finished the test, you can read the results from the display window. The meter will automatically store the date, time, and results of the test.

COLLECTING A URINE SPECIMEN: FOR MALES

Dear Patient:
Your doctor wants you to have your urine tested. A urine test can tell whether you have an infection or too much or too little of certain substances in your body. To make sure that test results are accurate, your urine shouldn't contain "outside germs" from your hands or penis.

Follow these directions carefully. Read them through to the end before collecting the specimen.

1. Wash your hands thoroughly. Open the package of disposable wipes that the nurse gave you, and place it on a clean, dry surface nearby.

2. Remove the lid from the specimen cup and place it flat side down. Don't touch the inside of the cup or lid.

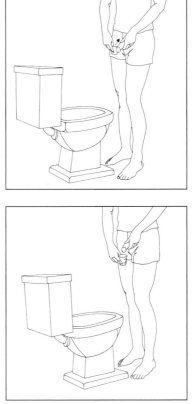

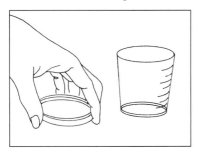

3. Prepare to urinate. (If you're uncircumcised, first pull back your foreskin.) Using a disposable wipe, clean the head of your penis from the urethral opening toward you (as shown at the top of the next column). Then discard the used wipe.

4. Urinate a small amount into the toilet. After 1 or 2 seconds, catch about 1 oz (30 ml) of urine in the specimen cup. The nurse will tell you how far to fill the cup. As a rule, you'll fill it about one-fourth or more full. Don't allow the cup to touch your penis at any time.

When you're done, place the lid on the cup and return it to the nurse.
Note: Don't drink a lot of water before the test. This could affect the accuracy of the test results.

COLLECTING A URINE SPECIMEN: FOR FEMALES

Dear Patient:
Your doctor has asked you to provide a urine specimen for testing. The specimen can tell whether you have an infection or too much or too little of certain substances in your body. To make sure that the test results are accurate, your urine shouldn't contain "outside germs" from your hands, labia, or urethral opening.

Follow these directions carefully. Read them through to the end before collecting the specimen.
1. Wash your hands thoroughly. Open the package of disposable wipes that the nurse gave you, and place it on a clean, dry, surface nearby.
2. Remove the lid from the specimen cup and place it flat side down. Don't touch the inside of the cup or lid.
3. Sit as far back on the toilet as possible. Spread your labia apart with one hand (as shown below), keeping the folds separated for the rest of the procedure

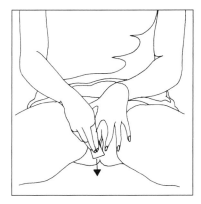

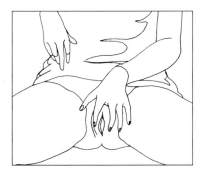

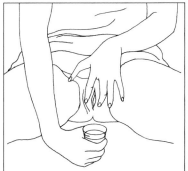

4. Using the disposable wipes, clean the area between the labia and around the urethra thoroughly from front to back (as shown at the top of the next column). Use a new wipe for each stroke. Discard the used wipes
5. Urinate a small amount into the toilet. After 1 or 2 seconds, hold the specimen cup below your urine stream

(as shown above) and catch about 1 oz (30 ml) of urine in the cup. Don't allow the cup to touch your skin at any time.
6. When you're done, place the lid on the cup and return it to the nurse.
Note: Don't drink a lot of water before the test. This could affect the accuracy of the test results.

TESTING FOR BLOOD IN YOUR STOOL

Dear Patient:
A home fecal occult blood test is an easy, inexpensive way to detect blood in your stool. For accurate results, follow the directions given by the nurse or doctor, read the instructions included with the test kit, and review these guidelines.

Getting ready
Don't eat red meat or raw fruits or vegetables for 3 days before you take the test and during the test period. Also avoid diet supplements containing iron or vitamin C and painkillers containing aspirin or ibuprofen (such as Advil and Nuprin) for the same time period. All of these substances can affect test results.

Increase your intake of high-fiber foods, such as whole grain breads and cereals. Your doctor may also ask you to eat popcorn or nuts.

Performing the test
1. Make sure all your supplies are in one place. They may include your test cards (or slides), a chemical developer, a wooden applicator, and a watch with a second hand.
2. Obtain a stool sample. You can do this by laying a long sheet of clear plastic wrap across the toilet bowl to catch the stool, or by removing stool from the bowl. Flush the remaining stool down the toilet.

Use the applicator to smear a thin film of the sample onto the slot marked "A" on the front of the test card. Smear a thin film of a second sample from a *different area of the same stool* onto the slot marked "B" on the same side of the card.
3. *If the doctor or a laboratory will be analyzing the test samples,* close slots A and B, put your name and the date on the test kit, and return the card (or slide) to the doctor or laboratory as soon as possible.

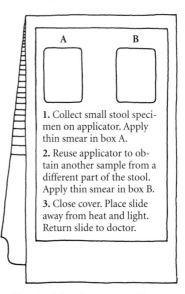

1. Collect small stool specimen on applicator. Apply thin smear in box A.
2. Reuse applicator to obtain another sample from a different part of the stool. Apply thin smear in box B.
3. Close cover. Place slide away from heat and light. Return slide to doctor.

If you're doing the test yourself, turn the card over and open the back window. Apply two drops of the chemical developer to the paper covering each sample. Wait 1 minute; then read the results.

If either slot has a bluish tint, the test results are positive for blood in the stool. *If neither slot looks blue,* the test results are normal. Write down the results. Discard the used applicator and wash your hands thoroughly.
4. Repeat the test on your next two bowel movements. Report the results of all of the tests to the doctor. Even if only one of the six test results is positive, the doctor may recommend other tests.

USING A HOLTER MONITOR

Dear Patient:
Your doctor has ordered you to wear a Holter monitor for 24 hours. It works like a continuous electrocardiogram (ECG) by recording irregular heartbeats you may have. The information from this recording will help your doctor determine if abnormal heartbeats are causing your symptoms, such as chest pain or discomfort, dizziness, or weakness. If you're taking a heart medication, the Holter monitor can also help your doctor evaluate how well the medication is working.

The monitor has adhesive patches (called *leads*) that the nurse will attach to your skin. She'll also show you how to wear the monitor on a belt or over your shoulder. If one of the leads becomes loose, secure it with a piece of tape.

While wearing the monitor, you can perform most of your usual activities. You'll even wear it to bed.

Practice these safety measures while wearing the Holter monitor:
■ Don't get the monitor wet — don't shower, bathe, or swim with it on.
■ Avoid high-voltage areas, strong magnetic fields, and microwave ovens.

While you're wearing the monitor, you'll write down your activities and feelings. This diary will help your doctor establish a connection between your monitor tracing and your activities and feelings. Jot down the time of day when you perform any activity, such as taking medication, eating, drinking, moving your bowels, urinating, engaging in sexual activity, exercising, and sleeping, or experience any strong emotions, such as anger or fear. (See the sample entries below.)

If your monitor has an event button, the nurse will show you how to press it in case you experience anything unusual such as a sudden, rapid heartbeat.

Tuesday	10:30 am	Rode from hospital in car	Legs tired, some shortness of breath
	11:30 am	Watched TV in living room	Comfortable
	12:15 pm	Ate lunch, took Inderal	Indigestion
	1:30 pm	Walked next door to see neighbor	Shortness of breath
	2:45 pm	Walked home	Very tired, legs hurt
	3:00-4:00pm	Urinated, took nap	Comfortable
	5:30 pm	Ate dinner, slowly	Comfortable
	7:20 pm	Had bowel movement	Shortness of breath
	9:00 pm	Watched TV-drank I beer	Heart beating fast for about one minute, no pain
	11:00 pm	Took Inderal, urinated, went to bed	Tired
Wednesday	8:15 am	Awoke, urinated, washed face and arms	Very tired, rapid heartbeat for about 30 seconds
	10:30 am	Returned to hospital	Felt better

CHECKING YOUR PACEMAKER BY TELEPHONE

Dear Patient:
Your doctor wants to check your pacemaker regularly by telephone. Doing this helps him monitor how well the pacemaker is working and the strength of the battery while you stay at home. Here's how to use your pacemaker's transmitter.

Inserting the battery
Before using your transmitter for the first time, remove the battery cover and insert the battery supplied by the manufacturer. You'll need to replace the battery every 2 to 3 months, according to the manufacturer's instructions.

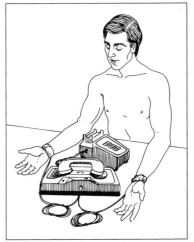

Setting up the transmitter
When you're ready, take the transmitter out of its case. Also remove the electrode cable from the case, and plug the cable into the jack on the transmitter.

Place the electrodes on your fingers or on your wrists. Then turn on the transmitter and listen for the tones indicating that the power is on.

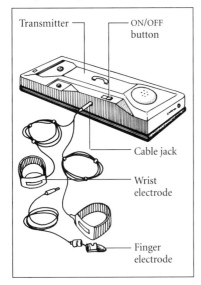

Transmitter — ON/OFF button
— Cable jack
Wrist electrode
Finger electrode

Phoning in your electrocardiogram
Dial the telephone number of your doctor's office or the pacemaker clinic, and listen for instructions.

When directed, place the telephone handset in the pacemaker transmitter. Stay still (for up to 60 seconds) to minimize interference with the signals from your heart.

Wait for further instructions. For example, the doctor may ask you to use a special magnet that's in the transmitter's case. To do so, simply hold the magnet over the pacemaker and transmit your electrocardiogram as before.

When you finish transmitting, take off the electrodes and turn off the transmitter. Place the equipment in the storage case until the next time you use it.

CHECKING YOUR BLOOD CHOLESTEROL LEVEL

Dear Patient:

Testing your blood cholesterol level can tell you whether you're at risk for heart disease. If you take cholesterol-lowering medication or are on a low-cholesterol diet, testing your blood cholesterol level will help you determine if your cholesterol is under control. If you have any questions about test results or the risk factors associated with heart disease, always consult your doctor.

Follow these steps to learn how to obtain a blood sample and how to perform the test. Remember, because cholesterol levels can change from day to day and can be affected by stress, weight loss, illness, or pregnancy, one cholesterol reading may not be final.

Getting ready

1. Begin by assembling the necessary equipment included in the packet: the test device, the test result chart, and a lancet, plus an alcohol pad and gauze pads.
2. Read the instructions thoroughly.

Obtaining blood

1. Wash your hands thoroughly and dry them. Choose a site on the end or side of any fingertip. To enhance blood flow, hold your finger under warm water for a minute or two.
2. Hold your hand below your heart, and press the blood toward the fingertip you plan to pierce by squeezing that fingertip with the thumb of the same hand. Wipe the designated fingertip with an alcohol pad, and dry it with a gauze pad. Place your fingertip (with your thumb still pressed against it) on a firm surface such as a table.

3. Twist off the lancet's protective cap. Then grasp the lancet and quickly pierce your fingertip just to the side of the finger pad, where you have more blood vessels and fewer nerve endings.
4. Push the sharp end of the lancet into the protective cap to avoid accidental sticks. Place the device in a sharps container (such as a coffee can or a 2-L plastic soda bottle).
5. Remove your thumb from your fingertip to permit blood flow. Apply gentle pressure to your finger until you get a large, hanging drop of blood.
6. Point your finger down directly over the blood well, and place the hanging drop of blood into the blood well, making sure that you fill the black circle completely. Then wait at least 2 but no more than 4 minutes. Press the puncture site with a dry gauze pad to stop the bleeding.

Reading the results

When the display windows indicate that the test is complete, read the results. Compare the reading on the testing device with the chart included in the packet for your cholesterol level. Remember to inform your doctor about the results.

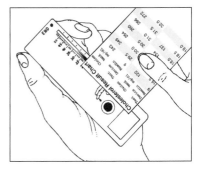

PERFORMING A HOME OVULATION TEST

Dear Patient:
A home ovulation test helps you determine the best time to try to become pregnant. It works by monitoring the amount of luteinizing hormone (LH) that's found in your urine.

Normally, during each menstrual cycle, levels of this hormone rise suddenly (LH surge), causing an egg to be released from the ovary 24 to 36 hours later. The release of the egg is known as *ovulation*. Ovulation normally occurs once a month, about 2 weeks before your period, and lasts about 24 hours.

This is your most fertile period—the only time each month that you can become pregnant.

Follow these directions to test your urine for the presence of LH and to determine when you're most likely to become pregnant. To know when to begin testing, you'll need to know the length of your menstrual cycle. Count from the beginning of one period to the beginning of the next period. (Count the first day of bleeding as day 1). Use this chart to determine when to begin testing.

Length of cycle	Start test this many days after your last period begins	Length of cycle	Start test this many days after your last period begins
21	5	31	14
22	5	32	15
23	6	33	16
24	7	34	17
25	8	35	18
26	9	36	19
27	10	37	20
28	11	38	21
29	12	39	22
30	13	40	23

PERFORMING A HOME OVULATION TEST *(continued)*

Getting ready
1. Read the instructions thoroughly before you perform the test. This test can be performed any time of the day or night but should be performed at the same time each day.

Note: Don't urinate for at least 4 hours before taking this test, and don't drink a lot of liquids for several hours before testing.

2. Remove the test stick from the package and remove the cap.

Performing the test
1. Sit on the toilet. Direct the absorbent tip of the test stick downward and directly into your urine stream for at least 5 seconds or until it's thoroughly wet. *Don't urinate on the windows of the stick.* You can also urinate into a clean, dry cup or container and dip the test stick (absorbent tip only) into the urine for at least 5 seconds.

2. Lay the test stick on a clean, dry, flat surface.

Reading the results
1. Wait at least 5 minutes to read the results. When the test is finished, a line will appear in the small window (control window).

2. *If there's no line in the large rectangular window (test window) or if the line is lighter than the line in the small rectangular window,* you haven't begun your LH surge. You should continue with daily testing.

3. *If you see one line in the large window that's similar to or darker than the line in the small window* (as shown at right), you've detected an LH surge. This means that you should ovulate within the next 24 to 36 hours.

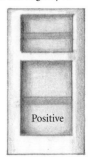

Once you've determined that you're about to ovulate, you know you're at the start of the most fertile time of your cycle.

PERFORMING A HOME HIV TEST

Dear Patient:

Human immunodeficiency virus (HIV) is a virus that attacks your immune system and causes acquired immunodeficiency syndrome (AIDS). By testing your blood, you can determine if you've been infected with HIV. Remember that even if you've been exposed to the HIV virus, it may not become evident in your blood for 6 months. If you have any questions about your test results or the risk factors associated with HIV, *always* consult a doctor.

Follow these steps to learn how to obtain a blood sample and how to perform the test.

Getting ready

1. Begin by assembling the necessary equipment included in the packet: a lancet, a test card with your personal identification number (to receive the confidential and anonymous test results), and the envelope in which to send the test card to the laboratory. Also gather an alcohol pad and gauze pads.
2. Read the instructions thoroughly before you stick your finger. Remove the personal identification card from the bottom of the test card, and place it in a safe place.

Obtaining blood

1. Wash your hands thoroughly and dry them. Choose a site on the end or side of any fingertip. To enhance blood flow, hold your finger under warm water for a minute or two.
2. Hold your hand below your heart, and press the blood toward the fingertip you plan to pierce by squeezing that fingertip with the thumb of the same hand. Wipe the designated fingertip with an alcohol pad, and dry it with a gauze pad. Place your fingertip (with

your thumb still pressed against it) on a firm surface such as a table.
3. Twist off the lancet's protective cap. Then grasp the lancet and quickly pierce your fingertip just to the side of the finger pad, where you have more blood vessels and fewer nerve endings.

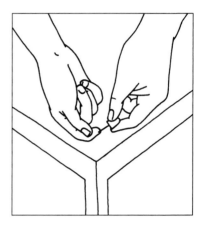

4. Push the sharp end of the lancet into the protective cap to avoid accidental sticks.
5. Remove your thumb from your fingertip to permit blood flow. Then apply gentle pressure to your finger until you get a large, hanging drop of blood.

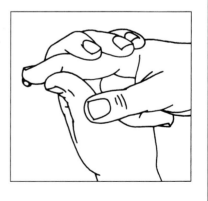

PERFORMING A HOME HIV TEST *(continued)*

6. Point your finger down directly over the three circles on the test card (as shown at right). Completely fill each circle with blood from your finger.

7. Place used lancets in the containers attached to the mailing card. Slip the test card into the postage-paid mailer, seal the mailer, and send it to the address printed on the front. Save the part of the card that lists the toll-free number to call for results.

Obtaining the results

In about 1 week, call the toll-free number on the identification card. Give your identification number to the person who answers, and wait for the results. *If your test is positive for HIV,* a specially trained counselor will advise you what to do next and will tell you about HIV and AIDS organizations nationwide. *If your test results are negative for HIV,* the trained counselor will advise you how to maintain your negative HIV status.

Remember, a negative test result doesn't necessarily mean you're free from HIV infection. It may simply mean that the antibodies aren't yet present in your blood. To be certain, repeat the test with a new package in 6 months.

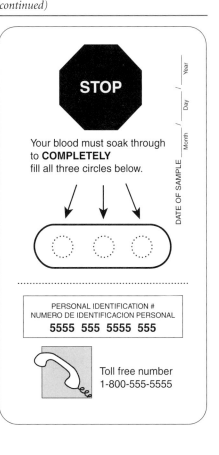

STOP

Your blood must soak through to **COMPLETELY** fill all three circles below.

DATE OF SAMPLE — Month / Day / Year

PERSONAL IDENTIFICATION #
NUMERO DE IDENTIFICACION PERSONAL
5555 555 5555 555

Toll free number
1-800-555-5555

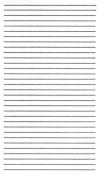

Crisis values of laboratory tests

The abnormal laboratory test values listed here have immediate life-or-death significance to the patient. Report such values to the patient's physician immediately.

Test	Low value	Common causes and effects	High value	Common causes and effects
Ammonia	< 15 µg/dl (SI,< 8.8 µmol/ L)	Renal failure	> 50 µg/dl (SI, > 29.3 µmol/ L)	Severe hepatic disease: hepatic coma, Reye's syndrome, GI hemorrhage, heart failure
Calcium, serum	< 7 mg/dl (SI, < 1.75 mmol/ L)	Vitamin D or parathyroid hormone deficiency; tetany, seizures	> 12 mg/dl (SI, > 0.3 mmol/L)	Hyperparathyroidism: coma
Carbon dioxide and bicarbonate, blood	< 10 mEq/L (SI,< 10 mmol/ L)	Complex pattern of metabolic and respiratory factors	> 40 mEq/L (SI, > 40 mmol/ L)	Complex pattern of metabolic and respiratory factors
Creatine kinase isoenzymes (CK-MB)			> 5%	Acute myocardial infarction (MI)
Creatinine, serum			> 4 mg/dl (SI, > 353.6 µmol/ L)	Renal failure: coma
D-dimer, serum or cerebrospinal fluid (CSF)			> 250 µg/ml	Disseminated intravascular coagulation (DIC), pulmonary embolism, arterial or venous thrombosis, subarachnoid hemorrhage (CSF only), secondary fibrinolysis

Test	Low value	Common causes and effects	High value	Common causes and effects
Glucose, blood	< 40 mg/dl (SI, < 2.2 mmol/L)	Excessive insulin administration: brain damage	> 300 mg/dl (SI, > 16.6 mmol/L) (with ketonemia and electrolyte imbalance)	Diabetes: diabetic coma
Gram stain, CSF			Gram-positive or gram-negative	Bacterial meningitis
Hemoglobin	< 8 g/dl (SI, < 80 g/L)	Hemorrhage or vitamin B_{12} or iron deficiency; heart failure	> 18 g/dl (SI, > 180 g/L)	Chronic obstructive pulmonary disease: thrombosis, polycythemia vera
International Normalized Ratio			> 3.0	DIC, uncontrolled oral anticoagulation
Partial pressure of carbon dioxide, in arterial blood	< 20 mm Hg	Complex pattern of metabolic and respiratory factors	> 70 mm Hg	Complex pattern of metabolic and respiratory factors
Partial pressure of oxygen, in arterial blood	< 50 mm Hg	Complex pattern of metabolic and respiratory factors		
Partial thromboplastin time			> 40 seconds (> 70 seconds for patient on heparin)	Anticoagulation factor deficiency: hemorrhage
pH, arterial blood	< 7.2 (SI, < 7.2)	Complex pattern of metabolic and respiratory factors	> 7.6 (SI, > 7.6)	Complex pattern of metabolic and respiratory factors
Platelet count	< 50,000/μl (SI, < 50 × 10⁹/L)	Bone marrow suppression; hemorrhage	> 500,000/μl (SI, 500 × 10⁹/L)	Leukemia, reaction to acute bleeding: hemorrhage
Potassium, serum	< 3 mEq/L (SI, < 3 mmol/L)	Vomiting and diarrhea, diuretic therapy: cardiotoxicity, arrhythmia, cardiac arrest	> 6 mEq/L (SI, > 6 mmol/L)	Renal disease, diuretic therapy: cardiotoxicity, arrhythmia

Test	Low value	Common causes and effects	High value	Common causes and effects
Prothrombin time			> 14 seconds (> 20 seconds for patient on warfarin)	Anticoagulant therapy, anticoagulation factor deficiency: hemorrhage
Sodium serum	< 120 mEq/L (SI, < 120 mmol/L)	Diuretic therapy: cardiac failure	> 160 mEq/L (SI, > 160 mmol/L)	Dehydration: vascular collapse
Troponin			> 2 μg/ml (SI, > 2 mcg/L)	Acute MI
White blood cell (WBC) count	< 2,000/μl (SI, < 2 × 10^9/L)	Bone marrow suppression: infection	> 20,000/μl (SI, > 20 × 10^9/L)	Leukemia: infection
WBC count, CSF			> 10/μl (SI, > 0.001 × 10^9/L)	Meningitis, encephalitis: infection

Blood tests requiring immediate transport of the sample

ABO blood typing
Acetylcholine receptor antibodies
Acid phosphatase
ACTH, plasma
Activated partial thromboplastin time
Aldosterone
Alkaline phosphatase
Ammonia, plasma
Androstenedione
Angiotensin-converting enzyme
Antibodies to extractable nuclear antigen
Antibody screening test
Antidiuretic hormone
Antiglobulin, direct (direct Coombs')
Arginine test
Arterial blood gas analysis
Aspartate aminotransferase
Bilirubin, serum
Calcitonin, plasma
Carbon dioxide, total
Carcinoembryonic antigen
Catecholamines, plasma
Ceruloplasmin, serum
Cholesterol, total
Cholinesterase

Coagulation, extrinsic system
Coagulation, intrinsic system
Cold agglutinins
Complement assays
Cortisol
Creatine, serum
Creatine kinase
Creatinine, serum
Crossmatching
Cryoglobulins
Erythrocyte sedimentation rate
Erythrocyte total porphyrins
Estrogens, serum
Euglobulin lysis time
Febrile agglutination tests
Fibrin split products
Fibrinogen, plasma
Folic acid, serum
Fungal serology
Galactose-1-phosphate uridyltransferase
Gastrin, serum
Glucose, fasting plasma
Glucose, plasma, 2-hour postprandial
Glucose tolerance, oral
Growth hormone, serum

Growth hormone suppression
Heinz bodies
Hematocrit
Human chorionic gonadotropin, serum
Human placental lactogen, serum
Hydroxybutyric dehydrogenase
Immune complex assays, serum
Immunoglobulins G, A, and M
Insulin, serum
Insulin tolerance
Iron, serum
Iron-binding capacity, total
Isocitrate dehydrogenase
Lactate dehydrogenase
Lactic acid and pyruvic acid (lactate and pyruvate)
Lipoprotein-cholesterol fractionation
Lymphocyte transformation
Manganese, serum
Microbiology culture
Neonatal thyroid-stimulating hormone
Parathyroid hormone, serum

Phenylalanine, serum
  (Guthrie test)
Phospholipids
Plasma thrombin time
Plasminogen
Progesterone, plasma
Prothrombin consumption
  time
Prothrombin time
Renin, plasma
Rh typing
Serum glucagon
T- and B-lymphocyte counts
Transferrin, serum
Triglycerides
Vitamin A and carotene,
  serum
Vitamin B_{12}, serum
Vitamin C, plasma
Zinc, serum

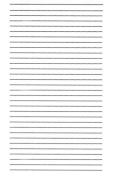

Imaging guide

COMMON RADIOGRAPHIC VIEWS

The following illustrations show the area
of radiographic coverage for each view

Frontal

This is performed with the X-ray beam
positioned posteriorly and anteriorly and
with the patient in an upright position.
The posteroanterior (PA) view is the most
common frontal view; it's preferred over
the anteroposterior (AP) view because the
heart is anteriorly situated in the thorax
and magnified less in a PA view than in an
AP view. The frontal views show greater
lung area than the other views because of
the lower diaphragm position.

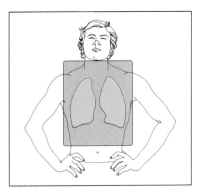

Lateral

This is performed with the X-ray beam directed toward the patient's side. The left
lateral (LL) view is the most common lateral view; it's preferred over the right lateral (RL) view because the heart is left of
midline and magnified less in an LL view
than in an RL view. Lateral views visualize
lesions not apparent on a PA view.

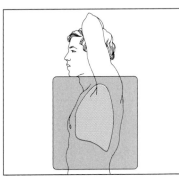

Recumbent

This is performed with the X-ray beam
overhead and with the patient supine. The
recumbent view helps distinguish free fluid from encapsulated fluid and from an elevated diaphragm.

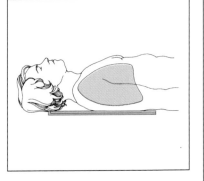

COMMON RADIOGRAPHIC VIEWS *(continued)*

Oblique

This is performed with the X-ray beam angled between the frontal and lateral views. The oblique view helps evaluate intrathoracic disorders, pleural disease, esophageal abnormalities, hilar masses, and mediastinal masses. Occasionally, it's also used to localize lesions with the chest.

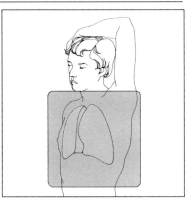

Lordotic

This is performed with the X-ray beam directed through the axis of the middle thoracic lobe and with the patient leaning back against the film plate. The lordotic view evaluates the apices of the lungs, which are usually obscured by bony structures, and helps localize sites of tuberculosis.

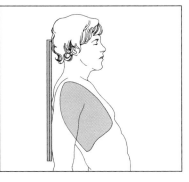

Decubitus

This is performed with the X-ray beam parallel to the floor and with the patient in one of several horizontal positions (supine, prone, or side). The decubitus view demonstrates the extent of pulmonary abscess or cavity, the presence of free pleural fluid or pneumothorax, and the mobility of mediastinal mass when the patient changes positions.

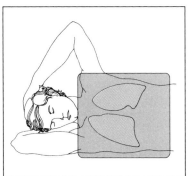

Respiratory system imaging

COMPARING NORMAL AND ABNORMAL LUNG VENTILATION SCANS

The normal ventilation scan on the left, taken 30 minutes to 1 hour after the wash-out phase, shows equal gas distribution. The abnormal scan on the right, taken 1½ to 2 hours after the start of the wash-out phase, shows unequal gas distribution, represented by the area of poor wash-out on both the left and right sides.

Normal scan

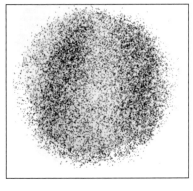

Abnormal scan

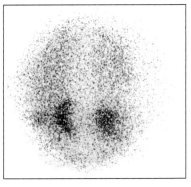

COMPARING NORMAL AND ABNORMAL THORACIC CT SCANS

In the abnormal thoracic computed tomography (CT) scan (top), note atelectasis in the right middle lobe and cancer in the right hilum. The normal scan (bottom) shows no such deviations.

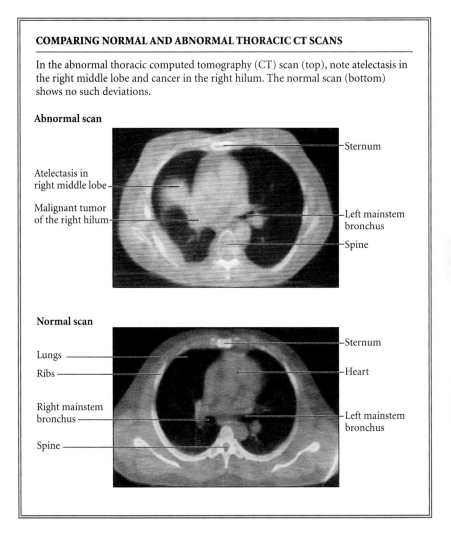

Skeletal system imaging

COMPARING NORMAL AND ABNORMAL ARTHROGRAMS

The arthrogram on the left shows a normal medial meniscus. The view on the right shows a torn medial meniscus.

Normal arthrogram of knee

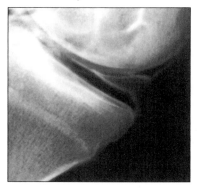

Abnormal arthrogram of knee

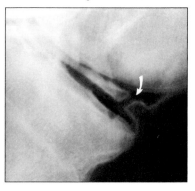

The arthrogram on the left shows a normal shoulder. The arthrogram on the right shows a shoulder with a ruptured rotator cuff. Contrast medium has collected in the subacromial bursa (indicated by the arrows).

Normal arthrogram of shoulder

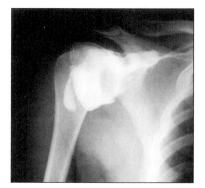

Abnormal arthrogram of shoulder

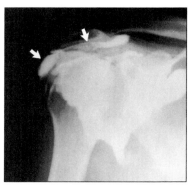

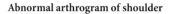

COMPARING NORMAL AND ABNORMAL BONE SCANS

The scans below compare a normal bone scan with an abnormal scan. The scan on the left is normal because the isotope is distributed evenly throughout the skeletal tissue. The scan on the right is abnormal because the isotope has accumulated in multiple metastases in the ribs and spine.

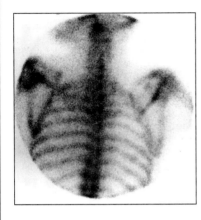 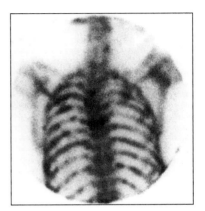

Nervous system imaging

COMPARING NORMAL AND ABNORMAL CEREBRAL ANGIOGRAMS

The angiograms below show the differences between normal and abnormal cerebral vasculature. The cerebral angiogram on the left is normal. The cerebral angiogram on the right shows occluded blood vessels caused by a large arteriovenous malformation.

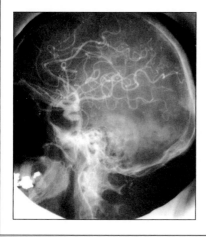 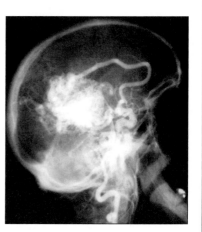

COMPARING NORMAL AND ABNORMAL CT SCANS

Shown here are two intracranial computed tomography (CT) scans. The scan on the left is normal. The scan on the right shows a large meningioma in the frontal region, represented by the white area.

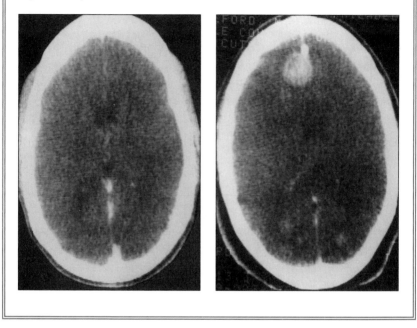

GI system imaging

COMPARING NORMAL AND ABNORMAL COLONOSCOPIC VIEWS

These two views, taken with a fiber-optic colonoscope, show a normal descending colon (left) and a colon with cancer (right).

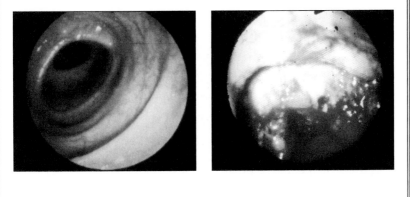

ABNORMAL PERCUTANEOUS CHOLANGIOGRAM

In this percutaneous cholangiogram, the dilated hepatic ducts indicate obstruction of the common bile duct by a tumor. The catheter tip has been passed through the tumor into the duodenum.

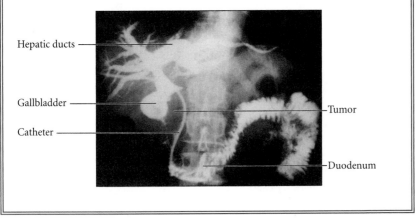

NORMAL T-TUBE CHOLANGIOGRAM

This T-tube cholangiogram shows homogeneous filling of biliary ducts. The ducts are of normal diameter, and the presence of contrast medium in the duodenum shows that the ducts are also patent.

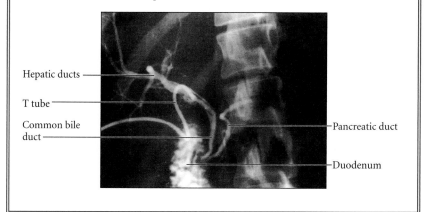

COLON ABNORMALITIES

These abnormal views of the colon were taken with a proctosigmoidoscope. The view on the left demonstrates familial polyposis — multiple adenomatous growths and high malignancy potential. The view on the right shows diverticular orifices of the colon associated with muscle hypertrophy, which almost obscures the slitlike lumen (far right).

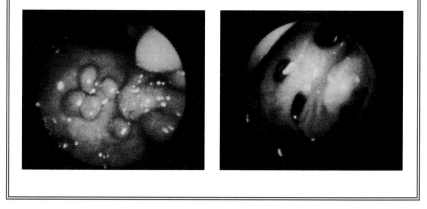

ABNORMAL ERCP

This endoscopic retrograde cholangiopancreatographic (ERCP) view shows a dilated pancreatic duct secondary to stenosis. Stenosis was cased by carcinoma at the head of the pancreas.

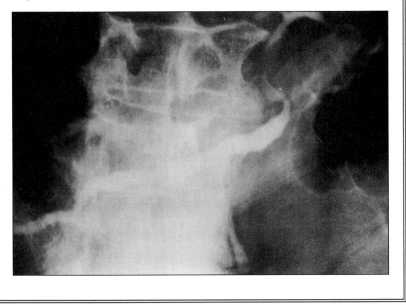

COMPARING NORMAL AND ABNORMAL IMAGES OF THE PANCREAS

The ultrasound view on the top shows a normal pancreas (outlined in color). The ultrasound view on the bottom shows a diffusely enlarged pancreas due to pancreatitis. The color outline indicates the extent of enlargement.

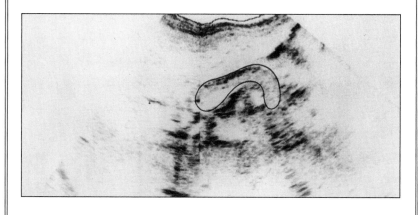

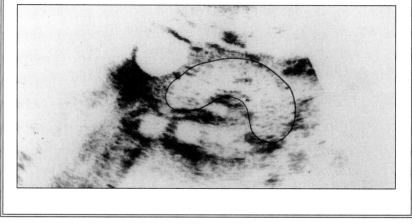

Cardiovascular system imaging

ABNORMAL VENOGRAMS

The venogram image of the lower extremities below show some filling defects as well as incompetent veins.

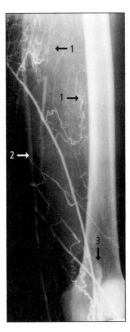
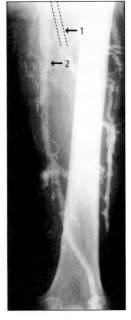

This venogram of the calf shows incompetent veins (arrows).

This venogram of the thigh shows development of collateral veins (1), filling of some superficial veins (2), and obstruction of the popliteal vein (3).

This venogram of the thigh shows a filling defect caused by a thrombus (1) and backflow from a blockage of the iliac veins (2).

REAL-TIME ECHOCARDIOGRAMS

The real-time (showing motion) echocardiograms shown below are short-axis, cross-sectional views of the mitral valve from a normal patient (top) and a patient with mitral stenosis (bottom). In the latter, note the greatly reduced mitral valve orifice caused by stenotic, calcified valve leaflets.

Normal

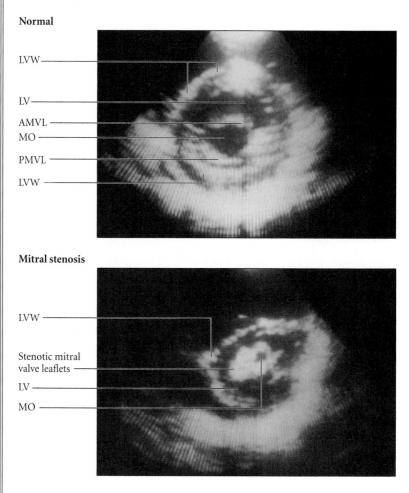

Mitral stenosis

Key:

AMVL = Anterior mitral valve leaflet
LV = Left ventricle
LVW = Left ventricular wall

MO = Mitral orifice
PMVL = Posterior mitral valve leaflet

REAL-TIME ECHOCARDIOGRAMS *(continued)*

The echocardiograms shown below are long-axis, cross-sectional views of the mitral valve from a normal patient (top) and a patient with hypertrophic cardiomyopathy, also known as idiopathic hypertrophic stenosis (bottom). Note the markedly thickened left ventricular wall in the latter.

Normal

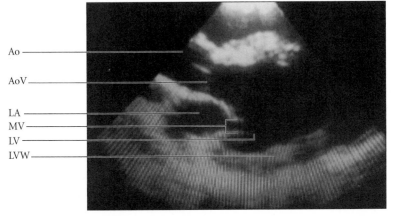

Hypertrophic cardiomyopathy

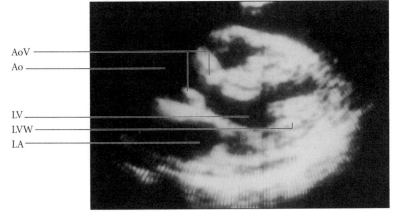

Key:

Ao = Aorta
AoV = Aortic valve
LA = Left atrium

LV = Left ventricle
LVW = Left ventricular wall
MV = Mitral valve

ABNORMAL CORONARY ARTERIOGRAM

This arteriogram taken from the right anterior oblique position shows occlusion of the left anterior descending artery

Catheter

Site of occlusion

Left circumflex branch

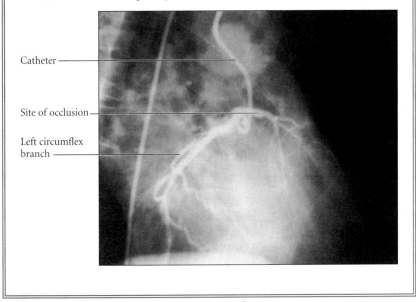

DIAGNOSING PERICARDIAL EFFUSION

Various tests, such as chest X-ray and M-mode echocardiography, aid diagnosis of pericardial effusion. In the chest X-ray shown below (top), the bulging white area in the center represents an enlarged pericardial sac resulting from pericardial effusion.

In the M-mode echocardiogram shown below (bottom), the wide light area at the bottom indicates accumulation of pericardial effusion. Pericardiocentesis followed by pericardial fluid analysis can determine the cause of such accumulation.

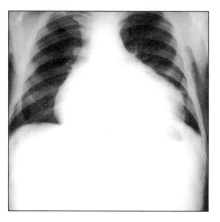

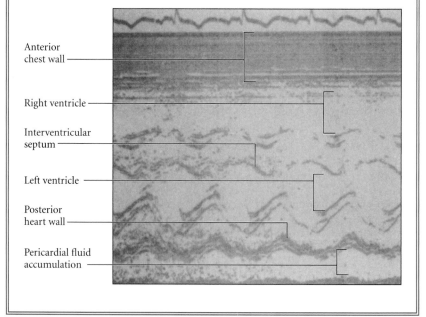

Anterior
chest wall

Right ventricle

Interventricular
septum

Left ventricle

Posterior
heart wall

Pericardial fluid
accumulation

Urinary system imaging

ABNORMAL RENAL CT SCAN

This photograph of a renal computed tomography (CT) scan reveals a renal adeno-carcinoma that has displaced and distorted the right kidney and that now exceeds the kidney in size. The left kidney appears normal, the spine is sharp and white in the center of the photography, and the stomach is equally clear at the top.

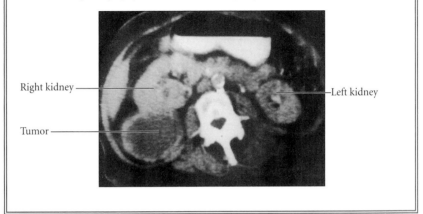

Right kidney —

—Left kidney

Tumor —

NORMAL AND ABNORMAL RETROGRADE CYSTOGRAMS

A normal retrograde cystogram (left) contrasts sharply with one showing a ruptured bladder (right). In the photograph on the right, the bladder, usually smooth and rounded when filled, has collapsed downward on itself, against the pelvic floor, and contrast material has extravasated upward into the peritoneal cavity from the tear in the bladder wall.

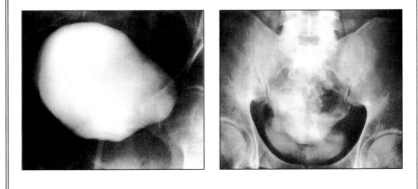

ABNORMAL EXCRETORY UROGRAM

In a patient with suspected renal hypertension, an excretory urogram taken 8 minutes after injection of a contrast medium shows normal filling of the right kidney but delayed filling of the left kidney and ureter (see below). This impaired excretion of the contrast material commonly results from narrowing of the renal artery feeding the subject kidney. Constriction hinders blood flow to the glomerulus and leads to increased renal absorption of water and decreased urine output. Demonstration of delayed filling can distinguish unilateral renal hypertension from essential hypertension.

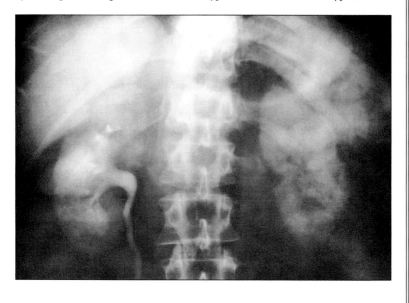

NORMAL AND ABNORMAL CYSTOURETHROGRAMS

In the oblique view of a normal cystourethrogram (left), the clear outline of the bladder and urethra shows normal structure. The oblique view of an abnormal cystourethrogram (right) shows abscesses in the prostate and proximal urethra.

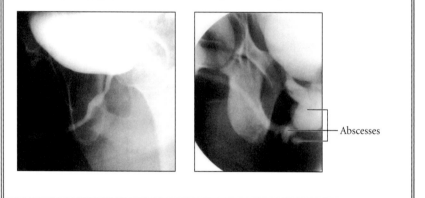

Abscesses

Index

i refers to an illustration; t refers to a table; **bold text** refers to main entries.

i refers to an illustration; t refers to a table; **bold text** refers to main entries.

i refers to an illustration; t refers to a table; **bold text** refers to main entries.

i refers to an illustration; t refers to a table; **bold text** refers to main entries.

i refers to an illustration; t refers to a table; **bold text** refers to main entries.

i refers to an illustration; t refers to a table; **bold text** refers to main entries.

i refers to an illustration; t refers to a table; **bold text** refers to main entries.

i refers to an illustration; t refers to a table; **bold text** refers to main entries.

i refers to an illustration; t refers to a table; **bold text** refers to main entries.

i refers to an illustration; t refers to a table; **bold text** refers to main entries.

.

i refers to an illustration; t refers to a table; **bold text** refers to main entries.

i refers to an illustration; t refers to a table; **bold text** refers to main entries.

i refers to an illustration; t refers to a table; **bold text** refers to main entries.

Erythroblastosis fetalis. *See also* Hemolytic disease of the newborn.
amniotic fluid analysis in, 675
plasma ammonia in, 214
urine human chorionic gonadotropin in, 375
Erythrocyte count, **11-12**
Erythrocyte indices, **14-15**
Erythrocytes. *See* Red blood cells.
Erythrocyte sedimentation rate, **15-16**
Erythropoiesis
factors that affect, 5-6, 5i
increased, protoporphyrin in, 219
Erythropoietic porphyria
coproporphyrin in, 219
urine porphyrin in, 405t
uroporphyrin in, 219
Erythropoietic porphyrins. *See* Fractionated erythrocyte porphyrins.
Erythropoietic protoporphyria
coproporphyrin in, 219
protoporphyrin in, 219
urine porphyrin in, 405t
uroporphyrin in, 219
Erythropoietin, **176-177**
Erythropoietin, red cell production and, 5, 6
Esophageal acidity, **749-750**
Esophageal atresia, amniotic fluid analysis in, 673, 675
Esophageal cancer
chest X-ray in, 614t
mediastinoscopy in, 611
Esophageal contents, analysis of, 746
Esophageal disorders, Bravo System and, 749
Esophageal motility disorders
barium swallow in, 776
gastroesophageal reflux scanning in, 774
upper gastrointestinal and small-bowel series in, 779
Esophageal spasm
barium swallow in, 776
upper gastrointestinal and small-bowel series in, 779
Esophageal stenoses, esophagogastro-duodenoscopy in, 766-767

Esophageal strictures
barium swallow in, 776
upper gastrointestinal and small-bowel series in, 778
Esophagitis
acid perfusion in, 752
endoscopic biopsy of gastrointestinal tract for, 449
esophageal acidity in, 750
esophagogastroduodenoscopy in, 766
Esophagogastroduodenoscopy, **764-767**
ESR. *See* Erythrocyte sedimentation rate.
Estrogens, **184-186**
menstrual cycle and, 187i
Estrogen therapy, testosterone in, 190
Ethylene glycol ingestion
routine urinalysis in, 347
urine oxalate in, 432
Euglobulin lysis time, **61-62**
Eunuchoidism, 17-KS in, 379
Eustachian tube, nonfunctional, otoscopic examination in, 559, 559t
Evoked potential studies, **712, 715-716**
auditory brain stem, 712
somatosensory, 712, 714i, 715, 716
visual, 712, 713i, 715
Ewing's sarcoma, bone biopsy in, 463
Excisional biopsy, 435, 436-437i
Excretory urography, **909-911**
abnormal, 1035i
Exercise
pulmonary function in, 597t
routine urinalysis in, 347
urine myoglobin in, 403-404
white blood cell differential in, 35t
Exercise electrocardiography, **836-840**
for bicycle ergometer test, 837
tracings from, 839i
on treadmill, 837
Exomphalos, amniotic fluid analysis in, 673, 675
Exophthalmometry, **537-538**
Exophthalmos
exophthalmometry in, 538
orbital computed tomography in, 550
thyroid-stimulating immunoglobulins in, 293

i refers to an illustration; t refers to a table; **bold text** refers to main entries.

i refers to an illustration; t refers to a table; **bold text** refers to main entries.

i refers to an illustration; t refers to a table; **bold text** refers to main entries.

i refers to an illustration; t refers to a table; **bold text** refers to main entries.

i refers to an illustration; t refers to a table; **bold text** refers to main entries.

i refers to an illustration; t refers to a table; **bold text** refers to main entries.

i refers to an illustration; t refers to a table; **bold text** refers to main entries.

i refers to an illustration; t refers to a table; **bold text** refers to main entries.

i refers to an illustration; t refers to a table; **bold text** refers to main entries.

i refers to an illustration; t refers to a table; **bold text** refers to main entries.

i refers to an illustration; t refers to a table; **bold text** refers to main entries.

i refers to an illustration; t refers to a table; **bold text** refers to main entries.

i refers to an illustration; t refers to a table; **bold text** refers to main entries.

i refers to an illustration; t refers to a table; **bold text** refers to main entries.

i refers to an illustration; t refers to a table; **bold text** refers to main entries.

i refers to an illustration; t refers to a table; **bold text** refers to main entries.

i refers to an illustration; t refers to a table; **bold text** refers to main entries.

i refers to an illustration; t refers to a table; **bold text** refers to main entries.

i refers to an illustration; t refers to a table; **bold text** refers to main entries.

i refers to an illustration; t refers to a table; **bold text** refers to main entries.

i refers to an illustration; t refers to a table; **bold text** refers to main entries.

i refers to an illustration; t refers to a table; **bold text** refers to main entries.

i refers to an illustration; t refers to a table; **bold text** refers to main entries.

i refers to an illustration; t refers to a table; **bold text** refers to main entries.

i refers to an illustration; t refers to a table; **bold text** refers to main entries.

i refers to an illustration; t refers to a table; **bold text** refers to main entries.

i refers to an illustration; t refers to a table; **bold text** refers to main entries.

Salpingitis, white blood cell differential in, 35t
Salt-losing nephritis, urine sodium in, 425
Salt-losing syndrome
  aldosterone in, 171
  urine aldosterone in, 368
Sandhoff's disease, hexosaminidase in, 126, 127
Sarcoidosis
  angiotensin-converting enzyme in, 131
  albumin in, 208i
  delayed hypersensitivity skin tests in, 936
  evoked potential studies in, 715
  Persantine-thallium imaging in, 865
  pulmonary function in, 600t
  synovial membrane biopsy in, 471
  urine calcium in, 428t
  urine phosphate in, 428t
  vitamin D$_3$ in, 243
Sarcomas, gallium scanning in, 940
Scarlatina, cold agglutinins in, 299
Scarlet fever, capillary fragility in, 47
Schirmer's tearing, **539-541**
  filter placement in, 539i
Schönlein-Henoch purpura, bleeding time in, 44
Schwabach tuning fork test, 559-561
Schwannomas, ear magnetic resonance imaging in, 579
Scleroderma
  antinuclear antibodies in, 286t, 287
  cold agglutinins in, 299
  fecal lipids in, 763
  lupus erythematosus cell preparation in, 294
Scoliosis
  chest X-ray in, 614t
  vertebral radiography in, 634
Scotoma
  Amsler's grid in, 529, 530i
  tangent screen examination in, 532
Scurvy. *See also* Vitamin C deficiency.
  capillary fragility in, 47
  routine urinalysis in, 347
Seborrheic keratoses, skin biopsy in, 447
Secretin test, 749

Seizure disorders. *See also* Epilepsy.
  creatine kinase in, 97
  electroencephalography in, 710, 711i
  fasting plasma glucose in, 224
  2-hour postprandial plasma glucose in, 225-226
Semen analysis, **658-662**
  for medicolegal purposes, 659
Seminoma, follicle-stimulating hormone in, 147
Sensitivity, 90
Sensitivity testing, 473-474
Sensorineural hearing loss, 556
  pure tone audiometry in, 564
  tuning fork test in, 561
Sensory organization test, 587-588
Sentinel lymph node biopsy, **445-446**. *See also* Lymph node biopsy.
Sepsis
  direct antiglobulin in, 256
  fasting plasma glucose in, 224
  2-hour postprandial plasma glucose in, 225-226
Septic arthritis, synovial fluid analysis in, 648
Septicemia
  blood culture in, 490
  blood lactate in, 232
  gastric culture in, 494
  urine catecholamine in, 371
  white blood cell differential in, 35t
Serotonin, 366
Serum electrolytes, 68-69. *See also specific electrolyte.*
  functions of, 68t
Serum ferritin, **30**
Serum iron, **27-30**
Serum sickness
  complement assays in, 282
  white blood cell differential in, 35t
Sex chromosome anomalies, 663, 664-665t
Sex chromosome tests, **662-664**
Sex hormones, 366
Sexual development, premature, in children, androstenedione in, 176
Shake test, 672i
Shaving as biopsy type, 436-437i

i refers to an illustration; t refers to a table; **bold text** refers to main entries.

i refers to an illustration; t refers to a table; **bold text** refers to main entries.

i refers to an illustration; t refers to a table; **bold text** refers to main entries.

i refers to an illustration; t refers to a table; **bold text** refers to main entries.

i refers to an illustration; t refers to a table; **bold text** refers to main entries.

i refers to an illustration; t refers to a table; **bold text** refers to main entries.

i refers to an illustration; t refers to a table; **bold text** refers to main entries.

i refers to an illustration; t refers to a table; **bold text** refers to main entries.

i refers to an illustration; t refers to a table; **bold text** refers to main entries.

i refers to an illustration; t refers to a table; **bold text** refers to main entries.

i refers to an illustration; t refers to a table; **bold text** refers to main entries.